Short Textbook of Physiology

Short Textbook of Physiology

A Concised Book for All Medical Professionals

K.C. Mathur
MBBS MD
Associate Professor
Department of Physiology
Sardar Patel Medical College
Bikaner (Rajasthan) - 334 003

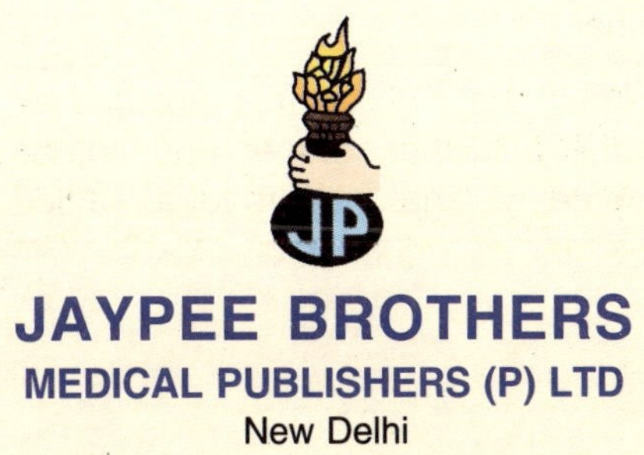

JAYPEE BROTHERS
MEDICAL PUBLISHERS (P) LTD
New Delhi

Published by

Jitendar P Vij
Jaypee Brothers Medical Publishers (P) Ltd
EMCA House, 23/23B Ansari Road, Daryaganj
New Delhi 110 002, India
Phones: +91-11-23272143, +91-11-23272703, +91-11-23282021, +91-11-23245672
Fax: +91-11-23276490, +91-11-23245683
e-mail: jaypee@jaypeebrothers.com
Visit our website: www.jaypeebrothers.com

Branches

- 2/B, Akruti Society, Jodhpur Gam Road Satellite
  Ahmedabad 380 015 Phones: +91-079-30988717, +91-079-26926233
  e-mail: jpamdvd@rediffmail.com
- 202 Batavia Chambers, 8 Kumara Krupa Road, Kumara Park East
  Bangalore 560 001, Phones: +91-80-22285971, +91-80-22382956, +91-80-30614073
  Tele Fax: +91-80-22281761 e-mail: jaypeemedpubbgl@eth.net
- 282 IIIrd Floor, Khaleel Shirazi Estate, Fountain Plaza, Pantheon Road
  Chennai 600 008, Phones: +91-44-28262665, +91-44-28259897, +91-44-30972089
  Fax: +91-44-28262331 e-mail: jpchen@eth.net
- 4-2-1067/1-3, Ist Floor, Balaji Building, Ramkote Cross Road
  Hyderabad 500 095, Phones: +91-40-55610020, +91-40-24758498, +91-40-30940929
  Fax: +91-40-24758499 e-mail: jpmedpub@rediffmail.com
- 1A Indian Mirror Street, Wellington Square, **Kolkata** 700 013
  Phones: +91-33-22456075, +91-33-22451926, +91-33-30901926 Fax: +91-33-22456075
  e-mail: jpbcal@cal.vsnl.net.in
- 106 Amit Industrial Estate, 61 Dr SS Rao Road, Near MGM Hospital Parel
  Mumbai 400 012 Phones: +91-22-24124863, +91-22-24104532, +91-22-30926896
  Fax: +91-22-24160828 e-mail: jpmedpub@bom7.vsnl.net.in
- "KAMALPUSHPA" 38, Reshimbag, Opp. Mohota Science College
  Umred Road, **Nagpur** 440 009 (MS) Phone: +91-712-3945220
  Fax: +91-712-2704275 e-mail: jpmednagpur @rediffmail.com

Short Textbook of Physiology

First Edition : **2006**

ISBN 81-8061-770-X

Typeset at JPBMP typesetting unit
Printed at Sanat Printers, Kundli.

Om Shri Krishna-R-Panam-Astoo

In loving memory of:

- *My father (late) Shri MC Mathur*
- *My elder father (late) Shri RC Mathur*
- *My elder mother (late) Smt. Anand Kanwar Mathur*

Dedicated to all Readers

Resigning all your duties to Me, the all powerful and all supporting Lord, take refuge in Me alone. I shall absolve you of all sins, Worry not.

Shri Madbhagwat Geeta 18/66

Om Shri Krishna-R-Panam-Astoo

Prof. Dr. D.P. Punia
M.D.

Principal & Controller
Professor & Head
Department of Radiotherapy
S.P. Medical College
& Associated Group of Hospitals,
Bikaner

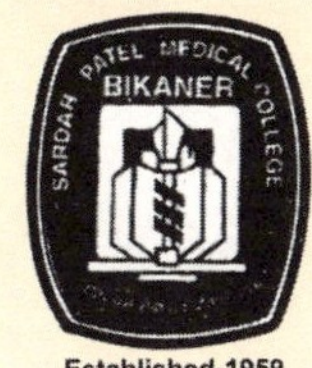

Gram:BIKMEDCOLL

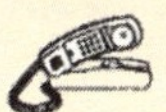

College : 523443, 202931-33
Hospital : 200851, 202931-33
Resi. : 520252

Residence:
Bungalow No. 28, Civil Lines
Bikaner-334 003 (Raj.)

FOREWORD

It gives me an immense sense of pleasure to constitute the foreword of this important book"Short Textbook of Physiology" compiled and constituted by Dr. KC Mathur — one of our staff members.

The staff members having a long association with the subject must compile such books; since they are regularly dealing with the subject along with changing trends. Author has taken this task to compile this book - which is of the subject classed as building block of medicine.

I congratulate the author and hope this book will be useful for all medical professionals to revise and refresh the memories.

I wish it a success and good luck.

Dr DP Punia
(Principal and Controller and Patron)

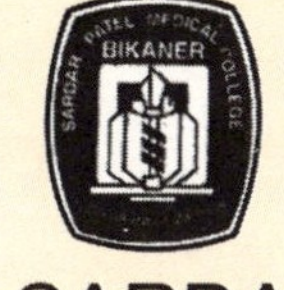

DEPARTMENT OF PHYSIOLOGY

Gram : BIKMEDCOLL
College : 523443
Hospital : 61851
EPABX : 61931-33

SARDAR PATEL MEDICAL COLLEGE, BIKANER-334 003 (RAJ.)

Ref. No........... Date ....

FOREWORD

It gives me a great sense of pleasure, privilege and honour to write foreword of this book written by my staff member and an accomplished teacher—Dr. KC Mathur.

I am sure, this book will fulfil the needs of both under and postgraduate students since the author has tried to accommodate all the relevant information for them. The question bank, multiple choice questions, viva voce questions after every unit along with glossary will further help them in assimilating the logical sequence.

I wish him good luck.

Dr Sushila Gahlot
(Professor and Head)

PREFACE

Long teaching career inspires a man to compile — a book which is his feelings, his teachings, his profession, etc. and one must do it since as a teacher it is his duty to impart the knowledge. Same is true and applicable for me. So I took the challenge and now this compilation is in your hands.

At many places attention has been paid on language, flow along with presentation. I hope readers will appreciate it.

Many chapters have been included for postgraduates in "appendix" and within various units. It is for them to get all these things at one place.

For students, question bank, (questions which have appeared in various examinations) objective and viva-voce questions have been compiled immediately at the end of one respective unit. I am sure, it will be of much benefit for my readers.

I am thankful to my Principal, Dr. DP Punia for his constant encouragement, Head of Department, Dr. (Mrs) Sushila Gahlot for her valuable suggestions, Dr. BK Jain, Professor and Head, Department of Pharmacology for his constant help in compiling some of the topics of his domine, and my other departmental colleagues — Dr. DK Srivastava, Dr. Rajesh Pathak, Dr. (Mrs) Nalini Kiri, Dr. Kailash Ojha, Dr. DK Devra, and Dr. BK Binawara, Miss Reshu Gupta, Miss Poornima Sharma for their help, moral support and valuable advises to compile this book.

I will be failing in my duties if thanks are not conveyed to my wife Manju, son Gaurav, daughter Garima, niece Deepti for sparing me for long hours to compile this book.

I am sure my readers will be satisfied and excuse me for any deficiency. It is worth recalling that these deficiencies will be covered in subsequent editions.

I express my sincere thanks to Shri JP Vij, CMD, Mr Tarun Duneja, General Manager, Publishing, Mr PS Ghuman, Senior Production Manager of M/s Jaypee Brothers Medical Publishers (P) Ltd. for publishing this book and thus converting my dreams into truth. I am also grateful to Ms Mubeen Bano, Md Shakiluzzaman, Mr. Bharat Bhushan, Mr. Deepak Goel, for their hard work in this book.

I cannot forget the homely and sincere services rendered to me by Shri Ravi Prakash Agrawal of M/s Agrawal Computers and Photostate, Bikaner for typing this script. Above all, by giving respectful thanks to my mother — 'Lalita Mathur' who is my constant inspirer, I dedicate this book to you all.

With warm regards

K.C. Mathur

CONTENTS

UNIT FOUR — RESPIRATION

UNIT FIVE — EXCRETION

UNIT SIX — SPECIAL SENSES

UNIT SEVEN — ENDOCRINES

UNIT EIGHT — REPRODUCTION

UNIT NINE — BLOOD

UNIT THIRTEEN — METABOLISM

UNIT FOURTEEN — CENTRAL NERVOUS SYSTEM

UNIT 1

Getting Introduced

"Just by reading this basic subject of medical science one has to say that oh? the supreme creation of Nature is human body and nothing else. So this is the correct time to get introduced with it and all this is—JUST BY THE WAY."

Just by the way

1 Scope: Field of Physiology

CONTROL SYSTEM (BODY MECHANICS)

Physiology and philosophy can be considered as a single unit. It means 'study of different functions and mechanism of various body organs and systems in a normal body.' Furthermore, it gives the answer of 'How, when, why and what?' in a normal body. Its range also reaches to onset of a disease and its treatment, since a 'disease' is nothing but an 'altered or impaired function.' By reading this subject we are actually opening the lock of 'suspense' and realising the fact that, human body is finest creation of God.

CONTROL OF BODY FUNCTIONS

Negative Feedback System

Let us consider following examples

- A high concentration of CO_2 in extracellular fluid causes increased pulmonary ventilation which eliminates excess CO_2 out of the body.
- When blood pressure of a person becomes high, the baroreceptors are stimulated which lowers the raised blood pressure.
- During normal menstrual cycle, when oestrogen level reaches at its peak then almost on 14th day, the controlling hormone. FSH from adenohypophysis is inhibited so level of oestrogen becomes zero or lowest.

So in nutshell it is clear that, "if some factors become excessive, or too little, a control system initiate negative feedback which consists of series of changes that return the factor towards mean/normal/average values/level.

Positive Feedback System

Let us consider following examples:

- During delivery of a child, the head of foetus irritates the wall of uterus which responds by contraction; and, each contraction will push the baby downwards: Thus the uterine contractions stretch the cervix which causes more contractions (Mechanical irritation theory of delivery).
- When membrane of a nerve is stimulated, it leads to slight leakage of sodium ions through sodium channel in the interior of nerve fibre. This influx of sodium ion will change the membrane potential which will open more sodium channel. So with smallest beginning of sodium ion there occurred bombardment of these ions.

This is positive feedback or 'vicious cycle.' This mechanism creates instability; not at all stability.

SERVO MECHANISM

- Stretch reflex which regulates muscle length is its example. In different positions of the limb, the resting muscle length of a given skeletal muscle changes. So set point at which length is regulated varies according to position of limb.
- Explanation
  - — On simultaneous stimulation of alpha and gamma motor neurones; the degree of stimulation of muscle spindle will be considered unchanged (mean neither increase nor decrease); if extra- and intrafusal fibres contract in equal amounts.
  - — If muscle is contracting against a load; then extrafusal muscle fibres contract less as compared with intrafusal fibres; then receptor portion of spindle will be contracted; which will terminate into elicitation of stretch reflex, and, because of this, there will be extra excitation of extrafusal fibres.
- Advantages
  - — Muscle can contract against a load. Less expenditure of nervous energy by brain.
  - — Between successive contractions, if the load is increased or decreased, then muscle contracts to desired length.

Jean Fernol (1542) for the first time introduced the term physiology.

— Compensation for fatigue/other muscular abnormalities occur.

Control by Coupling

During hypoxia, the respiration is stimulated. Since respiration and vasomotor centres are lying very close to each other in brain, so blood pressure also rises, along with respiration. This coupling (respiration + B. P.) is essential because it increases blood flow through these organs.

ANTICIPATORY CONTROL SYSTEM

Hypothalamus controls the body temperature but it is in close touch with environmental temperature via cutaneous thermoreceptors. So by this it manages body temperature before environmental temperature disturbs it.

So by having this much knowledge we can appreciate that how enumerable body cells are working in a harmonious way in normal body to maintain homeostasis and when this hormony is lost, disease process starts.

ELECTROPHYSIOLOGY STUDY (EPS) AND RFA PROCEDURE

Electrophysiology is a sub-speciality of cardiology and deals with electrical properties of the heart. Improved understanding of the mechanism of arrhythmia and radio-frequency ablation (RFA) has revolutionised the management of tachycardia.

EPS is the study of the electrical properties of the heart and helps to diagnose the mechanism of arrhythmias. The procedure is performed after all arrhythmic drugs are withdrawn for at least five half-lives in a cardiac catheterisation laboratory under local anaesthesia and mild sedation. Through the femoral veins, electrode catheters are advanced into cardiac chambers, i.e. right atrium, right ventricle, his bundle region and the coronary sinus. X-ray guidance is used to manipulate the catheters within the cardiac chambers. These electrode catheters help to record electrogram from within the cardiac chambers and electrical stimulation through them helps to initiate and terminate tachycardias. This helps to identify the mechanism of arrhythmia and to locate the abnormal focus or connection responsible for the tachycardia. A special electrode catheter called the radiofrequency or ablation (RFA) catheter is then introduced at that spot and the external end of the catheter is connected to RF generator. Delivery of RF energy creates sufficient heat at the local site to charge the abnormal tissue. The energy is delivered through a 4 mm tip electrode and this results in a 2 mm × 4 mm × 6 mm lesion, not damaging the surrounding cardiac structures. The EPS procedure takes one and a half to two hours. However, the RF energy delivered to destroy the abnormal tissue is given only for 45 to 60 seconds. After the procedure, electrical stimulating is performed for nearly 30 minutes to be sure that the tachycardia is no longer inducible and there are no other mechanisms of tachycardia. The electrode catheters are then removed and the groin manually compressed to achieve haemostasis. Immediately after the procedure, the patient is asked to take oral liquids and after 4-6 hours rest period, patient is mobilised and is ready for discharge the next morning. All drugs are withdrawn at discharge and only low dosage of aspirin is prescribed for three months to promote endocardial healing.

(*Source:*- ALMA MATER SPMC; SPMC CLUB INTERNATIONAL Vol. XIII, No. 11, 2003 June; p-4-5.)

GLOSSARY

1. *Morphology:* Study of external form, structure and relative position of various organs of living beings. It is required in accurate description of organism for identification.
2. *Molecular biology:* Branch of biology concerned with study of nature, physico-chemical-organisation, synthesis. Working and interaction of bio-molecules which bring about and control various activities of protoplasm.
3. *Biogeography:* Distribution of organism in various parts of the earth.
4. *Exobiology:* The branch of scientific enquiry dealing with possibility of life in outer space.
5. *Eugenics:* Science dealing with factors related to improvement/impairment of races, specially of human beings.
6. *Genetic engineering:* It deals with production of organism with combination of new heritable characters at will (gene manipulation).
7. *Anthropology:* Study of physical, cultural, mental and social nature of primitive and modern man.
8. *DNA finger printing:* By this technique, a person can be identified on the basis of his genes, as no two persons have identical sub-genetic make up.
9. *Euthenics:* Study of environment and its influence on mankind.
10. *Electron microscope:* Magnification 1,00,000 times. Used for ultra structure of nucleus and cell organelles. Stream of high speed electrons.

BIBLIOGRAPHY

1. Adolph EF. Physiologist. Physiological integration in action, 1982, 25 (supp.): I.
2. Gann DS, et al. Neural interaction in control of adeno-corticotrophin. Fed Proc. 1985;44:161.
3. Rusak B, et al. Neural regulation of circadian rhythms. Phy Rev 1979;59:449.
4. Stein JF. Role of cerebellum in visual guidance of movement. Nature 1986;323:217.
5. Thompson RF. The neuro biology of learning and memory, Science 1986;233:941.

2 Organisation: Human Body

HOMEOSTASIS

Homeo=Alike or Similar and Stasis = Standstill

In other words there is a balance—A constancy of internal state of human being, (Milieu-interieur coined by Walter B. Cannon of Harvard university). This word has become a part of the regular vocabulary of every physiologist.

Life began as a unicellular organism in the primordial sea. The salt content of the ancient sea was very different from the present day ocean, which became concentrated by evaporation and by the addition of minerals from the land leached out by rains and rivers over countless ages. Then the animal left this sea water but then it had to exchange for air and the saline fluid with which its cells were well adapted. So this sea environment, was carried with it, which is internal environment (salt water) without which the individual cells could not exist. However, air is the external environment. So today's organism has enclosed himself in a kind of hot house. The perpetual changes of external conditions cannot reach it—it is not subjected to them but is rather free and independent.

The mechanism by which the constancy of internal environment is maintained and ensured is called homeostasis by Cannon. The chief instrument in this orchestra is kidney along with endocrine glands

Common examples/illustrations: (According to L. L. Langley and E. Cheraksin):

i. Imagine a swimming pool with five feet of water in it and with water running into it at one end and out of it at the other but staying almost at five foot level all the time—perhaps rising an inch or two at times and lowering an inch or so at other times, but quickly coming back down to five feet level after it rises and back up to five feet level after it lowers. This is an illustration of state of dynamic equilibrium—an expression often used to describe essential, paradoxical characteristic of homeostasis. Dynamic means moving/changing/not static while equilibrium means constancy/stability/balance. Similarly human cells require a fairly uniform or stable environment in order to maintain their life and health.

The body must maintain relative constancy of its chemicals and processes in order to survive. Health and survival depend upon the body's maintaining or quickly restoring, homeostasis—it is main theme of physiology.

—Claude Bernard

ii. Every mother knows that her child's temperature should be about 98.6°F (37°C). If it is more than that she apprehensively summons the doctor. She does not stop to think whether it is any icy December morning or a hot and humid August afternoon. She expects her child's temperature to be about the same at all times and she is correct. A human being may be exposed to wide variations of climate and yet the temperature of inside of body remains remarkably close to 98.6°F.

iii. Another example of homeostasis is the constancy of blood sugar level. It can be easily demonstrated that the blood sugar is rapidly returned to within the normal range despite the fact that one eats, e.g. chocolate cake at one meal. On the contrary, if one starves for several days the blood sugar would still be close to its average value.

iv. Another example is of exercise. The net result here is, to allow the athlete to expend energy at a high rate with a medium of fatigue and with strikingly small deviations in the internal environment.

v. Other examples are—regulation of blood volume, heart rate and blood pressure, respiration, acid-base balance and ionic balance, etc.

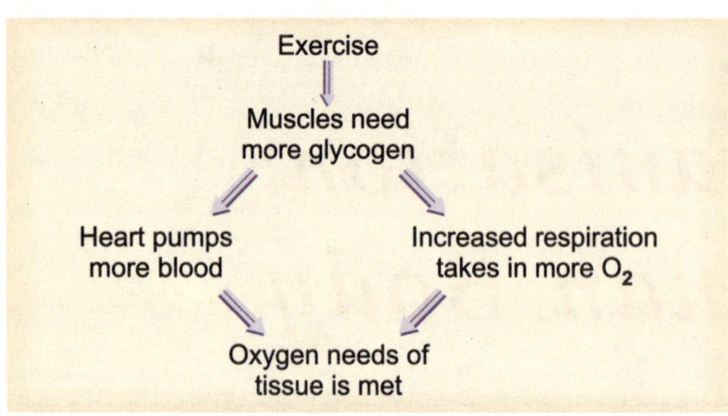

Diagram 2.1: Example of homeostasis

Table 2.1: Differences

Constituents	*Sea water (gm/litre)*	*Blood (gm/litre)*
1. Na	10.7	3.2–3.4
2. K	0.39	0.15–0.21
3. Chloride	19.3	3.5–3.8
4. CO_2 (Carbonate)	0.073	1.5–1.9
5. Ca	0.42	0.09–0.11

PHYSIOLOGY OF STRESS

Think of a pregnant lady; she is always worried about the birth and then further development of her child who is still unborn; a businessman is always worried of income tax raids; a student is always under pressure because of his examinations, an office clerk is always tense because of huge number of files to be dealt; a doctor can be called even in midnight under the title 'emergency.' *So as Hens Selye remarks 'stress is the spice of life, every class of persons is under stress, no one can escape stress.'*

> The stress and strain are increasing day by day with advancement of civilisation. In stress, chain of glandular and hormonal reactions take place to keep our body adapted for changing circumstances
>
> *Hens Selye*

- Now think of a mother who gets the information that her only son has died in the war. She gets shock, she is worried, she weeps; this is Distress - certainly and cent percent harmful. Now after sometime her son comes back to house suddenly in his full spirit/ vigour/and health and tells that the news of his death was wrong. The mother is filled with joy/happiness/ over crowded with laughters. This is *eustress*—of course not so harmful but not cent percent safe. *So this further proves that stress moves with the individual both in sad as well as jolly atmosphere.*
- The single word stress includes—mental tension, worries, inferiority complex/superiority complex, anger, frustration, desire to take revenge, jealousy emotions, excitement, etc.
- It is the single cause of many fatal diseases like heart attacks, hypertension, diabetes mellitus, migraine, peptic ulcer, other GIT disorders and even cancer, etc. ***During pregnancy stress is a double edged sword—on one side it is doing harm to mother while on another side the growth and development of foetus is impaired.***

Stress and Stomach

Hypothalamo-hypophyseal-adrenal axis has been found to be involved in mechanism through which an increase in gastric secretory activity occurs as a result of stress. Due to stress adrenal activity is increased which in turn leads to increased gastric activity. The adrenal corticoids by themselves increase the gastric secretion particularly the acid formation.

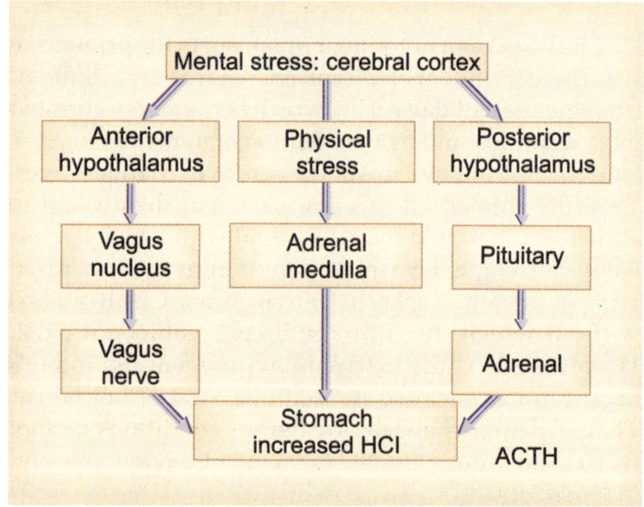

Diagram 2.2: Stress-oriented stomach diseases

STRESS V/S BODY MECHANICS: GENERAL ADAPTATION SYNDROME

The stages have been described as :

a. ***Alarm reaction:*** The changes come within 6–24 hours. It is characterised by fatigue, loss of muscle tone, diminished urine, fall of blood sugar and NaCl, together with lymphopenia. Adrenal gland is shrunken while thymus and lymphoid tissue involute. Animal may die if stress is severe otherwise it may pass into next stage.

Mass Discharge: Large Sympathetic Mass Discharging

1. Increased arterial pressure
2. Increased blood glucose concentration
3. Increased muscle strength
4. Increased mental activity
5. Increased glycolysis in liver
6. Increased rate of cellular metabolism

b. ***Stage of resistance:*** Recovery. Urine increases, blood, sugar and NaCl becomes normal. Granules reappear in cells.

c. ***Stage of exhaustion***: If stress is severe the animal cannot withstand and may die.

CAUSES: STRESS

1. Marital separation
2. Death of close family member
3. Personal injury/illness
4. Change in financial state
5. Any loan/mortgage
6. Trouble with boss
7. Minor violence
8. Failure in examination/love affair.

CATECHOLAMINE-RELEASED DURING STRESS

Sympathomimetic or adrenergic drugs are agents that mimic the responses obtained as a result of stimulation of the sympathetic or adrenergic nerves. Majority of these substances contain an intact or partially substituted amino (NH_2) group and hence are also called 'sympathomimetic amines.'

The catecholamine includes sympathetic neurohumoral transmitter noradrenaline, adrenaline, dopamine, isoprenaline and N-methyl adrenaline. Catecholamine of adrenal medulla is normally 85 per cent adrenaline and 15 per cent nor-adrenaline.

PHYSIOLOGICAL ACTIONS

Heart

- Rate is increased by increasing the slope of slow diastolic depolarisation of cells in SA node. It also activates latent pacemakers in AV node and Purkinje fibres.
- Force of cardiac contraction is increased, development of tension and relaxation are accelerated. Oxygen consumption and cardiac output are markedly increased.
- Conduction velocity through AV node, bundle of His, atrial and ventricular fibres is increased. It increases myocardial metabolism with increased oxygen consumption, thus decreasing the cardiac efficiency. Adrenaline abolishes the reflex vagal bradycardia in response to carotid sinus compression. It stimulates predominant β receptors of the heart.

Respiration

It is potent bronchodilator and this action is more marked when bronchi are constricted. It can directly stimulate respiratory centre. Its rapid intravenous administration in animals causes transient apnoea due to reflex inhibition of respiratory centre. Its administration in very high doses may lead to pulmonary oedema by shifting blood from systemic to pulmonary circuit. It is a weak stimulant of respiration.

Blood Pressure

Adrenaline given by slow intravenous infusion or subcutaneously causes a rise in systolic but fall in diastolic pressure. Peripheral resistance decreases because vascular β_2 receptors are more sensitive than α receptors. Generally mean blood pressure rises and pulse pressure is also increased.

Rapid intravenous administration in animals produces a marked increase in both systolic and diastolic blood pressure which returns to normal levels within a few minutes and a secondary fall in mean blood pressure follows.

Noradrenaline leads to rise in systolic, diastolic, mean BP. It does not cause vasodilatation (no β_2 action), peripheral resistance increased due to α action.

Adrenaline activates both α and β receptors. By stimulating α receptor it produces rise in blood pressure (α being dominant in number). Its action on β receptor is more persistent so when action on α receptor wears off, action on β receptor is unmasked producing fall of blood pressure.

Although adrenaline raises systolic blood pressure by its cardiac action, but it lowers diastolic blood pressure by its peripheral action, so it is not suitable in hypotensive shock.

VASOMOTOR REVERSAL OF DALE

Adrenaline produces a biphasic response on systolic blood pressure. There is rise of blood pressure followed by fall of blood pressure. This is attributed to α adrenergic receptor stimulation (rise of blood pressure) followed by β adrenergic receptor activity (fall of blood pressure) respectively. It goes to credit of Henry Dale who for the first time showed that if adrenaline is given after blockade of α adrenergic receptors by ergot alkaloids, it produces only fall of blood pressure due to β receptor activity. This phenomenon is also described as vasomotor reversal of Dale.

iv. *GIT (smooth muscles):* In isolated preparations of gut, relaxation occurs through activation of both alpha and beta receptors. Motility is reduced.

v. *CNS:* Adrenaline in clinically used doses does not produce any marked CNS effects because of poor penetration in brain (does not cross blood-brain-barrier) but restlessness, apprehension and tremor may occur. Activation of alpha$_2$ receptors in the brainstem results in decreased sympathetic outflow which leads to bradycardia and hypotension.

vi. *Metabolic*: Glycogenolysis—hyperglycaemia (β_2), hyperlactacidaemia, lipolysis, rise in plasma free fatty acid, calorigenesis (β_2+β_3)and hyperkalaemia followed by hypokalaemia by direct action on liver muscle, adipose tissue cells. In addition metabolic effects results due to reduction of insulin (α_2) and augmentation of glucagon (β_2) secretion.

vii. *Eye:* Mydriasis due to contraction of radial muscles of iris (α_1) but this is minimal after topical application because it penetrates cornea poorly. The intraocular tension tends to fall, specially in wide angle glaucoma. Exophthalmos may also result due to contraction of orbital muscles. Nictitating membrane contracts (lower animals).

viii. *Skeletal muscles:* It stimulates their contraction by acting on both sides of neuromuscular junction. The α effect on motor nerve ending increases the amount of acetylcholine and is probably the main factor in the improvement of neuromuscular transmission by adrenaline. The β action on the muscle fibres probably contributes to improvement of muscle contraction and tremor, sometimes observed following its administration.

Blood Vessels

- Blood vessels of skin and mucous membrane are constricted by adrenaline and noradrenaline. This is followed by after congestion. Adrenaline dilates the blood vessels of skeletal muscles on account of preponderance of β_2 receptors. It finally results into total decrease in peripheral resistance.
- Both these catecholamines constrict the mesenteric blood vessels and raise the portal venous pressure. Both raise pulmonary arterial and venous pressure but more by adrenaline. It is due to pulmonary vasoconstriction and partly as a result of increase in left atrial pressure.
- Constriction of musculature of great systemic veins tends to push the blood from periphery into pulmonary circulation which may occasionally result in pulmonary oedema.
- Adrenaline in moderate doses increases the cerebral blood flow and oxygen consumption probably by increasing the systemic blood pressure.
- It increases the coronary blood flow by a complex mechanism.
- Both of them lead to significant reduction in renal blood flow (vasoconstriction). Urinary excretion of sodium, potassium and chloride is decreased while renin secretion is increased.

Smooth Muscles

- Adrenaline is a powerful relaxant of bronchial smooth muscle.
- The human non-pregnant uterus is stimulated to contract by adrenaline. In the last month of pregnancy adrenaline relaxes the human uterus.

Miscellaneous

- Adrenaline contracts pilomotor muscle of hair follicle.
- It also produces a contraction of vesicle sphincter and trigone, while relaxing detrusor muscle.
- Both of these produce contraction of splenic capsule leading a release of RBC into the peripheral circulation. It is a protective measure against stress like hypoxia, haemorrhage, etc. (via alpha receptors)
- Thick viscid secretion from salivary glands (via alpha and beta$_2$ receptors)
- Leucocytosis and eosinopenia accelerating blood coagulation
- Stimulates platelet aggregation through alpha receptor in platelets.
- Inhibit cellular anaphylactic mechanism, preventing the release of mediators of allergic bronchospasm, e.g. histamine from tissue mast cells.
- Secretory activity of lacrimal gland is increased via alpha receptors.
- Secretion of apocrine sweat gland is increased via beta$_2$ receptors.
- Adrenaline decreases the latency of action potential in nerve fibres via alpha receptors.
- Renin secretion is increased from JG apparatus of kidney by adrenaline through beta receptors.

METABOLISM

Adrenaline is mainly metabolised by two enzymes—catechol-o-methyl-transferase (COMT), and monoamine-oxidase (MAO)—the former is situated outside and later inside the mitochondria of the adrenergic neurones. COMT changes adrenaline into metanephrine and noradrenaline to normetanephrine. MAO oxidizes these products into 3-methoxy-4 hydroxy mandelic acid (VMA - Vanilylmandelic acid) which is excreted in urine.

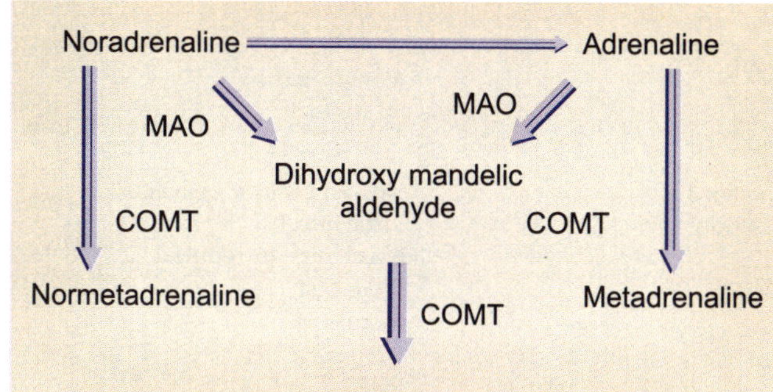

Diagram 2.3: Metabolism of adrenaline and noradrenaline

The normal 24 hour urinary excretion of VMA and free catecholamines is 4–8 mg and 50–100 µg respectively. A significant increase in these values is considered diagnostic of pheochromocytoma—an adrenal medullary tumour, producing excessive catecholamines.

NORADRENALINE

- Predominantly acts on α receptors (alpha agonist), minimal effect on cardiac beta receptors.

On Cardiovascular System

- Through vasoconstriction raises systolic blood pressure and diastolic also, due to increase in total peripheral resistance. Cardiac output little changed or unaffected. Produces bradycardia through baroreceptor and increased reflex vagal activity. So bradycardia is secondary to hypertension. Cardiac oxygen consumption is increased. Coronary flow is increased due to raised mean arterial blood pressure and due to production of a vasodilator substance "adenosine." Positive ionotropic effect on heart. Rate is usually slow.
- It is used in treatment of hypotensive states (surgical shock/myocardial infarction/cardiogenic shock).

ACETYLCHOLINE

Muscarinic actions

- Slowing of heart, vasodilatation in slightly higher doses and fall in blood pressure.
- Stimulation of smooth muscle of bronchi, GIT/gall-bladder and bile duct, ureter and bladder.
- Relaxation of sphincters in GIT/urinary tract.
- Constriction of pupil (miosis) and accommodation of lens for near vision.
- Stimulation of salivary/sweat/lacrimal/naso-pharyngeal, stomach, pancreas, intestine.
- Bradycardia, negative ionotropic effects.

Nicotinic Action

- Stimulation of skeletal muscle
- Stimulation of adrenal medulla
- Stimulation of sympathetic and parasympathetic ganglia.

DOPAMINE

- Secreted by adrenal medulla + dopaminergic neurones of CNS.
- Its effects include: Vasoconstriction, vasodilatation in mesentery, increase in heart rate through β receptors, increase in systolic blood pressure but not diastolic blood pressure.

ADRENAL MEDULLA

1. **Embryology:** Develops from ectodermal tissue, neural crest.
2. **Structure:** Irregular cells, take $K_2Cr_2O_7$ to give chromaffine reaction, arranged in short cords enclosed by sinusoids. Ill-defined boundary with cortex.
3. **Active principles:**
   a. ***Adrenaline:*** β hydroxy- 3:4 dihydroxy phenyl N. Methyl-ethylamine -
   b. ***Noradrenaline*** - β-hydroxy- 3:4 dihydroxy-phenyl-ethyl alanine.
   c. ***Normal concentration*:** Noradrenaline - 0.09 mg/gm, Adrenaline = 0.49 mg/gm.
4. **Secretion:**
   a. *Basal:* 0.2 µg/kg/min is adrenaline; 0.05 µg/kg/min is noradrenaline
   b. *Splanchnic or reflex stimulation* via carotid sinus
   c. More effective is hypothalamic stimulation
   d. Insulin hypoglycaemia may provoke its secretion (of adrenaline only)
   e. Hyperglycaemia inhibit medullary secretion of adrenaline.
5. **Hyperadrenia:** Paroxysmal hypertension, hyperglycaemia + glycosurea, dyspnoea, sweating, tremor, nervousness, due to pheochromocytoma
6. **Demedullation:** has no effect except recovery from hypoglycaemia
7. Inactive per os, IV infusion generally done.
8. **Importance:**
   a. Adrenaline and noradrenaline are having two sources of production—first from adrenal medulla, and second from activation of sympathetics. If sympathetics are removed/diseased then the part will receive adrenaline from adrenal medulla still, and it will serve the purpose or acts as a substitute. Conversely, if adrenal medulla is

Table 2.2: Main actions of adrenaline and noradrenaline

Effect on	*Adrenaline (alpha + beta)*	*Noradrenaline (alpha)*
Heart		
Rate	Increased (direct action)	Slowed reflexly via vagus
Force of contraction	Increased (direct action)	Little effect
Cardiac output	Increased	No change or reduced
Excitability and conductivity	Markedly increased	Increased
Coronary blood flow	Increased	Increased
Blood pressure		
Systolic	Rise	Rise
Diastolic	Fall	Rise
Mean arterial	Slight rise	Marked rise
Metabolic		
O_2 consumption	Increased	Little effect
Blood glucose	Increased	Little effect
Smooth Muscles		
Bronchi	Relaxed	Little effect
Intestines	Relaxed	Relaxed
Urinary bladder	Relaxed	Relaxed
Sphincters	Constricted	Constricted
Pregnant uterus	Inhibited	Stimulated
CNS	Stimulated	Little effect
Capillary permeability Vascular Beds	Reduced	Little effect
Skin and viscera	Constricted	Constricted
Skeletal muscle	Dilated	Constricted
Heart	Dilated	Dilated
Kidney	Constricted	Constricted
Brain	Dilated	No change/constricted
Total peripheral resistance	Decreased	Increased

diseased/destructed then even, the part will get adrenaline, etc. from sympathetics. This means that both these sources are acting as a substitute of each other.

b. Adrenaline and noradrenaline are capable to stimulate body structures which are not innervated by direct sympathetic fibres.

SUMMARY AND HIGHLIGHTS

So to meet with stress, face it but don't escape from it. Be natural in all the fields like living/dressing/thinking etc. Since 'Nature is fountain head of all our problems and solution, closer we keep to it better we realise it'.

Hens Selye

GLOSSARY

1. *Health:* A state of complete physical. Mental, social and spiritual well-being; not merely the absence of disease.
2. *Disease:* Is a condition in which normal state of well-being is impaired.
3. *Virulence:* Is the relative ability of pathogens to damage the host.
4. *Adaptation:* Any structural and functional modification occurring in an organism to adjust itself to the environment in which it lives and reproduces successfully is adaptation. It helps in successful survival. Short-term adaptation develops due to temporary/small changes in environment, while long-term adaptations are evolved gradually over hundred/thousand of years in response to some permanent changes in the environment.

BIBLIOGRAPHY

1. French, et al. Hypothalamic influences on HCl secretion of stomach. Surg 1953;33:875.
2. Gray: The adrenal glands and peptic ulcer, Gastroenterology 1960;39:533.
3. Gray, et al. Hormonal influences upon stomach, Amer J Gastroent 1955;24:244.
3. LL Langley and E. Cheraskin. Physiology of man, McGrew Hill book company. Inc. New York, Toronto London. Second edition, 1958.
4. Selye Hens: Stress. Journal Probe Quarternally J of Himalaya drug Co. Publication 1980;6-12.

3 Unit of Body Mechanics: The Cell

Each cell which is really a biological machine, contains physical and chemical mechanisms, designed to obtain from its environment, the various materials, to satisfy nutritional and energy requirements of the organ concerned, when these mechanisms which involve structure and functional relationship, are impaired the result is sickness, or death even.

The basic unit of all living organisms is the cell. Some forms such as amoeba, consist of a single cell. In more complex forms, there are millions of these units of various types; and in these organisms, the cells are arranged into aggregates known as ***tissues*** (Fig. 3.1).

CELL: HISTORICAL ASPECTS

- Term 'cell' coined by Robert Hook (1665).
- The name was given as utricle and saccules by Malpighi (1661).
- He observed cell before Hook.
- Plants are formed by membranous cellular tissue - Mirabel 1802.

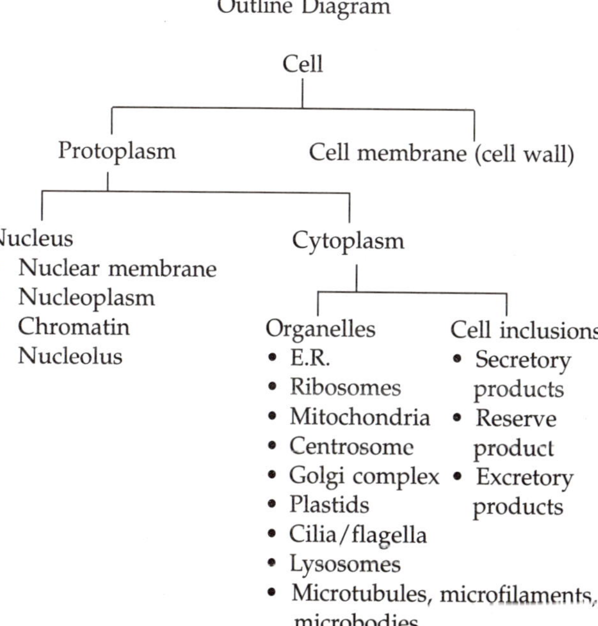

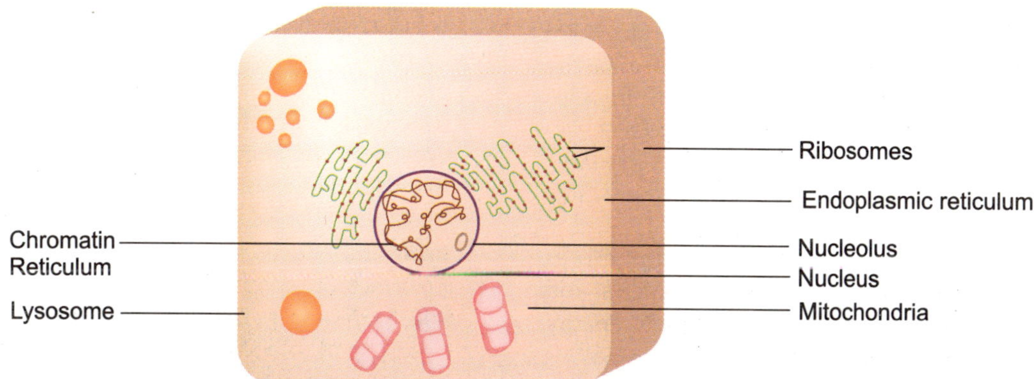

Fig. 3.1: Normal cell

- Robert Brown (1831) discovered nucleus in orchid root.
- Purkinje (1839) discovered protoplasm.
- Max Schultze (1861)—Protoplasmic theory.
- Sachs (1874)—organismal theory.

PROTOPLASM

i. This term is difficult to define. It is the stuff of which all living tissue is formed. It is living material of cell.

   It consists of basic elements carbon, hydrogen, oxygen and nitrogen which predominate. Other elements like calcium, potassium, sulphur, etc. collectively don't make more than 3 to 4 per cent of protoplasm. In most, water is present.

ii. In 1835, Dujardin described it as a homogenous, gelatinous substance. Purkinje and Von Mohl (1840) gave it the name of protoplasm. In 1861, Schutz described the famous Protoplasm theory which states that cell is an accumulation of living substances having a nucleus and a limiting cell membrane.

iii. Generally—water 85 to 90 per cent; Proteins 7 to 10 per cent; lipids 1 to 2 per cent, carbohydrates and others organic constituents 1 to 1.5 per cent; Inorganic constituents 1 to 1.5 per cent.

> Protoplasm is a viscid, gelatinous, semifluid substance heavier than water but its viscosity varies under different conditions. It is a colourless, translucent, jelly like substance in which there are small molecular suspensions. It may be reticular or fibrillar, or granular or a homogenous structure.

iv. Proteins: are found only in protoplasm and are made of C, O_2, H_2, N_2 and traces of P, S, Mg and Fe. They constitute the framework of protoplasm. They are in a colloidal state. They form amino acid on being broken down. Amino acids are called building blocks of protoplasm. There are about 20 amino acids and every protein is a complex combination of these building blocks. They coagulate on heating. They are most important constituent of cell protoplasm and membrane, they are indispensable in the maintenance of vital processes in a cell. Besides proteins—other compounds like mucopolysaccharides, mucoproteins, glycoproteins are also present in matrix of connective tissue where they act as binding and protective agents.

v. Lipids: are made of C, H, O. They are insoluble in water. They are present as stored food material and also as a part of protoplasm. They supply energy though not as readily as glucose.

vi. Water: occurs in the greatest amount in tissues. It is a medium of dispersion for colloids of protoplasm. High surface tension of water provides a consistency to protoplasm and, it affords protection against sudden temperature changes. Water exists in free and bound form within an organism; free water is miscible with protoplasm where it is the chief solvent for metabolic processes. Bound water has its molecules tied to proteins by hydrogen bonds, e.g. in gelatine each molecule of amino acid is capable of binding 2.6 molecules of water. It serves as a natural solvent for mineral ions and many other substances so that chemical reaction can take place. It is indispensable in metabolic processes since enzymatic activity takes place exclusively in the presence of water.

vii. Carbohydrates: are made of C, H and O; with hydrogen and oxygen in a 2:1 ratio. When they are broken down, they form glucose which supplies energy and forms glycogen for storage. Glycogen can be reconverted into glucose when needed. Mono, di and polysaccharides are their divisions of biological significance.

viii. Inorganic salts: less than 1% are inorganic salts, yet they are essential in regulating metabolism and maintenance of proteins in solution. Mineral ions of sodium, sulphur, iron and magnesium are present in protoplasm; they form chloride, phosphate, carbonates, bicarbonates and sulphates. Gases present in protoplasm are O_2 and CO_2 which are used in respiration. In general, the inorganic components maintain acid base balance and regulate osmotic pressure; the phosphate bond plays an important role as the source of energy. Inorganic component of the cell's protoplasm are present either in the form of salt or in combination with proteins/lipids/or carbohydrates. In some cases, they combine with amino acids to form hormones (e.g. thyroxin), or with proteins to form important compounds (e.g. haemoglobin), haemocyanin (copper), and cytochrome (iron).

ix. Hormones: are organic chemical secretions of the protoplasm of endocrine glands. They affect the functions of organs and metabolic processes with great rapidity. They are produced in minute quantity in one part of an organism and are then transported by blood to other parts where they exert some profound effects.

x. Enzymes: are complex proteins which form colloidal solution when dissolved; they are found in protoplasm, blood and the digestive system. They are organic catalytic agents present in minute amounts; they bring about chemical reactions of metabolism with great speed. A cell is a minute laboratory capable of synthesis and breakdown of various substances at normal body temperature, and all the chemical reactions involved are carried out by the intervention of enzymes which are biological catalysts for speeding up chemical reaction necessary for vital activities. Enzymes are named by adding the suffix "ase" to the name of the substance on which they act. An enzyme acts on a substance by combining with it and activating it in some known or unknown way. So that the substance undergoes further chemical change, and at the same time it separates from its enzyme, and enzyme is not consumed, but is free to deal with more of that substance. Enzymes are unstable substances and can be easily destroyed or inactivated by high temperature, or by a great range of chemical substances.

xi. Vitamins: They are complex organic substances, which though present in the protoplasm are obtained by the organism from its environment. Vitamins are essential for growth, metabolism, and maintenance of health. Their deficiency reduces the rate of metabolism and may result in a deficiency disease, and stunt the growth.

CELL MEMBRANE

- If amoeba is cut with a sharp knife the thick protoplasm will be seen to escape (microscopically). This indicates that protoplasmic mass must be normally contained by a very thin envelope. Actually the membrane itself is made up of protoplasm, but this protoplasm has been altered some what so as to perform some special functions. Firstly, it imprisons the cell protoplasm to give a particular shape to a structure. Secondly, it permits many substances to pass through, while at the same time it becomes barrier for many others; or in better way it is a semi-permeable membrane. So cytoplasm is enclosed within a fine retaining sheath called cell membrane; it is living part of the cell, and all substances entering or leaving a cell must pass through it; it has some very minute pores.
- It is about 2μ in thickness and is a dense double layered membrane having large amount of phospholipids forming long molecules. It has layers of lipid molecules with protein molecules sandwiched together.
- The lipid molecules are long and consist of a part with lipid property of being insoluble in water, and a group at one end with polar properties, i.e. with a tendency to dissolve in water, the lipid parts are turned inwards and polar groups in opposite direction.
- The cell membrane possesses true surface tension properties. The lipid molecules form a film which lowers surface tension and the protein layer is elastic.
- The cell membrane keeps the intracellular fluid of the cell from mixing with the surrounding liquids; thus it maintains a stable state of the cell which has a constant internal environment, and composition.
- As told earlier, it is semi-permeable in nature. Glucose, amino acid, hormones, vitamins, water, oxygen, carbon dioxide pass easily through it. Potassium passes rapidly but sodium cannot. Urea, fatty acids, glycerol pass less easily; while inorganic salts, protein, fats and carbohydrates cannot pass through it. Some water with dissolved salts certainly passes in and out of cells from between the lipid chains.
- The lipid bilayer serves as a transport medium for lipid soluble molecules to gain entry into the cell whereas protein lined hydrophilic pores probably provide channel for diffusion of polar entities, e.g. water and ions. The permeability to water seems to be inversely related to the proportion of cholesterol in the phospholipid membrane.
- Functions of proteins: (a) They act as 'pumps' (actively transports ions across the membrane. (b) They function as carriers - transporting substances down electrochemical gradients by facilitated diffusion. (c) They are ionic channels—permit the passage of ions across the cell membrane. (d) They act as receptor or binding hormones and neurotransmitters. (e) They also function as enzymes—catalysing reaction. (f) They as glycoprotein serve in processing of antibody.
- Underlying most cells, there exists basement membrane (basal lamina) which is made up of many proteins that hold cells together and control their growth and development. It consists of collagens, laminins fibronectin and proteoglycans.

CYTOPLASM

The protoplasm of a cell lying outside the nucleus is known as cytoplasm. It is a clear fluid in which float many small particles.

- It is concerned largely with the relation of cell with its environment.
- It is the main assembly and production centre of the cell and its endoplasmic reticulum is the site of protein synthesis.

- It is concerned with obtaining food and changing it into chemical energy. It extracts chemical energy from fats and sugars and transfers it to special energy rich molecules which circulates in the cell. It is concerned with synthesis of large molecules needed either by the cell or for export outside the cell.
- It contains numerous objects referred as organelles or cytoplasmic inclusions which are responsible for special functions in a cell and are briefly described below:

  a. ***Centrosome:*** Lying near the nucleus in the cytoplasm is a clear area free from granules, is centrosome, it contains one or two minute but darkly staining centriole—(short cylinders). They are located at right angles to each other. Structurally, it looks like that of cilium—a barrel like cylinder whose wall has nine longitudinal fibrils in a circle, fibrils are often double (and in some cells it also has two central fibrils); all the fibrils are held together by two girdles, each girdle has nine round spheres or macromolecules which are joined to the fibrils by thin threads.

  b. ***Mitochondria (Synonym = chondriosomes)***

  - 0.2 - 0.3μ in size. They have an outer cortex of lipid and an inner core of protein. Each mitochondria is a bag whose wall is made up of two lipo-protein membranes—the outer membrane is elastic and is covered with small particles; the inner membrane bears particles and is thrown into folds called cristae which project into the lumen of the mitochondrion and increase the surface area. The lumen of mitochondria is filled with fluid. It contains numerous enzymes either on cristae of the inner membrane or dissolved in the fluid. These are actually hundreds of filaments, rods or spheres in the cytoplasm and they are constantly in motion.
  - They perform two main functions—first is that they breakdown fats/carbohydrate/proteins into small molecules, and secondly they transfer their chemical energy into complex molecules—the most important of which is ATP which is the carrier of chemical energy and most of it is formed within mitochondria. The ATP molecules are then secreted by mitochondria and are used in the cell wherever energy is needed. Thus, they are power houses of a cell because they produce most of the usable energy. In them food molecules are burnt to form CO_2 and H_2O to release energy. In a cell energy does not escape as heat but is used directly to synthesise ATP which is a store of high energy.
  - Within the inner membrane, there is a matrix containing the granules, RNA and DNA. The DNA provides necessary information for replication of the mitochondria while RNA is responsible for synthesis of a few of the proteins of the mitochondrion. Respiratory enzymes and components of oxidative phosphorylation are associated in an ordered array on the inner membrane. This order tends to promote the sequential interaction of substrates and enzymes in these multi-enzyme system with conservation of energy.
  - The outer membrane of the mitochondrion has a different enzyme content, a large percentage of lipids, and is more permeable to simple sugars than the inner membrane.
  - Besides the above mentioned enzymes, (in both inner and outer membrane) certain enzymes (e.g. of tricarboxylic acid cycle) are found in matrix or they may be loosely attached to a mitochondrial membrane and they are solubilized after disruption of mitochondria.

  c. ***Golgi body (Lipochondria):***

  - It is particularly well developed in secretory gland cells. It is made of lipid and protein material. It consists of series of densely coiled and flattened double membranes of variable shapes and surrounded by vacuoles. It is involved in storing secretion or in transport of substances from one place to another within cell. It may serve in the modification of lipids and may play a role in maintaining a proper concentration of water in protoplasm. Smooth, non-granular membranes of the endoplasmic—reticulum run into the area of Golgi bodies. It is suggested that Golgi body gives rise to the membranes of the endoplasmic reticulum. It is a site for the concentration of protein and polysaccharides and is also a site for completion of synthesis of carbohydrate moiety of glycoprotein (thyroglobulin; immunoglobulin). These products are packed as granules within Golgi-vesicles which then migrate away from Golgi apparatus.
  - Synthetic functions: (i) Certain carbohydrates which cannot be formed in endoplasmic reticulum, e.g. sialic acid, galactose, etc.
  - Large saccharide polymer bound with small amount of protein, e.g. hyaluronic acid and chondroitin sulphate etc.
  - Processing of secretion from ER to Golgi body.

- A substance (protein) formed in ER transported through tubules towards its smooth portion which is near to Golgi body. Here, these small transport vesicles break away and diffuse to deeper parts of Golgi apparatus. Here, these transport vesicles fuse with Golgi apparatus and empty their contents into vesicular spaces of Golgi apparatus. Here, they are mixed with additional carbohydrates. As secretion pass towards outermost layer of Golgi apparatus, the compactness follows. Finally both vesicles break away from it, carrying with them secretory substance and diffuse throughout the cell.
- This is the mechanism of exocytosis. Another way is:- specialised portion of Golgi apparatus form lysosome—the membrane of which contain chemical receptor which causes attachment of acid hydrolase. So enzymes are concentrated and released from Golgi apparatus in the form of lysosomal vesicles.
- Many of the vesicles formed by Golgi apparatus finally fuse with cell membrane or with the membrane of other intracellular structure. This leads to an increase in the expanse of these membranes and thereby replenishes the membrane as they are destroyed.

d. ***Ribosomes:*** These are small granules which are attached to the membranes of the endoplasmic reticulum in very large numbers. They play an important role in protein synthesis from amino acids. They contain protein and bear small particles of RNA on their outer surface and the number of these particles is related to amount of synthesis of proteins and enzymes taking place there. The ribosomes attached to ER, synthesise protein, e.g. hormones that are secreted by cell, proteins that are segregated in lysosomes, and proteins that are inserted in cell membrane.

e. ***Endoplasmic Reticulum (ER):***
- It is a complex series of tubules in the cytoplasm.
- Rough ER provides attachment for ribosomes. So this is concerned with protein synthesis and the initial folding of polypeptide chains with the formation of disulfide bonds.
- Smooth ER (agranular) lacks ribosomes. It is the site of steroid synthesis in steroid secreting cells and the site of detoxification process in other cells. It also plays an important role in contraction process of cardiac and skeletal muscle.
- So ER is a network of tubular and vesicular structures, constructed of a system of unit membranes. The endoplasmic matrix is a fluid medium filling the space inside the tubules and vesicles.

ENDOPLASMIC RETICULUM

Cytoplasm is made of a complete system of interconnected network of membranes called endoplasmic reticulum. The membranes are double between which substances from the cell can pass out. Some of the membranes of the endoplasmic reticulum open on the surface of the plasma membrane and some are connected to the nuclear membrane. The membrane provides extensive surfaces on which various enzymes may be localised in an orderly fashion. It may be of two types—granular and agranular. Granular or ribosomes are attached to cytoplasmic side of the membrane and is concerned with protein synthesis and the initial folding of polypeptide chains with the formation of disulfide bonds. Another, agranular type is site of steroid synthesis in the steroid secreting cells and the site of detoxification process in other cells.

NUCLEUS

- A cell has round, ovoid or discoidal nucleus enclosed in a nuclear membrane. It is a controlling centre of a cell. It does not have a constant appearance because it undergoes a cycle of profound changes.
- Nuclear membrane is similar to cell membrane being a two layered structure made of protein and lipids. It is perforated by extremely minute rounded pores. It is semipermeable and some substances associated with gene activity can pass through it. It is 7.8 mm thick (7-8 mm).
- Nucleoplasm is a protein solution of low viscosity, but it can gelate at times; it completely fills the nucleus. It has a high proportion of proteins, large amount of phosphorus and some nucleic acid.
- The main mass of nucleus in a stained cell is seen as a fine network of threads having beaded granules; the threads and granules are made of chromatin which is made of DNA and proteins. The coarse granules of chromatin are known as chromo centres which stain darkly. It contains a poly acid of very high molecular weight called *DNA*.
- Chromosomes are having strongly acidic material. Their deep staining is due to two factors; firstly they lose some water and secondly they receive a quantity of DNA which is condensed with proteins, then they become clearly visible and are coiled, then they gradually become shorter and thicker. DNA is not added uniformly to chromosomes but at intervals along their lengths, so that darkly staining regions alternate with lightly staining ones. The darkly

staining regions are chromomeres and are site of genes generally, the genes have hereditary powers. The lightly staining regions are made of proteins. One of the lightly staining region is centromere by which the chromosome will get attached to spindle during cell division.

- Each nucleus also contains one or more nucleoli which is composed largely of RNA. Its function is not clear but it is manufacturing proteins and is also said to provide a means for passing genetic information and substances from nucleus to cytoplasm.

Nucleus, thus, contains genetic apparatus of a cell which ensures that on division each daughter cell has the necessary information to remake an exact copy of the mother cell. Chromosomes and their genes guide and determine the character, activities and destiny of each cell. So nucleus is considered as heart of a cell and is essential for the continued survival of the entire cell.

- The nuclear membrane appears like a sac with an enclosed perinuclear space. The granules (which are said to be ribosomes) are found on cytoplasmic surface of outer (cytoplasmic) nuclear membrane. Certain enzymes have been reported in both perinuclear space and cisternae of endoplasmic reticulum. Of course continuity has been reported between cytoplasmic portion of nuclear membrane and endoplasmic reticulum. Most gene products (mRNA) must leave the nucleus and enter the cytoplasm to show their effects and this movement is facilitated through pores or through membrane of perinuclear sac.

Nucleic Acids

Are mainly DNA (Deoxy-ribonucleic acid) and RNA (ribonucleic acid). These are having very large molecules with a complex chemical structure, yet they are made up of just a few kinds of smaller molecules. The molecules of nucleic acid are a pentose sugar, phosphoric acid (usually called phosphate in a chemical combination) and nitrogen containing bases of purines and pyrimidines held by hydrogen bonds. Pyrimidines have four carbon and two nitrogen atoms arranged in a hexagon, while purines have the same hexagon plus a side ring of one carbon and two nitrogen atoms.

DNA

Is found only in nucleus from where it controls and guides the cellular activities. It is a compound of very high molecular weight, having a giant molecule made of smaller molecule linked together. Its molecule consists of a pentose sugar called deoxy ribose, and phosphoric acid to which are joined four bases of pyrimidines and purines. The bases of purines are A (adenine) and G (guanine), while those of pyrimidine are C (cytosine) and thymine (T). The bases are always paired; G is paired with C in equal quantities and so also A with T and these pairs are tied to each other by hydrogen bonds. When a sugar molecule is linked to a phosphate and a pyrimidine or a purine base is attached to this sugar, then this new molecule made of three parts is called a nucleotide. A nucleotide is a single unit of nucleic acid and is made of phosphate sugar base. Only four kinds of nucleotide (A, C, G, T) are possible.

DNA never leaves the nucleus, it directs the activities of the cell from the nucleus. It has the power of self duplication by splitting longitudinally into two chains along its hydrogen bonds, after separation each of the two chains builds another exactly like its partner from which it has separated. Thus, it can make a copy of itself due to which a cell divides into two. DNA molecules have the unique property of adhering to each other forming an orderly structural pile.

The mitochondria contain DNA and are able to synthesise protein and so it presents as second genetic system in the cell. Of course it alone is not capable of containing enough genetic information to code for all mitochondrial components (Fig. 3.1).

DNA is the component of chromosomes that carries genetic message—the blue print for all the heritable characteristics of the cell and its descendants.

RNA

i. Is first formed by DNA in the nucleus where it may be stored in nucleolus, but most of it passes out into the cytoplasm either directly or after being stored in the nucleolus.
ii. It has the same constituents as DNA except that it contains ribose sugar which has one more atom of oxygen than in deoxy ribose sugar of DNA and its bases are adenine, cytosine, guanine and uracil.
    - Messanger RNA: Passes out through the pores of nuclear membrane into the cytoplasm and becomes associated with ribosomes, then this messanger RNA becomes a template.
    - Transfer RNA: are already present in cytoplasm. This picks up individual amino acid and takes them to the ribosomes. Various transfer RNAs along with their amino acids get aligned on the RNA of ribosomes in a specific order to form a new polypeptide chain which is a part of a protein

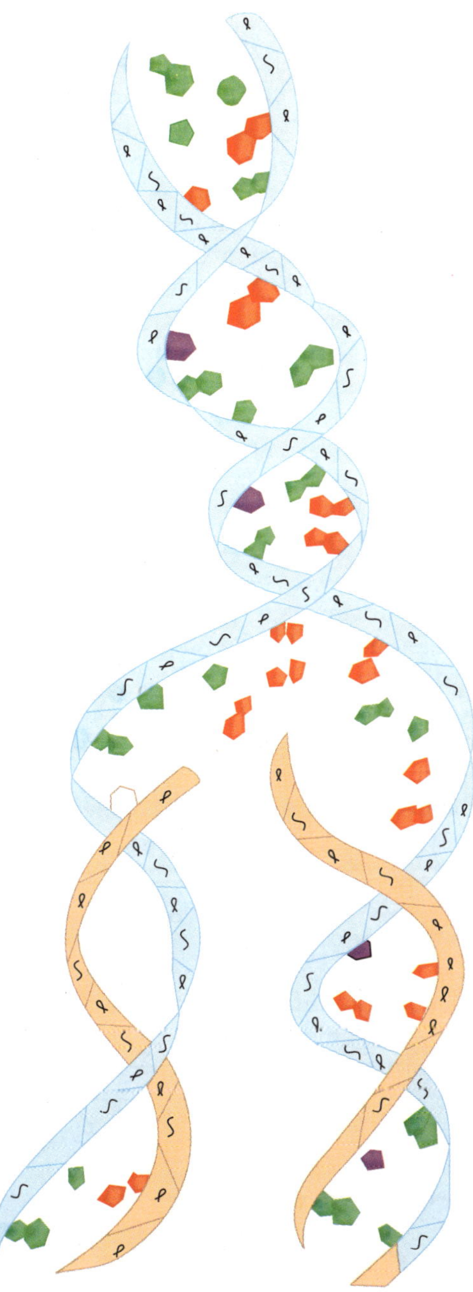

Fig. 3.2: DNA helix

molecule. The transfer RNA molecules are now freed and each becomes available to again pick up an amino acid of a particular kind. Such a control of nucleic acids over synthesis of proteins is an indirect control over all the chemical reactions of a cell.

- Ribosomal RNA: Several ribosomes attach to mRNA via their smaller subunits and this combination is called Polysome. Each ribosome of a polysome synthesise a polypeptide chain so that several chains will be produced simultaneously by a polysome.
- The interphase nucleus is seen under microscope as a spheroid body. The DNA containing material can be stained specifically. The nuclear chromatin is of two types, viz.
  * Euchromatin: loosely coiled and is more active in transcription process, i.e. there is little demonstrable RNA synthesis in chromosomes. This may account for some of the selective genetic expression associated with characteristic chromosomal uncoiling pattern found in different tissues within the same organism or at different developmental stages in the same tissue; and
  * Heterochromatin: compact one.
- Chromosome consists of DNA associated with basic proteins (histones) and with non-histone protein. Isolated chromosome appears as masses of fibres around 25 nm in diameter.

- Single chromosome contains one or very few extremely elongated DNA molecules complexed with protein and coiled into a fibre structure as seen in electron microscope.

- The main functions of nucleus include—replication of DNA and synthesis of RNA (ribosomal, transfer and messanger).
- The cytoplasmic surface of the outer nuclear membrane has granules which resemble ribosomes. The direct continuity is seen between the cytoplasmic portion of nuclear membrane and the endoplasmic reticulum. Certain enzymes have been reported in both perinuclear space and cisternae of endoplasmic reticulum. The inner surface of nuclear membrane is having chromatin and a dense lamella. The inner and outer membrane of this nuclear envelope join at intervals to form pores, which are not simple holes but are organised regions.

SIMILARITIES

Each have adenine, guanine, cytosine.

The nucleotides are linked together by phosphodiester-bonds

The bonding is in 3′-5′ direction

Main function is protein biosynthesis

CELL DIVISION - MITOSIS

Table 3.1: Difference between DNA and RNA

	DNA	*RNA*
1.	Mostly present inside nucleus	Mostly present in cytoplasm
2.	Double stranded	Single stranded
3.	Deoxyribose sugar	Ribose sugar
4.	Only one type	Three major types
5.	Bases are adenine, guanine, cytosine and thymine	Adenine, guanine, cytosine, and uracil
6.	It undergoes replication	No replication
7.	It synthesises RNA	It cannot synthesise DNA
8.	A genetic material	It is not genetic material
9.	It composed of more than four million nucleotides	Is composed of 12,000 nucleotides

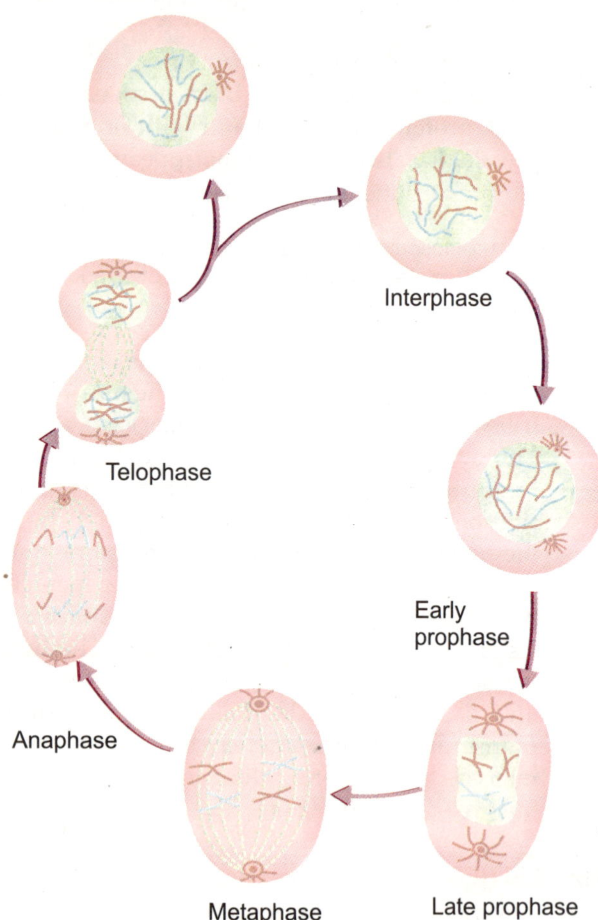

Fig. 3.3: Mitosis—Cell division

Cell divides by mitosis or amitosis. In mitosis there is differentiation and halving of chromosomes before the cytoplasmic fission. The following are mitotic stages.

i. *The prophase:* The activity centre is centriole. Radiating fibres called astral rays appear. Now the centriole begin to move away from each other and ultimately reach opposite sides of the cell. During this stage, the chromosomes appear as distinct and separate entities. They seem to be paired, each member of the pair being named a chromatid. At the end of prophase, the nuclear membrane disappears.
ii. *The metaphase:* This is a very short period during which the chromosomes become aligned in an orderly fashion. Arrangement is such that half the chromatids face one centriole while their partners face the other one. They are in a position to separate.
iii. *The anaphase:* The chromatids then separate, half migrating towards one centriole, the other half heading for other one. As they move to opposite poles they assume a V shape with the point of V facing the centrioles.
iv. *The telophase:* The chromatids reach the opposite centriole and once again called chromosomes. Cell membrane is seen to form a constriction which ultimately separates the cell into two distinct units. A nuclear membrane forms around each chromosomal mass. Simultaneously the individual centriole return to their original position. The new cells grow rapidly.

During interphase each chromosome duplicates itself and splits longitudinally into two chromatids that say attached to each other at only one point (the centromere). The centriole starts moving away from each other, and a spindle begins to form between them.

The reported time for this whole process is from 30 minutes to several hours which depends on temperature, presence or absence of specific enzymes etc.

The important factor here is the retention of original number of chromosomes in each cell. As soon as the chromosomes become differentiated at the beginning of the process they divide longitudinally so as to present a pair of chromatids. Accordingly if the cell begins with, e.g. 48 chromosomes, each cell resulting from mitotic division will also contain 48 chromosomes.

Motive Forces for Cell Division

- It is difficult to explain that one cell in a tissue divides and another does not. The cells producing erythrocytes divide at a rapid rate, while nerve cells

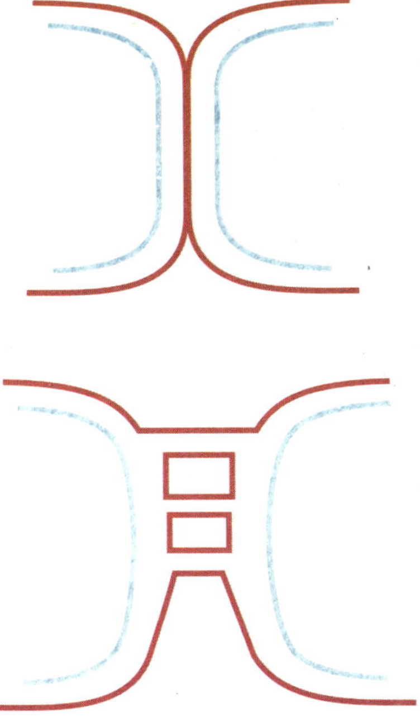

Fig. 3.4: Cellular junctions

are never replaced if destroyed. Cancer is the uncontrolled growth and division of cells.

- The surface to volume ratio declines as the cells enlarge, and this may serve as a stimulus for cells to divide. The surface area may become insufficient to handle the supply of food and oxygen necessary to the cell's needs. Similarly surface area of the nucleus may become inadequate to supply the needs of cytoplasm. Cell division may be the means by which a more favourable ratio is restored.
- Mitotic rate is directly proportional to the temperature; until an optimum temperature is reached; above this optimum, higher temperature decreases the rate of division and become destructive. Mechanical stimuli can increase growth rate. Other effects are probably influential in prompting cell to divide—gravity, pressure, etc. but very little detail is understood about how such mechanisms cause mitosis.

Significance of Mitosis

1. Extremely regular process.
2. It maintains the quantitative and qualitative distribution of hereditary material to daughter cells.
3. It maintains constancy of diploid number of chromosomes.
4. It maintains nuclear and cytoplasmic volume in the cell.
5. It ensures repair and replacement of dead cells.
6. It causes growth and development of organism.
7. It plays an important role in asexual reproduction.

Table 3.2: Cell and its functions

Cell-organelle	*Functions*
Plasma membrane	Differentially permeable membrane through which extracellular substances may be selectively sampled.
Cytoplasm	It contains machinery for carrying out the instructions sent from the nucleus
Microtubules	Transportation of water, ions, small molecules of various substances, form structural unit of centrioles. Assist in movement of chromosomes during cell division
Centrioles	They form the spindle. Have significant role in movement of chromosomes during cell division
ER	It provides greatly expanded surface area of biochemical reactions which normally occurs across membrane surface. Also having transport business of extra + intracellular chemical molecules
Ribosomes	Site of protein synthesis
Golgi complex	Synthesis, packaging and distribution of chemicals
Lysosomes	Digestion and waste removal, discharge, playing a role in cellular death
Vacuoles	Digestion and storage
Nucleolus	To assemble ribosomes
Cilia and flagella	Locomotion and generation of currents that draw in food

INTERCELLULAR JUNCTIONS (INTERCELLULAR COMMUNICATION)

Two functions are more important—one is to provide stability and strength to tissues and second is to permit the passage of ions and molecules from one cell to the next. For this purpose these structures have been designed.

Tight Junctions

- Since they are performing important functions like:-
  - — Providing strength and stability to the tissues;
  - — Prevention of ionic movement from one cell to another, and
  - — Prevention of lateral movement of proteins in cell membrane in order to keep them towards apical region of the cell membrane which will maintain cellular polarity.

- So they are constituted by a ridge which is having two halves which are fusing with each other very strongly and so occupy whole space between two cells. Of course ridge is constituted by proteins (cingulin, ZO-1)
- Synonym: Zonula occludens.
- Example: Intestinal mucosa (apical margins of epithelial cells), wall of renal tubule, capillary wall and in choroid plexus.

Gap Junctions

- Since there are gaps to provide passage of some important substances like glucose, amino acids, ions (of molecular weight 1,000), to exchange chemical messengers between cells, to rapidly propagate the action potential from one cell to another.
- So intercellular space is reduced and the cytoplasm of the two cells is connected by channels formed by membranes of both the cells. This channel facilitates the movements of molecules without making a contact with extracellular fluid. This channel consists of two halves; one half for each cell. Each half is surrounded by 6 sub-units of proteins.

Desmosome

The membrane between two cells is thick and having spot like patches. They function like tight junction. This thickened membrane is made up of cytoplasmic fibrils which are again made up of proteins.

Hemi or Half Desmosomes

Only one cell's membrane is thickened but not the opposite cell.

SUMMARY AND HIGHLIGHTS

- He was Robert Hook (1665) who coined the word cell. Each cell is composed of a discrete body enclosed by a membrane which separates it from environment, and contains the living material or protoplasm, included in which is nuclei. A cell is a very small body of protoplasm surrounded by a membrane and containing a nucleus.
- The physiological properties of protoplasm includes—contractility, absorption and assimilation, excretion, respiration, growth, secretion and reproduction.
- Protoplasm is the physical basis of life and is the general term to describe the stuff of which the cells are made.
- The nerve cells designed for conductivity, develop long strands of protoplasm—the nerve fibres. Just like contractility has developed in muscular tissue (so elongated form), similarly irritability and conductivity are highly developed in nervous tissue.
- Cell—the fundamental unit of living material. Every cell has a plasma membrane—a semipermeable covering that encloses the cellular contents and functions in the regulation of incoming food and water and outgoing wastes and secretions. Typically it is 10 nm thick (nanometer, 10–4 meter) and is formed like a sandwich of lipids between layers of protein molecules.
- The nucleus—a spherical or oval body act as a chemical controller of the cell. It is enveloped by a porous nuclear membrane which controls the chemical messengers that proceed in and out of the nucleus. Inside it, are one or more smaller bodies each of which is called 'nucleolus' which is the site at which ribosomes are formed. The ribosomes are small bodies rich in nucleic acids, that leave the nucleus and become attached to structures in cytoplasm; there they play an important role in protein synthesis. Nucleoli tend to disappear when a cell begins to divide, and later reappear.
- The medium outside the nucleus including plasma membrane-cytoplasm. Throughout the cytoplasm is a tortuous system of tubules which have a ribbon like appearance. These tubules are having membranous material that interconnect among themselves and the plasma membrane. They are collectively called 'endoplasmic reticulum' (network within the fluid), which enhances the cell's efficiency in carrying on its metabolism. The tubules also transport certain cellular fluids to the plasma membrane where they are secreted.

BIBLIOGRAPHY

1. Gloner DM, et al. The centrosome. Sc Am 1993;268:62.
2. Luna EJ, Hitt AL. Cyto-skeleton, plasma membrane interactions. Science 1992;258:955.
3. McIntosh JR, et al. Mitosis. Science 1989;246:622.
4. Neher E. Ion channels for communication between and within cells. Science 1992;256:498.
5. Verkman A. Water channel in cell membrane. Ann Rev Phy 1992;54:97.

4

Structure in Relation to Functions

EXCRETORY SYSTEM

- Urinary system consists of paired kidney, the paired ureter, which connects it to bladder and the urethra which opens to exterior.
- Capsule
  Kidney surface is covered by thin, tough connective tissue capsule. It is made up of outer layer of fibroblasts and inner of myofibroblasts. It passes inwards towards the hilum where it forms connective tissue covering of sinus, and becomes continuous with connective tissue forming the walls of calyces and renal pelvis.
- Cortex and medulla
  i. Outer reddish brown coloured part is cortex, while inner much lighter part is medulla.
  ii. Cortex is characterised by renal corpuscles and their tubules + collecting tubules and having extensive vascular supply. The corpuscles are spherical and comprise beginning segment of nephron, having unique capillary network the glomerulus.
  iii. Medullary rays are series of vertical striations that appear to emanate from medulla. Each medullary ray contains straight collecting tubules. Each nephron and its collecting tubule forms a functional unit of the kidney—the uriniferous tubule and there are 400–500 rays projecting into cortex from each pyramid. The region between medullary rays contain convoluted tubule of nephron and renal capsule and these areas are called cortical labyrinths.
  iv. The medulla is characterised by straight tubules, collecting ducts and a special capillary network, which continues from cortex to medulla. They are accompanied by a capillary network vasa recta which runs parallel with various tubules.

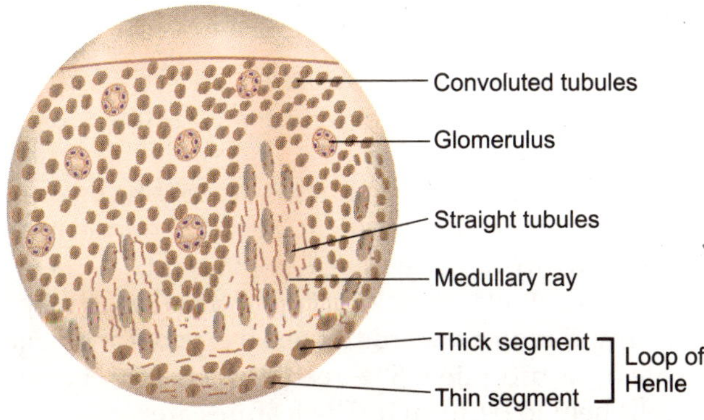

Fig. 4.1: Kidney

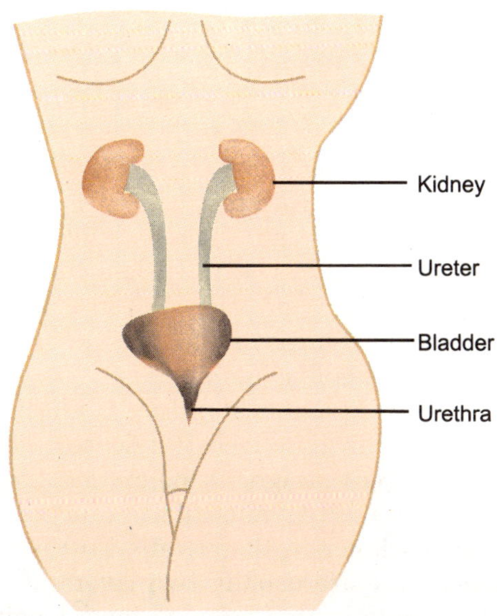

Fig. 4.2: Urinary system: General organisation

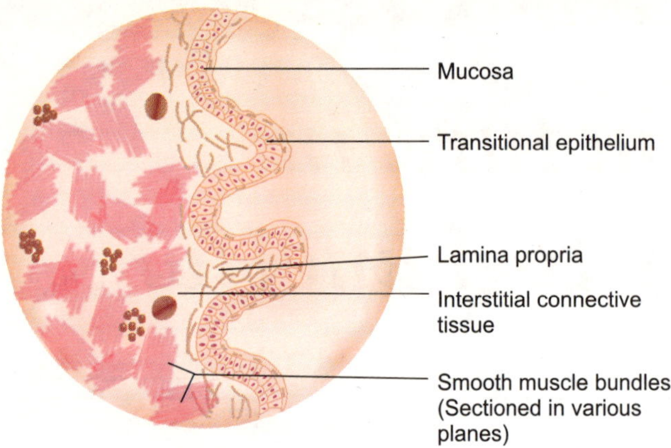

Fig. 4.3: Structure of urinary bladder

- The tubules in the medulla collectively form a number of conical structure called pyramids (usually 8–18 in number). Each pyramid is divided into outer medulla (adjacent to cortex) and inner medulla.
- The caps of cortical tissue lying over the pyramids are extensive and extending peripherally around lateral portion of pyramid forming renal columns of Bertin. The apical portion of each pyramid called papilla projects into minor calyx—a cup shaped structure which are branches of 2 or 3 major calyces—which are major divisions of renal pelvis.

EXCRETORY PASSAGES

Urine excreted at area cribrosa $\xrightarrow{to}$ minor calyx of papilla → to a major calyx → to renal pelvis → the ureter → to bladder → through urethra where voided.

Histological Stand Points

- All structures have same general structures like mucosa, muscularis, and an adventitia or serosa.
- Transitional epithelium lines entire passage :- Is selected by the nature because—It is essentially impermeable to salt and water, Its ability to become thinner and flatter allows distensibility of the lining of all these excretory passages. The structure of each cell of this epithelium is adapted to accommodate the distensibility of epithelium.
- Connective tissue and muscle :- Underlying the transitional epithelium there is a dense collagenous lamina propria throughout the excretory passage. There exists neither muscularis mucosae nor a submucous layer in their walls—In ureter and bladder, there are usually two layers of smooth muscle beneath laming propria—inner longitudinal and outer circular (opposite to that of muscularis externa of intestinal tract).
- Peristaltic contraction of smooth muscle move the urine from minor calyces through the ureter to bladder.
- Smooth muscle of bladder wall is less regularly arranged. Their contraction compresses the whole viscus and forces the urine into urethra.
- In terminal portion of ureter, a thick outer layer of longitudinal muscle is described in addition to above two layers.
- Urinary bladder contains 3 openings, two for the ureters, and one for urethra. The smooth muscle of bladder wall forms internal sphincter—a ring like arrangement of the muscle around the opening of urethra. The triangular region defined by these three openings—trigone is relatively smooth and constant in thickness. Bladder nerve supply is important:-
  - Sympathetic fibres—plexus in adventitia innervate blood vessels
  - Para sympathetic fibres—efferent fibres of micturition reflex—end in ganglia in muscle bundles and adventitia.
  - Sensory fibres from bladder to sacral spinal cord are afferent fibres for micturition reflex.

Nephron—The Functional Unit of Kidney

In human there are 2 millions nephrons in each kidney. Renal corpuscle is the beginning of nephron. It consists of glomerulus—a tuft of capillaries composed of 10 to 20 capillary loops, surrounded by double layer epithelial cup. Bowman's capsule which is the initial portion of nephron where blood which is flowing undergoes filtration. It is supplied by an afferent arteriole and drained by efferent arteriole which then branches forming a new capillary network to supply the kidney tubules. This is then an arterial portal system. Vascular pole is the name given to point where afferent and efferent arteriole penetrate and exist from parietal layer of Bowman's capsule; opposite to this is urinary pole.

- *Proximal segment:* begins as the proximal convoluted tubule at Bowman's capsule. It makes a short turn towards cortex and then returns to its site of origin where it follows a tortuous course. It then enters meduallary ray and continues as descending proximal straight tubule into pyramid. Next the thin segment descends towards the apex of pyramid, but before reaching at apex- say in between it makes a hairpin turn and return towards cortex. It is initial and major site of reabsorption, 80% reabsorption. The cuboidal cells help to perform it. The features are:
  - a brush border composed of numerous long micro villi.

— a terminal bar apparatus comprising narrow tight junctions and zonula adherens.
— Plicae or folds, i.e. large flattened processes on lateral surface of cells.
— Extensive inter digitisation of basal processes of adjacent cells.
— Basal striations—having elongated mitochondria concentrated in basal processes.
— Proteins and large peptides are reabsorbed by endocytosis in proximal tubules.

The Distal Segment

— The thick descending limb—cells are shorter with a less well defined brush border, few complex/lateral basal processes; smaller mitochondria randomly distributed in cytoplasm; few apical invagination, few lysosomes.
— It ascends through pyramid and medullary ray to the vicinity of its renal corpuscles of origin. It then leaves it and makes contact with vascular pole of its parent renal corpuscle. At this point tubule adjacent to afferent arteriole of glomerulus are modified to form macula densa. It then leaves the region and becomes distal convoluted tubule, which is less tortuous than proximal one. It empties into arched collecting tubule/connecting tubule.

Loop of Henle (U shaped)

— Descending limb of proximal thick segment + thin segment and its hairpin turn + ascending limb of distal thick segment = Loop of Henle

This part is performing counter current exchange, i.e. concentrating urine.

Distal thick segment: Third part of loop of Henle - includes both medullary and cortical portions. Its straight segment transports ion from tubular lumen to interstitium. Large cuboidal cells have extensive basal lateral plications with numerous large mitochondria; few less well defined microvilli than proximal tubule, nucleus located at apical portion of cell causing cell to bulge into lumen.

The short distal convoluted tubule located at cortical labyrinth is responsible for

- Reabsorption of Na^+ and secretion of K^+
- Continued reabsorption of HCO_3^- with secretion of H^+ leading to urine acidification.
- Conversion of ammonia to ammonium ion.

Collecting ducts and tubular ducts: They are composed of simple epithelium. Arched and cortical collecting tubules have flat cells (some that squamous to cuboid). Medullary collecting ducts have cuboidal cell with a transition to columnar cells. Two types of cells are seen:-

- Light cells (collecting duct CD cells, principal cells) Single cilium having few short microvilli, small spherical mitochondria.
- Intercalated cells (IC; Dark cells):- Small number, many mitochondria, dense cytoplasm. Microvilli and micro plicae, cytoplasmic folds are present in apical surface, numerous vesicles are present.

Types of Nephrone

1. *Cortical/subcapsular:* Renal corpuscle located in outer part of cortex. Short loops of Henle extended only into outer region of pyramid.
2. *Juxta medullary:* Have renal corpuscle in proximity to base of medullary pyramid. Long loops of Henle and long thin segments that extend well into inner region of pyramid. Essential feature of urine concentration.
3. *Intermediate:* Renal corpuscles in their mid region of cortex. Loops of Henle of intermediate length.
   - The straight collecting tubule empty into large ducts in medullary ray, the cortical collecting ducts, which in turn continue into medulla or pyramid. These ducts travel to the apex of pyramid where they join to form large collecting ducts called ducts of Bellini that open into calyx. The area on the papillae contains opening of these collecting ducts is called *area cribrosa*.

Renal corpuscle (Filtration apparatus)—Enclosed by parietal layer of Bowman's apparatus, consists of

— Endothelium of glomerular capillaries
— Viscreal layer of Bowman's capsule
— Basal lamina between these two

a. The endothelium has numerous fenestrations, 70 to 90 nm in diameter, more numerous and irregular.
b. Visceral layer is characterised by Podocytes—The cells of inner layer extend processes called foot or secondary processes which intermingle with neighbouring podocytes. Elongated spaces between interdigitating foot processes called filtration slits (25 nm wide allow filtrate from blood to enter Bowman's space). Numerous microfilaments (actin) have been reported in foot processes having role in regulating size and potency of filtration slits. A filtration slit membrane also reported.

The thick basal lamina is the joint product of endothelium and podocytes and is the main component of filtration barrier. This is called glomerular basement membrane (GBM)—which acts as a physical barrier and ion selective filter and is made up of:

- Lamina rara interna—adjacent to capillary endothelium.
- Lamina rara externa—near podocyte process
- Both are rich in poly anions, e.g. heparan sulphate
- Lamina densa—sand-witched between two sialo glycoproteins are involved

Why not Protein/Hb Pass Normally?

1. Poly anionic glycoaminoglycans of lamina rara restrict the movement of cationic particles and molecules across GBM.
2. Narrow slit pores formed by pedicels and filtration slit membrane also act as a physical barrier to free diffusion.
3. Fenestrae of capillary endothelium restrict the movement of blood cells from capillaries.

Blood Supply

- Each kidney receives a large branch of abdominal aorta "renal artery." It branches within renal sinus sending interlobar branches into substance of the kidney. They travel between pyramids as far as cortex and then follow an arched course along the base of pyramid between medulla and cortex. So it is called arcuate artery.
- Interlobar arteries branch from arcuate arteries, ascend through the cortex towards the capsule. As they traverse the cortex towards capsule, interlobar arteries give off branches afferent arterioles with one to each glomerulus. These give rise to glomerular tuft of capillaries which reunite to form an efferent arteriole, which in turn give rise to peritubular capillaries.
- Efferent arterioles from cortical glomeruli lead into peritubular capillary network surrounds the local uriniferous tubule.
- Efferent arterioles from Juxta medullary glomeruli descend into medulla alongside loop of Henle. They break up into smaller vessels that continue towards the apex of pyramid but make hairpin turns at various levels to return again as straight vessels towards the base of pyramid. This is the origin of *vasa recta*.

Lacis/Mesangium Cells—Part of JG Apparatus

(Additional group of cells in renal corpuscle). They constitute mesangium commonly seen at vascular stalk of glomerulus and at interstices of adjoining glomerular capillaries.

They are enclosed in basal lamina of glomerular capillaries. Confined to renal corpuscle. Functions are:

- Phagocytic - remove trapped residues and aggregated proteins from GBM (glomerular basement membrane).
- Provide structural support for podocytes.
- Cleaning of GBM (glomerular basement membrane).
- These cells are contractile so they play a role in regulating glomerular blood flow.
- They are derived from smooth muscle cell precursors.

Interstitial Cells

- In cortex—two types of cells resembling fibroblasts found between basement membrane of tubules and adjacent peritubular capillaries. They secrete + synthesise collagen and glycosaminoglycans of extracellular matrix of interstitium.
- In medulla—the main cells resemble myofibroblasts. They may compress tubular structures. They contain bundles of actin filaments, rough endoplasmic reticulum, a well developed Golgi apparatus, a lysosomes. They may secrete a hormone like material which may reduce blood pressure. In interstitium prostaglandins and prostacyclines are synthesised.

ENDOCRINE

Adenohypophysis

"Bandmaster of endocrine Orchestra." The cells are organised in clumps and cords that are separated by fenestrated sinusoidal capillaries of relatively large diameter.

a. ***Pars distalis:*** Three types of cells according to staining characters like eosinophil or alpha cell (acidophil 40%), basophil or beta cell (10%), and chromophobes (50%)—precursors of alpha and beta cells.
b. ***Pars intermedia:*** Here the endocrine cells surround the colloid filled cysts. It contains chromophobes and basophilic cells which further extend into pars nervosa. Basophil is said to contain granules in their cytoplasm rich in α or β-endorphin (a morphine related compound). Basophils also produce MSH.
c. ***Pars tuberalis:*** Highly vascular region containing hypothalamo-hypophyseal-portal-vessels (veins). Endocrinal cells are arranged in short clusters. Some gonadotropes have been reported.

Neurohypophysis (Posterior pituitary)

Is a nerve tract. Its terminals store and release secretory product from hypothalamus. It consists of following parts:

a. ***Pars nervosa (neural lobe):*** made up of non-myelinated axons and nerve endings of many neuro-secretory neurones whose cells bodies lie in hypothalamus (supraoptic and paraventricular nuclei). Neurones contain secretory granules in all parts of cell.

b. ***Infundibulum:*** which connects it with hypothalamus.

The nerve terminals contain vesicles which has got acetylcholine. Neurosecretory granules causes dilatation of a part of axon near the terminal which is called ***Herring bodies***. The membrane bounded neurosecretory granules that aggregate to form *Herring bodies* contain oxytocin or ADH. Each granule contains ATP and a neurophysin—a specific hormone binding protein that is bound to the hormone by non-covalent bonds.

It also contains mast cells, fibroblasts, fenestrated capillaries and pituicytes—which are the only cell types specific to neuro-hypophysis. They resemble glial cells, round/oval nuclei, pigmented granules in cytoplasm—serving a role like astrocyte of CNS.

Thyroid

Follicle

Is the structural unit of this gland. It is roughly spheroidal cyst like compartment with a wall lined by cuboidal epithelium—i.e. follicular epithelium. Hundreds/thousands of such follicle (0.2 - 1 mm diameter) constitute this gland. Lumen of follicle or the follicular cavity is filled with a gel like mass colloid. The apical surfaces of follicular epithelial cell are in contact with colloid.

Cells

a. ***Follicular (principal) cells:*** secrete T_4 (90% of total secretion) and T_3 (10% only)
b. ***Parafollicular cells:*** Secrete calcitonin.
   — The nuclei of follicular cells are spherical containing prominent nucleoli. Colloid contains thyroglobulin—the inactive storage form of thyroid hormone from which synthesis of thyroid hormones takes place.

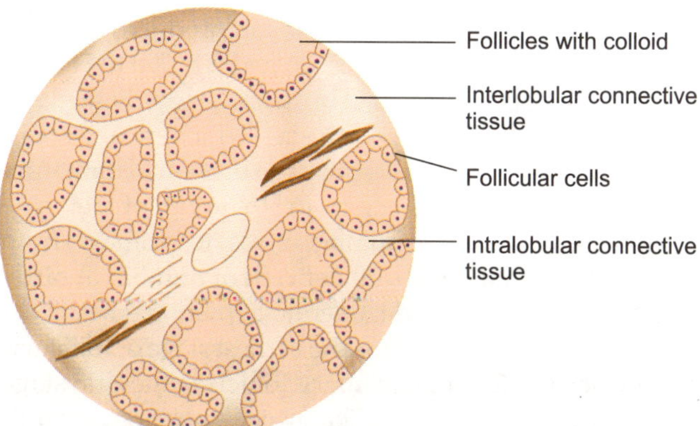

Fig. 4.4: Thyroid gland

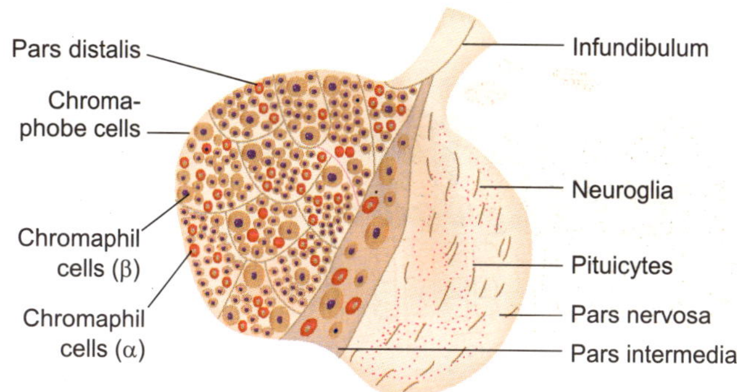

Fig. 4.5: Pituitary gland

   — The parafollicular cells are present within follicular epithelium and are scattered in connective tissue. They are pale staining cells present in clusters in the wall of follicle or in interfollicular space. In the follicle their location is near basal lamina but they don't extend to contact colloid. They are characterised by numerous secretory granules.

Parathyroid Gland

Cells

a. ***Principal cells or chief cells:*** more numerous, secrete parathormone. Are small polygonal cells (7–10 μm diameter), centrally placed nucleus. Pale staining slightly acidophilic cytoplasm having lipofuscin granules.
b. ***Oxyphil cells:*** minor number, secretory role not known. Larger than principal cells; distinct acidophilic cytoplasm. No secretory granules, mitochondria fill the cytoplasm.

Adrenal Gland

Cortex: *3 zones*

a. ***Zona glomerulosa:*** Outer most layer, very thin cells, arrange in ovoid shaped clusters/curved columns. Small columnar/pyramidal cells with spherical nuclei. Smooth ER, large mitochondria, multiple Golgi complex present. Secretes aldosterone.
b. ***Zona fasciculata:*** Middle layer cells are large and polyhedral, arranged in long straight cords. Light stained spherical nucleus. Acidophilic cytoplasm contains neutral fat, cholesterol lipid droplets etc. Highly developed mitochondria and smooth ER. It secretes mostly glucocorticoids and to a slight extent sex hormones.
c. ***Zona reticularis:*** Inner most layer, principally it secretes weak androgens along with gluco-corticoids.

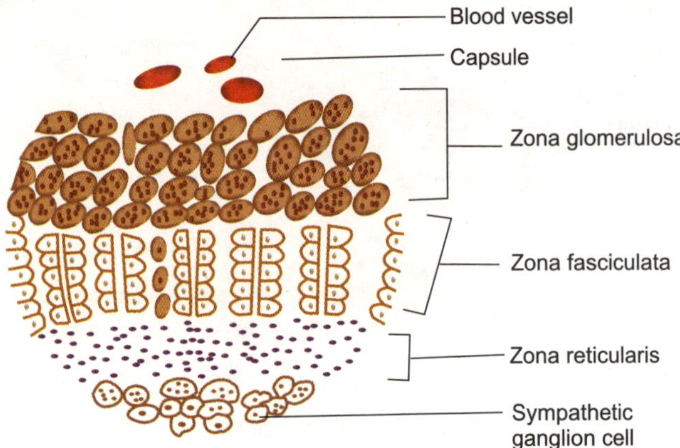

Fig. 4.6: Adrenal gland

Cells are comparatively smaller with deeply stained nuclei. Arranged in anastomosing cords, well developed SER and numerous mitochondria with tubular cristae.

Medulla (Forms 20% mass of adrenal gland)
Here cells are modified postganglionic neuronal cells having secretory function.

Chromaffin Cells

- — Pale-staining epithelial cells, arranged as oval clusters with short interconnecting cords. Characterised by membrane bounded secretory granules, profile of rER, well developed Golgi complex.
- — One type of cells secrete norepinephrine and they contain dense core-granules (10% cells).
- — Another type of cells secrete epinephrine and so contain granules which are smaller, less dense but more homogenous (90% cells).

Endocrine Pancreas (A diffuse organ)

A. *Islets of Langerhans:* Constitutes 1 to 2 per cent of pancreatic volume, numerous towards the tail. Polygonal cells are arranged in short, irregular cords with a network of fenestrated capillaries.
   a. *B cells (or beta cells):* 70 per cent population, secrete insulin. Contain numerous secretory granules (300 nm diameter) with dense polyhedral core and a pale matrix (believed to be crystallised insulin).
   b. *A cells (or alpha cells):* secrete glucagon, 15 to 20 per cent population, located towards periphery, secretory granules present which are densely packed in cytoplasm.
   c. *D cells (or delta cells):* 5 to 10 per cent population, produce somatostatin, located towards periphery. Secretory granules are comparatively larger.
   d. *F (or PP) cells:* which secrete pancreatic polypeptide.

ISLET ACTIVITY

- Blood glucose below 70 mg per cent stimulate release of glucagon while above level inhibits its release.
- Islets cells are innervated by both sympathetic and parasympathetics. There exists well developed gap junctions between islet cells. Ionic events triggered by synaptic transmitters at nerve endings are carried from cell to cell across these junctions.

FEMALE REPRODUCTIVE SYSTEM

- It consists of internal sex organs and external genital structures. The internals are: ovary, oviduct, uterus and vagina.

Ovary: meant for production of gametes and steroid hormones. It is paired/almond shaped/pinkish white structure/ 3 cm (length) × 1.5 cm (width) × 1 cm (thick) in dimension: Its superior/(tubal) pole is attached to pelvic wall by suspensory ligament of ovary, carrying nerves and vessels. The inferior/uterine pole is attached to uterus by the ovarian ligament.

- It consists of cortex and medulla.
   a. ***Medulla:*** present in its central part. Is having loose connective tissue, blood vessels, lymphatics and nerves.
   b. ***Cortex:*** Peripheral portion. Contains ovarian follicles embedded in connective tissue. Around the follicles is stroma having smooth muscle fibres.
- Ovarian surface is covered by single layer of cuboidal epithelium (in some parts - squamous cells). Germinal epithelium is an old term thought to be site of germ cell formation. A dense connective tissue layer tunica albuginea exists between the germinal epithelium and underlying cortex.
- During reproductive life a woman produces only 400 mature ova. Most of the estimated 600,000 to 800,000 primary oocyte present at birth fail to complete maturation and lost—called atresia—which means spontaneous death and subsequent resorption of immature oocyte. This process begins in 5th month of foetal life and thus reduces the number of oocyte (primary) from 5 millions in foetus to 20 per cent of number at birth. The remaining few degenerate at menopause.
- The primordial follicle, is the earliest stage of follicular development, while primary follicle is the first stage of growing follicle. Follicular cells undergo stratifi-

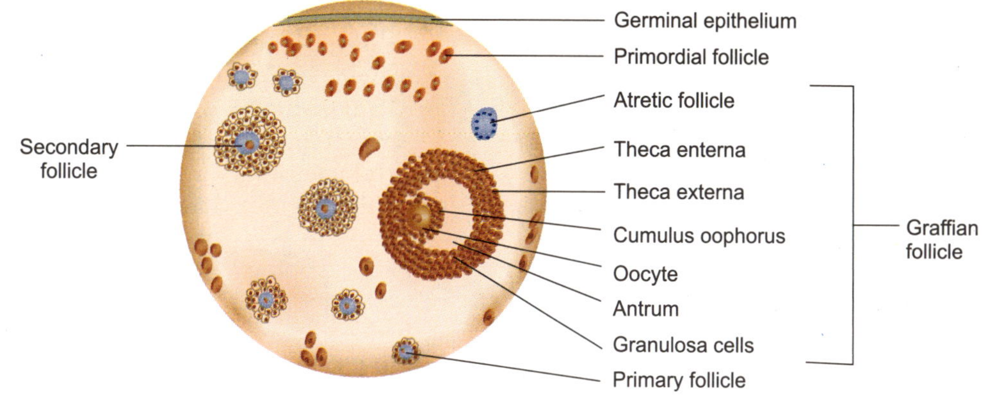

Fig. 4.7: Ovary

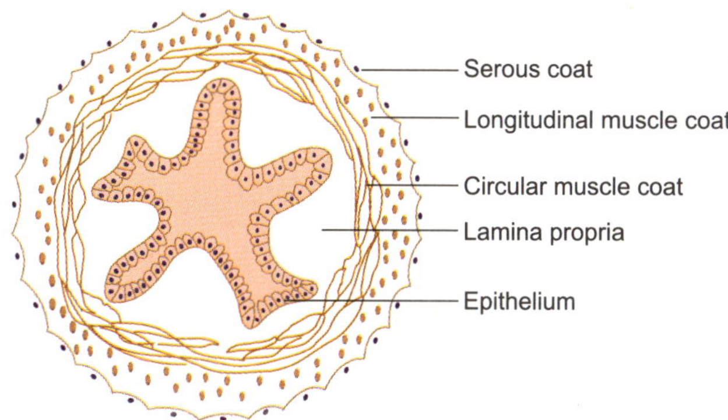

Fig. 4.8: Uterine tube

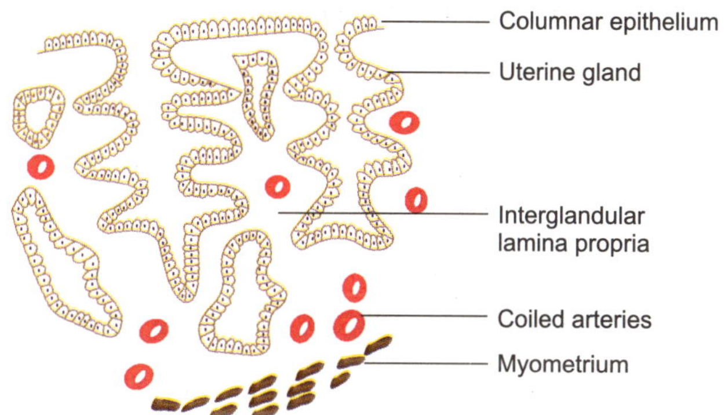

Fig. 4.9: Uterus: (Secretory phase)

cation to form granulosa layer of primary follicle. The connective tissue cells form the theca layers of primary follicle. Maturation of oocyte occurs in primary follicle, while antrum is the characteristic of secondary follicle. Cells of cumulus oophorous form corona radiata around the secretory follicle oocyte. The Graffian follicle contains the mature secondary oocyte.

- Ovulation is a hormone mediated process resulting in the release of secondary oocyte. The factors involved are:
  1. Increased volume and pressure of follicular fluid,
  2. Proteolysis of follicular wall by activated plasminogen,
  3. Deposition of glycosaminoglycans between oocyte—cumulus complex and stratum granulosumm,
  4. Contraction of smooth muscle fibres in theca external layer, stimulated by prostaglandin.
- ***Fertilisation:*** Occurs in Ampulla of oviduct or Fallopian tube. Only one sperm succeeds in fertilising ovum while others are prevented by following events:-
  1. Fast block - achieved by depolarisation of oolemma which creates a transient electrical block to polyspermy.
  2. Changes in polarity of oolemma → release of Ca^{2+} from ooplasmic stores → cortical granules move to the surface and fuse with oolemma leading to reorganisation of the membrane → released enzyme of cortical granules degrade glycoprotein. Oocyte-plasma membrane receptor for sperm binding + formation of perivitelline barrier by cross linking protein on the surface of zona pellucida → permanent block to polyspermy.
- Collapsed follicle undergoes re-organisation which is now called 'corpus luteum' after ovulation. Two types of luteal cells:-
  1. Granulosa lutein cells—large, 30μm diameter, centrally located, derived from granulosa cells.
  2. Theca lutein cells—Smaller (15μm), peripherally located derived from theca interna cells.

- *Atresia*

  Most ovarian follicles are lost. Sequential events are:

1. Cessation of mitosis.
2. Expression of endonucleases.
3. Neutrophil and macrophage invade the granulosa layer
4. Vascularised connective tissue further invades granulosa layer
5. Granulosa layer sloughs into antrum of follicle
6. Hypertrophy of theca interna cells
7. Follicle collapses as degeneration continues
8. Invasion of connective tissue into cavity of follicle. Interstitial gland arises from theca interna of atretic follicle.

Uterine or Fallopian Tube (Oviduct)

Paired tubes extending bilaterally from uterus towards the ovaries. 10-12 cm long wall composed of :

1. ***Serosa:*** consists of mesothelium and a thin layer of connective tissue
2. ***Muscularis:*** inner thick circular and outer thin longitudinal layer
3. ***Mucosa:*** exhibits thin longitudinal folds projecting into lumen of oviduct, throughout its length folds are numerous in ampulla, becoming smaller in isthmus. It is lined by simple columnar epithelium composed of ciliated and non-ciliated cells
   — Ciliated one are in plenty in infundibulum and ampulla and its wave is directed towards uterus: non-ciliated cells are secretory which provides nutrition to ovum.

- Its parts are:
  1. *Infundibulum:* Funnel shaped, adjacent to ovary, distally opening into peritoneal cavity, fimbria extends from mouth of infundibulum towards the ovary.
  2. *Ampulla:* Longest, site of fertilisation
  3. *Isthmus:* Narrow medial segment adjacent to uterus.
  4. *Uterine/intramural:* 1 cm long lies within uterine wall, opening into uterine cavity.

Uterus (Receiving Morula from Tube)

Hollow, pear shaped. Three layers from lumen outward

1. Endometrium: Mucosa two layers viz.
   - stratum functionale:- thick, sloughed off on menstruation. Simple columnar epithelium with secretory + ciliated cells. This surface epithelium invaginates into, underlying lamina propria—endometrial stroma forming uterine glands which are tubular glands with few ciliated cells with abundant ground substance.
   - Stratum basale:- Retained during menstruation and so is a source of regeneration of above layer.
2. Following are the arteries in endometrium
   - Radial arteries:- enter the basal layer where they branch into small straight arteries which supply endometrium.
   - Spiral arteries:- It is the coiled termination of main radial artery. Various arterioles are derived and thus forming a rich capillary bed.

Cervix: Mucosa 2 to 3 mm thick and having large branched glands. No spiral arteries. Not sloughed during menstruation. Its portion projecting into vagina is covered with stratified squamous epithelium. Cervical external os is the site of transition between vaginal stratified squamous epithelium and cervical simple columnar epithelium.

Vagina (a fibro-muscular tube lined by non-keratinised stratified squamous epithelium)

- *Mucosa:* numerous transverse folds (rugae), no glands but lubricated by mucus produced by cervical glands.
- *Lamina propria:* two regions—outer is highly cellular + loose connective tissue—inner is just like submucosa and is more dense.
- *Muscularis:* Outer longitudinal and inner circular (much thicker)
- *Adventitia:* Inner dense connective tissue layer and outer loose connective tissue layer.
- Vagina is having few sensory nerve endings in its lower third having sensitive towards pain and stretch.

MALE REPRODUCTION

Consists of testes, epididymis, genital ducts, accessory reproductive glands and penis. Accessory glands are: seminal vesicles, prostate, bulbourethral glands.

Testis

- Produce sperms and androgens (testosterone produced by its interstitial cells).

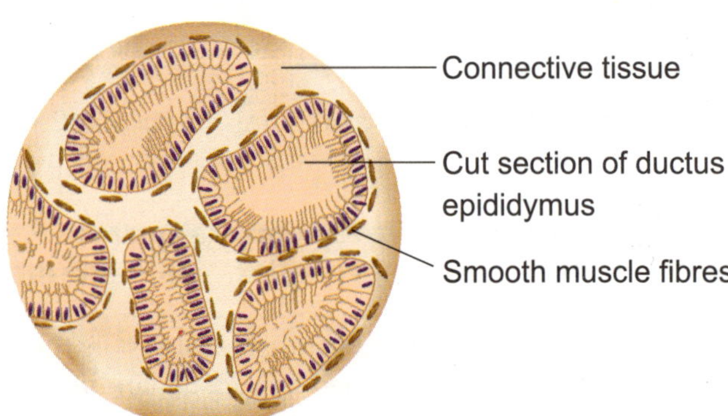

Fig. 4.10: Epididymus

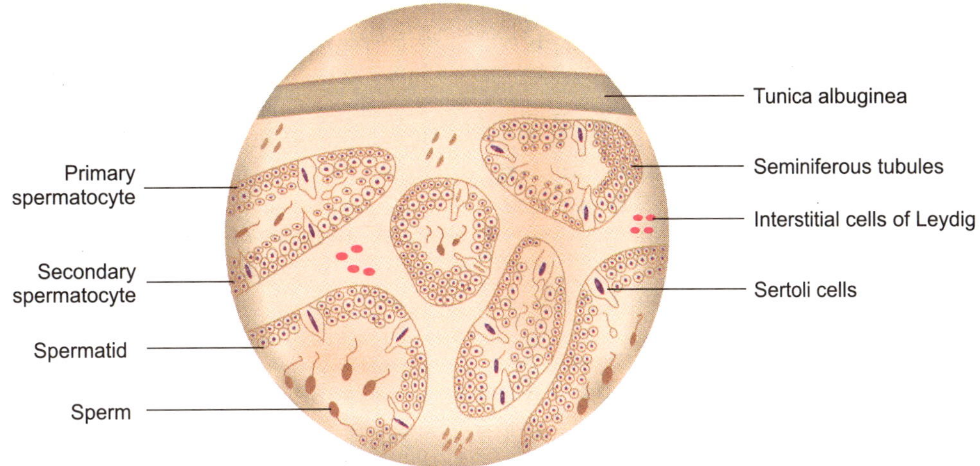

Fig. 4.11: Testis

- They descend from abdominal cavity into scrotum through inguinal canal, shortly before birth, along with extension of peritoneum called 'tunica vaginalis'. In scrotum the temperature is 2 to 3°C below the body temperature which is essential/beneficial/needed for sperm production. *Cryptorchidism* means failure to descend into scrotum.
- As said *tunica albuginea* is its covering which is thick fibrous connective tissue capsule. *Tunica vasculosa* is the name given to its inner layer containing blood vessels. These are connective tissue septa which divides testes into 250 lobules, which projects from capsule.
- Each lobule contains 1 to 4 seminiferous tubules (which produce the sperm) along with connective tissue stroma in which lie interstitial Leydig cell. Each tubule within the lobule forms a loop and is highly convoluted because of its length, it is folding on itself. The ends of the loop assume a short straight course which is called *tubuli recti* and is continuous with *rete-testis*–an anastomosing channel system with mediastinum.
- Each seminiferous tubule is 50 cm long (30-80 cm) and 150–250μm in diameter. It is a complex stratified epithelium having two cells - namely
  - — Spermatogenic cells—which differentiate into mature sperm
  - — Sertoli cells do not undergo replication (supporting sustentacular cells) once puberty is reached.

These are columnar cells, provide structural organisation to tubules.

Leydig Cells

Large, polygonal, acidophilic contain lipid droplets, lipochrome pigment is contained, smooth ER, which contains enzyme necessary for synthesis of testosterone from cholesterol. They secrete this testosterone from early foetal life.

Sertoli Cells

Tall, columnar, non-replicating epithelial cells resting on thick multi-layered basal lamina. Supporting cells for developing sperm, spherical and elongated mitochondria, well defined Golgi complex, characteristic inclusion bodies in cytoplasm. They are bound to one another by an unusual junctional complex (tight junctions); and this divides seminiferous epithelium into basal and luminal compartments.

- — In both these compartments, spermatogenic cells are surrounded by complex processes of sertoli cells.
- — Sertoli cell phagocytize/breaking down the residual bodies formed in last stages of spermatogenesis.
- — This junction is the site for blood-testis barrier. The exocrine secretory product of sertoli cells-ABP (androgen binding protein) is concentrated in the lumen, and it is necessary to concentrate testosterone in lumen of seminiferous tubule.
- — Sertoli cells also secrete *inhibin* which regulate FSH of anterior pituitary.

- *Straight tubules* (Tubula Recti), join the seminiferous tubules with rete-testis of mediastinum. A simple cuboidal or low columnar epithelium lines the channel of rete testis.

- The efferent ductules (20 in No.) connect rete testis to epididymis. As it exists the testis, it becomes highly coiled, forming 6 to 10 conical masses (coni vasculosi). The coni vasculosi contain highly convoluted ducts (15 to 20 cm measurement). At the base of cones the efferent ducts open into a single channel *ductus epididymis*. These efferent ducts are lined with pseudostratified columnar epithelium giving a saw-tooth appearance. Tall columnar cells are ciliated. Most of the fluid secreted in seminiferous tubules is reabsorbed in efferent ductules.
- Transport of sperm in efferent ductules is effected largely by ciliary action + contraction of its fibro-muscular layer.

Epididymis **(Lying over posterior surface of testis)**

- It is lined with pseudostratified columnar epithelium.
- *Principal cells:* 80μm height at head, 40μm height at tail.

Numerous *stereo cilia* (long, modified micro villi) extend from luminal surface of these cells. (25μm height at head, 10μm height at tail)

- *Basal cells:* Small, round, resting on basal lamina. Are stem cells of duct epithelium.
- *Halo cells:* Found in epithelium and are intraepithelial lymphocytes
- The smooth muscle coat consists of thin layer of circular smooth muscle. In tail two layers are added viz. inner and outer longitudinal layer. These three layers are continuous with three smooth muscle layers of vas deferens.

Functions

1. Fluid which is not absorbed by efferent ductules is reabsorbed in proximal part of epididymis.
2. Principal cells secrete glyco-phosphocholine, sialic acid and glycoproteins which leads to sperm maturation.
3. In its head and body spontaneous/rhythmic peristaltic contractions causes sperm movement along the duct. Few peristaltic contraction in tail- cause reservoir of sperm.

Vas (Ductus) Deferens

- Direct continuation of tail of epididymis. Its distal end enlarges to form *ampulla*. Is joined by duct of seminal vesicle and continues through prostate gland to urethra as ejaculatory duct.
- Lined by pseudostratified columnar epithelium. Cells have microvilli extending into lumen. Thrown into deep longitudinal folds due to contraction of muscular coat.
- Ampulla is taller having mucosal folds. Its epithelium is secretory (yellow pigment granules). No muscularis layer in the wall of ejaculatory duct.
- The three smooth muscle layers of epididymis by their intense contraction, forces the sperm into vas deferens.

Seminal Vesicles (Accessory Sex gland)

- Paired, highly folded glands have a muscular and fibrous coat, resembling ampulla.
- Mucosa is thrown into folds (primary, secondary, tertiary)
- Pseudostratified columnar epithelium contains tall ciliated cells resting on basal lamina.
- Its secretion is whitish yellow, viscous contain fructose + amino acid + ascorbic acid + prostaglandins.
- Contraction of its smooth muscle coat discharge their secretion into ejaculatory ducts, flushing sperm out of urethra.

Prostate (Largest accessory gland)

- Consists of 30 to 50 tubulo-alveolar glands surrounding proximal urethra. Glands are in 3 layers
  - — mucosal layer—secrete directly into urethra
  - — submucous layer
  - — Peripheral layer—containing main prostaglandins.
- Epithelium is columnar but may have patches of cuboidal, pseudostratified/squamous.
- It secretes protein enzymes (acid phosphates, and fibrinolysin, citric acid).
- Due to contraction of fibromuscular tissue the secretions are pumped into urethra.
- Prostatic alveoli, often contain—corpora amylacea)—2 mm diameter.

Bullo Urethral Glands (Cowper's glands)

- Secretes preseminal fluid, lubricating penile urethra.
- Paired structure; pea sized located in urogenital diaphragm; duct of each gland join initial portion of penile urethra.
- Glands are compound tubulo-alveolar gland structurally resemble mucus secretory glands.
- Epithelium is simple columnar.
- Clear mucus secretion contain galactose, galactosamine, sialic acid, methylpentose.

MUSCLE—TISSUE

- Two principal types:-
  - — Striated—cells exhibit cross striations
  - — Smooth—No cross striations

Striated further classified as:-

i. *Skeletal:* attached to bone and responsible for movements of axial and peripheral skeleton.

ii. *Visceral striated:* restricted to soft tissues (tongue, pharynx, diaphragm, oesophagus)

iii. *Cardiac:* muscle of heart

Skeletal Muscle

- Major component of body, responsible for gross and fine movements, maintenance of body posture.
- Each muscle cell called muscle fibre consists of multinucleated syncytium. Is formed by fusion of small muscle cells *myoblasts* during development. Nuclei of muscle fibre located immediately, under plasma membrane called *sarcolemma* which jointly represents basal or external lamina and surrounding reticular lamina.
- Skeletal muscle is made up of striated muscle fibres, held together by connective tissue: Connective tissue associated with muscle are named as:
  1. ***Endomysium:*** reticular fibres which immediately surrounds individual muscle fibres.
  2. ***Perimysium:*** thicker layer, form a bundle called fascicle.
  3. ***Epimysium:*** surrounds the fascicle which constitute the muscle, dense connective tissue.

Type of Fibres

1. *Red:* Small fibres, large amount of myoglobin + cytochromes + mitochondria. Make up slow twitch motor units.
2. *White:* Large fibres, less amount of myoglobin + few mitochondria + less cytochromes
3. *Intermediate:* Contain in between mitochondria etc., intermediate size

- Structural and functional sub-unit of muscle fibre is *myofibril* (stippled appearance). Two types are associated with cell contraction.
  1. *Actin:* 6 to 8 nm diameter, thin filament protein.
  2. *Myosin:* protein, 15 nm diameter, thick filament.
     - The bundles of myofilaments which constitute myofibril are surrounded by sER called Sarcoplasmic reticulum—which forms a highly organised tubular network around the contractile elements in all striated muscles.
- *Cross striations:* are characteristic feature of striated muscle. Alternating light and dark bands are evident viz. A, I, and Z line.
  — Dark bands are anisotropic, i.e. they alter the plane of polarised light, so A band is the name given.
  — Light bands are monorifringent, i.e. they don't alter the plane of polarised light, I band is the name given i.e. isotropic.
  — The *Z line* or zone (Ger. Zwischenscheibe = a between disc)—is a dense zone which bisects I band
  — The *H Zone* (Ger. Helle-light) light zone bisecting A band.
  — The *M line*—in middle of H band.
- *Sarcomere* is the basic contractile unit of striated muscle. Entire muscle exhibits cross striations. It is the segment of myofibril between two Z disc.
- Thin (actin filaments) composed of actin + troponin + tropomyosin and are associated with α-actin at Z disc.
  — Thick filaments are about 1.5μm long and are restricted to A band. They attach to Z line and extend into A band to the edge of H Zone.

Table 4.1: Difference between red and white muscles

	Red	*White*
1.	Make slow twitch motor units	Make fast twitch motor units
2.	Generate less muscle tension	Generate large muscle tension
3.	Don't fatigue early	Fatigue rapidly
4.	Adapted to long, slow contraction required for maintenance of posture	Adapted for rapid contractions and precise fine movements
5.	E.g. principal fibres of long muscles of back, limb muscles of mammals, breast muscles of migrating birds	E.g. fibres of extraocular muscles, and muscles controlling movements of digits

Contractile Mechanism

- When muscle contracts sarcomere shortens and these become thick, but length of myofilaments is unchanged.
- I band shortens during contraction while A band is unchanged in length, H zone becomes narrower and thin filaments penetrate H Zone. So thin filaments slide past the thick filament during contraction.
- ***Actin:*** F actin (filamentous) of the thin filament is composed of two strands of G-actin (globular) manomer forming a double helix. Each G-actin molecule is having a binding site for myosin.
- ***Myosin:*** Composed of two polypeptide chains arranged as a double helix. This has got a globular head which has a specific ATP binding site and ATP-ase activity of myosin. It is arranged tail to tail to constitute thick filament.

- ***Tropomyosin and Troponin:*** It consists of double helix to run in groove between F-actin molecules in thin filament. In resting state, tropomyosin + troponin mask a myosin binding site on actin molecules.
  - — Troponin T—binds to tropomyosin
  - — Troponin C—binds calcium ions
  - — Troponin I—Inhibits actin myosin interaction.
- ***Sliding filament:*** In resting state ADP and P (organic phosphate) which are breakdown product of ATP, remain bound to ATP-ase of globular head of myosin.
  - — They are released on binding between actin and myosin.
- ***Role of Calcium ion (Ca^{2+}):*** On addition of Ca^{2+}, troponin C is binding with it which drives tropomyosin molecule deeper into cleft between F-actin chains. It leads to exposure of myosin binding site on G-actin. So myosin-actin binding occurs; ADP and P, are released, myosin rod bends towards H Zone, this part of myosin is now bound to actin, so actin filaments is driven in the same direction.
- ***Step further:*** All this leads to re-exposure of ATP binding site in head where ATP binds to ATP-ase, thus releasing myosin head from actin, so myosin head is released from actin filament, ATP is split, myosin head is resumed the original position and now ready for next contraction.
- ***Rigor mortis: basis:*** This action pulls thin filament into A band—this leads to shortening of sarcomere. This process will continue as long as ATP and Ca^{2+} are present; this will be a continuous procedure. If they are not present thin binding will not release, so muscle cannot relax, this is the basis of rigor mortis—the muscles rigidity developing after death.
- ***Ca^{2+} the important faculty:***
  - — It should be available for action between actin and myosin and after completion of contraction it must be removed.
  - — This task is achieved by combined work of saroplasmic reticulum and transverse tubular system (T system) derived from plasma membrane.
  - — Sarcoplasmic reticulum is arranged in net works around or between a group of myofilaments, i.e. one network of it surrounds A band while another surrounds I band, and at their junction, there exists *terminal cisterna*—a ring like channel.
  - — Invagination of plasma membrane of muscle cell form T system, i.e. T tubules penetrate to all levels of muscle fibres.
  - — Sarcoplasmic reticulum is the reservoir and regulator of Ca^{2+}
- ***Sequence of events: A briefing:***
  Nerve impulse transmitted to muscle cells → depolarisation + development of action potential → here the triad (complex of T tubule + two terminal cisternae) is in close contact with sarcoplasmic reticulum → Ca^{2+} released from sarcoplasmic reticulum into cytoplasmic matrix → activation of contractile proteins → at the end, Ca^{2+} returns to cisterna of sarcoplasmic reticulum
  - — Influx of Na^+ into muscle cell triggers the Ca^{2+} release.
  - — Ca^{2+} interact with Troponin C to initiate contraction.
  - — Ca^{2+} activated ATPase in membrane of sarcoplasmic reticulum. Transport Ca^{2+} back into terminal cisternae.
  - — The resting concentration of Ca^{2+} is restored in cytosol within 30 millisecond, i.e. cessation of contraction.

MYASTHENIA GRAVIS

- It is an autoimmune disease.
- Acetylcholine receptors on sarcolemma becomes blocked by antibodies to the receptor protein.
- This reduces the number of functional receptor sites.
- All this leads to extreme muscular weakness, i.e. muscle fibre can be responded to nerve stimulus very feebly.

Smooth Muscle

- Is the intrinsic muscle of alimentary canal, blood vessel genitourinary and respiratory tract; along with other hollow and tubular organs, + iris and ciliary body of eye + isolation fibre in association with hair follicle etc.
- They generally occurs as bundles/sheets of elongated fusiform cells. Cytoplasm contains actin and myosin. Nucleus located in centre with a cork screw appearance. Cytoplasmic densities or ***Dense bodies*** are seen among the filaments and in relation to plasma membrane.
- Dense bodies + intermediate filaments are serving skeletal function here, just like Z disc of striated muscle. So bundles of contractile filaments containing actin + myosin are anchoring dense bodies on plasma membrane, at one end, and to dense bodies associated with bundles of intermediate filaments on cytoskeleton at the other end.
- Smooth muscle cell myosin hydrolyse ATP at less rate in comparison of skeletal muscle, thus a slow cross bridging cycle is produced which gives a slow contraction/sustained contraction , over long period of times, (using only 10% ATP).

- No T system reported here. Then source of Ca^{2+} are large number of pinocytic vesicles sER which sequester the calcium.
- Smooth muscle contracts in a wave like manner, producing peristaltic movements (in GIT) etc. They remain contracted for long periods without fatigue (spontaneous contractile activity).
- Their contraction is under control of ANS. They are innervated by sympathetic + parasympathetic nerve along with enteric branch in GIT.
- Hormones (ADH; oxytocin) are potent stimulators.
- Smooth muscle cells secrete connective tissue matrix (renin from JG apparatus- Kidney)
- Smooth muscle cells may respond to injury by undergoing mitosis.

Cardiac Muscle

- Is the type of striated muscle found in wall of heart and in the base of large veins which empty into heart. Fibres are formed by individual non-nucleated cardiac muscle cells which are joined to one another in linear array.
- Cardiac muscle fibres exhibit densely staining cross bands called *Intercalated discs* that cross the fibre in linear fashion. This disc is a representation of site of attachment of a cardiac muscle cell to its neighbours.
- Nucleus occupies central position in cell.
- In artria, granules are found (0.3-0.4μ in diameter) and they are also concentrated in juxta nuclear cytoplasm. These granules contain two polypeptide hormone, viz.
  — *ANF* (atrial - natriuretic factor)
  BNF (Brain-natriuretic factor)
- Both are diuretic and inhibit renin secretion in kidney and aldosterone secretion in adrenals. They stimulate relaxation of vascular smooth muscle. In CHF; circulating BNF increases.
- Very large mitochondria, are characteristic feature, which are densely packed between myofibrils; they extend for full length of a sarcomere and have numerous cristae. There are also associated concentration of glycogen granules between myofibrils.
- The T tubules penetrate into myosin filament bundles at the level of Z disc, between ends of sER network. So only one T tubule per sarcomere in cardiac muscle. A *diad* is formed by union of T tubule + small terminal cisternae of sER. They are less numerous in atrial muscle than in ventricular muscles.

CENTRAL NERVOUS SYSTEM

Organization of Spinal Cord

- It is a flattened cylindrical structure that is directly continuous with brain. It is divided into 31 segments (8 cervical + 12 thoracic + 5 lumbar + 5 sacral + 1 coccygeal) and each segment is connected to a pair of spinal nerves. Each spinal nerve is joined to its segment of the cord by a number of roots, grouped as, posterior (dorsal), or anterior (ventral) roots.
- In cross-section, it appears as butterfly, inner substance ***grey matter*** - surrounding the *central canal*, and a whitish peripheral substance—***white matter***. White matter contains myelinated and un-myelinated axons travelling to and from other parts of spinal cord, as well as, to and from the brain. Functionally related bundles of axons are called ***tracts***.
- Grey matter contain nuclei—i.e. neuronal cell bodies and their dendrites along with axons and neuroglia. Synapses occur only in grey matter. The term nucleus means a cluster or group of neuronal cell bodies + fibres and neuroglia.

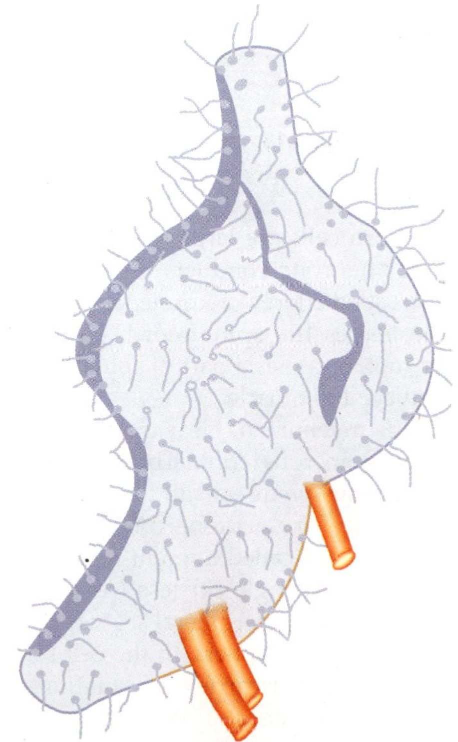

Fig. 4.12: Axon terminal

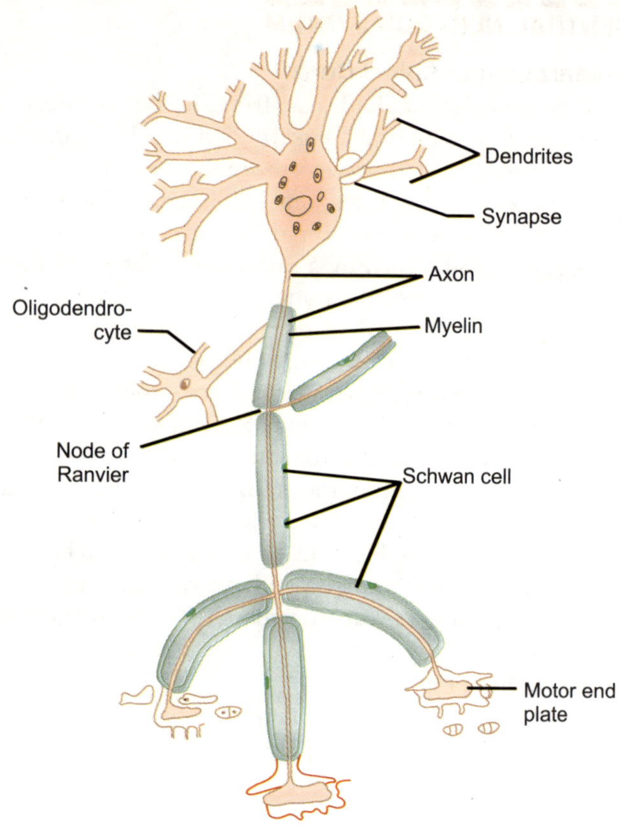

Fig. 4.13: Motor neuron

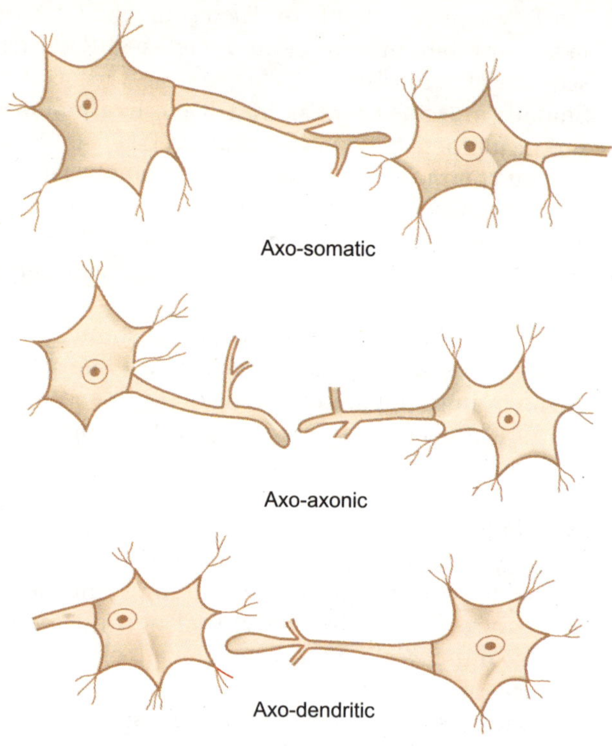

Fig. 4.14: Synapse

- Anterior horn cells are large basophilic cells. Since this motor neurone conducts impulse away from CNS, it is called efferent neurone. The axon of motor neurone leaves the spinal cord, passes through anterior root, becomes a part of spinal nerve and as such conveyed to muscle.
- The axon is myelinated. Near the muscle cell axon divides into numerous terminal branches which forms neuro-muscular synapses with the muscle cells.
- Because the sensory neurone conducts impulses to the CNS, they are called afferent neurone. Sensory neurones have a single process (pseudounipolar) which divides into a peripheral segment that brings information from periphery to the cell body and a central segment that carries information from cell body into grey matter of spinal cord.

Afferent (sensory) receptors Receptors are able to initiate a nerve impulse in response to a nerve stimulus. Following are types:

— Exteroceptors: Reacting to stimuli from external environment, e.g. touch, temperature, smell, vision, sound etc.

— Enteroceptors: Reacting to stimuli from within the body, e.g. degree of filling/stretching of alimentary canal, bladder and blood vessels.

— Proprioceptors: Reacting to stimuli from within the body—providing sensation of body position, muscle tone and movement.

— The simple receptor is a bare axon called free nerve ending found in epithelia/connective tissue.

Synapses

- These are specialised junctions between neurones which facilitate transmission of impulses from one neurone to another.
- Classification:

  a. ***Morphological***
     1. Axo-dendritic—between axons and dendrites
     2. Axo-somatic—between axons and cell body
     3. Axo-axonic—between axons and axons.
     4. Dendro-dendritic—between dendrites and dendrites.

  b. ***Chemical:*** There is:
     1. Presynaptic knob:- end of neurone process from which neuro-transmitter released.
     2. Synaptic cleft:- 20 to 30 nm space which is to be crossed by neuro-transmitter.

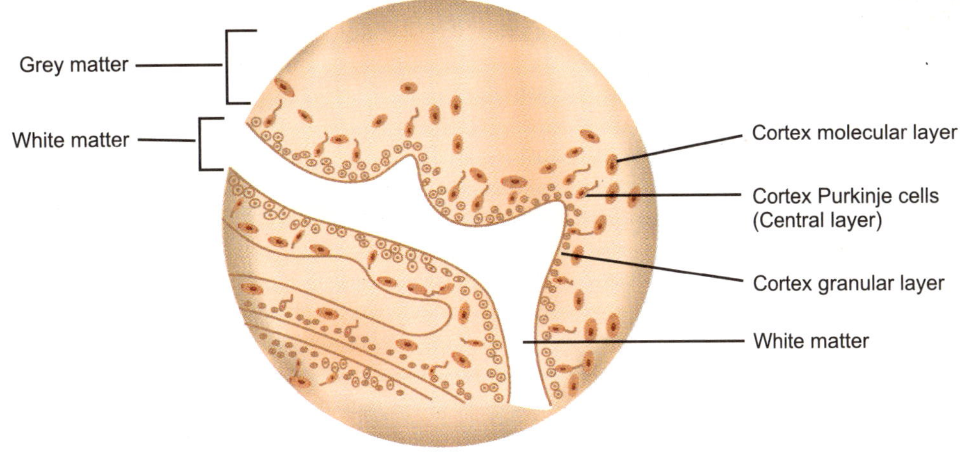

Fig. 4.15: Cerebellum

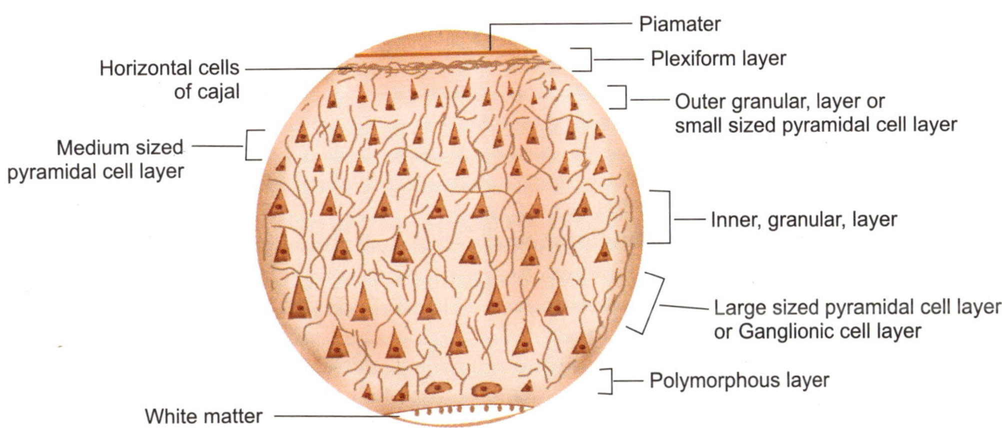

Fig. 4.16: Cerebrum

3. Postsynaptic membrane:- Have receptor site on plasma membrane with which neuro-transmitter interacts.

- In coming neurone travels along the surface of neurone, making several synaptic contact called ***boutons***. The axon then continues to end finally as a terminal twig with an enlarged tip—*bouton terminal*.
- Presynaptic component is separated from post-synaptic component by synaptic cleft. The plasma membrane of second neurone is characterised by presence of dense material layer called presynaptic density.
- Synaptic vesicles- a membrane limiting structure (30-100 nm diameter) contain the neuro-transmitter. It is bouton ending of axon.

Synaptic Transmission

- A nerve impulse reaches bouton → production of voltage reversal across the membrane → opening of voltage gated calcium channels → fusion of synaptic vesicles with presynaptic membrane → release of neuro-transmitter into synaptic cleft by exocytosis → diffusion of transmitter in cleft → binding of transmitter + receptor on postsynaptic membrane → ions enter the neurone → voltage reversal (depolarisation) in postsynaptic membrane → generation of second nerve impulse.
- This may produce:
  — excitatory synapses—leads to initiation of nerve impulse.
  — Inhibitory synapses—more difficulty in generation of nerve impulse.

NERVOUS TISSUE

- It consists of two principal cells, viz. nerve cells, i.e. neurones and supporting cells. Former is its functional unit.
- Neurones: are specialised to receive stimuli and to conduct electrical impulses to other parts of the system. Several neurones are in a chain like fashion (integrated communication network).
  - — Types:
    1. *Sensory:* carry impulses from receptor to central nervous system.
    2. *Motor:* carry impulses from CNS to effector cells,
    3. *Interneurones:* (internuncial or intercalated) - network between sensory and motor. Ninety-nine per cent population is of this variety.
  - — All neurones have a cell body and processes - the axon and dendrite. According to this they are classified as:
    1. Multipolar—one axon and more than two dendrites.
    2. Bipolar—one axon and one dendrite
    3. Unipolar—one process—the axon which divides into two long processes—close to the cell body. Sensory neurones are unipolar. The cell body of a sensory neurone is situated in dorsal root ganglia close to CNS—one axonal branch extends to periphery while another to CNS. Both axonal branches are conducting units.

  Motor neurones and interneurones are multipolar.
  - — Neurones don't divide—they are lasting for a life time. They don't replicate.
  - — The cell body (perikaryon) is a large dilated part of the cell containing large nucleus with prominent nucleolus. *Nissl bodies* are the main inclusions.
  - — Dendrites are neuronal processes which receive stimuli from other nerve cells/environment. They are unmyelinated, tapered forming extensive arborisation called dendritic trees which increase the receptor surface of neurone.
  - — Axons are neuronal processes which transmit stimuli to other neurones or to effector cells. There is one axon for each neurone. It originates from a conical projection of the cell body called *axon hillock.* Its region between apex of axon hillock and beginning of myelin sheath is initial segment which is the site of generation of action potential. Axons in CNS may be insulated by myelin sheath, specially in the tracts that constitute white matter; or may be unmyelinated in grey matter.
- Supporting cells of Nervous system:-

a. ***Schwann cells:***
  1. Myelinated axons are surrounded by layer called myelin sheath which is rich in lipids. Located externally to it is *sheath of Schwann or neurilemma* which consists of nucleus and most of organelles of Schwann cell. It is this structure which insulate the axon from surrounding extracellular compartment. Myelin sheath is not present at axon hillock and at terminal arborization where axon arborizes with its target cell.
  2. Each Schwann cell wraps in a spiral wound a short segment of myelin on an axon, in order to produce myelin sheath. During axon wrapping cytoplasm is squeezed out of concentric layers of Schwann cell.
  3. The myelin sheath is segmented because it is formed by numerous Schwann cells arrayed sequentially along the axon. The junction where two adjacent Schwann cells meet is devoid of myelin and this site is called *node of Ranvier.*
     - — The myelin is lipid rich because, as the schwann cell winds around axon, its cytoplasm is extruded from between opposing layers of plasma membranes.
     - — The nerves in peripheral nervous system are unmyelinated.

b. ***Satellite cells:*** The neural cell bodies of ganglia are surrounded by a layer of small cuboidal cell called satellite cells. They form a complete layer around the cell body. They also originate from neural crest cells. They are also responsible to establish and maintain controlled micro-environment around the neuronal body in the ganglion. So it is analogous to Schwann cell except that it does not make myelin.

Impulse Conduction

a. The nerve impulse which is an electrochemical process which propagates along the nerve fibre—is called action potential.

b. This action potential is due to changes in permeability of axolemma, which leads to influx of sodium ions into axoplasm and so voltage reversal across the membrane.

   Initially resting potential is—90 mV; after influx of Na^+ it becomes + 50 mV. Rapid efflux of potassium ions is associated with return of original polarity. Certainly it is Na^+K^+ activated ATP ase of axolemma which pumps sodium from axoplasm in exchange for potassium.

c. The nerve impulse is jumping from node to node along the myelinated axon which is described as *saltatory conduction*. Its speed is related to thickness of myelin as well as to thickness of axon—it is more rapid in thick axons than in thin one. It is also to be noted that large diameter myelinated axons conduct impulses more rapidly then small diameter myelinated axons.

Cerebral Cortex

(Pallium) Total area is of 220,000 sq. mm. Total number of nerve cells - $7X10^9$. The usual six layers from surface inwards given by Economo, are:-

a. ***Molecular (plexiform) layer:*** most superficial layer. Cells are sparse, small (4–6μ), cells are pear shaped or fusiform, dense network.
b. ***External granular layer:*** Large number of small, round, polygonal/triangular cells which are closely packed. Afferents pass to overlying layer; axons mainly end in deeper layers; Some may enter to white substance.
c. ***Pyramidal cell layer:*** Medium sized pyramidal cells are present in its outer part, while such large cells are present in deeper layers. May be divided into outer and inner parts.
d. ***Internal granular layer:*** Composed of densely packed masses of stellate cells, rich in nerve fibres. It contains many horizontal fibres looking like white stripe/line of Ballarger - which is well marked in calcarine cortex.
e. ***Ganglionic layer:*** (Internal pyramidal layer):- Well developed in precentral cortex (motor) where giant pyramidal cells are conspicuous. Cells of Martinotti are present and their axons pass out wards towards the surface of cortex. Its deeper part contains dense network of cells.
f. ***Fusiform cell layer:*** In contact with white matter. Composed of spindle shaped cells which are closely packed with their long diameters perpendicular.

The Cerebellum

- Cortex is a large folded sheet (17 cm wide by 120 cm long). Each fold is called *folium*.
- Functional unit
  — ***Purkinje cell:*** 30 million in number lying in cortex. Three major layers have been explained in cortex viz. molecular layer, Purkinje cell layer, granular cell layer. Far beneath these layers, in centre of cerebellar mass are deep nuclei.
  — ***Deep nuclear cell:*** It is under both excitatory and inhibitory influences. Former arise from direct connection with afferent fibres that enter the cerebellum from brain or periphery. The inhibitory influences arise from Purkinje cell.
- The afferent fibres are: climbing and mossy type
  — ***Climbing fibres:*** originate from inferior olivary nucleus. There is one such fibre for every ten Purkinje cells. They project to cerebral cortex (molecular layer) where various synapses are made with soma and dendrite of each Purkinje cell. Its characteristic feature is—Complex spike, i.e. a single impulse travelling through it will cause a single prolonged and peculiar oscillatory type of action potential in each Purkinje cell.
  — ***Mossy fibres:***
    1. Enter the cerebellum from spinal cord, brain stem and higher brain. Collaterals are also found to excite deep nuclear cells from where they project to granular cells.
    2. The granular cells send very small axons which extends 1–2 mm in each direction parallel to folia. Dendrites of Purkinje cells project into this molecular layer.
    3. The synapses of these fibres is very weak. This means in order to alter the activation of Purkinje cell, large numbers of mossy fibres are to be stimulated, i.e. simple spike.
- ***Firing:***
  — Purkinje cell fires at 50 to 100 action potential per second, while the rate of firing of deep nuclear cells is still more higher
  — Decrease in firing rate of deep nuclear cells → inhibitory output signal to motor system.
  — Increase in firing rate → excitatory output signal. In this way cerebellum acts as a brake for motor activities, i.e. excitation or inhibition as per circumstance.
  — Normally a balance between excitation and inhibition exists (identical with homeostasis) but a little so called partiality exists towards excitation because:-
    1. In execution of rapid motor movements, the timing of the two effects on deep nuclei is so that excitation comes first and then the inhibition.

2. This inhibitory signal acts as a negative feedback to stop the motor movement, otherwise it will overshoot its mark—and which when occurs give rise to tremors. Whole this phenomenon is ***damping***.

Direct stimulation of deep nuclear cells by both climbing and mossy fibres excite them. Signals arriving from Purkinje cells inhibit them.

The movement functions: Role of cerebellum

1. At the beginning of a movement—it sends *turn-on-signals* to agonists and *turn-off- signals* to antagonists muscles.
2. Just reverse occurs in the end of a movement. All mossy fibres transmit signals to cerebellar cortex and thence to Purkinje cells (through granular cells) which inhibit the deep nuclear cells. It will turn off the cerebellar excitation of the agonist muscles.
3. For excitation: Signals from cerebral cortex passes to agonist/antagonist muscle to begin contraction. At the same time parallel signals are sent by cerebellum through mossy fibres, dentate nucleus, etc. So *turn-on-signal* becomes very powerful since it is a mixture of cerebrum + cerebellar orders. Now if the cerebellum is diseased this extra support is lost.
4. For antagonists; few other cells are responsible which are present in cerebellum, viz. basket cells, stellate cells, Golgi cells, etc. which are inhibitory in function.
5. When a person first performs a new motor movement, it depends on:-
   — A degree of motor enhancement provided by cerebellum to the onset agonist contraction.
   — Degree of onset inhibition of antagonists.
   — Timing of offset,
   — The extent of inhibition of agonist at offset and
   — Extent of contraction of antagonist at offset.
6. Inferior olivary complex receives full information from corticospinal tracts and motor centres of brain stem which decide the intent of every motor movement. In other words, it acts as a comparator/decision maker—to test how well the actual performance matches the intended performance.

   So if every thing matches then no change in firing of climbing fibres occur. On any mismatching climbing fibres will be either inhibited or stimulated as per need—which will change the sensitivity of Purkinje cell till no further mismatch occurs - and in this way the things go on.

Autonomic Nervous System

- It is that portion of peripheral system which conducts impulses to smooth muscles/cardiac muscle and glandular epithelium. These effectors are the functional units in the organs that respond to regulation by nervous tissue.
- Sensory neurones leave the organ to convey impulse to CNS—these are visceral afferents and their cell bodies are in sensory ganglia and they possess long peripheral and central axon. There is a synaptic station in a ganglion outside of CNS where a preganglionic neurone makes contact with postganglionic neurone.
- The presynaptic neurones send axons from thoracic and upper lumbar spinal cord to vertebral and paravertebral ganglion. This is for sympathetic division.
- The presynaptic neurones of parasympathetic division are located in brainstem and sacral spinal cord.
- The enteric division of ANS consists of ganglia and postganglionic neuronal net works of the alimentary canal.
- A ganglia contains clusters of neuronal cell bodies and nerve fibres.

DIGESTIVE SYSTEMS

Salivary Glands

Parotid glands

- Totally serous; largest of all salivary glands.
- Its striated ducts are large and conspicuous.
- Large amount of adipose tissue is its distinguishing feature.
- Facial nerve (VII Cranial) passes through it. Mumps (Viral infection) may damage it.
- Parotid duct located below and in front of the ear.

Submandibular Gland (submaxillary)

- Mixed glands, mostly serous in humans.
- Located under either side of floor of mouth close to mandible.
- Intercalated duct are less extensive comparatively.

Sublingual Gland

- Mixed glands, mostly mucus secreting in humans.
- Smallest of all. Located in floor of mouth anterior to submandibular glands.
- Mucus secreting unit is more tubular than purely acinar.

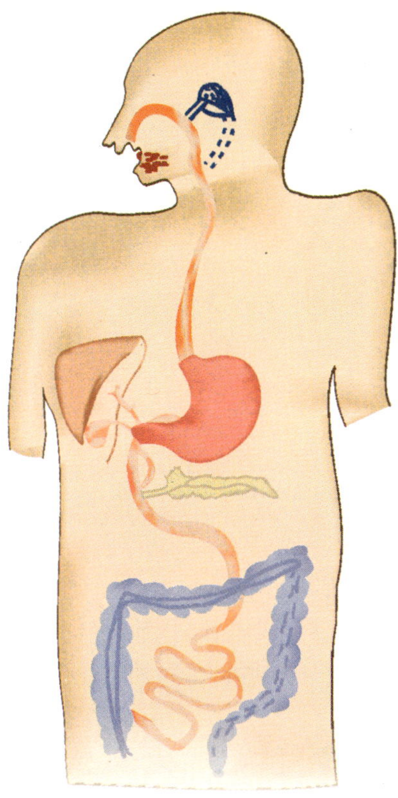

Fig. 4.17: Scheme: Digestive tube

Table 4.2: Secretory gland- Acini (Acinus = grape/berry, Latin)
1. *Serous acini:* spherical and are more tubular.
2. *Mixed acini:* Mucous acini have a cap of serous cells which secretes into highly convoluted intercellular space between mucous cells.
— *Serous cells:* Contain numerous secretory granules, rER, free ribosomes.
— *Mucous cells:* Undergo cycles of activity. During part, mucus is synthesised and stored within the cell as mucinogen granules. When the secretion is discharged, again synthesis starts.

- Multiple small duct of this gland empty into submandibular duct as well as directly onto floor of mouth.

Tongue

- Is a muscular organ projecting into oral cavity from its inferior surface. Its dorsal surface is divided into anterior two-third and posterior one-third by a 'V' shaped depression called sulcus terminalis.
- *Tongue papilla* are of four types:
  - *Filiform:* Most numerous and smallest. Conical and elongated projections of connective tissue covered with keratinised stratified squamous epithelium. Spread entirely over its anterior dorsal surface.
  - *Fungiform*: mushroom shaped projections on dorsal tongue surface and most numerous near its tip. They are characterised by the presence of taste buds on its dorsal surface with stratified squamous epithelium.
  - *Circumvallate:* Large, dome-shaped. contain taste buds and are with stratified squamous epithelium.
  - *Foliate:* on lateral edge of tongue contain many taste buds.

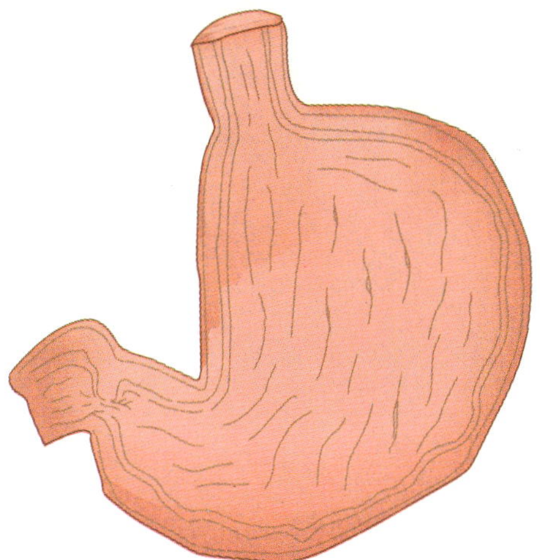

Fig. 4.18: Stomach

Taste Buds

- Present on above papillae
- Oval pale staining bodies extending through the thickness of epithelium, taste pore is the name given to a small opening onto the epithelial surface at the apex of taste bud.
- Three cells are found:
  - Neuroepithelial cell and supporting cells are mature elongated cells extending from basal lamina of epithelium to taste pore, through which apical cellular surface extends micro villi
  - The basal cells are located at periphery of taste buds, near basal lamina and are classed as stem cells for two other cell types
  - Taste buds at tip of tongue detect sweet
  - Taste buds at postero-lateral to tip detect salt
  - Taste buds at circumvallate paoillae detect bitter
  - Taste buds are also present on glosso palatine arch, the soft palate, posterior surface of epiglottis, posterior wall of pharynx down to the level of cricoid cartilage.

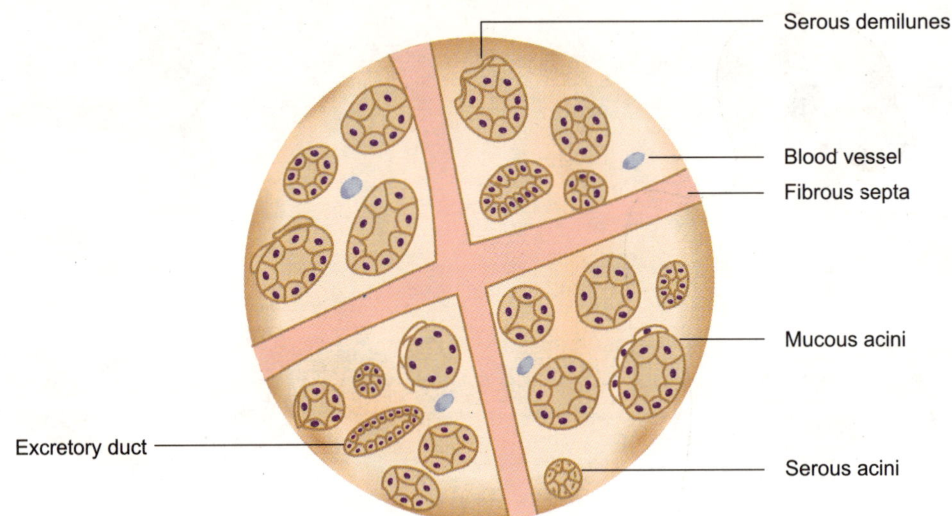

Fig. 4.19: Sublingual gland

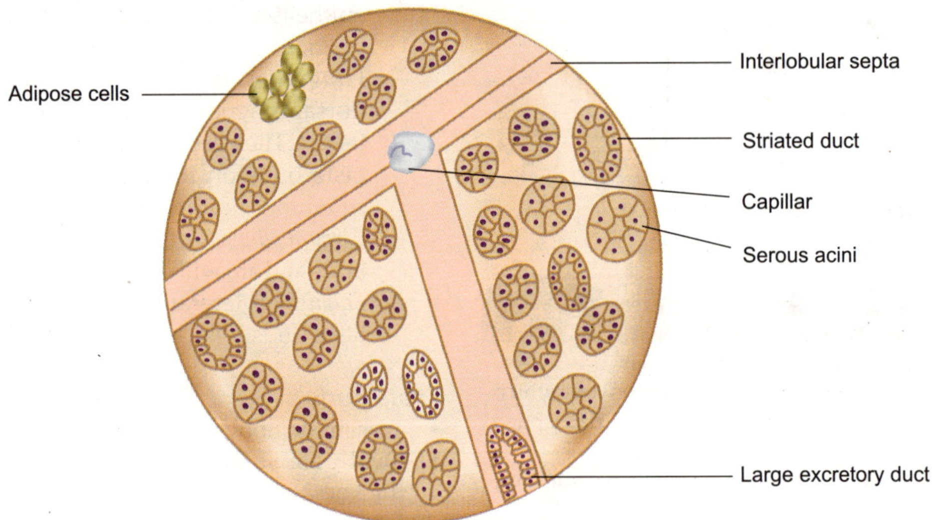

Fig. 4.20: Parotid gland

- Nerve fibres are found in between taste buds which are of VII, IX, X cranial nerve.

Stomach

- Expanded part of digestive tube lying under the diaphragm, receiving food bolus from oesophagus.
- It is having a number of longitudinal folds or ridges called *rugae* which are poorly developed in upper portions but prominent in its narrow regions.
- Small regions of mucosa are formed by grooves or shallow trenches which divide its surface into irregular areas called mamillated areas. Numerous openings are also observed in mucosal surface called *gastric pits*/foveolae.
- Histologically three parts:
  — Cardia – Part near oesophagus having cardiac glands.
  — Pylorus – Part proximal to pyloric sphinctre having pyloric glands
  — Fundus – (body) - Between these two having fundic or gastric glands.
- Gastric mucosa: Simple columnar epithelium lines the surface and gastric pits. These cells are called surface mucus cells having an apical cup of mucinogen

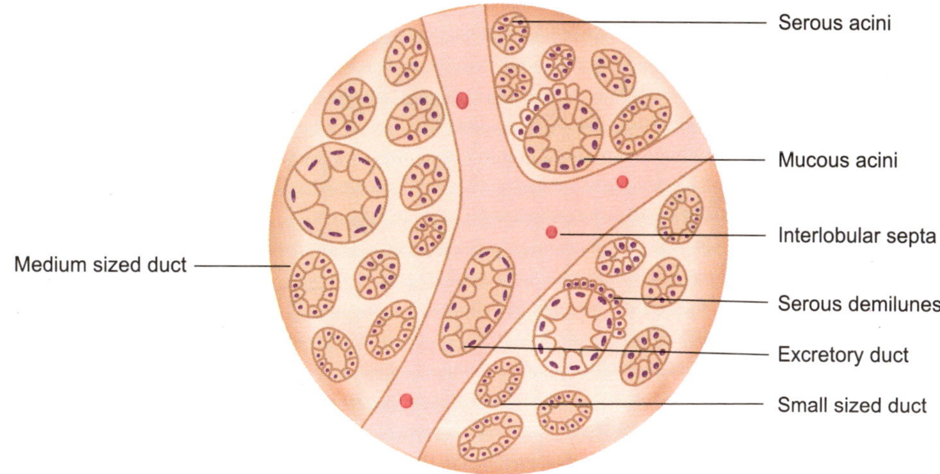

Fig. 4.21: Submandibular gland

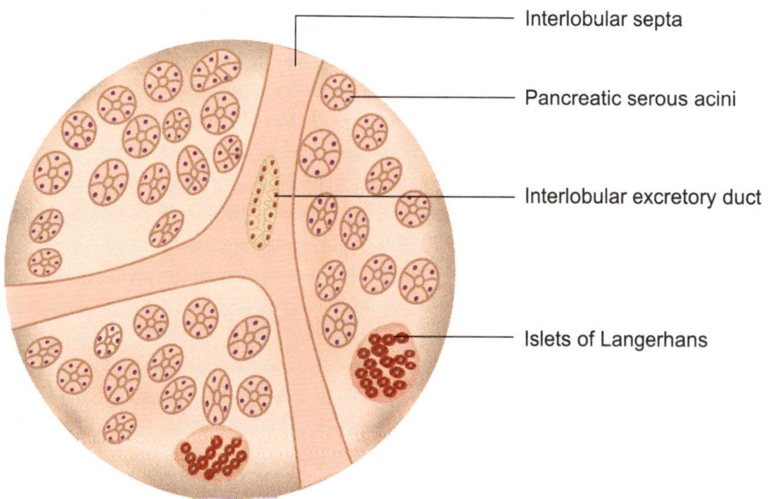

Fig. 4.22: Pancreas

granules. Its secretion is visible mucus due to its cloudy appearance.

- Fundic/gastric glands are present throughout mucosa, which produce gastric secretion. They are simple, branched tubular glands extending from bottom of gastric pits to muscularis mucosae.
- The different cells present in these glands are mucus neck cells, chief cells, parietal/oxyntic cell, entero endocrine cell, undifferentiated cells. Every 3–5 days surface mucus cells are renewed and cells of gastric glands are renewed once a year.
- *Mucus neck cells* is much shorter which secret soluble mucus.
- *Chief cells* are located in deepest part of fundic glands. They are protein secreting cells, i.e. pepsin from its inactive precursor pepsinogen.
- *Parietal/oxyntic cells* are found in neck of fundic glands, secreting HCl. Most numerous in upper and middle portions. Large binucleate cells.
- ***Enteroendocrine cells:*** found at any level of fundic glands. Small cells resting on basal lamina, don't reach to lumen.
- ***Lamina propria:*** composed of reticular fibres + smooth muscles + fibroblasts, lymphocyte, plasma cells, macrophages + eosinophil.

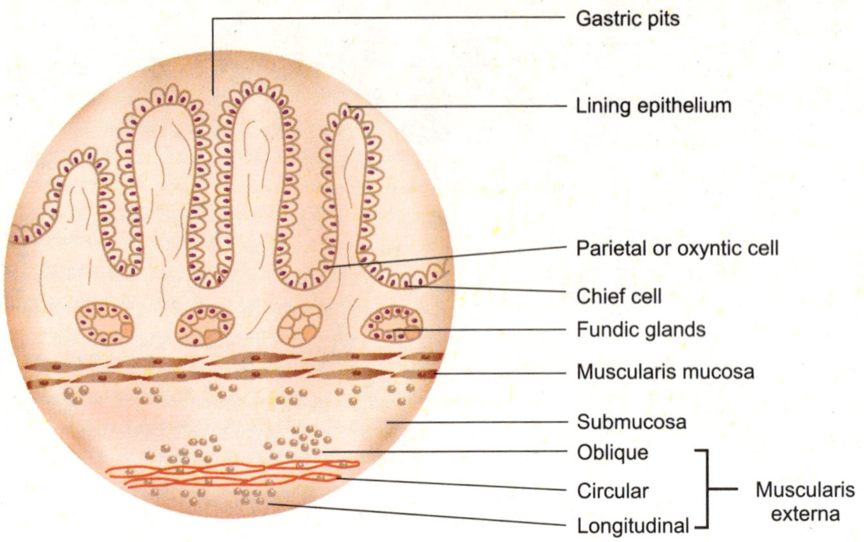

Fig. 4.23: Stomach

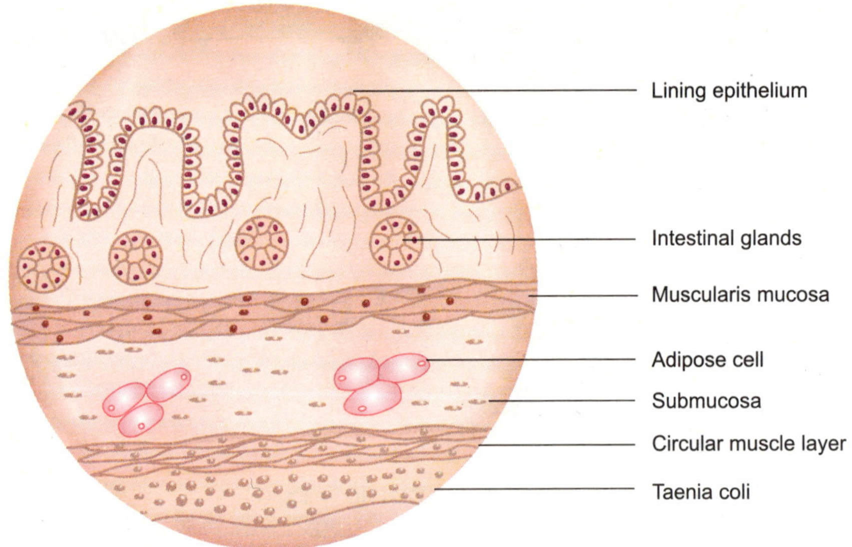

Fig. 4.24: Large intestine (Colon)

- ***Muscularis mucosae:*** Inner circular and outer longitudinal. They play a role in facilitating outflow of gastric gland secretion.
- ***Submucosa:*** Made of dense connective tissue + adipose tissue, blood vessels, nerve fibre and Meissner's plexus.
- ***Muscularis externa:*** Outer longitudinal, middle circular and inner oblique layer.
- ***Serosa:*** It is continuous with peritoneum of abdominal cavity.

Pancreas (Exocrine)

- Serous gland resembling parotid.
- Secretory units are acinar in shape, lined by simple epithelium of pyramidal serous cells.
- The Acinar cells—characterised by acidophilic zymogen granules in apical cytoplasm. Zymogen granules contain a variety of digestive enzymes in an inactive form.
- The ***centro acinar cells*** are the beginning of duct system, having a centrally placed nucleus (squamous

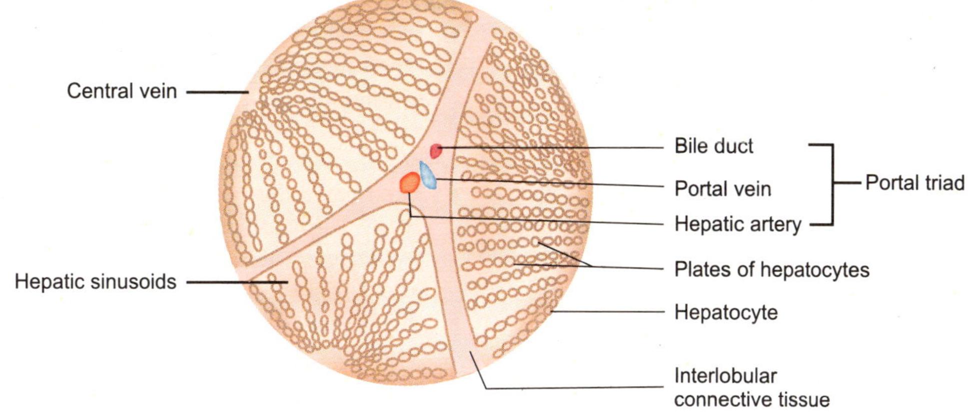

Fig. 4.25: Liver

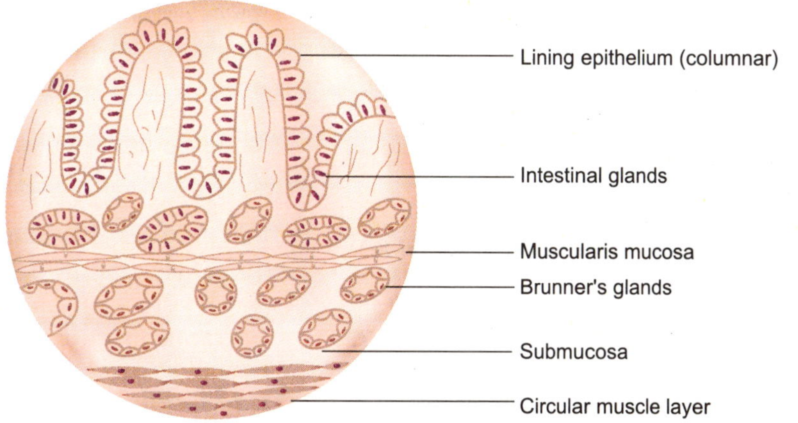

Fig. 4.26: Duodenum

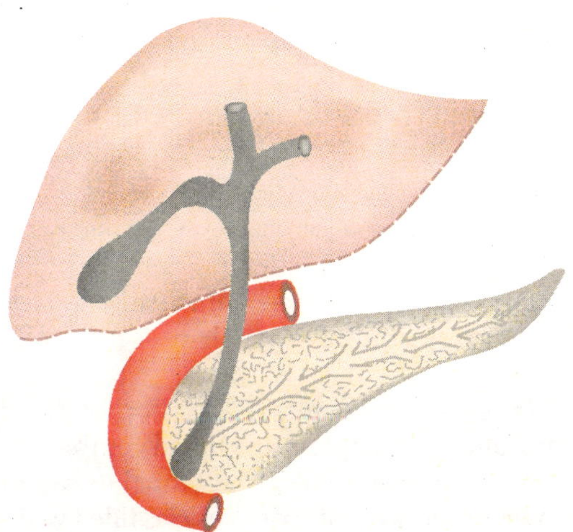

Fig. 4.27: Hepatobiliary system

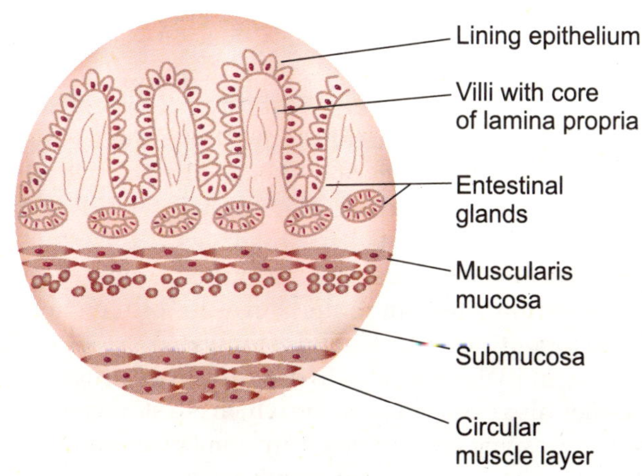

Fig. 4.28: Jejunum

cell). These are intercalated duct cells located in acinus.

- Intercalated ducts $\xrightarrow{\text{drain to}}$ intralobular collecting ducts $\xrightarrow{\text{drain into}}$ inter-lobular collecting duct $\xrightarrow{\text{drain into}}$ main pancreatic duct. Sometimes an accessory pancreatic duct arises in head of pancreas.
- The intercalated ducts add bicarbonate and water to pancreatic secretion.

Liver

- Largest internal organ. Receives major blood supply from hepatic portal vein.
- Its functional unit is lobule/classic/liver acinus.
- Classic hepatic lobule is hexagonal in shape. It consists of stacks of anastomosing plates of hepatic cells. At centre of lobule, there is large venule (central vein) into which sinusoids drain. At the angles of hexagon are portal areas, loose stromal connective tissue characterised by portal triads.
- The portal lobule performs the exocrine function, i.e. bile secretion. Interlobular bile duct of portal triad is classic lobule.
- The liver acinus is the smallest functional unit in hepatic parenchyma. The hepatocytes are arranged in their concentric elliptical zones.
- Hepatic sinusoids are lined with a thin endothelium which is discontinuous. It is provided with a ***Kupffer cell*** (stellate-sinusoidal macrophage)—and it is a difference from other sinusoids. Its processes may even occlude to the lumen. They are derived from monocytes. They form a part of lining of the sinusoid. They are concerned with final breakdown of senile red cells which reach here from spleen.
- Eighty per cent of cellular population of liver is constituted by ***Hepatocytes*** (20–30 μm in diameter) and are large polygonal cells. Nucleus lie in centre and is spherical. Cytoplasm is acidophilic. These cells are rich in peroxisomes which is involved in gluconeogenesis, purine- alcohol and lipid metabolism. Catalase and D amino oxidase, alcohol dehydrogenase are found in peroxisomes. It is the sER which fights against the challenges of drugs, toxins, etc. The sER hypertrophies after administering ethanol, phenobarbital, anabolic steroids, other chemotherapeutic agents. If sER is stimulated by one drug, its activity is enhanced to detoxify other drugs.

They also contain lysosome which is a storage site for iron. Lysosome are increased in number in conditions like biliary stasis, viral hepatitis, anaemia etc.

Biliary Tree

- The system of conduits of increasing diameter that bile flows through hepatocytes to gall bladder as well as intestine is called biliary tree. Its smallest branches are canaliculi into which bile is secreted by hepatocytes.
- The *canaliculus* is provided with irregular microvilli from hepatocyte. It is enveloped by *Zonule occludents*. They constitute a network which drains into small bile ducts—the *canals of Hering*.
- Bile canaliculi may form a complete loop around four sides of six sided hepatocytes. Their diameter is 0.5 to 1.5μm and are separated from rest of intercellular compartment by gap and tight junctions, desmosomes. Microvilli processes of two adjacent hepatocytes extend into lumen of canaliculi.
- The flow of bile is in opposite direction to the blood flow, i.e. from region of central vein toward the portal canal. Bile canaliculi join to form small ductules—the canals of Hering which is lined with cuboidal cells.
- The *ductules* carry the bile through boundary of lobule to interlobular bile ducts that form part of portal triad. These ducts are lined by cuboidal epithelium near the lobules but become columnar as the ducts reach near the porta hepatis. Interlobular ducts join to form right and left lobar ducts which join at hilum to form common hepatic duct.
- ***Common bile duct*** is lined with tall columnar epithelium. The cystic duct connects the common hepatic duct to the gall bladder and carries bile both into and out of gall bladder. Distal to junction with cystic duct, the fused duct is called common bile duct extending upto wall of duodenum at ***ampulla of Vater. Sphincter of Oddi*** is nothing but a thickening of muscularis externa of the duodenum at ampulla and it surrounds both opening, i.e. pancreatic duct and common bile duct. By this, flow of bile and pancreatic juice into duodenum is regulated.

Gall Bladder

- Pear shaped, distensible sac with a capacity of 50 ml. It is attached to posterio-inferior surface of the liver.
- ***Mucosa:*** Numerous deep mucosal folds. Simple columnar epithelium which presents following features:
  - — Many developed microvilli, mitochondria, lateral plications and apical junctional complexes.
  - — Na^+K^+ activated ATP ase on lateral plasma membrane and secretory vesicles filled with glycoproteins in apical cytoplasm are seen.

- ***Lamina propria:*** cellular, rich in fenestrated capillaries and small venules. Mucin secreting cells are sometimes seen
- ***Muscularis externa:*** having numerous. Collagen and elastic fibres.
- It does not have a submucosa or muscularis mucosae.
- ***Adventitia*** is external to muscularis externa containing blood vessels + lymphatics.

Small Intestine

- Longest component of GIT.
- Principle site for digestion and absorption of food stuffs.
- Mainly three parts—duodenum, jejunum and ileum.
- Chyme is received by it from stomach.

ENTERO-ENDOCRINE CELLS

Present in most of digestive tract viz. ducts of pancreas and liver, and in respiratory system.

They are:-

a. Gastro-entero-pancreatic-endocrine cells (GEP) - closely resemble CNS - neuro-secretory cell- OR diffuse neuro-endocrine system.
b. APUD cells (Amine precursor-uptake and decarboxylation cells). They produce biogenic amines and have appropriate enzyme systems. They also produce paracrine substances/ a candidate hormone along with various hormones of GIT. A paracrine substance differs from hormone in the way that it diffuses locally to its target cells instead of being carried in blood stream to target cells. The famous example is of somatostatin which inhibits other GIT and pancreatic islet endocrine cells.

- ***Mucosa:*** Its essential features include—Villi, intestinal glands (crypts of Lieberkuhn) are its characteristic features.
  - — ***Villi*** are finger like projections extending from mucosal surface to lumen, giving a velvety appearance. Lacteal is the name given to blind ending lymphatic capillary which lies in lamina propria of villus. Two types of cells are present, viz. smooth muscle cell and myofibroblasts.
  - — The cells are many. ***Enterocytes*** - are mainly responsible for transport of substances from lumen to circulatory system. Tall columnar cells. They are bound with other cells with Junctional complexes. The Na^+K^+ activated ATP-ase pump is located in lateral plasma membrane. They are also serving the secretory function and so produces necessary enzymes required for digestion and absorption.

ENTEROCYTES: AN OVERVIEW

- Plasma membrane of microvilli of the enterocyte plays a role in digestion and absorption.
- The end products of digestion are close to the site for their absorption; because digestive enzymes are anchored in the plasma membrane, and their functional groups extend outward to become a part of glycocalyx.
- Enzyme enterokinase is also contained in plasma membrane of apical microvilli. It is of special importance in duodenum where trypsin is formed from trypsinogen.
- Triglycerides are digested into glycerol/monoglycerides; which are emulsified by bile salts and pass into apical portion of enterocyte. Here resynthesis of triglycerides takes place which appear first in apical vesicles of sER → Golgi body → finally into vesicles which discharge chylomicrons into intercellular space.
- The final digestion of carbohydrate space.
- The final digestion of carbohydrate is brought about by enzymes bound to microvilli of the entrocytes.
- Amino acids (the end products of protein digestion) are absorbed by enterocytes.

  - — ***Goblet cells*** are interposed among other cells. Most numerous in terminal ileum. They produce mucus. They have microvilli (theca).
  - — ***Paneth cells*** - found in bases of mucosal glands occasionally seen in normal colon. It contains anti-bacterial enzyme lysozyme, other glycoproteins. They also play a role in regulating the normal bacterial flora of intestine.
  - — ***Enteroendocrine cells:*** Concentrated at lower part of intestinal crypt. CCK, GIP, Secretin etc. are released in this part of the GIT.
  - — ***M cells:*** are epithelial cells overlying Peyer's patches and lymphatic nodules. They have microfolds on their apical surface.
  - — ***Intermediate cells***: are in majority at lower half of intestinal crypt. They have short and irregular microvilli.
- ***Submucosa:*** In duodenum, *Brunner's glands* are characteristic which is both zymogen and mucous secreting. Their secretion is rich in bicarbonate and glycoproteins which neutralizes the acid chyme.
- ***Muscularis externa:*** Inner circular and outer longitudinal arranged smooth muscle cells. Between these two is myenteric plexus—a local nerve plexus. Segmentation and peristalsis are due to these muscular contractions; former by circular and later through longitudinal muscles.
- ***Serosa:*** Adventitia is the name given to attach loose connective tissue.

Large Intestine

- Is composed of caecum, ascending colon, transverse colon, descending sigmoid colon, rectum and anal canal.
- *Mucosa:*
  - — Contains straight tubular glands- crypts of Lieberkuhn extending throughout its full thickness. Simple columnar epithelium lines the glands. It operates Na^+K^+ activated ATPase transport system.
  - — Paneth cells are usually absent in adult human.
  - — Columnar absorptive cells predominant over goblet cells in most of the colon.
  - — Goblet cell may mature deep in the crypt. Continuously mucus is secreted by them. These are thin tall having small number of mucinogen droplets in central apical cytoplasm.
- ***Lamina Propria:*** includes a thick layer of collagen and ground substance, GALT, a well developed fibroblast sheath and absence of lymphatic vessels.
- ***Musculacis externa:*** Outer longitudinal called *taenia coli* and between these bands longitudinal muscle layer forms a thin sheet. *Haustrations* (saccules) are formed in the wall of colon by discontinuities in muscularis externa which allows intestinal segments to contract independently. This layer is causing segmentation, peristalsis and mass peristalsis movements.
- ***Submucosa*** *and* ***serosa,*** i.e. adventitia.
- ***Caecum:*** Caecum forms a blind pouch just distal to ileo caecal valve.
- The ***appendix:*** is thin finger like extension of this pouch. It is having a complete layer of longitudinal muscle in muscularis externa. It is characterised by the presence of large number of lymphatic nodules in submucosa.
- ***Rectum:*** is dilated distal portion of alimentary canal characterised by transverse rectal folds. The most distal part of GI tract is anal canal extending from anorectal junction to anus. Anal columns are nothing but longitudinal folds in upper part of anal canal. Depression between anal column are called anal sinuses.
- In ***anal canal*** there are anal glands extending into sub-mucosa and into muscularis externa. They secrete mucus and are lined with stratified columnar epithelium and same type of epithelium lines the distal part of it.
- ***Circum anal glands:*** are present in skin surrounding anal orifice; along with hair follicles + sebaceous glands.
- ***Submucosa:*** contains veins, superior rectal artery which may sometimes enlarge to constitute internal haemorrhoids.
- The circular layer of muscularis externa thickens to form ***internal anal sphincter*** while ***external anal sphincter*** is formed by striated muscles of perineum.

GALT—A VIEW (GUT ASSOCIATED-LYMPHATIC TISSUE)

- It responds to antigenic stimuli as well as it functions in a monitoring capacity.
- This is performed by lymphatic nodules of gut which contains M cell having microvilli.
- M cells performs pinocytosis for proteins from intestinal lumen, → transport the pinocytic vesicle through the cell → discharge the protein by exocytosis into deep recesses of adjacent extracellular space.
- Lymphocytes are able to produce antibodies against antigens.

RESPIRATORY SYSTEM

1. *Trachea:* Its wall consists of:
   - ***Mucosa:*** having ciliated pseudostratified epithelium with elastic fibre rich lamina propria.
   - ***Submucosa:*** more dense connective tissue than lamina propria
   - ***Cartilaginous layer:*** C-shaped hyaline cartilage
   - ***Adventitia:*** binds trachea to other structures. Fibroelastic tissue and smooth muscles (trachealis muscle) bridge gap between free ends of c-shaped cartilage at posterior end of trachea adjacent to oesophagus.
   - ***Ciliated cells:*** Most numerous extend through full thickness of epithelium. Cilia appear as short hair like processes from apical surface. Ciliated cell provide a co-ordinate sweeping motion of mucous coat, serving an important protective mechanism for removing small inhaled particles from lungs.
   - ***Mucous cells (goblet):*** Extend through full thickness of epithelium.
   - ***Brush cells:*** Columnar cells having microvilli regarded as a receptor cell.
   - ***Small granular cells:*** nucleus located near the basement membrane - more extensive cytoplasm which contain granules which secrete catecholamine, polypeptide hormone. They are thought to function in reflexes regulating the airway.
   - ***Basal cells:*** Nuclei form a row in close proximity to basal lamina.
   - The thick basement membrane is characteristics of tracheal epithelium and is located below it. 25 to 40 μm in thickness. In smokers, this layer is thick

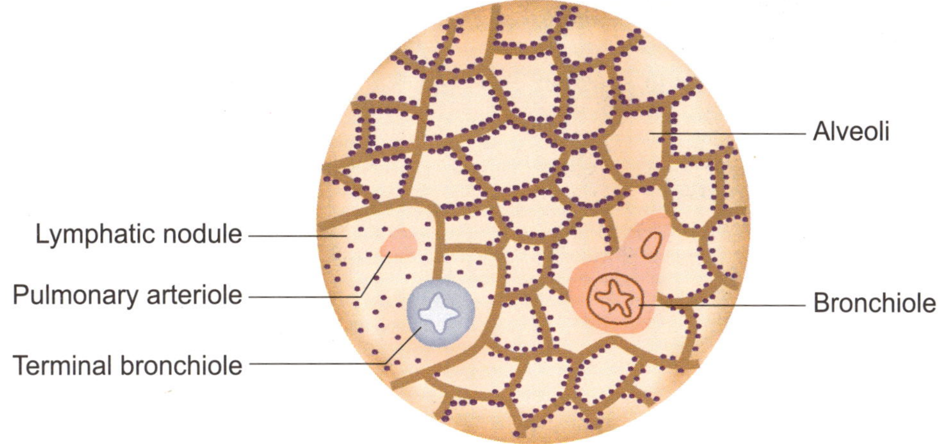

Fig. 4.29: Lungs (Panoramic view)

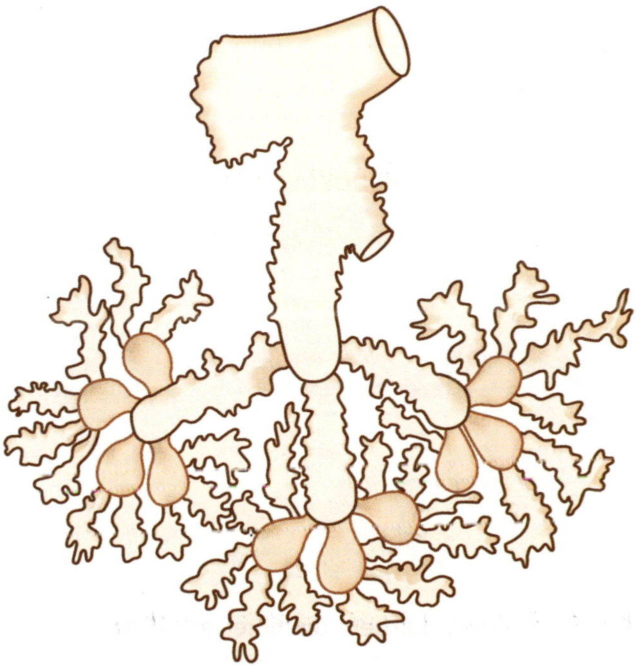

Fig. 4.30: Respiration tube

due to irritation of mucus. Lamina propria appears as collection of loose connective tissue + cellular + lymphocytes, + plasma cells + eosinophils + mast cells + fibroblasts

- Among the cartilaginous fibres are elastic fibres called band of elastic membrane. In submucosa it is dense layer. Submucosal glands composed of mucus secreting acini are present. These are specially numerous in cartilage free gap on posterior part of trachea.

Bronchus

- Can be identified by their cartilage plates and a circular layer of muscles (smooth) which becomes an increasing conspicuous layer as amount of cartilage diminishes.
- Following are the layers

Mucosa: pseudostratified epithelium, Basement membrane is conspicuous in primary bronchi but quickly diminishes in thickness and disappears as a discrete structure. Lamina propria is diminished in amount in proportion to diameter of bronchi

Muscularis: of smooth muscle, whose contraction maintains the appropriate diameter of airway

Submucosa: loose connective tissue glands + adipose tissues are present

Cartilage Layer

Adventitia: dense connective tissue—continuous with pulmonary structures, e.g. lung parenchyma and pulmonary artery.

- *Other peculiarities:*
  - Cartilage and glands are not present in bronchioles.
  - The large diameter bronchioles have ciliated pseudostratified columnar epithelium which transforms gradually to simple ciliated columnar epithelium as the duct narrows.
- Respiratory bronchioles are the first part of bronchial tree that allows gaseous exchange to occur.

EPITHELIAL ALTERATION: RESPIRATORY TRACT (METAPLASIA)

- Changes from ciliated pseudostratified to stratified squamous. This change may occur when pattern of air flow is altered or when there is a forceful air flow, e.g. chronic coughing, bronchiectasis, chronic bronchitis, etc.
- This altered/new epithelium is more resistant to stress. In smokers, ciliary beating is lost due to noxious elements of smoke which results into impaired removal of mucus. For its compensation, one coughs, which facilitates the expulsion of accumulated mucus in the airway.

Alveoli (the site of gas exchange) 100 millions alveoli are found in each lung. Each alveolus is a thin walled polyhedral chamber. 0.2 mm in diameter. Its epithelium composed of:

a. Type I alveolar cells (pneumocytes)—thin squamous cells lining most of alveolar surface (95%)
b. Type II (septal cells) secretory cells/cuboidal cells - cover only 5 per cent. Alveolar surface covered by them. Tend to bulge into air spaces. The parallel membrane lamella is rich in phospholipid among which is surface active agent surfactant which forms a mono molecular layer over alveolar epithelium, thus reducing the surface tension at air-epithelium interface. Very few brush cells present in alveolar wall.
   - Alveolar ducts are elongated airways having no walls. Alveolar air sacs are spaces surrounded by clusters of alveoli. Surrounding alveoli open into these spaces. The tissue between adjacent alveolar air spaces is called alveolar septum which is the site of air blood barrier and its components are alveolar epithelium cells, basal lamina of alveolar epithelium, endothelial cells of rich capillary network, other connective tissue elements, e.g. fibroblast, macrophages, elastic fibres.

EMPHYSEMA: AT A GLANCE

- Is a condition of the lung characterised by permanent enlargement of air spaces distal to terminal bronchiole and is caused by chronic obstruction of air flow, and narrowing of bronchioles. It leads to destruction of wall of alveoli. All this reduces the gaseous exchange.
- It is further associated with excess lysis of elastin and other structure protein in alveolar septa.

GENERAL FEATURES OF ARTERIES

Composed of three layers called Tunics. The three layers from lumen outwards are:

1. *Tunica intima:* innermost including endothelial lining.
2. *Tunica media:* middle muscular layer
3. *Tunica adventitia:* outer most connective tissue layer.
   - *Tunica intima* consists of single layer of squamous epithelial cells. The subendothelial layer consists of connective tissue, arteries and arterioles; a layer of fenesterated elastic tissue called internal elastic lamina. It may contain occasional smooth muscle cells.
   - *Tunica media*—circumferentially arranged smooth muscle cells. In arteries it is thick extending from internal to external elastic lamina. External layer contains elastin which separates tunica media from tunica adventitia. It also contains reticular fibres, proteoglycans etc.
   - *Tunica adventitia*—composed of longitudinally arranged collagenous tissue and a few elastic fibres which merges with loose connective tissue. Thin in arteries while thick in veins.
   - Large arteries/veins may also have
     —Vasa vasorum to supply vessels themselves.
     —Nervi-vascularis-network of autonomic nerves to control smooth muscle contraction.

ATHEROSCLEROSIS

- Most common abnormality.
- Characteristics are: accumulation of lipids and proliferation of smooth muscle cells.
- The lesions develop in intima.
- Thick layer of fibrous connective tissue and a necrotic mass of lipid in middle of lesion.
- As the lesion progresses there is a loss of integrity of the endothelium.
- In advanced lesions, blood stasis and clotting associated with fibrous capsule may lead to occlusion of the vessel.
- Other changes include—thinning of tunica media, calcification within fibrous capsule and necrotic mass, ulceration of fibrous capsule.

Elastic Arteries (Largest diameter arteries)

- e.g. Aorta and pulmonary arteries and their branches like subclavian, brachiocephalic, common iliac etc.
- They have sheets of elastic tissue in their wall. Not conspicuous internal elastic lamina because it is one of the many elastic layers in the wall of vessel.
- Endothelium is a simple squamous epithelium. Cells are flat elongated with their long axis parallel to the direction of blood flow in artery.
- The cells are joined by tight junctions serving as a barrier to transendothelial diffusion. The pinocytic vesicles move these substances from vascular lumen to the basal surface of endothelial cell and to lateral surface also. Thus, nutrients and regulatory

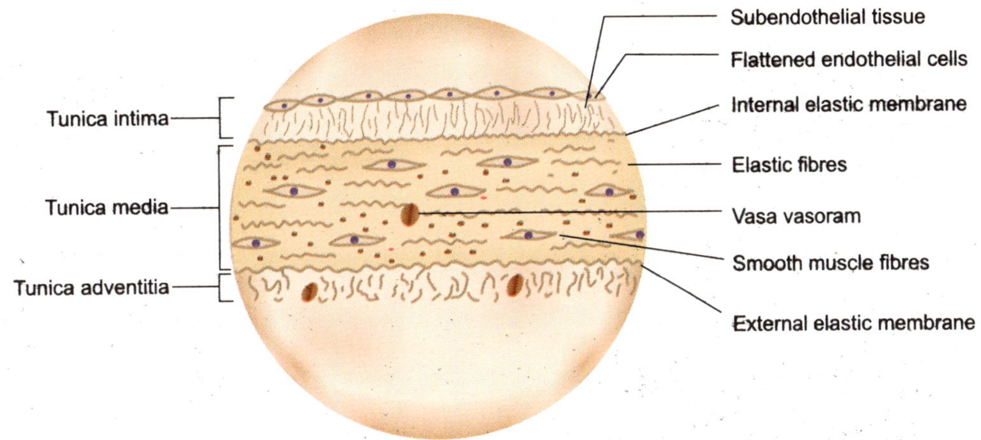

Fig. 4.31: Elastic artery

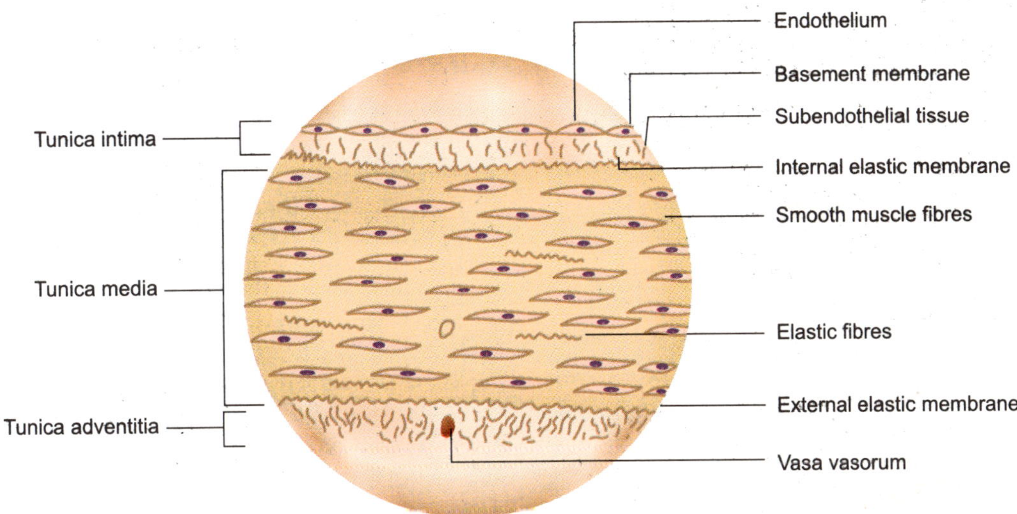

Fig. 4.32: Muscular artery

substances pass through such vesicles to the cells of intima and media. In endothelial cells clotting factor VIII is found to be present, (secretory function of cells).

- The number and thickness of elastic lamina in media layer is depending on age and blood pressure. At birth aorta is devoid of lamellae, in adult 40 to 70 lamellae and in hypertensive individuals their number increases.
- They serve like a conducting tube, facilitating continuous movement of blood along tube.
- The ventricle pump the blood into elastic arteries during systole. Pressure generated by systole moves the blood through elastic arteries and along arterial tree. It also causes their walls to distend which is limited by network of collagenous fibres in ***tunica media*** and ***tunica adventitia***. During relaxation, no pressure is generated by heart, recoil of distended arteries serves to maintain arterial B.P. and sustained flow of blood within the vessels. Initial elastic recoil forces blood both away from and back towards the heart. The blood flow towards the heart leads to closure of aortic and pulmonary valve. Continued elastic recoil then maintains continuous flow of blood away from the heart.

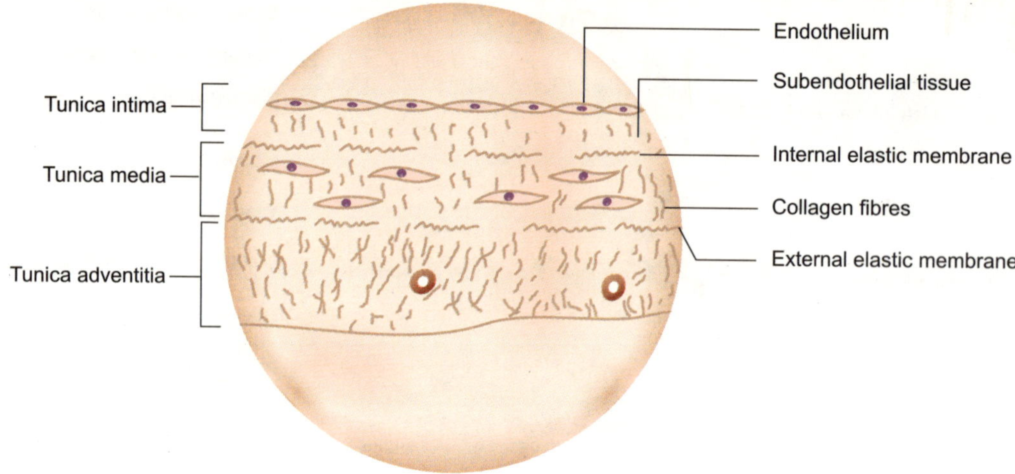

Fig. 4.33: Vein

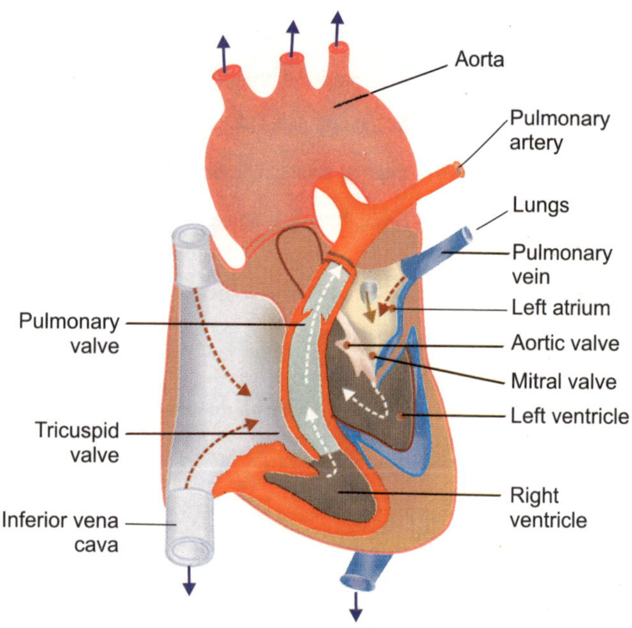

Fig. 4.34: Structure of heart

Muscular Arteries

- Have more smooth muscles and less elastin in tunica media than elastic arteries.
- In young adult, tunica intima accounts for about one sixth of total wall thickness. In older adults, the tunica intima may be grossly expanded by lipid deposits, often in the form of irregular fatty streaks. So its thickness varies with age, etc. Processes of endothelial cells penetrate through basal lamina and make junctional contacts with processes extending towards the lumen from smooth muscle cells of the media.
- Smooth muscles of media assist in maintaining blood pressure. No fibroblasts in this layer.

CHANGES IN HYPERTENSION

- Common cause of death—a silent killer.
- The central lesion is—decrease in size of lumen of small muscular arteries and arterioles. This may also result from active contraction of smooth muscle in the vessel wall, an increase in amount of smooth muscle in the wall, or both.
- In patients of high blood pressure, smooth muscle division increases, which increases the thickness of tunica media. Some smooth muscle cells accumulate lipid.

Arterioles

Acts as flow regulator to the capillary beds. Contraction of smooth muscle in the arteriolar wall shuts off the blood going to the capillaries. A slight thickening of smooth muscle at the origin of capillary bed from arteriole is called precapillary sphincter.

Heart

Consists of three layers viz.

1. ***Epicardium:*** Consists of layer of mesothelial cells on the outer surface of heart and its underlying connective tissues. Vessels and nerves are surrounded by adipose tissue which cushions the heart in the pericardial cavity.
2. ***Myocardium:*** (the cardiac muscle main component) Ventricular myocardium thicker than atrial one, because of large amount of cardiac muscle here.
3. ***Endocardium:*** Inner layer of endothelium and subendothelial connective tissue.
   - middle layer—connective tissue + smooth muscle cells

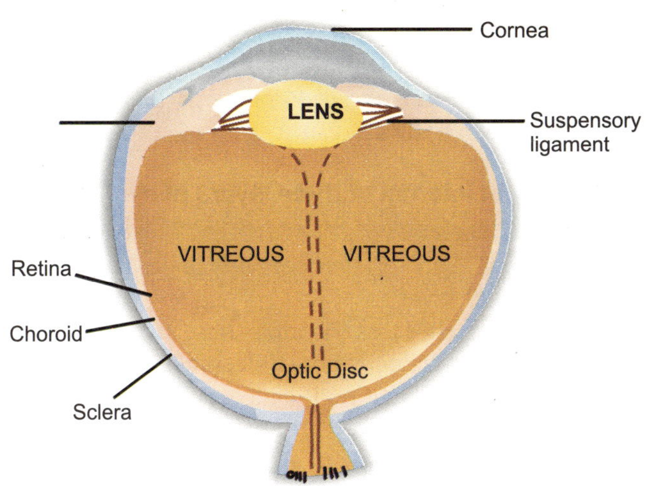

Fig. 4.35: Structure of eye

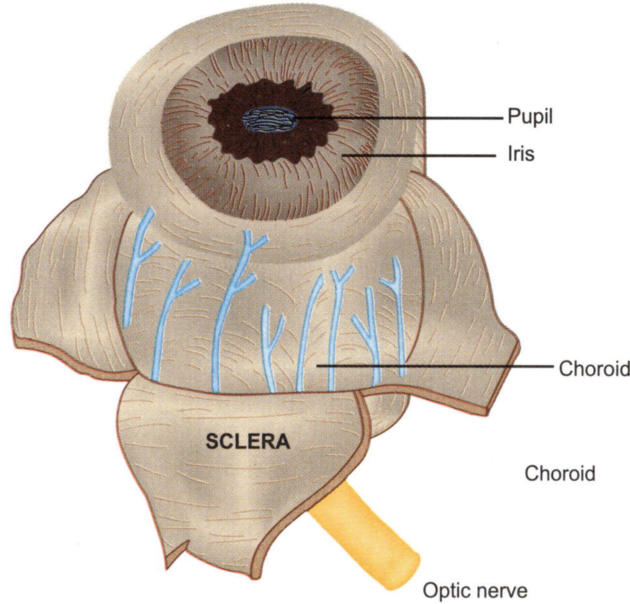

Fig. 4.36: Eyeball

- deeper (subendocardial layer)—connective tissue. Here the impulse conducting system present.

EYE

Complex sensory organs provide us the sensation of light. It is compared with a camera.

Layers

1. *Corneo-scleral coat:* Outer fibrous layer having cornea + sclera.
2. *Uvea:* middle layer/vascular coat—including choroid and stroma of ciliary body + iris
3. *Retina:* inner layer - outer pigment epithelium and inner neural retina and epithelium of ciliary body and iris.

- *Cornea:* covers anterior one sixth of eye, a window like region. It is continuous with sclera (Greek - Skleros = hard) which is white of the eye—a slightly blue in children due to thinness. Sclera provides attachment to extrinsic muscles of the eye.
- *Uvea consists of choroid:* the vascular layer which provides nutrition to retina. It is melanin pigment + blood vessels which give it a dark brown colour. This pigment absorbs the scattered light. Its anterior rim continues forwards where it forms stroma of ciliary body and iris.
- *Ciliary body:* a ring like thickening extending inwards just posterior to level of corneoscleral junction. It contains ciliary muscle—a smooth muscle meant for accommodation of lens.
- *Iris:* is a contractile diaphragm extending over the anterior surface of lens. It also contains melanin pigment cells + smooth muscles. Pupil is the central circular aperture of iris; It varies in size to control the amount of light passing through the lens to reach to retina. It appears black since one looks through the lens towards pigmented back of the eye.

Eye Chambers

1. *Anterior:* Occupy space between cornea and iris,
2. *Posterior:* between posterior surface of iris and anterior surface of lens
3. *Vitreous:* between posterior surface of lens and neural retina. Vitreous body is contained here which is composed of transparent gel substance. It also contains hyaluronic acid + Collagen fibrils + glycoproteins.

- ***The Refractile media:***
  1. ***Cornea:*** anterior window of eye.
  2. ***Aqueous humor:*** watery fluid in anterior and posterior chamber.
  3. ***Lens:*** Transparent, crystalline, bi-convex suspended from ciliary body by a ring of radial fibres - the Zonule of Zinn.
  4. ***Vitreous humor.***

CORNEA

a. ***Epithelium:*** Non-keratinized stratified squamous. 50µm thick, continuous with conjunctival epithelium that overlies adjacent sclera. Remarkable regenerative capacity. Numerous free nerve endings make it sensitive to touch in the form of blinking, tearing, pain etc. Drying may lead to ulceration.

b. ***Bowman's membrane:*** Is homogenous lamina over which epithelium rests. 8μm thick. It ends at limbus which is corneo-scleral junction. It does not regenerate. It provides strength to cornea and is a barrier for infection to spread. If damaged a opaque scar may be left which may interfere the vision.
c. ***Corneal stroma:*** Constitutes major corneal thickness. Made up by collagen fibrils which form lamella. Ground substance contain corneal proteoglycans, chondroitin sulphate etc. All this is giving it transparency. No blood vessels or pigments in cornea.
d. ***Descemet's membrane:*** Is unusual thick basal lamina. 10μm thick. Readily regenerates after injury. With age slowly increases in thickness.
e. ***Corneal endothelium:*** Single layer of flat cells that faces anterior chamber. All metabolic exchange occurs here. Its damage may lead to corneal opacity.

SCLERA (OPAQUE LAYER)

a. *Episclera:* external layer; loose connective tissue adjacent to periorbital fat.
b. *Sclera proper:* investing fascia of eye—dense network of thick collagen fibres.
c. *Lamina fusca:* Inner aspect; located adjacent to choroid. Have pigment cells + elastic fibres + thin collagen fibres.

Its opacity is due to its structural irregularities. It is pierced by blood vessels + nerves (optic).

IRIS

Five layers viz. (from anterior to posterior)

1. Discontinuous layer marked with ridges and grooves, of fibroblasts and melanocytes.
2. *Thin:* avascular layer of stroma anterior stromal sheat/lamella.
3. Loose connective tissue layer containing blood vessels.
4. Posterior membrane - discontinuous layer of smooth muscle.
5. Double layer of pigmented epithelial cells.
   - It arises from anterior border of ciliary body and pupil is its central aperture.
   - It forms contractile diaphragm anterior to lens surface.
   - The ciliary body is a thickened anterior portion of tunica vasculosa located between iris and choroid
   - The ciliary epithelium covers the ciliary body and secretes aqueous humour.
   - The choroid is the portion of vascular layer that lies deep to retina.

Retina (most internal of three layers of eye)

- Two basic layers:
  — Neural .... inner layer contains photo receptors
  — Pigment layer
  — In some diseases/trauma these two layers are separated called retinal detachment.
- In neural layer - two regions seen:
  — non-photosensitive regions - anterior to ora serrata.
  — photosensitive region :- posterior to ora serrata.
- The site where optic nerve joins the retina is optic disc. Since it is devoid of photo receptors so it is a blind spot. The *fovea centralis* is a shallow depression located 2.5 cm lateral to optic disc. It is area of greatest visual activity. *Macula lutea* is a yellow pigmented zone surrounding fovea. Fovea is the region having highest concentration and precisely ordered arrangement of visual elements.
- Following are the layers of retina from outside inwards.
  1. ***Pigment epithelium (RPE):*** Outer layer. Not a part of neural retina. Single layer of cuboidal cells. Cells tallest in fovea. Rests on Bruch's membrane of choroid layer. Adjacent to this layer is a junctional complex which is the site of blood retinal barrier. The cells have extensions which surround the process of rods and cones. Its functions are:-
     — Absorption of light passing through neural retina to prevent reflection and glare.
     — Isolation of retinal cells from blood borne-substances.
     — The metabolic apparatus for visual pigment synthesis is present in these cells.
     — Phagocytosis and disposal of membranous disc from rods and cones of retinal photo receptor cells.
  2. ***Layer of rod and cones***:- Outer segment of photo receptor cells. Rods and cones are arranged in a palisade manner. 120 million rods and 7 million cones. Rods are 2μm thick and 50μm long. The cones are 85μm long at fovea while 25μm long at periphery.

     Rods are more sensitive towards light and are the receptors used during long periods of low intensity (during night)—or a black and a white picture. Cones are having maximal sensitivity towards red, green and blue region of visual spectrum so permit better visual acuity.

3. ***External limiting membrane*** (Müller's cells). It is a row of zonula adherens between the apical ends of Müller's cells, i.e. the end that faces the pigment epithelium, with each other and with rods and cones.
4. ***Outer nuclear layer:*** Contain cell bodies of rods and cones.
5. ***Outer plexiform layer:*** Contains the processes of retinal rods and cones as well as processes of horizontal, amacrine and bipolar cells that connect to them. Many photo receptors converge onto one bipolar cell forming interconnecting neural networks. Cones located in fovea synapse with a single bipolar cell.
6. ***Inner nuclear layer:*** Contains cell bodies of horizontal amacrine, bipolar and Müller's cells.
7. ***Inner plexiform layer:*** Contain processes of bipolar, amacrine, horizontal as well as ganglion cells that connect to each other.
8. ***Ganglion cell layer:*** Contains cell bodies of ganglion cells. Scattered among them are neuroglial cells.
9. ***Layer of optic nerve fibres:*** Contain axon of ganglion cells.
10. ***Internal limiting membrane***: Composed of basal lamina of Müller's cells.

Crystalline Lens

Transparent, avascular, biconvex. 3 components

1. Capsule thick basal lamina measuring 10 to 20 μm, elastic, thickest at equator.
2. Subcapsular epithelium :- cuboidal on anterior surface of lens. Connected by gap junctions.
3. Lens fibres: derived from epithelial cells.

EAR

Three chambered sensory structure (auditory system) functioning as perception of sound + vestibular system functioning as maintenance of balance.

External Ear

i. Composed of an auricle (pinna) and external auditory meatus. Pinna is oval shaped appendage projecting from lateral surface of head. It is covered by thin skin with hair follicles, sweat and sebaceous glands. Considered as vestigial but is an essential component in sound localisation and amplification.

External Auditory Canal

Air filled tubular space following S shaped course to the tympanic membrane (ear drum). Its lateral part is lined by skin which contain hair follicles, Sebaceous glands and ceruminous glands (producing ear wax) which lubricates the skin and coat the meatal hairs to impede the entry of foreign particles into ear. However, its excessive accumulation can plug the meatus resulting in conducting hearing loss.

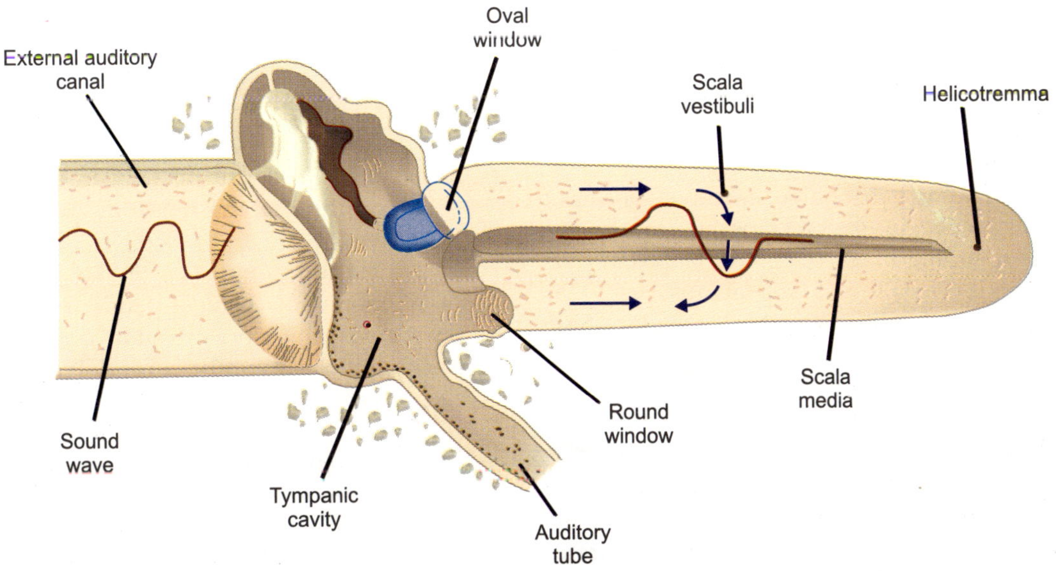

Fig. 4.37: Ear

Middle Ear

- It is an air filled space containing three small bones, the ossicles.
- The tympanic membrane (ear drum) separates the external auditory canal from middle ear.
- The layers of tympanic membrane from outside to inside are:
  - — Skin of external auditory canal.
  - — Collagen fibres: radially and circularly arranged
  - — Epithelial lining
- Three *ossicles* are:
  - — Malleus (hammer): attached to tympanic membrane
  - — Stapes (stirrup): foot plate fits into oval window
  - — Incus (anvil) - linking malleus to stapes
  - — These bones help to convert sound waves in air to mechanical vibrations in tissues and fluid filled chambers
- Two *openings* in its medial wall
  - — Oval window (vestibular)
  - — Round window (cochlear)
  - — Since primary function of middle ear is to convert sound waves (air vibrations) arriving from external auditory meatus, into mechanical vibration that are transmitted to inner ear. These two openings are essential components in this conversion process. Sound in the form of air waves leads to vibrations in tympanic membrane which are transmitted to attached auditory ossicles which links external to inner ear. Its perforation may lead to hearing impairment.
- *Muscles* attached to ossicles are:
  - — *Tensor tympani:* lying in bony canal above the auditory tube, its tendon inserts on malleus. Its contraction increases tension on tympanic membrane
  - — *Stapedius:* lies in bony eminencies on its posterior wall; its tendon inserts on stapes. Its contraction causes damping of movement of stapes at oval window. It is smallest of skeletal muscle.
  - — Contraction of muscles makes ossicular chain more rigid, thus reducing transmission of vibrations to inner ear. This protects ear drum from damaging effects of very loud sound.
- *The Eustachian tube* (auditory tube) connects middle ear to nasopharynx. It is narrow, flat channel lined by pseudostratified columnar epithelium 3.5 cm long. Its walls are normally pressed together but separates during yawning/swallowing. It vents the middle ear so its pressure is equalised with atmospheric pressure.
- The mastoid air cells are extending from middle ear into temporal bone.

Inner Ear

- *Two labyrinthine* compartments:
  - — Bony (osseous): complex system in petrous part of temporal bone.
  - — membranous: lies within bony labyrinth having small sacs and tubules which form a continuous space enclosed within a wall of epithelium.
- ***Fluid filled spaces are:***
  - — Endolymphatic—within membranous labyrinth
  - — Perilymph—between wall of bony labyrinth and membranous labyrinth
  - — Corticolymphatic—within organ of Corti
- The bony labyrinth consists of three connected spaces within the temporal bone namely semi circular canals, vestibule, cochlea.
- Vestibule is the central space of bony labyrinth. The auricle and saccule of membranous labyrinth lie in elliptical recess. The vestibular window (oval) into which footplate of stapes inserts lies in lateral wall of vestibule.
- The semicircular canals are bony walled tubes that lie at right angles to each other. Each forms about three quarters of a circle extend from wall of vestibule. They are lying at superior/posterior/horizontal planes. Ampulla is a dilatation at the lateral end of each semi circular canal, close to the vestibule.

Cochlea

Lumen of cochlea is continuous with that of vestibule.

Cochlea makes about $2\frac{3}{4}$ turns around a central bony core called 'mediolus' in which a sensory ganglion lies called 'spiral ganglion.' So cochlea, is a conical shaped helix connected to the vestibule.

- *Membranous labyrinth:* Its subcompartments are:-
  - — Membranous semicircular ducts (Vestibular system)
  - — Utricle and saccule (Vestibular system)
  - — Membranous cochlea—(auditory system)
- Six regions of sensory receptors project from wall of membranous labyrinth into endolymphatic space in each inner ear as:
  - — Three crysta ampullaris—present at ampulla of semi circular ducts and are sensitive to angular acceleration of head, i.e. its turning.
  - — Two macular—one in utricle and other in saccule, sense the position of head and linear movement
  - — The organ of Corti—projects into endolymph of cochlear duct. They are sound receptors

- ***Hair cell*** is the common receptor cell of vestibulo cochlear system. Important characteristics of hair cells include -
  1. All are epithelial cells
  2. Each projects modified microvilli called sensory hairs
  3. In vestibular system each hair cell possesses a single cilium called kino cilium, but In auditory system this is replaced by residual basal body
  4. All hair cells are associated with afferent and efferent nerve endings
  5. All hair cells are transducers which means mechanical energy is converted into electrical energy which is transmitted to the brain through vestibulo-cochlear nerve.
- In vestibular system—two types of hair cells—
  — Type I: piriform shaped, rounded base, surrounded by efferent nerve fibre
  — Type II: cylindrical, have afferent and efferent nerve endings synapsing basally.
- There are 50 to 100 stereocilia/cell in vestibular system and on inner hair cell of organ of Corti while 100 to 300 stereocilia in outer hair cell of organ of Corti.
- Common basis of receptor cell function (Hair):-

Bending/flexing of stereocilia (sensory hair) → stretching of plasma membrane → transmembrane potential changes in receptor cell → afferent nerve ending stimulated.

It is to be remembered that stereocilia that are bent away from kino cilium cause hyperpolarisation of receptor cell; while stereocilia bending towards kino-cilium leads to depolarisation of receptor cell and generation of action potential.

Organ of Corti

- Is the sensor of sound vibrations.
- Three parallel compartments, viz. Scala media, Scala vestibuli and scala tympani.
- Scala media:- triangular space; its acute angle attached to bony protrusion of modiolus - osseous spiral lamina. It is the vestibular membrane (Reissner's) which separates it from scala vestibuli. Its lateral/ outer wall is stria-vascularis. Lined with thick pseudostratified epithelium which synthesises endolymph. Its lower wall floor is basilar membrane.

Organ of Corti is being sheltered by tectorial membrane while it rests on basilar membrane.

- Perilymph is contained in space between scala vestibuli and tympani and communicate with each other through a small channel helicotremma.
  Scala-vestibule taken as beginning at oval window
  Scala tympani taken as ending at round window.
- ***Organ of Corti*** is formed by:
  — Inner and outer hair cells
  — Inner and outer supporting cells (phalangeal)
  — Pillar cells
- Hair cells are arranged in an inner and outer row of cells (single row). Pillar and supporting cells provide support to hair cells. The apical end of phalangeal cells are tightly bound to one another, forming reticular lamina which seals the endolymphatic compartment. It contains cortilymph.
- Pillar cells are of two types
  — Inner - rest on tympanic tip of spiral lamina
  — Outer - rest on basilar membrane
  — Between these two there is triangular space called tunnel of Corti.
- Tectorial membrane is a keratin like layer which is attached to organ of Corti by stereocilia of hair cells.

Balancing Apparatus

- Each of the three *cristae ampullaris* is the sensory region of one of the semi circular ducts in the semicircular canal. *Cupula* is a gelatinous structure attached to hair cells of each crista. Cupula is surrounded by endolymph and projecting into lumen.
- Bending of sterocilia in the narrow space between hair cells and cupula lead to generation of nerve impulse in associated nerve endings. During rotational movement of head, the walls of semicircular canal and its membranous ducts move but endolymph contained within ducts lag behind due to inertia.
- Maculae are innervated sensory thickenings of epithelium in vestibular utricle and saccule.
- Macula of utricle and saccule are oriented at right angles to one another. When one stands macula utricle is in horizontal plane while macula sacculi is in vertical plane.
- *Otolith membrane* is a gelatinous material over lying macula. It contains *otoconia* on outer surface which are particles of $CaCO_3$ and protein. Stereocilia of hair cells are bent by gravity in stationary position while otolith membrane pull on stereocilia.

BIBLIOGRAPHY

1. Leeson C Roland, Thomas S. Leason. Anthomy A Paparo Atlas of Histology 2nd ed. W.B. Saunders Co, 1985.
2. Michael H, Ross, Lynn J Romrell, Gordon I. Kaye-Hisotlogy: Text and Atlas, Williams and Wilkins. Third edition, 1995.
3. Roland Leeson, Thomas S. Leason - Histology, 3rd ed., W.B. Saunders Company.
4. William Bloom, Don W. Fawcatt A Text book of Histology, 10th edition, W.B. Saundars company.

5 Fundamental of Progress: Physiology of Growth

An adequate supply of food material, certain essential amino acids and vitamins are necessary for growth but entire factors responsible for it are yet unknown. Man reaches the zenith of his physical powers at the age of 20 years or so, and sooner or later his body tissues, even if they are not effected by disease, begin to deteriorate gradually. The maximum life span of a man is 110 years (average 70 years; 68 years for males and 74 years for females).

It is a complex phenomenon which is normally accompanied by an orderly sequence of maturational changes, and it involves protein use and increase in size and length. It should not be confused with obesity which may be due to deposition of fat or retention of salt and water in the body.

The word Growth refers to increase in physical size of the body which we measure in kilograms or centimetres; while the word development refers to increase in skill and function, which is measured or compared by milestone.

FACTORS INFLUENCING GROWTH

i. *Genetic:* Due to inherent gene of the spermatozoa or ovum, growth is effected. This genetic factor is responsible for racial tallness or shortness. This genetic factor according to its nature either reduces or increases the responsiveness of the tissues towards hormones like growth hormone, etc.
ii. *Nutritional:* Next to genetic factor, this is probably the important factor. The diet must be adequate in vitamins, minerals, calories, etc. besides the main building blocks, i.e. proteins. Any injury or disease retard the growth since these factors enhance protein catabolism. It is a common belief that maternal malnutrition affects growth of the foetus. Inadequate diet and infection slow down the rate of growth.
iii. ***Hormones:*** Growth hormone (adenohypophysis), thyroxin (thyroid), insulin (pancreas-islet cells of Langarhan's b type), adrenocortical hormones other than androgens are effecting the growth by their mechanism of action.
iv. ***Psychological*:** Love, emotional attachment, proper care and attention by the parents towards child are important growth stimulatory factors.
v. ***Age and sex:*** Growth is said to be maximum during foetal life, during first year and then at puberty. About the age of 10 to 12 years female child shows a sudden increase in height and weight.
vi. ***Other factors:***
   - Infections (diarrhoea, measles), parasitic worm infestation in intestine slow down growth and development process.
   - Economic status of family also influences growth in children.

Growth is the most fundamental of all physiological functions. It is brought about by multiplication of cells, not by increase in their size. Cells not only grow (multiply), they also differentiate and both are antagonistic.

PATHOPHYSIOLOGY OF GROWTH

a. *Metaplasia:* Is the transformation of one type of tissue into another type. It is best seen in closely related connective tissues, as when cartilage is converted into bones.
b. *Anaplasia:* Is merely the reversion of a more highly to a less highly differentiated form. So it is also named as reversionary atrophy.
c. *Atrophy:* Is a diminution in size, a shrinking of cell or fibres that have reached their full development. Hypoplasia indicates a failure of full development. Some of the important causes are old age, lack of nourishment, action of toxins, disease, pressure and interference with nerve supply, disuse of a structure etc.

d. *Hypertrophy:* Is an increase in size of individual cells or fibres as a result of which the organ may become enlarged.
   - *Physiological hypertrophy:* Occurs apart altogether from disease, example is pregnancy at the end of which the muscles fibres are ten times as long and four times as broad as in the non-pregnant uterus. This hypertrophy is called Black Smith's arm.
   - *Adaptive hypertrophy:* Is best seen in hollow muscular organs when outlet is partially obstructed. The wall of the organ becomes thickened owing to an increase in the size of the muscle fibres, e.g. left ventricle in stenosis of aortic valve, high blood pressure with its increased peripheral resistance, the stomach in pyloric obstruction, bowel in chronic intestinal obstruction, the bladder in stricture of urethra.
   - *Compensatory hypertrophy:* Is an increase in size to compensate for loss of tissue and is best seen in paired organs. When one kidney is removed or atrophies because of disease the remaining kidney does the work of the two and becomes correspondingly enlarged. There is no formation of new elements, but merely an increase in the size of the existing tubules and glomeruli.

e. *Hyperplasia:* Means an increase in the number of cells of a part. It is often the result of irritation. It gradually merges into the process of neoplasia or tumour formation.
   - *Compensatory hyperplasia:* Seen in bone marrow which becomes hyperplastic when there is demand for more blood. When a portion of thyroid gland is removed, the remaining tissues undergo hyperplasia so as to compensate for loss.

GROWTH PARAMETERS

Height-weight charts, head circumference charts, skeletal bone age chart are the main parameters.

GROWTH FACTOR IN HEALING WOUNDS

i. *Epidermal growth factor (EGF):* Leads to growth of epidermis and is mitogenic for fibroblasts. It is bounded with specific receptors on cell membrane, and then causes epidermal proliferation. It is a 6045 Dalton polypeptide, purified from sub-maxillary gland of mice or from human urine (urogastrone).

ii. *Platelet derived growth factor (PDGF):* It is released when platelets are activated since it is stored in alphagranules of platelets. It is a mitogen for fibroblasts and smooth muscle cell. It is a chemotactic agent for leucocyte and fibroblast *in vitro*.

iii. *Fibroblast growth factor:* Is a polypeptide which stimulates fibroblast and smooth muscle proliferation in culture.

iv. *Macrophage derived growth factors*: Macrophages when activated by stimuli leads to connective tissue growth in inflammation.

v. Presence of fibrin is associated with influx of fibroblasts and new vessels and formation of granulation tissue in wound healing. Fibrinogen and fibrin degradation products appear to be chemotectic to WBC including monocytes. Thrombin might be directly mitogenic to fibroblasts and endothelial cells.

NOTES

- The circumference of the head grows very fast till the end of first year of life. Then after it is slow and does not rise in puberty.
- After birth there is no increase in number of nerve cells. But individual neurone grows in length and thickness and myelination continues, which increases total weight of neural tissues. Growth of brain and other neural tissue is fast in second year of life.
- Thyroxin is necessary for the growth of brain.
- The lymphoid tissues grow fast till 10 to 12 years of life. Then they begin to involute.
- It is frequently stated that nervous system is not fully functional at birth. The cerebral cortex and its associated mechanism require several months after birth for significant functional development. Behavioural growth is a problem of maturity of nervous system.
- In females, puberty begins at 11 years of age or up to 13 years. Regular ovulatory menstrual cycles are established after 2 to 3 years of menarche. This linear growth ceases at the age of 16 to 17 years.
- In males, testicular size begin to increase at the age of 12 years which is followed one year after it by enlargement of the penis. Secondary sexual characters occur at 14 to 15 years of age and growth ceases at the age of 18 years.

GROWTH INHIBITORS (SYNONYM—CHALONES)

i. *Tumour-growth-factor (TGF-β)* Its major source is platelets. It inhibits growth of epithelial, mesenchymal, and immunological cells. It is involved in development and synthesis of extracellular matrix proteins. It acts through a transmembrane receptor which is widely distributed on many cell types. It is composed of 112 amino acids linked by disulphide bonds.

ii. *Tumour-necrosis-factor (TNF; Cachectin)* It is produced by macrophages in response to endotoxin. It causes necrosis of tumours, inhibition of lipoprotein lipase, stimulation of growth of fibroblasts. It is a polypeptide of 157 amino acids. It is said to induce β_2 interferon (they are antiviral in action inhibiting growth of various cells).

CLONING

- It is a group of plants or organism produced asexually from a common ancestor. By cloning, a gene which is a part of DNA, we get its many copies and a large quantity of useful products.
- Genetic engineering or cloning is the introduction of genetic material from one organism into another where it may be expressed.
- A large population of identical molecules/cells/bacteria arising from a common ancestor is called a 'clone'.
- Introduction of small foreign DNA molecules into circular DNA molecules of bacteria will cause foreign DNA molecules to be replicated along with circular DNA and a large number of foreign DNA molecules can be harvested in a small time. This procedure is cloning.

History:

— Dr. Ian Wilmut et al (Edinburgh US, Roslin institute) has produced clone of adult lap, "Dolly" from a Dorsat Lamb (Young sheep); it was just like its mother.

— Dr. Don Wolf et al (US, Beaverton oregon; after a weak of above discovery) have cloned monkeys.

- *Process:* They have taken a cell from 'udder' (a bag like milk secreting organ of cow, goat, etc.) of an adult sheep and fused with an egg from another sheep from which nucleus containing DNA has been removed. The fused cell developed into embryo which was then planted into uterus of another sheep who acted as "surrogate mother" (woman who bears a child on behalf of another). It was a strange enough that embryo developed into a lamb and it was genetically an identical copy of sheep from which the cell had been taken.

GLOSSARY

1. **Growth:** Increase in size and weight of organism due to synthesis of protoplasmic substances. Anabolism is dominant.
2. **Growth curve:** The growth of an organ for a definite period of time when plotted against time is S shaped sigmoid/growth curve.
3. **Phases**
   a. *Lag period:* Animal prepares for growth and adapt for different environment.
   b. *Exponential growth*: Initially growth is slower and then rate increases.
   c. *Deacceleration:* Growth is now completely checked up.
4. **Regeneration:** Process of repair, replacement or revival of damaged or severed body parts or reconstruction of the whole body from a small fragment of it during postembryonic period of multicellular organism.
5. **Epimorphosis:** It takes place by proliferation of new tissue cells from the surface of wound, e.g. regeneration of limb and tail.
6. **Death:** Most important biological fact. Cellular activity is ceased. End result of old age.
7. **Auxetic growth:** Volume of body increases without any increase in number of cells (In nematodes and early chordates).
8. **Multiplicative growth:** Number of cells increases, and average cellular size remains same. It is mitotic division (in prenatal growth of higher vertebrates).
9. **Accretionary growth:** Mitotic division of reserve cells to re-inforce and replace the worn out differentiated cells. (In formation of epidermal cells from malpighian layer).
10. **Degrowth:** Catabolism dominates over anabolism.

AVERAGE LIFE SPAN: DIFFERENT CELLS

Bone cells	-	25–30 years
Brain cells	-	Life time
Skin cells	-	15–35 days
Spermatozoa	-	2–3 days
Colon cells	-	3–4 days

BIBLIOGRAPHY

1. Carpevter G, Cohen S. Epidermal growth factor. Ann Rev Biochem 1979;48:193.
2. Deuel TF, et al. Human platelet derived growth factor-purification and resolution into two active protein fraction. J Biol Chem. 1981;256:8896.
3. Deuel TF, et al. Chemotaxis of monocytes and neutrophil to platelet derived growth factor. J Clin Invest. 1982;69:1046.
4. Doolitle, et al. Computer based characterisation of EGF. Nature. 1984;307:558-60.
5. EKB, et al. Stimulation of tyrosine specific phosphorylation by P. DGF, Nature. 1982;295:419-20.
6. Fox F, et al. Receptor remodelling and regulation in action of epidermal growth factor, Fed. Proc. 1982;41:2889.
7. Gospodarowicz, et al. Structural characterisation and biological function of FGF, End. Rev. 1987;8:95-114.
8. Grigory H. Isolatum and structure of inogastione and its relationship to EGF. Nature. 1975;257:325-27.

9. Ignotz RA, Massague E. Transforming growth factor β stimulates the expression of fibronectin and collagen and their incorporation into extracellular matrix. J Biol Chem. 1988;261:4337.
10. Liebovich SJ, Ross R. Role of macrophage in wound repair, a study with hydrocortisone and anti macrophage snim. Amer. J Path. 1975;78:71.
11. Ross R, Vogel A. The platelet derived growth factor. Cell. 1978;14:203.
12. Russell DW, et al. Domain map of LDL receptor: sequence homology with epidermal growth factor precursor. Cell. 1984;37:577-85.
13. Seppa H, et al. Platelets derived growth factor is chemotactic for fibroblasts. J Cell Biol. 1982;92:584.
14. Spom MB, et al. Transforming growth factor - biological function and chemical structure. Science. 1986;233:532-34.
15. Yarden Y, et al. Structures of receptor for platelet derived growth factor helps define a faculty of closely related growth factor receptors. Nature 323:226-32.

Ageing: Senescence

The changes in structure and function occurring in persons after the attainment of sexual maturity constitute ageing. With advancing age the adaptability to overcome environmental or internal challenges decreases and probability of death increases.

The discipline of geriatrics deals with the diagnosis and treatment of persons aged 65 years and above. The age of 65 as the commencement of senescence has been accepted arbitrarily. It is better to call senescence as the period when there is commencement of loss of vigor, skin changes of old age, slowed activity of musculo-skeletal system and onset of deterioration of mental functions. Ageing stands for growing old while senescence stands for an expression used for the deterioration in the vitality or the biological efficiency that accompanies the ageing. The ageing is the process of merely growing older, or 'It is the sum total loss of functions and structures when a person grows older'.

THE PROCESS OF AGEING

Heart

- As far as efficiency is concerned, old heart is more efficient than young. This is because of the fact that anastomosis throughout the coronary circulation become more effective and extensive with advancing years. This also explains the fact that old man can withstand the effects of coronary occlusion better than a young man.
- Cardiac output is usually normal during rest but cannot cope with the demands of stress.

Blood

- PCV declines in both the sexes at 70 or more years of age.
- There is decrease of haemoglobin in old age and colour index is more than normal. In most of the cases in old age (50%) MCHC increases.
- NPN in old age is 40 per cent higher than young.
- Uric acid is 30 per cent higher in old age.
- Slight fall in white cell count mainly lymphocyte. Platelet number unaltered.
- There is sharp fall of cholesterol level in women between 50 to 60 years due to menopause, of course there occurs no relationship between blood cholesterol and blood pressure.
- ESR also tends to increase with advancement of age more significantly in females than males.
- A small decline in serum Vitamin A level occurs with advancement of age.

In young women about 30 per cent of body weight is fat; in old women fat makes up 45 per cent, since the body weight increases with age the total fat content may increase by 50 per cent. In healthy men fat forms 30 per cent of total body weight at all ages. In young woman 52 per cent of body weight may be water; In old woman it declines to 42. In men total body water declines very little with advancing age.

Blood Pressure

- At birth blood pressure measurement has given values of 80/46 (systolic's range 60-90 mmHg.). At the age of 10, it rises to 100 mm. mercury systolic and at puberty to 120 mm mercury.
- Systolic blood pressure in mm mercury is roughly equal to 100 + age. Diastolic pressure is half the systolic + 10 or 20 mm. But after 50 years of age figure above 150 mm are certainly too high.
- In old people systolic and diastolic pressures tend to decrease after 65 to 70 years age. This is attributed to a progressively diminishing cardiac efficiency.
- There is a gradual rise in systolic blood pressure up to the age of 70 years. After this age systolic pressure remains constant in men and declines in women. There is only a small rise in diastolic pressure. The increase in blood pressure with age may be a physiological adjustment to the large rise in peripheral

resistance and the fall in cardiac output. With increased general peripheral resistance, blood pressure in aged may be adjusted to higher levels in order to maintain flow in the regions which exhibit a greater than average increase in vascular resistance. Therefore, the increase in blood pressure in aged may not be detrimental.

- Old subjects increase their systolic blood pressure and heart rate more after exercise and require a longer time to return to pre-exercise levels than do young.
- When subjects are tilted from supine to upright position, older subjects show a great decrease and slower recovery of diastolic BP and smaller increase in heart rate than young.
- Large number of elderly hypertensives have isolated elevation of systolic blood pressure which has greater predictability of stroke, IHD, CHF, renal failure and morbidity than diastolic blood pressure in old age.
- Blunted baroreceptor response as a result of sclerotic changes in carotid sinus. So there is central/peripheral failure of vasoconstrictor response to falling blood pressure.
- Decrease in elasticity of aorta + accumulation of lipofuschin in myocardial fibres.

Body Temperature

- A newborn child has a slightly higher temperature than an adult. Body temperature of a young child is more variable due to lack of control exercised by nervous system over blood vessels and other organs operative in temperature regulation. In old age temperature tends to be lower. It is not stable in new born. Heat production in old people is normal but heat loss is increased.
- They are at a greater risk of hypothermia.
- Sweat glands are decreased in number in old age.

Muscular Efficiency

- It gradually lessens with age. There is generalised atrophy of muscles, myotonia and loss of power. The output of creatine, which may be taken as an index of muscle mass, declines very little in old women but quite markedly in old men.
- Loss of muscle strength due to irreversible loss of motor unit and muscle fibres.

Pain Threshold

- Young people seem to be more sensitive to pain than the aged.
- Number of neurones decline with age (motoneurones of spinal cord, Purkinje cell of cerebellum, neocortical cells).

Bones

- The composition of bone tissue changes with advancing years. There is an increase in the mineral contents and a decrease in the organic matrix which normally gives bones elasticity and toughness; as a consequence they become more brittle and fracture more readily and when fractured they heal more slowly.
- This increase in calcium is not limited to bones, but it occurs in many tissues. In arteriosclerosis, it may be deposited in the walls of the arteries. The increased concentration of calcium in the cortex of the cell decreases the permeability of the cell membranes and thereby hinders the proper exchange of material between the cell and its environment. The retention of waste products may have deleterious effects upon the cell. This is an important factor in ageing; the depositing of calcium may indicate a dying condition of the structure. Osteoporosis may occur as the age advances. The reduction in bone thickness causes delayed healing of fractures.
- Loss of bone mass (minerals, proteins and tissues) more common among woman.

Cardiac Output

- Rising rapidly to a level greater than 4 litres per minute per square meter at 10 years of age the cardiac index declines to only slightly above 2 litres per minute at the age of 80. There is a gradual reduction in cardiac output as the age advances.

Respiration

i. From birth to maturity (upto 35 years of age) vital capacity gradually increases, but because of the stiffening of the costal cartilages it may decrease materially in old age and thereby lessen the ability to carry on vigorous muscular work. The capacity to ventilate pulmonary blood is also slightly impaired.
ii. Rate varies with age. At birth—40–70/minute, 5 years—25/minute, 15 years—20/minute; 30 years 16/minute.
iii. Reduction in alveolar surface for gas exchange.
iv. Decline in respiratory muscle strength and stiffening of thoracic cage.
v. Decreased lung elasticity.
vi. Residual volume increases.

Vision

a. The power of accommodation depends upon the elasticity of the lens. Greater the elasticity, greater is the power of accommodation and closer the near point of vision is situated to the eye. With increasing years the gradual loss of elasticity reduces the accommodative power and causes the near point to recede. In consequence, the book/news paper must be held progressively further away, until finally the images of the letters on the retina become too small to be recognised. This is Presbyopia—a sign of old age appearing after the age of 45 years. The waning accommodative power can be supplemented by properly fitted convex glasses. Myopia is also common.

b. Intraocular pressure diminishes gradually throughout life from childhood to old age (Normal 10–20 or 25 mmHg).
c. Cataracts are quite frequent. Eyelashes may fall off. There may be ptosis or enophthalmos.

Skin

- Becomes wrinkled, hyperkeratotic and atrophic, with diminishing sweat and sebaceous glands, leads to loss of elasticity. Due to smaller amount of dopa oxidase and tyrosinase in hair follicles greying of hair occurs since both of them are required for synthesis of melanin. Greying of hair shows strong genetic predisposition. It becomes thin and inelastic with reduction in subcutaneous fat and all these are making skin more vulnerable to chronic decubitus ulcer. Paresthesia and pruritus are common, skin loses its elasticity.

Lymphatic Organs

- The spleen undergoes atrophy. There is increase in number of plasma cells. Above 70 years, serum globulins are increased and amyloidosis may develop. There is generalised impairment of immune process and so infection takes a fatal turn.

Endocrines

- The gonads, thyroid and adrenal cortex show generalised hypofunction. Myxoedema is not uncommon.
- Decline in circadian rhythm.
- Impaired glucose tolerance due to impaired insulin secretion and glucose utilisation.
- Very little evidence of hypofunctions of pituitary, parathyroid or adrenals in old age. It responds to stress.

Psychological

- The elderly become irritable and less adaptable to surroundings. Change in social behaviour emotional instability, loss of self-confidence, mental depression, hallucinations and paranoid and per security fears result in social isolation.
- Impaired memory, rigidity of outlook and dislike of change are important mental changes in aged.
- Emotional disorders result from social maladjustment. The aged is often failure to adapt suffers from depression, bitterness, etc. which may terminate into fatal results like suicide, etc. *It is better to say that, years wrinkle the skin but worry/doubt/anxiety/depression, i.e. stress wrinkle the soul.* The tendency for some old people to live in the past, to be overcautious or timed is well known. Old man may not perform the work hurriedly as young does. However on another end, many intelligent old persons keep themselves in contact with external world and retain their interest and lead a live life with full grace and dignity.

Gastrointestinal System

- Oral cavity—Atrophy of mucous membrane, loss of teeth
- Oesophagus—defective swallowing mechanism due to weak oesophageal peristalsis.
- Stomach—delay in gastric emptying.
- Liver—Reduction in liver volume, blood flow, perfusion and regenerative capacity.

Urinary System

- Reduction in the number of nephrones and kidney size.
- Reduction in renal blood flow.
- Decline in GFR.
- Decrease bladder capacity.
- Increase size of the prostate in male.

Miscellaneous

- The fat content of body tissue increases with advancement of age. It is 30 per cent in young female and increases up to 50 per cent at the age of 50 years. This makes the arteries nonelastic with increase in calcium content along with cholesterol deposition in arteries, lens and cornea.
- Negative nitrogen balance in old is due to deficient intake of protein. The quality of protein becomes important during later years of life.
- Resistance to infection diminishes.
- The permeability of cellular wall increases with age.
- Urine is of high specific gravity. There may be low urinary output. There is also diminished excretion of creatinine. Blood urea tends to rise. After the age of 40 years there is a progressive reduction in renal blood flow, creatinine clearance and GFR.

- The rigidity of blood vessels increases with age, with an attendant increase in pulse wave velocity. The elastin of the aorta undergoes an increases in specific gravity, calcium content and proportion of amino acids containing free carboxyl groups. The amino acids-aspartic and glutamic acid increases while glycine, proline and valine decrease. The deposition of collagen increases in the intimal and medial layers of blood vessels. The collagen in the old blood vessels increases in resistance to solubilisation by chemical treatment. Certain aldehydes present in the blood accelerate the formation of chemical cross linkages in the collagen of blood vessels. Large blood vessels become more rigid.
- Between 25 to 95 years of age average fall in blood flow to brain is approximately 25 per cent of mean value at 25 years of age. Kidney blood flow determined by clearance of diodrast or PAH falls by about 60 per cent of the mean value at age 25 years, between ages of 25 and 90 years. Arteriosclerosis may explain this reduction in blood flow, along with functional vasoconstriction. In the aged person, under resting conditions, a functional increase in vascular resistance reduces blood flow to the kidney.
- The reduced capacity in the aged is related to their inability to increase their heart rate and thereby to increase cardiac output to meet the increased tissue demand for oxygen. The rate of recovery of heart rate, O_2 uptake and CO_2 elimination after exercise, is slower in old, than young.
- Ischaemic and hypertensive diseases often supervene as age advances. Above the age of 75 years interstitial fibrosis and fatty infiltration of myocardium develop. Endocardium and valves are thickened. Loss of elasticity leads to widening and tortuosity of aorta.
- Age related reduction in conduction velocity of nerves.
- Changes in autonomic functions include - alteration in heart rate and abnormalities of temperature regulation.

CLASSIFICATION

- Young old ...... 65 to 75 years
- Old old .... 75 to 85 years
- Very old .... above 85 years

PROGERIA

1. Means premature old age.
2. Hutchinson-Gilford syndrome—ageing starts around 4 years age, or 10 to 12 years. The affected child shows grey hair, baldness, loss of fat, atherosclerosis etc. Death results at puberty.
3. Werner's syndrome (adult progeria)—starts in early adult life, follow rapid progression.

ALZHEIMER'S DISEASE

1. A progressive condition in which nerve cells in brain degenerate and brain substance shrinks.
2. Three stages:
   First: Person becomes forgetful.
   Second: He experiences severe memory loss and disorientation, lack of concentration, loss of ability to express thoughts, anxiety and so sudden personality changes.
   Third: Patient is severely disoriented and confused, with hallucination, delusion, memory loss. Require hospital care since he may be violent. Nervous system declines with regression into infantile behaviour.

GLOSSARY

1. Study of ageing is *Gerontology*.
2. Theories
   a. ***Codon restriction***: Accuracy of translation which depends upon cellular ability to decode the triplet codon in mRNA molecule is impaired with ageing.
   b. ***Wear and tear***: A continuous process throughout life takes place in all the cells. Increased metabolic rate may shorten the life.
   c. ***Gene regulation:*** Ageing from changes in expression of genes after maturity is reached.
   d. ***Error theory***: Errors in transmission of information through RNA to protein may be responsible for cellular ageing. Initially its rate is low but with advancement of time it increases.
   e. ***System level theories:*** The effectiveness of homeostatic mechanism declines with failure of adaptive mechanism which may lead to ageing and death.

SUMMARY AND HIGHLIGHTS

Wear and tear occurs throughout the life. At the end of given duration of protoplasmic activity, degeneration and death supervene since nature is wise and it always pours new wine in an old bottle. Changes of old age are not very sudden or very striking. The social, psychological and medical problems of old persons (Geriatrics) are becoming increasingly important.

BIBLIOGRAPHY

1. Amery A, Schaepdryver AD. Introduction: The European working party on High B.P. in elderly. Amer J Med 1991;90 (suppl 3A):3.

2. Hendley DD, et al. Gerontol 1963;18:144, 250.
3. Hiss, et al. Amer J Cardiol 1960;6:200.
4. Lansing AI (Ed). The Arterial Wall. The William and Wilkins Co. Baltimore 1959.
5. Leblond CP, Walker BE. Renewal of cell population. Physiol Rev 1956;36:255-276.
6. Milch RA. Gerontologia (Basel) 1963;7:129.
7. NIH Consensus Development Panel: Diagnosis and treatment of depression in late life. JAMA 1992;268:1018.
8. Prinz PN, et al. Sleep disorders and ageing. New Eng J Med 1990;323:520.
9. Resnik NM, Greenspan SL. Senile osteoporosis reconsidered. JAMA 1989;261:1025.
10. SIU-A . Screening for dementia and assessing its causes. Ann Int Med 1991;115:122.
11. Welford AT. On changes of performance with age. Lancet i, 1962;335-339.

7 May I Help You? The Receptors: Detectors

Just like any big official complex is having a "receptionist" who detects the problem of every visitor and guide him in right direction; similarly our body is full of "receptors" which serves the same functions. Protein which is binding neurotransmitters and hormones initiating physiological changes, are receptors.

ADRENERGIC

- The idea was first introduced by James Langley (1905) and in 1948 Alhquist showed that they do exist.
- Broadly they are of two types alpha (α) and beta (β). α receptor occurs both at all membrane of smooth muscle and cardiac muscle as well as in some selective nerve terminals; while β receptors occur in cell membrane of smooth and cardiac muscle.
- Nor-adrenaline has high affinity for α receptors, moderate or low affinity for β_1 receptor and no affinity for β_2 receptor; whereas adrenaline has moderate to good affinity for α receptors, high for β_1 receptors and moderate for β_2 receptors.

Blockers (propranolol, metoprolol, atenolol, etc.)

i. β blockers cause inhibition of both β_1 and β_2 receptors thereby lowering the contractility and rate of heart and reduction of cardiac output and work load on heart. They are used in or to treat angina pectoris. This reduces demand of O_2 supply of heart thus patient is benefited. Atenolol is a selective β_1 blocker.

ii. α blockers are used for diagnosis of pheochromocytoma. After their administration only β receptors remain active and adrenaline released by tumour can cause sharp fall of BP by acting on β_2 receptors of skeletal blood vessels.

BETA RECEPTORS

β_1 Found in heart, JG cells of kidney. Drug atenolol is selective antagonist

β_2 Found in bronchi, blood vessels, uterus, urinary tract and GIT Drug propranolol a non-specific beta blocker antagonise these, while salbutamol is an agonist

β_3 Recently described. Low affinity for standard α blockers. Found on adipocytes. Mediate lipolysis.

ALPHA RECEPTORS

α_1 Location is post-junctional on effector organs. On stimulation they cause Smooth muscle contraction, glandular secretion and gut relaxation. It acts by IP_3/DAG pathway

α_2 Location is prejunctional on nerve ending as well as post-junctionally in brain. Drug clonidine is agonist. Inhibition of cAMP-; stimulation of K^+ channel are mechanism of action. The actions are—inhibition of transmitter release. Vasoconstriction and decreased central sympathetic flow.

ADRENERGIC RECEPTORS

These are membrane bound G-protein coupled receptors, which function primarily by increasing or decreasing the intracellular production of second messenger cAMP, or IP_3/DAG. In some cases G-protein itself K^+ or Ca^{++} channels, or increases prostaglandin production.

NOTES

- Clonidine is α_2 stimulant which are present in synapse of VMC as well as periphery. It causes its inhibition by acting on α_2 receptor of VMC.
- β_2 stimulators (Salbutamol and terbutaline) cause broncho-dilatation thus relieving bronchial asthma Isoprenaline by stimulating both β_1 and β_2 receptor cause broncho-dilatation so used in asthma; and by stimulating β receptors, it stimulates conductivity of heart so used in heart block.
- Both alpha and beta receptors are existing in coronaries. Epicardial coronary vessels have a preponderance of alpha receptors whereas intramuscular

arteries may have a preponderance of β receptors. Sympathetic stimulation can cause much constriction which may lead to vasospastic myocardial ischaemia, and, is common during excess sympathetic drive.

- Alpha receptors give more response to nor-adrenaline. Alpha one receptors act by activating second messenger—IP_3 (Inositol tri-phosphate) via phospholipase C.
- $Alpha_2$ receptors exert their effect by inhibiting adenyl cyclase and reducing cAMP (intracellular).
- $Beta_1$ receptors give response to both adrenaline and nor-adrenaline.
- $Beta_2$ receptors show more response to adrenaline than nor-adrenaline. They respond by activating adenyl cyclase through G proteins and by increasing intra-cellular cAMP.

Table 7.1: Actions

Alpha (α) receptor	*Beta (β) receptor*
Vasoconstriction, iris dilatation, intestinal relaxation, pilomotor contraction, bladder sphincter contraction, intestinal sphincter contraction	Vasodilatation, (β_2) cardio-acceleration (β_1) intestinal relaxation (β_2) calorigenesis (β_2) Bladder wall relaxation (β_2) uterus relaxation (β_2)

ACETYLCHOLINE RECEPTORS

Muscarine

- The alkaloid responsible for toxicity of toadstool, has little effect on the receptors in autonomic ganglia but mimics the stimulatory action of acetylcholine on smooth muscle and glands. These actions of acetylcholine are called muscarinic action and receptors are muscarinic receptors. They are blocked by atropine.
- In sympathetic ganglia small amounts of acetylcholine stimulate post-ganglionic neurones and large amount blocks transmission of impulses from pre- to post-ganglionic neurones. These actions are unaffected by atropine but mimicked by nicotine so these actions are called nicotinic actions and receptors are called nicotinic receptors.
  - — M_1 receptor abundant in brain.
  - — M_2 receptor abundant in heart.
  - — M_4 receptor pancreatic acinar and islet tissue
  - — M_2 and M_4 both found in smooth muscle.
  - — M_3 - present in smooth muscle and exocrine glands except gastric glands.
- **Nicotine receptors: Subtypes**
  (Rosette like pentameric structure)
  N_M N_N
  (Previously called N_1 and N_2)

N_M: Found at neuromuscular junction. They cause depolarisation of muscle end-plate which leads to contraction of skeletal muscle. Its agonist is nicotine while antagonist is tubocurarine. It has intrinsic ion channel.

N_N: Found at autonomic ganglia. Through the process of depolarisation post-ganglionic impulse arises which releases catecholamine from adrenal medulla. Nicotine is agonist while is antagonized by hexamethonium. It has intrinsic ion channel. It opens cation channel.

Table 7.2: Cholinesterase

True (Acetyl)	*Pseudo (Butyryl)*
1. Distributed at all cholinergic sites, RBC, grey matter	1. Plasma, liver, intestine white matter
2. Hydrolysis of acetylcholine is done very fast	2. Slow hydrolysis
3. It causes termination of acetylcholine's action	3. Not known
4. Inhibited by physostigmine	4. More sensitive to organo-phosphates

RECEPTORS: SYNAPTIC AND JUNCTIONAL TRANSMISSION

Dopamine Receptors

- Five have been cloned and all are G protein. D_1 and D_5 both increase cyclic AMP levels. D_2, D_3, D_4 all decrease cyclic AMP levels.
- D_4 receptors are increased in number in disease schizophrenia. Drug clozapine- antischizoprenic drug is having greater affinity for D_4 receptors.

Serotonin (5HT): Seven have been recognised $5HT_1$ again are of four types and are presynaptic

- — $5HT_2$ ... mediate platelet aggregation, smooth muscle contraction.
- — $5HT_3$ ... present in peripheral tissues and brain
- — $5HT_4$ ... Serpentine receptor acting via G protein to affect adenyl cyclase.

Histamine: H_1, H_2, H_3 receptors are found in brain and peripheral tissues. H_1 receptor activate phospholipase C, H_2 receptor increase intracellular cyclic AMP concentration, H_3 receptors are presynaptic and they mediate inhibition of release of histamine and other transmitters via a G protein.

Glutamate receptors: Two types

- Metabotropic .... are serpentine G proteins coupled receptors which decrease cyclic AMP level (intracellular).
- Ionotropic ....Resemble nicotine receptors.

Glycine receptor: Is a Cl^- channel.

Purinergic Receptors

A_1 ... Inhibits adenyl cyclase.

A_2 ... Activates it ... Found in brain (striatum, olfactory tubercle and nucleus accumbens)

CARDIOVASCULAR-RESPIRATORY RECEPTORS

Baro-receptors

- Synonym- pressure/mechano-receptors because they are sensitive towards pressure or mechanical handling, i.e. stimulated when stretched.
- They are abundant in carotid sinus, and wall of aortic arch.
- Their main characteristics are:
  - — They are rapidly acting
  - — They act on rising blood pressure and not on stationary.
  - — They adapt rapidly
- So they are rapid control system of blood pressure
- Mechanical stretch (high blood pressure) → stimulation of receptors → glossopharyngeal nerve (from carotid sinus) and vagus nerve (from aorticarch)

→ highest centre in medulla —Vasodilatation / decreased heart rate and strength of contraction→ lowering of blood pressure

Conversely low pressure exerts opposite effect, i.e. rise in blood pressure.

Chemo-receptors

- Lie in carotid body and aortic body. They are sensitive to change in hydrogen ion concentration and saturation of CO_2 and O_2.
- If CO_2 tension goes above 35 mm Hg.; or O_2 tension below 85 per cent then they are activated.
- This comes into action when blood pressure falls below 80 mm Hg.

J Receptor (AS Paintal 1955)

- Located in close relation to pulmonary capillaries (in walls of alveoli).
- When stimulated they cause bradycardia, hypotension, apnoea followed by hyperpnoea. It also causes weakness of skeletal muscles (inhibition of contraction)
- They are stimulated when small emboli lie in pulmonary vessels and pulmonary oedema.
- Afferent fibres from these receptors are carried by vagus
- Muscular exercise → congestion of pulmonary capillaries + accumulation of interstitial fluid → stimulation of J receptors → muscular weakness → natural brake on exercise.

Lung Irritant Receptors

- Lie in epithelial layer in tracheo-bronchi. They are stimulated by smoking, irritants, pollutants, etc. During asthma they are stimulated by histamine.

Atrial Receptors (AS Paintal 1950)

- Two types A and B.
- From here afferent fibres run to join vagus nerve and then to 'nucleus tractus solitareus'. From here fibres reach RAS of medulla where they terminate in sympathetic centres.
- Receptor A is stimulated during atrial systole
- Receptor B is stimulated when volume of blood rises in atrium.
- Hypervolaemia leads to atrial distension, which causes release of ANP (atrial natriuretic peptide) which results into diuresis (sodium excretion). All this corrects atrial distension by reducing blood volume.

PAINTAL'S RECEPTORS

- These are characterised by:
  - — Rapid adaptation
  - — Smallest action potential
  - — Stimulation by congestion and embolization of lungs
  - — No activity caused by deflation receptors during normal breathing state
- *Type I :* located juxtacapillary. On stimulation, deflation receptors cause shallow, rapid respiration
- *Lung irritant receptor:* located in between epithelial lining of bronchi and bronchiole. On stimulation they cause hyperventilation + bronchiolar constriction
- *Inspiration inhibitory reflex:* is caused by stimulation of proprioceptors (e.g. stretch receptor in alveolar wall).

BIBLIOGRAPHY

1. Julius D. Ann Rev Neurosc. Molecular biology of serotonin receptors. 1991;14:335.
2. Levitzki A. β adrenergic receptors and their mode of coupling to adenylate cyclase. Phy Rev 1986;66:819.
3. Luetje CM, et al. Nicotinic receptors in mammalian brain. FASEB J. 1990;4:2753.
4. Macdonald RL, et al. $GABA_A$ receptor channels. Ann Rev Neurosc 1994;17:569.
5. Nakanishi S. Molecular diversity of glutamate receptors and implications for brain function. Science 1992;258:597.
6. Nicoll RA, et al. Functional comparison of neurotransmitter receptor subtypes in mammalian CNS. Phy Rev 1990;70:513.
7. Stiles GL, et al. β adrenergic receptors. Biochemical mechanism of physiological regulation. Phy Rev 1984;64:661.

8 Basis of Life: Medical Genetics

Gregor Mendel did his work in a garden plot (30 by 7 feet) in a small country town. He crossed a red and a white pea. In the second generation four plants bore red flowers but in the third generation three were red while one was white. He put forwarded the concept of dominant (red) and a recessive (white) character, the latter being hidden but present in second generation. This was the birth of science of genetics. Mendel's work was given attention when T. H. Morgan (1907) began his work on Drosophilia (fruit fly). All this proves that men are not created free and equal but handicapped from the beginning.

The science of the transmission and distribution of hereditary traits from parent organisms to their progeny is called "Genetics." The fundamentals of this are due to the classical work of Gregor Mendel (1822–1884).

CHROMOSOMES

- During cell division (mitosis), instead of chromatin, some thread/rod like bodies are found in nucleus. They are chromosomes (chrome = colour; soma = body).
- Each chromosome consists of two parallel and identical filament *chromatids*, which are joined together at a narrowed region *primary constriction*, within which is a pale, staining region the *centromere*. A *secondary constriction* has been reported in some chromosomes, near one end of each chromatid, dividing of terminal knobs the *satellite bodies*; and, these are believed to be associated with the organisation of nucleoli.
- Each cell contains a fixed number of chromosomes characteristic for that species/organism. In human somatic cells this number is 46 called *diploid number*. Half number of chromosomes is called *haploid number*.
- Out of 23 pairs of diploid set of human chromosomes, one pair of chromosome is not always identical and these are called *sex chromosomes* and are distinct from remaining 22 pairs of chromosomes called *autosomes* in males. While in females the sex chromosomes are identical, each being called an X chromosome, so giving 44 autosomes plus two X chromosomes, i.e. 44 + X + X. In males, two sex chromosomes are not identical but there is only one X chromosome and another y chromosome, i.e. 44 + X + Y. So at fertilisation - following situation can come:

(22 + X) spermatozoan	+	(22 + X) ovum	=	44 + X + X (female zygote)
(22 + Y) spermatozoan	+	(22 + X) ovum	=	44 + X + Y (male zygote)

CHROMOSOME NUMBER

a. *Monoploidy:* Not known in man. Normal human somatic cells contain diploid number (46) of chromosomes. Monoploidy will occur if somatic cells of body will contain haploid number (23) of chromosomes. It is common in plants and male honey bee.

b. *Polyploidy:* Further multiples of chromosomes if found then the manifestation is called polyploidy; e.g. in some instances 69 chromosomes are found (66 + X + X + Y; it is called *triploidy* since this number is three times of haploid number of chromosomes; and *tetraploidy* means four times the haploid number).

c. *Monosomy:* Here, the individual has one less number of chromosome, e.g. in males (43 + X + Y); and in females 43 + X + X.

d. *Trisomy:* Usually the chromosomes are in pairs, but when they are in triplicate the situation is called trisomy, e.g. 45 + X+ Y or 45 + X + X = 47 chromosomes. Its interesting examples are -

   i. *Down's syndrome (Mongolism):* Was first described by Langdon Down of London Hospital

(1866). The key substance here is an extra autosome in every cell; so that chromosome count is 47 instead of 46. This is an acrocentric chromosome in the smallest size range, thus resembling the Y sex chromosome. It is an example of trisomy, i.e. the presence of a Mongol autosome, no. 21, in triplicate, probably due to non-disjunction or failure of a pair of homologous chromosomes to segregate during meiosis. Now two possibilities are there -

— One is trisomy *Mongol* — extra chromosome (no. 21) is a separate entity and individual is having 47 chromosomes. Thus, two kinds of *zygotes* are possible — triplo 21's and haplo — 21's. The probability of *Mongoloid* children increases with age of the mother while age of the father has no relation with it, for the simple reason. In man, the spermatogenesis occurs every day almost throughout life but a woman has all the ova she is ever going to have at the time she is born. Hence on one end, the sperms of an old man are still young; but on another end, the old woman's ova may be 40 to 45 years old before she stops being able to become pregnant. As the age of ovum increases, it becomes more difficult for its chromosomes to be accurately distributed resulting in chromosomal anomalies like *mongolism.*

— Another is *Translocational Mongolism* which is running in families. It has been shown that one of them have only (parents of translocated Mongoloids) 45 chromosomes, including one 21, one 15, and a fused 15 to 21. Here exchange of material between two chromosomes had occurred rather than a true fusion.

— Here the newborn child has *Mongoloid* (slanted) eyes, hyperextensibility of finger joints, imbecile facies and an imbecile mind. There is a high incidence of leukaemia in mongolism.

ii. *Klinefelter's syndrome* (*1942*) : These persons are sex chromatin positive due to one extra X chromosome, so 44 + X + X + Y = 47 chromosomes instead of normal 46 number. 48 chromosomes have also been reported, e.g. 44 + X + X + X + Y = 48.

This is the commonest of sex anomaly and is said to occur about once in every 500 males. Testes are much smaller than normal and spermatogenesis is minimal and azoospermia is constant because seminiferous tubules are abnormal, i.e. seminiferous tubule dysgenesis. This is presence of feminine stigma in an apparent male. So this condition is an important cause of male sterility. In some cases, there is gynaecomastia and eunuchoid traits (long limb, scanty facial hair) and urinary gonadotropins are usually elevated. Tubular fibrosis and hyalinisation along with preservation of Leydig cell is a salient feature. Presence of more than two X chromosomes leads to severe mental deficiency.

iii. *Turner's syndrome (1938, 1960)*:

— Such persons have only one X chromosome in their somatic cell. The somatic cell contains 45 chromosomes 44 + X or 44 + X + O instead of normal 46 chromosomes. This single chromosome present in somatic cell remains extended so it does not appear as Barr body resulting in a negative sex chromatin test.

— Ovarian dysgenesis, i.e. associated with absence of gonads.

— Delayed puberty, diminished sexual development of female type. Shortness of stature, webbing of neck, primary amenorrhoea.

— Males and females can be distinguished without a chromosomal analysis, because of the presence of a stainable body found on the edge of the nuclear membrane of a cell called *Barr body.* The cells of the male don't show Barr bodies, but the cells of normal females exhibit one. The sex of unborn foetuses can be determined by examining cells from the amniotic fluid (the fluid surrounding a foetus) for the presence of Barr bodies. So we must be thankful to Murray Barr (1949; University of *Western Ontario*). Such cells (for examination of Barr bodies) can be obtained from various sources, e.g. skin, blood (WBC) but the most convenient method is to make a smear from oral mucous membrane.

— The size of sex chromatin varies between 0.8 to 1.1 microns. It may be spherical, triangular, disc shaped or sigmoid shaped; moreover its shape depends on its position in relation to other components of the nucleus. It is usually present on the inner surface of the nuclear membrane with the exception of nerve cell. In neutrophil, it occurs as a knob about 1.5μ in diameter and is called drumstick. The drumstick is an additional small lobe of the nucleus of neutrophil and is found in about 1 in 40 neutrophils in normal females. This sex chromatin can be studied with basic dyes like haematoxylin, crystal violet, thionin, fuschin, etc.

READ AND DIGEST: SEX CHROMOSOME ABNORMALITIES

1. *Harry Fitch Klinefelter's Syndrome (1942 American; 47XXY).* In females two XX chromosomes do not separate but remain together. When such an abnormal egg (XX) is fertilised by normal sperm (Y) an abnormal zygote is formed (XXY in addition to autosomes); so total 47 chromosomes instead of 46. This male has undeveloped sex organs with their size reduced. Slight development of breast so body contours will be like that of female. External genitalia normal, testes small, sperms not produced, mental retardness, arms longer than average, positive sex chromatin. Frequency is one out of 500 male births.
2. *Henry Hurbert Turner Syndrome (1938, American endocrinologist; 45X)* when two X chromosomes stick together during oogenesis, both sex chromosomes go to the polar body leaving behind the egg without any sex chromosome. If this egg is fertilised with a normal sperm (X), the zygote produced will be with 45 chromosomes instead of 46. Sterile females, short stature, slight mental retardness, absence of breast, reduced pubic hair. Negative sex chromatin having only one X chromosome. Frequency is one in 5,000 female births. Absence of Y chromosome results in female embryo. Confirmed by Ford et al (1959).
3. *John Langdon Haydon Down Syndrome (English physician, 1828–1896, Mongolism).* 47 chromosomes are found instead of 46. Short body stature (dwarf), mental faculties are not properly developed. Autosomes fail to separate during meiosis, sloping forehead, below average height. Frequency is one out of 770.

THE GENES

- These are segments of DNA molecule (the key to genetics or master word of heredity, in nucleus) and they being 100,000 per cell.
- Genetic information is encoded in DNA, which is replicated in its own image and also directs the synthesis of messenger RNA, which in turn controls synthesis of right kind of protein. The gene acts as a biochemical carrier of biological information from one generation to the next.
- The *genotype* is an individual's full set of genes. The *phenotype* is the entire physical, physiological and biochemical nature of an individual, as determined by his genotype and the environment in which he develops.
- They are arranged in a linear fashion along the chromosome; each gene having its own location or locus. Like chromosomes, the genes are in pairs. All alternative forms of a gene found at one locus are called *alleles* (allelon = one another), but chromosome bears only one allele for a given locus. Alleles segregate at meiosis, and a child receives only one of each pair of alleles from each parent.
- We are now identifying specific genes relative to specific enzyme defects and disease resulting due to this. If any mutation takes place in the structure of a gene, there will be a corresponding modification of the gene product and this in turn will result in a functional disturbance somewhere in the body. This is the theme or basis of hereditary molecular disease.
- Genes are of different grades of potency, the more powerful being called *Dominant* and weaker - *Recessive*.
- A homozygous is an organism with two genes of the same kind, one on each of its homologous chromosomes. Thus, TT and tt are both homozygous and the organism to which they refer are said to be *homozygous*. Tt combination (one dominant and one recessive or different alleles on each of chromosome) is said to be *heterozygous*.
- Crosses or mating are made among organism that have been bred true with respect to a particular characteristic. The parental generation includes the organism of an initial cross in a genetic experiment. The first generation produced by the parent is called F_1 (*first filial generation*), and second generation is called F_2 (*second filial generation*) and so on.

FIVE POSSIBLE RESULTS OF MATING DOMINANT WITH RECESSIVE GENES

1. DD × DD = DD
2. dd × dd = dd
3. DD × dd = Dd
4. DD × Dd = ½ DD + ½ Dd.
5. Dd × Dd = ¼ DD + ½ Dd + ¼ dd.

MUTATION

i. These are sudden changes in genotype, involving qualitative or quantitative alternations in genetic material itself. It is of two types:
   Chromosomal: Abression produces alterations in amount or position of genetic material.
   Point mutation: Are changes within DNA molecule.
ii. Each gene is made up of millions of atoms. Occasionally a rearrangement of the atoms may occur, giving the gene fresh properties; such a change is called mutation. So mutation is one of the great driving forces of evolution which creates new variations in living.
iii. Mutation may involve colour, shape and many other characteristics. Colour mutation plays a major role in horticulture and in fancy breeding of animals, for mutants are inherited just as normal genes.

iv. Mutation may be caused by a number of means :-
- — Thermal agitation of molecules may cause an energetic molecule to strike DNA and produce a chemical change.
- — Mutagenic chemicals can cause mutation, if they penetrate the gonads, e.g. formaldehyde.
- — Ionizing radiation: is a well established mutagenic agent. Gamma and X-rays produce mutation.

HEREDITARY DEFECTS/DISEASES

i. *Metabolic:* Inborn errors of metabolism, e.g. lipid storage disease like Gaucher's disease, Niemann-Pick disease, etc.; Wilson's disease, vonGierke's disease, phenyl ketonurea (disorder of protein metabolism), hereditary fructose intolerance, galactosaemia, gout, cystinurea, porphyria, alkaptonurea, diabetes insipidus, diabetes mellitus.

ii. *Blood diseases:* Haemophilia, sickle cell anaemia, pernicious anaemia, favism, haemorrhagic telengiectasia, hypertension, heart diseases.

iii. *Skeletal defects:* Multiple cartilaginous exostoses, brachydactyly (short fingers), fragility ossium.

iv. *Neuromuscular:* Progressive muscular atrophy, Friedreich's ataxia, myotonia and amyotonia congenita.

v. *Skin:* Baldness, xeroderma pigmentosum, Von-Recklinghausen's disease.

vi. *Eye:* Retinitis pigmentosa, hereditary optic atrophy blue sclerotic, colour blindness, coloboma of iris, some forms of night blindness, retinoblastoma, strabismus, myopia.

vii. *Mental:* Dementia, Huntington's chorea, Mongolian idiocy.

viii. *Cancer:* Polyposis of rectum and colon with its marked tendency to become malignant.

ix. Susceptibility to infection depends on genetic basis. There is a question of inherited susceptibility or resistance to specific infectious disease.

RNA : PROTEIN SYNTHESIS

i. Some functions of the cell are carried out by cytoplasm, and DNA is located in the nucleus. So RNA is formed under the control of DNA of the nucleus and genetic code transferred to RNA (this process is called *transcription*). The RNA so formed diffuses through nuclear pores into cytoplasm, where it controls the synthesis of proteins.

ii. RNA molecule is having only three differences from DNA molecule as:
   a. It is single stranded.
   b. Among four bases — three (adenine, cytosine and guanine) are common and fourth is uracil instead of thymine.
   c. In place of sugar deoxyribose, ribose is used.

iii. Above mentioned nucleotides (adenine, cytosine, guanine and uracil) are activated by addition of two phosphate radicals with the addition of high energy phosphate bonds derived from cellular ATP.

iv. Functional typing
   a. ***Messenger RNA (mRNA):*** Conveys the information encoded in DNA base sequence to the site of protein synthesis. It itself is encoded and this is accomplished at the time of its transcription. It is a linear chain of ribonucleotides, the length of which depends on complexity of the protein for which it is the encoded messenger. The molecules of mRNA carry an inscription of the sequences arranged along DNA molecules, but with 3 letter words written from four alphabets — A, C, G, U. Thus DNA triplets are transcribed into complementary triplets or codons of mRNA. When the whole DNA master band has been transcribed the codon bearing mRNA separates from master band and moves to the cytoplasm through nuclear pore.
      - mRNA molecules are long single RNA strands that are suspended in cytoplasm.

   b. ***Transfer RNA (tRNA):*** All tRNA molecules have molecular weight of about 25,000 and consists of about 80 nucleotides. It is mentioned here that the codon (the unit composed of a number of bases on mRNA template that specifies a specific amino acid) is a triplet i.e. it consists of three bases such as ACU. The three bases of tRNA that attach to a codon are called anticodons the complementary base pairs of the codon; e.g. for the codon ACU the anticodon is UGA. This anticodon is located in the middle of tRNA molecule. tRNA combines specifically with one of the 20 amino acids that are to be incorporated into proteins. tRNA then acts as a carrier to transport its specific amino acid to the ribosomes where protein molecules are formed. In ribosomes, each specific tRNA recognises a particular codon on mRNA and delivers appropriate amino acid to appropriate place in the chain of newly forming protein molecule.

   c. ***Ribosomal RNA (rRNA):*** Carries no genetic information. Ribosomes are composed of roughly half protein and half rRNA. It constitutes about 60 per cent of ribosome. *mRNA* provides the information necessary for sequencing the amino acid in proper order for each specific type of protein to be manufactured; while tRNA transports amino acids to the ribosome for incorporation into the developing protein molecule.

v. In transcription, the two strands of DNA molecule separate locally to expose a particular cistron, on one of them — the master strand (the other strand being complementary). Upon this master strand of DNA, a strand of RNA (mRNA) is constructed with the aid of RNA polymerase and ATP. mRNA is synthesised in much the same way as a new strand of DNA is formed besides an old strand in replication. The synthesis of mRNA in association with DNA is called transcription. The DNA triplets are transcribed into complementary triplets, or codons of mRNA.
   - When whole cistron (of DNA master band) has been transcribed, the codon bearing mRNA separates from master band and moves to the cytoplasm through the nuclear pore. In the cytoplasm, mRNA attaches to a ribosome, which are essential to serve as sites where three letter words code (triplet codons) along the molecule of mRNA becomes specifically attached to the three letter code words (anticodons) of the tRNA.
   - Each molecule of tRNA is capable of recognising on one hand a single mRNA codon, and on the other hand, a corresponding amino acid. Each ribosome moves along the strands of mRNA, reading its codes, so that a corresponding sequence of amino acids is formed each being linked with the other by a peptide bond. After completion of decoding, the ribosome detaches itself and both mRNA and protein are released.
   - The energy for protein synthesis process is supplied by GTP (*Guanadine*—triphosphate) which is similar to ATP, except that *guanadine* replaces adenine. It takes about one minute to make a typical protein.
   - Several ribosomes may attach to same mRNA (and they are called polyribosomes) and produce identical proteins simultaneously.
   - When process of protein synthesis is complete, the ribonucleotides of mRNA are broken apart by the enzyme ribonuclease and are reused in the transcription process on DNA molecules to make more mRNA with a different code. The tRNA molecules are recombined with appropriate amino acids and repeat their role of transporting the amino acids to the site of protein synthesis. The energy for recombination is provided by ATP. Ribosomal subunits are separated until they rejoin on a new mRNA molecule to begin the synthesis process a new.

Table 8.1: Difference between m-RNA and t-RNA

m-RNA	*t-RNA*
• Large molecule weight	• Low molecule weight
• Acts as a template for protein synthesis	• Acts as a carrier for amino acid
• Carries codons	• Carries anticodons
• Shape and size not constant	• It is constant
• Stem and loop structure not found	• It is a consistent feature

GENETIC REGULATION

A structural gene, which is a section of DNA responsible for the production of a particular enzyme, or a group of structural gene are considered to be under the influence of an operator gene or simply on *operator*. This may stimulate one or more structural genes into activity under proper conditions and the operator is situated immediately adjacent to the structural genes under its influence. The operator and its associated structural genes are collectively called an *operon*. The entire operon is controlled by a substance called *repressor* which is a protein whose production is directed by still another section of DNA (on the same chromosome) called *regulator gene*.

- The repressor has two functional states—active or inactive, and it assumes one or the other of these states by combining with either a *copressor*, which activates the repressor, or an *inducer* which inactivates the repressor. Copressor and inducers are external molecules that are absent or present depending on the nutritional or metabolic state of the cell. When repressor is activated it can bind to the operator, which in turn prevents the binding of RNA polymerase and thus specifically prohibits the initiation of mRNA synthesis. If the repressor is combined with an inducer, it cannot bind to the operator and so cannot inhibit mRNA synthesis.

Other Mechanism for Control of Transcription by Operon

i. By regulatory gene; which leads to the formation of regulatory protein which acts as activator/repressor substance.
ii. Sometimes initial control is lacking. The process is controlled during processing of RNA molecules in the nucleus before they are released into cytoplasm. The control may occur at level of RNA translation by ribosomes.

There are 100,000 different genes in each human cell so large number of control system may be available.

Operon = Formation of all the enzymes needed for the synthetic process is often controlled by a sequence of genes located in series one after other on the same chromosomal DNA strand. This area of DNA strand is called operon and genes responsible for forming respective enzymes are called structural genes.

Promoter = Is a segment on DNA strand, which is a series of nucleotides having special affinity for RNA polymerase. It is an essential element for activation of operon, since polymerase RNA must bind with promoter before it travels along DNA strand to synthesise RNA.

Repressor protein = Is an additional band of nucleotides located in middle of promoter. A regulatory protein can bind here and prevent attachment of RNA polymerase to the promoter, thereby blocking transcription of the genes. Such a regulatory protein is called "repressor protein."

Inhibitor substance = Various non-protein substances in the cell, e.g. some of cell metabolites can bind with repressor protein to change its state. A substance that causes it to change so that it will bind with the operator and stop transcription is called inhibitor or repressor substance.

Activator/inducer substance = It activates the transcription process.

Still another means by which cellular metabolism may be controlled is *end product inhibition.*

- In above sequence threonine → Isoleucine by different pathway if isoleucine is added (exogenous) to this; the cell uses this exogenous isoleucine and stops their own synthesis of isoleucine. This inhibition occurs at the very first step as shown above.
- It is thought that inhibitors can bind to completed enzymes at a location other than the active site of the enzyme. The enzyme slightly changes its shape as a result of the binding of the inhibitor, so that its active site no longer accepts its substrates and is temporarily

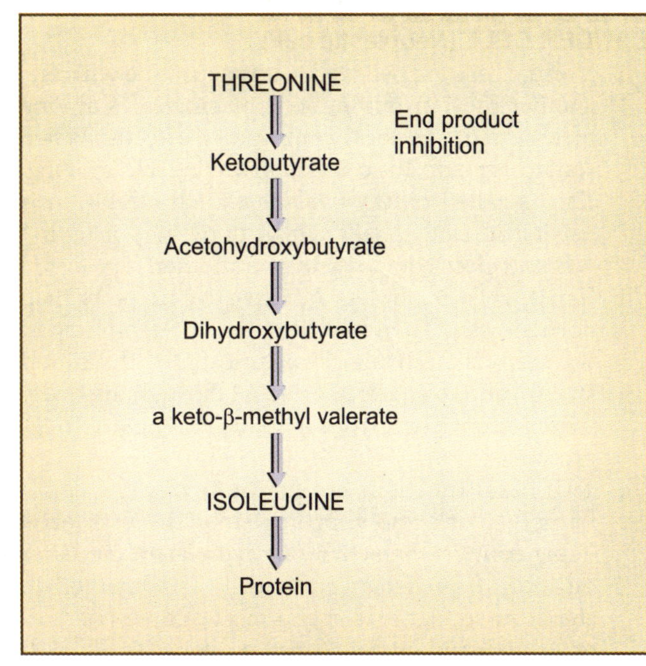

inactive. Proteins that change shape as a result of combination with another molecule are *allosteric proteins*.

Enzyme activation

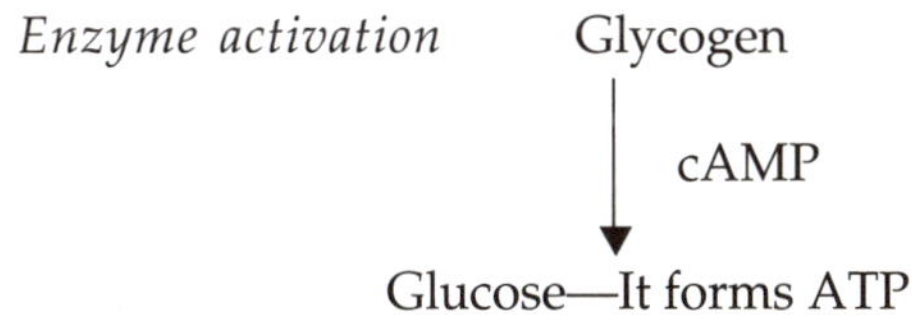

- When most of ATP has been depleted in a cell, a considerable amount of cAMP begins to be formed as a breakdown product of ATP. This cAMP shows that cellular reserves of ATP are at low level. However, cAMP immediately activates the glycogen-splitting enzyme phosphorylase, liberating glucose molecules that are rapidly metabolised and their energy used for replenishment of the ATP stores. So cAMP acts as an enzyme activator and so helps to control intracellular ATP concentration.
- DNA is not only the governing force controlling the life of a cell, but it also controls the genetics of the organism by virtue of genes which are in essence composed of DNA. As the double helix DNA molecules are thousands of turns long and are arranged by thousands in each chromosome, it is evident that a structure of such complexity may well become damaged and it is believed that carcinogens (poly cyclic hydrocarbons, viruses, ionising radiations) may bring about such derangement.

CANCER CELL (Neoplastic cell)

i. Normal cells are believed to communicate with one another by transmitting ions or molecules among members of the local community of cells. When contact is made, the cells stop growing and moving. This is called *contact inhibition*. Such inhibition is lacking in cancer cells which don't stop growing when in close contact with one another.
ii. Cancer cells are far less adhesive to each other than normal cells. Therefore, they have a tendency to wander through the tissues, to enter the blood stream, and to be transported all through the body, where they constitute a locus for new cancer growths.
iii. Two main functions are performed by the cell—namely work and reproduction; the former is dependent on the activity of cytoplasm, the latter on that of nucleus. Cancer cells are changed in character so that they spend most of their energies on growth and little on function.
iv. The tumour cell is a modified normal cell.
v. Metabolic superiority of the tumour cell is largely due to its enhanced amino acid concentration power.
vi. Since cancer cells are continuously multiplying; so they will demand essentially all the nutrition available to the body. So normal tissues suffer from nutritive death.

CANCER

- Some cells of the body (often of stem cell type) undergoes a genetic change of such a nature that the genetically altered cell is much less susceptible than its neighbours to factors which control cell population in the body. It multiplies under conditions in which multiplication of the normal cells of the body would be restrained.
- Cancer continues to grow and multiplying cells thus invade other tissues and organs. So it generally spreads through blood, lymphatics and the phenomenon is called *metastasis*.
- Cancer is a disorder of growth control. A cell is growing in an unrestrained fashion and supportive cells and blood vessels are also growing. Cancer arises from previous normal cells through genetic mutations which are both dominant and recessive in type. These mutant genes termed *oncogenes* arising through mutation of cellular genes called proto-oncogenes, are involved in controlling normal cell growth and differentiation. Dominant mutation affect genes by either removing normal structural controlling elements which regulate their function or by enhancing their expression by gene amplification or enhanced transcription. Recessive oncogenes result in deletion of genetic loci which encode growth-restraining proteins.

MEIOSIS

- It consists of two successive divisions each with its own prophase, metaphase, anaphase and the telophase; it thereby results in four daughter nuclei instead of two as in mitosis.
- In meiosis I, the chromosome number is halved to the original haploid value. In meiosis II, there is no reduction in the chromosome number.

Meiosis I

a. *Prophase I*: long and complex phase divided into following stages
   i. *Leptotene stage:* Chromosome becomes visible as individual threads attached at one end to the nuclear membrane. Each chromatid shows characteristic beads called chromomeres throughout its length.
   ii. *Zygotene stage*: Chromosomes come together side by side in homologous pairs (zygo-pair) so that corresponding regions of pairing chromosomes lie in contact. This is called pairing/conjugation/synapsis; each chromosome pair is now called bivalent. In X and Y male chromosomes only limited segments are homologous.
   iii. *Pachytene stage:* Chromosome shorten and thicken further. The two *chromatids*, one from each bivalent chromosome become partially coiled around each other (i.e. crossing over).
   iv. *Diplotene stage:* The chromosomes of homologous pair now move slightly apart except at the site of crossing over. These cross connections between two non-sister chromatids break, causing an exchange of segments of the non-sister chromatids beyond the break. Normally at least one chiasmata is formed between each pair of homologous chromosomes. There occurs an exchange of genetic material between maternal and paternal chromosomes.
   v. *Diakinesis:* The chromosomes which still form bivalent become even shorter and thicker. The bivalent pairs of chromosomes move away from each other and become spread out against the nuclear membrane.
   So during termination of Prophase I; the characteristics are viz. - breakdown of nuclear membrane and movements of bivalent chromosomes towards the equatorial plane of the cell; disappearance of nucleoli.

b. *Metaphase I:* It is characterised by following which are differences from metaphase of mitosis.
  i. Homologous pairs of chromosomes lie parallel to equatorial plane with one member on either side.
  ii. The bodies attaching to the spindle tubules (spindle microtubule) are bivalent and not single chromosomes.
c. *Anaphase I:* Whereas anaphase of mitosis is marked by the separation of sister chromatids, this anaphase I of meiosis is characterised by separation of homologous entire chromosomes. This is because of the fact that division of centromere is delayed until Anaphase II while in mitosis centromere divides in anaphase.

  Two longitudinally double chromosomes of each pair, each made up of two joined chromatids depart to opposite poles, so that each pole receives either a paternal or a maternal longitudinally double chromosomes of each pair. This leads to change in chromosome number from diploid to haploid in the resultant reorganised daughter nuclei.
d. *Telophase I:* its beginning is marked by arrival of chromosomes at the poles of spindle. The nucleolus and nuclear membrane are reconstituted and cytokinesis occurs as in mitosis to produce two daughter cells each with a haploid number of chromosomes.

Meiosis II: It starts only after a short interval during which no synthesis of DNA occurs. It is similar to mitosis passing through its own stages, with separation of chromatids by the division of centromere during anaphase. Unlike mitosis the separating chromatids during meiosis II are dissimilar genetically.

Significance of Meiosis

1. It helps to maintain constant number of chromosomes in the organisms.
2. The genetic crossing over brings about varied combination of genetic material. This brings about variations.
3. The random distribution and combination of chromosomes in the gametes give rise to different combination of parental characters in offsprings.

GENETIC CODE

- The genetic code is the relationship between the sequence of bases in DNA (or its mRNA transcript) and the sequence of amino acid in a protein. In the nucleotide sequence of mRNA molecule, code words are present for each amino acid. This is referred as genetic code.
- We are thankful to Nirenberg, H. G. Khorana, Crick and their co-workers for remarkable work in this field.
- The basic problem of such a genetic code is to indicate how information written in a four letter language (four nucleotides of DNA) can be translated into a twenty letter language (twenty amino acids of protein). The group of nucleotides that specifies one

Table 8.2: Difference between mitosis and meiosis

	Mitosis	*Meiosis*
A. Prophase	• Chromomeres not visible	• Visible
	• Homologous chromosomes	• They pair up
	• No crossing over	• May occur
	• No chiasmata formation	• occurs
	• Pairs of chromatids live up	• Line up only in second meiotic division
B. Metaphase	• Centromeres line up on the same plane on the equator of spindle	• They lie equidistant above and below the equator in first division
C. Anaphase	• Centromeres divide	• Divide only during second division
	• Chromatids separate	• Separate only in second division
	• Separating chromatids identical	• May not be identical due to crossing over
D. Telophase	• Same number of chromosomes present in daughter cell as parent cell	• Half the number of chromosomes present in daughter cell
	• Both homologous chromosomes present in daughter cell if diploid	• Only one of each pair of homologous chromosomes present in daughter cell
E. Occurrence	• May occur in haploid, diploid or polyploid cell	• Only in diploid or *poly-ploid* cell
	• occurs during formation of somatic cells/gametes in plants	• In formation of gamete cells or spores

MENDEL'S LAW : FOLLOWING ARE ITS COMPONENTS

a. *The law of Dominance :* The offspring of parents which are pure for contrasting characteristics will resemble one parent only. The hereditary unit (gene), for one characteristic, the dominant prevents the other - the recessive, from expressing itself when the two are combined in the same organism.

b. *The law of segregation :* When hybrids are crossed with other hybrids or with individuals showing either the dominant or recessive characteristic, the dominant and recessive both appear in offspring, in a definite ratio.

c. *The law of unit characters :* Each pair of characteristics operates independently of others, following the laws of dominance and segregation.

Incomplete Dominance : Some contradiction have been reported since the timing of Mendelian era. Here, neither of the contrasting genes appear to be strictly dominant or recessive in heterozygous condition. The result is an apparent blending of characteristics so as to produce an intermediate condition.

amino acid is a code word or codon. The simplest possible code is a singlet code (a code of single letter) in which there is one nucleotide code for one amino acid. Such a code is inadequate for only four amino acid — could be specified, e.g.

A
G
C
U

Singlet code = 4 × 1 = 4

- A doublet code (a code of two letters) is also inadequate because it could specify only sixteen amino acids 4 × 4 = 16, e.g.

	A	G	C	U
A	AA	AG	AC	AU
G	GA	GG	GC	GU
C	CA	CG	CC	CU
U	UA	UG	UC	UU

4 × 4 = 16 Doublet code

- Now a triplet code (4 × 4 × 4 = 64 amino acids for 20 amino acids) can satisfy the need.

This clearly states that each code word (termed as codon) consists of a sequence of three nucleotides, i.e. it is a triplet code (Crick 1961, Mathei and Nirinberg, and Gamow) — 1954.

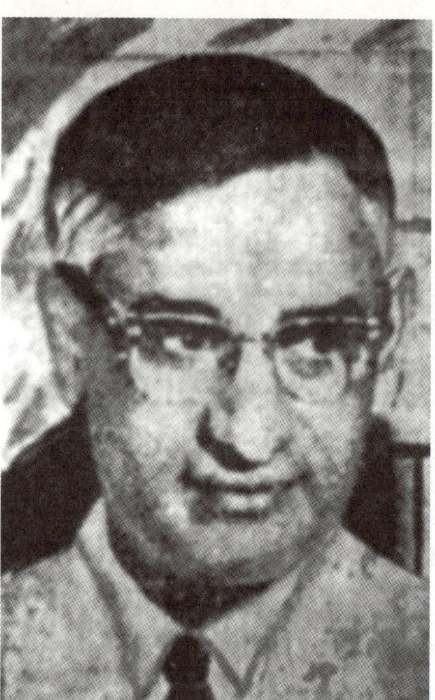

Fig. 8.1: Dr HG Khurana

Genetic Code Dictionary

Total 64 codes are constructed (i.e. 4 × 4 × 4 = 64). There are more than 20 amino acids to be coded.

- **Contribution of Hargovind Khurana (Nobel Prize 1968)**
  — He and his colleagues artificially synthesised mRNA of known nucleotide sequences. They provided experimental evidence for codon sequences.
  — Two series of polyribo-nucleotides are:-

i. Poly CUC UCU CUC UCU: (Here they are two codons namely CUC and UCU. They are distributed in one single chain in series. It facilitates/regularise the manufacture of two amino acids viz. leucine and serine.

ii. Poly CUA CUA CUA CUA: (It is an example of co-polymer chain. It is constituted by repeated involvement of CUA codon. This helps in manufacturing polypeptide chain having leucine amino acid.

GENETIC CODE OF FEW AMINO ACIDS

1. *Serine...* UCU, UCC, UCA, UCG, AGU, ACU
2. *Arginine...* CGU, CGC, CGA, UCG, AGA, AGG.
3. *Leucine...* CUU, CUC, CUA, CUG, UUA, UUG.
4. *Valine.....* GUU, GUC, GUA, GUG.

SECOND BASE

FIRST BASE		U		C		A		G		THIRD BASE
U		UUU		UCU		UAU		UGU		U
		UUC	Phe	UCC		UAC	Tyr	UGC	Cys	C
		UUA		UCA	Ser	UAA		UGA		A
		UUG	Leu	UCG		UAG		UGG	Tyr	G
C		CUU		CCU		CAU		CGU		U
		CUC		CCC		CAC	His	CGC		C
		CUA	Leu	CCA	Pro	CAA		CGA	Arg	A
		CUG		CCG		CAO		CGG		G
A		AUU		ACU		AAU		AGU		U
		AUC		ACC		AAC		AGC	Ser	C
		AUA	I Leu	ACA	Thr	AAA		AGA		A
		AUG	Met	ACG		AAG	Lys	AGG	Arg	G
G		GUU		GUU		GAU		GGU		U
		GUC		GCC		GAC		GGC		C
		GUA	Val	GCA		GAA	Asp	GGA	Gly	A
		GUG		GCG	Ala	GAG	Glu	GGG		G

Properties of Genetic Code

1. *It is composed of nucleotide triplet:* Three nucleotides in mRNA specify one amino acid in polypeptide product thus each codon contains three nucleotides.
2. *Genetic code is non-overlapping:* Each nucleotide in mRNA belongs to just one codon except in rare cases where genes overlap; e.g. ACCGCU represent 2 codons only viz. ACC & GCU and not CCG or CGC etc.
3. *Genetic code is comma free:* There are no commas or other forms of punctuations within coding regions of mRNA molecules. There is no blank space in between two codons.
4. *Genetic code is degenerate*: All but two of amino acids are specified by more than one codon.
5. *Genetic code is ordered:* Multiple codons for a given amino acids and codons for amino acid with similar chemical properties are closely related usually differing by a single nucleotide.
6. *Genetic code contains start and stop codons:* specific codons are used to initiate and terminate polypeptide chains.
7. *Genetic code is nearly universal:* The codons have the same meaning in all living organisms, e.g. from virus to human beings.
8. *Ambiguity:* One specific codon indicates specifically towards one specific amino acid. (One codon don't code two different amino acid). But in some special circumstances this may be possible.

Explanation

1. *Triplet:* Three code letters from one code word which code for one amino acid.
2. *Commaless:* UUU CCC GGG AAA has four code words and upon translation we will have a tetrapeptide chain of phe-pro-gly-lys. So all these letters are used to code for one or other amino acid.
3. *Degenerate:* There are 4 codons (GCU, GCC, GCA, GCG) for alanine. The first two position of triplet codon on mRNA pair precisely.

SUMMARY AND HIGHLIGHTS

- As it became evident that genes controlled the structure of polypeptides, attention focussed on how the sequence of different nucleotides in DNA could control the game of 20 amino acids present in proteins, with discovery of mRNA intermediary the question became how the sequence of the four bases present in mRNA molecules could specify the amino acid sequence of a polypeptide.
- Genetic code is the relationship between the sequence of bases in DNA (or its mRNA transcript) and sequence of amino acid in a protein. In the nucleotide sequence of mRNA molecule code words are present for each amino acid. This is called as genetic code.

OR

- Genetic code is concerned with the processes involved in translating or decoding the information contained in primary structure of DNA. Genetic information flows from gene (DNA) to RNA to protein. RNA thus serves as an intermediate between DNA and proteins. These genetic code processes are the basis of life or is fundamental secret of nature. The basic question that we try to answer is which DNA code words specify which amino acid? Answer to this comes from genetic code dictionary.

BIBLIOGRAPHY

1. Barr ML. Sex chromatin and sex anomalies. Science 1959;130:679.
2. Barr ML, Bertram EG. A morphologic distinction between neurones of the male and female and behaviour of the nucleolar satellite during accelerates nueleo protein synthesis.Nature (Lond) 1949;163:676-78.
3. Beckwith JR. Regulation of the lac operon, Science 1967;156:597-604.
4. Book JA, Saniession B. Lancet 1960;i,858.
5. Burns GW. The science of Genetics. Macmillan: New York (1969).
6. Cooper GM, et al. Transforming activity of DNA of chemically transformed and normal cells. Nature 1986;233:1050;284:418-21.
7. Echols. Multiple DNA protein interaction governing high precision DNA transactions. Science 1986;233:1050.
8. Edivard JH, et al. Trisomic syndromes. Lancet 1960;1:787.
9. Ford CE, et al. Mongolism and Klinefelter's syndrome, Lancet 1959;1:709.
10. Friend SH, et al. Oncogenes and tumour suppressing genes New Eng J Med 1988;318:618-22.
11. Ham AW. Histology. Lippincott, Philadelphia, Torronto 1969.
12. Hamilton WJ, Boyd JD, Moosman HW. Human Embryology. W. Heffer: Cambridge 1964.
13. Hisa DYY. Medical Genetics. New Eng J Med 1960;262:1172.
14. Holley RW, et al. Structure of a RNA. Science 1965;147:162-65.
15. Lake JA, et al. Yeast transfer. RNA science. 1967;156:1371-73.
16. Lennox B. Chromosomes for beginer. Laoncet 1961;1:1046.
17. Macara IG. Oncogenes and cellular signal transduction. Phy Rev 1989;69:797.
18. Madison JT, et al. Nucleotide sequence of a yeast tyrosine transfer RNA. Science 1966;153:531-34.
19. Muzammil Ullah. Histology and genetics. Aryan Press. Merrut.
20. Nomura M, et al. Regulation of synthesis of ribosomes and ribosomal components. Ann Rev Biochem 1984;53:75.
21. Pabo CO, et al. Protein DNA recognition. Ann Rev Biochem 1984;53:293.
22. Roberts JAF. An Introduction to medical genetics. 2nd ed. London 1959.
23. Shih et al. Transforming genes of carcinomas and neuroblastomas introduced in mouse fibroblasts. Nature 1981;290:261-64.
24. Sorsby A. Clinical Genetics. St. Louis 1958.
25. Sutow WW, Welsch VC. Acute leukaemia and mongolism. J Paed 1958;52:176-81.
26. Teir H, Rytomaa T. Control of cellular growth in adult organism, academic press, New York. London 1967.
27. Thompson JS, Thompson MW. Genetics in Medicine; Philadelphia 1966.
28. Ullrich, et al. Human insulin receptors and its relationship to tyrosine kinase family of oncognes. Nature 1985;313:756-61.
29. Varmus HE. Oncogenes and transcriptional control. Science 1987;238:1337.

9 Clock and the Health Circadian Rhythm: Biological Rhythm

A person is subjected to many biological rhythms. These rhythms developed during the course of evolution in response to environmental processes and now are inherent in every organism. The environmental periodicity no longer causes biological rhythm but it acts as a synchronising agent for the self-sustained cycle within organism.

- Menstrual cycle follows a lunar cycle (28 days), while body temperature, hormone levels, periods of rest and activity exhibit circadian rhythm (1 day). As a result of circadian rhythm a person is a different physiologically and psychologically at each hour of the day.
- Both T_3 and T_4 show circadian rhythmicity but the amplitude of variation is very low. With usual activity the plasma level of T_3 is highest in early morning and gradually decreases during the day and evening. Plasma T_4 concentration show two peaks one occurring in early morning and a smaller peak occurring in mid afternoon. Normal rhythm is re-established when activity is resumed.
- During normal activity, insulin level reflect the pattern of food intake, with large increase following breakfast and midday meal and a smaller but more prolonged increase after the evening meal.
- The diurnal variation occurring significantly in the levels of glucose, insulin, growth hormone suggest that prolonged bed-rest leads to instability of these homeostatic mechanisms. The mean daily glucose concentration in blood is not altered by 30 days of bed-rest, but amplitude of diurnal variation is increased, i.e. fluctuations at different times throughout the day are more pronounced.
- In myocardial ischaemia. Sudden cardiac death is precipitated by abrupt plaque change followed by thrombosis. The initiating event is disruption of previously stenosing plaques with (a) haemorrhage into atheroma expending its volume, (b) rupture or fissuring which exposes highly thrombogenic plaque constituents, (c) erosion or ulceration exposing thrombogenic subendothelial basement membrane to blood.

  The adrenergic stimulation associated with awakening induces a pronounced circadian periodicity for the time of onset of acute MI, with a peak incidence at 6 am to 12 noon with a surge in BP and immediately following heightened platelet reactivity. Aspirin - a drug famous to interfere with platelet function depresses the morning peak in the incidence of acute MI.
- ACTH is secreted in irregular bursts through out the day, and plasma cortisol tends to rise and fall in response to these bursts. Seventy-five per cent of daily cortisol production occurs between 4 am to 10 am, and frequency is least in the evening. This circadian rhythm in ACTH secretion is found in patients with adrenal insufficiency receiving glucocorticoids.
- The suprachiasmatic nuclei are the main pacemakers for many circadian rhythms in the body, e.g. ACTH and melatonin secretion, sleep-wake cycle, body temperature rhythm, etc. The nuclei receives input from eyes through retinohypothalamic fibres, from lateral geniculate body and their function is to synchronise the various body rhythms to 24 hours light-dark cycle.
- The melatonin synthesis and secretion is increased during dark period of the day and maintained at low levels during daylight. This diurnal is brought by noradrenaline secreted by sympathetics (postganglionic fibres) which innervate the pineal.

- RBC: The values are highest in the morning and lowest in the evening. It is more marked in woman.
- Day to day variation (ranging between 0.8 to 3.0 g/dl, with an average of 1.75 g/dl) in haemoglobin values is due to fluctuation in plasma volume and fall which may occur at about the time of menstruation is due to hydraemia which commonly precedes the onset of menstruation.
- WBC: Undergoes minor diurnal variation. It increases slightly in afternoon — called "afternoon tide".

10 The Secret of Health: Physiology of Exercise

The term physical exercise is restricted to the mechanical phenomenon accompanying the activity of the organs of locomotion, but efficiency in exercise demands the correlated co-operation of all the organs and systems in the body. It is, therefore, necessary to consider the organism as a whole made up of integrated parts, the actions of which combine with admirable precision.

Of all the normal activities that make up the regular daily life of a man, severe exercise probably imposes the greatest physiological stress on the body.

Physical exercise is the doing of work, and the severity of exercise is determined by the rate at which the work is done. It has become customary to express the rate at which work is being done by the body in terms of the amount of oxygen the body is consuming per minute.

CATEGORIES OF WORK

i. *Mild work:* The oxygen consumption is increased only a little as well as the total metabolic rate. So it leads to minor physiological changes.

ii. *Moderate work:* Here, the oxygen consumption is increased upto 0.8 L/min. The metabolic rate in this work range is about 240 Cal/hr and a man working at such a rate for 8 hr/day uses about 3800 cal/da.

iii. *Hard work:* Here, the oxygen consumption may be 1-2 L/min. The metabolic rate may be typically 360 cal./hr. and the daily caloric usage of a man working at this rate for 8 hr/day would be about 4300 cal.

iv. *Maximal work:* It is so hard work which cannot be sustained indefinitely. Any thing can set the limit like rise in body temperature, exhaustion of carbohydrate store (hypoglycaemia), circulatory failure, inadequate supply of oxygen.

The physiological changes associated with work would also be expected to vary with the work rate and with time. Let us study them.

BODY CHANGES OCCURRING IN EXERCISE

Oxygen Consumption

- Muscular contraction is accompanied by an increase in oxygen consumption, because when working, the muscles require a supplement of energy which is obtained by burning a larger amount of foodstuffs. This increase in combustion causes an increase in oxygen consumption of the whole organism, and several adjustments in the respiratory and circulatory functions must be made to assure the arrival of more oxygen to the active muscles.
- During first few minutes of exercise, O_2 consumption rises, but O_2 absorbed is less than that needed to oxidise the metabolic products of muscular contraction, and it is because of delayed adaptation of cardio-pulmonary apparatus to greater demand of oxygen by the tissues. Of course, due to energy set free by anaerobic chemical reaction the muscles continue to contract. Because of O_2 deficiency; complete resynthesis of lactic acid, into glycogen is prevented which leads to lactacidaemia (more lactic acid in blood). During steady state the amount of lactic acid accumulated neither increases nor decreases. During recovery, the rate of O_2 consumption should fall suddenly to the resting level, but it does not happen, because the lactic acid which is accumulated during the first stages and which is not removed during steady state must be disposed of during the period of recovery. This means contraction has taken place in state of 'oxygen debt' which means - the amount of oxygen in litres necessary for the removal of metabolic products accumulated while the supply of oxygen is below the needs of the organism.
- On this basis, the above classification of exercise can be narrated as :
  — *Moderate* : When O_2 consumption is upto three times the basal rate.

— *Heavy* : When it is three to eight times the basal rate.
— *Maximum* : When it is more than eight times.

- The exercising muscle is not only more liberally supplied with blood but the low O_2 tension in the cells, the increased formation of CO_2 and acid metabolites—all favour an increased uptake of O_2 from the blood. More O_2 is taken out of each ml of blood so that arterio-venous. O_2 difference is greater in exercise than at rest.
- R. Q. at rest is about 0.85 on the average and it is raised on vigorous exercise. This suggests that a slightly larger proportion of carbohydrate is being oxidised

Heart Rate

i. When a bout of exercise begins, it takes sometime for the heart rate to rise to its maximum value, and after the exercise is stopped, it takes time for the heart rate to return to normal.
ii. The greatest heart rate response occurs in speed contests, e.g. sprinting; the next greatest response occurs in endurance contests, e.g. distance running, and the least response occurs in strength contests, e.g. weight lifting.
iii. Explanation
   - Adrenaline poured into blood stream during exercise increases heart rate.
   - Changes in chemical composition of blood during exercise may result in cardiac acceleration.
   - The rise in body temperature during exercise may also lead to increase in heart rate.
   - This increased heart rate may be due to decreased vagal tone, and this is brought about through alteration of activity of the cardiovascular centres under the influence of the muscle-joint reflexes. The 'Bain-bridge reflex' presumably brings about an increase in heart rate by stimulation of receptors in the large veins and the right atrium. These receptors would be stimulated by an increase in venous pressure, which occurs because of the large increase of venous return due to muscular message, increased pressure in capillaries associated with reduction of peripheral resistance, etc.
iv. The pulse is accelerated as soon as exercise commences, the first cardiac cycle already shows a shortening of the diastole. Probably this is due to a psychic effect on the vagal tone.
v. The most important factor is the intensity of exercise; the heart rate increases with the intensity of effort made. Exercise of the same intensity causes a greater increase in heart rate in young subjects than in older ones.
vi. The barometric pressure influences the heart rate in exercise mainly because of a decrease in partial pressure of oxygen causing varying degrees of anoxia.
vii. After exercise has come to an end, the heart rate diminishes at first rapidly, then gradually until it falls to the resting level. The continuing tachycardia after exercise is due to the effect of local metabolites in the exercising muscles, hormones and temperature.
viii. During short bouts of near maximal exercise heart rate as high as 240 to 270 per minute has been recorded in young persons. Initial rapid increase in heart rate (160–180 per minute) is probably due to vagal withdrawal as well as a rapid reflex from mechano-receptors in the active muscles. Further increase in heart rate is probably due to sympathetic discharge or release of catecholamines as well as activation of pulmonary stretch receptors.

CHANGES DURING MUSCULAR ACTIVITY

1. *Circulation:* Increase in blood volume due to blood discharge from spleen. Red cell count increases. Due to increase in stroke volume, cardiac output increases. Heart rate and systolic blood pressure rises.
2. *Respiration:* Direct relationship exists between rate and depth of respiration and muscle work done. Rising blood CO_2 stimulates the respiratory centre. O_2 consumption per minute increases and slight rise in body temperature may occur.
3. *Body fluids:* Loss of NaCl and water through perspiration; so approximately 8 to 10 pounds body weight may decrease.
4. Others
   i. Increased heat loss, some rise in body temperature.
   ii. During and after exercise urine volume is lower than normal and urine is acidic and dark in colour,
   iii. Exercise seems to be beneficial to digestion,
   iv. Urine contains significant amounts of lactic acid in moderate and severe exercise.

Cardiac output + O_2 consumption in exercise

Exercise	*Cardiac output l/min*	*Total O_2 consumption of Body l/min.*	*Arterio venous O_2 difference ml/100 ml.*
Rest	5	0.25	5
Walking 2 mph	10	0.8	8
Walking 5 mph	20	2.5	12
Running 7 mph	25	3.0	12
Very severe exercise (max. athletic effort)	34	4.0	13

Blood Pressure—Cardiac Output

i. The systolic blood pressure rises rapidly as soon as exercise is begun and reaches a maximum conditioned by the intensity of the exercise. This is due to an increase in the cardiac minute volume; therefore systolic and pulse pressure increase more than the diastolic pressure. Stabilisation at a level slightly below the maximum observed at the beginning of exercise is probably due to compensatory mechanism, e.g. mechanical stimulation of presso-receptors of the aorta and carotid sinus, and stimulation of chemo-receptors in the carotid and aortic bodies, by variations in the pH and other changes in blood.

ii. Mere thinking of exercise may raise the blood pressure due to stimulation of sympathetic system and pouring of adrenaline hormone (psychic stimuli).

iii. Once the exercise is ended, the cardiac minute volume diminishes and therefore the systolic and diastolic pressure fall. The rise in diastolic pressure a few minutes after the end of exercise has been attributed to constriction of the vascular territories which were dilated during the exercise. It is, therefore, said that diastolic pressure shows less marked fluctuations; and after exercise it drops rapidly and then again rises.

iv. In very light exercise, there may be no change in arterial pressure, or there may even be a slight drop in systolic pressure.

v. There is usually an increase in the cardiac output. The minute volume may rise to 35 litres from resting 4 to 5 litres. The systolic output may increase to 100 to 150 cc from resting 60 to 70 cc and it is dependent on venous return. All this is having possible under mentioned mechanism -
   - There is an increased circulating blood volume produced by evacuation of stored blood in skin, splanchnic area and liver spleen.
   - The venous return is increased by the contraction of skeletal muscles, the more frequent and ample respiratory movements and contraction of abdominal muscles that accelerate the circulation in the large veins of abdomen and thorax (increased thoracic pump).
   - This greater venous return increases the strength of systolic contraction, as the heart muscles-fibres are distended by the greater diastolic filling of heart (Starling law), and distension of right auricle reflexly increases the heart rate (Bain bridge reflex).

INCREASED VENOUS RETURN DURING EXERCISE : CAUSES

- Great increase in muscular activity and thoracic pump.
- Mobilisation of blood from viscera.
- Increased pressure transmitted through the dilated arterioles to the veins.
- Increase in amount of blood in arteries which is mobilised from splanchnic area and other reservoirs.

Circulatory Changes

i. Active muscles need a greater blood flow. This increased blood flow is produced by many mechanisms, viz. local vasodilatation and a rise in blood pressure. Local vasodilatation of arterioles and capillaries is always accompanied by the opening of a large number of capillaries that were closed in the resting muscle. In one of the studies it was shown that an area in a skeletal muscle containing 1690 muscle fibres had at rest 1050 open capillaries. In the exercise condition, the same area had 2010 open capillaries and these capillaries were of greater diameter; Arterioles were dilated and capillary pressure was greater. According to some general agreeable concept, the number of open capillaries in an active muscle can be upto 10 times those open in a resting muscle. Thus, oxygen pressure in the tissues is raised and oxygen consumption by the muscle increases between 30 to 90 per cent.

ii. There is increased blood flow in the lungs and brain during exercise and a decreased blood flow in the viscera. Visceral vasoconstriction is probably due to both nervous and hormonal influences, and adrenaline brings about this action which is released into blood stream during exercise. It is muscle-joint reflex and other associated exercise reflexes which shifts blood flow from viscera to skeletal muscle. The increased blood flow through lungs and brain is thought to be primary passive and due to increase in pressure in the central arterial reservoir.

iii. During exercise the increased CO_2 tension, decreased O_2 tension and pH, local accumulation of metabolic product like lactic acid, adenyl pyrophosphate, etc. cause local vasodilatation in the active muscles and thus increase the local blood flow. Nervous mechanism for vasodilatation consists in a diminished vasoconstrictor tone, produced reflexly by the action of high blood pressure on the carotid sinus.

iv. The coronary arteries are dilated during exercise which leads to increased blood flow through heart muscle. This is due to (vasodilatation of coronaries)
- Decreased parasympathetic discharge;
- Local chemical conditions;
- Increased temperature.

v. In isotonic muscle contraction there is a marked increase in stroke volume but in addition there is a net fall in total peripheral resistance due to vasodilatation in exercising muscles. So systolic pressure rises only moderately and diastolic pressure either remains unchanged or falls.

- Fall in tissue PO_2; and rise in PCO_2 and accumulation of K^+ and other metabolites which are vasodilators.
- Temperature rises in active muscles.
- Dilatation of arterioles and pre-capillary sphincters causes many fold increase in number of open capillaries.
- Lymph flow is greatly increased.
- Shifting of O_2 dissociation curve towards right, due to increased temperature and decreased pH.
- Decreased O_2 affinity for haemoglobin due to increased concentration of 2–3 DPG, in RBC.

vi. *Exercise and muscle blood flow*

vii. Exercise induces positive ionotropic effect which shortens ejection and increases the rate of relaxation, which along with increased atrial contraction, enhances ventricular filling. Thus with mild to moderate exercise, stroke volume increases (due to Frank Starling Mechanism and increased myocardial contractility), which leads to decreased ventricular end systolic volume and increased ejection fraction.

viii. During normal strenuous exercise when the heart rate is very high, the large number of systolic contractions per minute tends to abbreviate the duration of diastole markedly. A forceful atrial contraction between each ventricular beat under such conditions greatly improves the transport of blood through the ventricles.

Increased Blood Lactic Acid Level (Lactacidaemia)

- Blood lactic acid level in resting state is 15 mg per cent, which increases to 100 to 200 mg per cent in moderate or maximum exercise.
- The source of lactic acid is by glycolysis (which increases in alkalosis and also when the blood passes through lungs), and muscular contraction. During strong or sustained muscular contraction, the insufficiency of oxygen supply causes the accumulation of lactic acid which diffuses into blood stream.
- Effects of Lactacidaemia:
  1. Urinary lactic acid and ammonia level increases during and after exercise, since part of excess lactic acid is excreted by the kidney.
  2. It also causes an increased output of CO_2 and a fall in alkali reserve. It is because of the fact that lactic acid displaces CO_2 from the base with which it is combined and forms lactates.
  3. Lactacidaemia increases the hydrogen ion concentration which results into stimulation of respiratory centre, which provoke hyperpnoea and which terminates into speedy elimination of CO_2.
  4. Respiratory distress (dyspnoea) at the beginning of exercise has been said to be due to lactacidaemia and this dyspnoea disappears suddenly (second wind) due to adaptation and partly due to readjustments in cardio-pulmonary apparatus.
- The lactic acid level in the blood during mild exercise (walking) does not rise above the resting value of 15 mg/100 ml. This means that it is disposed of as quickly as it is formed. It does not accumulate in muscle tissue. In vigorous exercise its level increases up to 50 to 200 mg/100 ml and it is because of the fact that mechanism for oxidising it or reconverting it to glycogen are overloaded.

Respiratory Changes

1. Violent breathing is the primary effect. The first event is increase in frequency and depth of breathing; from normal resting 16–22 to 50 or more per minute. In untrained persons the dyspnoea often limits the ability to perform hard work. Athletic training is partly a matter of development of respiratory responses to exercise. The ventilatory response to exercise often begins before the exercise starts which is due to cortical stimulation of the breathing. Almost as soon as the exercise actually starts, there is a sharp rise in the minute ventilation, after which it levels off if the exercise is moderate. After the exercise ceases, the minute ventilation begins to decline until it reaches the resting level.

2. Physical exercise $\xrightarrow{\text{Blood changes}}$ Hyperpnoea
Thus rise in CO_2 tension; the fall in O_2 tension and decrease in pH are factors which stimulate respiratory centre and peripheral chemo-receptor

which causes increase in depth and frequency of the respiratory movements.

3. Hyperventilation seen in beginning and during the exercise may also be due to afferent nerve signals from exercising joints and muscles.
4. The rise in ventilation which occurs in steady state of exercise is closely related to the increase in metabolic rate. The fact that in moderate exercise the arterial blood gas pressure don't alter appreciably from their resting values suggests that the hyperpnoea of exercise can be thought of as a compensating device tending to minimise the changes that the higher metabolic rate would otherwise cause.
5. Second wind: At the beginning of moderate-severe exercise (long distance run); the breathing becomes difficult, but after sometime this discomfort disappears so called 'subject has taken second wind.' At the same time sweating may occur and body temperature may rise, but RQ usually falls.
6. Exercise effect is due to increase in metabolic CO_2 and partly due to liberation of lactic acid which displaces CO_2 from bicarbonate and this additional CO_2 causes stimulation of respiratory centre. In time, when this additional CO_2 is eliminated by this vigorous breathing and the circulatory adjustments to meet the demands of exercise are completed, less lactic acid reaches the blood, and body reaches a steady state in which least discomfort is felt in respiration.

Other Changes

- In moderate and severe exercise the body temperature rises. After cessation of exercise, the body temperature drops back slowly. In moderate exercise the rise may be 1–2°C while in maximal exercise it may rise to several degrees and fever so produced can limit the exercise.
- Heat loss is increased by
  - i. Evaporation of water in the expired air by increased pulmonary ventilation;
  - ii. Evaporation of water on skin (sweating),
  - iii. Increased convection by the movement of exercising parts.
- The increase in body temperature facilitates the dissociation of oxyhaemoglobin and accelerates metabolic processes, thereby aiding the adaptation of subject to the conditions of exercise.
- Sweat secretion is also increased during exercise and this sweat is vaporised which constitutes the major path for heat loss.
- Body temperature rises due to activation of hypothalamic centre. Probably it cannot adjust the situation which is produced due to increased heat production.
- Glucagon level tends to rise during exercise.
- The increased energy output during exercise give rise to an increased production of heat since only some 25 per cent of the energy liberated is converted into mechanical work. The raised blood temperature results in cutaneous vasodilatation and an increased heat loss. In strenuous exercise the increased heat loss may be incapable of balancing the increased production of heat and body temperature may rise in several degrees, during the exercise.
- During exercise muscle working undergoes hypertrophy (but not hyperplasia). If workload on muscle is increased continuously; it causes persistence of hypertrophy. If this load is below maximum there is an increase in the density of the network of blood capillaries which are extending between the muscle fibres.
- The hyperaemia which accompanies the muscular contraction is due to some causative factors like increased PCO_2 tension, lactic acid, hydrogen ions, bradykinin, histamine, potassium ions, acetylcholine, adenosine, etc. Hyperaemia may occur also following a period of complete occlusion of arterial supply to a limb or following vigorous contractions (During exercise/vigorous contractions the blood flow increases markedly at rest but later on returns to control level; this phenomenon is called reactive hyperaemia).
- In 88 per cent of athletes, protein is found in urine during strenuous exercise. Since proteins are not normally found in urine, their presence suggests that during exercise, the glomerular capillary membrane becomes more permeable; which may be due to oxygen lack attendant on the decreased blood flow through the kidney.
- In moderate and severe exercise, lactic acid is found in significant amount in urine, in the form of sodium lactate. Large amounts of ammonia and phosphates and even erythrocytes have been found in the urine after exercise.
- In the resting subject plasma NEFA level is 500 μEq/l; moderate exercise doubles this value (non-esterified-fatty acids). If glucose is taken at half hourly interval during exercise; then these changes do not occur. Thus, if exogenous carbohydrate is not available, the muscle use NEFA released from fat stores by HGH (Human-growth-hormone).

- At rest, skeletal muscles receive about one litre of blood per minute (1/5th of cardiac output). During maximal exercise it may exceed upto 20 L/minute particularly to exercising muscles.

Sympatho-adrenal discharge induces an increase in muscle blood flow in anticipation of exercise, and adrenaline sustains the increased blood flow during and beyond the exercise. The response is augmented firstly by intrinsic nerves and then by accumulating metabolites, which also maintains some increase in blood flow during recovery from the exercise.

- Blood flow through the skin is controlled by the requirements of temperature regulation and may increase in heavy exercise to dissipate the heat generated by the exercising muscles. Renal and splanchnic vessels have only sympathetic nor-adrenergic vasoconstrictor fibres and they respond to adrenaline with vasoconstriction because they are provided with alpha-adrenergic receptors.

BODY CHANGES DURING MODERATE EXERCISE

1. *CVS:* Heart rate, cardiac output venous return increased, blood pressure raised because of vasoconstriction caused by stimulation of vasomotor centre.
2. *Respiration:* Increases/stimulated, After stopping exercise, it comes to normal level.
3. *Blood*: Cell count rises, acidosis, reduced alkali reserve, less than normal O_2 content.
4. *Urine:* Less volume, reaction acidic
5. *Skin:* Constriction of vessels and later on dilatation. Sweat-first reduced and then increased.
6. *Miscellaneous :* Quick recovery, fatigue delayed, oxygen debt nil, can be continued for a longer time.
7. *Notes:*
   - In late stages of moderate exercise the person feels more comfortable and respiratory distress passes away. This is second wind.
   - As exercise continues, rate of O_2 consumption rises along with blood supply. A state/time can come when the rate of O_2 supply exactly equalises the rate of lactic acid formation and two processes assume an uniform rate called 'steady state'.

ENDOCRINES AND EXERCISE

ADH

From hypothalamus/neurohypophysis is increased which makes more fluid and electrolyte available to meet with situation like excess sweating.

Pituitary

- Growth hormone increased which causes more protein synthesis in muscle.
- ACTH increased in endurance. Is needed for mobilisation of fats to provide energy.
- Prolactin increased. Needed to act like ADH on kidneys and to mobilise fats.
- Endorphins are released from several areas of brain. They stimulate food intake and relieve pain. It relieves mental stress and creates a sense of well-being.

Adrenal Cortex

Secretion of aldosterone is increased. It reduces loss of salt, and water in urine so fluid balance is maintained.

In prolonged and heavy exercise cortisol secretion is increased. It prepares the individual against stress by mobilising fats and amino acid.

Adrenal Medulla

Release of adrenaline and nor-adrenaline is increased when exercise is intense to raise the O_2 consumption by 60 per cent. They also mobilise fats and glucose and so fuel is kept available.

METABOLIC ADJUSTMENTS

- Immediate source of energy is ATP and its whatever amount which is consumed, is replenished by oxidative phosphorylation.
- For short episodes of intense activity (e.g. 100 meter sprint or weight lifting) almost entire energy comes from ATP and creatine phosphate during exercise (Breaking down of these substances is an anaerobic process). If this exercise is further continued or if it has become more intense then glycogen is also broken down during exercise but it is an aerobic process. If it is further continued then extent of aerobic metabolism increases and quantity of lipids as fuel increases.
- At any given glucose concentration, the rate of glucose uptake into muscle is enhanced by muscular contraction and this effect does not depend on an increase in insulin concentration. This phenomenon is of practical importance in the management of diabetes mellitus.

FITNESS V/S UNFITNESS

- Physiologically a person is fit who has. Lower O_2 consumption for a given task, low pulse rate during work, large stroke volume, low blood lactate, quick return of BP and heart rate to normal levels after completion of exercise, Late onset of exhaustion, etc. Opposite is true for unfit person.
- Anatomical fitness may require a person to be of a certain height or weight, or have specified dimensions of various parts of the body.

At present time physical fitness measures merely the ability to pass physical fitness tests.

We have methods of measuring the maximum efforts that may be tolerated for a short time, we can determine what constitutes an overload, but we are unable to predict how long the human machine will be able to carry a normal load, we cannot even say how long it can carry a moderate over load. The best we can hope for is a measure for actual accomplishment and present perfection of adjustment—Schneider 1923.

BIBLIOGRAPHY

1. Bernardo A. Houssay Human Physiology.
2. Bevegard BS, Shephered JT. Regulation of circulation during exercise. Phy Rev 1967;47:178-213.
3. Blmoqvist CG, B Saltin. Cardiovascular adaptation to physical training. Ann Rev Phy 1983;45:169-89.
4. Bristow JD, et al. The influence of ventilation CO_2 and hypoxia on Baroceptor reflex in man. J Phy 1968;198:102-103P.
5. Bristow JD, et al. Changes in baroceptor cardiac reflex exercise. J Phy 1969;201:106-107P.
6. CCN VASS. A synopsis of Physiology, Fifth edition. 1961.
7. Chapman CB (Ed) Physiology of Muscular Exercise. American Heart Association Monograms No. 15-Circulation Research 1967;22: Suppl 1-11 to 1-28.
8. Clausen JP. Effect of physical training on cardiovascular adjustments to exercise. Phy Rev 1977;57:779-815.
9. Cunningham JC. Some quantitative aspects of regulation of human respiration in exercise. British Medical Bulletin 1963;19:25-30.
10. De Vries HA. Physiology of exercise London Staplas press 1967.
11. Dexter L, et al. J applied physiol 1951;3:439.
12. Donald DE. Myocardial performance after excision of extrinsic cardiac nerves in dog. Cir Res 1974;34:417-24.
13. Donald DE, Shephord JT. Response to exercise in dogs with cardiac denervation. Amer J Phy 1963;205:393-400.
14. Dripps RD, JH Comroe. Amer J of Physiol 1947;149:43.
15. Falls HB (Ed.). Exercise physiology. New York. Academic press 1968.
16. Frick MH. Coronary implication of haemodynamic changes caused by physical training. Amer J Cardiology 1968;22:417.
17. Gollnick PD, et al. Enzyme activity and fibre composition in skeletal muscle of untrained and trained men. J APP Phy 1972;33:312-19.
18. Hammond HLFC, et al. Association of decreased myocardial β receptors and chronotropic response to isoproterenol and exercise in pigs following chronic dynamic exercise. Cir Res 1987;60:720-26.
19. Higginbotham MB, et al. Regulation of stroke volume during submaximal and maximal upright exercise in normal man. Cir Res 1986;58:281-91.
20. Margaria R (Ed). Exercise at altitude Amsterdam: Excerpta Medica foundation 1967.
21. Morehouse LE, Miller At. Physiology of exercise (4th ed) St. Louis Mosby 1963.
22. Nicholas Sperelakis, Robert O. Banks (Ed) Physiology - Little Brown and Co. Boston/Toronto/London 1993.
23. Ogden E, Shock N. Proc Soc Exper Biol and Med 1935;33:5.
24. Plotnick GD, et al. Use of the Frank Starling Law during submaximal versus maximal upright. Exercise. Amer J Phy 1986;251:H. 1107-5.
25. Willmore JH. Acute and chronic physiological responses to exercise. In E.A. Amsterdam, JH Wilmore and A Ndemaria (Eds), Exercise in Cardiovascular Health and Disease. New York, Yorke Medical Books 1977;53-69.

UNIT 2

Just Going Through

The study of physics and very simple biochemical processes is deeply involved in medical science. This is correct time to just go through them.

General Physiology

11 Basic: Biophysical Concepts

OSMOSIS

i. If a layer of water separated from sugar solution by a semi-permeable membrane (which will allow only water molecules to pass but not the sugar molecules; so it acts like semi-permeable one), it is observed that (sugar molecules being impermeable) more water molecules will pass from water layer into sugar solution. Due to this, the volume and level of sugar solution will rise, which will raise the hydrostatic pressure of the sugar solution and this increased pressure, will force more and more water molecules to pass out of the sugar solution. Thus, a time comes when movement of water molecule on either side will be same, so that no further alteration of volume will take place. More clearly, at this stage the hydrostatic pressure of sugar solution exactly neutralises the attractive force of solution for water molecules. This force is osmotic or oncotic pressure. So osmosis means, *diffusion of water through a semi permeable membrane or distribution of water across cell membranes in living organisms.* It is depending on the number of solute particles in the solvent. Osmotic pressure means, *the amount of pressure which has to be applied on sugar solution in above example to prevent the movement of water molecule or, the force under which a solvent moves from a solution of lower solute concentration to a solution of higher solute concentration when a selective permeable membrane separates these solution or, osmotic pressure of a solution is the hydrostatic pressure which must be applied to that solution to exactly balance the osmotic transfer of solvent from body of pure solvent into the solution across a membrane which is permeable to the solvent but not to the solute.*

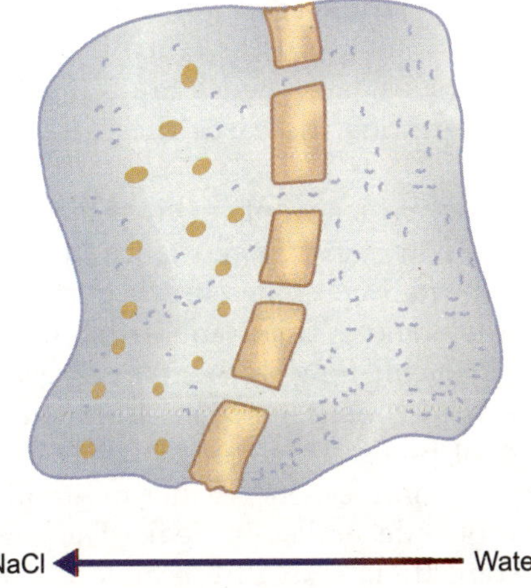

Fig. 11.1: Osmosis

ii. Osmosis is a simple diffusion process resulting from a difference in the chemical potential of the solvent (usually water) on the two sides of a membrane. The only usefulness of osmotic pressure in connection with osmosis is as a measure of the tendency for osmosis to occur; so it should be noted that the osmotic pressure is in no way responsible for osmosis. If two solutions of the same osmotic pressure are placed in contact across a membrane, osmosis will not take place; if the osmotic pressure are different, osmosis will occur, and the flow will be from the solution of lower osmotic pressure to that of higher osmotic pressure and will be in general proportional to the difference in osmotic pressure. For many biological purposes it is preferred to use the term 'osmolar concentration' which is defined as, the concentration, in moles per litre, of an ideal solution of a non-electrolyte which would have the same osmotic pressure.

iii. Osmotic pressure does not depend upon the size of molecules but upon the total number of discrete particles per unit volume.

If two solutions separated by a membrane have the same osmotic pressure, they are called ***iso-osmotic***, one having lesser osmotic pressure is ***hypotonic***, while that having higher osmotic pressure is ***hypertonic***. The solution in which the size of the cell remains unchanged is called ***isotonic***.

Examples

1. Absorption from intestine.
2. Exchange, in capillary bed.
3. Reabsorption of cerebro-spinal fluid.
4. Regulation of urine formation.
5. Continuous osmotic exchange between plasma and red cells.
6. NaCl and other solutions are used for different purposes.

SHIFTING OF FLUID BETWEEN EXTRA AND INTRA-CELLULAR COMPARTMENTS : BASIC PRINCIPLES OF OSMOSIS

i. Let us assume a condition that—pure water on one side of cell membrane and a solution of sodium chloride on another side. This membrane is said to be semi permeable, i.e. water molecule pass through the cell membrane with ease while sodium chloride ions can pass with difficulty. In fact sodium chloride solution is a mixture of permeant water molecules and non-permeant sodium and chloride ions. So water is the most abundant substance to diffuse through cell membrane.

ii. In normal circumstances the balance on both the sides of membrane is nicely balanced and volume of the cell is maintained.

iii. Under some abnormal circumstances, a concentration difference exists for water so the cell either swells up because of entry of water into it, or it can be shrinked because of exit of water from it.

iv. In above example more water molecules will pass from water layer towards sodium chloride layer. This process of net movement of water caused by a concentration difference of water is called osmosis.

v. After sometime a pressure difference develops between these two sides and because of which either osmosis is stopped, or slowed, or reversed. This is called osmotic pressure.

vi. This osmotic pressure is determined by the number of particles per unit volume of the fluid and not the mass of the particle. So unit 'osmole is used to express the concentration and not the grams (one osmole is one gm molecular weight of undissociate solute).

A solution that has one osmole of solute dissolved in each kilogram of water is said to have an osmolality of one osmole per kilogram; and a solution having 1/1000 osmole dissolved per kilogram has an osmolality of one milliosmole per kilogram. The normal osmolality of extra- and intracellular fluid is about 300 milliosmoles per kilogram.

The term osmolarity is used which is osmolar concentration expressed as osmoles per litre of solution rather than osmoles per kilogram of water (osmolality). It is used because of the fact that there exists difficulty of measuring kilograms of water in a solution.

DIFFUSION

- The continual movement of molecules among each other in liquids or in gases is called diffusion. This occurs in the way that in a solution; one moving molecule strikes with a stationary molecule; so this gets kinetic energy to move and this second molecule strikes with the third and so on.
- As we already know, the cell membrane consists of lipid bi-layer with large number of protein molecules floating in the lipid. It is the lipid solubility of the substance which determines how rapidly a substance will move through the lipid bi-layer and also through protein channels. Water molecules are diffusing through the cell membrane in large amounts simply because of two reasons—one is water molecule is of small size and second is its kinetic energy is large enough.
- Now there are certain substances like sodium-potassium-hydrogen ions which penetrate this lipid layer less rapidly than water. Because cell also need these substances so they are entering the cell by crossing the cell membrane through a carrier and the process is called *'facilitated diffusion'* (*carrier mediated*). By this process glucose, amino acid are important substances which are diffused; of course insulin hormone increases the rate of facilitated diffusion.
- A substance which wants to cross the cell wall; first combines with a carrier substance (the substance to be transported combines itself on receptor site of carrier substance). This combination of substance + carrier molecule now crosses the cell wall and enter the cell. There the substance is dissociated from carrier because of two reasons—one is weak binding force of receptor and, second is thermal motion of attached molecule makes it weak. The carrier again comes outside to take a fresh molecule of the same substance.

- Factors affecting permeability of cell membrane :
  - Greater the thickness—less is diffusion.
  - Rate is directly proportional to number of channels per unit area.
  - Diffusion increases directly in proportion to temperature since greater is the temperature more is the thermal motion of molecules.
  - Greater is the lipid solubility—more is the diffusion rate.
  - The rate at which substances diffuse inward is proportional to the concentration of molecules outside. This further depends on concentration of molecules inside and number of molecules striking outside.
  - Another factor is area of membrane
    D = P X A
    D = Diffusion coefficient
    P = Permeability
    A = Total area
- Another way of diffusion is *simple diffusion* which is constituted by
  - *Selective permeability*, e.g. sodium channels (0.3 by 0.5 nanometer size)—their inner surface is strongly electronegative because of this they are pulled strongly as well as because of their small ionic diameter. So this channel is specifically selective for passage of sodium ions.
  - Another ion which transports is the potassium ion (0.3 by 0.3 nanometer, smaller than sodium) which is not negatively charged like sodium ions so they are not pulled away from water molecules that hydrate them.

Importance

- Mixing of food with digestive juices
- Exchange between plasma and red cells
- Intestinal absorption
- Exchange in capillary bed
- Admixture of gases in lungs
- Exchange in lung capillaries

GLOSSARY PART

Biological membranes: plasma membrane and intracellular. They are semi permeable and are dynamic too. They are made up of lipid and protein molecules held together by non-covalent interactions.

Diffusion: The movement of molecules from higher to lower concentration—or physical process which involves the transport of materials from a region of higher to a region of lower concentration to spread uniformly.

Osmosis: Diffusion of water through a differentially permeable membrane.

Isotonic solution: A solution equal in solute concentration to that of a cytoplasm of a cell. "No loss no gain for the cell."

Hypotonic solution: Lower solute (more water) concentration than cytoplasm of a cell. Leads to gain of water by the cell.

Hypertonic solution: Higher solute concentration (less water) than the cytoplasm of cell. Leads to loss of water from cell.

Active transport: Use of plasma membrane carrier protein to move particle from a region of lower to higher concentration. It requires energy because it opposes equilibrium.

Passive transport: It is a physical process which neither requires energy nor O_2 for transport of substances by the cell.

Sodium potassium pump: A transport protein in plasma membrane that moves sodium ion out of and potassium ion into animal cells. Important in nerve-muscle cells.

SUMMARY HIGHLIGHTS

The spontaneous admixture of the molecules of two substances in contact due to inherent molecular movement is diffusion.

ACTIVE TRANSPORT

- Generally the substances move from higher to lower concentration. But in some situations, large concentration of a substance is required in intracellular fluid inspite of the fact that it is present in minute quantity in extracellular fluid. This is true for potassium ions.
- Sodium is present in large quantity in extracellular fluid than in intracellular fluid. So it is necessary to keep low concentration of sodium inside.
- Now say if potassium ions are entering the cell from ECF; or sodium is coming out in ECF; this is say something against the motion/electric differences/pressure difference/concentration difference or uphill movement and so it certainly requires energy. This phenomenon is active transport.
- In "Primary active transport" the energy is obtained from breakdown of ATP, or some other high energy phosphate compounds. It is 'sodium-potassium-pump' which is functioning here. Through this potassium ions are moving from outside to inside; and sodium ions are moving from inside to outside.

This pump is responsible for maintaining sodium-potassium concentration difference across the cell membrane as well as for establishing a negative electrical potential inside the cell. It is essential to control the volume of cell, otherwise cell would have been burst.

- In secondary active transport the energy is obtained secondarily from ionic concentration gradient.
- This transport depends upon 'carrier protein.' It has receptor sites for binding sodium ions on inner side two receptor sites for binding potassium ions on outside; there is also binding sites for ATPase activity.
- This, pumps, three sodium ions (Na^+) to the outside of the cell; for every two potassium ions pumped to the interior. This pump is said to be electrogenic because it creates an electrical potential across the cell membrane as it pumps. When potassium moves outside which means more positivity is going out so negativity is created inside.
- Calcium pump has also been reported. Their concentration is extremely low in intracellular cytosol. There are two calcium pumps viz. (a) One pump Ca^{2+} outside the cell; and (b) Second, pumps Ca^{2+} into internal cellular organelles like mitochondria, or sarcoplasmic reticulum.
- As per requirement of body, to maintain homeostasis this active transport also gets saturated.
- Energy is obtained by breakdown of ATP and is generated by separate carrier proteins.

Primary Active Transport: At A Glance

- Carrier protein for Na-K-pump:- Following are the sites.

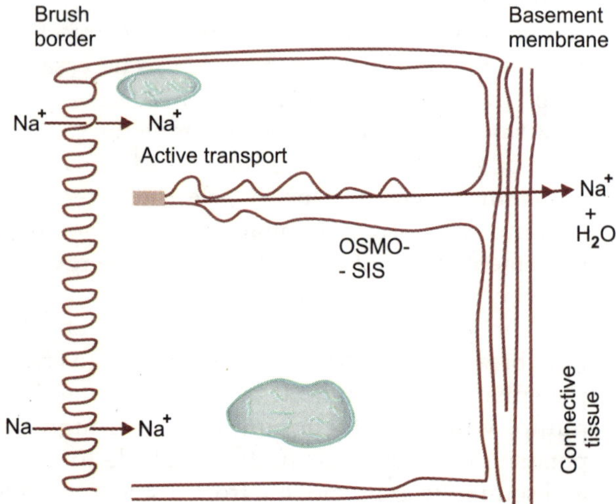

Fig. 11.2: Mechanism of active transport through cell

— 3 receptor sites for binding 3 sodium ions, on inner cytoplasmic surface of protein molecule.
— 2 receptor sites for binding 2 potassium ions, on outer surface of protein molecule.
— 1 site for ATP, near to sodium sites.

- *Mechanism:* Sodium and potassium ions get themselves attached to their binding sites. This activates ATPase which breaks ATP $\rightarrow$ ADP. This energy which is released leads to some positional change in the molecule of carrier protein. This causes dissociation and release of the ions causing potassium ion release inside cell while sodium ions outside the cell.
- Why sodium ion outside and potassium ion inside cell.... As mentioned above, the released energy leads to positional changes in carrier protein molecule. So by virtue of it, outer surface of molecule (potassium ions) now faces inner side of the cell, while inner surface of molecule (sodium ions) faces towards extra-cellular fluid.

Secondary Active Transport: At A Glance

- Carrier protein for sodium co-transport has two receptor sites on outer surface; one is for itself and another for molecule of other substances.
- The other substances which are carried by sodium include glucose, amino acid, chloride, urate, iron etc.
- Sodium amino acid transport—has five sets of carrier proteins in the cell membrane and each one carries different amino acids according to molecular weight.
- The mechanism is same as in primary active transport.

Sodium Counter Transport

- Calcium: In sodium calcium counter transport, both these ions move in opposite direction owing to some carrier proteins, i.e., sodium inwards and calcium outwards the cell.
- Hydrogen: In sodium–hydrogen–counter transport (in renal tubules) both are moving in opposite direction, i.e., sodium from lumen to tubular cell, hydrogen from tubular cell to lumen.
- Other counter transports are: "Sodium potassium," "calcium magnesium," "calcium potassium," "chloride bicarboante," "chloride-sulphate," "sodium-magnesium."

READ AND DIGEST

Q. In what way diffusion differs from active transport?

Ans.

- Diffusion means random molecular movement of substances; molecule by molecule. The energy is coming from normal kinetic motion of matter.

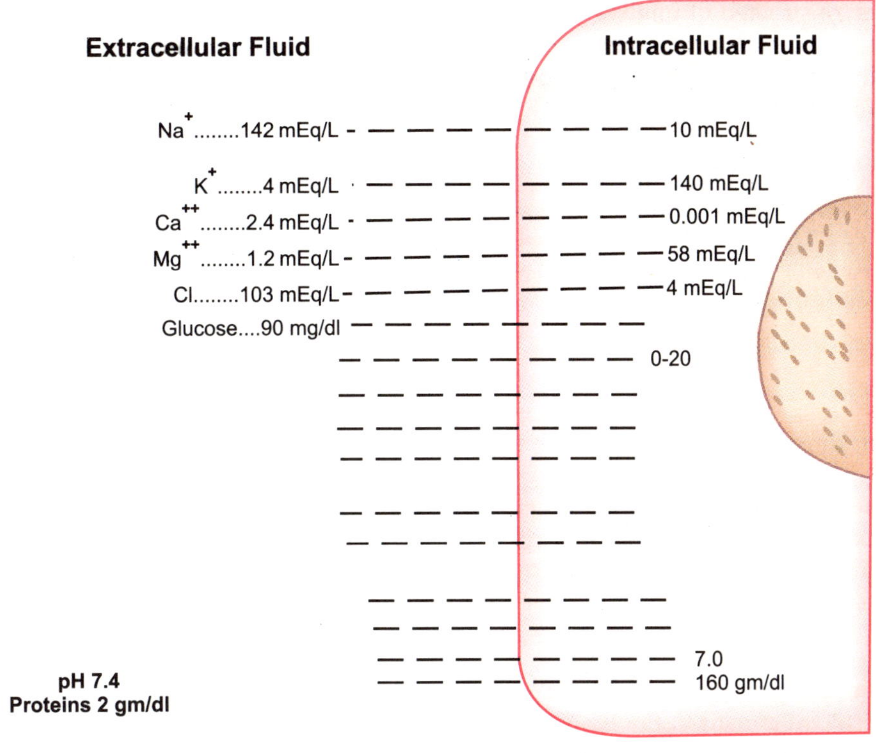

Fig. 11.3: Extra v/s intracellular fluid

- Active transport means movement of ions across the membrane, against an energy gradient, e.g. from a low concentration state to high concentration state.

Q. What do you mean by saturation of active transport?

Ans. Saturation means—limitation of rates at which chemical reactions take place. At large concentration of a substance, transport reaches to a maximum.

Q. Simple diffusion occurs through protein channels. It is said that gating of protein channels provides a means for controlling the permeability of channel. How?

Ans.

- When there exists strong negative charge inside the cell membrane, sodium gates remain closed. When this inside negative charge is lost then these gates open. This results into entry of large quantities of sodium ions inwards via sodium pores. Now the atmosphere of inside becomes positive, so potassium gates also open but the response is much slower (voltage-gating).
- The protein combines with another molecule. This combination leads to a conformational change in protein molecule; which acts on gate, i.e. closure or opening (ligand gating; substance binding is called ligand) Example is effect of acetylcholine on acetylcholine channel.

FILTRATION

i. Means, The passage of a substance in solution through a membrane by a mechanical force. By means of it, suspended materials can be separated from the fluid in which they are suspended.

ii. When a mixture of sand in a water solution of NaCl is placed upon a sheet of filter paper, the hydrostatic pressure forces the water and the NaCl dissolved in it through the pores of the filter, but the suspended matter sand, is retained by the filter.

Greater the hydrostatic pressure and larger the surface of the filter to which the material is exposed, the more fluid is squeezed through in a unit time.

iii. Filters differ in the size of their pores. In filter paper the holes are fairly large and allow suspended particles of minute size (e.g. bacteria) to pass through. Filters constructed of unglazed porcelain or similar material, e.g. Pasteur and the Berkfeld filters, through which the material is forced by a considerable amount of pressure, retain all bacteria with the exception of very smallest. But the pores of these filters are sufficiently large to allow the particles of a colloidal solution to pass through. Filters with exceedingly small pores that are able to restrain these last named particles can be made from collodion or cellophane; these are known as ultrafilters.

ULTRAFILTRATION

Is a kind of filtration through a jelly filter or any ultra-filter which serves to separate colloid solution from crystalloids and to separate particles of different size in a colloid mixture. It results from the exertion of a pressure on a solution. This pressure forces the solution through a membrane impermeable to one or more of the solutes.

Example

Absorption from small intestine, passage of water/salts/ foodstuffs, etc. from blood stream to the tissue fluid—hydrostatic pressure in the capillaries being higher than in the latter.

SURFACE TENSION

Always exists at the surface of separation between a liquid and a gas, between two immiscible liquids (e.g. water and oil) and between a liquid and a solid.

It is the manifestation of attracting forces in between atoms or molecules OR the energy with which the surface molecules closely adhere together is called surface tension.

Physiological Importance

- The formation of pseudopodia and process of phagocytosis by WBC are among those biological activities which can be explained on this basis.
- Bile salts reduce the surface tension of fat, converting it into an emulsion in intestine, which helps in digestion and absorption of fats.
- The globular shape of an oil drop in water, of the fat particles in milk, etc. is due to surface tension.

ADSORPTION

i. When a coloured solution of congo red or Methylene blue is allowed to pass slowly through bone black, glass wool, or absorbent cotton, the fluid loses its colour to a greater or lesser extent; the pigment clings to the surface of these substances; this is adsorption.

So

It is a sort of union by surface contact; or a form of combination in which substances adhere together on their surfaces.

ii. It is a reversible process. In the absorption of gas by liquid, the gas is uniformly distributed throughout the liquid; while in adsorption there is a local condensation of the adsorbed material upon the surface of the adsorber. Absorption involves the penetration of molecules into the body of a mass, whereas adsorption involves only their adherence to the surface.

iii. *Mechanism* involves following facts
   - Surface tension .. manifests adsorption which is developed from attraction of dissimilar molecules of two substances.
   - Electrical state : Similar electric charge repel two molecules while opposite charge attract each other. During adsorption process much kinetic energy is lost which appears as heat of adsorption.

     Furthermore residual valency is another factor governing adsorption process.

Physiological Importance

1. The combination of toxin and antitoxin by which they neutralise each other.
2. Enzyme and substrate are both colloid in nature and by this process they come in closer contact and interaction is hastened.
3. Various adsorption compounds are formed like lecithin with protein; blue compound formed by adding iodine with starch.

HYDROTROPY

- It is the property of making water insoluble substances soluble in water.
- Such hydrotropic substances form loose compounds with insoluble substances; and so they are made soluble and diffusible through membrane.
- Such substances include:- Bile salts and other compounds of cholic acid, lecithin and soaps of higher fatty acids; such substances are found in intestinal juice, blood plasma and in body fluids.
- Importance:- (a) cholesterol is kept in solution in bile, (b) In intestine insoluble soaps, fatty acids etc. make hydrotropic compounds with bile salts.

CHARACTERISTICS OF COLLOIDS

Gelation

Certain colloids are known as *emulsoids;* of these we may use the well known gelatin as an example. When solid gelatin is stirred up in hot water, a colloidal solution is formed; this is *hydrosol*. On cooling, the sol sets, or gels to a more or less firm mass, it is now called *hydrogel or gel*. In the apparently structureless gel, there is a more solid, or continuous, phase which forms a meshwork, in the interstices of this a more fluid, or dispersed, phase is held. In cream, an emulsion, the droplets of fat constitute a dispersed phase in water, the continuous phase; In butter, a colloid, water forms a dispersed phase in continuous phase of fat. Churning cream into butter is a phase reversal.

The gel of gelatin has a great affinity for the enclosed water; it requires heating at a temperature of 120°C for a considerable length of time or great mechanical pressure to drive the water from the gel. Some gels (e.g. gelatin) are reversible; other gels are irreversible in that the gel cannot be transformed into sol.

Diffusibility

Crystalloid like NaCl or cane sugar diffuses rapidly in water. In contrast, it is a familiar fact that a piece of soap left in a basin of water dissolves very slowly and an exceedingly long time is needed for the complete diffusion of the soap throughout the entire body of water. The same holds true for egg albumin. NaCl diffuses about 20 times faster than albumin. This is due to the larger size of the albumin molecule (34,000) as compared with that of NaCl (58.5). While crystalloids in solution (sugar/NaCl) diffuse as freely through gels as through water, colloids in solution don't; that is, a gel is impermeable to colloids in solution. This difference enables us to separate crystalloids in solution from colloids.

Dialysis

In a container, the bottom of which is formed by an irreversible gel (e.g. collodion, parchment or cellophane), let us place a water solution of sugar (or NaCl) and egg albumin. The membrane is freely permeable (allowing passage through) to water and sugar molecules, but it is impermeable to albumin. This vessel is properly suspended in a large vessel of water, which is essentially being renewed. After a sufficient length of time, practically all the sugar disappears and only albumin remains. By this process of dialysis the more diffusible material (dialyzable) is separated from the less diffusible and non-dialyzable. Graham called the former compounds crystalloids and latter colloids (kolla = glue).

The above property of a membrane is generally designated as semi-permeability. Some define a semi-permeable membrane as one permeable to the solvent and not to the material in solution, or the solute. Permeability, however, depends on - the nature of substance (size of molecule/substance) and nature of membrane. For any substance a membrane can be found to which this particular substance is impermeable and other membranes to which it is permeable. Hence, the term selective permeability is more appropriate.

OTHER WAYS OF TRANSPORT

Exocytosis

- Process by which substances are expelled out from cell, without passing through cell membrane.
- Hypothetically → secretory vesicles in cytoplasm have a secretory substance. This vesicle approach the cell membrane and fuse with it. Then contents of the vesicles are released out of the cell.

Endocytosis

- Process by which substances enter the cell without passing through the cell membrane.
- In the pits, present in surface of cell membrane there is receptor protein (clathrin) and this whole is called "receptor coated pits."
  — *Pinocytosis*: (a type of endocytosis/cell drinking)
    ⇒ It's the only means by which most large macromolecules (e.g. protein molecule) can enter the cell.
    ⇒ The protein molecules attach to specialised receptors on the surface of membrane. Once protein molecule bind with receptor, surface property of membrane changes. This causes invagination of entire pit, which then breaks away from surface of the cell forming a pinocytic vesicle inside cytoplasm. Energy is supplied by ATP and calcium ions are also required which are present in extracellular fluid.
  — *Phagocytosis:* described with section dealing with blood.

ISOTOPES

These are substances, which, though differing in masses, occupy the same place in the periodic classification of elements and are chemically indistinguishable.

Definition

Isotopes are atom of chemical element which have the same number of planetary electrons as the normal atom but more or less neutrons in the nucleus. They have the same chemical properties, because these are dependent upon the number of electrons, which is the same in all atoms. The physical properties on the other hand are different because the atomic mass of each isotope differs from that of the normal atom because of different number of neutrons in the nucleus.

Isotopes are atoms of the same elements whose nuclei contains different number of neutrons, but the same number of protons (Iso = equal; topos = space).

Radioactive Isotopes

Can be prepared by bombarding an atom on a cyclotron, or by bombarding a normal atom with neutrons in an atomic pile so as to eliminate one or more neutrons from its nucleus. These isotopes emit β or γ radiation, or positrons. By measuring the intensity of radiation in a Geiger-Muller counter or some other device, it is possible to detect and to estimate the concentration of isotope. The stability of radioactive isotope is measured by time taken for its radiation to lose half its initial activity, this is known as half life. Thus, half life of P^{32} is 14.3 days and K^{42} is 12.4 hours; C^{14} is 5.720 years, ^{11}C is 21 minutes.

PHYSIOLOGICAL APPLICATION

A. Therapeutic
B. Diagnostic

Therapeutic (Treating Cancer)

i. Teletherapy sets = Co^{60}, Ir^{192}
ii. Needles and tubes = Ra^{226}, Co^{60}, Au^{198}, tantalum wire
iii. Solution I^{131}, for Hyperthyroidism and cancer thyroid P^{32} Leukaemia, Polycythaemia vera.
iv. Colloidal solution—Gold^{198}—for pleural and peritoneal effusion
v. Yitrium 90—Pallets for pituitary implant
vi. Strontium 90—for eye applicator
vii. Cobalt 60—for Retinoblastoma (eye tumour)

> Any substance which emits out ionising radiations like α, β or γ rays is called radioactive. An isotope which is radioactive is called a radioactive isotope.

Diagnostic

History

Schoenheimer is pioneer in this study. Urey (1932) is said to be the discoverer of deuterium D. Havesy (1923) realised first of all the importance of isotopes in various investigatory procedures.

Importance

i. They are used in study of metabolic processes.
ii. Radio-nuclides are commonly used in radiotherapy. But the difficulties are:
   a. They are prepared with a difficulty,
   b. The forms in which they are prepared are very limited;
   c. Special skills are required.

- The principal use of isotopes in biological work has been as *labels*. If it is desired to trace the fate of a particular atom in a compound, or of a particular compound, that atom or compound may be labelled by replacing it with or incorporating into it an identifiable isotope. Thus, in one of the early applications of tracer technique, fatty acid molecules were labelled by incorporating deuterium into their structure. They were then fed to animals and deuterium was traced by analysing tissues and excreta for deuterium. Similar experiments have been performed with C^{14}, N^{14}, O^{18}, P^{32}, S^{35} and other isotopes.
- The success of tracer technique depends on the enrichment of a compound or a solution in a particular isotope, i.e., the isotope must be present in a concentration significantly greater than its usual one. When a stable isotope occurs in relatively large amount (Cl^{37}), its usefulness as a tracer is correspondingly reduced.
- The success of tracer technique also depends on detectability of the isotope. In the case of radioactive isotopes, detection depends on the emission of radiation, which may be detected by the ionisation it produces, or by its action on a photographic plate. The most widely used device for the detection of radiation is the Geiger-Muller counter.

QUALITIES OF AN ISOTOPE FOR EFFECTIVE RADIOACTIVE TRACER:

i. It must produce radiation in sufficient intensity for counting.
ii. Isotope must be sufficiently stable to be present in appreciable concentration at the end of an experiment. Stability is expressed in terms of half life which means the time required for one half of the particle to undergo disintegration. Many isotopes are known with half lives so short as to render them useless as tracers. C^{14} having long half life permits extensive manipulations without fear of loss, and its radiations are sufficiently strong to count.

BIBLIOGRAPHY

1. Agnew WS. Voltage regulated sodium channel molecules. Ann Rev Phy 1984;46:517.
2. Finkelstein A, et al. Ann Rev Phy Osmotic swelling of vesicles. 1986.

Table 11.1: Diagnostic isotopes

Functions		*Isotope used*
1. Thyroid functions		I^{131}, I^{132}
2. Haematology	RBC survival	Cr^{51}
	Blood volume	Cr^{51}
	Iron utilisation	Fe^{59}
	vitamin B_{12} in pernicious anaemia	Co^{60}, Co^{58}
3. GIT	Bleeding	Cr^{51}
	Fat absorption in malabsorption	I^{131}
	Ascites	Na^{24}
4. CVS	Blood flow	Na^{24}
	Cardiac output	Cr^{51}
5. Tumour localisation	Thyroid	I^{131}
	Brain	I^{131}
	Bone secondaries	Ca^{45}
	Skin melanoma	P^{32}
Miscellaneous	Kidney function	I^{131}

Table 11.2: Isotope and half-life

Radioactive Isotope		*Half-life*
1. Hydrogen	H^3	25 years
2. Carbon	C^{11}	20 minutes
	C^{14}	6×10^3 years
3. Potassium	K^{42}	12.4 hours
4. Iron	Fe^{59}	47 days
5. Sodium	Na^{29}	14 hours
6. Gold	Au^{198}	2.7 days
7. Radium	Ra^{226}	1600 years
8. Iodine	I^{131}	8 days
	I^{132}	2 hours
9. Calcium	Ca^{45}	153 days
	Ca^{47}	47 days

3. Haas M. Properties and diversity of Na-K-Cl cotransporters. Ann. Rev Phy 1989;51:443.
4. Haynes DH, et al. Computer modelling of Ca^{2+} pump function of Ca^{2+} Mg^{2+} ATPase of sarcoplasmic reticulum. Phy Rev 1987;67:244.
5. Jackobson K, et al. Lateral diffusion of protein in membrane. Ann Rev Phy 1987;49:163.
6. Kaplan JH. Ion movements through sodium pump. Ann Rev Phy 1985;47:535.
7. Lauger P. Dynamics of ion transport system in membrane. Phy Rev 1987.
8. Lauger P. Dynamics of ion transport system in membranes. Phy Rev 1987;67:1296.
9. Macey RL. Amer J Phy 1984;246:C 195.
10. Schatzmam HJ. Calcium pump of surface membrane and of sarcoplasmic reticulum. Ann Rev Phy 1989;51:473.
11. Verner K, et al. Protein translocution across membrane. Science 1988;241:1307.

12 Membrane Physiology

The physiologist is most concerned with action potential because the electrical phenomenon which accompanies the stimulation of cells and tissues enables him to visualise and study such activity.

- Towards the end of eighteenth century *Galvani* demonstrated the existence of electrical phenomenon in living tissues.
- When a nerve or muscle is injured and the damaged part is joined to the intact surface by a circuit in which there is a sufficient but a sensitive galvanometer, the injured part is found to be electronegative with respect to the parts that are undamaged. This is the injury or demarcation potential. It is due to the existence of an electromotive force in the intact membrane *the membrane resting potential*, the protoplasm being negative and external fluid positive. It diminishes in approximately exponential form with distance from injury.
- When a cell is stimulated and an excitatory state is evoked, the point stimulated becomes electronegative with respect to the parts at rest. A negative variation spreads like a wave over the whole surface of a cell; this is *action potential*, or more precisely the *spike potential*, of the propagated excitatory state. It travels at a definite speed-100 m/sec.
- When an excitable cell is stimulated and enters into activity, the membrane potential is reversed. The inside of resting cell is negative to the external fluid by 50 to 100 mV. This reversal is attributed to a sudden change in the membrane which becomes highly and specifically permeable to sodium during rising phase of spike potential. During the falling phase permeability for potassium increases and cell loses K^+. During the recovery period the membrane is repolarised but cell cannot respond to stimulation until repolarisation has reached to a certain level (*refractory period*).
- The axons are cylindrical fibres capable of conducting electrical impulses. In resting state it is in a highly polarised state; 75 mV (negative) inside. This is because K^+ is 20 to 50 times more concentrated in the axon and Na^+ is only about 1/20th of plasma. Na^+, K^+ and Ca^{++} are permeable through the membrane, but in the resting state, they don't show much movement in either direction. The principal anions inside - proteins and nucleic acids are impermeable. To maintain this differential concentration, the sodium pump operates. Na^+, K^+, -ATPase on the axon membrane pumps out $3Na^+$ for every $2K^+$ which enter the cell. One ATP molecule is broken during the process.
- Any stimulus which can cause a depolarisation and reduce the electric potential at a point to below - 50 mV (from - 75 mV) will trigger a series of event which will result in an action potential. The permeability of membrane to Na^+ greatly increases and Na^+ rushes into the cell due to its higher concentration in the plasma. It may actually cause an overshoot so that electric charge may become + 30 mV. This +ve charge will repel further entry of Na^+ into the cells, the permeability of membrane to Na^+ falls rapidly and Na^+, K^+, -ATPase is stimulated to pump out Na^+ to restore electric potential to the basal level.
- The resting membrane potential is due to the polarised condition of the membrane separating the inside negative charge from the positive charge outside. It is represented by minus (-) sign which shows inside negativity in relation to positivity outside the cell membrane.
- Then begins depolarisation, during which the membrane suddenly begins to be very much permeable to sodium ions which leads to influx of sodium ions to interior of axon.
- Within 10,000th of a second of sodium permeability, the sodium channels begin to close and potassium

channels open more than normal. The rapid diffusion of potassium ions to the exterior re-establishes the normal negative resting membrane potential. This is repolarisation.

- When sodium channel opens, it is increasing the sodium permeability of the membrane from 500 to 5000 folds.
- Membrane potential becomes even more negative than the original resting membrane potential for a few milliseconds after the action potential is over. This is called *positive after potential*. Its causes lie in the fact that many potassium channels remain open for several milliseconds after completion of repolarisation process. This allows excess potassium ions to diffuse out of the nerve fibre, leaving an extra deficit of positive ions inside, which means more negativity.
- A calcium pump also exists besides sodium pump. Voltage gated calcium channels have been reported. When these open, both calcium and sodium ions flow to the interior of the fibre (so they are sometimes called calcium-sodium channels). They are called slow channels because they require 10 to 20 times more to be activated as compared with fast sodium channels.
- When there is deficiency of calcium ions, the sodium channels are activated by very little increase of the membrane potential above the normal resting level. So the nerve fibre becomes highly excitable, discharging repetitively without any provocation rather than remaining in resting state.
- The calcium ion bind to the exterior surfaces of the sodium channel protein molecule. Their positive charge alter the electrical state of channel protein itself, and thus increasing the voltage level required to open the gate.
- Calcium channels are numerous in smooth and cardiac muscles.
- Like above mentioned ions; the chloride ions also leak through the resting membrane. Their diffusion is about one half as great as diffusion of potassium ions. They function passively in this process. It has been also evident that permeability of chloride leak channels does not change significantly during the action potential.
- The vicious cycle (positive feedback) ... Whenever there is an initial rise in membrane potential from -90 mV upwards towards zero level; the voltage gated sodium channels are opened up. This results into rapid inflow of sodium ions, which causes still further rise of membrane potential—which further opens more sodium channels, and in this way this vicious cycle proceeds. After sometime of course, these channels are inactivated and potassium channels are opened up. There exists a particular threshold for stimulation, i.e. an action potential will not occur until initial rise in membrane potential is great enough to create the above mentioned vicious cycle. Usually a sudden increase in membrane potential of 15 to 30 mV is required.
- It has been already stated that during depolarisation, influx of sodium ions takes place; while repolarisation consists of efflux of potassium ions. The number of impulses depend on various factors like size of nerve fibre, etc. The sodium influx and potassium efflux are returned to their original state by Na^+ K^+ pump which requires energy and that is supplied from ATP. The degree of activity of Na^+ K^+ ATPase pump is strongly stimulated when excess sodium ions accumulate inside the cell membrane.
- The velocity of conduction in nerve fibre varies from 0.5 m/sec. to 120 m/sec. It varies with fibre diameter (myelinated nerves); and with square root of fibre diameter (unmyelinated fibres).
- In saltatory conduction; the insulance is afforded by myelin membrane and membrane capacitance is decreased which allows repolarisation process to take

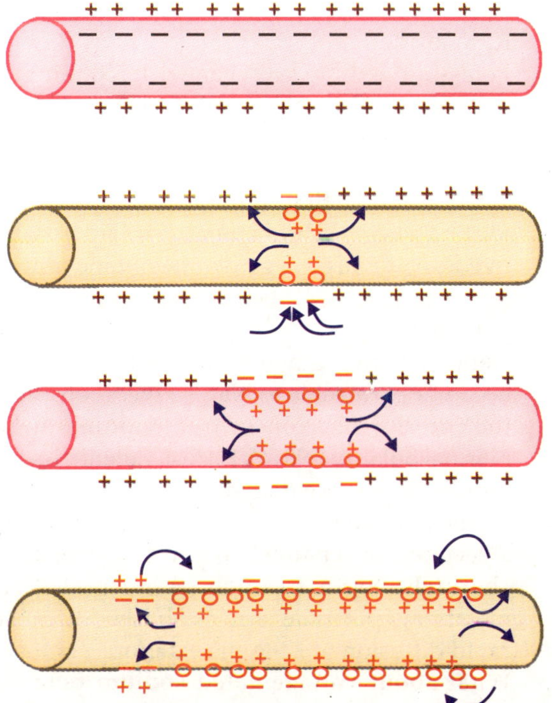
Propagation of Action Potential

Fig. 12.1: Propagation of action potential

place with little transfer of ions. This explains the occurrence of repolarisation rapidly even before beginning of efflux of potassium ions. This further explains conduction of nerve impulse in myelinated fibre accompanied by voltage gated Na^+ channels.

- Factors inhibiting excitability include:
  - Low potassium ion concentration in extracellular fluid since it directly affects permeability of K^+ channels.
  - High calcium ion concentration in extracellular fluid; since it decreases permeability.
  - Local anaesthetics (procaine, tetracain) by causing difficulty in opening of Na^+ channels.
- The only common type of meter that is capable of responding accurately to the very rapid membrane potential changes is cathode ray oscilloscope.

To record monophasic action potential a micro pipette electrode is inserted into interior of the fibre. The changes in potential inside the fibre are recorded as the action potential spreads.

READ AND DIGEST: MEMBRANE POTENTIAL

1. **What makes the resting membrane potential?**
   a. Sodium potassium pump: This powerful electrogenic pump; is pumping more positive charges outside than inside (3 Na^+ to outside for each two K^+ to inside).
   b. Potassium sodium leak channel: It is one hundred times more permeable for K^+ than Na^+. This RMP in skeletal muscle fiber is about the same as that in large nerve fiber - 90 mV.
2. **What about 'action' potential?**
   a. Resting stage — The membrane is said to be polarized due to large negative membrane potential. Actually it is RMP before beginning of action potential.
   b. Depolarization stage — Membrane suddenly becomes permeable to Na^+, so these ions flow to the interior of axon in tremendous number. Normal polarity (-90 mV) is lost. Potential is rising rapidly in positive direction.
   c. Repolarization stage — Within a few, 10,000th of a second Na^+ channels begin to close, and K^+ channels begin to open. A normal resting membrane potential is re-established because of rapid diffusion of K^+ to the exterior.
3. **What about voltage gated sodium potassium channels?**
   a. Na^+ channel has got two gates; (i) activation gate near the outside of channel and (ii) inactivation gate near the inside. When -90 mV potential rising toward zero and reaches some where -70 and -50 mV; conformational change occurs and activated gates are opened, leading to pouring of Na^+ inwards, leading to increased sodium permeability many times.
   b. After 10,000th of a second, the above channel is closed or inactivated gate' will not re-open till membrane potential returns to original resting membrane potential.
   c. K^+ channels is closed during resting state. When RMP rises from -90 mV towards zero, these channels open just at the same time that Na^+ channels begin to close because of inactivation.
4. **What is 'Electrotonic potential'?**
   The principle is that sub-threshold stimuli do not produce an action potential, but they have an effect on membrane potential. This can be demonstrated by placing recording electrodes within a few mm of a stimulating electrode and then sub-threshold stimuli is applied. Such a procedure with cathode caused localised depolarising potential change which rises and decays with time, conversely an anodal current produces a hyperpolarising potential change of similar duration. These changes are called 'Electrotonic potential' (Catelectrotonic - means produced at cathode; and anelectrotonic means those at anode).
5. **What is compound action potential?**
   In mixed nerves, (contrast to single axon), there appears multiple peaks in the action potential.
   Its shape is because of the fact that a mixed nerve is made up of different fibers having different speed of conduction. So on stimulating all the fibers, the activity in fast conducting fibers arrives at recording electrodes sooner than the activity in slower fibers.
6. **The term positive after potential is misnomer. Explain?**
   It is even more negative than original resting membrane potential. The answer lies in 'history' when first potential measurements were made on outside of the nerve fiber membrane, than inside. On recording it on outside, the potential is of positive record.

BIBLIOGRAPHY

1. Agnew SW. Voltage regulated Na^+ channels molecules. Ann Rev Phy 1984;45:517.
2. Armstrong CM. Sodium channels and gating currents. Phy Rev 1981;61:644.
3. Bretag AH. Muscle chloride channels. Phy Rev 1987; 67.

4. Deweer P, et al. The voltage dependence of Na^+K^+ pump. Ann Rev Phy 1980;50:225.
5. DiPolr R, Beauge L. The Ca^+ pump and Na^+ Ca^+ exchange in squired axons. Ann Rev Phy 1983;45:313.
6. Hodgkin AL, Huxley AF. Quantitative description of membrane current and its application to conduction and excitations in nerve. J Phy (Lond) 1952;117:500.
7. Kaplan JH. Ion movements through Na^+ pump. Ann Rev Phy 1985;47:535.
8. Latorre R, et al. Voltage dependent channels in lipid bilayer membrane. Phy Rev 1981;61:77.
9. Latorre R, et al. K^+ channels gated by voltage and ions. Ann Rev Phy 1984;46:485.
10. Miller RJ. Mutiple Ca^+ channels and neuronal functions. Science 1987;235:46.
11. Rogarh R. Sodium channels in nerve and muscle membrane. Ann Rev Phy 1981;43:711.
12. Ross WN. Changes in intracellular Ca^{2+} during neuron activity. Ann Rev Phy 1989;51:491.
13. Schwartz W, et al. Calcium activated K^+ channels in erythrocytes and excitable cells. Ann Rev Phy 1983;45:359.
14. Tsiea RW. Calcium channel in excitable cell membrane. Ann Rev Phy 1983;45:341.
15. Windhager EE, Taylor A. Regulatory role of intracellular calcium ions in epithelial Na transport. Ann Rev Phy 1983;45:519.
16. Zigmond RE, et al. Influence of nerve activity on macromolecular content of neurones and then effector organs. Ann Rev Phy 1981;43:673.

QUESTION BANK

1. **Define threshold, spike and action potential. Discuss their ionic basis. Give difference between receptor and action potential.** (Raj. Univ. 1981 M.D.)
2. **What is Gibb's Donnan equilibrium. Mention various physiological phenomenon based on it.** (Raj. Univ. 1994, M.D.)
3. **Enumerate the various forces, producing movement of substances across cell membrane.** (Raj. Univ. 1980, 1997, M.D.)
4. **Short notes**
   a. Ageing (Raj. Univ. 1996, M.D.)
   b. Nerve growth factor (Raj. Univ. 1995, M.D.)
   c. G. protein (Raj. Univ. 1995, M.D.)
   d. Biological rhythm (Raj. Univ. 1981, 1992, 2000, M.D.)
   e. Carriage of genetic information (Raj. Univ. 1990, M.D.)
   f. Samson Wright
   g. I. P. Pavlov
   h. Von Bekesy
   i. Sherrington
   j. Genetic code (Raj. Univ. M. D. 1985)
   k. Osmosis (Raj. Univ. 1984, M.D.)
   l. Stress Syndrome (Raj. Univ. 1983, M.D.)
   m. Standard deviation, (Raj. Univ. 1982, M.D.)
   Use of "P" value in statistical analysis (Raj. Univ. 2000, M.D.)
   n. Polarisation microscopy (Raj. Univ. 1980)
   o. Resting membrane potential (Raj. Univ. 1980, 2000, M.D.)
   p. Turner syndrome
   q. Surface tension (Raj. Univ. 1985, M.D.)
   r. Computers in medicine (Raj. Univ. 1979, M.D.)
   s. Cyclic AMP (Raj. Univ. 1979, M.D.)
   t. Mean, mode, median (Raj. Univ. 1989, M.D.)
   u. Hereditary diseases (Raj. Univ. 1986, M.D.)
   v. tRNA (Raj. Univ. 1989, M.D.)
   w. Axonal transport (Raj. Univ. 1986, M.D.)
5. **Show diagrammatically organization of a gene. Write briefly about transcription and post-transcriptional modification. Write a note on human-genome concepts.**
6. **Discuss various feedback mechanism of body.** (Raj. Univ. 1992, M.D.)
7. **Discuss the physiology of ageing.** (Raj. Univ. 1980, 1991, M.D.)
8. **Give an account of concept of homeostasis and its control.** (Raj. Univ. 1989, M.D.)
9. **Discuss the factors responsible for development of sexual characteristics. What is sexual differentiation. Describe biological fractions of sex chromosomes.** (Raj. Univ. 1988, M.D.)
10. **Describe Handerson-Hasselbach equation. Discuss various conditions which lead to acidosis and compensatory mechanism of the body for regulating pH in those situation.**
11. **Write an essay on normal and aberrant sex differentiation.**
12. **How diseases are produced due to genetic defects** (Raj. Univ. 1979, M.D.)
13. **Describe**
    a. Physiology of growth and its disorders (Raj. Univ. 1983, 1985, M.D.)
    b. Genetic control of protein synthesis in cells (Raj. Univ. 1986, M.D.)
14. **Write an essay on, Physiology is a synthetic science which applies physical and chemical methods to biology.** (Raj. Univ. 1984 M.D.)
15. **Write an essay on, Role of physiology in primary health care.** (Raj. Univ. 1983, M.D.)
16. **Discuss the mechanism of bio-electric potential.** (Raj. Univ. 1982, M.D.)
17. **Describe contribution of I.P. Pavlov to our knowledge of physiology.** (Raj. Univ. 1976, M.D.)
18. **Briefly describe the life and work of any one Indian physiologist who is internationally known, reputed and recognised.** (Raj. Univ. 2000, M.D.)
19. **Describe various ion channels. Discuss the single channel recording technique and give the advantages of the technique. Write briefly about some diseases caused by altered ion channels.** (BF, 2003/08, M.D.)

20. **Write short notes on:**
    a. Dihydropyridine receptor
    b. Resting membrane potential
    c. Microtubules. (BF, 2003/08, M.D.)
21. a. Describe the structure and functions of Lysosomes
    b. Endocytosis
    c. Amoeboid movement (BF, 2003/08, M.D.)
22. a. Codons and Anticodons
    b. Operon of the cell and its control
    c. Gating of protein channels. (BF, 2003/08, M.D.)

VIVA VOCE : BIOPHYSICS AND GENERAL PHYSIOLOGY

1. **What is diffusion ?**
   Molecules of gases (maximum), liquid (intermediate) and solids (least) are regularly in motion. When two substances are kept in contact the molecules of these substances will pass into each other till uniform admixture is attained. This spontaneous admixture of the molecules of the two substances in contact due to inherent molecular movement is named as diffusion.
2. **What are the factors effecting rate of diffusion ?**
   a. Concentration difference is directly related to diffusion rate.
   b. Diffusion rate is greater as the distance is short.
   c. Cross section area of site of diffusion is directly related to diffusion rate.
   d. Increase in temperature increases diffusion rate.
   e. Diffusion rate is inversely proportional to molecular weight.
3. **Can you give some examples of diffusion process ?**
   a. Mixing of food with digestive juices.
   b. Intestinal absorption of foodstuffs.
   c. Admixture of gases in lungs.
   d. Exchange in capillary bed.
   e. Exchange in lung capillary.
   f. Exchange between plasma and red cells.
4. **What is facilitated diffusion ?**
   Mentioned earlier, some substances which are not soluble in lipid matrix of cell membrane they diffuse through this process. Among this glucose (sugar) is the main substance. This process occurs through 'carrier substance', whose main function is to render glucose soluble in membrane. Amount of 'carrier substance' and 'rapidity of chemical reaction' are the two major factors governing this phenomenon.
5. **What is the main difference between 'facilitated diffusion' and 'active transport' ?**
   In facilitated diffusion phenomenon; substances are moving through carrier from high concentration to low concentration side; while in 'active transport' phenomenon opposite movement is also possible, i.e. active transport is a process of moving molecules uphill against a concentration gradient, which occurs by expanding metabolic energy taken from ATP mol.
6. **Name the hormone; increasing rate of glucose transport?**
   Insulin from islets of Langerhans of pancreas.
7. **What is 'osmosis' ?**
   Process of net diffusion of water molecules caused by a concentration difference through a semipermeable membrane is called osmosis.
8. **Process of osmosis is of great physiological importance. Give some examples?**
   a. Absorption process by intestine.
   b. Reabsorption of CSF.
   c. Regulation of process of urine formation.
   d. Principle of osmosis is playing a leading role in administration of iso-hypo and hypertonic solutions, saline purgatives, saline diuretics, etc.
9. **What do you understand by term 'adsorption' ?**
   It is actually union of two substances by contacting through their surfaces. So it is a form of combination in which substances adhere together on their surfaces.
10. **What do you understand by phenomenon of 'hydrotropy' ?**
    Some substances have the property of making water insoluble substances soluble in water. This is known as hydrotrophy.
11. **What is pinocytosis ?**
    It is the process by which cell membrane gets the ability to imbibe small amounts of substances from extracellular fluid. (intake of liquid material by the cell).
12. **Why phenomenon of sodium pump is said to be useful?**
    It is important because it prevents continual swelling of cells otherwise eventually cell may burst.

MULTIPLE CHOICE QUESTIONS : BIOPHYSICS AND GENERAL PHYSIOLOGY

1. **The facilitated diffusion of glucose is greatly increased by:**
   a. ADH
   b. Excess calcium ions
   c. Insulin
   d. Water [ ]
2. **The process of moving molecules uphill against a concentration difference is called:**
   a. Facilitated diffusion
   b. Active transport
   c. Osmosis
   d. Filtration [ ]
3. **Active transport of sugar mainly depends on -**
   a. Active transport of sodium
   b. Phagocytosis
   c. Pinocytosis
   d. Transport of amino acid [ ]

4. **Following hormones are controlling amino acid transport *except:***
   a. Insulin
   b. Glucocorticoids
   c. Estradiol
   d. Thymic hormone [ ]
5. **The process by which cell membrane acquires the ability to imbibe small amount of substances from extracellular fluid is known as:**
   a. Phagocytosis
   b. Pinocytosis
   c. Active transport
   d. Sodium pump [ ]
6. **Following are the causes of resting membrane potential *except:***
   a. Active transport of Na and K ions through membrane.
   b. Diffusion of Na and K ions through membrane.
   c. Imbalance of negative and positive charges on sides of membrane
   d. Hydrotrophy [ ]
7. **The membrane potential is returned back to its normal level after depolarisation. The main cause is:**
   a. Sodium pump
   b. Efflux of potassium ions
   c. Influx of K^+
   d. Release of Ca^{++} [ ]
8. **In cardiac muscle after depolarisation the potential remains in a steady state before repolarisation, for a little time which is called:**
   a. Spike potential
   b. After potential
   c. Rhythmicity
   d. Plateau [ ]
9. **The following are considered as transmitter substances *except:***
   a. Acetylcholine
   b. Norepinephrine
   c. Serotonin
   d. Acetyl cholinesterase [ ]
10. **Which of the following drugs is blocking transmission at neuro-muscular junction:**
    a. Epinephrine
    b. Norepinephrine
    c. Acetylcholine
    d. Curariform drugs [ ]
11. **Disease in which end-plate is unable to secrete sufficient quantity of acetylcholine is known as:**
    a. Poleomyelitis
    b. Parkinson disease
    c. Myaesthenia gravis
    d. Hydrocephalus [ ]

ANSWERS: MCQs

1 c 2 b 3 a 4 d 5 b 6 d 7 b 8 d 9 d 10 d 11 c

UNIT

3 Glamour of the Life

"Yes, it is the nerve which like a postman delivers the order of brain to the respective muscle—which is better classed as-effector. By its response (contraction/relaxation), it gives grace and glamour to the individual—Principles controlling neuromuscular system presents a paradox to patho-physiologists. Muscle is a unique organ since it is capable of converting stored chemical energy into mechanical energy to perform work in the cell. So now is the correct time to study—LOCOMOTION."

Locomotion

13 Contractile Tissue: Skeletal Muscle

There is no life without movement. The function of all muscle tissue is contraction and relaxation which brings about movement or work. These organs not only serve for locomotion but also carry out all major displacements of mass within the body. It has provided one of the best biological systems for understanding the relation between structure and function at the molecular level.

In adjusting the body to environmental changes, muscles as responding organs play a major part. All vital processes are dependent more or less upon muscular activity. By their contractile power, either the whole body is moved from one point in space to another as the need arises, or the adjustment is made by the movement of a limited part of the body in respect to the body itself or to the environment. Their importance is readily appreciated by the fact that they constitute 43 per cent of total body weight, contain more than one-third of all body proteins, and contributes about one half of the metabolic activity of the resting body.

Agonists: One set of muscles give the power for a particular movement (synonym = prime movers)

Antagonists: They oppose the agonists

Synergists : Group of muscles which assist the agonists.

CLASSES OF MUSCLES

A muscle consists of a large or smaller number of muscle fibres, or cells which constitute the structural units of a muscle.

Striated/skeletal or Voluntary Muscles

Here, the fibres are cross-striated. Their innervation is derived from somatic nerves and to a large extent they are under voluntary control. They account for some 43 per cent of the total body mass of an average man. It exhibits no automaticity. It contracts and relaxes much more rapidly than the other two types.

Unstriated or Smooth, or Visceral or Involuntary

Their fibres are devoid of cross striations. They are not subjected to the will and receive their innervation via autonomic nervous system. They are found in the walls of internal, or visceral organs (generally hollow organs).

They contain a reticular membrane system, which in terms of its ability is made to store and release Ca^{2+} and is analogous to the sarcoplasmic reticulum of skeletal muscle.

Smooth muscle cell contain thick myosin and thin actin containing filaments. However, here the thick and thin filaments are not organised into myofibrils or regular sarcomeres. There are no Z bands, but specialised cytoskeleton regions known as 'dense bodies or patches,' appear to serve as comparable structure for the attachment of thin filaments. The ratio of thin to thick filaments in smooth muscle (15 : 1) is considerably higher than that of striated muscle.

Most impressive characteristic of smooth muscle is its ability to maintain large forces at relatively low energy cost.

It is the most primitive. Its contraction is very slow and it contracts automatically (without need for stimuli from nervous system). It is associated with vegetative processes of the body, e.g. contraction of GIT, closing down of blood vessels, contraction of urinary bladder, stretching of eye lens in focussing.

Cardiac Muscle

This is involuntary and innervated by ANS and its fibres are imperfectly cross striated. It is a specialised muscle making up the mass of the heart. Individual cells are connected by protoplasmic bridges to form a *'syncytium,'* so that all the cells of heart muscle act together. It is also automatic and does not require an external nerve supply for its contraction.

A muscle is a mechanical device — it is an engine, capable of converting chemical energy into mechanical energy.

Table 13.1: Composition of muscle tissue

Component	%
Water	75%
Protein	20%
Fats	2%
Salts	1%
Nitrogenous material + carbohydrates...	2%

Protein

These are myosin, myoglobin and myogen. Myoglobin resembles 'haemoglobin.' It is found in sarcoplasm and imparts a red colour to it—so called dark muscles. The most abundant and of great interest is 'myosin' and is said to exist with another protein actin (actomyosin) and is main constituent of myofibrils.

Actomyosin is the contractile machinery of muscles. Protein molecule is made up of large number of amino acids.

Minerals

Na, Ca and Mg. Potassium phosphate is the principal salt. Others include ADP, ATP, hexose phosphate, certain phosphates etc.

SKELETAL MUSCLE : CIRCULATION

- Normally 4–7 ml/100 gm of muscle tissue/minute blood flows through the muscle. During exercise this may go as high as 30 ml/100 gm/minute.
- By application of plethysmographic techniques muscle blood flow can be measured;

Factors Affecting

i. *Nerves:* Innervated by both vasoconstrictor (coming from postganglionic sympathetics) and vasodilator fibres (coming from both parasympathetic and sympathetic postganglionic fibres). These effects are mediated by α, β, γ receptors.

ii. *Chemical:* Excess CO_2 leads to diminished blood flow. Hyperventilation increases forearm blood flow (5-10% CO_2 inhalation = no effect; only 30% is effective).

iii. Intra-arterial administration of potassium and magnesium ions increase forearm blood flow *(ionic effect)*.

iv. Administration of ADP, ATP, AMP increases forearm blood flow (effect of *metabolites*).

v. Administration of acetate, citrate and pyruvate increases forearm blood flow *(anions effect)*

vi. Bradykinin increases muscle blood flow

vii. Increased temperature, low O_2, local increase of CO_2, increased production of metabolites, high blood pressure, high potassium, etc. increase local muscle blood flow (*Local agents* - exercise)

viii. Muscle blood flow increases faithfully with increasing perfusion pressure.

ix. Adrenaline—both vasodilator (β receptor), vasoconstrictor (α receptor)
- Nor-adrenaline has only constrictor effect.
- Acetylcholine dilates muscle blood vessels.
- Muscle is supplied by branches of main artery. The arterioles give rise to meta-arterioles which break up into capillaries, which ultimately form venules and veins.

RED AND PALE MUSCLES

- There are two types of stripped muscle fibres—the white and the red. White fibres are thick, poor in sarcoplasm with nuclei exclusively under the sarcolemma and in large numbers near the end plate, cross striation is regular and well marked and longitudinal striation is not easily distinguished.
- The red fibres have abundant sarcoplasm with nuclei distributed all through the fibre; cross striation is irregular and poorly marked and longitudinal striation is outstanding. Red fibres have got more myoglobin and less cytochrome than white fibres.
- In man, both types are found in all muscles, but in certain muscles one or the other type predominates.
- The red fibres are considerably slower in their action and undergo fatigue less rapidly than the white fibres do. By these two characteristics the red fibres are well adapted for static, or postural contractions. Postural contractions are sustained contractions chiefly concerned in maintaining, for a considerable length of time, the position of the body in space (as in standing), or maintaining the position of a part of the body. Body posture is largely mediated by extensor muscles (antigravity of lower limb), they are well supplied with red fibres. On the other hand, phasic contraction, by which changes in position of body or a limb are brought about, are better served by the more rapidly acting white fibres. These fibres predominate in the flexor muscles.

The motor unit: All the muscle fibres innervated by a single motor nerve fibre are called motor unit. An average figure for all the muscles of the body can be considered to be about 100 muscle fibres to the motor unit.

Muscle tone: A certain amount of tautness (tension) has been observed in skeletal muscles even at rest. This is muscle tone. It results entirely from nerve impulses (Asynchronous γ-motor discharge) coming from spinal cord since skeletal muscles don't contract without an action potential.

Table 13.2: Differences between fast fibres and slow fibres

Fast fibres (White)	*Slow fibres (Red)*
• Much larger and longer fibres; so great strength of contraction.	• Small and short fibres and nerves innervating are also smaller.
• Contain extensive sarcoplasmic reticulum for discharge of Ca^{+2}. Less number of mitochondria.	• Greatly increased number of mitochondria
• Less extensive blood supply	• More extensive blood supply to supply extra oxygen.
• No such combination exists	• It is its combination with myoglobin which gives red appearance. Myoglobin $+O_2$ = reddish appearance.
• Adapted for rapid and powerful muscle contractions (jumping, running etc.)	• Adapted for prolonged and continuous muscular activity (athletes)

STRUCTURAL ASPECT: MUSCLE FIBRES

- Muscle fibres are giant cells formed by fusion of several mesenchymatic cells—the 'myoblasts'. They are enclosed in a thin structureless membrane–*sarcolemma*. This membrane is exclusively formed by myoblasts without participation of connective tissue cells (Sarco = muscle) (lemma = sheath).
- The myofibrils are surrounded by a network of filament which have a tendency to unite and form continuous sheets. They contribute greatly to the stability and elastic properties of muscle.
- The nucleus of myoblast divides several times, but the cell does not divide, thus the adult fibre has several nuclei situated mainly under sarcolemma. The protoplasm is made up of fibrils and sarcoplasm, which is found between the fibrils and under the sarcolemma. In the neighbourhood of nuclei, a Golgi apparatus, mitochondria and lipid inclusions are seen. The myoblast forms a fibril which later divides into bundles of fibrils, the *sarcostyles*, the outer layer of which behaves as a semi Z= Zwischenchcibe permeable membrane.
- The sarcostyles are made up of segments—the *sarcomeres*. A relatively thick, resistant and impermeable membrane separates one sarcomere from another and it is called *Z disc or Krause's membrane*. It and neighbouring sarcostyles are joined together and finally inserted in the sarcolemma. Thus, they form partitions which hold at the same level all sarcostyles of a muscle fibre. This division of sarcostyles into segments gives the fibre the cross striated aspect particular to skeletal/striated muscle. Longitudinal striations due to the fibrillar constitution is common to all type of muscles.

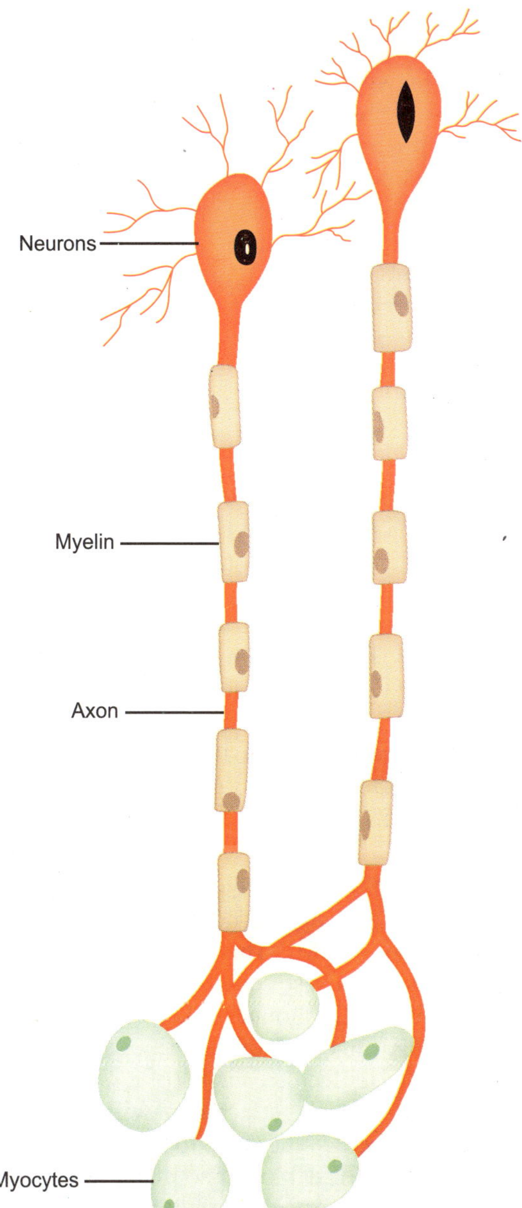

Fig. 13.1: Normal motor units

- The middle part of sarcomere, which is dark is called *Q OR A Disc/Brucke's disc*. It is separated from Krause's membrane by a clear, hyalin substance called *'J or I disc'*. A clear disc - *the line of Hensen (H)* divides Q into two equal parts. In a stretched fibre, a fine membrane - *Heidenhan's membrane* (M) can be seen in middle of H. The J disc shows a dark line about halfway between the membrane of Krause (Z) and the Q disc - this is *Engelmann's - accessory disc* (N) which is probably an artefact. There is also another dark line close to Z known as *terminal disc.*

- The sarcomere is about 2.5μ in length. I band contains only actin molecules which run from Z to Z band; In the A band they are intermixed with myosin molecules. The H band seems to be connected by very small filaments to the actin molecules.
- It has been suggested that myofibril has a tube like structure, the walls containing the filaments and an A substance surrounding an aqueous core. During contraction the A substance in the Q disc shifts towards Z membrane and the M band is widened, becoming the most transparent part of the fibril. The dense substance on each side of Z membrane forms so called contraction band. The sarcomeres shortens to half the resting length and becomes much wider.
- *Sarcolemma:* This is the outermost coat of the muscle cell or is the cell membrane of the muscle fibre. It consists of true cell membrane called plasma membrane and an outer coat made up of thin layer of polysaccharide material containing numerous thin collagen fibrils.

MYOSIN

- Myosin also acts as a deaminase, splitting off the amino groups of AMP. This enzymatic activity is not dependent on ATPase activity.
- Myosin is one of the families of fibrous proteins, which includes keratin, epidermin, fibrinogen, fibrin etc.
- Each myosin molecule consists of a tail and a head. The head is the site for attachment with actin filament and ATP molecule. The tail is made up of two chains intertwined with each other so that a double helix is formed. At its one end, the tail turns up, becomes expanded and globular. This globular part is head. The central part of myosin filament which is present in H-zone does not have any myosin head.
- Each thick myosin filament is 1.6μm long and have 200 molecules called myosin molecules.
- *Filament* is composed of multiple myosin molecules, each having a molecular weight of 480,000. There are no cross bridge heads in the centre of filament but there are only tails of myosin molecules in the centre. It is made up of 200 or more individual myosin molecules.
- *Molecule* is composed of six polypeptide chain, two heavy chains (molecule weight 200,000), four light chains (molecule weight 20,000). Both the heavy chains wrap around each other in a spiral way to form a double helix.
- Myosin head functions as an ATPase enzyme. This is essential in cleavage of ATP by head and the energy so liberated is used for muscular contraction.
- Myosin filament is twisted, so that each successive set of cross bridges is displaced axially from previous set by 120°. Cross bridges extend in all directions around filament.

Troponin

A protein molecule attached to near one end of each tropomyosin molecule. Three sub-units:-
Troponin I ... strong affinity for actin
Troponin T ... strong affinity for tropomyosin.
Troponin C .... Strong affinity for calcium ions.

ACTIN

It forms 12 to 15 per cent of total protein in the muscle. It is having molecular weight of 70,000.

Its main component is double stranded F-actin protein molecule. Each strand is composed of polymerised G-actin molecules, having a molecular weight of 42,000. Attached to each one of G molecule is one molecule of ADP; which are the active sites on actin filaments with which the cross bridges of myosin filaments interact to cause contraction. Each actin filament is 1 micrometer long and their bases are inserted strongly into Z discs while other ends protrude into adjacent sarcomeres in both the direction to lie in spaces between myosin molecules.

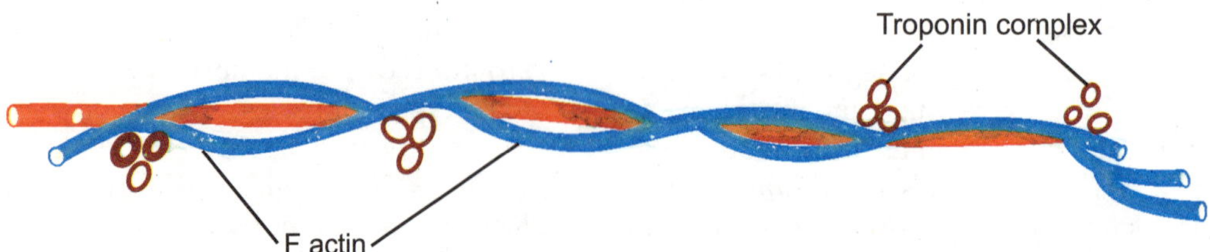

Fig. 13.2: Actin filament

ACTOMYOSIN

Myosin and F-actin in appropriate condition of ionic equilibrium unite to form an F-actomyosin ATP complex- a colloid of high viscosity. This complex contains 1 part of actin to 2.5-3 parts of myosin.

TROPOMYOSIN

Is a prototype of myosin; perhaps one of the units from which the myosin filament is made. It, in relaxed state of muscle, is situated in such a way that the active sites remain covered by tropomyosin. It is a protein contained by actin filament with a molecular weight of 70,000. These molecules are connected loosely with F-actin strands, wrapped spirally around the sides of F-actin-helix.

GLYCOGEN

Is found in close association with myosin. Its total amount is 500 mg per cent in resting muscle; red fibres have two-third to three fifths the glycogen content of white fibres. It diminishes in the course of contraction and falls to about 100 mg per cent in fatigued muscle; when the glycogen store has been exhausted, the muscle goes into contracture. It is rapidly restored during the period of recovery after exercise.

PHOSPHOCREATINE

(Creatine phosphate; phosphagen) It acts as a phosphate donor, on being split into creatine and phosphate. A great amount of energy is liberated, from 10,000 to 12,000 cal. per mol.; as Lipman designated it as an, energy rich phosphate bond. It is a stronger acid than phosphoric acid.

ATP (ADENOSINE-TRIPHOSPHATE; ADENYL PYRO-PHOSPHORIC ACID)

Is an important phosphate donor acting as a co-enzyme in phosphorylation reactions. ATP $\rightarrow$ ADP $\rightarrow$ AMP.

MYO-HAEMOGLOBIN

Is present in higher concentration in red fibres (700-800 mg %) than in white fibres. It increases after birth and decreases a little in senility. Its molecular weight is 16,800. Its affinity for oxygen is greater than that of haemoglobin. At 40 mmHg oxygen partial pressure haemoglobin is only 38 per cent saturated. The relative affinities for oxygen are such that it acts as an oxygen carrier, taking O_2 from the blood and giving it up to the muscle enzyme system.

BASIC PROPERTIES

The Muscle Twitch: Simple Muscle Curve (SMC)

Muscle responds to each of four types of stimulus namely electrical, thermal, mechanical or chemical. It may be stimulated directly by placing electrodes on its surface, or indirectly through its nerves, as occurs normally in body. On stimulation the muscle contracts and then relaxes and all this can be obtained in the form of a curve on a smoked drum, called muscle twitch. It is due to shortening (contraction) in unison of numerous fibres of which the muscle is composed. A simple muscle curve does not occur in living animal under ordinary physiological condition, but the reflex contraction of the extensor muscle of thigh caused by a tap on patellar tendon (knee jerk) is of this nature. It is composed of .-

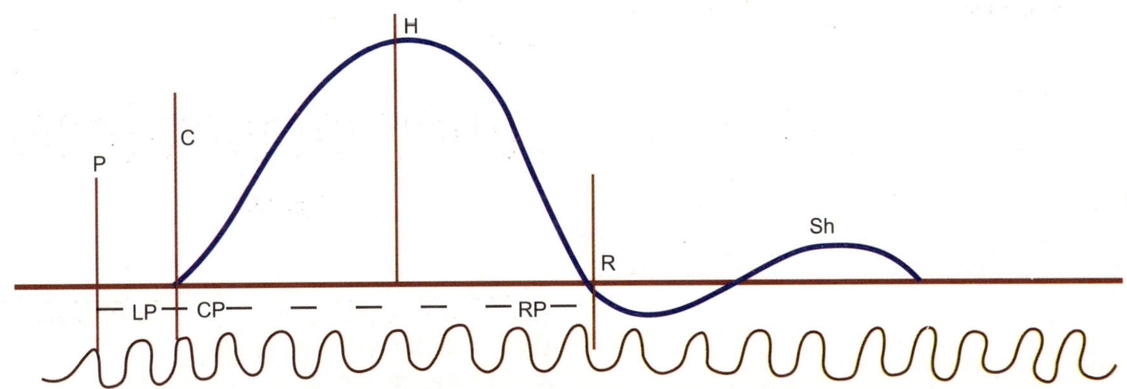

Fig. 13.3: Simple muscle curve

P = Point of stimulation
C = Point of contraction
LP = Latent period
CP = Contraction period
RP = Relaxation period
H = Height of contraction
R = Point of relaxation
Sh = Shatter's of physiological curve (due to inertia of lever)

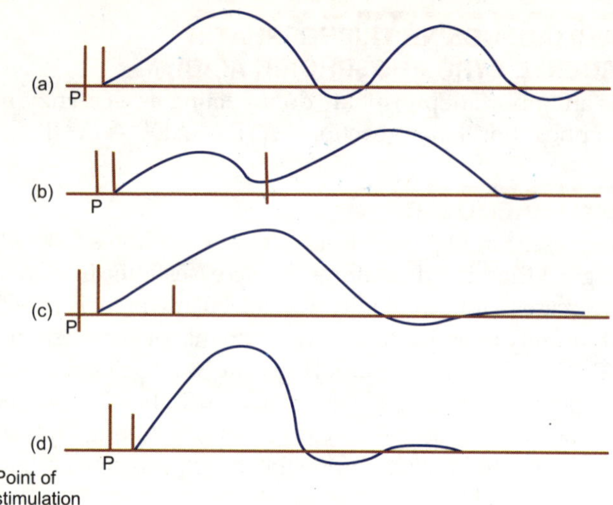

Fig. 13.4: Effect of two successive stimuli
a. Second stimulus applied after sufficient intervals
b. Second stimulus applied in relaxation period of first
c. Second stimulus applied in contraction period of first
d. Second stimulus applied in latent period of first

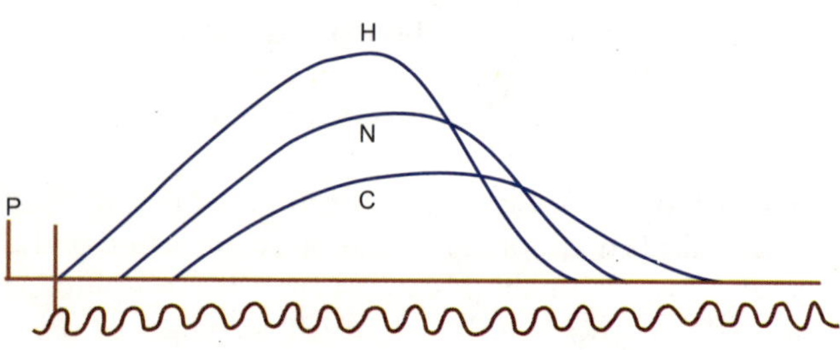

Fig. 13.5: Effect of temperature
P = Point of stimulation H = Effect of heat
N = Normal C = Effect of cold

Latent Period (LP)

Period elapsing from the application of stimulus to the commencement of contraction. Its duration is about 0.01 second.

Contraction Period (CP)

At the end of LP the muscle begins to shorten. Time interval from point of contraction to summit of the curve (peak) is the contraction period which lasts for about 0.04 second.

Relaxation Period (RP)

Relaxation period (RP) from height of contraction to base line. Duration 0.05 second.

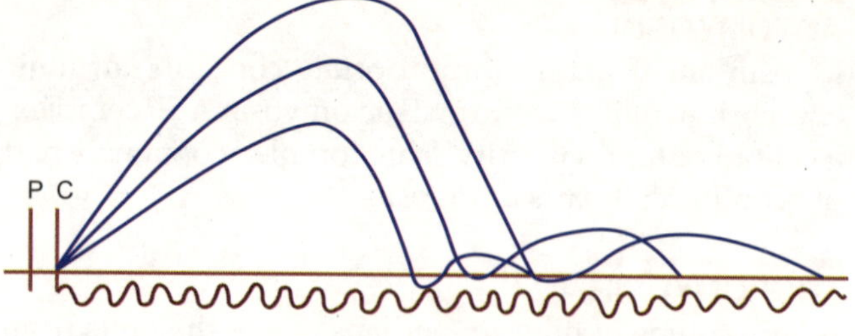

Fig. 13.6: Effect of load

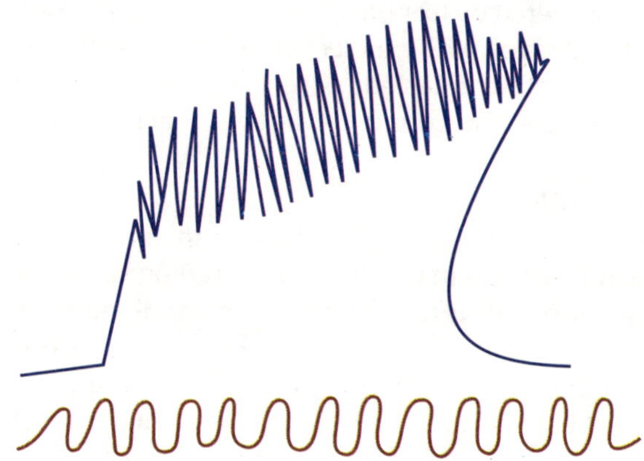

Fig. 13.7: Clonus

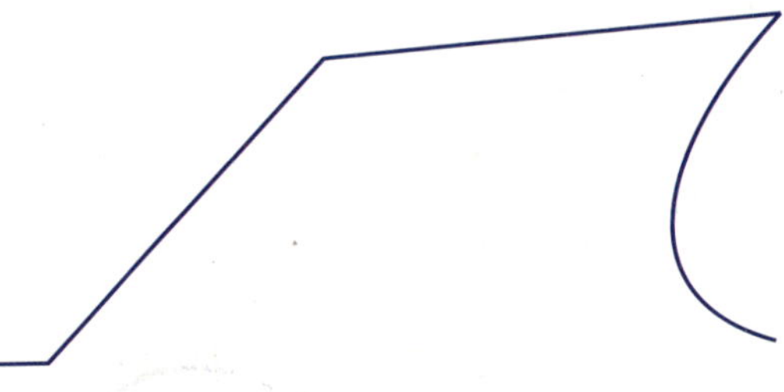

Fig. 13.8: Tetanus

ISOTONIC Vs ISOMETRIC CONTRACTION
(Iso = same; metric = length)

- In isometric contraction, there is no change in the length of the muscle, but there is a sharp augmentation of tension.
- In isotonic contraction, on the other hand, the tension remains constant while the length of the fibre shortens.
- In both instances energy is utilised.

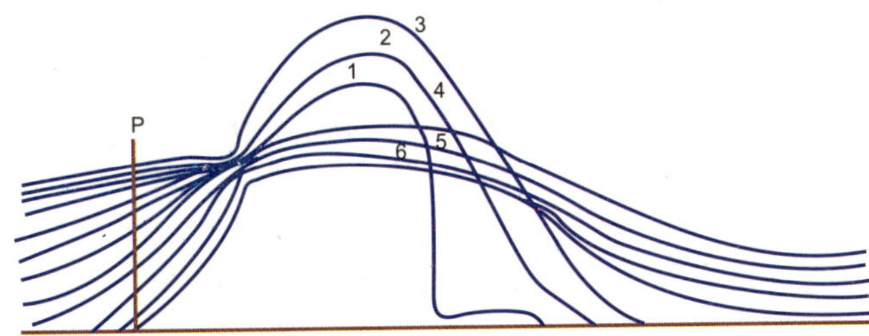

Fig. 13.9: Effect of fatigue muscle

- The muscles of the hands and arms in holding an object and the muscles of the trunk and legs in supporting the body in its erect position against the force of gravity are in isometric contraction. When these last mentioned muscles by alternate contraction and relaxation propel the body, as in walking, these contractions are isotonic.

DIFFERENCES BETWEEN TWO CONTRACTIONS

Isometric contraction	*Isotonic contraction*
• Muscle is not allowed to shorten	• Muscle shortens in length
• Great tension develops	• Less tension develops
• Strength of stimulus decides development of tension	• Tension depends on load applied; not on strength of stimulus
• Heat production is less	• Great production of heat
• No external work performed by muscle	• Muscle performs external work
• SMC represents (a) long C.P., (b) long relaxation period, (c) little change in latent period	• SMC represents (a) no change in latent period, shorter contraction period, shorter relaxation period

INITIAL HEAT

Heat produced during the mechanical response in a single twitch is composed of :

- *Heat of activation:* Begins during the latent period of the mechanical response well before shortening, or the rise in tension commences. It starts at a maximum rate then diminishes in rate continuously as contraction proceeds.
- *Heat of shortening:* Begins when the muscle commences to shorten and is proportional to the amount of shortening. It is not dependent on the load, speed of shortening. If the muscle does not shorten the heat observed is equal to the heat of activation.
- *Heat of maintenance:* In a tetanic contraction is the sum of heat of activation produced by each one of the successive shocks of stimulus.
- *Recovery heat:* Heat continues to be produced after the mechanical response is ended at a low rate and for a long time. The absence of oxygen does not modify the output of initial heat, but diminishes considerably the heat of recovery. In the presence of oxygen, total recovery heat is about equal to total initial energy as heat and work together.

FATIGUE

i. On continuing the stimulation, the contraction may show a constant height for some time, but soon, if the work is at all severe, they gradually decrease in height and finally no more twitches can be elicited, no matter how strong the stimulus is. This is fatigue. It is characterised by decreased irritability, contractility and conductivity. It is a transitory loss of these properties because recovery is possible under proper conditions.

ii. Causes of muscle fatigue are (a) the accumulation of intermediate or final waste products and (b) the deficiency in energy furnishing materials.

iii. The intermediate waste products — lactic acid, pyruvic acid are either oxidised into CO_2+H_2O, or by expenditure of energy, built up into higher compounds like glycogen. Lactic acid formed in the muscle may be removed by blood circulation and carried to the heart where it is used as such in the production of energy for cardiac activity. The CO_2 is carried to the lungs and acid salts to the kidneys for elimination. To prevent fatigue, not only O_2 but also food must be brought to the muscles from the organs of supply. All these activities depend upon the circulation of blood and upon respiration. Any interference with blood supply hastens the onset of fatigue.

iv. Seat of fatigue is myo-neural-junction. It is evidenced by the fact that on stimulating the motor nerve of a muscle nerve preparation for a sufficient long time, the muscle refuses to contract which means fatigue has set in. If now the muscle is stimulated directly contractions are obtained, hence the fatigue shown when nerve was stimulated cannot be referred to the muscle and nerve fibre is practically incapable of experiencing fatigue. So out of three sites (muscle, nerve, myoneural junction) the myo-neural junction is the most susceptible site for fatigue.

v. Drugs affecting:
   — Caffeine is increasing work output and therefore delays the fatigue.

— Glycine (amino acid) increases the working power and delays the fatigue.
— Tobacco smoking reduces capacity to work and physical fitness too.
— Benzedrine delays the fatigue.

vi. Contracture: As fatigue develops, the muscle curve shows changes in that the shortening and relaxation process becomes slower, this is essentially true for latter. Due to the slowness of relaxation, the muscle fails to attain its full length before the next stimulation is thrown in, and so it remains in what is known as contracture. This is an early sign of fatigue.

It is a reversible process and therefore differs from cadaveric rigidity and from rigidity due to coagulation of muscle proteins. In contracture there is an increase in the metabolism of muscle, heat production is considerably greater than at rest and there are glycolysis and lactic acid formation.

STRENGTH OF STIMULI

- When a gastrocnemius muscle is arranged so that contraction may be recorded on a moving kymograph, the strength of stimulation can be studied. If the muscle is stimulated with a stimulus too weak to cause a contraction and then stimulus is increased in strength with each successive stimuli, the muscle will finally show its maximal contraction.
- The weak stimulation that does not cause contraction is called *'subliminal or subthreshold'* stimulus; while the stimulus of just sufficient strength to cause a response is *threshold stimulus*. If stimulus is further increased in intensity to give a gradual increase in the power of contraction, then it is *submaximal* and if it is continued until a maximum response is obtained then it is *maximal*.
- No further increase in strength of stimulus will increase the size of response, then it is *supramaximal*.
- So as strength of successive stimuli is increased the height of contraction will increase to a given height and then show no more increase. This demonstrates graded response to graded stimulus and it is directly related to the principle that as strength of stimulus is increased, an increased number of motor units are involved; therefore more muscle fibres respond and greater shortening occurs. Each muscle fibre, if it responds to stimulus at all, responds to its maximal ability.

TETANUS

- When a large number of stimuli are applied to a muscle in rapid succession, so that little time is given for the relaxation between the successive contraction, there is more or less, fusion of twitches. Greater the frequency of stimuli, the more nearly complete is the fusion (incomplete tetanus). On the contrary complete tetanus is defined as a sustained contraction of a muscle due to the fusion of many twitches following each other in rapid succession; the external cause lies in the large number of stimuli sent into the muscle in a unit of time. Due to summation, the height of the tetanic contraction is generally considerably greater than that of the twitch produced by a single stimulus of the same intensity.
- The rapidity of stimulation required to induce complete tetanus varies with the nature of the muscle; for the fast acting external eye muscle, this is about 350/second; for the frog gastrocnemius 30. The condition of the muscle (temperature, fatigue) also greatly influences.

REFRACTORY PERIOD

- When muscle is stimulated and contraction occurs, it loses its irritability for a short time, so that if a second stimulus is applied within that period, there will be no second contraction. During this very brief lapse of time, known as *absolute refractory period*, the muscle will not respond to any stimulus, however strong. This is followed by relative refractory period, during which time the muscle slowly regains its irritability and will respond to a stimulus. Skeletal muscle has a relatively short, smooth muscle longest and cardiac muscle in between the two, refractory period. It seems that the activity of all protoplasm is associated with a loss of irritability during a certain phase of the activity.
- The duration of absolute refractory period may vary from 5 to 50 m sec.
- In skeletal muscles, the refractory period occupies a fractional part of the latent period.
- The relative and absolute refractory period, taken together constitute total refractory period. Its first portion is absolute refractory period and remaining is relative refractory period.

RHEOBASE-CHRONAXIE

1. Rheobase is defined as minimal galvanic current which when allowed to flow indefinitely will excite the tissue.

2. Chronaxie is defined as the shortest duration of current *twice as great as rheobase,* which will excite a tissue. It is a definite measure of its excitability, i.e. a less excitable tissue has a longer chronaxie while more excitable tissue has a shorter one.

ELECTROMYOGRAPHY

- Is a study of action potential in human skeletal muscle.
- Electric current generated is transmitted to outer surface of the body, the changes in action potential can be studied by either putting electrodes at the surface of active muscle area or inserting them directly into concerned muscle.
- It is helping in diagnosis of various neuromuscular disorders in which either the rate or rhythm of nerve impulse is influenced.

RIGOR MORTIS

- Is state of rigidity developing after death. The muscle loses excitability and translucency. It increases in thickness, gradually becomes stiff and of course pH becomes acidic (5.8). Its glycogen disappears.
- It is a state of permanent irreversible contraction associated with loss of ATP and establishment of permanent link between actin and myosin.
- Here, muscle proteins are denatured.
- Order is ... lower jaw, face, neck, thorax, abdomen upper extremity and lastly lower extremity.
- It disappears 24 to 36 hours after death due to autolysis.
- Factors hastening are:- caffeine, chloroform vapour, increased temperature, acidity etc.

MUSCULO-TENDINOUS-ENDINGS

a. Muscle spindles
b. Golgi tendon organs
c. Pacinian corpuscles

Muscle Spindle

1. Is a special type of receptor present within the muscle.
2. Each muscle consists of a bundle of two to ten slender striated muscle fibres enveloped in a thin connective tissue capsule. This capsule is tapered at both the ends.
3. The slender muscle fibres within capsule are intrafusal fibres, which are arranged in parallel with the extrafusal fibres.
4. The intrafusal fibres at their terminal end (polar) are striated and so contractile, while central end of each fibre is unstriated and non-contractile and filled with multiple nuclei-called nuclear bag region.

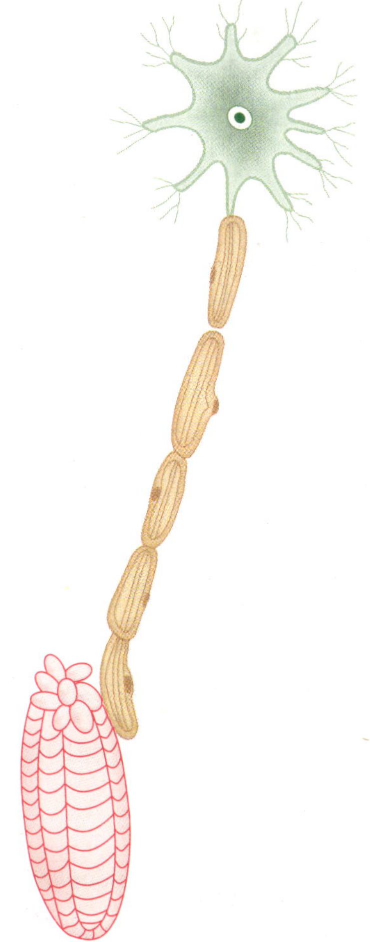

Fig. 13.10: Contraction of skeletal muscle

5. At a distance, the space on either side of nuclear bag region — primary annulo-spiral region is nuclear chain region — nuclei arranged in central core.
6. Nerve fibres-innervating.... Three types of fibres:-
   - Large *afferent* -8-12μ diameter, primary afference fibres, end in nuclear bag region. Before ending in intrafusal fibres, they loose their myelin sheath and wind round the muscle fibres forming a spiral ending.
   - Secondary afferent 6-9μ in diameter, called flower spray endings because they enter the spindle to form a small ring which coils or sprays like varicosities on either side of nuclear bag regions.
   - Third set of fibres — gamma efferent - 3-7μ diameter, entering the spindle and ending at motor end plates of contractile and striated ends of intrafusal fibres. The extrafusal fibres are supplied by alpha motor fibres.

- Afferent fibre from this muscle spindle enter the spinal cord and synapse in alpha motor *neurone*, from which the alpha efferent fibres arise, then a monosynaptic path is established which act as stretch or myotatic reflex.

PART IN ACTION

SARCOTUBULAR SYSTEM

i. It is the striking feature of skeletal muscle—a series of tubules and cisterns equivalent to a modified endoplasmic reticulum.
ii. This system has a dual character and may be divided into a *Transverse T system* organised in relation to Z band, and a *Longitudinal system* - consisting of a series of tubules closely applied to the surface of the myofibrils.
iii. From one Z line to the next, the longitudinal system is a continuous structure with both transversely and longitudinally arranged elements, whilst at Z line the transverse, or T system, intrudes between the two terminal sacs of the longitudinal system.
iv. When the two systems come together there is apparently no connection, but the respective membranes come in close apposition to give the appearance of a triad.
v. It would seem that longitudinal system of tubules is the strict analogue of the endoplasmic reticulum of other cells, while the transverse T system is a development connected with the activation process of muscular contraction. Thus, there is a little doubt that T-system opens on to the surface of the muscle fibre, its wall being continuous with the sarcolemma, and is thus in direct connection with the extra-cellular fluid of the tissue—this is in contrast with the longitudinal L system. It is through the transverse T system that the individual myofilaments are activated rapidly during the contractile process. It causes rapid transmission of the action potential from the cell membrane to all the fibrils in the muscle.

MUSCLE ACTION POTENTIAL : AT A GLANCE

- Resting membrane potential — -80 to -90 mV (Skeletal) velocity of conduction - 3 to 5 m/sec. Duration of action potential 1 to 5 milliseconds.
- Transverse (T) tubules penetrate all the way through the muscle fibre from one side to other. Action potential passes through these tubules. This leads to release of Ca^{2+} from sarcoplasmic reticulum, which causes contraction and entire process is called 'excitation contraction coupling.
- T tubules run transverse to the myofibrils. Where T tubules originate from cell membrane they are open to the exterior. Thus, they communicate with the fluid surrounding the muscle fibre and contain extracellular fluid in their lumen, so they are internal extension of the cell membrane.
- Sarcoplasmic reticulum — composed of (1) Long longitudinal tubules — running parallel to myofibrils and terminate into (2) terminal cisternae. It contains Ca^{2+} in abundance.
- Action potential of T tubule leads to flow of current through the tips of cisternae. At these points each cisternae projects *junctional feet* that attach to the

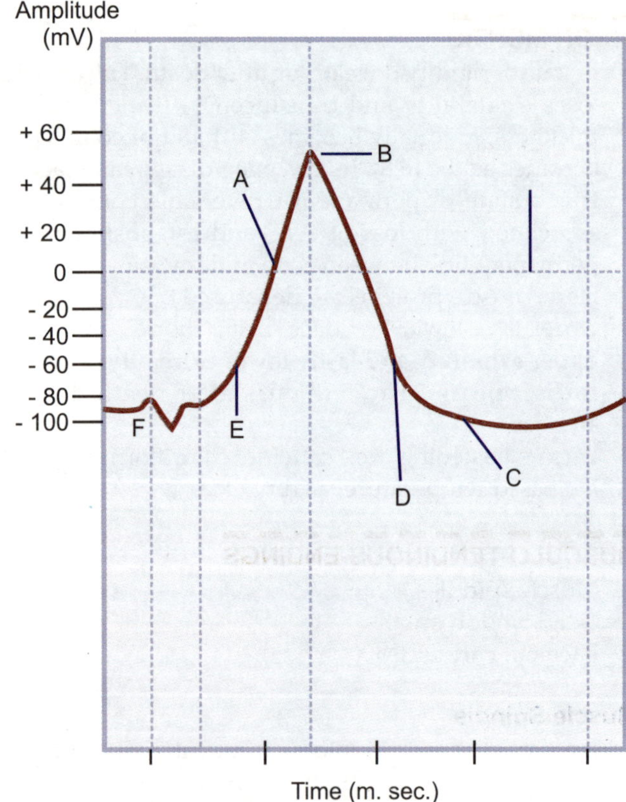

A = Over shoot
B = Spike potential
C = Positive after potential
(After hyperpolarisation)
D = Negative after potential
(After depolarisation)
E= Firing level
F = Stimulus artifact

Fig. 13.11: Action potential: skeletal muscle

membrane of T tubule. This action potential (signal) leads to rapid opening of large number of Ca^{2+} channels which remain open for a few milliseconds. These Ca^{2+} diffuse to the adjacent myofibrils, where they bind strongly with troponin C which elicits muscular contraction.

- At the same time there exists an active pump in the walls of sarcoplasmic reticulum which pumps Ca^{2+} out of sarcoplasmic fluid back into sarcoplasmic tubules. Besides this, there exists a protein calsequestrin which can bind Ca^{2+} forty times. By both these mechanisms, there exists a total depletion of Ca^{2+} in fluid of myofibrils. So contraction ceases. In resting state troponin — tropomyosin complex keeps actin filaments inhibited thus maintaining a relaxed state. This is calcium pulse (total duration is 1/20 of a second).

EXCITATION—CONTRACTION COUPLING

- The process by which depolarisation of muscle fibre initiates contraction is excitation contraction coupling.
- The action potential is transmitted to all the fibrils in the fibre through T system which triggers the release of Ca^{2+} from terminal cisterns and this Ca^{2+} initiates contraction. Ca^{2+} also affects excitability.
- The increased Ca^{2+} concentration is translated into increased actin-myosin-interaction by the regulatory proteins—troponin and tropomyosin, which are located on the thin filament. A subunit of troponin is the intracellular receptor protein for Ca^{2+}. The Ca^{2+} released from 'sarcoplasmic reticulum' rapidly diffuses to and binds to troponin-C. The conformational change elicited by this binding is propagated along the thin filament by tropomyosin and releases the inhibition on the interaction between actin and myosin. When Ca^{2+} is bound to troponin C, actin and myosin interact, slide past one another and generate force. The bound ATP is released as ADP and phosphate. The heads of myosin molecules contain ATPase activity.
- Very shortly after releasing Ca^{2+}, the sarcoplasmic reticulum begins to re-accumulate it by actively transporting it into the longitudinal portion of the reticulum. From here it diffuses into the terminal cisterns, where it is stored until released by the next action potential. All this reduces Ca^{2+} concentration outside the reticulum, which leads to cessation of chemical interaction between myosin and actin and the muscle then relaxes.
- So, contraction stops when Ca^{2+} is re-accumulated in sarcoplasmic reticulum by Ca^{2+} -ATPase transport proteins on sarcoplasmic-reticulum-membrane and intracellular free Ca^{2+} concentration returns to resting levels.
- Relaxation is brought about when Ca^{2+} moves back from sarcoplasm into sarcoplasmic reticulum.
- When calcium ions combine with troponin C, each molecule of which can bind strongly with up to four calcium ions. The troponin complex undergoes a conformational change which tugs on the tropomyosin molecule and moves it deeper into the groove between two actin strands. It leads to uncovering of active sites of actin, which causes the contraction to proceed.

Differences between EPP and AP

EPP (End-plate Potential)	*AP (Action Potential)*
1. It is a highly local event. It does not propagate. It is confined within motor end plate.	If developes, then propagates
2. It does not show all or none phenomenon	An adequate stimulus is enough.
3. It is fore runner of A.P.	It develops by the development of EPP.
4. It belongs to graded potential i.e. its intensity can be changed/graded.	—
5. MEPP = miniature end plate potential. Even at rest some acetylcholine vesicles burst giving rise to EPP.	—

EXCITATION CONTRACTION COUPLING—AT A GLANCE

1. When a muscle is stimulated, it develops action potential, i.e. excitation—an electrical phenomenon.
2. When it is excited it contracts—a mechanical phenomenon.
3. Excitation → development of action potential → it travels into interior of muscle fibres through T tubules → action potential reaches to cisterna which is close to L system and Ca^{2+} are abundantly present there → L system releases Ca^{2+} as action potential reaches into fibrils → contraction develops.
   Then Ca^{2+} go back into L system → relaxation.

RATCHET THEORY (WALK ALONG THEORY)

- On activation of actin filament by calcium ions the heads of cross bridges from the myosin filaments immediately is attracted to the active sites of actin filament which leads to contraction.
- When head attaches to an active site, this leads to changes in intramolecular forces between head and

arm of cross bridge. This causes the head to tilt towards the arm and thus actin filament is dragged along with it (power stroke).

- After this, head automatically breaks away from active site.
- In the next phase head returns to its normal direction where it combines with a new active site further down along the actin filament, then the head tilts again to cause a new power stroke.
- Greater the number of cross bridges in contact with actin filaments at any given time, greater is the force of contraction. So heads of cross bridges bend back and forth along actin filament towards the centre of myosin filament.

ENZYME SYSTEM FOUND IN THE MUSCLE

1. *Cytochrome-cytochrome-oxidase:* found in higher concentration in white than in red fibres.
2. *Flavoproteins:* its prosthetic group is flavin-di-nucleotide (synonym—Warburg's yellow respiratory pigment)
3. *Dehydrogenases:* for lactate, succinate, malate, tartrate, glycerophosphate, triose phosphate, isocitrate, hydroxybutyrate, glutamate.
4. *ATPase:* ATPase activity of myosin inhibited by Mg^{++} with an optimum at pH 9.
5. *Phosphorylase:* which activates the reversible hydrolysis (phosphorolysis) of glucose-1-phosphate (Cori's ester) in the synthesis and breakdown of glycogen.
6. *Phosphopherases:* enzyme that catalyzes transfer of phosphate from one compound to another, e.g. hexokinases which transfer phosphate from ATP to glucose giving Glucose-6-phosphate (*Robison's* ester) and to fructose, giving fructose-6-phosphate (Neuberg's ester). It also transfers phosphate from creatine phosphate to ADP and AMP and from ATP to Neuberg's ester, giving Fructose 1:6-diphosphate.
7. *Myokinase:* which dismutates ADP activating the reaction : $2ADP \rightleftarrows ATP + AMP$
8. *Phosphoglucomutase:* It catalyses the following reaction Glucose 1-phosphate + glucose 1:6 diphosphate → Glucose-6-phosphate + Glucose 1:6 diphosphate
9. *Phosphohexose Isomerase:* Catalyses the equilibrium found in resting muscle between *Robison's* ester (70%) and Neuberg ester (30%). The mixture of the two is 'Embden's Ester.'
10. *Aldolase:* Catalyses the reversible cleavage of Fructose 1:6 diphosphate into glyceraldehyde -3-phosphate and dihydroxy-acetone phosphate.

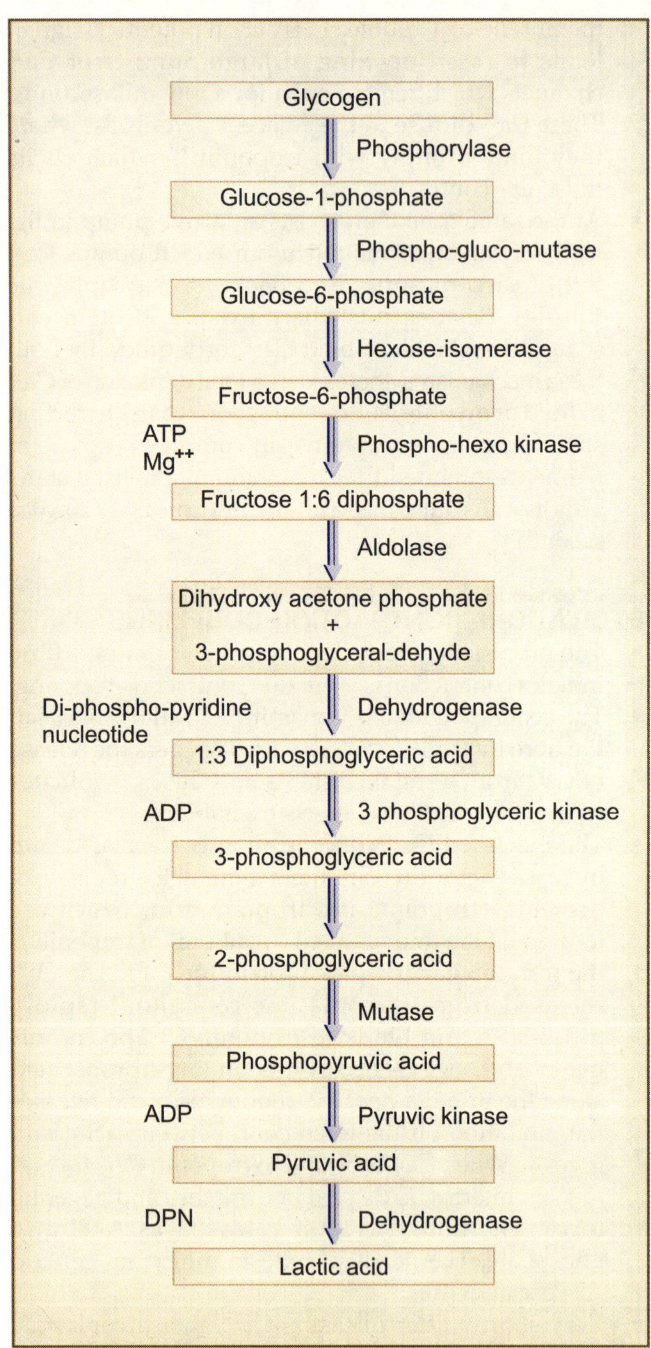

METABOLIC PROCESS

a. Aerobic process (respiratory metabolism)
   Muscle oxygen consumption increases considerably on contraction and increase is proportional to the activity developed. The excess oxygen consumption of activity begins early in contraction and there is an increased reduction of haemoglobin, therefore the muscle takes up more O_2. The excess O_2 consumption

persisting after the activity is ceased has been called the 'oxygen debt.' Recovery of the initial resting condition requires the energy set free by oxidation, and although the oxygen consumption diminishes rapidly after activity has ended, it remains for a long-time above the resting level.

b. Muscle can contract in an atmosphere free of oxygen. The capacity to perform work is considerably diminished. In muscle kept in anaerobiosis, glycolysis occurs, glycogen diminishes and lactic acid is formed.

c. Maximum efficiency can be realised when muscle contracts at a moderate velocity. If muscle contracts very slowly, large amount of maintenance heat are released during contraction process, thus decreasing the efficiency. If contraction is too rapid, large proportion of energy is used to overcome viscous friction.

CHEMICAL EVENTS : MOTION OF MYOSIN HEADS

- ATP → ADP + Pi. Before contraction begins the heads of cross bridges bind with ATP.
- By release of calcium ions, there occurs inhibition of inhibitory effect of troponin - tropomyosin - complex, which leads to uncovering of actin filament for binding with myosin heads.
- This is followed by power stroke as mentioned.
- On tilting the head, ADP and Pi are released which were previously attached to the head. A new molecule of ATP is bound at the site of release of ADP. This binding act terminates into detachment of head from actin.
- The new molecule of ATP is cleaved after detachment of head from actin; the head is back to its perpendicular condition to begin with a new cycle.
- Once again power stroke begins.
- The process proceeds again and again until actin filament pulls Z membrane up against the ends of myosin filament.

CHEMICAL REACTION ACCOMPANYING MUSCULAR CONTRACTION

- In a second phase pyruvic acid may follow one of the two paths, according to availability of oxygen. If there is oxygen deficiency (an aerobiosis), pyruvic acid accepts H_2 from reduced DPN and lactic acid is formed which is a reversible reaction catalysed by a special dehydrogenase. Lactic acid passes into the blood and in the liver is reconverted into glycogen, which by glycogenolysis is transformed into glucose, which is taken back to the muscle by the blood and there synthesised into muscle glycogen, which on being broken down again gives lactic acid. This series of reaction is *Cori cycle.*
- If on the contrary, there is abundance of oxygen (aerobiosis), pyruvic acid is oxidised to CO_2 and H_2O possibly along the path of citric acid or tricarboxylic acid cycle.

MUSCLE CONTRACTION: ENERGY SOURCE

1. Muscle contraction depends upon energy supplied by ATP. Most of it is required for contraction but small amounts are required for:
   - Pumping calcium into sarcoplasmic reticulum from sarcoplasm after completion of contraction.
   - Appropriate ionic environment is required for propagation of action potential. So energy is also required for pumping sodium and potassium ions through muscle fibre membrane.
2. $\text{ATP} \rightarrow \text{ADP} \xrightarrow[\text{rylation}]{\text{Re-phospho}} \text{ATP}$ (new molecule)
3. The sources of energy for rephosphorylation (construction of new molecule of ATP) are:-
   - Phosphocreatine
   - Glycogen. Its importance in glycolysis is
     - —It can occur even in absence of oxygen
     - —Rate of formation of ATP is 2 times great
     - —Process of oxidative metabolism, i.e. combination of oxygen with various cellular foodstuffs to liberate ATP.

MUSCULAR CONTRACTION—AT A GLANCE

- Action potential is generated travelling along a motor nerve to its endings on muscle fibres.
- Secretion of acetylcholine—a neurotransmitter at each ending.
- Acetylcholine, further opens multiple acetylcholine gated protein channels in the muscle fibre membrane.
- The action potential travel along muscle fibre membrane—It depolarises the muscle fibre membrane and travel deeply. Under its effect, large quantities of calcium ions are released from sarcoplasmic reticulum.
- The calcium ions so released act as an attractive medium between actin and myosin filaments causing them to slide together.
- These calcium ions are pumped back into sarcoplasmic reticulum after a fraction of second, where they remain stored.

ELECTROMYOGRAPHY (EMG): A VIEW

1. Definition: It is a non-invasive technique through which electrical activity of muscle is studied.
2. Requisites: Electrodes, high gain amplifier (10-5000 Hz. frequencies), recorder of output, specially constructed and shielded room to avoid extra-electromagnetic and electrostatic forces.

3. Principle: Motor unit potential (MUP) or motor unit action potential (MUAP)
   i. It is the basic unit of EMG signal. The unit of activation of a muscle is 'Motor Unit', while unit of activation within a motor unit is muscle fibre. Here it is worth mentioning that on stimulation of motor unit, all muscles fibres are not simultaneously activated, because the nerve impulse has to travel a variable distance so activation of muscle fibre → action potential → generation of electromagnetic field around it → action potential detected by electrode present in field.
   ii. The magnitude of an action potential is 100mV but amplitude of a motor unit potential is 0.5-3.00 mV. This is because of the fact that EMG electrodes are little away from muscle fibres. This means that electrodes are exposed only to electric field generated by action potential. The action potential lasts for 1-2 ms, but this period is extended to 5-12 ms in MUP.
4. Analysis:
   i. Visual inspection of record.
   ii. Quantitative analysis—amplitude, duration and frequency with help of computer.
   iii. Power spectrum analysis—determining 'power' of waves at selected frequencies.
   iv. 'Integrator' may be used.
5. Uses:
   i. To study the degree and sequence of contraction of various muscles involved in a movement.
   ii. It shows the mechanism for grading the force of muscular contraction.
   iii. To diagnose and follow-up myopathies along with response of muscle/nerve towards injury.
   iv. Fibrillation: 'Contraction of individual muscle fibres', invisible through skin (10-100 microV potential, 1-2 ms duration, 10 Hz frequency).
      - Fasciculation: 'Coarse contraction of individual motor units visible through the skin 50-500 microV potential, 2-4 ms duration, 2-20 Hz frequency.
6. Notes:
   i. EMG signals: There may be signal at the time of insertion of electrode as well as on any movement of electrode. Sometimes signals are observed even at rest which is an indication of neuromuscular activity which is considered as basis of muscle tone. Signals are there with voluntary contraction. Its basic unit is MUP/MUAP.
   ii. Biphasic Vs/Monophasic record.

- Two electrodes A and B are used

↓

A muscle fibre is polarised—both electrodes are at some potential

↓

Impulse then reaches to 'A' electrode which makes it negative as compared with 'B'. This produces 'excursion' in the record

↓

Impulse reaches to 'B electrode'. So both A and B are at depolarisation potential. So record returns to base line

↓

Wave of repolarisation

↓

A first repolarises, B still depolarised; so 'excursion' just opposite to previous occurs.

↓

Then 'B' repolarises, so record returns to base line.

- ECG electrodes are equally satisfactory with EMG also.

   iii. Hypertonicity: Increased muscle tone; occurring in upper motor neuron lesion → gamma motor neurons are not inhibited → exaggerated discharge from these neurons → muscle tone increased. High resistance to stretch is presented by muscles (spasticity).
   iv. Hypotonicity: Decreased tone in voluntary muscle, occurring in lower motor neuron lesion. Very little resistance to stretch is offered by muscles (flaccid paralysis).
   v. Myotonia: Inherited disease continuous contraction of muscle after completion of voluntary act. Ionic channels in sarcolemma are affected.
   vi. Muscular dystrophy: Progressive degeneration of muscle fibres without involving nervous system. Hereditory origin.
      - One variety is inherited sex link recessive disorder due to the absence of a gene product in X-chromosome called 'dystrophine'. There occurs degeneration and necrosis, of muscle fibre first which is followed by replacement with fat and fibrous tissue. Respiratory muscles are commonly involved making breathing difficult (Duchenne muscular dystrophy).
      - Second variety is again a sex linked heredity disorder due to alteration of 'dystrophin'. Fatigue, difficulty in walking, mental retardness are usual symptoms (Becker's muscular dystrophy).

14 Contractile Tissue: Muscle; Myoneural Junction

FUNCTIONAL ANATOMY

- The skeletal muscle fibres are innervated by large myelinated nerve fibres that originate in large motor neurones of anterior horns of spinal cord.
- The nerve fibre branches at its end to form a complex of branching nerve terminals which invaginate into muscle fibre. It lies completely outside the muscle fibre membrane. This is called *motor end-plate,* which is covered by Schwann cells. This invagination is called *synaptic gutter* and the space between terminal and fibre membrane is *synaptic cleft*. At the bottom of this gutter are smaller folds of muscle membrane—*sub-neural clefts*.
- Many mitochondria are present in axon terminal. The neurotransmitter acetylcholine is synthesised in the cytoplasm of the terminal. Enzyme acetyl choline-esterase which destroys acetylcholine is present attached to matrix of basal lamina.

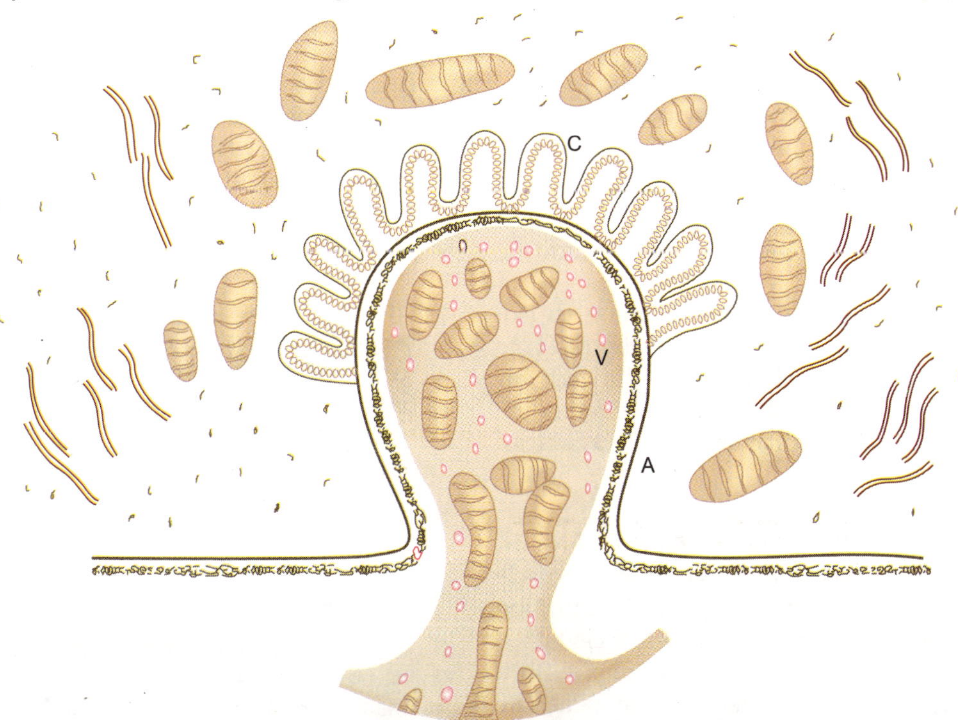

Fig. 14.1: Motor end-plate
V = Synaptic vesicles (Acetylcholine)
C = Subneural clefts
A = Axon terminal in synaptic trough

SEQUENCE OF EVENTS

- Voltage gated calcium channels are present inside the neural membrane.
- When action potential develops these channels open up allowing large quantities of calcium to diffuse to interior of the terminal.
- These Ca^{2+} attract acetylcholine vesicles. So some of the vesicles fuse with the membrane and empty their contents, i.e. acetylcholine into synaptic cleft by a process of exocytosis.
- Near the mouth of subneural cleft, many acetylcholine receptors are found which are nothing but acetylcholine gated ion channels. These acetylcholine channels allow all positive ions (Na^+, K^+, Ca^{2+}) to move easily; out of which Na^+ moves readily because it is present in extracellular fluid in plenty. This influx of sodium ions causes the development of what is called *end-plate potential*. It is increased up to 50 to 75 mV. This causes muscular contraction.
- The acetylcholine so liberated is destroyed by enzyme 'cholinesterase,' together with the fact that its small amount diffuses out of 'synaptic gutter' which is then no longer available to act on muscle fibre membrane.

PHARMACOLOGY

- Drugs like methacholine, carbachol, nicotine are having similar action as that of acetylcholine with the difference that they are not destroyed by cholinesterase enzyme.
- Curare (a drug of curariform group) blocks the transmission at myoneural junction by competing with acetylcholine for the receptor site of membrane. It prevents passage of impulses from end-plate into the muscle.
- Many drugs (neostigmine, physostigmine, di-iso-propyl-fluorophosphate) inactivate the enzyme cholinesterase so acetylcholine is not destroyed; this leads to excessive accumulation of acetylcholine which keeps muscle in contracting state. This causes a muscular spasm.

NEUROMUSCULAR PHYSIOLOGY : AT A GLANCE

- There are many acetylcholine receptors in muscle membrane, which are actually acetylcholine gated ion channels located near mouth of subneural clefts.
- Each receptor is a large protein complex with a molecular weight of 2,75,000. These proteins penetrate all the way through the membrane lying side by side in a circle to constitute a tubular channel. This channel is having enough diameter to allow the passage of all important ions, e.g. Na^+, K^+, Ca^{++}, Cl^- etc.
- So on secretion of acetylcholine, the constriction of channel is removed and it is opened up, allowing ionic exchange.
- More sodium ions flow through these channels because: (1) Na^+ is more in extra and K^+ is more in intracellular fluid (2) Very negative potential (-80 to -90 mV) pulls positively charged sodium ions to inside of fibre while efflux of K^+ is prevented.
- This entry of Na^+ inside, creates 'end-plate potential' which causes muscular contraction (50 – 75 mV).
- Artificial stimulation of nerve fibres more than 100 times per second for several minutes often diminishes the number of vesicles of acetylcholine released with each impulse so that impulse fails to pass through muscle fibres. This is fatigue.

ACETYLCHOLINE : MOLECULAR LEVEL

- Very small vesicles are formed by Golgi apparatus in cell body of motor neurone of spinal cord. They are then carried to neuro-muscular junction.
- It is synthesised in cytosol of terminal nerve fibre. Then it is transported to interior, where it is stored in highly concentrated form.
- On arrival of an action potential at nerve terminal calcium channels are opened up, which increases Ca^{2+} concentration which increases rate of fusion of acetyl choline vesicles with terminal membrane. On this fusion its outer surface ruptures, leading to exocytosis of acetyl choline into synaptic cleft, (approximately 200/300 vesicles rupture/one action potential). Soon enzyme cholinesterase comes into action; dissociating acetylcholine into acetate ion and choline; this choline is reabsorbed back into neural terminal for re-synthesis of acetylcholine.
- On release of acetylcholine, the membrane of vesicle becomes part of the cell membrane. For continued functioning of myoneural junction vesicles need to be retrieved from nerve membrane, which is achieved by process of endocytosis. Within a very short time of completion of action potential, pits appear on the surface of terminal nerve membrane which is due to contractile protein of cytosol. After a short while, pit breaks due to contraction of proteins and thus a new vesicle is formed and a new cycle begins.

MYAESTHENIA GRAVIS

In this disease; there is very weak end-plate potential which is unable to stimulate muscle fibre. Patient is paralysed specially of respiratory muscles. Drug neostigmine is the drug of choice. This is an autoimmune disease. It occurs in about one of every 20,000 persons. By this therapy the patient can begin to function almost normally.

15 Contractile Tissue: Smooth Muscle

INTRODUCTION

They are made up of elongated, spindle shaped cells, with a central nucleus and a thin membrane. The fibres are much shorter than those of striated muscle. The protoplasm is differentiated into slender fibrils which have no transverse striations. In some smooth muscles, the fibrils pass from one cell to another, the protoplasmic bridges endow these muscles with some of the characteristics of syncytium. They fall into two categories namely -

a. *Multiunit group:* e.g. nictitating membrane, piloerectors, muscles of blood vessels. They are usually activated by motor nerves (similarity with skeletal group).
   Discrete smooth muscle fibres. Each fibre contracts independently of the others. They rarely perform spontaneous contraction. Their outer surface is covered by a thin layer of basement membrane like substances viz. a mixture of fine collagen and glycoprotein fibrillae.
b. *Visceral:* e.g. muscles of intestinal tract, uterus etc. syncytial character with well developed automatism, less dependent on nervous system (similarity with cardiac muscle).
   The cell membranes are joined by many gap junctions through which ions can flow freely from one cell to another which facilitates action potential to travel and thus causing muscular contraction.

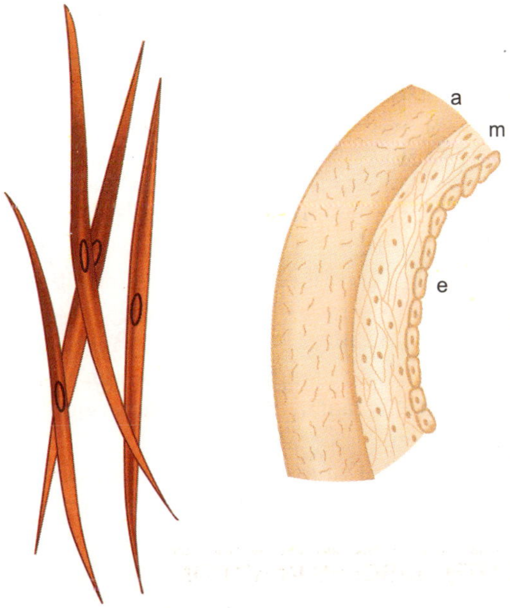

(A) (B)

a m e

Fig. 15.1: Smooth muscle: An outlook
(A) Multiunit smooth muscle
(B) Unitary smooth muscle
a = Adventitia, m = medial muscle fibres, e = endothelium

INNERVATION

They are innervated by sympathetic and parasympathetic postganglionic fibres which are fine, nonmyelinated fibres, with the exception of those from the ciliary ganglion which have a myelin sheath up to their ending in the intrinsic musculature of the eye. Most smooth muscles have a double nerve supply — one for excitation and one for inhibition. The nictitating membrane and piloerectors are innervated exclusively by the sympathetics and ciliary muscle by parasympathetic.

TONUS

This is an outstanding feature of smooth muscles. Smooth muscles exhibit tonic activity but extent of contraction of the muscle fibres may vary greatly. By this the viscera organ resists more or less the effort to be stretched. Thus when stomach is empty, its cavity is virtually obliterated by the tonus of gastric muscles. As food is put into the stomach, the wall yields and stretches; for this reason, intra-gastric pressure remains fairly constant as stomach

Table 15.1. Characteristics of smooth muscle

i. Individual fibres are fusiform cells with a centrally placed oval nucleus and structureless protoplasm which contains less soluble protein, glycogen, potassium, phosphate but more sodium than striated muscle.
ii. Supplied by ANS with motor and inhibitory nerves, the ganglia of which are contained in nerve nets near to or on the muscle cells they supply. Denervated smooth muscle may show tonic or intermittent rhythmic contraction.
iii. A single stimulus is often subliminal. They respond to make and break of a constant current, with a long latent period of 0.2-2.0 sec.; contraction period of 0.5 sec. - few minutes, with a corresponding period of relaxation.
iv. Decreased pH causes increased tonus; increased pH decreased tonus. Eserine, lead salts, barium salts, histamine, acetylcholine, pilocarpine may cause contraction.
v. Shows extensibility in oxygenated Ringer solution the degree depends on initial tonus. Acetylcholine and histamine increases while adrenaline reduces the tone.

is being filled. The same principle applies to urinary bladder. Therefore, the walls of hollow organs accommodate themselves by their tonus to the volume of the contents without any marked alteration in the internal pressure or in the tension of the wall.

Tonus in smooth muscle is therefore not an exclusively reflex phenomenon, which can be suppressed by denervation, like the tonus of striated muscle.

CHEMICAL PHENOMENON

- Myosin is the principal protein but it is not similar with the myosin of skeletal muscle.
- There is less potassium than in striated muscle; the Na/K ratio is 1 : 1.5 instead of 1:5.
- Creatine phosphate is found in a quantity approximately one tenth that of striated muscle.
- Oxygen consumption rises and falls with the activity of the muscle; there is therefore no strictly basal oxygen consumption.
- Glycogen is found in a concentration of about 150 mg per cent. Inorganic phosphate makes up half the total phosphorus; a large quantity of P is bound in nucleoproteins.

CONTRACTION

- Contraction in response to any stimuli is very slow and frequently rhythmical. The contraction time of a single twitch is 10 to 15 times that of slow striated muscle. Relaxation is even slower.
- The maximum tension developed in contraction increases with the resting length up to an optimum as in the striated muscle; but this optimum initial length varies considerably and is influenced by previous condition of the muscle.
- When a smooth muscle is stretched, it lengthens, at first rapidly and then more slowly, taking a long time to reach the final length, owing to its internal fraction or so called "viscosity." Tension also increases on stretching, but after quickly arriving at a maximum, it decreases slowly following an exponential curve, similar in its time course, to that of relaxation. This release of tension without change in length gives great 'plasticity' to smooth muscles — a property of importance in visceral functions.
- Repeated stimulation provokes fatigue; contraction and relaxation are shortened and finally there is complete relaxation instead of contracture such as occurs in fatigued striated muscles.

FACTORS AFFECTING

- An increase in temperature diminishes excitability and tonus — between 45 to 50°C, relaxation is complete; the thermic contracture seen in striated muscle at 45°C temperature is not observed. Cold increases tonus and prolongs its survival.
- Acidity provokes contracture in striated muscle but in smooth muscles it produces relaxation and quiescence while alkalinity increases tonus and spontaneous rhythmic activity.
- Ionic Equilibrium - A decrease in total concentration of salts increases excitability and amplitude of rhythmic movements; an increase has the opposing effects. K^+ in adequate concentration increases tone and contraction; Ca^{++} has opposite and antagonistic effect of K^+. The whole response is conditioned by K : Ca ratio.
- Previous activity .... A contracted muscle or one that is in a condition of high tonus will relax when excited by a stimulus that in other conditions would provoke contraction.
- Stimulation of vagus usually produces an increase in tonus and in rhythmic movements of intestine.

SMOOTH MUSCLES IN ACTION

Membrane Potential

a. Resting

The resting membrane potential of smooth muscle is ranging between - 40 to - 70 mV (average - 55 -ve) depending on the location of smooth muscle. It is lower

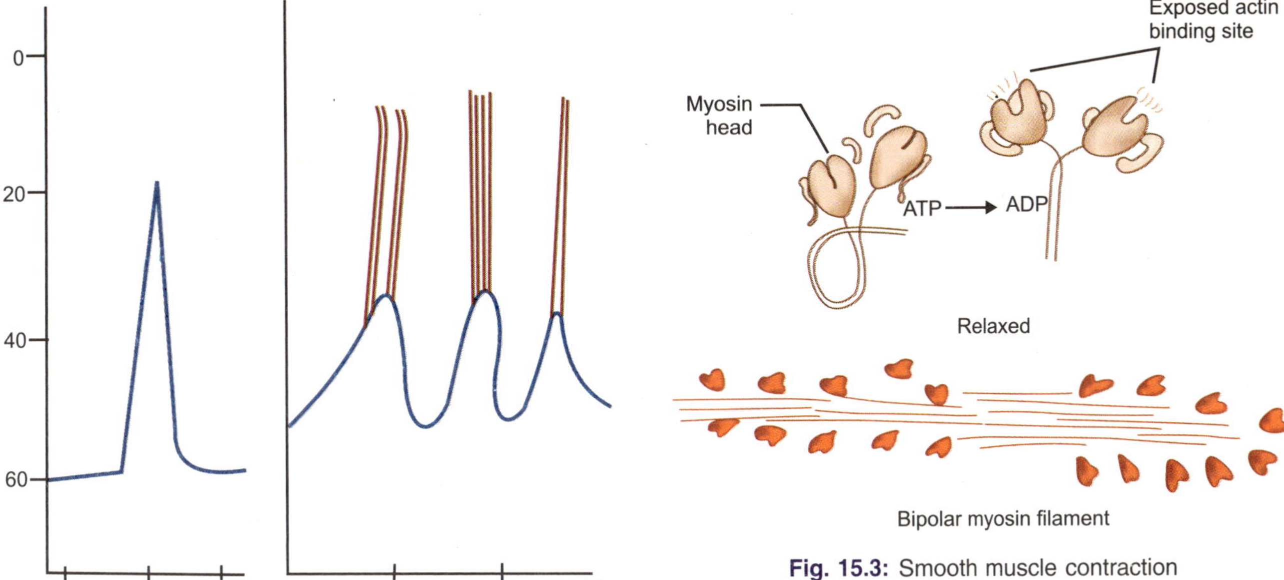

Fig. 15.2: Smooth muscle in action

Fig. 15.3: Smooth muscle contraction

than cardiac or skeletal muscle because of a higher ratio of Na^+ to K^+ permeability (30 mV less negative than skeletal muscle).

b. Action Potential (AP)

- Typical spike action potential occurs in most type of single unit smooth muscle and duration of which is 10 to 50 milliseconds.
- However, some vascular smooth muscles (e.g. rat's aorta) exhibit a prolonged plateau component that follows the spike. The importance of plateau is that it can account for the prolonged periods of contraction that occur in some type of smooth muscles such as ureter, uterus and vascular.
- Sodium participates very little in generation of action potential in smooth muscle.

c. Spontaneous Activity and Slow Wave Potential

i. Many smooth muscles have spontaneous contractions and electric activity, i.e. they possess 'automaticity' which means that action potential arise within smooth muscle without an extrinsic stimulus. Automaticity is produced by pacemaker potential that depolarise the cell to its threshold potential.

ii. Some smooth muscles (e.g. longitudinal layer of small intestine) have a peculiar type of pacemaker potential called 'slow waves' which are slow oscillations in the membrane potential with a periodicity of several seconds. These slow waves are caused by waxing and waning of pumping of sodium ions outward through the muscle fibre membrane; the membrane potential becomes more negative when sodium is pumped rapidly and less negative when the sodium pump becomes less active.

iii. Another cause of slow wave is that conductance of the ion channels increase and decrease rhythmically. Anyway, during their depolarisation phase, a train of action potential is elicited, the frequency of the burst gradually diminishes and action potential stops when re-polarising phase of the slow wave is underway. Therefore, action potential occurs in bursts during successive slow wave oscillations and the peak to peak amplitude of slow wave is about 15 to 30 mV. Therefore, the slow waves are called 'pace maker waves' and this type of activity controls the rhythmical contractions of the gut.

iv. Another hypothetic cause of slow wave is based on K^+ channel whose activity is stimulated by Ca^{2+} giving rise to a Ca^{2+} activated K^+ conductance or current. The gain in Ca during an action potential burst would activate this current, which would then hyperpolarise and shut off the burst. When Ca is lowered again, the cell would depolarise and initiate a new burst.

v. The slow waves are called pacemaker because they can initiate action potentials. The slow waves themselves cannot cause muscle contraction, but when their potential rises above the level of - 35 mV an action potential develops and spreads over the muscle mass, causing contraction.

d. Stretch Response

Some smooth muscles behave like stretch receptors, in that stretch (increased longitudinal applied tension) of the muscle leads to partial depolarisation and initiation of action potential bursts and contractions. Thus, a load applied to such a smooth muscles causes it to contract actively to counteract the deforming strain. The common such examples are longitudinal muscle layer of GIT, smooth muscles of urinary bladder, uterus, blood vessels etc. The above mentioned response is due to a combination of normal slow wave potentials plus a decrease in negativity of the membrane potential caused by the stretch itself.

e. Control by Nerves

Some smooth muscles (notably multiunit muscles) are controlled by ANS. Majority of smooth muscle cells are affected by diffusion of a neuro-transmitter; which is capable of causing contraction or relaxation of concerned smooth muscle and this action depends on type of neurone and released neuro-transmitter. Because of cell to cell propagation of action potential, the effect of neurone can be quickly reflected over greater distances than the diffusion of the neuro-transmitter alone would predict. The common such neuro-transmitters are acetylcholine and nor-epinephrine and both of these cause depolarisation of the smooth muscle membrane which elicit the muscular contraction. According to these facts, this local depolarisation generates what is called "junctional potential" which spreads "electrotonically over the entire fibre which finally leads to muscular contraction. It is to be remembered here that fibres are too small to generate an action potential.

f. Calcium: Controlling Factor

- Elevation of calcium initiates contraction and lowered calcium produces relaxation.
- In skeletal muscles, excitation-contraction coupling is mediated by calcium ions. But here in smooth muscles, calcium ions may not be released from sarcoplasmic reticulum and furthermore, there is no troponin for calcium to react.
- *Contractility:* Smooth muscles are devoid of troponin and in its place they contain regulatory protein called *calmodulin* which is a Ca^{2+} binding protein.
- Ca^{2+} binds with calmodulin → Ca^{2+} calmodulin complex activates myosin kinase (phosphorylating enzyme) → phosphroylated myosin head interacts with actin which causes contraction

Relaxation

- Is produced by lowering calcium ion concentration which is accomplished by turning off Ca^{2+} influx and Ca^{2+} release coupled with stimulation of sarcolemmal Ca^{2+} pump.

Cessation of Contraction

i. Reduction in Ca^{2+} level of extracellular fluid
ii. It leads to activation of an enzyme called, myosin phosphatase → dephosphorylation of myosin head → termination of actin — myosin — interaction → relaxation.

The Latch Mechanism

i. Once the smooth muscle is at its full bloom means fully contracted; the degree of activation of muscle can usually be reduced to far less than the initial level and yet the muscle is able to maintain its full strength of contraction. Furthermore, the energy consumed to maintain contraction is very little as compared with energy required for continuation of contraction of skeletal muscles. This is Latch mechanism which means, state of maintaining force despite reduced velocities.
ii. It is due to prolonged attachment of the myosin cross bridges to the actin filaments.
iii. Due to this property, muscle is capable of maintaining prolonged tonic contraction by using very little energy and that too for hours together.
iv. Very little energy is used by the muscle because ATP is not degraded to ADP (exception - detachment of head).

LATCH MECHANISM : AT A GLANCE

- Strong activation of enzyme myosin kinase and myosin phosphatase → velocity of contraction is great.
- Decreased enzymatic activation → decreased cyclic frequency → myosin heads to remain attached to actin filament for long period → number of heads attached to actin filament large → tension still maintained or latched.
- This mechanism maintains the tone in many smooth muscle organs.

STRESS RELAXATION IN SMOOTH MUSCLE: AT A GLANCE

- When there occurs sudden increase in volume of fluid in urinary bladder, this leads to large increase in pressure here. But during next little time the pressure returns to original level despite of continuous stretch. This is stress relaxation.
- So this is nothing but ability of a hollow organ (visceral type of smooth muscle) to return nearly to its original force of contraction; within a short time of its elongation/shortening.
- Stretching of muscle → Latch phenomenon resists.
- Successive recycling → head release and attach further along actin filament myosin cross bridges is very nearly the same → length of muscle changes while tension returns to original value.

CA^{2+} AND CONTRACTIONS

1. Elevation of calcium is produced by :
   - *Ca^{2+} influx:* through voltage dependent slow and fast Ca^{2+} channels.
   - *Ca^{2+} release:* from sarcoplasmic reticulum stores through activation of Ca^{2+} release channels in sarcoplasmic reticulum membrane by Ca^{2+} (trigger Ca^{2+}) or by IP_3, or both.
   - Ca^{2+} - Na exchange
   - Inhibition of sarcolemmal Ca^{2+} - ATPase - Ca^{2+} pump.
   - Receptor operated ion channels (not voltage gated)
2. In most smooth muscles, the number of fast Ca^{2+} channels is relatively small compared with the number of slow Ca^{2+} channels. Even then Ca^{2+} influx is existing and causing muscular contraction because of the occurrence of Ca^{2+} triggering of Ca^{2+} release phenomenon from sarcoplasmic reticulum which further depends on absolute calcium level. In this way, this Ca^{2+} current serves as second messenger involved in initiating contraction.
3. Therefore, there are two sources from which calcium may enter the sarcoplasm following excitation - one is sarcoplasmic reticulum; and another is extracellular fluid.
   a. Extracellular fluid : calcium source ..... It supplies in following ways -
      i. First mechanism is voltage dependent. Threshold depolarisation leads to opening up of voltage-gated calcium channels in the sarcolemma. Due to this the Ca^{2+} enter the muscle cell leading to depolarisation phase of the action potential. Therefore, calcium is responsible for action potential as well as it initiates the contractile process by raising sarcoplasmic calcium level.
      ii. Neurotransmitter/hormone which can excite smooth muscle combines with its receptor on sarcolemma. The receptor is coupled to G-protein which in turn is coupled to calcium channel in the sarcolemma. These channels are chemically gated and opening of these channels leads to influx of extracellular calcium into the muscle cell, and thus also raising sarcoplasmic calcium level.
4. So in nutshell, "All the calcium ions that cause contraction enter the muscle cell from extracellular fluid at the time of action potential and another source of calcium ion, i.e. sarcoplasmic reticulum is almost considered as a rudimentary source. There is reasonably a high concentration of Ca^{2+} in extra-cellular space - greater than 10^{-3} molar in comparison with less than 10^{-7} molar in cell sarcoplasm."
5. When there occurs a reduction in Ca^{2+} concentration in extracellular fluid, the contraction of smooth muscles ceases. Therefore, the force of contraction of smooth muscle is highly dependent on extracellular fluid Ca^{2+} concentration.
6. The above mentioned reduction in Ca^{2+} level is achieved in two ways — one is throwing Ca^{2+} back into extracellular fluid from smooth muscle fibre and second is by pumping the Ca^{2+} into sarcoplasmic reticulum. Whatever the means, it is said that these pumps are very slow acting as compared with skeletal muscles and this explains that the duration of smooth muscle contraction is often in order of seconds rather than 100th to 10th of a second, as occurs for skeletal muscle.
7. Factors affecting ...
   i. Lack of O_2 in local tissues causes smooth muscle relaxation; excess CO_2 causes vasodilatation; excess H^+ concentration causes increased vasodilatation.
8. For relaxation, the elevated calcium level must revert to the resting level of about 1×10^{-7} M. This is accomplished by following mechanisms :
   - Intracellular Ca^{2+} - extracellular Na+ exchange across the sarcolemma.
   - Stimulation of sarcolemmal Ca^{2+}-ATPase - Ca^{2+} pump due to higher Ca^{2+} concentration during action potential.
   - Stimulation of sarcoplasmic reticulum Ca^{2+} ATPase - Ca^{2+} pump.
   - The high calcium during action potential stimulates the Ca^{2+} - Na exchange to operate in forward direction - internal Ca^{2+} for external Na^+.

9. Smooth muscle metabolism is oxidative. The density of mitochondria is low. Due to low contractile energy requirement, oxidative ATP synthesis generally matches energy demand. Therefore, inspite of low phosphocreatine pools compared to skeletal muscles little change in phosphocreatine or ATP concentration can be measured during contraction, because increase in oxidative phosphorylation provide ATP as needed. Hence, oxygen debt phenomenon does not exist for smooth muscles. When a smooth muscle is fully oxygenated, it produces substantial amounts of lactate.

SMOOTH MUSCLE CONTRACTION : HUMORAL AND LOCAL FACTORS

- Hypoxia in local tissues → smooth muscle relaxation → vasodilatation
- Hypercapnia → vasodilatation
- Increased H ion concentration → vasodilatation.
- Blood-borne hormones affecting contractions are noradrenaline, acetylcholine, vasopressin, angiotensin histamine, oxytocin, serotonin, etc.
- Muscle cell membrane contains excitatory as well as inhibitory receptors and action depends on respective activation. These receptors on activation opens ionic channels (Na^+, Ca^{2+}) which leads to depolarisation of membrane leading to development of action potential which promote contraction. Closing the entry of these two ions and by opening the potassium channels inhibits contraction.
- Sometimes - hormone activates membrane receptor → release of Ca^{2+} from sarcoplasmic reticulum → contraction. Conversely

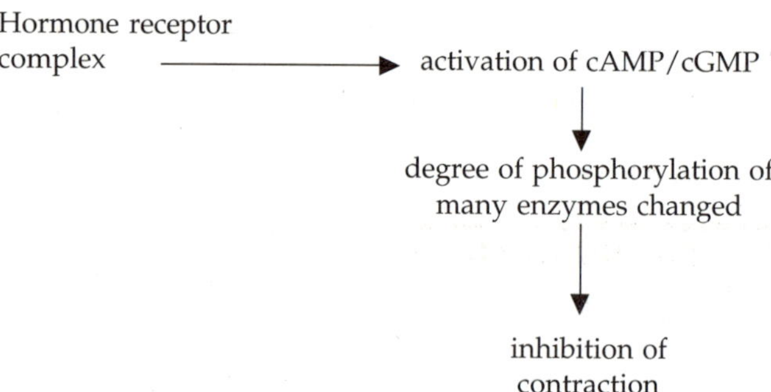

16 Contractile Tissue Cardiac Muscle—In Action

Calcium is the key intracellular messenger for the regulation of contraction. The force of contraction depends on extra cellular Ca^{2+} concentration. When calcium concentration goes below the normal level the contractile force is diminished and when its concentration is elevated, contractile force is augmented.

INTRODUCTION

i. The calcium required for contraction is coming from following sources.
   a. The extracellular Ca^{2+} pool, as a Ca^{2+} influx through voltage gated slow Ca^{2+} channels;
   b. Ca^{2+} pool in the sarcoplasmic reticulum lumen. Calcium from first source triggers the release of Ca^{2+} from the second source. Ninety per cent contribution is derived from Ca^{2+} release from sarcoplasmic reticulum.
ii. The release of calcium ion (Ca^{2+}) from sarcoplasmic reticulum occurs through Ca^{2+} release channels embedded in sarcoplasmic reticulum membrane. These are not voltage gated but are gated by Ca^{2+} and IP_3 and ATP is also required for its release.
iii. The Ca^{2+} concentration in sarcoplasmic reticulum lumen is much higher than that of myoplasm and therefore there is a large concentration gradient for the transport of Ca^{2+} from sarcoplasmic lumen into the myoplasm. The existence of membrane potential across sarcoplasmic reticulum membrane is doubtful.

- In cardiac muscle, the action potential is caused by opening of two channels viz.
   a. Fast sodium channels — identical with skeletal muscle. They are called fast channels because they allow tremendous number of sodium ions to enter the muscle fibres, and they remain open for only 10,000th of a second, and then they suddenly close, and this closure is associated with process of repolarisation
   b. Slow calcium channels or calcium sodium channels.

Cause of Plateau and Prolonged Action Potential

Because of entry of sodium and calcium ions the membrane remain depolarised for sometime which means the graph stays for sometime called "plateau." These two ions prevent potassium ion outflux which is another "cause of plateau." When sodium calcium channel closes, potassium outflux starts which marks repolarisation.

i. Action potential → decreased permeability for potassium → decreases outflux of K ions → prevention of early recovery
   (Decreased permeability for K^+ may be due to excess Ca^{2+} influx through calcium channels)
   Conversely:
   Slow Ca^{2+} channels close → influx of Ca^{2+} and Na^+ decreases → membrane permeability for K^+ increases → rapid loss of potassium from fibre → resting membrane potential + cessation of action potential

Slow Ca^{2+} Channels

The main characteristics are:

i. Their activity depends on metabolic energy, in the form of ATP. This is the reason that in condition of hypoxia or ischaemia (which are known to inhibit metabolism and lower ATP level), these channels are selectively inhibited.
ii. Their activity is selectively inhibited by acidosis. This permits normal action potential to be generated, continuously, of course contractions are greatly depressed.

iii. Their activity is regulated by cyclic nucleotides. It is stimulated by cAMP and inhibited by cGMP; So these messengers are acting as antagonists to each other.
- cAMP → activates cAMP-PK → Increases the permeability of Ca^{2+} channels being opened at a given voltage and the mean open time is increased.
- cGMP →activates cGMP-PK phosphorylation Inhibits (Protein kinase) channel activity

iv. Their activity is blocked by calcium antagonists or slow channel blockers. (e.g. nifedipine, verapamil, bepridil, diltiazem).

v. They protect the heart
- Vasospasm → resultant acidosis → shutting of Ca^{2+} channel →heart cells stop contraction.
- Ca^{2+} influx is indirectly controlled by regulating the activity of one type of K^+ channel.

Table 16.1. Differences between two calcium channels

Slow channel	*Fast channel*
• High threshold	• Low threshold
• Regulated by cAMP and cGMP	• Such regulation does not exist
• Regulated by phosphory lation	• No such regulation
• Blocked by Ca^{2+} antagonist drugs	• No such blockage
• Can be opened by Ca^{2+} agonist drugs	• No such opening
• Kinetically slower	• Kinetically faster

Ca^{2+} - Na^+ Exchange Reversal

- This exchange reaction contributes to the removal of Ca^{2+} from the cell. The exchange in a resting cell is directed to trade one intracellular Ca^{2+} for three extracellular Na^+. Therefore this exchange reaction contributes to the relaxation of cardiac muscle, immediately after action potential and it requires rapid lowering of elevated calcium level.
- This exchange also contributes to excitation-contraction coupling.
- Anything that causes Na level to rise will also cause Ca level to rise secondarily, thereby leading a more forceful contraction called 'positive ionotropic effect.' This is the basis of action of drugs like digitalis and ouabain-the cardiac glycosides — the drugs given in failing hearts.

EXERCISE

If muscles are worked too hard, the cells run out of oxygen. This causes accumulation of lactic acid due to fermentation. It leads to soreness and stiffness.

MUSCLE — GLOSSARY

Muscle: Is a contractile tissue which brings about movements. Forty to fifty per cent body mass is muscles. Muscle cells are slender-elongated.

Fatigue: Exhaustion/tiredness. Due to prolonged contraction lactic acid accumulates and because of this muscle does not or no more responds to stimulus.

Actin: Secondary filament present in myofibril. Mol. wt. 70,000. Associated with Ca^{2+}.

Myosin: Contractile element in myofibril. Mol. wt. 4,80,000. Associated with Mg^{++}.

Myofibril: Protein fibrils present in sarcoplasm of a myofibre.

Myofibre: Muscle cell (myocyte).

Muscle twitch: Response by a muscle to a stimulus.

Sarcolemma: Cell membrane present over muscle cell.

Sarcoplasm: Cytoplasm of a muscle cell.

Sarcomere: Functional unit of a myofibril space in between two Z lines of a myofibril.

Sarcosome: Mitochondrium of a muscle cell.

Hensen's disc: H band present at centre of anisotropic band. Myosin filaments seen.

Isotropic band: I band/light band present on myofibril. Only actin filaments seen.

Muscle tone: Some degree of contractility seen even during rest. This type of slight contractility seen is tone. It may be due to nerve impulses coming from spinal cord.

Krause's membrane: Membrane present at the middle of I band of a myofibril. Represented as Z.

Ratchet mechanism: by which actin filaments move in one direction.

Tropomyosin and Troponin: Proteins present on actin filament, prevent formation of actomyosin complex.

Isometric contraction: Does not require much sliding of actin filaments, e.g. while standing leg muscles become stiff.

Isotonic contraction: Muscle does not shorten during contraction. It requires much sliding over, e.g. weight lifting. During running both types of contractions are seen.

He was ***Szent-Gyorgyi*** who first studied chemical changes during contraction.

Wasting: Reduction in size of muscle.

Hypertrophy: Excessive development of a muscle due to its overuse.

Table 16.2: Different type of muscle

Part	*Smooth*	*Striated*	*Cardiac*
1. Muscle fibre	Spindle shaped, 15-500 µm size	Cylindrical unbranched 10 cm	Short 100 µm cylindrical branched
2. Sarcolemma	Thin indistinct	Distinct	Thin
3. Sarcoplasm	Less abundant	Plenty	Abundant
4. Nucleus	Single, centrally located	Many	Single, centrally placed
5. Myofibrils	Not distinctly visible	Larger distinct	Less distinct
6. Striations	Absent	Present	Faint
7. Intercalated disc	Absent	Absent	Present
8. Contraction	Slow, no fatigue	Rapid, undergo fatigue	Strong, No fatigue
9. Control	Involuntary	Voluntary	Involuntary
10. Distribution	GIT, Respiratory tube, blood vessels, urogenital system	Attached to bones	Heart
11. Blood supply	Moderate	High	Very high

Disused atrophy: When a muscle is not used for a longer time it becomes weak.
Muscular spasm: Painful pulling of a muscle.
Paralysis: Loss of motor power.
Schwann cell: Internodal part nodular on axon. It secretes myelin.
Ranvier's node: Wherever myelin is absent neurolemma touches the axon giving appearance of a node called Ranvier's node.
Nissl's granules: Basophilic. Present in neuroplasm of a cyton. They contain RNA Provide necessary energy for impulse conduction.
Myelin: Fat material enclosing axon. Gives support to axon. Prevents leakage of information.

BIBLIOGRAPHY

1. Bessman SP, Geiger PS. The phosphoryl creatine shuttle. Science 1981;211:448.
2. Blinks JR. Intracellular (Ca^{2+}) measurements. In: The Heart and CVS Edited by HA Fozzard et al. New York, Raven Press 1986;671-702.
3. Bohr DF, Webb RC. Vascular smooth muscle function and its changes in hypertension. Amer J Med 1984;77:3.
4. Brady AJ. Electrophysiology of cardiac muscle: In mammalian myocardium Edited by GA Langer and AJ Brady, New York, John Wiley and Sons 1974;135-161.
5. Branuwald EJ, et al. Mechanism of cardiac contraction and relaxation: In heart diseases, edited by E. Braunwald. Philadelphia, WB Saunders Co. 1988;383-25.
6. Braunwald EJ, Ross Jr. EH. Sonnenblick Mechanism of contraction of normal and failing heart. 2nd ed. Boston. Little Brown, 1976.
7. Bulbring E, Tomita T. Catecholamine action on smooth muscle. Pharm Rev 1987;39:49.
8. Butler TM, et al. High energy phosphate metabolism in vascular smooth muscle. Ann Rev Phy 1985;47:629.
9. Edward R. Perl, Somatosensory mechanism. Ann Rev Phy 1963;25:459.
10. Fitts RH. Cellular mechanism of muscle fatigue. Phy Rev 1994;74:49.
11. Franzini Armstrong C, et al. Structure and development of E.C. coupling unit in skeletal muscle. Ann Rev Phy 1994;56:509.
12. Gabella G. Structural apparatus for force transmission in smooth muscle. Phy Rev 1984;64:455.
13. Hartshorne DJ, et al. Regulation of smooth muscle actomyosin. Ann Rev Phy 1981;43:519.
14. Homsher E. Muscle enthalpy production and its relationship to actomyosin ATPase. Ann Rev Phy 1987;49:673.
15. Huxley AF, Gordon AM. Nature (Ld.) Striation pattern in active and passive shortening of muscle. 1962;193:280.
16. Huxley AP. Muscular contraction. Ann Rev Phy 1988;50:1.
17. Janmey PA. Phosphoinositides and calcium as regulators of cellular actin assembly and disassembly. Ann Rev Phy 1994;56:169.
18. Kamm KE, et al. Regulation of smooth muscle contractile elements by second messengers. Ann Rev Phy 1989;51:299.
19. Katz AM. Cardiac ion channels. New Eng J Med 1993;328:1244.

17 Excitable Unit: Nerve

THE NEURONE

It is the essential unit of central nervous system, and is constituted by nerve cell and nerve fibre.

Nerve Cell

It can live for years together but if it is destroyed by any means, it cannot be replaced; any way, it is famous for its long life. It is also having characteristic quality of having great susceptibility to environmental and metabolic disturbances. *Nissl granules* are the most characteristic feature in the cytoplasm, appearing as ergastoplasmic structures through electron microscope. It is said to possess high class metabolic activity which is dependent upon adequate supply of oxygen and glucose. This is the reason that cerebral cortex cannot resist anoxia of five minutes duration as well as blood sugar level falling to 20 mg per cent; both the states are resulting in unconsciousness.

Nerve Fibre

- It is constituted by *axon* (axis cylinder) *myelin sheath* and *neurolemma* (nucleated sheath of Schwann).
- The myelin sheath is a lipid structure and is a characteristic feature. It should be remembered that 50 to 60 per cent of dry weight of brain is made up of lipid consisting of cholesterol, sphingomyelin and cerebrosides, gangliosides (sphingolipids); there is no esterified cholesterol.
- After giving off one or more collateral fibres, the larger axons may run for long distances in central nervous system, as they do in peripheral nerves, without branching. Near their termination, they lose their myelin sheath and break up into *a number of five terminal twigs* which either enter the peripheral end organ or make synaptic connection with the cell bodies of other neurones by ring like endings or with dendrites of these neurones.
- As told, neurone consists of body (soma) and two types of processes viz. *dendrites and axons.*
  - — Nerve fibres in which axon and dendrite arise by a common stem called unipolar -
  - — Nerve fibres in which axon and dendrite spring from opposite or at least different parts of soma, called bi or multipolar.
- Neurones are linked together to form conducting pathways and this phenomenon is *effected* by contact of axon terminal of one nerve cell with body or dendrite of another. Such a function is named as *synapse*.
- Within the grey matter, axis cylinders are enclosed only by plasma membrane, but upon leaving the grey substance they acquire a sheath of lipid material called myelin. Myelin sheath of somatic nerves is enveloped in turn by a delicate membrane of flat cells called sheath of *Schwann or neurilemma*. In these nerves, myelin is absent at certain points which gives the appearance like constricted at regular intervals and dipping inwards of neurilemma and it is named as *Nodes of Ranvier*. The usual internodal distance is considered to be 1 mm and each internodal segment of neurilemma consists of a single Schwann cell.

NEUROGLIA (GLIA = GLUE)

It is regarded as a type of putty serving the humble purpose of holding together the more noble neurones. It is a special type of interstitial tissue. Three types of cells can be distinguished within it namely — astrocytes, oligodendrocytes, and microglia.

Astrocytes

They are found surrounding blood vessels and are thought to make up blood brain barrier. They are of two types—protoplasmic (found entirely in grey matter specially in middle and deep layers of cerebral cortex and in cerebellum in its molecular layer) and fibrous (found in white matter but also arranged in a dense layer in most superficial zone of cortex immediately under the pia mater to form a superficial limiting membrane).

- They are involved in selection and transport of metabolites and fluid interchanges between vascular spaces and the nerve cells. They also play an active part in diseases since it is said that it is the astrocyte cell from which great majority of gliomas (brain tumour) arise.

Oligodendroglia

Is largest group of interstitial cells. They bear same relation to the myelin sheath of nerve fibres in central nervous system as the cells of sheath of Schwann do in peripheral nerves so it can be said that they are related with myelin's preservation. They are sensitive to noxious agents. They are not characteristically epithelial; they lack basal laminae.

Microglia

Are mesodermal in origin. They are not present at birth but invading the brain from pia mater in the course of a few weeks. They are phagocytic in function.

NEURONAL DEGENERATION

When any part of neurone is injured, the remainder of it will also show constant and characteristic changes.

Wallerian Degeneration: (Waller-1850)

These are the characteristic changes in distal part of nerve fibre when any level of it is divided. The axis cylinder becomes fibrillated and disintegrates, medullary sheath breaks up into droplets of myelin. Cells of Schwann sheath are converted into phagocytes. Since this sheath is not present in central nervous system which illustrates non-occurrence of healing after injury in brain and spinal cord. There are also changes occurring in proximal part of divided fibre like degeneration of medullary sheath up to the first node of Ranvier, etc. The B group fibres are failed first of all, then A and C comes in the last. Up to first three days of injury nerve continues to conduct impulse but after fifth day an impulse cannot be evoked.

Nissl's Degeneration

It occurs when the nerve fibre which arises from it is injured. It may also be due to viral originated or a bacterial toxin originated one. The cell becomes swollen and rounded, nucleus is eccentric, Nissl's granules of cytoplasm disintegrate and disappear, chromatolysis, are changes occurring.

About 3 weeks after nerve division, regeneration takes place with reappearance of granules. Its rate is 1 to 4 mm daily. There is a rapid proliferation of Schwann cells. A neuroma is a tumour like mass in which fibres are intermeshing forming a tumour like swelling.

STAGES: REGENERATION

1. Schwann cells from proximal and distal cut ends of the nerve grow out like fibrils (pseudopodia like). The fibrils at both extremes are in contact. This gap filling between two extremes leads to development of continuity of neurilemmal tube.
2. Full establishment of axis cylinder inside the neurilemmal tube.
3. Within one year, myelination is completed.
4. In nerve cell body, first Nissl's granules appear and then Golgi body.
5. Excess fluid is lost. Nucleus centrally placed.
6. Functional recovery occurs after a long time.

CLASSIFICATION OF NERVE FIBRE

a. Histologically

- Medullated (myelinated)
- Non-medullated (non-myelinated)

Nerve receives a white covering called myelin sheath which is an integral part of Schwann cell. It is composed of layers of mixed lipids arranged concentrically alternating with layers of neurokeratogenic protein. Its function is to insulate the nerve fibres and thus to prevent spread of nerve impulse to other adjacent fibres. Myelinated nerve fibres which are found in brain and spinal cord differ from those of peripheral nerve fibres in that the neurolemma is not present. In non-medullated fibres this sheath is absent, so fibre being directly invested with neurolemma.

b. Chemically

- Adrenergic (Producing nor-epinephrine)
- Cholinergic (Producing acetylcholine)

c. Functionally

- Motor (efferent)
- Sensory (afferent)

d. Diameter and Conduction Velocity

- A fibre — myelinated, somatic, afferent and efferent axons.
  - $A\alpha$ — nerve fibres with larger diameter and higher conduction velocity.
  - $A\delta$ — nerve fibres with least diameter and slowest conduction velocity.

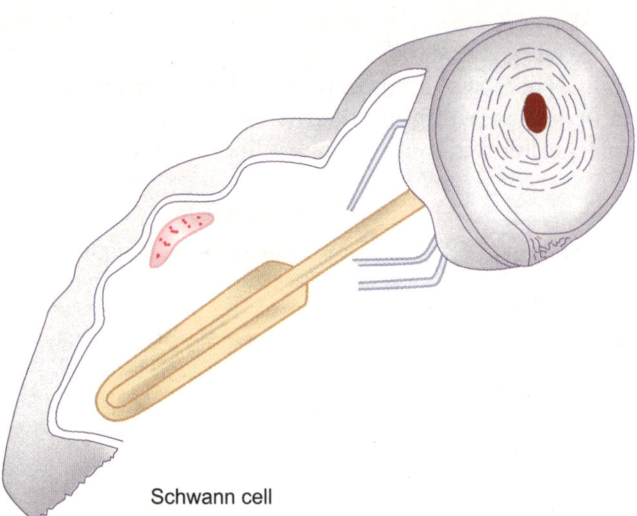

Fig. 17.1: Schwann cell

- B fibre — preganglionic, myelinated, efferent, sympathetic axons
- C fibres — Sympathetic and somatic, unmyelinated axons. Slow conduction velocity, long spike duration, high electrical threshold

e. Numerical Classification

- Ia — originating from muscle spindle and annulo-spiral-spindle ending. Its destination is spindle of extensor or flexor muscle. It reflexly responds as relaxation of antagonist muscle during myotatic contraction of agonist muscle.
- Ib — originating from Golgi tendon organ and destination is muscle of origin. It reflexly responds by lengthening reaction.
- II (A-β; A-γ)—originates from muscle spindle (flower spray ending, skin touch receptors). Its destination is extensor and flexor motoneurones. It reflexly responds by relaxation of extensor and excitation of flexors muscles (withdrawal flexor response).
- III (A-δ)—Originates from muscle and skin (pain temperature receptors). Its destination is extensor and flexor *motor neurones*. It reflexly responds by withdrawal flexor reflex and crossed extensor reflex of opposite limb.
- IV (Dorsal root C fibres)—Originates from muscle and skin pain receptors; otherwise similar with III.

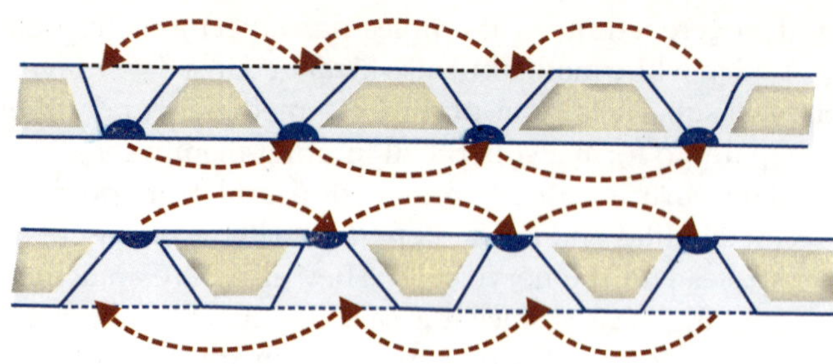

Fig. 17.2: Saltatory conduction (Myelinated nerve)

PHYSIOLOGICAL PROPERTIES

a. Excitability and Conductivity

i. A *neurone* must be excited (or stimulated) for transmitting information from one region to another - is excitation.
ii. The corresponding impulse is said to be conducted along the nerve fibre the property called conduction.
iii. Electrical, mechanical, thermal and chemical are usual types of stimuli known for excitation. Electrical stimuli are commonly used to study this property of excitation and conduction.
iv. Characteristics of stimulus are:
   a. It must be adequately intense
      - Threshold — intensity of a current of a stimulus adequate to cause an impulse.
      - Sub-minimal — Intensity below threshold.
   b. It must be having a sufficient duration. This gives rise to strength — duration relationship.
   c. Its rate of rise should be adequate.

b. Saltatory Conduction in Myelinated Fibres

- It means impulse jumps down the fibre. Electric current flow through the surrounding extracellular fluids and through axoplasm from node to node and in this way successive node are excited one after another.
- It is the reason for high velocity of nerve transmission in myelinated fibres since depolarisation process is jumping long intervals along the axis of nerve fibre.
- Only nodes of Ranvier are depolarised, it conserves energy for axons.
- So impulses are conducted from node to node by myelinated nerve rather than continuously along entire length of fibre.

INJURY CURRENT—ACTION CURRENT

- An excess of positively charged ions is present on the outer surface of the membrane while there is an excess of negatively charged ions on the interior. If the fibre is injured; the alignment of molecules along the membrane is destroyed, called *Depolarised membrane,* while normally it is polarised one. The normal end of the fibre which is still polarised is positive as compared with the injured end, and if the two regions are connected in a circuit, flow of current may be detected. The current recorded under these conditions is called *injury current.* A very sensitive galvanometer must be used or the current can be amplified until it is detectable by less sensitive instruments.
- On effective stimulation of nerve, the polarity of a portion of the fibre is altered. It seems probable that reversal of polarity occurs too. Once a section of fibre undergoes reversal of polarity, local currents are set up which are influencing the adjacent region on each side to cause them to show a similar change. This causes progressing of reversal of polarisation along the fibre in each direction from the site of stimulation. Therefore, shortly after application of single stimulus segments some what removed from the locus of stimulating electrode show reversal of polarity and the normal polarity has been restored at the site of stimulation.

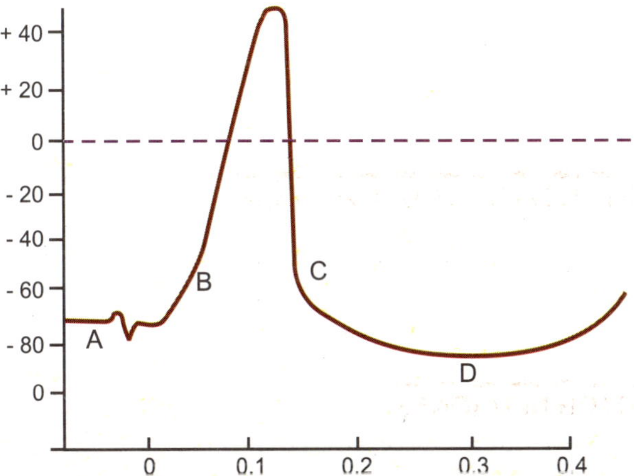

A = Stimulus artifact
B = Firing level
C = After depolarization (Negative after potential)
D = After hyperpolarization (Negative after potential)

Fig. 17.3: Action potential: Nerve fibres

- *Demarcation or injury potential:* It is the potential difference between the intact surface and an injured part. The injured segment provides a low resistance pathway between outside and inside of a nerve. When the nerve is excited, the demarcation current is decreased. Negative variation is propagated with a velocity equal to that of the nerve impulse.
- The spike potential commences from the firing level and is present till the beginning of the *negative after potential.*
- The ***negative after potential*** follows the spike potential till it returns to zero potential. It is succeeded by ***positive after potential.***
- Impulses are passing in one direction only which means from synaptic junctions or receptors along axons to their terminations. This is ***orthodromic*** *conduction* while its opposite term is ***antidromic*** means conduction in opposite direction.
- The story of resting and action potential is based on recording with two electrodes; one on the surface of axon and other inside it. It is better to connect the leads in such a way that when first electrode becomes negative, relative to second, an upward deflection is noted. So ultimately the record is showing an upward deflection followed by an isoelectric interval and then a downward deflection. This is ***biphasic action potential.***
- Factors which affect excitability of nerves and nerve fibres include disturbances of concentration ratios of sodium, calcium and potassium ions in the blood and tissue fluids. Sodium and calcium increase while potassium decreases the excitability. Anaesthetics and narcotics depress the activity due to direct action on protoplasm while local anaesthetics prevent the passage of nerve impulses. A decrease in pH lessens the excitability while opposite response is noticed with increased pH.

Conduction of Nerve Impulse

Nerve cell and its fibre are surrounded by a semi-permeable membrane which is polarised when cell is at rest. It means that on its outside there is a layer of cations while on inner surface, a layer of anions. During excitation the membrane of the axon changes its relative permeability to K^+, Na^+ and Cl^- (relatively impermeable to K^+ and more permeable to Na^+). Sodium ion rapidly moves from interstitial fluid into nerve fibre until sodium concentration inside fibre is greater than that outside the fibre. This reversal of resting ratio of external to internal Na^+ concentration reverses the sign of resting membrane polarisation. Thus, the membrane in active area has become polarised in the reverse direction.

Change in sodium permeability is short lived. It is, increase in K^+ permeability following increase in Na^+ permeability, which is responsible for producing repolarisation of the nerve membrane. This increase in permeability decreases all the barrier to K^+ diffusion, thus causing K^+ to leave the cell which terminates into transfer of positive charge out of cell, leading finally to *repolarisation.*

After depolarisation and *after hyperpolarisation* are representing restorative processes in the cell. Net flux of Na^+ to exterior hyperpolarises the membrane until equilibrium conditions are restored.

Events Causing Action Potential

i. There always occur a resting potential (inside negative and outside positive) whose magnitude varies from 50 to 100 -ve. During application of stimulus when impulse passes along cell membrane, the resting potential is reversed for a very short while and goes towards positivity of the order of +30 to +60 mV. Its duration varies — in mammals it is less than 1 m/sec while in amphibian cardiac muscle it is about 500 m/sec.
ii. As long as membrane of nerve fibre remains totally undisturbed, no action potential occurs in normal nerve. However if any event at all causes enough initial rise in the membrane potential from -90 mV up towards zero level the action potential develops. However, an action potential elicited at any one point on an excitable membrane usually excites adjacent portions of the membrane, resulting in propagation of the action potential.

Refractory Periods

- During the passage of an impulse along the nerve fibre, if a second stimulus is applied (which may be strong enough), it will be unable to produce a response. This interval is named as, absolute refractory period, which is 1.0 to 0.4 m/sec in large mammalian medullated nerve fibres while in sciatic nerve of frog, it has been measured as 2–3 m/sec (2500 impulses per second).
- The period following absolute refractory phase and during which the excitability gradually rises to normal is called *relative refractory period.* For large myelinated fibres it is one-fourth the duration of the refractory period.
- The refractory period is limiting the frequency of the impulses. It renders a continuous excitatory state of nerve *impossible.*
- After above both refractory periods, there exists so called period of *supranormal excitability* during which a stimulus of even less than threshold is capable of eliciting an impulse. It is lasting as long as *negative after potential*. It is followed by a period of subnormal excitability.
- The causes of relative refractory period includes (i) Potassium channels are widely open, causing a state of hyperpolarisation causing difficulty in stimulating fibre; (ii) Sodium channels have yet not been reversed from their state of inactivation.

All or None principle: When a nerve fibre is stimulated impulses are initiated and the impulse travels over the fibre at the same rate of speed regardless of strength of stimulus.

It is a well known fact that a strong stimulus causes an action current of greater amplitude along with a greater muscular response as compared with a weak stimulus. This is because of the fact that weak stimulus is capable of exciting only few fibres while strong stimulus is exciting almost all of them. To sum up, propagated disturbances in a nerve fibre cannot be graded, i.e. nerve fibre either gives a maximum response or nothing at all.

It is better to say that it is a fundamental law of cell physiology since every living cell has to follow it.

The existence of the refractory period follows from theory of nerve conduction which tells that irritability of a nerve fibre lies in its polarised state and impulse generation in its depolarisation. If a stimulus is thrown in during depolarised state of fibre, further depolarisation is impossible and hence, no impulse can be formed. Since the threshold stimulus is followed by an absolute refractory period, the depolarisation of the surface membrane must be complete and therefore, a stronger stimulus can have no greater effect than that produced by the threshold stimulus — this establishes the basis for all or nothing principle.

METABOLISM OF NERVE FIBRE

The energy for sodium potassium pump is derived from hydrolysis of ATP. While in activity it is having resting heat, during action potential it is having initial heat while recovery heat is following the activity.

MOTOR NEURONES

1. *Alpha fibres:* Axons having a diameter ranging between 12–20 μ are generally classified as alpha (α) fibres of A group, and innervate muscle fibres outside muscle spindle. These muscle fibres are called extra fusal fibres and are responsible for the tension a muscle exerts.
2. *B and C fibres:* Myelinated fibres leaving the ventral root in area of thoracic and lumbar cord, are "B" fibres

Table 17.1: Classification of nerve fibres

Group	Diameter (μ)	Rate (m/sec)	Origin	Spike duration (m/sec)
1. Aα	12–20	70–120	Muscle spindle	0.4
2. Aβ	6–12	40–70	Flower spray	0.5
3. Aγ	5–6	15–40	Touch, pressure	0.5
4. Aδ	2–5	12–30	Fast pain	0.5
5. B	< 3	< 3–14	Postganglionic sympathetic	1.2
6. C	0.5–2	0.5–2	Slow pain	2

having a diameter of 3μ (pre ganglionic sympathetic neurones). They synapt with unmyelinated "C" fibres in lateral chain of sympathetic ganglia on either side of the vertebral column or in collateral ganglia.

ACCOMMODATION

Nerves are not readily stimulated by the application of slowly rising currents, because they tend to 'accommodate' to this type of stimulus. This accommodation' arises because of:

i. Depolarisation brings about a long lasting rise in potassium permeability.
ii. Sustained depolarisation semi permanently inactivates the sodium permeability mechanism. Both changes take place with an appreciable time lag after the membrane potential is lowered, so that they are not effective when a constant current is first applied, but become important at long times.

AFTER POTENTIAL

In many types of nerve and muscle fibres the membrane potential does not immediately return to the base line at the end of spike, but undergoes further small and relatively slow variations called 'after potentials.' A variation of membrane potential in same direction as the spike itself is termed 'negative after potential' while a variation in opposite direction is positive after potential.

SUMMARY AND HIGHLIGHTS

Refractory Period

At the end of the spike, the membrane is left with its sodium permeability mechanism inactivated, and its potassium permeability appreciably greater than normal. Both changes help to raise the threshold for re-excitation above normal. The partial inactivation of the sodium permeability means that even to raise inward Na^+ current to the normal critical level requires more depolarisation than usual, and the raised potassium permeability means that the critical Na^+ current is actually greater than normal. Until the permeabilities for both ions have returned to their resting values and sodium mechanism is fully reactivated the shock necessary to trigger a second spike is above the normal threshold in size.

READ AND DIGEST

1. What is excitability of nerve fibres?

Ans. On application of stimulus, there occurs some physico-chemical changes. This is excitability. Following responses occur on adequate stimulus:
a. Action potential
b. Electrotonic potential

2. Comment on action potential?

Ans. It is propagated, biphasic. It obeys 'all or none law' and has refractory period. Normal RMP in nerve fibres is -70 mV; the firing level is at -55 mV; depolarisation ends at +35 mV. Action potential starts in initial segment of nerve fibres.

3. Comment on electrotonic potential? (local response)

Ans. It is non-propagating; and does not obey 'all or none law': on application of subthreshold stimulus, action potential is not produced but some changes are noticed in RMP.

4. Nerve fibres cannot be fatigued. Why?

Ans. Nerve fibres can conduct only one action potential at a time and at that time it is refractory and so does not conduct another action potential.

5. What is the mechanism of saltatory conduction?

Ans. a. Myelin sheath is not permeable to ions.
b. So, entry of Na^+ from extracellular fluid into nerve fibres occurs only at node of Ranvier because here myelin sheath is not present. So node is depolarized.
c. So action potential jumps from one node to another (saltare = jumping)

6. What are `Neurotrophins'?

Ans. a. These are substances, facilitating growth, survival and repair of nerve cells.
b. They are protein in nature.
c. They are nerve growth factor, ciliary neuro-trophic factor, glial cell derived neurotrophic factor, fibroblast growth factor, nurotrophin 3.

7. What is retrograde degeneration?

Ans. The degenerative changes taking place in distal part of the axon also develop in proximal part. The changes occur only upto first node of Ranvier, near the injury.

8. What is transneuronal degeneration?

Ans. If afferent fibres are cut, the degenerative changes occur in neuron with which afferent nerve fibres synapses.

9. What is strength duration relationship?

Ans. In general stronger a stimulus less is the duration required for it to excite an action potential. The weakest stimulus which is able to excite an action potential is `Rheobase.' The minimum duration for which the rheobase has to be applied for excitation is called `utilization time'.

BIBLIOGRAPHY

1. Bullock TH. Conduction and transmission of nerve impulses. BY Nervous control of cellular activities caroline E. Stackpole and Lutie Clemson Leavell Text book of Physiology Macmillan Co. 1953. New York. Ann Rev Physiol 1951;13:26.
2. Huxley. Excitation and conduction in nerve: Quantitative analysis. Science 1964;145:1154.
3. Hodgkin. Ionic basis of nervous conduction. Science 1964;145: 1148.
4. Robert S. Shepard JB Lippincott company Philadelphia Toronto. Human physiology. 1971.
5. Stampfli. Conduction and transmission in nervous system. Ann Rev Phy 1963;25:493.
6. VASS (ed.) A synopsis of physiology - Vth edition. Bristol John Wright and Sons. Ltd. 1961.
7. Watson. Physiology of neuroglia. Phy Review 1974;54(2) 245-71.
8. William D. Zoethout and WW Tuttle. C.V. Mosby company. Conductivity : Nerve physiology. Text book of physiology 13th ed. 1958.
9. Youmans. Basic medical physiology The year book publishers inc. Stimulation and response of muscle and nerve. 1953.

QUESTION BANK

1. **Short notes:**
   a. Latch mechanism of smooth muscle contraction.
   b. Sources of energy for muscle contraction.
   c. Electromyography
   d. Saltatory conduction (Raj. Univ. 1982, M.D.)
   e. Wallerian degeneration (Raj. Univ. 1981, M.D.)
   f. Reaction of degeneration (Raj. Univ. 1980, M.D.)
   g. Refractory period
   h. Rigor mortis (Raj. Univ. B. Sc. Nursing Part I., 1999)
   i. Nerve-impulse transmission (Raj. Univ. B. Sc. Nursing Part I., 1999)
2. **Write in brief:**
   a. End-plate potential and excitation of skeletal muscle fibre.
   b. Oxygen debt
   c. Chronaxie (Raj. Univ., 1992 M.D.)
   d. Excitation contraction coupling (Raj. Univ., 1991 M.D.)
3. **Describe microscopic structure of skeletal muscle. What is excitation - contraction coupling.** (Raj. Univ. 1992, 1994 M.D.)
4. **Describe:**
   a. Mechanism of skeletal muscle contraction
   b. Muscle fatigue
   c. Smooth and cardiac muscle (Raj Univ 1993, M.D.)
5. **Describe structure and transmission across neuromuscular junction. Explain physiological basis of drugs acting on it.** (Raj. Univ. 1992, M.D.)
6. **Describe physiological basis of myaesthenia gravis and rationale of its treatment.** (Raj. Univ. 1988 M.D.)
7. **How has electrophysiology helped in study of physiology? How does electroneurography and electromyography help us in the diagnosis of peripheral nerve injuries?**

UNIT 4

Nature's Obligation

"Respiration is the first essential of life. The lung is more a space than substance and it is the spaces which determine the confirmation of most pulmonary lesion."

Respiration

18

General Plan

Therefore respiratory system consists of organs of respiration (lungs) where gaseous exchange occurs together with various air passages which are meant to connect exterior with lungs. Oxygen is absorbed by the blood while carbon dioxide is eliminated back to the atmosphere.

GENERAL INTRODUCTION

i. It is an established fact that even in hibernation/ animation, exchange of respiratory gases is very much essential for survival. In this connection unicellular organisms are in advantage that they can utilise oxygen from atmosphere and eliminate carbon dioxide to the atmosphere directly. Since cells are deeply placed in multicellular organisms so they are not lying with direct contact with atmosphere. Hence exchange of gases for survival occurs through a specially designed system called 'respiratory passage which further requires a healthy nervous system (Figs 18.1 and 18.2).

ii. For better understanding it consists of (a) *Upper-respiratory passage* — which is constituted by nose, naso and oropharynx, larynx (upto vocal folds), (b) *Lower Respiratory tract* — constituted by trachea, larynx (below vocal folds), two bronchi, bronchioles, terminal bronchioles while, (c) *lung unit* comprises of respiratory bronchioles, alveolar ducts, air sacs.

iii. *General structural outline*: Nose is a median pyramid on face located above oral aperture and in between two eyes. Nostrils are its two elliptical openings. It is peripheral organ of smell together with provider of air passage connecting exterior to the pharynx. Its mucous membrane is highly vascular.

PHARYNX

- Epithelium of oropharynx is of stratified squamous type while nasopharynx is with ciliated columnar type. It is located behind nasal cavities, mouth and larynx. It is extending from cranial base to the level of 6th cervical vertebra and lower border of cricoid cartilage. It is better a musculo-membranous tube—12 to 15 cm long.
- Nasopharynx is behind nose and above soft palate. Its wall is static, cavity is not obliterated.
- *'Larynx'* the 'organ of voice' or it is also told as 'watch dog of respiratory tube, or may also be termed as 'organ of phonation' is extending from tongue to trachea. It is 44 mm long in males and 36 mm in females. It is continue with trachea below. Stratified squamous type of epithelium covers its upper part up to vocal folds while its lower part below vocal fold is covered by ciliary epithelium. In adult males it is lying at the level of 3rd to 6th cervical vertebra but a little higher in females and children.
- *Trachea* is in fact 10 to 12 cm long tube made up of cartilage and fibromuscular membrane. It descends from larynx (extending from level of 6th cervical to 5th thoracic vertebra's upper boarder where it divides into right and left pulmonary bronchi. It is mobile structure capable of altering in length.
- *Bronchi and further division:* As told above trachea terminates into right and left principal bronchi which further divides into secondary bronchi which then subdivides into tertiary bronchi. Each tertiary bronchus divides into several bronchioles which further ramify into terminal bronchioles (normally 50 to 80 in number in a lobule) which further divides into 'respiratory bronchiole' (one-two or even more in quantity) which ramify into alveolar ducts (may be 2 to 12 in number). These alveolar ducts finally meet at one place 'atrium' which is leading into alveolar sacs. Lung unit (primary lobule) is thus constituted by respiratory bronchiole with alveolar ducts — alveolar sacs and alveoli along with their blood vessels-nerves-lymphatic and connective tissue.

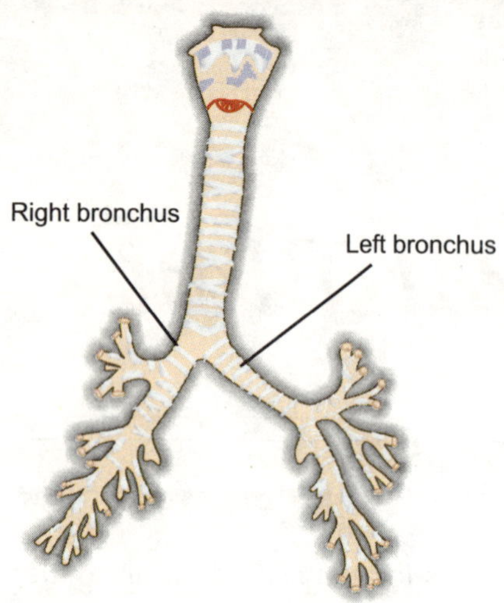

Fig. 18.1: General plan—structure of respiration tube

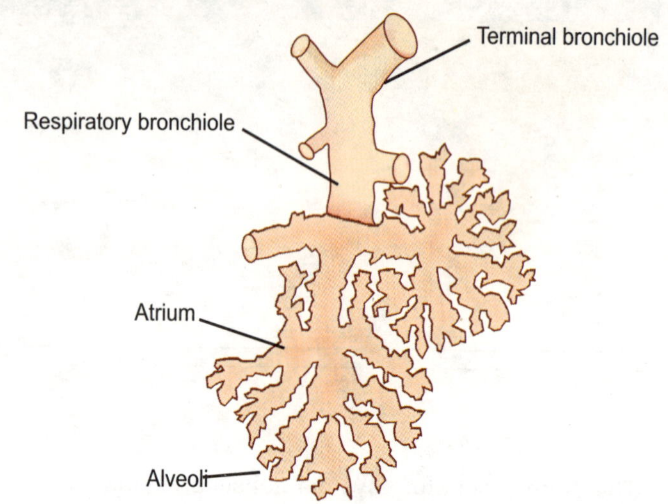

Fig. 18.2: Lung unit

- *Bronchioles:* Their first or initial branching is 1.5 mm long and 0.3 to 0.4 mm in diameter. As regards functions they may be divided into non-respiratory and respiratory; the former are extending from trachea to terminal bronchioles and are devoid of respiratory functions with columnar ciliated epithelium coverage, while later are capable of serving respiratory functions with non-cubical epithelium, which shows flattening towards alveolar sacs.
- Both sympathetic and parasympathetic (vagus) nerves are controlling bronchial muscle. Sympathetic are bronchodilator while vagus is broncho-constrictor. Effect of vagus is said to be a tonic one while bronchodilation is observed when tracheal pressure falls.
- *Broncho-pulmonary segment* is classed as a functionally independent unit of lung tissue having its own blood nerve lymphatic and connective tissue supply and is constituted by tertiary bronchus along with its ramifications and alveoli in connection. There are ten such segments in right lung while left lung is with only nine. They are in fact not broncho-vascular units and are surgically important.
- *The lungs:* At birth their colour is pink, changes to dark grey in adults and with advancement of age this becomes black due to deposition of inhaled carbonaceous material which deposits in loose connective tissue and is more marked among smokers. The weighs of adult right lung is 625 gm while left weighs about 565 gm. It being a spongy structure floats in water and due to air within alveoli it crepitates on handling and also it shows retraction when removed from thorax because of its elastic structure. It is almost conical in shape.
- Each lung is covered by a serous membrane like a closed invaginated sac called 'pleura'. It is of two types visceral and parietal; former adheres to pulmonary surface as well as its interlobular fissures while later is its continuation lining the corresponding half of thoracic wall, diaphragm as well as structures lying in middle thoracic region. The potential space between them is pleural cavity. Both of them are having sliding contact with each other at all phases of respiration.

LUNGS

The two lungs are not identical. Right lung is shorter than left by one inch however its total capacity is greater. The right lung has three lobes, the left lung has two. The maximum capacity of lung averages about 6,500 cubic cm or 1.7 gallons or 6.4 litres.

IMPORTANCE OR PURPOSE

- Respiration is better transport of gases meaning by transport of oxygen from atmosphere to cells together with carbon dioxide transport back to the atmosphere from the different body cells. So it is a mechanical process consisting of supply of oxygen to lung alveoli and removing carbon dioxide from alveoli. It is associated with flow of air both ways in and out of lungs with individual breath, and the process involves respiratory muscles for providing necessary force.

Oxygen is certainly needed for oxidation purposes which causes expenditure of energy together with energy stores as ATP — 'the currency of energy'.

- So functionally respiration is important because:
- Gaseous exchange takes place.
- Maintenance of normal acid-base balance. If there is any change in pH, respiration is altered (normal pH of extracellular fluid is 7.4)
- Maintenance of water balance. Normally during expiration 600 to 800 ml of water is lost as water vapour (frothing during summer in bulls/buffaloes).
- Metabolic products are eliminated through respiration; e.g. acetone breath in diabetic ketosis.
- Body temperature is stabilised. Panting in animals like dogs, cats (warm blooded) during summer is an example. Roughly about 10 per cent of body heat is changed in this way.
- It helps in elimination of some toxic substances like alcohol, etc.
- *So homeostasis is maintained.*

NON-RESPIRATORY FUNCTIONS: LUNGS

- They manufacture surfactant for local use.
- They are said to contain a fibrinolytic system which lyses clot in pulmonary vessels.
- The lungs activate angiotensin I to angiotensin II in pulmonary circulation. The angiotensin converting enzyme (ACE) is present in abundance in surfaces of endothelial cells of pulmonary capillaries and in small pits of vascular surfaces of these cells.
- Prostaglandins, histamine, and kallikrein are the substances which are synthesised/stored and then released into the blood.
- Prostaglandins, bradykinin, serotonin, noradrenaline, acetylcholine, etc. are the substances metabolised by the lungs and partially removed from the blood.

MECHANICS: PULMONARY VENTILATION

- The lungs can be expanded in two ways:
  - — By downward and upward movement of diaphragm to shorten or lengthen the chest cavity;
  - — By elevation or depression of the ribs to increase or decrease the antero-posterior diameter of chest cavity.
- Respiration consists of two phases - inspiration (process of inhaling air from atmosphere into the lungs) and expiration (process of exhaling air to the atmosphere from the lungs). During inspiration the thoracic cage is enlarged, intrapleural pressure falls, volume of lung enlarges with fall in pressure in alveoli, thus occurs a pressure gradient between atmospheric and alveolar air so air rushes into alveoli; while during expiration thoracic cage becomes smaller, pressure in intrapleural space rises, lungs recoil pressing on the alveoli which also shrink, this results in rise in pressure in alveolar air thus a reverse pressure gradient occurs forcing air to exit. The normal rate of respiration in adult is 10 to 18 per minute and the ratio between respiration and arterial pulse in health is 1:4.

Movements of Ribs

- — Bucket handle movement: Middle of rib is moved upwards and outward around the anteroposterior axis, causing increase in transverse diameter.
- — Pump handle movement: Anterior end of lower ribs are raised leading to increase in anterior posterior diameter along oblique axis.

- The ratio between respiration and pulse is 1 : 4 in normal health, altered in pneumonia (1 : 1), in narcotic poisoning 1 : 6.

Abdominal Muscles: Mechanics

- In the resting supine subject, abdominal muscles may be completely inactive throughout breathing cycle.
- In moderate hyperpnoea they become active during expiration. In severe hyperpnoea they exhibit a rapidly augmenting activity during early part of expiration with a decrease well before the beginning of next inspiration.
- They are active during expiration in standing position.
- Atrial mechano-receptors are concerned with reflex inhibition of tonus of abdominal muscles. Any decrease in volume of atria will lead to an increase in tonus of these muscles because of withdrawal of this inhibitory effect.
- The rise in intra-abdominal pressure reduce the capacity of venous system and hence promote better cardiac filling.
- Impulses from atrial mechano-receptors can be channelled to motor neurones which innervate the abdominal muscles without influencing the respiratory centre.
- Tonus of abdominal muscles may be influenced reflexly from receptors in circulatory system (abdominal or thoracic cavity).

Entrance of air into lungs: because of pressure gradient which is created due to:

- Contraction of inspiratory muscles which increases the thoracic cavity in all diameters.
- Then due to increased thoracic cavity, the air rushes due to

— Intrapleural pressure being more negative to intrapulmonary pressure.
— Lower alveolar surface tension due to surfactant.
— Hydraulic traction by fluid which maintains the contact of visceral and parietal pleura due to negative intrapleural pressure.

Inspiratory muscles: Diaphragm, external intercostal, scapular elevators, serratus anterior, erector muscles of spine, sternomastoid.

Expiration

- It is a passive process, while inspiration is an active process. During this act the inspiratory muscles are relaxed, and due to which leads to contraction of stretched lungs (due to its elastic recoil); as well as retraction of thorax (due to its own weight + elastic recoil of costal cartilages). There occurs contraction of anterior oblique muscle + transversus abdominis which raise the intra-abdominal pressure by drawing in of lower ribs downwards and medially to aid expiration.
- During quiet breathing abdominal muscles are not used. Viscera and diaphragm are kept in position because of elasticity of abdominal wall. During special circumstances like coughing, straining or high respiration rates, these muscles come into action. The accessory muscles of inspiration are sternomastoid and scaleni.
- The Diaphragm (muscle of respiration)
  — Quiet breathing results from alternate contraction and relaxation of diaphragm and intercostal muscles.
  — It is normally domeshaped. It is attached circumferentially to fixed structures, vertebra, sternum and to mobile structures - the lower ribs.
  — During inspiration there exists increased tension within it. So its central tendon is pulled down, increasing vertical dimension of thorax, while lower ribs are moved upwards. Thus, lateral and antero-posterior diameter of lower chest is increased.
  — Interruption of both phrenic nerves immobilises the diaphragm without changing its configuration.
  — If circumference of lower chest is increased due to any reason (e.g. obstructive pulmonary disease) then diaphragm will be flattened.
  — Normal breathing is predominantly diaphragmatic.
  — Abdominal pressure does not interfere with its mobility. But extreme obesity, advanced pregnancy, excessive flatulence, tight abdominal garments may interfere. Its descent is accomplished by displacement of abdominal contents.

Work of Breathing

Functionally, it depends upon the amount of energy required to overcome — (a) airway resistance (b) elastic resistance of lungs and thorax (c) non-elastic viscous resistance.

- The *pleural pressure* is the pressure in the narrow space between lung pleura and chest wall pleura. Normally it is - 5 cm of water at the beginning of respiration (inspiration). Then the pressure increases to - 7.5 cm of water.

INTRAPLEURAL PRESSURE: AT A GLANCE

— During inspiration .... - 5 to - 6 mmHg.
— During expiration .... - 2 mmHg.
— Thin layer of fluid derived from visceral pleura is filling intrapleural cavity. This fluid is constantly pumped into lymphatic vessels from intrapleural space. This creates negative pressure.
— Due to its negativity; the collapsing tendency of lung is prevented which is caused by elastic recoiling. Furthermore, due to its negativity larger veins are dilated which acts like a suction pump to suck blood from lower parts of the body towards the heart, i.e. it helps in venous return (respiratory pump).
— By introducing a needle into pleural cavity and connecting it to mercury manometer, it can be recorded directly.
— Indirect approach of its measurement is by introducing oesophageal balloon which is then connected by a mercury manometer.

- The *alveolar pressure* is the pressure inside the lung alveoli. It is equal to 0 cm of water, when no air is flowing in or out of lungs. During inspiration the pressure in alveoli must fall below it - (–1 to –4 mmHg). During expiration the situation is reversed (+ 1 to + 4 mmHg).

INTRA-ALVEOLAR PRESSURE: AT A GLANCE

— Pressure existing in alveoli; normally it is equal to atmospheric pressure (760 mmHg). During inspiration is – 4 mmHg (756 mmHg); During expiration is + 4 mmHg (764 mmHg).
— It maintains the respiratory rhythm. Since pressure in alveoli is negative during inspiration so air enters and it becomes positive during expiration, so air is expelled out. It is also helpful in exchange of gases between alveolar air and blood.

- The difference between above two pressure is *Transpulmonary pressure*, (pleural pressure - alveolar pressure). It is an index of elastic recoil tendency of lungs, so also called *recoil pressure*.

- The *compliance of the lung* means the extent to which the lungs expand for each unit increases in transpulmonary pressure. OR ability of the lungs and thorax to expand OR the expandability of lung and thorax OR change in volume per unit change in the pressure. Normally it is 200 ml/cm of water pressure; i.e. with increase in 1 cm water transmural pressure, the lungs expand 200 ml.
  - — The compliance of lung alone - 200 to 220 ml/cm.
  - — The compliance of lung + thorax - 110 to 130 ml/cm. The total compliance is reduced in conditions like fibrotic pleurisy, respiratory muscular paralysis, pleural effusion, deformities of thorax like kyphosis and scoliosis.
- *Surfactant:* Is secreted by epithelial cells of alveoli. They are granular containing lipid. It is a mixture of phospholipids, ions and proteins. It greatly reduces the surface tension. If an alveolus becomes smaller (or shrinks) the surfactant molecules on the alveolar surface are squeezed together, increasing their concentration and this reduces the surface tension further. So this prevents alveoli from collapsing.

The Cells secreting it (type II alveolar epithelial cells) are characterised by presence of microvilli on their alveolar surface. In its absence the alveoli collapse producing a disease called "adult respiratory distress syndrome" (ARDS) OR "Hyaline membrane disease of newborn."

FUNCTIONS OF SURFACTANT

- It reduces the surface tension in alveoli of lung thus preventing collapsing tendency.
- It stabilises the alveoli which are in a habit of deflation.
- It helps in lung inflation during birth.

- *The work of breathing* can be divided into:
  - — Compliance work—that required to expand the lung against the elastic forces.
  - — Tissue resistance work—that required to overcome the viscosity of lung and chest wall structures.
  - — That required to overcome airway resistance during the movement of air into lungs. It increases during bronchiolar constriction.
  - — The energy generated by respiratory muscles to overcome the resistance in thorax and respiratory tract is work of breathing.

Table 18.1: Mechanism/Mechanics of respiration

1. Air enters the lungs due to pressure gradient - Contraction of inspiratory muscle leading to enlargement of thoracic cavity in all direction.
   This causes air to enter in lungs.
2. Uniform distribution of air to all alveoli
3. Uniform alveolar ventilation perfusion ratio
4. Diffusion of gases.

Table 18.2: Collapsing tendency of lungs

- *Factors preventing collapse*:- Negative intrapleural pressure, surfactant.
- *Factors causing collapse* :- Elastic properties of lung, existing surface tension over the surface of lung alveoli.
- *Role of diaphragm* :- Before inspiration it is dome-shaped with upward convexity. During inspiration, because of contraction muscle fibres are shortened; but the central tendinous portion is drawn downwards. It is flattened which increases vertical diameter of thoracic cage.

VENTILATION

- *Pulmonary ventilation means*: Respiratory minute volume; while alveolar ventilation is the amount of air utilised for gaseous exchange every minute. So Alveolar ventilation =
  = Tidal volume - Dead space volume × Respiratory Rate
  = (500 - 150) × 12 = 4,200 ml or 4.2 litres/mt.
- *Dead Space*: The part of respiratory tract where gaseous exchange does not take place is dead space. From nose to terminal bronchiole is anatomical dead space.

Physiological dead space = anatomical dead space + air in those alveoli which are non-functioning + air in those alveoli which don't receive adequate blood flow. Normal value 150 ml.

- *Ventilation perfusion ratio*

V_A alveolar ventilation ratio

Q blood flow (perfusion)

$$= \frac{4,200}{5,000} = 0.84$$

It signifies the gaseous exchange.

Ratio increases, if ventilation increases without any change in blood flow. It decreases, if blood flow increases without any change in ventilation. It is drastically reduced in condition like emphysema (obstruction and destruction of alveolar membrane).

BREATH SOUNDS

- Vesicular breath sounds are heard through normal lungs. There is usually no distinct pause between end of inspiration and beginning of expiration. The attenuating and filtering effect of lung produces quiet and low pitched rustling sounds.
- Bronchial breathing are heard as a result of consolidation, fibrosis or collapse. Of course sounds are abnormal but can be heard normally on trachea. So they are also called as "tracheal sounds." It is harsh sound bearing higher frequency. It becomes inaudible just before the end of inspiration, so that there is a gap before the expiratory sound is heard.
- *Wheezes:* are added abnormal sounds. They are musical sounds associated with narrowing of airway. The most obvious and loudest is stridor associated with laryngeal spasm or tracheal stenosis.
- *Crackles:* are short, explosive sounds (bubbling or clicking noises). They are produced by sudden changes in gas pressure related to sudden opening of previously closed small airways. The sounds are low pitched, scanty and loud and may clear up with coughing.
- *Pleural rub:* characteristic of pleural effusion, having a rubbing character. It does not change its character after coughing and is associated with local pain (difference from crackles).

DIFFERENCES

Vesicular breathing	*Bronchial breathing*
1. Intensity is low	Louder sound
2. sounds are heard better during inspiration	These are heard better during expiration.
3. Inspiratory sound passes inperceptibly in the expiratory sound	Inspiratory sound becomes practically inaudible before expiratory sound starts
4. Inspiratory sounds much longer (twice as long as expiratory sound)	Duration of inspiratory and expiratory sounds are equal
5. Inspiratory sound is more intense than expiratory sound	Expiratory sound is not less intense than inspiratory sound
6. Inspiratory sound is like rustling of leaves by a gentle breeze, while expiratory sound is little hollow.	Both inspiratory and expiratory sounds are hollow (guttural character)

BREATH HOLDING

- We can voluntarily inhibit respiration for sometime.
- "Breaking point" means point at which breathing can no longer be voluntarily inhibited.
- This is due to rise in Pco_2 and fall in Po_2.
- Breaking point can be delayed by breathing 100 per cent pure O_2 which will increase Po_2.
- If such persons (breath holders voluntarily) are encouraged, then such subjects can hold their breath for a longer time. This is psychogenic effect.

19 Gaseous Exchange: Diffusion of Gases

The process of diffusion (O_2 from alveoli to pulmonary blood and CO_2 in opposite direction) is important step in respiratory physiology. It includes rate and mechanism of diffusion.

DIFFUSION: ASPECT FROM PHYSICS

- All the gases concerned in respiratory physiology are simple molecules which are free to move among each other and the process is called diffusion.
- For the diffusion to occur, energy is provided by the kinetic motion of the molecules.
- If a gas chamber or a solution has a high concentration of a gas at one end of chamber and a low concentration at the other end, net diffusion of the gas will occur from high concentration area to low concentration area.
- Pressure is caused by the constant impact of kinetically moving molecules against a surface. Total pressure is directly proportional to the concentration of the gas molecules. Now consider mixture of air having 79 per cent N_2 and 21 per cent O_2 and total normal pressure is 760 mmHg. To express this statement in some other way, it is better to say that 79 per cent of 760 mmHg pressure is caused by nitrogen (about 600 mmHg) and 21 per cent by oxygen (about 160 mmHg). So the partial pressure of nitrogen is 600 mmHg and of oxygen is 160 mmHg as designated by Po_2, Pco_2, PN_2 etc.
- Gas dissolved in water or the body tissues also exert pressure because the dissolved molecules are moving randomly and having kinetic energy.
- The partial pressure of each gas in alveolar respiratory gas mixture tends to force molecules of that gas into solution first in alveolar membrane and then in the blood of alveolar capillaries. On the contrary, molecules of gas already dissolved in the blood are bouncing in fluid of blood and some escape back into the alveoli. The rate at which they escape is directly proportional to their partial pressure in the blood.
- Gases of respiratory importance are all highly soluble in lipids as well as in cell membrane. Diffusion of gases through the tissues including through respiratory membrane, is almost equal to diffusion of gases through water.
- It is evident that atmospheric air is containing mainly nitrogen; almost no CO_2 and very little water vapour. This air becomes humidified as it enters the respiratory passage.
- As already stated; the functional residual capacity of the lung is amounting 2,300 ml. At the same time only 350 ml of new air is brought in alveoli and same amount of old alveolar air is expired. Looking to huge amount of functional residual capacity; the amount replaced is very less (one seventh). This slow replacement is important since:
  - — It prevents sudden changes in gaseous concentration of the blood.
  - — It makes control of respiration more stable.
  - — It prevents excessive increase and decrease in tissue oxygenation.

Table 19.1: Alveolar air: An overview

Gases	*Atmospheric air* Pressure (mmHg)	%	*Alveolar air* Pressure (mmHg)	%	*Expired air* Pressure (mmHg)	%
N_2	597.0	78.62	569	74.9	566	74.5
O_2	159.0	20.84	104	13.6	120	15.7
CO_2	0.3	0.04	40	5.3	27	3.6
H_2O	3.7	0.50	47	6.2	47	6.2

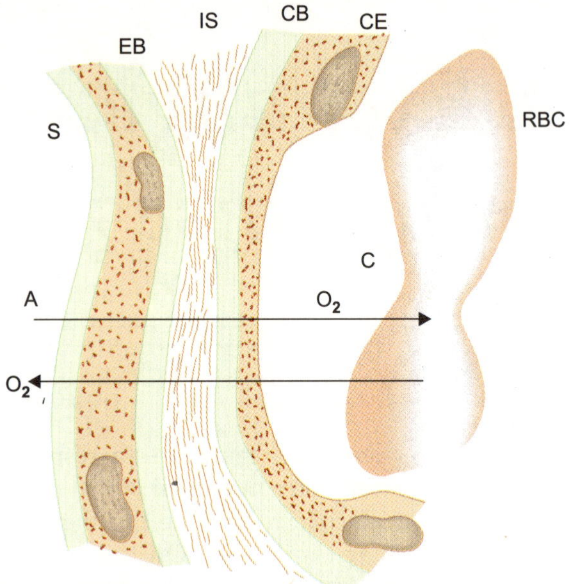

Fig. 19.1: Respiratory membrane (CB = Capillary basement membrane CE = Capillary endothelium, IS = Interstitial space, EB = Epithelial basement membrane, S = Fluid surfactant layer)

- The concentrations and partial pressure of both O_2 and CO_2 in the alveoli are determined by -
  — The rate of absorption, of two gases
  — The rate of excretion of two gases
  — Alveolar ventilation.
- Expired air is a combination of dead space air + alveolar air.

RESPIRATORY MEMBRANE: DIFFUSION

- Its layer-wise description is as:-
  — A layer of fluid lining the alveolus:- It contains surfactant which reduces the surface tension.
  — Alveolar epithelium (thin cells)
  — Epithelial basement membrane.
  — Between alveolar epithelium and capillary membrane there is a thin interstitial space.
  — A capillary basement membrane.
  — A capillary endothelial membrane.
- The diameter of pulmonary capillary - 5 microns. So RBC have to be squeezed while passing through them.
  — Its total surface area is 50 to 100 square meters.
  — The total quantity of blood in capillaries of the lung is 60 to 140 ml.
- Factors affecting

1. The rate of diffusion is inversely proportional to thickness of membrane. The thickness is said to be increased in accumulation of oedema fluid in interstitial space of membrane and alveoli; pulmonary diseases causing fibrosis. This may interfere with gaseous exchange.
2. It is the surface area which also means. When total surface area is decreased; then gaseous exchange is also reduced to a significant extent. The examples include - removal of one entire lung, emphysema etc.
3. CO_2 diffuses through the membrane twenty times as rapidly as O_2; and O_2 in turn diffuses twice as rapidly as N_2. All this depends on its ability to be soluble in the membrane and inversely on square root of its molecular weight.
4. *Partial pressure:* When partial pressure of a gas in the alveoli is greater than its pressure in the blood; then net diffusion from alveoli to blood occurs as seen with oxygen. On the contrary when pressure of a gas in blood is greater than alveoli, then net diffusion from blood towards alveoli is seen; as seen with CO_2.
5. Diffusion capacity of oxygen is 21 ml/minute/mmHg. During quiet breathing the mean oxygen pressure difference is 11 mmHg. So 11 × 21 = 230 ml of O_2 is diffusing through respiratory membrane per minute.
6. Diffusion capacity of CO_2 is 400 to 450 ml/minute/mmHg. Diffusion coefficient of CO_2 is twenty times as that of O_2. Since CO_2 diffuses through respiratory membrane very rapidly, so it is difficult to measure it.
7.
   — The diffusion capacity is defined as volume of a gas which diffuses through a membrane each minute for a pressure difference of 1 mmHg.
   — The partial pressure represents a measure of total number of molecules of a particular gas striking a unit area of alveolar surface of the membrane in a unit time. Pressure of a gas in the blood represents the number of molecules trying to escape from blood to opposite direction.
8. Diffusion Co-efficient—
   of oxygen is 1
   CO_2 ..... 20.3
   N_2 ..... 0.53
   Helium 0.95
   Diffusion coefficient of oxygen has been defined as the volume of a gas in ml diffusing 0.001 mm distance over a square cm surface area.
9. The O_2 diffusion capacity may be calculated by following data .... alveolar O_2 pressure, pulmonary blood oxygen pressure, and degree of O_2 utilisation.

10. CO diffusion capacity
    - O_2 diffusion capacity is 1.23 times more than that of CO diffusion capacity so 17 × 1.23 = 21 ml/ minute (The diffusion capacity of CO is 17 ml per minute in young adult man.
    - CO combines with haemoglobin, 210 times faster than that of oxygen. Thus at a CO tension of 0.46 mmHg. (equivalent to 0.065%), CO produces identical saturation of haemoglobin, as does a partial pressure of 100 mmHg of O_2.

BIBLIOGRAPHY

1. Guyton AC, et al. An arteriovenous oxygen difference recorder. J App Phy 1957;10:158.
2. Klocke RA. Velocity of CO_2 exchange in blood. Ann Rev Phy 1988;50:625.
3. Paiva M, et al. Theoretical studies of gas mixing and ventilation distribution in lung. Phy Rev 1987;67:750.
4. Wagner PD. Ventilation perfusion relationship. Ann Rev Phy 1980;42:235.
5. Wagner PD. Diffusion and chemical reaction in pulmonary gas exchange. Phy Rev 1977;57:257.

20 Gaseous Transport

OXYGEN CARRIAGE

The diffusing capacity for oxygen is 21 ml/minute in young healthy adults. Oxygen pressure gradient across respiratory membrane is 11 mmHg during quiet breathing so this whole amounts to be 250 ml of oxygen which is diffusing per minute through respiratory membrane. Now this holds to be true in normal sedentary states. During exercise, because of increase in surface area of respiratory membrane owing to dilatation of already opened pulmonary capillaries and opening of previously dormant pulmonary capillaries together with, stretching of alveolar membrane, the diffusion capacity for oxygen increases three or four times (i.e. up to 650 ml or so each minute). So it is worth mentioning that oxygenation of blood is increased during exercise due to both reasons—first by an increase in alveolar ventilation and secondly by more capacity for oxygen transmission into blood by respiratory membrane.

Haemoglobin—Oxygen Combination (Fig. 20.1)

a. The oxygen combines with heme portion of haemoglobin molecule and this combination is certainly reversible and hence a lose one.
b. It is an established fact that each gram of haemoglobin can bind 1.34 ml of oxygen
c. In this way 20 ml of oxygen is the maximum amount of it which can be bounded with haemoglobin and is expressed generally as 20 volumes per cent.
d. It is further evident that 5 ml of oxygen is transported by 100 ml of blood through the tissues in each cycle under all normal conditions. If normal cardiac output is considered as 5000 ml, the total amount of oxygen transported to tissues amounts to be 250 ml per minute (5/100 × 5000 cc). In heavy exercises this amount is raised to almost fifteen times or even more, and it may amount to be 3750 ml (15 × 250) in each minute.
e. When blood passes through the tissues it releases oxygen from oxygen haemoglobin combination.

Partial Pressure Oxygen

Primary contributing factor: The oxygen at arterial end is at 90 to 100 mmHg pressure while at tissue ends it is at 40 mmHg pressure. So there exists a net pressure difference of 50 to 60 mmHg, due to which the oxygen is diffused to tissues from blood haemoglobin. Reduced haemoglobin is the name given to that haemoglobin from which oxygen has been dissociated. This unloading of oxygen in tissues further depends on many factors the first being (a) Rate of blood flow; which means that if blood flow through a particular tissue is increased due to any reason greater quantities of oxygen are transported to that area in a given time, (b) Rate of tissue metabolism .... which means that increasing the oxygen consumption will significantly reduce the interstitial fluid Po_2 while decreasing oxygen consumption is going to raise Po_2, (c) Haemoglobin concentration by reducing haemoglobin concentration below normal standard also causes reduction in interstitial fluid Po_2 since oxygen to be transported is carried by haemoglobin.

The entire reverse changes occurs in lung alveoli. There oxygen is present with a partial pressure of 100 to 104 mmHg while at venous end it is only 40 mmHg so a net 60 to 64 mmHg pressure gradient exists which facilitates the oxygen diffusion into pulmonary capillaries.

Partial Pressure Carbon Dioxide

Important factor: The Pco_2 of venous blood is measured as 45 or 46 mmHg while CO_2 is present within alveoli at pressure of 40 mmHg establishing pressure gradient of 5 to 6 mmHg. Though this pressure difference is very small and tiny as compared with oxygen cases but since this is an established fact that carbon dioxide diffuses twenty times greater or more in comparison of oxygen, so carbon dioxide is transferred from venous end to alveoli. It is further evident that on increasing the metabolic rate Pco_2 is also increased while reverse effect is seen on inverting the situation.

Oxygen-Dissociation Curve

The curve if plotted, relating percentage saturation of oxygen carrying power of haemoglobin to partial pressure (Po_2) will attain a characteristic sigmoid shape. Its explanations are:

if we look on following combinations -

$Hb + O_2 \rightarrow HbO_2$

$Hb_4O_2 + O_2 \rightarrow Hb_4O_4$

$Hb_4O_4 + O_2 \rightarrow Hb_4O_6$

$Hb_4O_6 + O_2 \rightarrow Hb_4O_8$

Haemoglobin is having affinity with oxygen, the combination being lose and reversible. Each of four iron (heme) atoms are able to bind one oxygen molecule, but iron persists in ferrous state and the reaction hence is 'oxygenation' and not oxidation. Combination of first heme in entire haemoglobin molecule with oxygen increases affinity of second heme for oxygen, this increases affinity for third-fourth and so on. Affinity for fourth O_2 molecule of haemoglobin is many times more than first and this is sufficient to give characteristic shape sigmoid to the graph.

That fraction of haemoglobin which releases its oxygen on its passage through tissues and normally it amounts to be 27 per cent (one-fourth). This coefficient is increased to three quarters (77%) during severe exercise which is considered as highest of utilisation coefficient.

O_2-Hb Dissociation Curve: Effects of 2-3-DPG (Di-phospho-glycerate)

- The O_2-Hb dissociation curve is shifted to the right all the time by DPG.
- Due to hypoxia, its quantity increases which displaces this curve to more towards right. This causes O_2 to be released to tissues at least 10 mmHg higher O_2 pressure than without this increased DPG. It may be a means to adapt hypoxia.
- Excess DPG is also harmful because it makes difficult for haemoglobin to combine with O_2 in the lungs on reduction of PO_2.

O_2-Hb Dissociation Curve: Role of Exercise

- During exercise changes evident are:
  - — Release of large quantities of acid + CO_2 by exercising muscle.
  - — Increase in hydrogen ion concentration in muscle capillary blood.
  - — Rise in temperature of muscle (by 2-3°C).
  - — Release of phosphate compounds.
- All these factors shift this graph towards right.
- Under normal conditions the rate of O_2 utilisation is controlled by rate at which ATP breaks down to ADP.

Myoglobin

This is again a pigment containing iron but found in skeletal muscle. Myoglobin is capable of providing oxygen even when blood flow is cut off since blood supply of muscle is reduced or compressed during sustained contractions.

Oxygen Transport in Dissolved States

On the arterial end almost 0.29 to 0.30 ml. O_2 per 100 ml of blood is present as physical solution form. As pressure falls at tissue level (40 mmHg) 0.12 ml of oxygen remains in a dissolved state or 0.17 or 0.10 ml of oxygen is being transported to tissues by each 100 ml of blood. On the contrary only 0.15 ml of oxygen is present at venous end as physical solution per 100 ml of blood.

In total at arterial end 19 to 20 ml of oxygen per 100 ml of blood, while at venous end 14 to 15 ml of oxygen is present per 100 ml of blood.

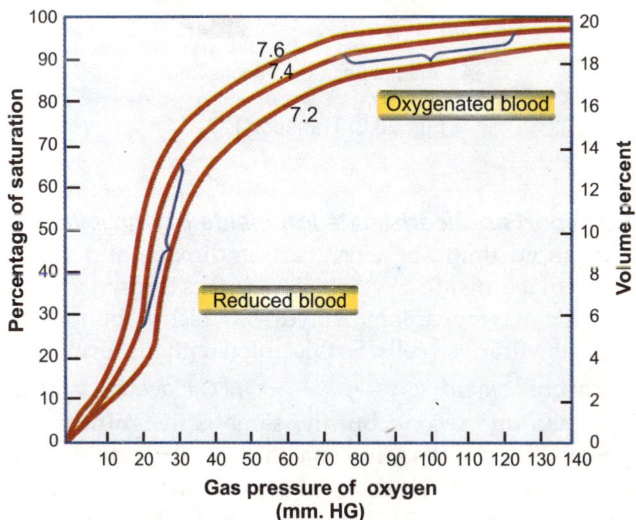

Fig. 20.1: Oxygen hemoglobin dissociation curve

At pH-7.4 — Normal (Sigmoid shape)

At pH-7.2 — Shift to right (Increased Co_2 temp. and DPG increased)

At pH-7.6 — Shift to left (Foetal Hb, Co_2 myoglobin decreased body temp.)

CARBON DIOXIDE CARRIAGE

This is important since carbon dioxide is chiefly concerned with acid base balance of body fluids.

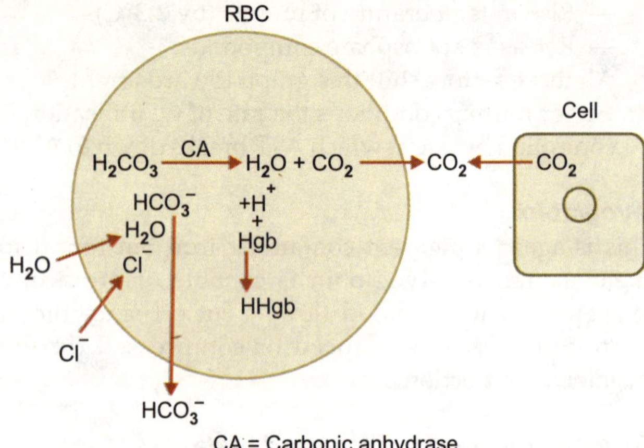

Fig. 20.2: Transport CO_2

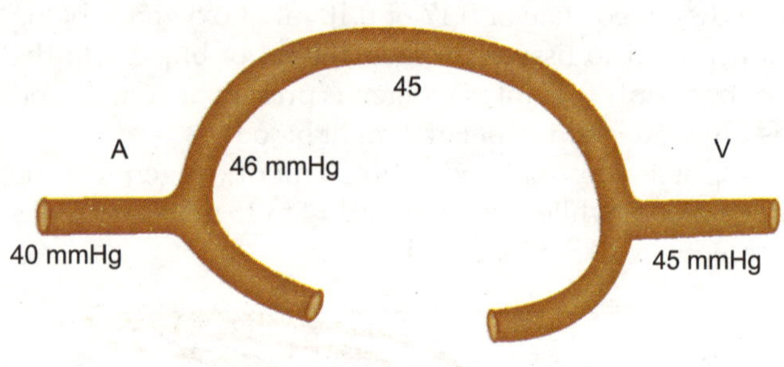

Fig. 20.3: Transport CO_2

Transport as Bicarbonate Ion Inside Erythrocyte

Very rapid union between carbon dioxide and water takes place inside erythrocytes in the presence of a catalytic enzyme carbonic anhydrase which is abundantly present within red cells. So this union with the formation of carbonic acid ($CO_2 + H_2O \xrightarrow{CA} H_2CO_3$) occurs within less than one second but the same is insignificant in plasma. Then this carbonic acid then, dissociates into hydrogen and bicarbonate ion within the cell ($H_2CO_3 \longrightarrow H^+ + HCO_3^-$) thus increasing the concentration of bicarbonate ions (HCO_3^-) within the cell as compared with plasma. So these bicarbonate ions diffuse from red cell to plasma through cell membrane (here it should be remembered that potassium ion cannot cross the cell membrane easily). This bicarbonate shift is followed by another diffusion of some negative ions to balance the situation and so chloride ions are present in abundance coming from dissociation of sodium chloride of plasma ($NaCl \longrightarrow Na^+ + Cl^-$) which then enters the cell constituting so called *chloride shift*. So this way of carbon dioxide transport is considered as most important, but if any carbonic anhydrase inhibitor, e.g. acetazolamide is given, the gaseous transport is seriously interfered up to the extent that it becomes very poor. However, most of the hydrogen ion ($H^+ + HCO_3^- \longrightarrow H_2CO_3$) combines with haemoglobin which too is a potent buffer. The above mechanism of chloride shift is capable to illustrate the fact that chloride in venous red cells is slightly higher than arterial red cells.

Diffusion from Tissues to the Blood and Transport to Lung

- 46 mmHg is the tension of carbon dioxide in tissues while at arterial end it is measured as 40 mmHg due to this pressure gradient the gas is passing actively from tissues to blood.
- 100 ml of venous blood is said to carry almost 52 ml of CO_2 while same quantity of arterial blood is carrying only 48 ml of CO_2. This means, that each 100 ml of arterial blood will take 4 ml of CO_2 and same quantity of blood on venous end will release 4 ml of CO_2 while passing through the lungs (52-48 = 4 ml is arterio-venous difference). In this way it is apparent that a constant charge of 48 ml. CO_2 per 100 ml of blood is carried by blood which is labelled as *alkali reserve*.
- Under normal physiological conditions. CO_2 is also carried in physical solution. This means that 2.6 ml of CO_2 is carried in physical solution in 100 ml of venous blood.
- Similarly CO_2 remains at a pressure of 46 mmHg at venous end while at alveolar site it is with 40 mmHg. Due to this pressure difference the gas enters alveoli from venous end.

Transport as Carbamino Compounds

- In addition to its transport as physical solution, bicarbonates etc. it also readily combines with haemoglobin constituting carbamino compounds and is said to be a very quick reaction and is not at all dependent upon enzyme carbonic anhydrase. It is said that reduced haemoglobin is having more affinity in regards with formation of carbamino compounds even at a low pressure, as compared with oxyhaemoglobin.
- CO_2 also readily combines with plasma proteins but it is less significant as compared with its combination with haemoglobin. In general, 3.6 ml of CO_2 is carried as carbamino compounds.
- An increase in Po_2 tends to displace CO_2 from blood and this is called *Haldane effect*. First cause is, combination of oxygen with haemoglobin makes Hb, a stronger acid which decreases affinity of haemoglobin

for combining with CO_2 to carbamino haemoglobin. Second cause is increased acidity of haemoglobin increases the acidity of the fluids both in plasma and RBC. It leads to conversion of bicarbonate ions into carbonic acid which then dissociates releasing CO_2 from blood. 100 ml of venous blood carrying 52 ml of CO_2 at a tension 46 mmHg is exposed to alveolar CO_2 tension of 40 mmHg and O_2 tension 100 mmHg. Due to difference in CO_2 tension, CO_2 diffuses from the alveoli with lowering of CO_2 tension.

- On the contrary, when Pco_2 rises, pH of blood decreases and there exists increased combination of CO_2 and haemoglobin and both of which cause to have considerable less affinity for O_2. So CO_2 causes O_2 to dissociate from haemoglobin. It is called *Bohrís effect* and is much of academic interest than of practical significance.

Ordinarily blood pH is 7.40 and as blood acquires CO_2 in tissues, pH falls to 7.36 (difference of 0.04 units). Reverse occurs when CO_2 is released from blood in lungs, pH rising to arterial value once again. In the lungs, Pco_2 in alveoli is slightly less than that of blood causing CO_2 to diffuse from blood into alveoli. This decreases Pco_2 of RBC so carbonic acid of cells changes back into CO_2 + H_2O and carbamino haemoglobin also releases CO_2.

DOUBLE BOHR'S EFFECT: PREGNANCY

1. Hb can carry more O_2 at a low Pco_2.
2. The foetal blood entering placenta carries large amount of CO_2, but much of this excess CO_2 diffuses into maternal blood from foetal blood.
3. Loss of CO_2 makes blood alkaline (in foetus) while increased CO_2 on maternal side makes it acidic.
4. This causes increased combining capacity of foetal blood for O_2 while for maternal blood it is decreased.
5. This forces more oxygen from maternal blood while O_2 uptake by foetal blood is increased.
6. So in this way Bohr's effect during pregnancy works in two directions first in maternal and second in foetal blood.
7. This is double Bohr's effect: It becomes more important during pregnancy.

GASEOUS INTERCHANGE IN LUNGS

A. O_2 Exchange .....

a. O_2 secretion theory ... (Bohr, Doughlas and Haldane) In condition of low O_2 pressure in alveoli, O_2 is secreted to keep a high tension in arterial blood.

b. O_2 diffuses into the blood due to difference in partial pressure of O_2 between alveoli and the pulmonary capillaries fed by pulmonary venous blood coming into the lungs, ventilation-perfusion ratio and diffusion capacity.

c. The oxygenation of venous blood in pulmonary capillary blood is completed in about 0.3 second within pulmonary circulation time which is 0.75 second. This quick rate is because of:
— Higher pressure gradient.
— More surface area of alveoli.

B. CO_2 exchange ... In venous blood CO_2 tension - 46 mmHg while its pressure in alveoli. 40 mmHg. So CO_2 passes from venous blood to alveoli. It is also because of its high diffusion capacity.

OXYGEN UTILISATION: (A) DIFFUSION DISTANCE

- From capillary to cell:- the distance normally is 50 micrometers. Fortunately, diffusion of O_2 can take place within this distance normally.
- But in some pathologic states, this distance may be increased so oxygen utilisation by cell is diffusion limited.

OXYGEN UTILISATION: (B) BLOOD FLOW

- The factors determining total amount of oxygen are:
  — Quantity of O_2 transported in each decilitre of blood
  — Rate of blood flow
- Now if rate of blood flow is reduced to minimum then available oxygen will also be reduced to minimum.
- This is blood flow dependent O_2 utilisation.

21 Homeostasis: Regulation of Respiration

RESPIRATORY CENTRE

Is a widely dispersed group of neurons located bilaterally in reticular substance of medulla and pons. It is further subdivided into three main groups (a) Medullary rhythmicity area consisted by *inspiratory and expiratory neurons*, (b) the *apneustic* area and (c) *pneumotaxic* area 'Apneustic centre' is responsible for apneusis at the level of striae-acoustica. The pneumotaxic centre controls the apneustic centre in such a way that apneusis is converted into rhythmic respiratory movement. Inspiratory centre (situated in ventral reticular formation lying immediate over cephalic 4/5th of inferior olive at the level of entrance of vagus nerve) and expiratory centre (situated cephalic and dorsal to inspiratory centre, adjacent to spinal root of fifth nerve) are inhibiting each other. Most factors that increase the activity of vasomotor centre thereby increasing blood pressure, also elevate the pulmonary ventilation rate since these two centres are actually intermingled together in reticular substance of brainstem. Similarly many emotional states can affect the character of respiration. Respiratory centre automatically discharges impulses.

DORSAL RESPIRATORY GROUP OF NEURONS: A VIEW

- It is located in dorsal portion of medulla which mainly causes inspiration. This group of neurons emits the repetitive bursts of inspiratory action potential; even after sectioning peripheral nerves entering the medulla or transaction of brainstem both above and below the medulla.
- The nervous signal begins very weak at first and increases steadily in a "*ramp fashion*" for at least few seconds. Then it abruptly ceases for next few seconds, then begins again for another cycle.
- Control of this ramp signal is as follows:
  - — During very active respiration, the ramp increases rapidly filling the lungs rapidly.
  - — Checking the point where respiration ceases. "So earlier the ramp ceases, shorter is the duration of respiration."

VENTRAL RESPIRATORY GROUP OF NEURONS: AN OVERVIEW

- Located anterior and lateral to dorsal group of neurons found in nucleus ambiguous rostrally and nucleus retro-ambiguus caudally.
- It is totally inactive during normal quiet respiration, so that is purely controlled by dorsal neurons.
- They are not involved in basic rhythmic oscillation which controls respiration.
- On demand, i.e. when respiratory drive for increased pulmonary ventilation becomes greater than normal; then these neurons contribute their share; both in expiration as well as inspiration.

THE APNEUSTIC, PNEUMOTAXIC CENTRE: AT A GLANCE

- Apneustic centre is located at lower part of pons and is a strange one. When vagus nerve is sectioned and when its connection from pneumotaxic centre has been blocked by transacting the pons in its mid region then it gives signal to dorsal neurons to switch off the inspiratory ramp signal; which leads to occasional short expiratory grasp.
- The primary function of pneumotaxic centre is to limit inspiration plus increase in breathing rate since limitation of inspiration shortens the expiration a long with entire period of respiration.
- This centre is located in nucleus parabrachialis (dorsally) of upper pons transmitting signals to inspiratory area. It controls switch off point of inspiratory ramp.

RECEPTORS (A. S. PAINTAL—1955)

- The stretch receptor in alveolar wall. The inspiratory inhibitory reflex is initiated by stimulation of proprioceptors.

- The deflation receptors respond better to pulmonary congestion/embolism leading to shallow rapid respiration. These are type J receptors and they are located juxtacapillary.
- Another receptors are located in between epithelial lining of the bronchi and bronchiole. They lead to hyperventilation and bronchiolar constriction on stimulation. They are lung irritant receptors.
- These receptors are characterised by rapid adaptation, smallest action potential, no activity during normal breathing (by deflation receptors).
- When stimulated J receptors produce apnoea, followed by hyperpnoea, bradycardia and hypotension, inhibition of contraction of skeletal muscle, bronchospasm etc.

NERVOUS CONTROL

When the lungs become stretched, the stretch receptors especially those of bronchioles transmit impulses through vagus nerves into tractus solitarius of brainstem and thence into respiratory centre where they inhibit inspiration and thereby prevent further inflation; effect called *Hering-Breuer inflation reflex* which prevents over distension of lungs. Such type of deflation reflex occurs too, during expiration. The major effects of the reflex are (a) decrease in tidal volume and (b) compensatory increase in respiratory rate. Physiological role of it is that (a) It regulates lung inflation, (b) it helps to maintain tidal volume within certain range, (c) it helps filling and emptying of lungs inspite of considerable resistance, (d) it is a proprioceptive reflex forming a feedback. The reflex takes place through vagi. This reflex is not activated until tidal volume increases to 1.5 litres or more.

HERING-BREUER REFLEX: AT A GLANCE (1868)

- This is an effect on respiratory cycle elicited by inflation and deflation of lungs.
- The receptors concerned are in the lungs and afferent pathways in vagus nerve.
- Its function is to regulate the respiratory cycle rather than to alter significantly the pulmonary ventilation for prolonged period.
- Their observation was that inflation of lung causes arrest of inspiration.
- A physiological role of this reflex is to regulate the extent of lung inflation so that tidal volume tends to fall within a certain range. This also serves to insure filling and emptying of the lungs despite a considerable increase in resistance in airway.
- These reflexes are proprioceptive in nature.

Other Factors Adjusting Respiration

a. *Cough reflex:* Protective reflex. Sudden forcible expiratory act. Its purpose is to drive out the irritating substance. The sequence of events are some amount of air inspired → closure of epiglottis, shutting of vocal cords → forceful contraction of abdominal muscles pushing against diaphragm + contraction of other expiratory muscle → rise of pressure in lungs → sudden opening of vocal cords and epiglottis.

b. *Sneezing reflex:* Identical with cough but the outlet is through nose. Irritation of nasal mucosa produces it by stimulating the sensory nerves of trigeminal and olfactory nerves.

c. *Swallowing reflex:* During deglutition, respiration is momentarily inhibited.

d. *Afferents from joints* : Reflexly respiration is stimulated. Respiratory stimulation due to exercise is because of this effect. Similarly afferents from intercostal/diaphragm/abdominal muscles reflexly stimulate the respiratory centre.

e. During fever the respiration gets stimulated because thermo-receptors are present in hypothalamus as well as on peripheral part of the body and during fever these receptors are stimulated. Increased venous pressure in the great veins and right auricle may stimulate the respiration.

HUMORAL/CHEMICAL REGULATION

i. *Oxygen lack*: There is a little change in rate of respiration, till O_2 content of inspired air falls to 14 per cent or less even. If Po_2 of inspired air is lowered there exists stimulation of ventilation through sino-aortic mechanism, of course severe oxygen lack depress respiratory centre directly.

ii. *Effect of CO_2*: 1.5 per cent CO_2 in inspired air causes slight but measurable increase of pulmonary ventilation without awareness; 4 per cent CO_2 in inspired air leads to two times increase in pulmonary ventilation; 10 per cent CO_2 in inspired air leads to tremendous increase of ventilation with dyspnoea, 15 per cent CO_2 in inspired air leads to muscular rigidity, tremor, convulsion and loss of consciousness; 20 per cent CO_2 in inspired air leads to surgical anaesthesia (CO_2 narcosis).

iii. Raised Hydrogen ion concentration stimulates breathing while low hydrogen ion concentration depress respiration.

REVIEW: CHEMOSENSITIVITY—RESPIRATORY REGULATION

- A chemosensitive area is located bilaterally one-fifth millimetre beneath the ventral surface of the medulla. The above mentioned respiratory centres are not at all sensitive to chemical changes.
- For this area, hydrogen ions are the important direct stimulus since they are unable to cross blood brain barrier.
- CO_2 is having a potent indirect effect. $CO_2 + H_2O$ (of tissues) → Carbonic acid → $H^+ + HCO_3^-$. H^+ are then having potent direct effect of stimulation.
- CO_2 is a stronger stimulant because it is capable of crossing blood brain/blood CSF barrier while hydrogen ions cannot cross them. So Pco_2 increases → CO_2 crosses blood brain barrier → Pco_2 of medulla increases → CO_2 reacts with water to form hydrogen ions which are released into chemosensitive area → rapid excitation of respiration.
- After 1 to 3 hours to 1 to 2 days, this stimulatory effect comes to normal. The kidney plays a leading role by increasing blood bicarbonate, which bind hydrogen ion in cerebrospinal fluid to get their concentration reduced. After some time bicarbonate ions will themselves diffuse slowly through blood brain barrier. So CO_2 effect is characterised by quality of adaptation.
- Decreased blood Po_2 → excitation of chemoreceptors → increasing respiration → decrease Pco_2 and hydrogen ion concentration → depression of respiratory centre.

Despite its weak response to diminished oxygen chemoreceptor mechanism is very important, for it is the only mechanism by which low oxygen concentration in arterial blood can increase alveolar ventilation and this slight increase can sometimes be a life saver.

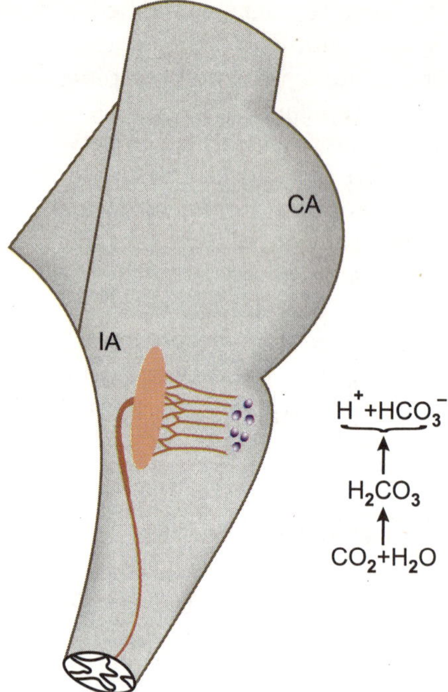

Fig. 21.1: Respiratory centre
IA = Inspiratory area
CA = Chemosensitive area

RESPIRATORY ADJUSTMENT: CO_2

- On breathing 4 per cent CO_2 RMV is doubled; on 4 to 10 per cent concentration, RMV may increase to 8 to 10 times. Symptoms of dizzines, faintness, headache may increase to 8 to 10 times. At its 20 per cent concentration RMV begins to decrease, with convulsions. Its site of action is the respiratory centre and its near surroundings. It has been suggested that both a rise in Pco_2 and hydrogen ion concentration (CH) in the respiratory centre, contribute and supplement each other in causing an increase in pulmonary ventilation. Chemorecepotrs are concerned with reflex drive of breathing even under resting conditions. These chemoreceptors are activated in significant degree only after considerable increase in arterial Pco_2.
- The lowering of Pco_2 in arterial blood is achieved by voluntary hyperventilation; after which apnoea is observed. Breathing is resumed when either PCO_2 rises to approximately the resting level or when Po_2 of arterial blood drops to a level sufficient to set up reflex drive of breathing on O_2 lack basis; whichever occurs first.
- When one has hyperventilated moderately with atmospheric air, oxygen lack develops quickly as store of O_2 in lung is absorbed and utilised quickly. Breathing is resumed in response to O_2 lack stimulus before Pco_2 has been restored and takes over as a sole drive. This is the physiology of few cycles of periodic breathing after hyperventilation.

RESPIRATORY ADJUSTMENT FOR OXYGEN

- Po_2 when lowered cause slight stimulation of breathing. When it is reduced to 10 per cent or below, breathing is stimulated but with irregularities.
- The only sensitive mechanism which responds to O_2 lack elicits an increase in RMV, is chemoreceptor reflex.

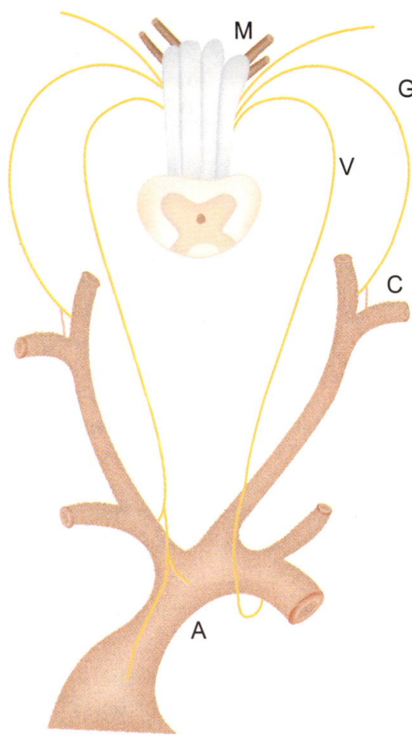

Fig. 21.2: Chemoreceptors: Control of respiratory C = Carotid body, A = Aortic body, V = Vagus, M = Medulla, G = Glosso-pharyngeal nerve

- The typical responses to significantly lowered oxygen tension in inspired air include—stimulation of breathing, cardiac acceleration, rise in arterial pressure. Chemoreceptors cause vasoconstriction which raises blood pressure. It is apparent that cardiac acceleration is secondary to respiratory stimulation.
- According to one concept, on stimulation of chemo-receptors; the stress machinery is stimulated which liberates ACTH/adrenaline/nor-adrenaline which causes above changes.
- Sodium cyanide if administered intravenously produce similar changes as of hypoxia. It is said that cyanide prevents utilisation of oxygen by tissues and thus produces hypoxia.

HYPERPNOEA: DURING EXERCISE

a. - During exercise pulmonary ventilation increases and the rise is quite proportionate to the amount of increase in muscular activity.
   - As a consequence of increased muscular activity there is an increased rate of production of CO_2 and acid metabolites along with increased rate of O_2 utilisation.
   - The causes include... (a) Respiration is stimulated reflexly by impulses arising in working muscles or the joints which are acted upon by these muscles.

b. During voluntary activity impulses are directed into respiratory centre to exert a stimulatory effect.

c. Accessory respiratory drives are brought into play during exercise so that increased ventilation may occur even before a change in Pco_2, Po_2 have had time to occur at the sites upon which these stimuli act (Cunningham and Lloyd—1963, Gradins—1950).

pH and Respiration (Reaction theory; Winterstein—1921)

- Cells of the respiratory centre are stimulated when there is a rise in intracellular H ions concentration. Cells continuously produce lactic acid which is removed by oxidation. Lactic acid cannot be removed if oxygen is deficient. As a result there is increase in hydrogen ion concentration, which leads to increased rate and depth of respiration.
- Acid + bicarbonate $\rightarrow H_2CO_3 \rightarrow H^+ + HCO_3^-$. H^+ diffuse into the cells of respiratory centre which causes the above effect.

EFFECT OF DRUGS ON RESPIRATION

- Adrenaline and nor-adrenaline stimulate breathing. Adrenaline increases blood pressure which stimulates baro-receptors and then apnoea may result (adrenaline - apnoea).
- Progesterone stimulates ventilation which may reduce Pco_2.
- Analeptic drugs like coramine, micoren etc. in large doses, increase the frequency of respiration.
- Morphine, barbiturates (sodium pentobarbital) tend to depress respiratory centre.
- Caffeine, theophylline stimulate the respiratory centre.

TERMS

a. *Eupnoea:* Normal breathing.
b. *Tachypnoea:* Rapid shallow breathing without increase in depth.
c. *Apnoea:* Temporary cessation of breathing e.g. voluntary, during periodical breathing, after voluntary hyperpnoea, reflex apnoea, deglutition apnoea (adrenaline).
d. *Dyspnoea:* (difficult breathing) means consciousness of necessity for increased respiratory effort). It occurs physiologically in stimulating the respiratory centre (reflexly, directly, impulses from higher centre,

asphyxial states), hyperactivity of Hering-Breuer reflex, decrease in breathing reserve or vital capacity, increased metabolic activity, muscular exercise, low mechanical efficiency of respiratory apparatus. It occurs pathologically in impaired blood oxygenation, deficient function of respiratory apparatus (muscle paralysis, kyphosis, etc.), acidosis, emotional disturbances, increased metabolism, impairment of O_2 transport (CHF, less vital capacity, pulmonary congestion, diminished lung elasticity), lung conditions (airway obstruction, structural lung lesions), cerebral conditions (tumour, haemorrhage, oedema).

PERIODIC BREATHING

Cheyne-Stokes

Characterised by slow waxing and waning of respiration occurring over and over again every 45 seconds to 3 minutes. Conditions where found are including raised intracranial pressure, drugs like morphine, uraemia and other toxic conditions, hypoxia at high altitude, voluntary hyperventilation and is found in healthy infants and healthy adults during deep sleep.

Biot's

Rhythm and depth of respiration are irregular with occasional sighs and irregular pauses. Period during which respiration takes place is of variable length. These alternate with apnoea of variable duration. Switch over to hyperpnoea to apnoea and back is abrupt. Respiration comes in couples, triples, quadruples and so forth. It is seen in meningitis, contusion, concussion of brain etc.

Periodic Breathing: Cheyne-Stokes Breathing

A. Basic mechanism → Say respiration becomes rapid and deep → Pco_2, in pulmonary blood decreases (hyperpnoeic phase) → inhibits respiration as this blood reaches the brain (apnoeic phase) → so pulmonary Pco_2 increases → respiration stimulated again as increased Pco_2 reaches centre.
An increase and decrease in blood concentration of oxygen also contributes.

B. Why not normally occur? Normally this does not occur because of damping mechanism.
   - Our body fluids, contain enough quantity of stored gases. So a long time of either hypo or hyperventilation is required to change the concentration of these gases up to a significant level. In normal circumstances, before the significant changes in gaseous concentration occur, the centre of respiration readjusts for breathing and so normality is maintained.
   - When one over breaths for some purpose, he will feel apnoea which will be followed by few damped cycles of Cheyne-Stoke breathing.
   - A simple one to two minutes delay in passage of blood from lungs to the brain leads to Cheyne-Stokes breathing.

Table 21.1: Differences between Biots and Cheyne-Stokes breathing

Biots	Cheyne-Stokes
• There are periods of variable length during which breathing is present; and these alternate with and these alternate different lengths.	Although, periods of respiratory activity alternate with apnoeic periods, the amplitude of breathing increases gradually to a maximum and then decreases gradually until next period of inactivity.
• Occurs in meningitis etc. where medulla is affected	Physiologically seen at high altitude as well as in normal sleeping infant. Morphine may induce, CHF.

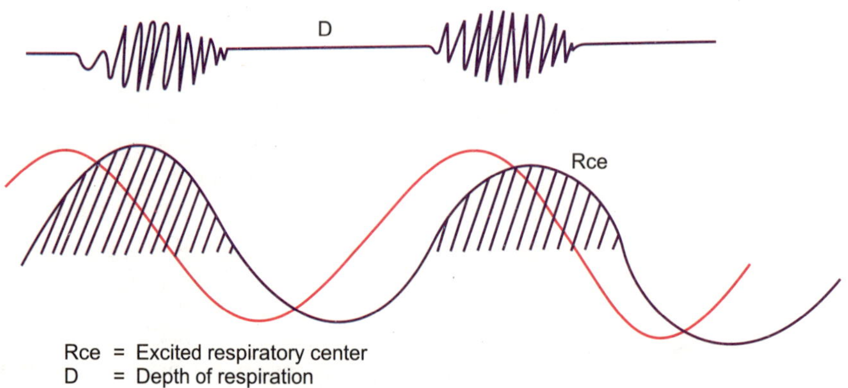

Fig. 21.3: Cheyne-Stokes breathing: Periodic breathing

C. Cardiac failure is associated with Cheyne-Stokes breathing because:
   i. Of slowed circulation
   ii. Sluggish rate of blood flow
   iii. Impaired O_2 uptake by oedematous lungs
   iv. left heart volume increases → increases circulation time.

Cyanosis

- It is a clinical condition characterised by diffuse blue or dusky colouration of skin and mucous membrane of body. Cause is excessive amount of deoxygenated haemoglobin (5 gm% or more). Common sites are lips, cheeks, nail beds, mucous membrane of tongue, nose tip, skin of ear lobule. Conditions giving rise to it include hypoxic hypoxia, stagnant hypoxia, increased meth-haemoglobin and sulf-haemoglobin content, polycythaemia. Factors determining are quantity of deoxygenated haemoglobin in arterial blood, rate of blood flow through skin and skin thickness.
- If haemoglobin is 5 gm or less, no cyanosis is possible, i.e. degree of unsaturation of haemoglobin is important factor. In polycythaemia, even slight degree of unsaturation may produce cyanosis. In cold, patients of polycythaemia exhibits cyanosis due to excess amount of blood in capillaries + sluggish circulation.
- Methoemoglobin is normally reduced in body by "lactic acid dehydrogenase - coenzyme I." When this is absent or deficient then methoemoglobin level will be raised (methoemoglobin aemia), which gives cyanotic hue.
- Similarly sulphhaemoglobinaemia also results into cyanosis.
- If skin is thick or pigmented (dark individuals) the cyanotic colour may not be distinctly visible.
- State of blood vessels specially the capillaries, must contain the reduced haemoglobin. If the vessels are constricted then because of less amount of blood travelling the cyanotic colour is not imparted.

Decompression Sickness (Dysbarism, Caisson's Disease)

- This happens in deep sea divers (caisson) who suddenly come to the surface and exposed to normal pressure after expanding some time in a high pressure zone.
- When he works underneath a sea, he is exposed to high pressure and he is equilibrated with gases at high pressure. When he comes back to the surface (or out of sealed cabin), he is now exposed to reduced pressure. Gases try to come out, O_2 and CO_2 are easily diffusible and moreover O_2 is used metabolically also. The problem is with N_2 which is less diffusible. N_2 is more soluble in adipose tissue and blood, the nitrogen bubbles tend to lodge in small blood vessels and impairs the circulation.
- It is a distressful condition in which the manifestations are due to sudden reduction of pressure of ambient gases in the body. Main symptoms include pain and anaesthesia (due to bubble within myelin sheath of sensory nerves), paresis or paralysis (due to bubble pressure inside motor nerves), dyspnoea (due to bubbles in pulmonary capillaries), cardiac damage (due to air bubble in coronary vessels), pain in bones (due to bubble in marrow), cerebral symptoms, shock like features (due to adrenal failure). If the subject is inadvertently decompressed, he should be quickly recompressed to original pressure and when the symptoms alleviate, gradually decompressed again.

22 Adjustment: Hypoxia, High Altitude

"Anoxia — hypoxia — oxygen lack — oxygen want are synonyms but more correct word is hypoxia. It not only stops the machinery but also wrecks the body machinery."

INTRODUCTION

- Due to any reason if body tissues are not getting adequate oxygen supply, the state is hypoxia. It may be also defined as deficiency of oxygen at tissue level. The common term 'Anoxaemia' is used as synonym of anoxic anoxia but it means diminished or low oxygen tension in arterial blood.'
- At sea level the barometeric pressure is 760 mmHg but at the height of 10,000 ft this pressure lowers down to be 523 mmHg and at the height of 50,000 ft it goes as down as 87 mmHg.
- Now, we must also look at this moment to oxygen content of air at different heights. At sea level it is 159 mmHg, while as one ascends to 10,000 ft height it lowers to 110 mmHg or so while at 50,000 ft height it reduces to only 18 mmHg.
- Now it is quite evident that on decreasing partial oxygen pressure in atmosphere at higher altitudes, alveolar oxygen tension will be also directly effected.
- So for any time, when barometric pressure decreases, oxygen pressure will also be decreased.

VARIETIES

a. Hypoxic-Hypoxia

Po_2 of arterial blood is (anoxic-anoxia) reduced. It is caused when -

i. Low oxygen tension in inspired air (high altitudes, mountain sickness), breathing in closed space
ii. *Pulmonary abnormalities:* (asthma, emphysema, water in lungs, pneumonia, respiratory muscle paralysis, respiratory centre depression by anaesthetics or narcotics).
iii. Communication of right and left side of heart-shunt.

b. Anemic Hypoxia

Amount of blood haemoglobin for oxygen carriage is reduced, otherwise arterial Po_2 is said to be normal. That's why anaemic patients feel difficulty during exercise owing to limited supply of oxygen to tissues as compared with demand. So it is lowered oxygen capacity of the blood. It is found in situations like -

i. All types of anaemia—haemoglobin content is less than normal.
ii. Carbon-monoxide poisoning.
iii. Chlorate, nitrites, ferricyanides poisoning.

Volume per cent of oxygen carried is reduced in proportion to decrease in haemoglobin.

c. Stagnant Or Hypokinetic Hypoxia Or Ischaemic

It is characterised by decreased blood flow rate. It is seen in:

i. Haemorrhage, shock, congestive cardiac failure.
ii. Thrombosis, embolism
iii. Myocardial infarction—localised hypoxia leading to generalised state of hypoxia.
Po_2 and volume per cent of oxygen in arterial blood are normal and due to slow circulation all vital organs (liver, heart, kidney, brain) are badly sufferer.

d. Histotoxic Hypoxia

Simply tissue itself is not capable to utilise oxygen although plenty of it is available. This occurs in cyanide poisoning which blocks the action of cytochrome oxidase enzyme. Methylene blue or even nitrites are used to reverse the condition by first forming 'methemoglobin' and then cyanmethemoglobin by combining with cyanides and it is said to be a non-toxic compound. Methylene blue may cause slight rise in body temperature due to increased metabolism.

SIGNS AND SYMPTOMS : EFFECTS OF HYPOXIA

Such effects collectively classed as mountain sickness are briefly summarised as follows:

i. Mental Changes

Hypoxia is said to cause a sequence of mental aberrations not unlike those classed as 'alcoholism'. It includes headache, drowsiness, - impaired judgement, disorientation, excitement, lassitude, mental fatigue, occasionally euphoria etc. All such symptoms usually make their appearance at height of 12,000 feet or so. As one further ascends the symptoms become still severe and convulsions may start terminating into coma as one ascends to more than 20,000 feet. other parameters of mental proficiency may decrease to 20 per cent from normal values as measured by reaction time, handwriting, etc. at height between 12,000 to 15,000 feet, further including memory tests, calculations, telling the time from mirror image of clock.

ii. Respiration

Increased breathing is the result of oxygen lack and due to increased breathing alveolar CO_2 tension is reduced since much of CO_2 is washed out during increased respiration which may tend to cause blood more and more alkaline so to compensate so called 'alkalosis' kidney starts excreting alkaline urine (or less acid excretion) together with fall in 'ammonia coefficient'. Now due to less CO_2 tension respiration depresses which results into increased CO_2 tension, which causes again stimulation of respiration, a pattern more or less like periodic breathing.

In severe hypoxic state (characterised by convulsions or coma) respiratory centre is depressed within few minutes due to metabolic deficiency of neurons.

iii. Vision

A little decrease in oxygen concentration of the arterial blood is capable enough to depress the function of rods in retina and thus night vision is seriously effected.

iv. Digestion

Nausea, vomiting and loss of appetite are the main problems existing with digestive system.

ACCLIMATISATION TO LOW Po_2

It is quite a natural aspect of the life that one adapts to newly changed situation or circumstance and so is the case here also. As one reaches the high altitude or remains there for couple of days or months his or her body will be acclimated so that minor bad effects take place. Those changes are summarised briefly-

i. The hypoxia at higher altitude is the best stimulus for release of erythropoietin from kidney tissue which stimulates bone marrow to produce more erythrocytes as much as 6 to 8 millions per cubic mm. blood, or more to cause polycythaemia haemoglobin level also rises from normal level and reaches to 20 gm per cent or even more. Hematocrit values also goes higher from 45 per cent normal to 60 to 72 per cent value. All this are sufficient to cause an increase in blood volume.
ii. Cardiac output is said to increase initially but due to acclimatisation it may tend to fall to normal levels. Of course blood supply to vital organs is increased like heart, brain, muscles etc. The anoxic tissue's vascularity is also increased.
iii. According to hypoxic effects, individual cells or tissue itself must be acclimatised to low Pco_2 by increasing its essential enzyme content concentrations of oxidative nature.
iii. Oxygen diffusion capacity is also rising higher from its normal value of 21 ml/minute. It is due to increase in lung volume together with increase in pulmonary capillary blood volume.

NATIVES: LIVING AT HIGH ALTITUDE

(17 to 19,000 feet height)

Acclimatisation begins in infancy. Chest size is increased but body size decreases. Right side of the heart is considerably larger. All this provides a high ventilatory capacity to body mass. The delivery of oxygen by blood to tissues is highly facilitated.

ACUTE MOUNTAIN SICKNESS: PATHOLOGY

- Hypoxia → local vasodilatation of cerebral vessels → increase in capillary pressure → leakage of fluid into cerebral tissues → cerebral oedema → various dysfunctions.
- Hypoxia → constriction of pulmonary arterioles → capillary pressure increased → pulmonary oedema → various dysfunctions.
- Red cell mass and haematocrit value high
- Congestive heart failure
- Fall in peripheral arterial pressure.

CARBON MONOXIDE POISONING

i. It is a gas formed by incomplete combustion of carbon. For criminal purposes it was used specially by Greek and Romans.
ii. It combines with blood haemoglobin to form 'carbon-monoxy haemoglobin - a toxic compound,

(CO Hb.). This compound is formed when alveolar Pco exceeds 0.4 mmHg. On the whole toxicity depends upon concentration and duration of exposure of gas. This is having two-fold difficulties; one is that compound CO Hb cannot take up oxygen and second is it liberates CO slowly. In the presence of this compound (CO Hb) the dissociation curve of remaining oxyhaemoglobin (HbO_2) shifts to left.

iii. This compound CO Hb is cherry red in colour. So its colouration is distinctly visible in skin and mucous membrane and nail buds, etc.

iv. The condition may be reversed by:
- getting rid of such atmosphere,
- adequate ventilation or artificial respiration if essential
- hyperbaric oxygenation is useful.

OXYGEN TREATMENT

i. Excepting in hypoxic hypoxia the oxygen treatment for hypoxia is of very limited value. In anaemic hypoxia, e.g. the defect is inadequacy of haemoglobin and oxygen content is within normal limits; so by oxygen treatment we can further increase oxygen concentration in body fluids but any alteration in haemoglobin is not possible. Similarly in stagnant hypoxic cases again the oxygen supply is not of much importance since the basic problem is slow circulation and not inadequate oxygen. Similarly in histotoxic hypoxia it is again doubtful that oxygen supply is of any use or not since the main fault is lying in utilisation by tissue itself and not in oxygen concentration.

ii. *Oxygen Toxicity*

a. If nearly 80 to 100 per cent pure oxygen is breathed by any individual for roughly 8 to 10 hours it may lead to some toxic manifestations. Headache, dizziness, sore throat, nasal congestion, coughing, substernal distress are usual symptoms. Muscular twitching, convulsions, ringing in ears and coma may also be added in severe poisoning.

b. Nitrogen gas is said to be eliminated on oxygen administration.

c. All above mentioned symptoms (other than nervous system's symptoms) are said to occur when O_2 is administered within 0.5–1 atmospheric pressure. Substernal pain appears within 4 to 12 hours of oxygen administration and is related to trachea-bronchitis. Fatigue, nausea, vomiting, anorexia, paraesthesia in hands and feet are other symptoms reported at this situation.

d. At 2 to 4 atmospheric pressure, if oxygen is administered it can lead to disturbances in higher mental function in the form of irritational apprehension, convulsions, mood changes, loss of judgement, etc. Death may result when one is exposed to an oxygen tension of 8 atmospheric. Vertigo is also said to exist in oxygen poisoning.

iii. A man of normal body weight is eliminating nearly 18 ml. N_2 per minute on breathing oxygen. The elimination rate of nitrogen is rapid in most vascular parts of body like brain and blood itself. Hence, it is provided to prevent from decompression.

iv. The usual methods of oxygen administration are through a nasal (or oronasal) tube or catheter, or through specially designed facial mask or by placing the patient in airtight cabinet where percentage of oxygen is maintained at required concentration, of course 5 to 10 per cent CO_2 may be added, to enhance lung expansion specially in conditions like CO poisoning, atelectasis, hiccough etc.

v. Air spaces of the lungs are directly exposed to high O_2 pressure, while O_2 delivery to other tissues is at normal Po_2 because of O_2 haemoglobin buffer system. This explains the symptoms occurring on exposure to 100 per cent O_2 at normal atmospheric pressure, (after 12 hours of exposure) in the form of pulmonary oedema, lung congestion, atelactasis etc.

vi. It is the excessive intracellular oxidation which is the cause of nervous system O_2 toxicity. The molecular O_2 is converted into active form of O_2 called oxygen free radicals, i.e. super oxide free radical O_2^-; and per-oxide radical as hydrogen per oxide. Normally these radicals are formed, but they are removed rapidly so long as oxy-Hb buffers functions normally. When this buffer fails, then these radicals accumulate and damage, as:-

a. oxidation of polyunsaturated fatty acids.

b. oxidation of some of the cellular enzymes.

c. nervous tissues are highly susceptible because of their increased lipid content.

23 Respiratory Insufficiencies

ATELACTASIS (GREEK - ATELES = INCOMPLETE EKTASIS = EXPANSION) (NOW SYNONYMOUS = COLLAPSE)

i. Any condition which lowers the pressure within the alveoli, or increase the pressure upon lung surface may lead to collapse of lung. Therefore, pleural effusion/pneumothorax or tumours pressing from without, or isolation of the alveoli from their air supply by the obstruction of a bronchus will lead to collapse of lung.

ii. *Congenital:* Alveoli have failed to expand. It is seen in stillborn child who has never breathed or in children who live only few days and never breathe well, the lung shows many area of atelactasis. The collapsed lung sinks in water—a common practical test to determine whether child has breathed.

Resorptive: Is found in infants who have breathed well so that the lungs have been fully expanded. Then due to some interference with respiration, the air is slowly absorbed from many of alveoli. In hyaline membrane disease of newborn the alveolar ducts are blocked with protein rich fluid as alveolar walls are lined with hyaline material.

iii. *Compression:* Pressure on the lung drives out the air and produces collapse. It may be complete when pressure is great and uniform (e.g. empyema, pneumothorax, massive pleural effusion); but it may be partial when pressure is more local (e.g. tumour, elevated diaphragm, enlarged heart). When pressure is removed the lung will expand again, but a thick cortex of fibrous tissue may be formed which may prevent re-expansion.

iv. *Obstructive: Here there are two key words—obstruction of a bronchus and weakening of respiratory movements.* If obstruction is due to a foreign body in a bronchus the second factor may not be present, but usually it is caused by accumulation of mucus in bronchioles associated with poor respiratory movements. If deep breathing and coughing were possible, the obstruction of bronchiole would be cleared away (e.g. debilitated children suffering from bronchitis/bronchopneumonia).

Above two key words are present after an abdominal operation, for anaesthetic stimulates the bronchial secretion, and abdominal section prevents the patient from breathing deeply. The frequent causes of this includes enlarged lymph nodes, tuberculous stenosis, tumours of bronchus.

In all these instances, the air in affected part of the lung is absorbed into the blood, no more air can enter on account of obstruction so that part of lung collapse.

Acute massive collapse—The two key words—bronchial obstruction and respiratory weakness.

The patient suddenly develops catastrophe, i.e. extreme dyspnoea, marked cyanosis and collapse. There exists no respiratory movement on affected side, the heart is displaced to that side and there are no physical sign of consolidation.

> Gairdner (1853) gave three chief causes of collapse in infancy — mucus in bronchi, weakness of respiratory power, and inability to cough and thus remove the mucus.

v. Effects on pulmonary functions

- Collapse occludes the alveoli.
- Resistance to blood flow is increased, through pulmonary vessels.
- Hypoxia in collapsed lung alveoli → vasoconstriction → blood flow through atelactic lung becomes slight → most of the blood is diverted through ventilated lung so well in aeration.
- When a large part of the lung is collapsed → decrease in lung volume → intrapleural pressure

becomes more negative with pulling the mediastinum to the affected side.

EMPHYSEMA (GREEK-EM+PHYSEMA; A BLOWING)

It is most crippling disease so most to be feared. Patient does not die quickly but drags out a miserable existence for years, a burden to himself, his family and his doctor. He suffers with every breath (20,000 times/day).

- Increased intra-alveolar pressure is the key word. Trapped air in alveoli constitutes great danger, which may be due to some obstruction of smaller bronchi and bronchioles. It is of checkvalve type, which allows:- air to be drawn in during inspiration, but prevents its passing out during expiration. Obstruction may be spasmodic or permanent which is exemplified by paroxysmal bronchial asthma—in which development of emphysema is a constant threat.
- Smoking runs parallel with emphysema. Where there is smoke there is likely to be cough and the cough associated with obstruction of airways spells trouble in the form of alveolar distension—namely emphysema.
- The respiratory bronchioles can become occluded by either inflammatory swelling or by plugging. The cough which accompanies chronic bronchitis intensifies the tension within alveoli and aggravates their distension. During each cough there is building up of pressure with glottis closed followed by sudden release with resulting stress on alveolar walls. The bronchioles leading to emphysematous lesion may have great collars of muscle and narrow lumina, perhaps adding an obstructive factor to the development of emphysema.
- Atrophy of alveolar walls and elastic framework is another key word justifying its cause. Impaired nutrition of the alveolar walls will impair their elasticity which may be due to ischaemia which may be further caused either by sclerosis of bronchiolar arterioles or by distension of alveoli with disruption of their walls.
- *Compensatory emphysema:* A portion of the lung becomes expanded in order to fill a space formerly occupied by pulmonary tissue. This is seen in atelactasis, and fibrosing conditions etc.
- *Atrophic emphysema (Senile):* In old age, and wasting disease. Not a true emphysema since there are no features like distension, lung enlargement, bullae on the surface. Only existing thing is atrophy and disappearance of walls of alveoli so that large spaces are formed. It is atrophied from defective nutrition.
- *Interstitial emphysema (air block):* The air escapes from alveoli and appearing into interstitial tissue of the lung along perivascular sheaths. It may be due to tearing of lungs, e.g. fracture rib or a wound. In children it may be due to over distension/rupture of alveoli during violent paroxysm of whooping cough.
- *Effects:* Chest has got barrel shaped appearance the ribs raised, sternum pushed forwards so that antero-posterior diameter equals to transverse one. The lungs are hyper-resonant, respiratory movements are diminished, expiration is prolonged and difficult. Pulmonary artery may show arteriosclerosis which may obstruct the pulmonary circulation (cor pulmonale) which leads to hypertrophy and dilatation of right ventricle along with general venous congestion. Dyspnoea and cyanosis are main troubling symptoms which leads to compensatory increase in erythrocyte number.
- The main physiological effect is hyperinflation of lung after expiration due to the obstruction caused by bronchospasm/permanent narrowing of bronchioles. It results into increased residual volume which is reflected in increased CO_2 content of arterial blood which makes respiratory centre refractory. So only chemoreceptors are left which can stimulate the respiratory centre.
- Is a fatal degenerative disease in which lungs lose their elasticity as a result of disruption of elastic tissue and walls between alveoli break down so that alveoli are replaced by large air sacs. Physiological dead space is greatly increased along with development of severe hypoxia owing to in adequate and uneven alveolar ventilation and perfusion of under ventilated alveoli. Inspiration and expiration are laboured along with development of hypercapnia.
- Heavy smoking → increase in number of pulmonary alveolar macrophages

Chemicals liberated → (elastase protease) Leucocytes are attracted towards lungs

Elastase protease → (in hibition of α_1 antitrypsin which normally inhibits elastase protease) elastic tissues are attacked upon increased destruction of lung tissue

- This α_1 antitrypsin may be congenitally absent.

Effects

- The smoking/infection/excess mucus/inflammatory oedema/irritate the bronchioles and bronchi and they are obstructed. It increases airway resistance, resulting into increased work of breathing.
- Smoking, etc. interferes with protective functions of lungs along with partial paralysis of cilia (loss of lung parenchyma). This causes a decrease in diffusing capacity of lung.
- This automatically reduces aeration of lungs by O_2 and removal of CO_2.
- This causes extremely abnormal ventilation/perfusion ratio with very low Va/Q in some parts, and very high Va/Q in some other parts of lung.

DYSPNOEA (AIR HUNGER)

- Difficulty in breathing OR subject is conscious of shortness of breath.
- When dyspnoeic index is less than about 70 per cent, dyspnoea is usually present. Dyspnoea may be produced by increased discharge in vagal afferents from lung receptors.

Increase in rate and depth of breathing regardless of subjective sensation, is hyperpnoea while tachypnoea is rapid shallow breathing.

Physiological Conditions—Dyspnoea

i. Stimulation of respiratory centre (by chemoreceptors, e.g. O_2 lack - CO_2 excess, asphyxia etc.)
ii. Impulses from higher centres, e.g. over activity of Hering-Breuer reflex
iii. Decrease in breathing reserve/vital capacity
iv. Low mechanical efficiency of respiratory apparatus
v. Muscular exercise
vi. Increased metabolic activity.

Dyspnoea—Pathological Causes

- Arterial hypoxia
- Impairment of transport of O_2 in blood e.g. pulmonary congestion, reduction of vital capacity, diminished elasticity of lung, increased Hering-Breuer reflex
- Acidosis
- Increased metabolism
- Emotional disturbances (hysteria)
- Respiratory muscle paralysis
- Lung conditions (e.g. airway obstruction, structural lesions, e.g. pneumonia, atelactasis fibrosis, emphysema etc.)

Dyspnoea: Pulmonary Diseases

a. In laryngeal/bronchial obstruction, asthma; dyspnoea is due to hypoxia + CO_2 retention.
b. Oedema terminates into reduced lung distensibility which causes dyspnoea. (inflammation, fibrosis, congestion)
c. In emphysema; there is loss of lung elasticity.

Dyspnoea: Cardiac

- In mitral stenosis there is dyspnoea on exertion.
- Pulmonary engorgement leading to diminished distensiblity of lung is the cause.
- Diminished distensibility → stiffness of the lung → greater inspiratory effort is expended in breathing the extra volume of air which is demanded by muscular exercise — or more force is required to distend it.
- The recoil tendency of the lung is moderately reduced, so expiration now requires the help of contraction of expiratory muscles to expel the air from lungs. So intra pleural pressure which is negative normally, now becomes positive towards the end of expiration. All this reduces the vital capacity. It also increases the sensitivity of Hering-Breuer reflex which produces shallow breathing.
- Dyspnoea is associated with hyperpnoea, which leads to reduction in cardiac output. So hyperpnoea and dyspnoea in cardiac patient at rest is due to reduced blood flow through the respiratory centre, resulting in high CO_2 tension as well as accumulation of acid products of its own metabolism.
- Cardiac asthma (paroxysmal nocturnal dyspnoea) - In CHF - dyspnoea may terminate into pulmonary oedema specially in the night, with a feeling of suffocation. Patient likes to go to the window or assumes an upright position.
- There occurs excessive engorgement of lungs with blood which increases pulmonary capillary pressure which then causes transudation into the alveoli. This increases the volume of blood in the lungs when one changes from upright to recumbent position.

Dyspnoea: Increased Metabolism

- Muscular exercise increases the metabolism and it leads to hyperpnoea. As the severity of exercise is increased hyperpnoea merges into dyspnoea. The main differences between athlete and untrained persons are:

1. *Vital capacity:* In a normal man, pulmonary ventilation increases four five times before the arrival of dyspnoeic point. Athlete because is having more

vital capacity, show a correspondingly greater increase in his pulmonary ventilation before dyspnoea comes into action.

2. *Circulation:* Circulatory rate of a trained man increases to a greater degree than an untrained person.
3. Pathological states like fever, hyperthyroidism, etc. does not cause dyspnoea at rest provided respiratory/ circulatory diseases should not exist. Of course on exertion dyspnoea is felt which causes no distress in a healthy person.

Dyspnoea: Anaemia

- At rest, there is no dyspnoea felt in anaemic subjects. The haemoglobin of course reduced in amount, becomes fully saturated with oxygen in the lungs. The oxygen tension and the quantity of gas in arterial blood are normal. The chemoreceptors are not apparently stimulated so the patient is not dyspnoeic while resting. To compensate cardiac output is increased along with re-distribution of blood flow. Skin vessels are constricted and great amount of total blood volume is driven through other regions. But during exertion, extra demand of O_2 is there which cannot be met.

ORTHOPNOEA

- Dyspnoea occurs at rest and is exaggerated when person lies down. He is slightly better in sitting position because:
  - — Pressure of enlarged liver on diaphragm is removed so facilitating its movements,
  - — Vital capacity is more (slight) in erect than in recumbent position

KUSSMAUL BREATHING

- More rapid and deep breathing than normal. Usually accompanied by "sigh" : Vital capacity is normal with increased tidal volume. Unaccompanied by apprehension—a difference from dyspnoea. Usually seen in acidosis (diabetes mellitus - uraemia) by stimulating chemoreceptors.

BRONCHIAL ASTHMA (GREEK-MEANING PANTING)

- Mainly allergic in origin, due to pollen grains, food, dust, bacteria, drugs etc.
- Smaller and medium sized bronchi are occluded with thick, tough and tenacious material mucus. Microscopically, the mucosa is thickened and oedematous infiltered with eosinophils, lymphocytes and plasma cells. The basement membrane shows a characteristic hyalianised thickening. There may be well marked hypertrophy of the bronchial muscle. Essential feature is bronchospasm which is revealed by wheezing and high pitched expiratory ronchi always accompanied by some degree of distension.
- The asthmatic suffers from recurring attacks of paroxysmal dyspnoea, a wheezing cough and a sense of constriction in the chest. Between the attacks patient may feel well but with the passage of time there is likely to be constant shortness of breath with characteristic expiratory wheezing.
- Prolongation of expiratory phase → reduction in vital capacity + diminution in tidal air → Increase in residual air + reduction in arterial oxygen saturation → retention of CO_2 → fatigue of respiratory centre → only chemoreceptors can stimulate the centre → so each breath is an effort.
- Because of allergy bronchial muscle undergoes spasmodic contraction, thus narrowing the lumen of bronchioles with resulting dyspnoea. The beneficial action of adrenaline may be explained by its action on oedematous mucosa rather than on muscle.
- Characterised by wheezing, cough and feeling of tightness in chest as a result of broncho-constriction.
- Three abnormalities—airway obstruction, airway inflammation and airway hyper-responsiveness to a variety of stimuli. Proteins released from eosinophils in inflammatory reaction may damage airway epithelium and contribute to hyper-responsiveness. Leukotriens are released from eosinophils and mast cells which cause vasoconstriction. Tachykinins and deficiency of VIP-a bronchodilator also contributes as causative agent.
- Attacks are more severe in early morning and late night since this is the period of maximal constriction. In circadian rhythm of bronchial tone β-adrenergic receptors mediate broncho-dilatation and treatment with inhaled β-adrenergic agonists is a standard therapy for asthma.
- When any allergen (allergy producing substance/ enters the body, it leads to formation of IgE antibodies, which causes allergic reactions.

  Mast cells are lying in lung interstitium. In this disease, antibodies attach themselves with these mast cells and many substances are released like histamine, SRS, eosinophilic chemotactic factor, bradykinin, etc. They lead to localised oedema in wall of small bronchioles, spasm of bronchiolar smooth muscle and overall increase in airway resistance.

- Because of difficulty in expiration, residual volume as well as functional residual capacity is increased during attack of disease. In time to come, chest becomes permanently enlarged—"barrel chest."
- During expiration, increased intrapulmonary pressure compresses the outer margin of bronchioles so they become more occluded. This makes expiration - a troublesome job while inspiration is normal.
- Disease is aggravated by stress/emotion. It is also having genetic basis. Infection is also reported as a cause of disease.

PNEUMONIA

- Inflammatory consolidation of lung. Lung is the organ which is in direct contact with outside air, so bacterial infection is frequent. The defensive mechanism includes sticky mucus of bronchial mucosa which entraps the invaders, and, cilia whose movements is directed upwards (cough reflex).

- Lobar pneumonia is caused by infection by *Pneumococcus* (It is captain of death as told by Wiliam Osler). This bacterial infection creates irritation which leads to outpouring of inflammatory exudate into alveoli, it fills alveoli, air is displaced and lung or its affected part is converted into solid and airless organ. This process is called *consolidation or hepatization* because lung becomes liver like. Process is a progressive one, beginning at hilus and sweeping out to the periphery, involving one or more lobes and sometimes both lungs.
- Resolution is the most remarkable phenomenon. The huge mass of solidified exudate consisting largely of fibrin which has converted the airy lump into something resembling to lung of flesh, is completely removed and lung is resorbed, uninjured to its former intact condition. The reason for it is that there is no necrosis of alveolar walls. The invading bacteria pass so readily into alveolar spaces and there is so little struggle in interstitial tissue that no destruction takes place.
- The physical signs like dullness, blowing breathing, increased vocal fremitus and resonance are caused by conversion of lung into a solid organ which conducts sound from large bronchi to the chest with readiness. Pain is due to pleurisy. Blood culture may be positive with leucocytosis.
- Lowered O_2 saturation (anoxaemia) - the leak that sinks the ship is the characteristic whose index is cyanosis.
- *Broncho-pneumonia* (postoperative, terminal pneumonia): Patchy character. It occurs principally in childhood and old age; pneumonia following measles/whooping cough, etc.
- This is bronchial as well as pulmonary infection and inflammation, bronchi being first to be involved. There exists a patchy consolidation of both lungs, sometimes patches fuse together. Collapsed areas dark purple in colour and depressed below the surface are seen on outside of lung. Infection begins in upper respiratory tract, descends in droplets of finer bronchioles which become inflamed and finally invades alveoli.

CONSOLIDATION: SERIES OF EVENTS

- Infection is the starting point. Pulmonary membrane is inflamed. Blood + fluid pass out of the blood into alveoli. So in this way infection spreads from alveolus to alveolus.
- The net results are:- Reduction in total surface area of respiratory membrane, decreased ventilation-perfusion ratio, all this reduces diffusing capacity, which ultimately results into low blood oxygen and high blood carbon-dioxide.

TUBERCULOSIS

- Of lungs is commonest of all. The re-infection usually comes from a primary infection that occurred in another part of the lung many years previously. The right lung is attacked much more commoner than the left and lesion is always at the apex.
- The explanation of remarkable localisation of lesion at apex is as follows:

  Low pulmonary arterial pressure at the apex owing to height of column of blood from right ventricle to the apex when patient is erect. Pressure at apex is practically nil when an adult is in erect posture. In tall long chested persons, the mean pressure is negative. As a consequence there is no production of tissue fluid/lymph in erect posture, immune bodies don't reach the part, removal of oxygen minimal from alveoli and tubercular bacilli find optimum atmosphere for growth. Patients with mitral stenosis are immune from apical tuberculosis and in them pulmonary arterial pressure is high to supply needs of the part. On the other hand disease is remarkably common in Congenital stenosis of pulmonary valve a condition that produces lowest known pulmonary arterial pressure. These considerations explain the importance of rest in recumbent posture in treatment of pulmonary tuberculosis.

It is the erect posture maintained for many consecutive hours which has given man an Achillis heel through which the acid fast arrow may pass—Dock

- The principal features of primary tuberculosis includes—lack of any constant site of the initial lesion, caseous involvement of lymph nodes, presence of liquefaction and cavity formation in lung—while in secondary infection it includes—healing with fibrosis, chronic fibrocaseous tuberculosis, acute tuberculus caseous pneumonia, acute miliary tuberculosis.
- Secondary pulmonary tuberculosis is classically localised to apex of one or both upper lobes. The reason is obscure but it may relate to high O_2 tension in the apices.
- The initial lesion is usually a small focus of consolidation, less than 2 cm in diameter, located within 1 to 2 cm of apical pleura.
- Typically the inhaled bacilli implant in distal air spaces of the lower part of upper lobe, or upper part of lower lobe, usually close to the pleura.

TUBERCULOSIS

- The infection by tubercular bacilli leads to invasion by macrophages, walling off lesion by fibrous tissue to form tubercle.
- Its main effects include:- increased work by respiratory muscles, reduced vital capacity, reduction in surface area of respiratory membrane, increase in thickness of respiratory membrane, abnormal ventilation-perfusion ratio and decreased pulmonary diffusing capacity.

CYANOSIS (GREEK-KYANOS = BLUE DISCOLOURATION/SUBSTANCE)

- Condition characterised by blue (dusky) colouration of skin and mucous membrane of body when reduced/deoxygenated haemoglobin level is 5 gm or more. Its common sites are — lips, cheeks, nail beds, mucous membrane of tongue and tip of nose, skin of ear lobule, fingers etc. where the skin is thin.
- *Conditions giving rise*
  1. *Hypoxic hypoxia*: (low Po_2 in inspired air, paralysis of muscles of respiration, airway obstruction, lung diseases like emphysema/pneumonia/cavity formation/fibrosis etc., impaired diffusion across alveolar membrane, hyaline membrane disease, venoarterial shunt.
  2. *Stagnant hypoxia*: e.g. congestive cardiac failure - venous obstruction.
  3. *Polycythaemia*: Only slight degree of unsaturation will produce cyanosis. It is because of excess amount of blood in capillaries as well as due to sluggish circulation.
  4. *Increased methaemoglobin content of blood* (it is normally reduced in the body by lactic acid dehydrogenase with help of co-enzyme I. In congenital cases this enzyme is absent which leads to cyanosis.
  5. *Due to intake of sulfa drugs* and intestinal putrefaction by bacteria leading to formation of H_2S. → sulphaemoglobinaemia → cyanosis (enterogenous).
- *Factors causing*
  i. Total amount of haemoglobin:- in extreme anaemia — no cyanosis, It should be 5 gm in each decilitre of blood.
  ii. Degree of unsaturation of haemoglobin.
  iii. State of blood vessels. Specially capillaries which must contain reduced haemoglobin. If vessels are constricted the amount of blood is not sufficient to impart cyanotic colour.
  iv. If skin is pigmented (dark complexion) and thick the colour may not be evident.
  v. Oxygenated blood is red in colour, while deoxygenated blood is blue coloured. If both are mixed deoxygenated blood's colour will be dominant over the colour of oxygenated blood.
  vi. In moderate cold cyanosis develops because of cutaneous arteriolar and venous constriction; which makes a slow blood flow through capillaries and so more oxygen is removed from capillaries. But cyanosis does not develop in very cold weather because decreased skin temperature inhibits the dissociation of oxyhaemoglobin. O_2 consumption of cold tissue is decreased.

BIBLIOGRAPHY

1. Auerbach O. Changes in bronchial epithelium in relation to cigarette smoking. New Eng J Med 1979;300:285.
2. Chan Yeung M. Cryptogenic fibrosing alveolitis. Lancet 1997;350:651.
3. Cosio MG, et al. The relationship between structural changes in small airways and pulmonary function tests. New Eng J Med 1978;298:1277.
4. Crapo JD. Morphological changes in pulmonary oxygen toxicity. Ann Rev Phy 1987;49:721.
5. Deneke SM, et al. Normobaric O_2 toxicity of lung. New Eng J Med 1980;303:76.
6. Fishman AP, et al (Ed.). Pulmonary Edema. American physiological society 1979.
7. Goerke J. Lung surfactant. Biochim, Biophys Acta 1974;344:241.
8. Hautami R, et al. Requirement for macrophage elastase for cigarette smoke-induced emphysema in mice. Science 1997;277:2002.
9. Hogg JC, et al. Site and nature of airway obstruction in chronic obstruction lung disease. New Eng J Med 1968;278:1355.
10. Imlay JA, et al. DNA damage and oxygen radical toxicity. Science 1988;240:1302.

24 Adjustments of Respiration: Abnormal Situations

AVIATION PHYSIOLOGY

- Changes occur due to accelerator forces as a result of changes in velocity and direction of the motion.
- Linear acceleration may occur in the beginning of the flight and at the end there is deceleration. Angular acceleration is felt when aeroplane takes the turn and is measured in terms of "*g*."
- A subject who is pressed against his seat with a force equal to his body weight which is equal to the pull of gravity it is called *positive (+) g*. If force is five times of his body weight it is 5g. If subject is held down of his seat belt then negative g is applied. If the force with which he is thrown against his belt is equal to his body weight, it is called *negative (-) g*.
- *Effects of positive (+) g:* Blood shifts from one part to another (being mobile) by angular acceleration. Organs being solid are slightly displaced. On positive g blood is centrifuged towards inferior extremity, force is 5 g and subject is standing then hydrostatic force in lower limb will be five times the normal pressure of 90 mmHg → deficient venous return → diminution in cardiac output → lowering of blood pressure. If angular acceleration is more than +5 g it may lead to symptoms of *black out* (dimness of vision, unconsciousness due to cerebral ischaemia). If this increases to +20g it may cause fracture of vertebra.
- *Effects of negative (-) g:* On pressure of -4/-5 g transient hyperpnoea, psychotic derangement due to brain oedema occur. Rupture (haemorrhage) of cerebral vessels may occur due to dilatation. Temporary blindness may occur due to hyperaemia (red out) since eyes are not protected by rigid cranium.
- *Effect of linear acceleration:* During "take off" of aeroplane this is evident. Subject tends to be pushed backward when the back rest hits the body of pilot, causing damage.
- *Deceleration:*

$$\frac{MV^2}{2}$$

M = Mass of body, V = Velocity

On landing of aeroplane these forces become important, e.g. in aeroplane crash. The force of impact is proportional to the kinetic energy divided by distance of stopping. It is rupture/tearing/disintegration of different structures which become cause of death.

- *Weightlessness in space:* Due to absence of the pull of the gravity, the subject will simply float in ship. The other consequences include demineralisation of bone, increased urinary excretion of minerals, reduction in blood volume, reduced muscle tone, visual + aural hallucination, fatigue, increased heart rate, after over of flight blood pressure falls.
- As far as temperature is concerned, temperature falls to -55°C several miles above the earth. In ionosphere at an altitude about 350 miles above earth the temperature is 3000°C. Because of sparsity of particles this temperature has no effect and more over space ship is so constructed to have no effect.

Greater Gamma than X radiations are found to occur at 20 miles above the earth.

During take off and landing effects of linear acceleration and deceleration may affect.

DYSBARISM (DIVING PHYSIOLOGY)

- These manifestations occur in deep sea Divers or Caisson workers who suddenly come to the surface and exposed to normal pressure after spending sometime in a high pressure zone.
- *Mechanism:* When divers work underneath the sea, he is exposed to high pressure. When he comes to the

surface (out of his sealed cabin), then due to reduction in pressure, gases try to come out because of fall in alveolar pressure of gases.

- At high pressure N_2 is dissolved more in the body than O_2 and CO_2. So on falling the pressure N_2 comes out as bubbles. Since O_2 and CO_2 are freely diffusible and O_2 can be metabolically used so problem remains with N_2.
  - — *Symptoms:* Pressure in myelin sheath of sensory nerves leading to pain, itching, paraesthesia.
  - — Pressure of bubbles on motor nerves lead to paresis or paralysis.
  - — Due to bubbles lodged in cerebral vessels, seizures/convulsions may ensue.
  - — Due to lodging of air bubble in bone marrow, pain in bones may be felt.

HIGH GASEOUS PRESSURE: NITROGEN NARCOSIS

- O_2, CO_2 and N_2 are the main gases by which the diver is exposed. Four fifth of air is N_2, which does not affect at sea level.
- Mild nitrogen narcosis appears at 120 feet depth, when the diver lose many of his cares. He becomes drowsy at 150 to 200 feet depth, at 200 to 250 feet depth, he loses his strength. More than this depth he becomes useless. These changes are also called raptures of depths.
- N_2 dissolves freely in body fats, i.e. also in membranes of neurones. It reduces their excitability by altering electrical conductance of membranes.
- Nitrogen narcosis: identical with alcohol intoxication.

LIFE SAVING MEASURE: ARTIFICIAL RESPIRATION

It should be given when respiration is failed but heart is still beating.

Manual Method

Schafer's Method

Patient is in prone position with a pillow or so under thorax/epigastrium. Doctor sits with his face towards head of the patient. Doctor puts his both hands on both sides of the chest. Then doctor puts his body weight by leaning forwards and pressing upon the loin of the patient → rise in intra-abdominal pressure → diaphragm is pushed up → expiration. After this the doctor resumes back the original position which causes inspiration. This is repeated 12 times per minute to start respiration. Because patient is in prone position so chances of dribbling of saliva is very thin but even then if it comes, it should be cleaned.

Holger-Nielson Method

Patient is in prone position with arms abducted at shoulders and elbow flexed. The face is turned to one side. Doctor sits by facing towards head of the patient. Now the doctor puts his hands on both sides of the back of the patient with thumbs and fingers quite spreaded. Now the doctor puts his body weight by leaning forwards upon the patient's back which causes expiration. Then he comes back in original position which causes inspiration. This is repeated 12 times/minute.

In Newborn Baby

1. Alternately put the child in cold and warm water which will reflexly stimulate the respiration.
2. Hold the baby upside down and back should be patted. More blood will go towards the brain and respiration will start reflexly.
3. Pump CO_2 forcibly through nostrils which will stimulate the respiratory centre.

Mouth to Mouth

The patient is first placed in supine position, and doctor puts his hand under the neck of patient, for lifting. Doctor covers the mouth of patient by his mouth and closes his nostrils by the fingers which are already on forehead. Doctor blows air in the mouth of patient 12 times/minute. The patient's neck is kept extended.

MECHANICAL METHODS: SOME OTHER TRIALS

a. *Sylvester's Methods:* The subject is placed in supine position. The doctor stands at the head end and holds the two arms of the patient. Doctor then raises the hands of patient above his head and then folds the hands back upon the chest, compressing the chest wall at the same time. By such movements thoracic cavity is alternately increased and decreased which leads to drawing air in as well as blowing out. It should be repeated 12 times/minute. Mucus from mouth cavity should be wiped out from time to time.

b. *Eve's Rocking Method:* In a stretcher, the patient is tied. Hand and feet are alternately tilted through an angle of 45°. Eight or nine such movements per minute (4 seconds head down and 3 seconds feet down). Head down → weight of abdominal viscera presses against diaphragm → air pushed out of lungs (expiration).
Feet down → diaphragm descends → air is drawn into lungs (inspiration).

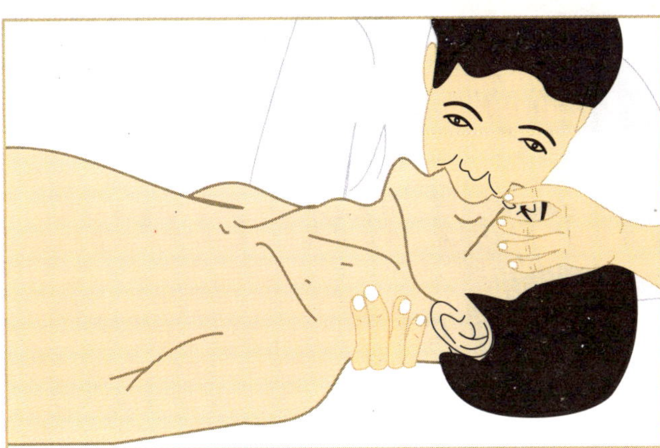

Fig. 24.1: Mouth to mouth respiration

INSTRUMENTAL METHODS

a. *Drinker's Method:* The patient is placed in air tight chamber and head remains out. By mechanically driven pumps the pressure in the chamber is alternately lowered and raised.
   Low pressure → chest wall swells up → air is drawn into lungs.
   High pressure → Chest is compressed → air is pushed out so the principle of working is alternate compressing and relaxing the chest wall. So it is useful when prolonged artificial respiration is required, e.g. paralysis of respiratory muscles, poliomyelitis, morphine poisoning.
b. *Braggpaul's Method:* A rubber bag is wrapped and by suitable pumps, pressure is lowered and increased thus compressing and relaxing the chest wall alternately which carries out the respiration.
c. *By introducing air directly into lungs:*
   A thin flexible tube is inserted in trachea up to its bifurcation and a constant stream of oxygen (with/without 5% CO_2) is allowed to pass into lungs so lungs remain slightly distended (continuous insufflation).
   In animals, a cannula is introduced and tied to the trachea. Warm moist air is driven into the lungs from a rhythmically acting pump. After each blast, the lung collapses and air is expelled through a side tube in cannula. (Intermittent inflation).

BIBLIOGRAPHY

1. Melamed Y, et al. Medical problems associated with underwater diving. New Eng J Med 1992;326:30.
2. Weinberger SE. Recent advances in pulmonary medicine. New Eng J Med 1993;328:1309.

25

Assessing Lungs: Pulmonary Function Tests

i. *Ventilatory functions*
   - Peak-expiratory flow rate
   - Spirometery

ii. *Respiratory gas exchange:* This measurement inform about overall ventilation and efficiency of gas exchange.
   - Estimation of blood CO_2 tension.
   - Gas exchange.
   - Transfer factor (TCO)

iii. *Exercise testing:* Maximal oxygen uptake (VO_2 max.)

iv. *Bronchoscopy*

v. *Laboratory investigations*

vi. *Response of bronchodilator drugs*

vii. *Biopsy*

viii. *Radiology:* Routine radiography scanning, pulmonary angiography, brochography, tomography.

PEAK EXPIRATORY FLOW (PEF)

Can be measured during forced expiration by a gauge or meter, which is simpler and cheaper than spirometer. Reduced values indicate airflow obstruction. This is of little value in restrictive ventilatory defects. The subject takes a maximal inspiration and then gives a maximum expiratory blast through the instrument. The pointer sticks at point of maximum excursion and PEFR can be read directly from the scale. Normal value — 400 litres per minute. It is measured by the instruments Wright's or mini peak flow meter.

EXERCISE TESTS

Bicycle, treadmill exercise are done and they are of value in detecting exercise hypoxaemia and in assessing disability due to respiratory diseases.

DIFFUSION CAPACITY

This so called 'gas transfer factor' constitutes a useful estimate of ability of lungs to exchange gases specially in states like sarcoidosis, emphysema, interstitial lung diseases etc. It is normally estimated by measuring the uptake of CO from a single breath of a 0.3 per cent mixture of air. Normal value is 20 to 30 ml/min/mmHg at rest.

PULMONARY VOLUMES

The various such volumes are:

a. *Tidal volume:* In normal young healthy adult it amounts to be 500 ml. It is the usual normal quiet breathing, i.e. volume of air inspired (taken in) and expired (given out) in each normal breath.

b. *Inspiratory-reserve-volume:* In normal adult individual it amounts to be 3000 ml. It is that volume of air inspired over and above the usual tidal volume.

c. *Expiratory reserve volume:* In normal healthy adult it is 1100 ml. It is the volume of air which can be expired after normal tidal expiration by forceful expiration.

d. *Residual volume:* In young healthy adult it is said to be normally 1200 ml. The volume of air remaining in the lungs after most forceful expiration is termed as residual volume. It is this residual air which is needed to aerate the blood in between breaths otherwise O_2 and CO_2 concentrations in blood may significantly alter leading to fatal consequences.

e. *Minute Respiratory volume:* It is the tidal volume multiplied by respiratory rate (tidal volume × respiratory rate). So 500 × 12 comes to be 6000 ml or 6 litres per minute, in a normal healthy adult individual. A person can survive up to 1.5 to 2 litres per minute's volume. So it is the total volume of new air passed through respiratory passages per minute.

It should be well remembered that all above mentioned lung volumes are little less in females and asthenic persons as compared with males and athletes respectively.

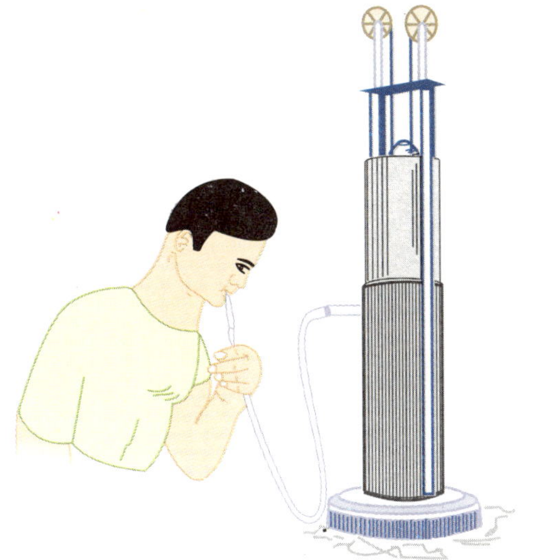

Fig. 25.1: Use of spirometer for measuring various lung capacities and volumes

PULMONARY CAPACITIES

The capacities are combination of two or even more volumes together as shown in following list (always active process):

a. *Inspiratory capacity:* It is the sum total of tidal volume and inspiratory reserve volume; so it comes out to be 500 + 3000 ml. So 3500 ml. More clearly it is that amount of air which one can breath up to expiratory level and then distending lungs up to maximum value.
b. *Functional residual capacity:* It is calculated by summing up expiratory reserve volume and residual volume. So it amounts to be 2300 ml (1100 + 1200 ml). In other words, it is that amount of air which persists within lungs even after normal expiration.
c. *Vital capacity:* It can be calculated by adding tidal, inspiratory reserve and expiratory reserve volume together. So it amounts to be 4600 ml in males (or 4.6 litres) while in females it is 3.1 litres. So in other words it is maximum amount of air expelled by an individual after first filling lungs to their maximum and then expiring to their maximum extent.

Few Facts

i. A tall and thin individual is having vital capacity towards higher side in comparison of an obese person.
ii. A trained athlete is having more vital capacity as compared with an individual of sedentary habits.
iii. If respiratory muscles are paralysed (bulbar poleomyelitis, spinal cord injuries etc.), vital capacity is decreased to a greater extent.
iv. Any condition decreasing 'lung compliance' also said to reduce vital capacity to a significant extent. It includes conditions like bronchial asthma, pulmonary tuberculosis, lung cancer, pleurisy, chronic bronchitis etc. Due to this reason vital capacity measurement is included in lung function tests.
v. Vital capacity is also said to be decreased when due to any reason, pulmonary vascular congestion results, and this further is due to reduced lung compliance owing to increased quantity of fluid in lung tissues.
vi. It is also affected by posture of individual.
vii. It is also said to be proportionate to surface area. It is 2–2.3 litres per square meter surface area in males while in females it is 1.8 to 2.1 litres per square meter surface area.
viii. *Timed vital capacity:* It is the fraction of vital capacity expired in first second. (FEV_1 = synonym - forced expiratory volume). Its measurement gives information additional to that given by vital capacity. In air way obstruction (acute asthma) the vital capacity remains normal but FEV_1 is reduced to 20 per cent of FVC.

FORCE EXPIRATORY VOLUME (FEV)

Normal values:-
FEV_1 = 83 per cent of total vital capacity
FEV_2 = 94 per cent of total vital capacity
FEV_3 = 97 per cent of total vital capacity
After third second = 100 per cent of total vital capacity.

- Significance: Great diagnostic value. Decreased significantly in some respiratory diseases e.g. obstructive disease (asthma, emphysema), restrictive diseases (fibrosis etc.).

d. *Total lung capacity:* It amounts to be 5800 ml. It is sum total of tidal, inspiratory, expiratory and residual volume. In more clear sense, it is a maximum volume to which lungs can be expanded by great inspiratory effort.
e. *Maximum Breathing capacity:* It usually equals to 90 to 170 litres per minute. We can easily appreciate the remarkable respiratory reserve but what a pity on our part is that the diseases are capable enough to decrease this capacity to a significant standard and can force one individual to fight for breath. Also called MVV (Maximum Voluntary Ventilation) Since it can be induced by voluntary hyperventilation, severe

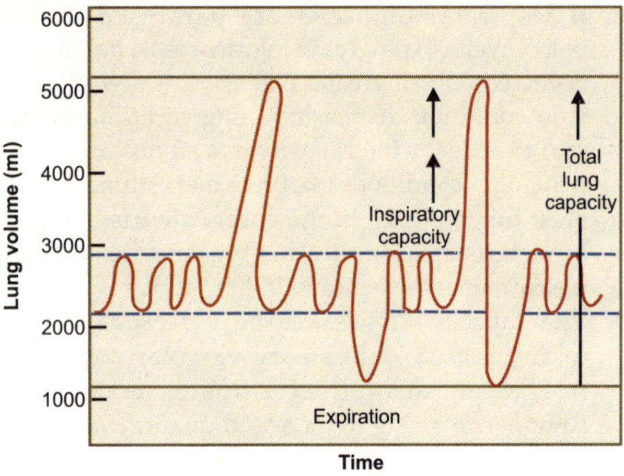

Fig. 25.2: Spirogram: Alterations in lung volumes

muscular exercise, inhalation of 7 per cent CO_2. It is "Maximum Volume of air a person could breathe in or out in one minute by maximum voluntary effort."

BRONCHODILATOR DRUGS

First FEV_1 and PEFR is measured. Then a bronchodilator in its suitable dose is administered. Both of above tests are repeated. Increased values are suggestive of bronchospasm, while in emphysema, the values are not changed.

LABORATORY INVESTIGATIONS

1. Blood—Haemoglobin, TLC, absolute eosinophil number.
2. Sputum—Culture for AFB (acid fast bacillus).
3. Cytological—for carcinoma cells.
4. Routine urine examination if suspicion of tuberculosis.

BRONCHOSCOPY

In bronchogenic carcinoma, foreign body. FOB (Fibre optic bronchoscopy) is needed for deeper penetration into bronchial tree and of easy visualisation of upper lobe division.

MAXIMAL OXYGEN UPTAKE (VO_2. MAX)

- Tidal volume is 500 ml.; Respiratory rate is 12/min., ventilation volume is 6000 ml./min. This contains roughly 1,200 ml. of O_2 and one consumes only about 250 ml O_2/minute so this 250 ml/min is oxygen uptake at rest.
- During physical work need for O_2 rises which gives rise to VO_2 max This may be as high as 3,000 ml in trained athletes.

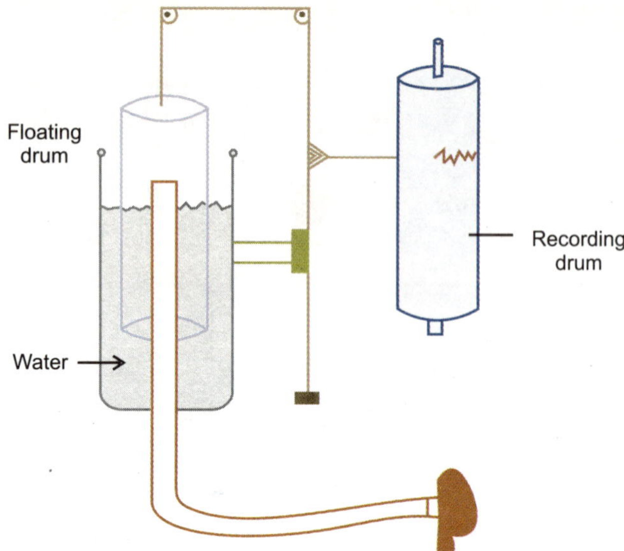

Fig. 25.3: Spirometer

- It is low in emphysema, pulmonary oedema, left ventricular insufficiency, etc.
- Determination—The subject works hard on bicycle ergometer/treadmill. During this expired air is collected in a Douglas bag. After 2 minutes work, O_2 percentage of expired air in Douglas bag is analysed and VO_2 is determined.
- It is routinely done in sportsman but procedure is very exhaustive. It is of value in lung disorders and assessment of fitness in sportsman.

SPIROGRAM

Recording of lung volumes and capacities is called spirogram. Downward deflection indicates expiration. We should note "normal end expiratory level, "normal end inspiratory level," "maximum expiratory and inspiratory level."

SPIROMETER

Metallic instrument. All volumes and capacities can be measured except total lung capacity, residual volume and functional residual capacity.

PEAK FLOW METER

A popular instrument is peak flow meter and still cheap simpler version is mini peak flow meter and is suitable for use at home. Most healthy people will achieve values upto 400 litres/minute. Patients with air flow obstruction are having reduced rates upto 200 and even 100 litres/minute is extremely severe. It actually measures maximal rate of flow achieved during forced expiration.

VENTILATION—PERFUSION RATIO (V_A/Q)

a. The Concept:

   i. The partial pressure of a gas (O_2.; CO_2) is chiefly determined by—the rate of alveolar ventilation; and; rate of transfer of O_2 and CO_2 through respiratory membrane. It is presumed that all the alveoli are ventilated equally and blood flow through the alveolar capillary is the same for each alveolus.

   ii. —Now in normal states, some areas of the lungs are well ventilated but almost have no blood flow then the ratio V_A/Q is infinity.

   —On the contrary, when ventilation is zero but perfusion of alveolus is existing; then the ventilation perfusion ratio is zero.

   —In either of the above cases, there exists no exchange of gases through the respiratory membrane of the affected alveoli. This is its importance.

b. *V_A/Q = Zero:* means ventilation is zero but perfusion exists. This means further that air in alveolus is in equilibrium with the blood gases CO_2 and O_2; this is because the venous blood comes here. These gases here are having partial pressure - 40 mm Hg of O_2 and 45 mm Hg of CO_2.

c. *V_A/Q = Infinity:* Means well ventilation but no blood flow. OR there is no capillary flow to carry O_2 away or to bring CO_2 to the alveoli. So now alveolar air becomes equal to humidified inspired air. So no O_2 is lost to the blood by inspired air neither; nor no CO_2 is gained. The inspired humidified air has Po_2 - 149 mm Hg and Pco_2 of 0 mm Hg which are the partial pressure of these two gases in the alveoli.

d. *Under Conditions of normal V_A/Q:* the exchange of O_2 and CO_2 through the respiratory membrane is nearly optimal. OR alveolar Po_2 is at 104 mm Hg (in between 149 and 40 mm Hg); and alveolar Pco_2 is at 40 mm Hg (between 45 and 0 mm Hg)

e. *Physiologic shunt:* In cases of V_A/Q below normal, the oxygen is less to oxygenate fully the alveolar capillaries. So a certain fraction of venous blood passing through the pulmonary capillaries does not become oxygenated. This fraction is called shunted blood. Its total quantity per minute is physiologic shunt.

f. Abnormal V_A/Q is seen in emphysema and in chronic obstructive lung diseases.

g. In conditions where perfusion is defective, oxygenation of the blood as well as evolution of CO_2 will be deranged, e.g. embolism/thrombosis of pulmonary vessels, mechanical obstruction of pulmonary vessels by effusion, reduction of pulmonary vascular bed by lung diseases, anatomical venous-arterial shunt.

OTHER INVESTIGATIONS

- CT scan
- X-Ray chest
- Radio-isotope imaging
- Ultrasound
- MRI (Magnetic resonance imaging)
- Bronchoscopy/thoracoscopy
- Lung biopsy
- Immunological tests

FEW MORE POINTS

1. *Dyspnoea index* $= \dfrac{\text{walking ventilation (1/minute)}}{\text{MVV or MBC in 1/minute}}$

   $= \dfrac{19}{100} = 0.19$

   Dyspnoea never occurs till index becomes 0.35
   Moderate dyspnoea - 0.45
   Severe dyspnoea - 0.50

2. *Forced expiratory flow*: ($FEF_{25\text{-}75\%}$) Normally 3001/min. "This is the mean expiratory flow rate during middle 50 per cent of FVC." The time taken for it is "Mid Expiratory Time (MET), which normally is 0.5 sec and it increases in obstructive lung disorders."

3. *Closing Volume (CV)*: It is the lung volume above residual volume at which airways in lower dependent part of lungs begin to close off due to lesser transmural pressure here.

4. *Douglas bag*: Is a closed canvas bag lined internally by rubber. A tube emerges from the bag throug which subject inspires. Through valves such arrangements are made that expired air collects in bag which can be measured and analysed. Its chief use is during mountain expedition.

5. *Forced Vital Capacity* (FVC): It is the largest volume of air measured on complete expiration after deepest inspiration; with expiration being as forceful and rapid as possible.

26 Pulmonary Circulation

- Pulmonary artery carries deoxygenated blood and pulmonary vein carries oxygenated blood.
- In systemic circulation capillary filtration takes place into tissue spaces but this does not occur in lungs. If it occurs here then fluid will be accumulated in the alveoli which will retard the oxygenation of blood. Pulmonary congestion from any cause will increase the local blood pressure leading to filtration and thus causing oedema.
- It (pulmonary vascular bed) is a low resistance circuit while systemic circulation is a high resistance circuit.
- Pulmonary vascular bed can accommodate a large volume of blood so it is called blood reservoir.
- It has to supply the blood to only one type of tissue while systemic circulation has to supply the blood to whole body, i.e. to different types of tissue.
- *Receptors*: Baro-receptors are located in pulmonary arch of aorta. An increase in pulmonary arterial pressure produces reflex bradycardia, hypotension and increased blood flow in splanchnic bed. This depends on vagus nerve, which if severed, no such response will be elicited.
- Increased blood volume in the thoracic cavity reflexly produces diuresis through inhibiting ADH.
- Multiple emboli if present will stimulate receptors in pulmonary vascular bed which leads to rapid shallow breathing.
- *Paintal AS* demonstrated the existence of pulmonary deflation receptors. On intravenous injection of phenyl diguanide he found bradycardia and hypotension.
- The Pulmonary vascular bed is innervated by both sympathetic and parasympathetic nerves, but their role in maintenance of circulation is less important as compared with systemic circulation.
- *Few facts*: Pressure in right ventricle .... 25 mm Hg Systolic

  ....0-1 mmHg diastolic

  Pressure in pulmonary artery .... 25 mmHg systolic

  ....8 mmHg diastolic

  mean pulmonary arterial pressure = 15 mmHg

  Pulmonary arterial pulse pressure = 17 mmHg

  Pulmonary capillary pressure = 7 mmHg.

  Left artial and pulmonary venous pressure = 2 mmHg (1-5 mmHg)
- The blood volume of the lung is 450 ml approximately (9% of total blood volume; 70 ml of this is in capillaries while remaining is distributed between veins and arteries).

BIBLIOGRAPHY

1. Acker H. Chemoreception in arterial chemoreceptors. Ann Rev Phy 1989;51:835.
2. Adamson JW, et al. Haemoglobin function, oxygen affinity and erythropoietin. Ann Rev Phy 1975;37:351.
3. Cohen MI. Central determinants of respiratory rhythm. Ann Rev Phy 1981;43:91.
4. Crapo JD. Morphologic changes in pulmonary oxygen toxicity. Ann Rev Phy, 1987.
5. Crapo RO. Pulmonary function testing. New Eng J Med 1994;331:25.
6. Deneke SM, et al. Normobaric oxygen toxicity. New Eng J Med 1980;303:76.
7. Fels AOS, et al. The alveolar macrophage. J App Phy 1986;60:353.
8. Gaar KA. Jr. Oxygen transport : A simple model for study and examination. Physiologist 1985;28:412.
9. Guyton AC, et al. Basic oscillating mechanism of Cheyne-Stokes breathing. Amer J Phy 1956;187:395.
10. Hadded GG, et al. Hypoxia and respiratory control in early life. Ann Rev Phy, 1984.
11. Jansen AH, et al. Development of respiratory control. Phy Rev 1983;63:437.

QUESTION BANK

1. Describe cardio-respiratory responses during isotonic and isometric exercises (Raj. Univ. 1993, M.D.)
2. Give an account of various problems of physiological importance encountered in aviation and space flights (Raj. Univ. 1989, M.D.).

3. Describe chemical and non-chemical mechanism which regulate pulmonary ventilation (Raj. Univ. 1988 M.D.).
4. What is forced expiratory volume. How you will measure it. What is its significance?
5. Discuss:
   a. Origin and control of respiratory rhythm
   b. O_2 therapy in various types of hypoxia (Raj. Univ. 1986, M.D.)
   c. Pathophysiology of chronic respiratory failure.
   d. The present concepts regarding neurogenesis of respiratory rhythm (Raj. Univ. 1982, M.D.).
   e. The role of chemoreceptors in regulation of respiration (Raj. Univ. 1992, M.D.).
   f. The integrative aspects of regulation of breathing (Raj. Univ. 1984, M.D.)
6. Show diagrammatically and explain - changes in intra-pleural pressure in quiet respiration, what are the consequences of increased intrapleural pressure?
7. Describe exchange of gases in lungs. Write briefly about O_2 dissociation curve (Raj. Univ. 1995).
8. Short Notes -
   a. Dysbarism (Raj. Univ. 1982, M.D.)
      Medical problems produced by diving and treatment (Raj. Univ. 2000, M.D.)
   b. Lung compliance (Raj. Univ. 1995)
   c. J receptor (Raj. Univ. 1991, M.D.)
   d. Cyanosis (Raj. Univ. First M.B.B.S., 2001)
   e. Regulation of pulmonary blood flow
   f. Ventilation perfusion ratio
   g. FEV_1 (Raj. Univ. 1992, 2001 M.D.)
   h. Hering-Breuer reflex (Raj. Univ. 1995, 2001)
   i. Respiratory centres (Raj. Univ. 1986)
   j. Lung surfactant (Raj. Univ. 1992, M.D.)
   k. O_2 dissociation curve
   l. Cardio-respiratory adjustments at high altitude [Raj. Univ. 2000, M.Sc. (Med. 1)]
   m. Sleep apnoea - BF/2003-M.D.
   n. Role of O_2 therapy in different types of hypoxia - BF/2003-M.D.
9. Locate respiratory centres and explain how it functions in control of breathing. Define emphysema and explain how it affects breathing (Raj. Univ. 1993, M.D.).
10. i. What are the components that contribute to the work of breathing? Discuss normal and pathologic conditions that cause alteration in each component. (Raj. Univ. 2000, M.D.)
    ii. Give an account of chemical regulation of respiration. Add note on periodic breathing. (M.B.B.S. 1st professional exam. 2004, Rohtak University)

MULTIPLE CHOICE QUESTIONS : RESPIRATION

1. The normal pressure of fluid in intrapleural space is:
   a. - 10 to - 12 mmHg
   b. + 10 to + 12 mmHg
   c. - 3 mmHg
   d. + 3 mmHg [ ]
2. Following are the muscles of inspiration except:
   a. Diaphragm
   b. Sternocleidomastoid
   c. Scapular elevators
   d. Abdominals [ ]
3. Method by which majority of respiratory volumes and capacity can be measured is:
   a. Phonogram
   b. Resuscitator
   c. Spirometer
   d. Under water breathing apparatus [ ]
4. Residual volume is important because it:
   a. Makes room for artificial respiration
   b. Stimulates respiration centre
   c. Provides air in alveoli to aerate blood even in between breaths
   d. Improves Hering-Breuer reflex [ ]
5. Tubercle bacilli sometimes are detected in stomach washing with the fact that they are absent from sputum; because:
   a. Bacilli of tuberculosis find favourable circumstances in stomach
   b. Mucous coated epithelium cilia are beating towards pharynx; and onwards
   c. Stomach provides a much more dimensional room for bacterias
   d. Enzyme pepsin of gastric juice is favourable for them [ ]
6. The diffusion capacity for oxygen in normal young adult is:
   a. - 10 ml per minute
   b. 100 ml per minute
   c. 21 ml per minute
   d. 50 ml per minute [ ]
7. Total amount of oxygen transported to tissues per minute amounts to be:
   a. 100 ml
   b. 5 ml
   c. 250 ml
   d. 400 ml [ ]
8. Number of molecules of a gas in a mixture when strike a unit surface area in a given time is known as:
   a. Respiratory quotient
   b. Diffusion coefficient
   c. Partial pressure
   d. Utilisation coefficient [ ]
9. Cyanosis is very common in polycythaemia because:
   a. Less availability of haemoglobin
   b. Skin becomes sensitive for blue colouration
   c. Antigen antibody of haemoglobin
   d. More availability of haemoglobin [ ]
10. The substance mainly responsible for blue colouration in cyanosis is:
    a. Sulfhaemoglobin
    b. Bilirubin
    c. Methoemoglobin
    d. De-oxygenated haemoglobin [ ]

11. Ratio between respiration and arterial pulse in health is:
    a. 10 : 20
    b. 1 : 4
    c. 1 : 1
    d. 0 : 3 [ ]

---

1 a 2 d 3 c 4 c 5 b 6 c 7 c 8 c 9 d 10 d 11 b

VIVA VOCE : RESPIRATION

1. Name the structures involved in upper and lower respiratory tract as well as lung unit ?
   a. Upper respiratory tract
      i. Nose
      ii. Nasopharynx
      iii. Oropharynx
      iv. Larynx, up to vocal cords
   b. Lower respiratory tract
      i. Larynx below vocal cords
      ii. Trachea
      iii. Two bronchi
      iv. Bronchioles
      v. Terminal bronchioles
   c. Lung unit
      i. Respiratory bronchioles
      ii. Alveolar ducts
      iii. Atria
      iv. Air sacs
2. Enumerate muscles concerned with inspiration act ?
   i. Diaphragm
   ii. External intercostal
   iii. Sternomastoid
   iv. Serratus anterior
   v. Errector muscles of spine
   vi. Scapular elevators
   vii. Scaleni
3. Enumerate muscles concerned with expiration ?
   i. Abdominal muscles
   ii. Internal intercostal
   iii. Serratus posterior inferior
   iv. Transverse thoracic
   v. Subcostalis
4. How much is normal respiratory rate?
   It is varying between 10–18 per minute (average 12). Its ratio with pulse is 1 : 4. In pneumonia it alters to 1 : 1 while it may change to 1 : 6 in narcotic poisoning.
5. Mention the different 'lung volumes' ?
   i. Tidal volume : In normal young adult it amounts to be 450 to 500 ml. It is a volume of air inspired in or expired out with each normal breath at resting state of subject.
   ii. Inspiratory reserve volume : It is an extra volume of air which can be inspired over and beyond normal tidal volume. It amounts to be 3000 ml in young healthy adult (2000–3200 ml).
   iii. Expiratory reserve volume : It is the amount of air that can be expired by forceful expiration after tidal expiration. In normal healthy adult it is 1100 ml (750–1000 ml).
   iv. Residual volume : Normally it amounts to be 1200 ml. It is the volume of air remaining in lungs after most forceful expiration.
   v. Minute respiratory volume
      Tidal volume × Respiratory rate
      500 × 12 = 6000 ml. or 6 litres per minute
      'It is the total amount of new air moved into respiratory passage each minute'.
6. What is the significance of residual volume ?
   It provides air in alveoli to aerate blood between breaths. In its absence there are bright chances of alternation in gaseous composition during each respiration.
7. Describe various 'lung capacities' ?
   i. Inspiratory capacity
      Tidal volume + Inspiratory reserve volume
      500 ml + 3000 ml = 3500 ml
      'It is amount of air that a person can breath beginning at normal expiratory level distending his lungs to maximum amount.'
   ii. Functional residual capacity
      Expiratory reserve volume + residual volume
      1100 + 1200 = 2300 ml.
      'So it is volume of air remaining in lungs at the end of normal expiration'.
   iii. Vital capacity
      Tidal volume + inspiratory reserve volume + expiratory reserve volume
      500 + 3000 + 1100 = 4600 ml.
      It is hence maximum amount of air that a person can expire after first filling his lungs to their maximum extent and then expiring to maximum extent. In females it is 3.1 litres normally.
   iv. Total lung capacity : Normally it amounts to be 5800 ml. It is maximum volume to which lungs can be expanded with greatest possible inspiratory effort.
   v. Maximum breathing capacity : it amounts to be 150–170 litres per minute (range 82–169 litres/minute) for about 15 second.

8. What is timed vital capacity ?
   Here, vital capacity is timed which means, percentage of vital capacity expired in one, two and third second is determined. It is denoted by FEV_1, FEV_2, FEV_3 forced expiratory volume of first second.
   (FEV_1) normally is 83 to 84 per cent, in second second (FEV_2) it is about 93 per cent while in third second (FEV_3) it is 97 per cent. Obstructive disease of lungs are expected when FEV_1 is less than 70 per cent.
9. Enumerate volumes or capacity which cannot be measured by spirometer ?
   Residual volume, functional residual capacity, and total lung capacity.
10. Mention the factors affecting vital capacity ?
    i. Posture : Less in lying down position.
    ii. Sex : Comparatively less in female
    iii. Surface area : It is proportional to body surface area.
    iv. Disease : It is decreased in diseases like disorders decreasing compliance, paralysis of respiratory muscles, pulmonary congestion, diaphragmatic diseases etc.
11. What is the function of nose ?
    i. Air is warmed
    ii. Air is moistened
    iii. Air is filtered
12. How inspiration and expiration acts are brought about ?
    i. During inspiration thoracic cage is expanded so fall in intrapleural pressure occurs, volume of lung enlarges with fall in pressure of alveoli. Air rushes into alveoli because a pressure gradient is established between atmosphere and alveolar air.
    ii. On expiration thoracic cage becomes smaller, rise occurs in intrapleural pressure, lungs recoil pressing alveoli causing them to shrink. Air expelled out because reverse pressure gradient is established.
13. What is Halden effect ?
    It suggests that increase in Po_2 is tending to displace CO_2 from blood. Following explanations have been put forwarded.
    i. When oxygen combines with haemoglobin, it is formed a more stronger acid which decreases its affinity for CO_2 to form carbamino haemoglobin.
    ii. When acidity of haemoglobin is increased it tends to increase the acidity of body fluids which convert bicarbonate ions into carbonic acid which releases CO_2 on dissociation.
14. What is meant by Bohr's effect ?
    It is opposite of above mentioned Haldane effect. It means that carbon dioxide causes oxygen to dissociate from haemoglobin. It is of academic interest only. When Pco_2 rises, blood pH is decreased leading to enhanced union between CO_2 and haemoglobin and less affinity for oxygen.
15. What is breath holding ?
    Inhibition of respiration voluntarily is known as breath holding. At some point it cannot longer be inhibited called 'breaking point'. Which may be due to
    i. rise in arterial Pco_2 and fall in Po_2
    ii. psychic factors.
16. What is oxygen toxicity ?
    i. On 8 hours or more administration of pure oxygen, symptoms are manifested like respiratory irritation, substernal distress, nasal congestion, coughing, sore throat. If administered for 20–48 hours it can lead to lung damage also.
    ii. The cause of O_2 toxicity are:
    a. Production of super oxide ion (O_2) and H_2O_2,
    b. Inhibition of ability of lung macrophages to kill bacteria,
    c. Reduction in production of surfactant.

UNIT 5

Out Go

It is better to consider kidney as a part of cardiovascular renal unit, disturbance of which results into cardiovascular renal diseases. The heart, arteries and kidney form one physiological whole.

Excretion

27 Homeostasis: Regulation of Water Balance

The more aware the student is of physiology of water and electrolyte distribution, the more appropriate and successful will be his therapy when he becomes a physician.

EXTRACELLULAR COMPARTMENT

This contains a heterogeneous collection of fluids and is not a continuous fluid phase.

It is composed of following subcompartments.

Transcellular water (2.5%)—It means the extracellular fluid separated from other extracellular fluid by an epithelial membrane; viz. CSF, joint or synovial fluid, intraocular fluid, fluids of pleural—pericardial—peritoneal cavity, fluids within the ducts of digestive glands, mucous membrane of GIT/nasorespiratory tract and intraluminal fluid of GIT.

From this fluid, the cells take up O_2 and nutrients into it, they discharge metabolic waste products. This is divided into two components—the interstitial fluid and the circulating plasma. Interstitial fluid is that part of extracellular fluid which is outside the vascular system, bathing the cells. Total body water consists of 2/3 intracellular fluid and remaining extracellular fluid.

INTRACELLULAR FLUID

This makes up 40 to 55 per cent of body weight, the bulk being contained in the muscle.

The supreme difference between the two great reservoirs of body water intra- and extracellular, is in potassium and sodium, both alkaline cations in identical concentration, only separated by the cell membrane. A simple but striking example of this statement is provided by the blood, where erythrocytes are rich in potassium, the plasma rich in sodium and this perfect balance is getting disturbed by massive haemorrhage.

It contains very low concentration of Na^+, Cl^- and HCO_3^-; of course predominant cation is K^+; while predominant anion is organic phosphate and proteins. The main causes responsible for it are :

- Na^+/K^+ ATPase in cell membrane actively transports Na^+ from and K^+ into cells
- The cell membrane separating intracellular fluid from interstitial fluid is provided with a limited permeability to organic phosphates and proteins, which establishes Gibbs—Donnan—equilibrium across the cell membrane.

Table 27.1: Different fluids

i. ICF = TBW - ECF
   or
   Interstitial fluid = ECF—Plasma

ii. Plasma volume = Blood volume (1 - Hct)
   ICF = Intracellular fluid; TBW = Total body water, ECF = Extracellular fluid
   Hct = Hematocrit

Table 27.2: Differences

	Intracellular fluid	*Interstitial fluid*
1.	Concentration of Na^+, K^+ is greater (diffusible cation)	Concentration of Cl^- is greater (small diffusible anions)
2.	Total concentration of equivalents of charge is greater	It is comparatively less.
3.	Electrical neutrality is maintained in	Each compartment

When extra fluid accumulates in extracellular spaces, (due to much intake and decreased kidney output) then almost 1/6th 1/3rd of it increases blood volume; while remainder is accumulated in interstitial spaces. If this accumulation is continued (almost 50%) then the extra fluid directly goes to interstitial spaces since its pressure rises. This leads to oedema (i.e. swelling of loose tissue). The interstitial spaces become an overflow reservoir for excess fluid.

Table 27.3: Water + three major ions: in GIT

Juice	*Vol./day (ml.)*	*Sodium mEq/day*	*Potassium mEq/day*	*Chloride mEq/day*
Saliva	1500	15	40	15
Gastric	2500	150	25	310
Bile	500	75	3	50
Pancreatic	700	100	4	50
Succuus entericus	3000	320	15	300
Total	8200	660	87	725

ECF VOLUME—REGULATION

- Amount of Na+ in ECF is most important determinant of volume of extracellular fluid, and next to it is Cl^-.
  - * Rise in ECF volume → Inhibits vasopressin secretion.
  - * Fall in ECF volume → Increased secretion of vasopressin.
  - * Osmotic regulation of ADH also exists.
  - * Angiotensin II stimulates aldosterone and vasopressin secretion. It causes constriction of blood vessels which maintain blood pressure.
- ECF volume decrease → blood pressure falls → fall in glomerular capillary pressure → GFR falls → amount of Na^+ filtered decrease → tubular reabsorption of Na^+ increased.
- Rising from supine to standing position increases aldosterone secretion.

Control of Extracellular Fluid Volume

- The fluid first goes into the blood, but it rapidly becomes distributed between interstitial spaces and the plasma. So without controlling extracellular fluid volume, blood volume cannot be controlled.
- When an extra amount of fluid accumulates in extra cellular fluid spaces (because of reasons like intake of too much fluid; or; decreased kidney output); then one-sixth to one-third of this extra fluid normally remains in blood while remainder gets distributed to interstitial spaces. If it rises more than this (50% above normal) then very little remains in blood and majority enters interstitial spaces. This makes them overflow (because pressure within them rises; from negative to positive) causing oedema.

INTERSTITIAL FLUID

This member of extracellular pair comprises the real internal environment. Including the lymph it constitutes 15 per cent of weight and measures 11 litres in a man weighing 150 pounds. Its volume and solutes contained by it are regulated by kidneys, lungs and endocrine glands and are influenced by the sweat glands and GIT. These regulators are connected with the interstitial fluid by the blood stream, the plasma being in equilibrium with the fluid in the interstitial compartment.

Table 27.4: Concentration of anion-cation in different compartments in mEq/L

Cation/Anion	*Plasma*	*ECF*	*ICF*
Sodium	142	145	10
Potassium	4	4	160
Calcium	5	2	2
Magnesium	5	2	26
Total	153		
Chloride	101	114	3
Bicarbonate	27	31	10
Phosphate	2	2	100
Sulphate	1	1	20
Organic acids	6	7	
Proteins	16	0.8	64
Total	153		

Plasma and interstitial fluid has similar composition, with Na^+ as the predominant cation and Cl^- and HCO_3^- as predominant anions. Of course plasma contains larger concentration of proteins (a point of difference).

INTRAVASCULAR FLUID

This compartment contains plasma and blood cells. The plasma constitutes 3 litres of fluid (5% of body weight). The plasma together with the cells determine the blood volume which amounts to be 5 litres in a man of average size.

Blood volume decreased ..... haemorrhage, dilatation of vascular bed which may result into shock.

Blood volume increased .... CHF, Polycythaemia

THE ELECTROLYTES

i. These are those substances which, when placed in water, conduct an electric current and become dissociated into electrically charged particles called *Ions* (Greek = to pass or go). These may be positively charged cations (Na^+, K^+, Ca^{++}, Mg^{++} etc.; they collect at negative or cathod pole) or negatively charged anions (Cl^-, HCO_3^-, PO_4^- etc.) and they pass to positive or anode pole.

ii. • The chief functions of electrolytes may be enumerated as—maintenance of proper osmolality and volume of body fluids -
- Maintenance of proper acid base equilibrium
- Specific effects, e.g. effect of Ca^{2+} on neuromuscular excitability.

iii. The total amount of electrolytes may determine the amount of body fluid and its osmotic tension. The chief electrolytes are Na^+, K^+, Cl^- and HCO_3^-. The total electrolyte concentration is essentially the same in all three phases of body fluids, but the relative amount of different electrolytes vary widely. Thus higher levels in plasma, tissue fluid and cell fluid for sodium in mEq/L. are 150, 150 and 5 whereas those for K^+ are 5, 5 and 110. In extracellular fluid (plasma + interstitial fluid) the important ions are Na^+, Cl^- and HCO_3^- and protein and out of these Na^+ is main cation, and $Cl^- + HCO_3^-$ are chief anions. In intracellular fluid potassium is the great cation and organic phosphate the corresponding anion. Changes in total electrolyte concentration is usually more important than changes in relative concentration of different electrolytes.

a. ***Sodium:*** It is of paramount importance in extracellular fluid. Its deficiency may be developing as a result of :
- Direct loss from body prolonged vomiting, diarrhoea. The most serious effects are seen in infants whose kidneys are less able to reabsorb sodium and when both sodium and water are lost but only water is replaced then salt depletion may be quite severe.
- Loss of power to retain salt it may be due to deficiency of hormone aldosterone, renal disease, Addison's disease. In water depletion there is a loss of intracellular fluid but in salt depletion there is an excess of this fluid. This is because water passes into the cells in order to lower their osmotic pressure to that of the extracellular fluid. Therefore, the patient is not thirsty. The net result of the combined loss of water into the cells and from the kidney is a reduction in the volume of extracellular fluid including the vascular compartment which may result into shock and circulatory collapse (untreated Addison's disease).

Sodium Retention: It is the chief component of the extracellular fluid on the basic side. Its concentration is regulated by its reabsorption from the glomerular filtrate as it passes along the renal tubules. If this reabsorption is increased (under the effect of aldosterone) the volume of extracellular fluid will increase which means 'oedema' in the interstitial compartment. It so happens in acute renal diseases, congestive heart failure, nephrotic syndrome, nutritional oedema, liver cirrhosis with ascites.

Sodium: Input... Actually daily input of Na^+ vary depending upon individual's dietary habits. Of course average diet of an adult American contains 100–400 m mol Na^+ per day.

Sodium: Output... Sweat, faeces and urine are the channels through which sodium is lost. On an average 100–400 m mol per day sodium is lost in urine. Under normal circumstances, faecal loss of sodium is negligible; but it increases in conditions like diarrhoea.

Sodium Excretion: At a Glance
- The average intake of sodium/day is 150 mEq. Glomerular filtrate contains 26,000 mEq./day.
- Approximately 65 per cent of it is reabsorbed by proximal tubule through active transport mechanism by its epithelial cells. It also attracts Cl^- (co-transport/passive diffusion).
- 27 per cent of it (approximately) is reabsorbed by thick ascending limb of loop of Henle. Only 8 per cent of it enters distal tubule. Here this portion is almost impermeable to water, so concentration of sodium ions falls before it enters the distal tubule; while proximal tubule is quite permeable to water. So any way its concentration falls to 30–40 mEq/L from normal 140 mEq/l.
- So these two parts (proximal + loop ascending thick) are capable of returning most of sodium to glomerular filtrate back to plasma and in this way it's consumed.
- In late distal tubules and cortical collecting, the rate of its absorption is controlled mainly by concentration of aldosterone in blood - from adrenal cortex. ADH-thirst system greatly overshadows the aldosterone system for sodium concentration control under normal condition.

b. ***Potassium:*** It is again of great importance. It is the chief basic ion of the body cells. It has been said that, "A normal adult has enough potassium in his body to kill 100 people, if it were injected into their blood, yet if he gets no potassium in his diet he would soon be paralysed and die." Again if as little as 6 per cent of cellular potassium could escape rapidly into the extracellular fluid, death would quickly follow. The kidney seems to be designed to retain sodium by tubular reabsorption and to excrete potassium and the entire process is under the control of hormone aldosterone.

Potassium Depletion is Much More Common

Causes: stress (postoperative etc.), primary aldosteronism, vomiting and diarrhoea, familial periodic paralysis, iatrogenic deficiency.

Symptoms: As the bulk of potassium is within muscle cells it is the muscle, which suffer most. Lack of muscular tone, flabbiness, weakness and finally paralysis which is attributed to blocking of nerve impulses to the muscles. Intestinal atony with abdominal distension in the post-operative patient is due to potassium depletion. Myocardial failure with cardiac dilatation are amongst serious consequences of hypokalaemia.

Potassium Retention (Hyperkalaemia): Is much less common. The major cause is inadequate excretion of potassium by the kidneys. The main symptom is again muscular weakness but heart suffers more in the form of bradycardia due to interference with the conducting system. Since K^+ and Ca^{2+} are antagonistic, so excess K^{++} leads to falling contraction of muscles.

Potassium: Input: This depends on food and water consumed by an individual. Its input may be limited by starvation or diseases. 50–100 m mol of K^+ per day is existing in diet of average adult American.

Potassium: Output: Its loss in faeces averages 5 – 10 m mol/day but may exceed in conditions like diarrhoea. It is mainly excreted in urine (49–90 m mol/day in American adult). Its loss in sweat is not significant.

Potassium Excretion: At A Glance

- Its amount entering glomerular filtrate is 800 mEq; while its daily intake is 100 mEq. So to keep balance, 1/8th of total tubular load of potassium must be excreted.
- In proximal tubules (through active transport) 65 per cent of K^+ reabsorbed; another 27 per cent in ascending loop of Henle, leaving about 8 per cent of original filtered K^+ to enter the distal tubules (potassium co-transport with sodium).
- Potassium is also secreted by principal cells in late distal tubule, cortical collecting ducts, and it is poured into tubular lumen. This secretion occurs only when extracellular fluid potassium concentration is higher than a critical value. When a person is on an extremely low intake of potassium, tubular secretion of K^+ is necessary to prevent death.
- Even a slight increase in extracellular potassium concentration will lead to a significant increase in potassium excretion into the urine.
- Potassium ion secretion is also controlled by hormone aldosterone as already described.

READ AND DIGEST: POTASSIUM REGULATION

1. What about potassium distribution?

Ans. a. For a 70 kg adult, who is having 28 litres of intracellular fluid (40% of body weight), and 14 litres of extracellular fluid (20% of body weight); there is 3920 mEq. of potassium are inside the cell and 59 mEq are in extracellular fluid (4.2 mEq/L × 14 L = 59 mEq; In ICF = 140 mEq/L × 28 L = 3920 mEq).

b. Its daily intake ranges between 50–200 mEq (average 100 mEq/day).

2. How much of it is filtered per day?

Ans. GFR × plasma potassium (i.e. 180 litres/day × 4.2 mEq). = 756 mEq/day or 800 mEq/day.

3. Something about its balance?

Ans. a. With its normal intake of 100 mEq daily, kidney must excrete 92 mEq daily, and remaining 8 mEq is excreted in faeces.

b. When its intake is high; then it should be excreted more. This target is achieved by increasing the secretion of potassium into distal and collecting tubules.

c. When its intake is below normal, its secretion at these sites is reduced. So its balance is regulated at the level of distal, cortical collecting tubules.

4. What is role of Principal cells?

Ans. a. They constitute 90 per cent of epithelial cells in distal and cortical collecting tubule, and of course, secrete potassium.

b. In first step, the Na^+K^+ ATP'ase pump located at basolateral membrane, drives one molecule of Na^+ into interstitium and at the same time, potassium (one molecule) to the interior of the cell.

c. In next step, there occurs passive diffusion of it, from interior of cell to tubular fluid. The high intracellular concentration of potassium created by this Na^+K^+ ATPase pump is the main driving force here.

d. The principal cells are highly permeable to potassium and the special channel present here make them highly permeable.

5. How its secretion by principal cells is controlled?

Ans. a. Activity of Na^+K^+ ATPase pump;

b. The electrochemical gradient for its secretion into tubular lumen from blood,

c. Permeability of luminal membrane for potassium.

6. Then, what is the role of intercalated cells?

Ans. In circumstances where potassium level is deficient (depletion) then through these cells, it is reabsorbed at late distal and collecting tubules through H^+K^+

ATPase transport mechanism located at luminal membrane. This potassium re-absorption is associated with secretion of one molecule of hydrogen which is secreted into lumen.

7. **Increased extracellular fluid potassium concentration stimulates potassium secretion. How?**

Ans. • Increased potassium in ECF → stimulation of Na^+K^+ ATPase pump → increased uptake of potassium by basolateral membrane → increased concentration of potassium ion intracellularly → more diffuse towards lumen.
- Increased potassium concentration → aldosterone secretion stimulation → stimulated potassium secretion.
- Increased extracellular potassium → increases potassium gradient from interstitial fluid to interior of cell → back leakage of these is prevented.

8. **Acidosis is having dual effect. How?**

Ans. • Acute acidosis → reduced activity of Na^+K^+ ATPase pump → decreased intracellular potassium concentration + passive diffusion of potassium across luminal membrane → reduced secretion of potassium.
- Prolonged acidosis → inhibition of Na^+, Cl^-, H_2O reabsorption by proximal tubules → more delivery of these substances at distal tubule level → potassium secretion stimulated by just over-riding the inhibition of Na^+K^+ ATPase pump.

9. **Increased distal tubular flow rate stimulate potassium secretion. How?**

Ans. High sodium intake (or diuretic) → decreased aldosterone secretion → decreased rate of potassium secretion reduced excretion of potassium in urine.

AND ALSO COUNTER EFFECT

High sodium intake → increased fluid delivery to cortical collecting duct → increased potassium secretion.

So because of this counter balance, there is little change in potassium excretion.

10. **What happens if aldosterone is blocked?**

Ans. This so happens in Addison's disease. Extracellular concentration of potassium becomes high due to impaired renal secretion of potassium, which leads to fatal results. Conversely, excess aldosterone (hyperaldosteronism) its secretion is greatly increased → more loss by kidney → hypokalaemia.

Calcium ion: Regulation

- Its day to day concentration remains within a few percentage of 2.4 mEq/L and is controlled by effect of parathyroid hormone on bone reabsorption; like
  - — Calcium concentration in blood falls → increased secretion of parathyroid hormone → increased reabsorption of bone salts → releasing large amount of calcium salts in extracellular fluid → elevating blood calcium level to normal.
  - — Calcium concentration in blood high → depressed production of parathyroid hormone → almost no bone reabsorption → reducing blood calcium level.
- Even in absence of parathormone it is reabsorbed in major amount by proximal tubule, loop of Henle, diluting segment of distal tubule; but least amount is also reabsorbed by late distal tubule.
- So in long-term regulation of this ion; the parathormone increases its reabsorption by kidney when its concentration is low in blood. In early kidney tubules calcium reabsorption is secondary to sodium transport (secondary active transport or passive reabsorption down an electro-chemical gradient).

Magnesium ion: Regulation

- These are absorbed by all parts of renal tubules.
- It is controlled by negative feed mechanism, i.e.
  - — When more Mg^{++} in extracellular fluid → more excretion
  - — When less Mg^{++} in extracellular fluid → more conservation

Phosphate ion : Regulation

- Its transport maximum (Tm) is 0.1 mmol./minute when load is less than this, all is absorbed, when more than this amount is present in glomerular filtrate then the excess is excreted. This is overflow mechanism. Its threshold value is 0.8 m mol/minute which gives Tm of 0.1 m mol/mt (tubular load).
- Role of parathormone:- When its concentration is less, then
  - — It encourages bone reabsorption so large amount of phosphate ions are poured into extracellular fluid.
  - — It decreases Tm for phosphate so its larger amount is excreted when its concentration is high.

Urea Excretion

- Its normal concentration is 25 to 40 mg per cent in blood. Each day 25 to 30 gm. urea is formed which requires to be excreted otherwise it will accumulate.
- Factors determining its rate of excretion are:- urea concentration in plasma and GFR.
- In kidney diseases → GFR reduced → decreased excretion of urea. But body continues to form it to increase its blood level; until blood level becomes very high → excretion of urea because.

  Urea filtered in glomerular filtrate = plasma urea concentration X GFR

- Because of its reabsorption in medullary portion into medullary interstitium, urea concentration is increased many folds. Its little amount absorbed into thin limb of loop so it passes upwards through distal tubule, through cortical collecting duct and back down through collecting duct again. So it recirculates many times before excretion which is necessary for economy of body fluids in persons who live in water deficient area.

INTERSTITIUM: INTERSTITIAL FLUID

1. Spaces between the cells called interstitium and fluid contained here is called interstitial fluid.
2. Structurally, it is composed of
   — Collagen fibre bundle—extend along long distances in interstitium and provide tension strength to the tissues.
   — Proteoglycan filaments—thin and coiled molecules composed of hyaluronic acid + protein. They form a mat of fine reticular filaments.
3. Interstitial fluid is having the same composition as plasma except for much lower concentration of proteins since proteins are not easily coming out of capillaries. Tissue gel is the name given to that fluid which is entrapped within proteoglycan filaments and it resembles gel in constituency. So the fluid moves molecules by molecules through gel from one place to another by kinetic motion.

Besides this, free fluid vesicles are also present, i.e. fluid free from proteoglycan and so it moves freely. Its amount is less than 1 per cent; of course, during oedema this amount is increased.

WATER BALANCE

i. When intake exceeds output of water it is called positive water balance; when subject loses more water than his intake it is negative water balance.

ii. Positive water balance occurs in infancy (growth period), recovery from a disease (convalescene), pregnancy, change from high fat to high protein diet etc. Negative water balance occurs in vomiting, diarrhoea, postoperative states, burns, haemorrhage, diabetes mellitus, diabetes insipidus, active intake of food is limited, unconsciousness, etc. For a healthy adult 1 ml./cal. of diet is sufficient. The total amount of intake for an adult amounts to be 2500 ml.

iii. The routes of water intake includes free drinks (water, soft drinks, beer, coffee, mineral water and it amounts to be 1,200 ml), semi solid or liquid (dal, milk, meat soup, and it amounts to be 1000 ml), and metabolic water.

The channels of water output includes urine, faeces, expired air, skin etc.

iv. The total amount of water in a man of average weight of 70 kg is 40 litres (approximately), i.e. 57 per cent of his total body weight. Obesity decreases the percentage of water in the body.

v. By choosing the appropriate marker substance, the fluid volume of almost any compartment of body can be measured using dilution principle.

Functions of Water

- It can form true solutions as well as colloidal solution. Water insoluble substances are made water soluble by hydrotropic action. So it is more suitable solvent.
- It is a good ionising medium. Opposite charged particles can coexist in water.
- All chemical reactions in the body proceed in presence of water only.
- Water has the highest latent heat of evaporation than any other liquid.
- Water acts as a lubricant in the body to prevent friction in joints, pleura, peritoneum and conjunctiva.
- If plasma proteins are decreased, water will flow into the tissues. More water is said to flow into the tissues if capillary pressure is increased.
- Excessive ingestion of water → lowering of osmotic pressure of plasma proteins → Increase capillary pressure.
- It is a good refractive medium (aquous humour)
- It acts as a great mechanical buffer (CSF)
- It is a medium for various biophysical processes like diffusion, filtration, etc.
- So it is an essential constituent of all cells.

Water Balance : Regulation

- The body fluids in three great compartments are not only free to move, but they do move ceaselessly and in great volume like the currents of ocean. The main factors responsible are:
  i. Hydrostatic pressure within the vessel, and
  ii. Osmotic pressure of electrolytes and proteins.
- The hydrostatic pressure drives fluid out of capillaries, while the osmotic pressure of plasma protein pulls it back. The resultant of these forces determines the end result. At the arterial end of the capillary the hydrostatic pressure exceeds the osmotic pressure of plasma protein, so that water and electrolytes pass from the vascular to the interstitial compartment. At the venous end of capillary the conditions are reversed and so also flow is reversed. Changes in electrolytes, by altering the osmotic

pressure, lead to a shift of water from intra cellular to extracellular compartment.

- Although the cell membranes and the capillary walls are both entirely permeable to water, they differ greatly in their permeability to electrolytes, the wall of the capillary being completely permeable, while the membrane of the cell is relatively impermeable. The result is that the composition of intra- and extracellular fluids differ profoundly from one another. Most of the Na^+ and Cl^- of the body (Nacl) are in extracellular fluid (internal environment), while most of the Potassium—Magnesium—and phosphate are in intracellular fluid. When osmotic pressure in extra cellular compartment is altered by a change either in its electrolyte or its water content, the osmotic equilibrium which is so essential to health is maintained by the passage of water from or into the intracellular compartment. Such a shift of water will of course change the volume of two compartments. As the capillary wall presents no barrier to the passage of inorganic ions, it follows that two divisions of extra cellular water are practically identical in inorganic content, the only chemical difference being the high protein content of the plasma.

Table 27.5: Water metabolism

Supply		*Loss*	
1. Drink	1,450 ml	1. Kidney	1,500 ml
2. Solid foods ...	800 ml	2. Skin ...	600 ml
3. Oxidation ...	350 ml	3. Lungs	400 ml
		4. Faeces	100 ml
Total	2,600 ml		2,600 ml

100 gm of fat gives .... 107 gm water

100 gm of starch gives ... 55 gm water

100 gm of alcohol gives .... 117 gm water

100 gm of protein gives ... 41 gm water

Table 27.6: Water content of various tissues

Skin ... 20%, muscle .... 75-80%; Heart 79%
Plasma ... 92%, Blood ... 76%, Lung..... 79%
Connective tissue ... 60%, Corpuscles 60% Brain ... 75%
Bones ... 25%, CSF 99% Liver ... 68%
White matter 70%, adipose tissue 20% Spleen 78%
Dentine 10%, kidney 80%, Pancreas - 73%
GIT 79%
Skeleton 22%; Skeletal muscle ... 76%

Regulation of Water Balance

Though mechanism is not a singular entity, but many factors are involved as follows:

i. *Posterior Pituitary:* Plays an important part by secreting ADH which increases reabsorption of water from distal renal tubule and thus reduces urine volume. Secretion of this hormone is controlled by water content of the body (negative feedback mechanism).

ii. *Adrenal:* Adrenaline hormone → constriction of renal vessels → reduction in renal circulation → decrease in urine volume
Aldosterone is an important hormone from adrenal cortex in maintaining water balance. It leads to water retention and ADH release.

iii. *Thyroid:* Thyroxin → raising BMR → increasing nitrogenous end products which exert diuretic effect → increase in urine volume along with increased elimination of salt. In myxoedema there is increased fluid retention in extracellular tissue.

iv. *Kidney:*
   - Excess water intake leads to more excretion of water. This is through
     Increased blood volume → rise of blood pressure → raised filtration pressure
     Increasing the number of active glomeruli
   - Dilution of plasma proteins → reduced colloid osmotic pressure → increasing filtration pressure.
   - Inhibition of secretion of ADH - reflexly through stimulation of stretch receptors present in left atrial wall.
   - Kidney produces Angiotensin II which regulates water balance through secretion of aldosterone.

v. Water is also excreted through lungs and skin.

vi. *Hypothalamus:*
   - Excess water in body → dilutes blood + reduction in osmotic pressure → depressed hypothalamus → less ADH secretion → diuresis
   - Reduced body water → increased osmotic pressure of blood → stimulation of hypothalamus → more secretion of ADH → reduced urine volume.

Water Excess (Water intoxication)

Kidneys are unable to discard the extra water. This leads to reduction in osmolality of extracellular fluid which causes migration of water into the cells. Hence intracellular fluid expands and become diluted causing deteriorated cellular functions specially of brain which leads to symptoms like convulsions, coma, headache dizziness and which follow death. Low plasma sodium concentration is revealed.

Pure Water Depletion

- Children are more susceptible
- Compensatory mechanism... loss of water from plasma → hyperosmolality of plasma → increased ADH secretion → conservation of body water.
- Symptoms include mental confusion owing to shrinkage of intracellular fluid of brain, highly concentrated urine, blood pressure remains normal due to compensatory mechanisms.

Thirst

i. Any depletion will lead to sensation of thirst and then the subject drinks water to maintain water balance. Slight fall in blood volume or extracellular fluid volume leads to a chain of events called 'thirst.' This is also assisted by diminution in salivary amount and so dried oral cavity which manifest into thirst.

ii. Injection of 850 mEq./L NaCl is capable of producing thirst by increasing the osmotic pressure of extra cellular fluid. This leads to passage of water from intra to extracellular fluid raising osmolarity in intra cellular fluid. This will stimulate thirst centre and therefore urge for water intake occurs. Salt depletion also produces thirst (vomiting, diarrhoea, etc.) through renin-angiotensin mechanism which results in intake of water. Potassium low level and high calcium level in blood plasma also stimulates thirst centre.

iii. Shortage of water causes more immediate and more intolerable distress than shortage of food. A person completely deprived of water soon feels his mouth dry and craving for fluid, saliva decreases in amount and swallowing of food becomes impossible. Finally delirium is followed by death within a day or two in a dry climate or little longer in moist one. The thirst sensation is to be regarded as the expression of a general bodily need for water.

iv. Thirst centres .. They are :
   - Area along the antero-ventral wall of third ventricle which promotes release of ADH.
   - Stimulation of area located antero-laterally in pre-optic nucleus produces thirst.
   - These neurones function as osmo-receptors.

v. Thirst stimulation

vi. Due to sensation of thirst, one drinks water which requires at least 30 minutes to one hour to be absorbed. During this period one gets temporary relief from thirst. On entry into stomach; this part along with upper GIT gets distended which provides this temporary relief.

Table 27.7: Factors affecting thirst

Increasing	*Decreasing*
Decreased blood volume	Increased blood volume
Decreased blood pressure	Increased blood pressure
Increased osmolality	Decreased osmolality
Increased angiotensin II	Decreased angiotensin II

READ AND DIGEST: THIRST

1. What is thirst?

Ans. It is conscious desire for water.

2. What are its causes?

Ans. a. Extracellular dehydration - means extracellular fluid volume is reduced. If low salt intake → fall in osmolar concentration of extracellular fluid → volume of extra cellular fluid decrease → balance will be maintained by taking salt and water, not water alone.

b. When haemorrhage is so severe to reduce the cardiac output, then thirst is felt.

c. dryness of mouth.

d. intracellular dehydration.

3. What is the basic stimulus for exciting the thirst centre?

Ans. Intracellular dehydration.

4. What is the possible mechanism?

Ans. a. Extracellular dehydration promote loss of fluid from inside cells; which in turn causes sufficient dehydration of neurones in thirst centre to promote thirst sensation;

b. In circulatory failure, inadequate supply of nutrients to the cells depresses active transport mechanism which maintain intracellular electrolyte composition, and if this channel is lost, intracellular dehydration may ensure.

DEHYDRATION

- There is a decrease in water content of the body, i.e. negative water balance.
- It may be due to little intake (dysphagia, mental weakness, desert travel, etc.), or excessive loss (vomiting, diarrhoea, sweat, diuresis, etc.)
- It leads to disturbed acid-base balance, rise in NPN of blood, increased pulse rate and cardiac output, dry and wrinkled loose skin, rise in body temperature due to reduction in circulating fluid, loss of weight due to reduction of tissue water, exhaustion and collapse.

It can be corrected by parenteral administration of NaCl. A mixture of two-third isotonic saline solution and one-third sodium lactate I.V. is also given in the cases of removal of fluid high in Na and HCO_3. Of course, dehydration is a problem in diabetes mellitus, Addison's disease, uraemia, burns and shock.

- When a person is dehydrated → extracellular fluid volume is decreased → concentration of sodium and other osmolar elements rise → stimulation of thirst centres (drinking threshold) → person drinks water and extracellular fluid volume comes to normal, i.e. satiety (tripping mechanism).

OEDEMA

a. It is an abnormal accumulation of fluid in the tissue spaces and serous cavities. When water collects in the tissue, it may be in free or combined form. When combined it is united with the protoplasm of the tissue elements. When free it lies between these elements and can be moved from one place to another. For this reason, a pit is left (between these elements) when oedematous part is pressed one which is called pitting oedema, and, when no such pitting on pressure exist it is classed as solid-oedema. It is only when 5 or 6 litres have collected in water depots; then oedema becomes evident.

b. **Causes:** *There are four main causes*
   i. Increased permeability of capillary walls
   ii. Decreased colloid osmotic pressure of plasma proteins
   iii. Increased blood hydrostatic pressure
   iv. Lymphatic obstruction

Secondary factors: There exists two such secondary factors–firstly, osmotic pressure in tissues and second is chloride retention due to renal insufficiency.

c. ***Cause-wise description:-***
   1. ***Cardiac oedema*:** The main cause is congestive heart failure (CHF). There occurs increase in extracellular fluid + salt retention. Therefore, it is treated by diuretics which improve the output of urine and by improving cardiac actions by agents like digitalis, etc.
   2. ***Renal diseases producing oedema*:** It is striking feature in Nephrotic syndrome, of course it is not so pronounced in glomerulo-nephritis. As loss of protein in urine there occurs reduction in plasma protein. This loss of protein in urine leads to passage of an abnormally large volume of fluid from capillaries. This is responsible for renal retention of salt + water.
   3. ***Inflammatory oedema*:** Many factors like slowing of blood stream/dilatation of vessel/thrombosis or obstruction in veins—leads to increased capillary pressure. This leads to increased filtering surface. The capillary walls are also seriously damaged by the bacterial toxin, or other injurious agents. This leads to escape of fluid of high protein content from the vessel. The oedema is localised to an area of varying extent surrounding the injured part.
   4. ***Heat eodema*:** It occurs in tropics. Heat leads to oedema. The factors stimulating include-enlargement of filtering surface because of opening of new capillaries, rise in capillary pressure, dilatation of previously patent capillaries, etc.
   5. ***Lymphatic obstruction oedema*:** Is readily produced in frogs. It is seen in infection with filarial parasite which resides in limb lymph vessels and block their lumen and thus giving birth to so called "elephantiasis." As a result of lymphatic obstruction accumulation of fluid may occur in pleural cavity. The milk leg of puerperium is in part due to lymphatic obstruction.
   6. ***Malnutrition/toxic oedema*:** On a diet deficient in protein/fat/vitamin the oedema may occur. The cause is marked lowering of plasma proteins—(more common—albumin). Many times amino acid deficiency is the cause rather than protein deficiency. Increased capillary permeability due to impaired nutrition of the vascular wall is the main cause. Certain chemicals act as capillary poisons and cause oedema. They include—arsenic, salts of heavy metals, acute nephritis, diphtheria, etc.
   7. ***Mechanical venous obstruction:*** *A cause of oedema*: Obstructions like new growth fibrous tissue, thrombosis, cirrhosis, etc. may increase the capillary pressure as well as its permeability and amount of filtering surface which can cause oedema.

SUMMARY AND HIGHLIGHTS

Water is by far, the most abundant component of the body. The total body water (TBW) is about 60 per cent of body weight in normal young adult male and 50 per cent of body weight in normal young adult female, who have larger amount of subcutaneous fat. The percentage of body weight, i.e. water will vary inversely with the body's fat content. TBW is distributed in two fluid compartments viz. ICF (55% TBW) and ECF (45% of TBW). The ECF is further distributed as:

Plasma (7.5% of TBW); interstitial fluid (20% TBW), which includes fluid in between cells, (interstitium) and in lymphatics; water cyrstallized in bond and fluid in dense connective tissue, i.e. cartilage (each 7.5%); fluid in GIT/intraocular tissue/urinary tract/CSF/serosal spaces viz. pleura, peritoneum/pericardium. This last category is popularly named as transcellular fluid.

BIBLIOGRAPHY

1. Boron WF, Sachkin H. Measurement of intracellular ionic composition and activities in renal tubules. Ann Rev Phy 1983;45:483.
2. Elkington JR, Danowski TS. The body fluids—basic physiology Practical therapeutics. London Bailcere Tudal and Cox, 1955.
3. Fitzsimons JT. Thirst Phy Rev 1972;52:468.
4. Fourman P et al. Thirst and polyurea Lancet i. 1959;268-70.
5. Gamble JL. Chemical Anatomy. Phy. Pathology of ECF 6th Ed. Cambridge Mass Harvard University Press. 1954.
6. Hardy JD. Fluid therapy London Henry Kimpton. 1954.

28 Kidney: Introduction

> The kidney alters the internal environment to fit the organism, much as the nervous system modifies the behaviour of the organism to fit the external environment.

Kidney is considered as the most challenging organ for medical personalities since it is famous as, organ with altered structure and disturbed function. Furthermore, its importance lies in the fact that it is directly linked with cardio-vascular system. If kidney fails, heart and vascular system also get disturbed and vice versa. Its main functions may be enumerated as :

Table 28.1: Functions of kidney—at a glance

i. Elimination of water not needed by body fluids.
ii. The excretion of certain substances normally present in plasma when their concentration rises above a certain level.
iii. Selective reabsorption of substances of certain importance to the body like glucose.
iv. Excretion of useless substances.
v. Regulation of acid-base balance.

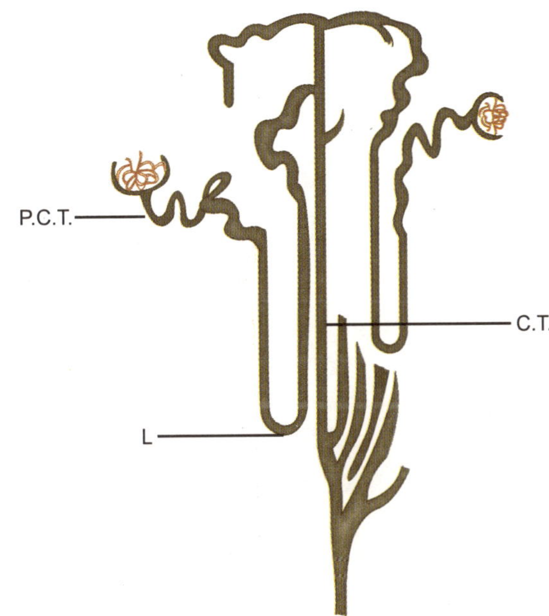

Fig. 28.1: Functional structure of nephron
PCT = Proximal convoluted tubule, CT = Collecting tubule, L = Loop of Henle

FUNCTIONAL STRUCTURAL CONSIDERATION

***Nephrons*:** These are units of kidney and said to be 1,000,000 in number. It further consists of four units namely—glomerulus, proximal convoluted tubule, the loop of Henle and the distal convoluted tubule.

***Glomerulus (Renal filter)*:** It is an filtration mechanism. It consists of tuft of capillaries which empty not into a vein but into artery. The diameter of efferent arteriole is only half that of afferent one which raises the pressure in glomerular capillaries and thus facilitate filtration. The afferent arteriole divides into three or four branches, which gives a lobulated appearance. The basement membrane covering the capillaries, is though continuous with capillaries but it does not enclose the entire circumference of any single capillary. The interluminal cell aggregates is the name given to endothelial cells lining the capillaries and forming small groups in the areas between capillary lumen but within basement membrane. They occupy intercapillary space. Basement membrane is the only continuous barrier between vascular and urinary spaces. It is in fact a combination of endothelium, true basement membrane and a portion of foot processes of the epithelial cells. It allows a huge volume of water to leave the blood temporarily as well as glucose, amino acids, sodium, chloride, potassium and calcium, all of which must be reabsorbed, because they are essential.

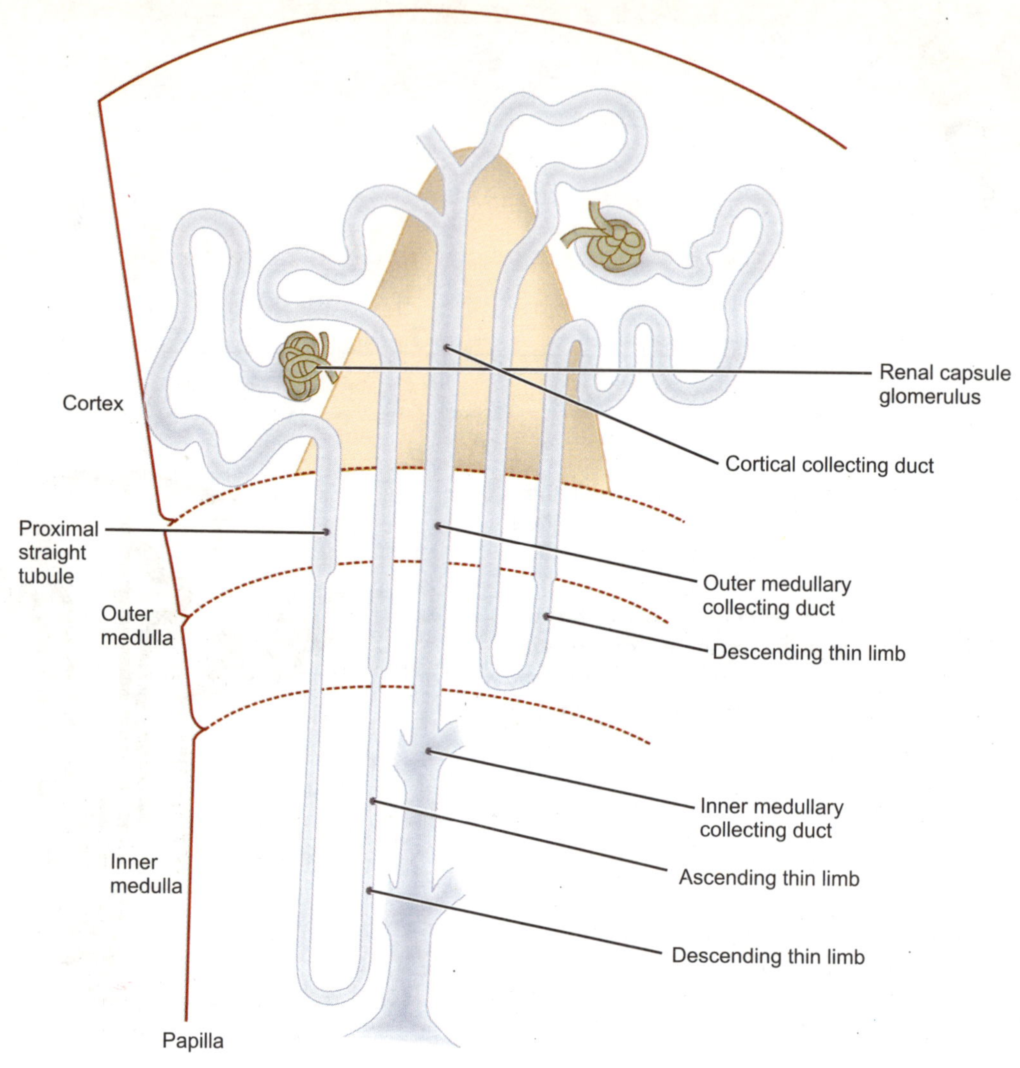

Fig. 28.2: Nephron

Bowman's capsule is the dilated blind end of the nephron, invaginated by the glomerular tuft. Histologically it is made up of two layers namely—visceral and parietal. Former consists of single layer of flattened cells with incomplete outline; while later is made of same type of cells but with the distinction that their outline is complete. The epithelium covering the capillaries (which is visceral layer) is presenting countless, villous processes which terminate as feet, the soles of which are firmly planted on basement membrane of capillary, like the tentacles of an octopus and for the same reason cells are called *foot cells or podocytes*. The main body of these cells is lifted from basement membrane by the processes, thus allowing filtration to occur without the fluid passing through the epithelial cell.

Renal tubules: The glomerulus is having two poles—At one pole the blood vessels are attached called 'vascular pole' while another is tubular pole where tubule begins. Just below glomerulus, the tubule is having a constricted portion called "neck" from where it is divided into -

First or Proximal: convoluted tubule—The large size of lining cells, marked granularity of cytoplasm due to numerous mitochondria and brush border are its characteristic features. The main feature of it is - the absorption and so it is having microvilli on the surface of the cells facing the lumen and thus absorptive surface is increased to enormous degree. The mitochondria are oriented perpendicular to the cell membrane. The cells present here are metabolically active containing a number of enzymes. These cells reabsorb about two thirds of water of the glomerular filtrate and all glucose, and a part of sodium, chloride and phosphate. Protein enzymes are also reported at brush border and canaliculi.

PROXIMAL TUBULES: FUNCTIONS AT A GLANCE

- Here the epithelial cells are highly metabolic having large number of mitochondria. This is natural gift to organise active transport process.
- These cells have an extensive brush border on apical (luminal) side of the membrane. Also extensive labyrinth of intercellular and basal channels. This is again natural arrangement to provide extensive surface area for rapid transport of ions and other substances, specially on luminal and basolateral sides of epithelium.
- This brush border epithelium is also loaded with protein carrier molecule which helps to organise transport and co-transport of many substances as will be discussed in proceeding discussions.

Loop of Henle: It is U shaped loop dipping for a variable length into medulla and anatomically it is divided into descending limb, thin walled ascending limb and thick walled ascending limb. The wall of bottom of loop of Henle is as thin as that of capillary, suggesting absorption of fluid and concentration of electrolytes.

LOOP OF HENLE: STRUCTURE V/S FUNCTIONS

- The thin limbs (descending + ascending) have thin epithelial membranes without brush borders, few mitochondria and minimum metabolic activity. Lower reabsorptive capacity.
- The descending thin segment is highly permeable to water and moderately permeable to most of other solutes (e.g. urea, Na). About 20 per cent of filtered water is reabsorbed here.
- Ascending limb (thin + thick) is virtually impermeable to water.
- Thick limb is having high metabolic activity so capable of actively reabsorbing sodium, potassium and chloride (25%) and calcium bicarbonate and magnesium.
- In thick ascending limb there exists sodium-potassium ATPase pump in the epithelial cell in basolateral membranes. This is also provided with sodium-hydrogen counter-transport in its luminal membrane which mediate sodium reabsorption and hydrogen secretion.
- Because thick ascending limb is impermeable to water so most of the water remains here as such making the urine dilute.

After passing through Loop of Henle, the fluid then enters ***"Distal Convoluted tubule"*** which is lacking true brush border and there exists extensive in folding of the cell membrane. It has got comparatively much smaller number of microvilli. This segment of the nephron is concerned both with reabsorption and with excretion. It lies in renal cortex.

DISTAL TUBULE: AT A GLANCE

- Thick ascending limb of Henle's loop empties into distal tubule. Its first part forms JG apparatus; the next part is highly convoluted which is impermeable to water so it is called diluting segment.
- Its second half and subsequent cortical collecting tubule is having two types of cells viz. principal cells (reabsorb sodium and water from lumen + secrete potassium ions into the lumen) and intercalated cells (reabsorb potassium ions and secrete hydrogen ions).
- Tubular membrane of both these segments are impermeable to urea. So all urea as such passes through to be excreted in urine.
- Both distal tubule + cortical collecting tubule reabsorb sodium ions which is controlled by aldosterone hormone which also controls potassium secretion into lumen. Sodium reabsorption is dependent on activity of sodium potassium ATPase pump in each cell's basolateral membrane.
- Intercalated cells secrete hydrogen ions by active hydrogen ATPase mechanism. It can secrete these ions against a large concentration gradient. So these structures are of use in acid-base balance maintenance.
- Permeability of this part of nephron is controlled by ADH; in its high concentration they are made permeable for water.

Many such types of tubules coalesce to form cortical collecting duct and passes downward in the medulla where it becomes 'medullary collecting duct,' but a common name *'collecting tubule'* is reserved for its description. It is lined by pale cuboidal cells. Several collecting tubules from different nephrons, join successively and form 'Duct of Bellini' which opens at the apex of renal pyramid. In each kidney there are about 250 of these very large collecting ducts, each of which transmits the urine from about 4000 nephrons.

MEDULLARY COLLECTING DUCT: AT A GLANCE

- Its permeability towards water is controlled by ADH.
- These are permeable to urea, so some of the urea is reabsorbed here.
- It is capable of secreting hydrogen ions against a large concentration gradient so it plays a leading role in acid base balance maintenance.

THE JUXTAGLOMERULAR APPARATUS

- The Juxtaglomerular body is a group of modified smooth muscle cells resembling epithelioid cells which replace the normal muscle of the afferent arterioles just before it enters the normal glomerulus. It is said to include macula densa, Juxtaglomerular cells and Polkissen.

- *Macula Densa*: It is the term applied to a concentration of nuclei in the commencement of distal convoluted tubule, the cells of which are columnar and rich in acid mucopolysaccharide. So it is a modified epithelial cell in the portion of distal convoluted tubule lying in contact of glomerular vessel of the same nephron.
- *Juxtaglomerular cells*: These are granular neuro-epithelioid cells situated in media of afferent glomerulus. Granulation is related with secretable renin.

READ AND DIGEST: JG APPARATUS

1. **Describe Juxtaglomerular apparatus (JG Apparatus)**

Ans. It is a composite of specialised tubular and vascular cells. It lies at vascular pole where afferent and efferent arterioles enter and leave the glomerulus. Its components include:

a. ***JG cells.*** They synthesise, store and release renin which is a proteolytic enzyme. They have provided with well developed Golgi apparatus and endoplasmic reticulum. These are myo-epithelioid cells present in the form of thickening in afferent arteriole just before entering the glomerulus. These are actually baro-receptors so responding towards pressure changes. Sympathetic nerve fibres innervate them. Renal perfusion pressure is assessed by these cells and so they are stimulated by hypovolemia.

b. ***Macula densa cells.*** These are located at the point where ascending thick segment of Henle's loop continues as distal covoluted tubule. They serve as chemoreceptors. They are stimulated by decreased NaCl load which leads to release of renin. They are neither innervated, nor adapted for reabsorption, nor secreting one.

c. ***Mesangial cells (Lacis cell).*** They are present between capillary loops. They are provided with contractility and in extreme stages of activity they show granulation to secrete renin. It regulates GFR.

Normal plasma renin → 200 ng/100 ml.

RENAL BLOOD FLOW

- There are two capillary beds in nephron:-
  a. *Glomerulus:* It receives blood from afferent arteriole and from here it goes to (b) peritubular capillaries - via efferent arteriole which offers considerable resistance to blood flow. So it is evident that 'glomerulus is a high pressure area while peritubular capillary bed' is a low pressure bed (functioning just like venous end of capillary and fluid being absorbed into the capillaries).

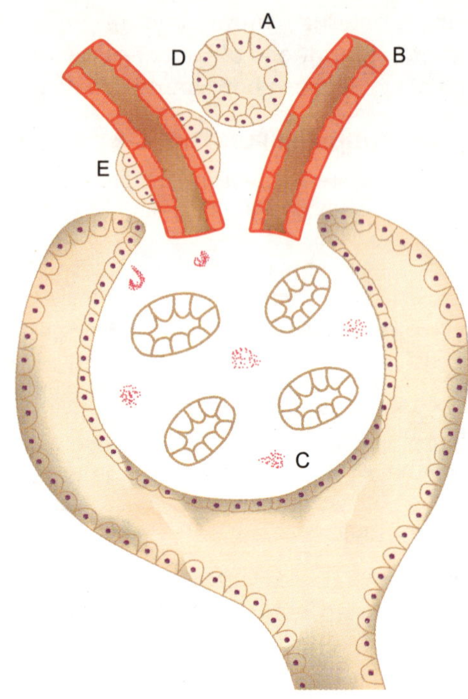

Fig. 28.3: JG apparatus
A = Distal convoluted tubule, B = Efferent arteriole, C = Glomerular mesangial cells, D = Macula densa, E = Juxtaglomerular cells

- Renal blood flow is further characterised by vasa recta—which are a network of capillaries that descend into medulla around the loop of Henle. These capillaries form loops in medulla of the kidney and then return to the cortex before emptying into veins, so they play a special role in urine concentration. Only 1-2 per cent blood flows through these vasa recta or blood flow is rapid in cortex while it is sluggish in medulla.
- *Autoregulation of renal blood flow*:
  i. *Myogenic concept*: Smooth muscles present in preglomerular blood vessels are capable of reacting to distension by shortening during elevation of perfusion pressure. These are site of autoregulation. Thus, the preglomerular vascular tone is increased due to this myogenic response to increased arterial blood pressure. If these smooth muscles are paralysed (potassium cyanide, procain, papaverin, etc.) then this reactivity is abolished.

ii. Both the intrarenal neurogenic component (axon reflex) and smooth muscles of preglomerular blood vessels are playing important role in autoregulation (intrarenal reflex).

iii. Any increase in perfusion pressure → increase in tissue pressure → clamping effect over renal vessels to flow → maintenance of constant blood flow (intrarenal tissue pressure - concept).

iv. Increase of pressure → viscosity in interlobular arteries and in cortex is increased → constancy in flow is maintained.

v. With mild hypoxia there is slight renal vaso dilatation due to reactive hyperaemia but if it is severe and prolonged it may cause vasoconstriction which may be a reflex chemoreceptor response.

Hypercapnia and acidosis reduce the renal blood flow which is a centrally mediated neurogenic action.

- *Hormones*
  - — adrenaline and noradrenaline - vasoconstriction
  - — 5HT (Serotonin) - On direct infusion in renal artery it leads to vasoconstriction (increase in vascular resistance)
  - — On I.V. administration - it causes renal hyperaemia which terminates into diuresis.
- *Nervous control*
- Mild stimulation of splanchnic nerve leads to vasodilatation in outer medulla with simultaneous vasoconstriction in outer cortical peritubular capillaries. But total blood flow to kidney remains constant.
- *Anaesthesia*: During deep anaesthesia renal blood flow is decreased. During light anaesthesia there is redistribution of blood from splanchnic beds to skin and muscles of extremity.
- *Other pharmacological agents:*
  - — Ephedrine, hydroxyamphetamine when injected directly into renal artery leads to vasoconstriction.
  - — Caffeine, theophylline increase GFR.
- *Posture*: In upright posture, there occurs reduction in central blood volume which may reflexly produce vasoconstriction in renal vascular bed.
- Different pressures:
  - — 100 mmHg in large arcuate arteries.
  - — 8 mmHg in veins into which blood finally drains.
- The pressure falls from 100 mmHg to 60 mmHg at small renal arteries and afferent arteriole.
- When blood passes to peritubular capillaries from glomerulus, through efferent arteriole, pressure further falls another 47 mmHg, so it remains with 13 mmHg. So glomerulus works at 60 mmHg pressure and peritubular capillaries functions at 13 mmHg pressure.

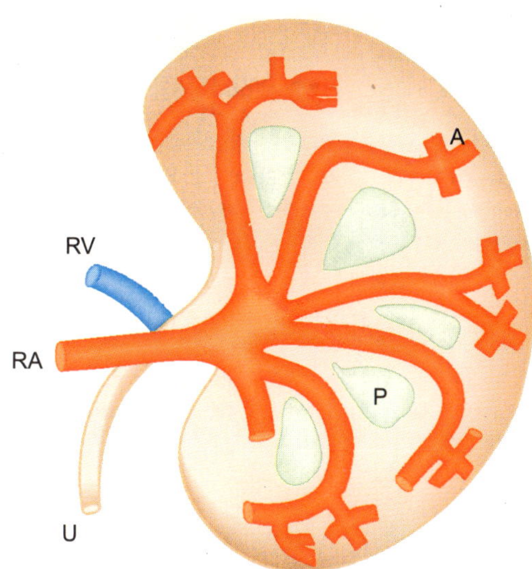

Fig. 28.4: Renal blood vessels
A = Afferent arterioles, B = Arcuate arteries, P = Medullary pyramid, U = Ureter, RV = Renal vein, RA = Renal artery

- Intrarenal pressure (or needle pressure) is ranging between 10–18 mmHg (average 13 mmHg).
- 180 litres/day- the fluid is filtered through glomeruli but only 1–1.5 litres/day is excreted as urine, rest is reabsorbed into renal interstitial spaces and then into peritubular capillaries.
- Peritubular capillaries are extremely porous, so extremely osmosis of fluid resulting from colloid osmotic pressure of plasma proteins can lead for rapid absorption which is required.

RENAL VASCULARITY: A VIEW

- Renal artery (branch of aorta) → interlobar arteries (ascending between medullary pyramids) → arcuate arteries (coursing between cortex and medulla) → inter lobular arteries running towards the surface) → afferent arterioles (short and thick walled having multiple capillary branches to form glomerulus) → glomerular capillaries (high pressure area) → efferent arteriole (smaller diameter than afferent + thin walled → they break up to form peritubular capillary plexus in cortical nephrons which surrounds all convoluted tubules + in juxta medullary region they form vasa recta which run parallel to all tubules in medulla → both, i.e. peritubular capillaries and vasa recta join to form stellate vein → draining into interlobular vein → arcuate vein → interlobar vein → renal vein.
- The volume of blood in renal capillaries is 30 to 40 ml.
- Total surface area of renal capillaries is 12 m^2.
- Glomerular capillaries are the only capillaries in the body that drain into arterioles. These arterial segments are portal system (portal gate).

Table 28.2: Renal blood flow

A. *Increased:* Cold, emotions, high protein diet, pregnancy, polycythaemia, hyperpyrexia.

B. *Decreased:* Upright posture, pain, exercise, low protein diet, hypothyroidism, hypopituitarism, senescence, anaemia, poisons like carbon tetrachloride, nitrites, propylene glycol.

SUMMARY AND HIGHLIGHTS

- The kidney forms the urine which is carried to urinary bladder by ureters. Urine is extruded from bladder to urethra and then to exterior.
- The kidney is divided into two zones—outer cortex and inner medulla. In medulla—pyramid shaped structures (4–14 in number) called renal pyramids are seen and its narrow apex is called papillae and individual papilla is fitted into calyx minor a tube like structure. In between two neighbouring pyramids, there exists column of Bertin—a mass of cortical tissue several minor calyces coalesce to form renal pelvis—the beginning of ureter.
- Nephron is the functional and structural unit of kidney consists of following parts:
  a. Malpighian or renal corpuscle which is having two viz. glomerulus and Bowman's capsule.
  b. Proximal tubule—subdivided into convoluted (PCT) part and straight part pars recta.
  c. Loop of Henle—Subdivided into descending and ascending limb.
  d. Distal nephron—made up of distal and collecting tubule.
- There are two types of nephrons. viz. cortical (85%) and Juxta medullary. Later is mainly concerned with concentration of tubular fluid and sodium conservation. There are about one million nephron in human kidney. The tubule portion of each nephron is further divided into 12 segments arranged in series; each segment has unique morphologic characteristics and transport functions. The individual nephron segments are made of epithelial cells arranged in cylindrical or tubular sheets.

29 Formation of Urine-I: Glomerulus as a Filter

The tubules serves three functions—reabsorption, secretion, and preservation of acid-base balance; while glomerulus is renal filter : the tubular reabsorption is just as important as glomerular filtration.

As said earlier glomerulus act as ultra filter.

WONDERS OF URINARY FORMATION

1. Each kidney is made of 1 to 2 million nephrons. Each is capable of formation of urine. There exists no power of regeneration of these nephrons. According to one data there is a decrease 10 per cent every 10 years in number of nephrons after the age of 40 years. Adaptive changes occur in remaining nephrons; so this loss does not produce any fatal effect.
2. Normally volume of filtrate is 180 litres daily; tubular reabsorption is 178.5 litres daily so total amount of urine which is excreted daily is 1.5 litres. Now if blood pressure increases from normal 100 mmHg to 125 mmHg; this must increase GFR also by 25 per cent, i.e. from 180 litres to 225 litres daily. This would increase urine volume from normal 1.5 litres to 46.5 litres daily (225-17.8 = 46.5 litres) means a 30 fold increase. This is quite a fatal condition. But this does not happen because of renal autoregulation.
3. Entire plasma volume is 3 litres; whereas GFR is 180 litres daily. This means entire plasma can be filtered and processed about 60 times daily (60 × 3 = 180). This process allows the kidney to rapidly remove waste products from the body and, also, allows the kidney to control the volume and composition of body fluids.
4. The process of glomerular filtration and tubular reabsorption are quantitatively very large relative to urinary excretion of many substances. If 10 per cent decrease in tubular reabsorption occurs (from normal 178.5 to 160.7 litres/day, then there may be 13-fold increase in volume, i.e. from normal 1.5 to 19.3 litres daily). But in reality, changes in tubular reabsorption and glomerular filtration are closely co-ordinated to avoid fluctuations in urinary excretion.
5. In kidney, changes in renal blood flow (RBF) are running parallel with renal VO_2. Here the key or master word is active sodium (Na^+) transport since (Na^+ reabsorption) is the main process, which causes largest expenditure of renal energy (VO_2). So decreased RBF → decreased GFR → decreased load of filtered NaCl to be reabsorbed. So there exists a linear relationship between VO_2 and RBF.

COMPOSITION OF FILTRATE

- Glomerular filtrate is having same composition as that of plasma except that it has no significant amount of proteins (plasma without colloids).
- It is said that glomerular filtrate has exactly the same composition as the fluid that filters from arterial ends of the capillaries into interstitial fluid.

Glomerular Filtration Rate (GFR): The quantity of glomerular filtrate formed each minute in all nephrons of both kidney is called GFR. In normal healthy persons it is 125 ml/minute or 7.5 L/h, or 180 L/d.

At the rate of 125 ml/mt, the kidney filters per day an amount of fluid equal to four times the total body water, 15 times the ECF volume and 60 times the plasma volume.

Table 29.1: True about kidney

Figures	*ml/minute*
1. Blood flow through kidney	1,200
2. Plasma flow through kidney (diodone clearance)	700
3. Glomerular filtrate (inulin clearance)	125
4. Filtration fraction (125/700)X100	18%
5. Urine	1

Variants of GFR-I: Glomerular filtration is a function of three variables, viz. glomerular membrane, intracapsular hydrostatic pressure, capillary blood pressure as well as colloid osmotic pressure of plasma proteins.

Table 29.2: GFR—Fall In

1. Severe haemorrhage with decrease in blood volume
2. Severe dehydration
3. Muscular exercise
4. Hypophysectomy
5. Thyroid deficiency
6. Sleep
7. Reduction in number of functioning glomeruli.

i. ***Glomerular membrane***: The permeability of the membrane is anatomical fact. The only physiological variation is that the diseased membrane may permit the passage of molecules larger than those which normally penetrate. Filtering pores are actually present in capillary basement membrane, and size of such pores is bigger than the size of the molecule. The normal glomerular membrane is completely impermeable to plasma proteins. The smallest of these is albumin (molecule weight 70,000; size 6-7 mili microns) which cannot pass. Serum globulin and fibrinogen (molecular weight 170,000) cannot pass, but haemoglobin (molecular weight 68,000) can freely pass out (its molecule is less elongated than albumin molecule). Gelatine, Bence Jones Proteose, egg albumin (molecular weight 35,000; size 4 milli-microns) can easily pass out. In certain pathological conditions (anoxia, heart failure) the filtering pores enlarge in size which leads to passage of large amount of serum albumin which ultimately appear in urine leading to what is known as ***'albumin urea.'*** The number of glomeruli active at any time and number of functioning capillaries in each glomerulus is another factor of importance. This constitutes the effective area available for filtration. Under physiological conditions, all glomeruli are continuously active.
   Increased pressure in the renal veins probably accounts for protein urea of pregnancy. Orthostatic albuminurea occurs only when the subject is erect, disappearing when he lies down.

ii. ***Capillary Blood pressure***: The major regulator of GFR is the pressure within glomerular capillaries.
   a. Constriction of afferent arteriole → decrease GFR and glomerular pressure. Dilatation of afferent arteriole → increase GFR and glomerular pressure
   b. Constriction of efferent arteriole → increases resistance to outflow from glomeruli → glomerular pressure + GFR increased
      If constriction is severe → blood flow through glomerulus becomes sluggish → rise in plasma colloid osmotic pressure → decreased GFR
   c. Mild sympathetic stimulation of both the kidneys → afferent and efferent arterioles constrict approximately proportionate to each other → GFR neither rises nor falls
      Strong sympathetic stimulation → glomerular blood flow reduced to zero → great reduction in GFR
   d. Increase in arterial pressure can greatly increase urinary output but GFR is affected only sluggish or slightly because of phenomenon of autoregulation. So GFR does not bear any particular relationship with cardiac output. If general arterial blood pressure shows extreme changes, this autoregulation fails and then GFR is affected. In general it may be mentioned that -
      Fall of blood pressure → fall of renal arterial per fusion pressure → fall of glomerular blood pressure → fall of effective filtration pressure → fall of renal filtration. Reverse may occur with rise in blood pressure.

iii. ***Intracapsular pressure***:
   a. The glomerular hydrostatic pressure is the average pressure in glomerular capillaries. It varies between 55 to 90 mmHg (average being 60 to 70 mmHg).
   b. Pressure in Bowman capsule has been measured as 14 mmHg (14–18 mmHg).
      Under ordinary conditions variations in the pressure within Bowman's capsule probably contribute little to changing GFR.

iv. ***Colloid osmotic pressure of plasma proteins***: An inverse relation is said to exist, i.e. higher the colloid osmotic pressure—less is GFR; and, lower the colloid osmotic pressure—higher is GFR. It has been found experimentally that sudden dilution of plasma proteins by administration of isotonic NaCl solution produces an increase in GFR and urine flow (dilution diuresis). Because approximately one-fifth of the plasma in capillaries filters into the capsule, the protein concentration increases about 20 per cent as blood passes from arterial to venous ends of the glomerular capillaries. Average colloid osmotic pressure is about 32 mmHg.

Filtration fraction: It is the ratio between the volume of glomerular filtrate and plasma flow per minute. It indicates the efficiency of filter bed.

It is 120/700 = 0.17

Filtration pressure (Net effective): It is the force upon which filtration depends. It is about 10 mmHg.

$P = P_g - P_{OP} - P_C$ (P = Effective filtration pressure, P_g = glomerular capillary pressure, P_{OP} = osmotic pressure by plasma protein P_C = Intracapsular hydrostatic pressure)

Table 29.3: Physiological, decrease in GFR

a. Glomerular hydrostatic pressure reduced, e.g. hypotension
b. Plasma oncotic pressure rises, e.g. dehydration, dysproteinaemias, multiple myeloma
c. Permeability or total surface area of filtration is reduced, e.g. glomerulonephritis
d. Tubule hydrostatic pressure increased, e.g. obstruction in ureter/bladder
e. Renal blood flow and plasma flow decreased, e.g. heart failure.

Autoregulation of GFR

1. Kidney possesses the ability to maintain constancy of renal blood flow and GFR over a wide range of renal perfusion pressures and this autoregulation phenomenon is seen also elsewhere like brain, myocardium, etc.
2. Tubulo-glomerular feedback is playing a role in maintenance of this autoregulation. It is also reported in the absence of macula densa-glomerulus feedback. Thus, myogenic factors intrinsic to renal vasculature and independent of renal nerves may play an important role in renal response to variations in perfusion pressure.
3. Sodium/Renin theory: Too rapid flow of glomerular filtrate through the tubules allow sodium concentration to rise in distal tubule. GFR decrease via afferent constriction which in turn causes conversion of angiotensinogen (present in tissue fluid) into angiotensin; which leads to constriction of afferent arterioles and due to this blood flow through glomerulus is cut down, leading ultimately to decrease in GFR back to normal.
4. Osmotic theory: Rapid formation of glomerular filtrate → decrease in osmolality of fluid at macula densa → fluid is diluted → constriction of afferent arteriole → decrease in GFR and glomerular blood flow.

   Now the chain ahead decreased GFR → excess osmolality of fluid at macula densa → dilatation of afferent arteriole → increased GFR and glomerular blood flow.
5. So it is an arrangement by which the organ concerned can ward off the effects of changing perfusion pressure, to itself, e.g. the arterial pressure can change from 70 mmHg to 200 mmHg but renal blood flow and GFR will change only a few percent. It is probably attributable to spontaneous adjustments of arteriolar resistances. When this autoregulation fails the patient enters the cardiovascular shock which is characterised by sharp fall of blood pressure which can even stop filtration resulting an urea constituting what is known as 'renal shut down.' The nerves are not essential to this autoregulation.
6. If GFR is very slight then tubular fluid will pass slowly through tubules. It will lead to hundred percent reabsorption. So kidney will fail to eliminate the necessary waste products.

On the other hand if GFR is too much high the fluid will pass so rapidly through the tubules so reabsorption will be impossible and necessary substances will not be conserved in the body.

So it is necessary that glomerular filtrate must flow into tubular system at an appropriate rate. This demands for autoregulation of GFR which is achieved by following two mechanisms which are jointly called 'tubulo-glomerular feedback; which occurs at juxtaglomerular complex.

1. The afferent arteriolar vasodilator feedback mechanism

   Too little flow of glomerular filtrate into tubules → decreased sodium and chloride ion concentration at macula densa → afferent arteriolar dilatation → increased blood flow into glomerulus → increased glomerular pressure.
2. The efferent arteriolar vasoconstrictor feedback mechanism

   Too low GFR → excess reabsorption of Na^+, Cl^- - reducing ionic concentration at macula densa → release of renin from JG apparatus → formation of angiotensin II → constriction of efferent arteriole.

This also controls renal blood flows as:

a. Afferent arteriolar vasodilator mechanism:
   Fall in renal blood flow → decreased GFR → dilatation of afferent arteriole → increased blood flow in glomerulus
b. Myogenic mechanism
   Rise in arterial pressure → stretching walls of arterioles → secondary contraction of arteriole → decrease in renal blood flow to normal.
c. Effect of sympathetic stimulation : Slight to moderate degree of sympathetic stimulation leads to only mild effect. Very strong acute sympathetic stimulation can constrict the renal arterioles greatly which tends to reduce the renal blood flow and thus decreasing urine volume. Within 20–30 minutes the situation is controlled because of diminished release of sympathetic neurotransmitter at sympathetic nerve endings.
d. Prostaglandins, increases blood flow in renal cortex and decreases in renal medulla. Acetylcholine causes renal vasodilatation. A high protein diet raises glomerular capillary pressure and increases renal blood flow.

Measurement of GFR :
Inulin Clearance as its Measure

i. • The difference between the rate at which a substance is filtered at the glomeruli; and the rate at which it is excreted in urine; represents the rate at which the substance is removed from or added to the urine as the later traverses the renal tubules.
 • The rate at which the substance is filtered is given by the product of its concentration in the plasma. The rate of excretions determined by its concentration in the urine.

ii. To select such substance; it must have some qualities like that (a) it should be freely filterable at glomeruli; (b) It should be neither reabsorbed nor secreted by tubules (c) It should not be toxic. *Inulin* - a polysaccharide with a molecular weight 5,200 fulfils all these qualities and therefore its clearance is taken as a measure of GFR.

iii. 10 gm of Inulin dissolved in 100 ml of normal saline is given intravenously at the rate of 10 ml/minute.

Clearance value is $\frac{U \quad V}{P}$ ml/minute

U = Inulin concentration in gm/100 ml. of urine
V = Volume of urine in ml/minute
P = its concentration in gm/100 ml of plasma
Normally it is 125 ml/minute which equals to GFR.

- Mannitol is another such polysaccharide which can be used instead of inulin. The mannitol clearance is about 10 per cent lower than clearance of inulin indicating that about 10 per cent of filtered mannitol is on the average reabsorbed. Another is "radioactive iothalamate."

iv. Thus if we assume that GFR is maintained at 125 ml/minute rate throughout the day, we may calculate that some 7.5 litres are filtered each hour or 180 litres/day in an individual of normal size and 99 per cent of it is reabsorbed.
The total body water is 4.5 litres in an average man of 70 kg body weight and all body water is filtered into renal tubules and reabsorbed four times each day.

Tubulo-glomerular feedback: The JG Apparatus is ideally suited for a feedback system whereby a stimulus received at macula densa would be transmitted to the arterioles of the same nephron to alter GFR. It has been shown that changes in composition of fluid flowing past the macula densa elicit rapid changes in glomerular filtration of the same nephron. Increase in delivery of fluid out of the proximal tubule result in decreases in filtration rate of the same nephron.

The glomerulotubular balance means the phenomenon by which effectiveness of the rise of GFR (for Na^+ excretion) due to plasma hypervolaemia is automatically cancelled.

Rise in GFR → Increase in colloid osmotic tension (COT) of blood leaving the glomerulus → COT of peritubular capillaries rise → It attracts more fluid and Na from peritubular space.

READ AND DIGEST: AUTOREGULATION

1. What is role of Tubulo-glomerular feedback in auto-regulation of GFR?

Ans. The key substance is changed in NaCl concentration at macula densa level.

a. Decreased GFR → slow flow rate in Henle's loop → increased reabsorption of NaCl at proximal tubule → reduced concentration of NaCl at macula densa

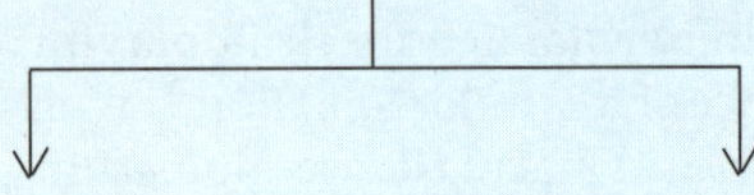

Decreased resistance of afferent arterioles → raised glomerular hydrostatic pressure → raised GFR	Renin released from JG cells → angiotensin I and II → constriction of efferent arterioles → raised glomerular hydrostatic pressure → raised GFR.

b. The persons taking ACE inhibitor drugs (angiotensin converting enzyme) for treatment of hypertension which is due to renal artery stenosis are exposed to fatal results since this may lead to severe reduction in GFR → acute renal failure.

c. Now think of a man on heavy diet of protein → increased release of amino acid → reabsorbed by proximal tubules with sodium (co-transport) → decreased NaCl level at macula densa → increased GFR as mentioned above.

d. Now think of a man on high blood glucose level → it is reabsorbed with Na^+ by proximal tubule → increased glucose causes more reabsorption of NaCl → less NaCl at macula densa → increased GFR as mentioned above.

e. Now the whole story is reversed if renal tubules are damaged (by tetracycline drugs, heavy metals etc.) → no or less reabsorption of NaCl → more NaCl at macula densa → opposite effect.

f. Myogenic theory → increased BP → more stretch of vascular wall → increased movement of Ca^{++} from extra cellular fluid to cells → contraction → prevention of overdistension.

(Source: Braam B et al, 1993. J. Am. Soc. Nephrology 41: 1275. Relevance of tubulo-glomerular feedback mechanism in pathophysiology. Quoted by Guyton and Hall Textbook of Medical Physiology - W.B. Saunders).

Glomerulotubular Balance : A Review (of sodium)

1. At 100 ml/minute GFR, the proximal tubules reabsorb 65 per cent (or 65 ml/min). When GFR is doubled (i.e. 200 ml per minute), then this rate will also be doubled, i.e. 130 ml per minute. This is a balance.
2. Its advantages are:-
   - It controls GFR.
   - Distal tubular segments are prevented from over loading. It is also necessary because here aldosterone and ADH acts but they have a limited range of control of sodium reabsorption.
   - So proximal tubules acts like a father who takes every extra burden on his head in order to keep his son (distal tubules) away or protected from extra burden.

SUMMARY AND HIGHLIGHTS

Filtration by glomerulus is essentially a physical process depending on such elements as hydrostatic pressure in capillaries, the pores in endothelial cells, the arrangement of podocytes and the permeability of basement membrane. When any of these become deranged because of any reason, the result becomes evident in urine. Glomerular function is expressed in terms of renal clearance; which is a quantitative description of the rate at which the kidney excretes various substances relative to their concentration in plasma. It gives GFR. It is measured by the use of such substances as 'inulin' which is neither secreted nor absorbed. The filtrate is identical with blood plasma except for protein and substances bound to protein.

Tubules: Re-absorption involves in particular—water, glucose, chloride, phosphate, sodium, potassium, calcium, bicarbonate as well as amino acid and probably albumin. The function of proximal convoluted tubule is conservation through re-absorption. Hence, microvilli are plentifully present which increase absorptive surface and capacity enormously. Water re-absorption is a passive phenomenon due to changes in hydrostatic and osmotic pressure in peritubular capillaries of the efferent arterioles. Absorption of glucose, sodium, potassium, calcium, chloride, etc. is active being mediated by energy of the cellular enzymes of proximal tubules.

30 Formation of Urine-II: The Tubular Functions

What are the physiological mechanisms by which the ultra-filtrate of plasma (primary urine) acquires the composition of final urine which is excreted from the body, while passing ahead glomerulus? The answer is lying within the tubules.

THEME OF EXCRETION

Urinary excretion rate = Filtration rate-reabsorption rate + secretlon rate

Now there are following possibilities

1. A substance is freely filtered by glomerulus, but is neither reabsorbed nor secreted. So its rate of excretion is equal to rate at which it is filtered; e.g. creatinine, inulin etc.
2. A substance is freely filtered, but is partly reabsorbed by tubules and returned to the blood so rate of excretion is equal to filtration rate minus rate of reabsorption; e.g. electrolytes.
3. A substance is freely filtered by glomerulus, but its entire amount is reabsorbed by tubules and returned to the blood; e.g. glucose and amino acids.
4. A substance is freely filtered by glomerulus and is not reabsorbed, but additional amount is secreted from peritubular capillaries blood into renal tubules. So excretion rate is equal to filtration rate plus tubular secretion rate.

A comparison between the composition of blood plasma, which is almost the same as that of glomerular ultra-filtrate, and that of urine obtained from the bladder, shows that some of the components of plasma (or glomerular ultrafiltrate) are not found in urine (e.g. glucose), others have been considerably concentrated, and others are in almost the same concentration in plasma and urine. For absence of glucose, it is necessary to admit that it has been reabsorbed as it passes down the renal tube. For others (a) the tubes excrete concentrated solutions of some substances which are added to glomerular ultrafiltrate; (b) the tubes besides water, reabsorb selectively some of the substances in glomerular filtrate, and the urine is the resulting residue of this filtrate.

***Proximal convoluted tubule*:** lined by truncated cubical epithelium whose luminal surface is covered with microvilli. Long characteristic mitochondria occupy basal end of cell, and acidophilic cytoplasm is filled with granules of ribose nucleic acid. It becomes -

***Loop of Henle*:** which runs more or less deeply into the medulla. The descending limb and the loop are lined by flattened epithelial cells (thin segment). The ascending limb is lined by cubical epithelium and ascends to glomerular root to form. *Distal convoluted tubule* which joins 'collecting tubule' which units with other such collecting tubules to form 'duct of Belline' which is lined by columnar cells and opens on the apex of one of the papillae into the renal pelvis.

Human proximal convoluted tubules are on average about 14 mm long and 60 μm in diameter. This means that surface area of tubule is about π (60/1000) × 14 mm^2 or about 2.5 mm^2.

TUBULAR REABSORPTION: ACTIVE PASSIVE TRANSPORT

- The tubular load of a substance is the total amount of a substance that filters through the glomerular membrane into the tubules each minute.
- For most actively reabsorbed substances there is a maximum rate at which each can be reabsorbed. This is called Tubular transport maximum (Tm).

Table 30.1: Tm of various substances

Substances	*Tm*
Glucose..............	320 mg/min
Plasma protein...........	20–30 mg/min
Haemoglobin..................	1 mg/min
Amino acid..................	1.5 mM/min
Lactate.......................	75 mg/min

- As per general biophysical law; any substance to be reabsorbed; it must first be transported across tubular epithelial membranes into renal interstitial fluid and then through the peritubular capillary membrane back into the blood.
- The transport of water and solutes may be through the cell membrane themselves (i.e. transcellular route); or through the junctional spaces between cells (i.e. para cellular route).
- The water and solutes are transported through peritubular capillary walls into the blood by ultrafiltration which is controlled by hydrostatic and colloid osmotic forces.

Primary Active Transport through Tubules: ATP Hydrolysis

(Example:- reabsorption of sodium ion across proximal tubules)

- Since this process requires energy because it takes place against electrochemical gradient. This comes from hydrolysis of ATP by way of membrane bound ATPase sodium potassium that energy is used to transport sodium ions out of the cell into the interstitium.
- At the same time potassium is transported from interstitium to inside of the cell.
- This ionic movement means - low intracellular sodium and high intracellular potassium, as well as -70 mV charge within the cell.
- Because of (i) tubular fluid sodium concentration is high (140 mEq/l) and low intracellular sodium concentration (12 mEq/l); and (ii) negative charge inside attracts the positive charged sodium ions; so passive diffusion of sodium occurs across luminal membrane of cell.
- In first half of proximal tubule, sodium is reabsorbed by co-transport along with other solutes like glucose, amino acids, etc. But in its second half little glucose and amino acids remain to be reabsorbed.

SUGAR TRANSPORT—REABSORPTION

i. Glucose is reabsorbed almost exclusively in the proximal tube; (first half).

ii. It is found, as with absorption from the intestine, that the rates of reabsorption are different in different specificities. For example; the absorption of L-glucose being much less than that of D-glucose. The reabsorption of these compounds shows competition; so that the more actively reabsorbed D-glucose tends to depress the reabsorption of D-fructose or xylose. The order of monosaccharides is:-
Glucose → Galactose → Mannose → Fructose → Xylose → Arabinose.

iii. Phlorhizin—a metabolic inhibitor inhibits this reabsorption process. The process is unaffected by insulin.

iv. Absorption of sugar and amino acid by the intestine is linked with active transport of Na^+; the same is true of tubular reabsorption.

v. A large rise in the concentration of glucose in the blood (due to any reason like heavy carbohydrate meal or diabetes mellitus) will increase the filtered load of glucose presented to proximal tubule, and if this load exceeds the Tm, some of glucose will spill over into the urine. Thus, the blood glucose can rise from an average resting value of about 100 mg/100 ml to over 150 mg/100 ml without any glucose appearing in the urine, the primary role in the homeostasis being, in fact, uptake by the liver.

vi. As far as the mechanism is concerned; glucose and Na^+ bind to a common carrier in the luminal membrane, and glucose is carried into the cell as Na^+ moves down its electrical and chemical gradient. The Na^+ is then pumped out of the cell into the lateral intercellular spaces, and glucose moves into the interstitial fluid by simple diffusion. So glucose transport here is an example of secondary active transport and the energy is provided by Na^+-K^+-ATPase that pumps the Na^+ out of the cell.

GLUCOSE REABSORPTION: SECONDARY ACTIVE REABSORPTION

- As with primary active reabsorption of sodium the energy released by hydrolysis of ATP is also used to drive some other substances (e.g. glucose, amino acid etc.) against electro-chemical gradient. These transport mechanisms are so efficient that they remove virtually all glucose and amino acid from the tubular lumen.
- It is to be noted that downhill diffusion of sodium to the interior of cell provides energy for uphill transport of glucose across the luminal membrane. So glucose reabsorption is secondary active transport because glucose itself is reabsorbed uphill against a chemical gradient; but it is secondary to primary active transport of sodium.

REABSORPTION OF WATER

i.

- The glomerular filtrate has the same osmotic pressure as the plasma except for the absence of the plasma proteins. As the fluid flows through proximal tubules, its volume is reduced to a fraction of that which enters the glomerular space. It is generally estimated that approximately 1/5th

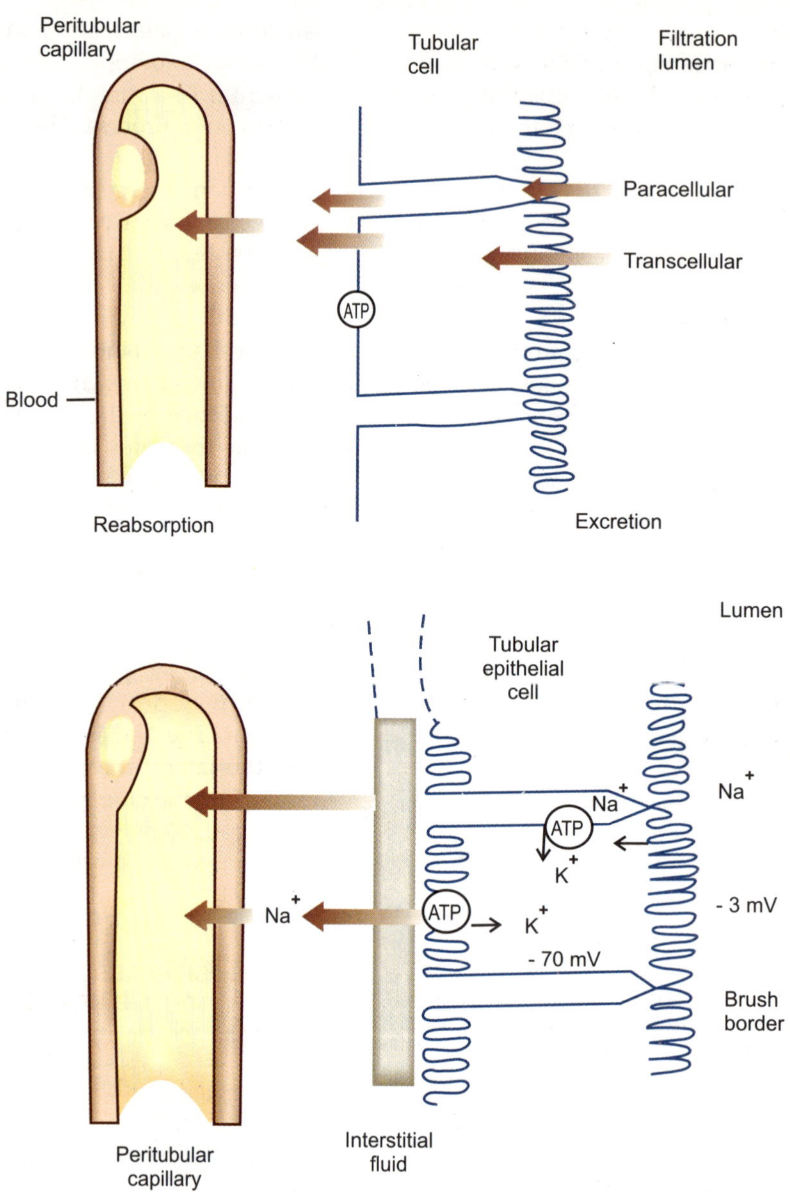

Fig. 30.1: Basic mechanism of reabsorption

of the filtered volume reaches the end of the proximal tubule and enters the loop of Henle. This reduction of volume occurs without change in osmotic pressure whether the urine being produced is dilute or concentrated. Thus, the large fraction of fluid reabsorbed in proximal tubule does not take part in concentration and dilution process, and in fact, is lost to the process of osmoregulation. The water thus reabsorbed in the proximal segment is *obligatory water reabsorption* and to distinguish it from *facultative water reabsorption* in the more distal portion of nephrone where water reabsorption is subject to regulation in accordance with excess or deficit of water in the body fluids.

- Out of 170 litres of water filtered by glomeruli per day, 168.5 litres are reabsorbed in the renal tubules. Only 1.5 litres are excreted as urine. The reabsorption of water occurs in proximal, distal and collecting tubules.

ii.

- Water reabsorption in proximal tubule is entirely a passive process and that the active process which underlies it is the transport of salt (Na) out of tubule lumen. As Na salts are transferred from lumen to peritubular fluid there is a tendency to produce dilution of tubule contents and hypertonicity of surroundings. The proximal tubule is highly permeable to water, and in response to the osmotic gradient, water follows the salt out of the tubule. Within the limits of determinations, the proximal tubule contents are always isotonic with the blood.
- Active reabsorption of sodium along with passive reabsorption of water takes place in proximal tubule. Here water and electrolytes are reabsorbed as *iso-osmotic* solution and do not take any part in dilution or concentration process. This is *obligatory water reabsorption*. Chloride reabsorption is passive, sodium and potassium active process while water is reabsorbed passively at osmotically equivalent rates and therefore the tubular fluid leaving the proximal tubule is *isotonic*.

iii.

- In the distal tubule *'Facultative water reabsorption'* occurs and is regulated by ADH, which increases the permeability of the distal tubule to water. There is active reabsorption of sodium and chloride in the distal tubule and the tubular fluid becomes isotonic. ADH may also stimulate the pumping of sodium in the loop of Henle.
- The epithelial cells of this part can establish a relatively high ion concentration gradient between the blood and tubular fluid which is altered with the change of blood content of ions and controlled by mineralocorticoid hormones. This portion can also establish relatively high osmolar concentration gradients between blood plasma and tubular fluid which is altered with the percentage of body fluid content.

iv. Now, the fluid passes into collecting ducts which are permeable to water, this passes through the duct walls with the osmotic gradient into medullary interstitium. Here, ADH has its effects in enhancing the movement of water, so producing a hyperosmolar urine. So *In the collecting ducts, the reabsorption of hyperosmotic fluid takes place.*

v. *Dilute urine formation* : The dilute fluid which enters the distal tubule is further diluted by the continual removal of salt and it probably continues through the collecting system. The urine is thus rendered hypotonic by the active reabsorption of salt in a region which clearly has a low permeability to water, otherwise the osmotic gradient would be dissipated, as it is in the proximal tubule, by the escape of water to the more concentrated surroundings. The low permeability to water which characterise the distal convoluted tubule and collecting system during the formation of diluted urine is dependent upon absence of ADH.

vi. *Concentrated urine formation*: The events are similar up to the point at which fluid enters the distal convoluted tubules. In the presence of ADH, the distal convoluted tubules and collecting ducts become permeable to water. As it flows through distal tubule the osmotic gradient, established by reabsorption of NaCl, is dissipated and despite additional salt removal in distal tubule the dilute character of urine is lost, so that it regains isotonicity before it enters collecting system.

- Reabsorption of water in distal tubule is facultative because the water may be either saved or discarded, and is under control of ADH of posterior lobe of pituitary which acts by increasing the permeability of the cells of distal tubules. Reabsorption of electrolytes is also under hormonal control.
- Tubular excretion—Is function of distal tubule, which is responsible for preservation of acid-base balance.

It is important to note that it enters collecting isotonic, never hypertonic. The additional water loss which renders the urine more concentrated than blood occurs in the collecting system.

PROXIMAL TUBULAR REABSORPTION OF NA^+

i. It is an active transport of Na^+ with its accompanying anions into the adjacent extracellular space surrounding the tubule; which consequently causes an increase in osmolality which causes the passage of water.

ii. Mechanism

a. Na^+ (in proximal convoluted tubular fluid) enter brush border epithelial cells by the process of passive diffusion which is further assisted by Na^+K^+ATPase system. Since on the basal and lateral surfaces of the tubular epithelial cells the cell membrane contains an extensive Na^+K^+ATPase system that is capable of cleaving ATP and this energy is utilised for the same purpose. In the membrane of this brush border epithelium there are sodium carrier proteins that bind with the sodium ions on the luminal surface of the membrane and release them inside the cell. This constitutes the facilitated diffusion of the sodium to the interior of the cell. This ensures rapid diffusion of sodium through the luminal border of the epithelial cell at the same time that the sodium ion is being actively transported out of the cell at the basolateral borders.

Sodium pumped from the tubule is absorbed into the peritubular capillary and carried away by blood. The excess Na^+ present in peritubular space (space in between renal tubules) raises the local osmotic tension which facilitates the entry of Na^+ into the capillary blood. Another factor assisting here is existing low blood pressure here at peri-tubular capillary and colloid osmotic pressure/tension remains constant at normal value (25 mm Hg). So indrawing forces become dominant and therefore Na^+ and fluid enter peritubular capillary. All this constitutes 'unidirectional Na^+ transport mechanism.'

b. As told above, 'if one substance moves to one direction then another substance move exactly in opposite direction. Glucose, amino acid and several other organic compounds are the examples and phenomenon is named as *co-transport*.

Chloride ions (Cl^-) are co-transported mainly in the thick segment of ascending limb of loop of Henle. Because of increasing concentration of Cl^- here (as compared with peritubular space), osmotic movement of Cl^- is set up and Cl^- moves to the peritubular space; which makes tubular lumen more positive (+ve) in respect to peritubular space. Now the movement of Na^+ towards peritubular space from tubular fluid becomes more facilitated as Na^+ are electrically repelled.

c. To conclude factors affecting Na^+ reabsorption are
   - If peritubular capillary blood pressure rises; Na^+ absorption is reduced.
   - Low plasma colloid osmotic pressure is also capable, of reducing Na^+ absorption.

iii. Out of 560 gm of Na^+ filtered by glomeruli per day, 490 gm reabsorbed in proximal tubule and 65 gm reabsorbed in distal tubule and 5 gm excreted in urine.

iv. *Sodium ion—speciality*
   - They don't exhibit Tm.
   - In proximal tubules the rate of sodium active transport by the basolateral membrane of tubular epithelial cell is more than rate of diffusion of sodium ions from tubular lumen into the cell through brush border. So rate of transport is maximum than diffusion or spread of these ions so it cannot be a limiting factor. Further more these sodium ions may be leaked back from interstitium to the tubular lumen through epithelial junctions. So this does not follow the Tm principle.
   - Furthermore, in distal tubules and beyond; epithelial cells are having tight junctions and transport less quantity of sodium. So here Tm for sodium is same as that of other actively transported substances and also it changes/varies with secretion of ADH and aldosterone.
   - So we mean that:
     —Greater the concentration of sodium in proximal tubules, greater is its re-absorption.
     —Greater is the time during which tubular fluid remains in proximal tubule—more is the re-absorption of sodium.

READ AND DIGEST: SOME MORE ABOUT SODIUM

1. **What is pressure diuresis/natriuresis?**

Ans. Increased fluid or salt intake → increased fluid volume + increased blood volume → increased venous return increased cardiac output → increased blood pressure increased urinary output + increased sodium output (natriuresis).

2. **Discuss integrated responses to changing intake of sodium?**

Ans. Suppose sodium intake is high then possibilities are:
   a. More sodium intake → slight increase in extracellular fluid volume → stretching of receptors in right atrium and pulmonary vessels → activation of brainstem inhibition of sympathetics → decreased sodium reabsorption by tubules.
   b. Increased sodium intake → slight rise of blood pressure increased sodium excretion (natriuresis).
   c. Increased sodium intake → increased arterial blood pressure → inhibition of formation of angiotensin II → decreased tubular reabsorption of sodium.
   d. Increased sodium intake → increased extracellular fluid volume → stimulate ANP → natriuresis.

SYNTHESIS OF NEW SUBSTANCES

Kidney has a power of synthesis of new substances which are metabolically important.

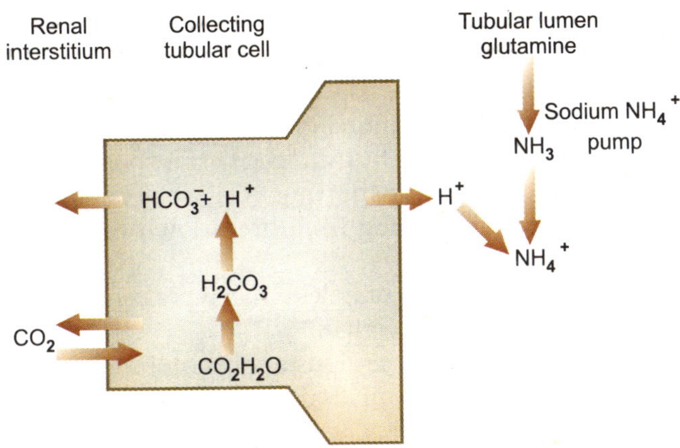

Fig. 30.2: Ammonia buffering: Glutamine metabolized - yield NH_4^+ and bicarbonate

i. It forms part of an antitoxic defensive mechanism, by synthesising hippuric acid. It is said that injection of benzoic acid (sodium benzoate) and glycine is followed by the accumulation of hippuric acid in the blood, but no hippuric acid is formed if renal blood vessels are first tied off. This confirms the synthesis of this substance by kidney.

ii. Kidney also synthesise ammonia which is produced and excreted by distal tube. When the ingestion of acids, or of foodstuffs that give acid, as end product, increases, the urinary excretion of ammonia also increases; on the contrary, when base or base forming foodstuffs are ingested, the production of ammonia diminishes. The principal precursor of urinary ammonia seem to be glutamic acid and its amide, glutamine. The conversion of glutamine into NH_3 increases with the degree of acidosis. Glycerine, D-L-alaine, L-leucine, and D-L-aspartic acid can also increase renal production of ammonia. The capacity of an amino acid to increase the formation of ammonia by the kidney is related to the facility with which it is deaminated by renal enzymes *in vitro* and to the readiness with which it is reabsorbed by the renal tubes.

Tables 30.2: Tubular secretion

i. Physiologically - H^+, NH_4^+, K^+
ii. Foreign substances—exogenous creatinine, phenol red, diodrast, penicillin, PAH (plasma clearance—700 ml/minute/1.8 sq.m., extraction rate—90%)
iii. Aglomerular kidney can secrete water, urea, uric acid, creatinine, Mg^{++}, K^+, Cl^-, SO_4^-.

SOME GENERAL CONSIDERATIONS: GOING THROUGH

1. **Secretion.** It is the transport of solutes from peritubular capillaries into the lumen of tubules. So it adds to glomerular filtrate.
2. **Filtered load.** GFR × plasma concentration of solute
   = ml/minute × mg/ml
   = mg/minute
   'It is the amount of solute transported across the glomerular membranes per unit time.'
3. **Reabsorption.**
   a. It means removal of a substance from the filtrate; OR; active transport of solutes and passive movement of water from tubular lumen into peritubular capillaries.
   b. ***Transport maximum (Tm).*** Highest attainable rate of reabsorption; OR; it refers to maximal amount to a given solute that can be transported (reabsorbed or secreted) per minute by renal tubules. For glucose it is 320 mg per cent.
   c. ***Threshold.*** It is the plasma concentration at which a solute begins to appear in urine. For glucose it is 220 mg per cent. It is to be noted that threshold of a substance reaches before Tm is reached. Since all nephrons are not having the same transport maximum for the same substance (e.g. glucose). So some of the nephrons excrete glucose before others have reached their Tm.
   d. ***Maximum tubular reabsorptive capacity (Tr).*** It is the highest attainable rate of reabsorption.
4. **Clearance.** It is measure of the volume of plasma completely freed of a given substance per minute by the kidney: or: It is the volume of plasma (in ml) that contains the amount of the substance which is excreted in the urine, in one minute.
5. **Counter current system.** It is a system in which the inflow runs parallel to, counter to, and in close proximity to outflow for some distance. The loop of Henle consists of two parallel limbs with tubular fluid flowing in opposite direction.

ACIDIFICATION OF URINE: SECRETION OF HYDROGEN IONS

Secondary Active Secretion

- As sodium is carried to the interior of the cell hydrogen ions are forced outward in the opposite direction into tubular lumen. This is by sodium hydrogen-counter transport.
- This further explains that, 'energy liberated from down hill movement of sodium ions, enables uphill movement of a second substance in opposite direction.
- Some organic acids and bases (e.g. bile salts, oxalate, urate catecholamines, etc.) are secreted from proximal

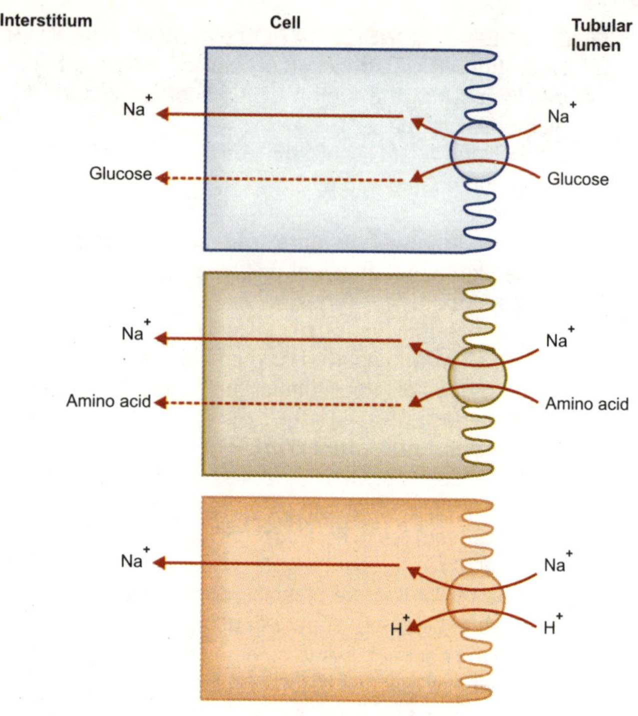

Fig. 30.3: Mechanism: Secondary active transport

tubules. These are end products of metabolism so must be removed.

- PAH (Para-amino-hippuric acid) is so rapidly secreted that normal person can clear about 90 per cent of it from plasma flowing through it and excrete it in urine.
- This explains its clearance can be used as an index of renal plasma flow.
- **Secondary active transport**
  - — $CO_2 + H_2O \xrightarrow{CA}$ Carbonic acid $\longrightarrow H^+ + HCO_3^-$
  - — Hydrogen ions are secreted into tubules by a mechanism of Na^+-H^+ counter transport
  - — This means, when a molecule of Na+ moves from lumen to tubular cell and thence to interstitium, it first combines with a carrier protein in luminal border of cell membrane. At the same time; a hydrogen ion combines at opposite pole of carrier protein. Then counter movement, i.e. movement in opposite direction takes place. Sodium moves towards the interstitium because concentration of sodium is much lower inside the cell than in lumen; and hydrogen ion moves in opposite direction by utilising same energy. Tremendous number of hydrogen ions are secreted in this manner.
- **Primary Active Transport: In late distal tubules**
  - — $CO_2 + H_2O \xrightarrow{CA} H_2CO_3 \longrightarrow H^+ + HCO_3^-$
  - — Now there at luminal side, Hydrogen ions are transported directly by a specific transport protein - Hydrogen transporting ATPase. The energy required is coming from breakdown of ATP to ADP.
  - — It amounts to be only less than 5 per cent of total hydrogen ion excreted.
  - — Here, the hydrogen ions are concentrated many times more as compared in proximal tubules.
  - — The dark or intercalated cells are responsible for H^+ secretion. They first appear in late distal tubules and then extend all the way.
- **Titration of H^+ and HCO_3^-**
  - — Normally 3.5 mmol/minute is the rate of H^+ secretion; while the rate of HCO_3^- secretion is very near/almost equal to it.... i.e. 3.46 mmol/minute. So both of them titrate each other. This very little excess of H^+ is because of metabolic effects.
- **Acidosis**
  - — In this state, the ratio of CO_2 to HCO_3^- in extra cellular fluid increases. So rate of H^+ secretion rises to more level than the rate of HCO_3^- secretion. So there are only few or less HCO_3^- to react with H^+ since diminished quantity of HCO_3^- enter the glomerular filtrate. The excess hydrogen ions are excreted in urine after combining with buffers in tubular fluid, to correct acidosis.
  - — With the formation of one H^+; one HCO_3^- is formed in tubular epithelial cell + a Na^+ is absorbed from tubule into epithelial cell. The Na^+ and HCO_3^- are both then transported from epithelial cell into extra cellular fluid. So by increasing bicarbonates in this way, acidosis is compensated.
- **Alkalosis: Role of kidney:**
  - — In this state, the ratio of bicarbonate ions to dissolved CO_2 molecules increase. Because almost no HCO_3^- can be reabsorbed without initially combining with H^+, so all excess HCO_3^- pass into urine carrying Na^+ with them. So $NaHCO_3$ is removed from extracellular fluid.

REABSORPTION OF CA^{2+} AND PHOSPHATE IONS

- Phosphate is reabsorbed by proximal tubule and the process is active; of course depressed by parathyroid hormone.
- Both are absorbed in such a way that normally about one-third of the filtered load reaches the urine.

BICARBONATE REABSORPTION

$$H_2O + CO_2 \xleftrightarrow{CA} H_2CO_3$$

$$H_2CO_3 \longleftrightarrow H^+ + HCO_3^-$$

H^+ are actively extruded in the lumen, where $NaHCO_3$ is abundant so-

$$NaHCO_3 + H^+ \longleftrightarrow Na^+ + H_2CO_3$$

$$H_2CO_3 \longrightarrow H_2O + CO_2$$

Water goes out as urine and CO_2 diffuses back into the cell. The Na^+ enters the cell (tubular) by passive diffusion and then actively pumped out into the peritubular fluid.

UREA-URIC ACID

- Proximal tubule is the site of reabsorption.
- Drug probenecid inhibits reabsorption.
- Only 10 per cent of the filtered load of uric acid is excreted. Uric acid stones are also found.
- Water reabsorption takes place in proximal tubule in great concentration. This leads to high concentration of urea in tubular fluid. This sets up a gradient between the tubular fluid and the peritubular fluid and so urea is reabsorbed.
- Urea is produced in the liver, as the end product of protein metabolism, and one of the functions of the kidney is to clear it from the body in the urine. Indeed plasma urea concentration is often used clinically in the assessment of renal function.

RE-ABSORPTION OF OTHER SOLUTES

- *Chlorides:*
  - — Transport of positively charged sodium ions out of the lumen leaves negative charge inside the lumen compared with interstitial fluid. This causes diffusion of chloride ions passively through paracellular pathway (between the cells).
  - — In lumen, chloride ions are also concentrated by water which is reabsorbed by osmosis. This leads to development of chloride concentration gradient which further helps in its reabsorption.
  - — The second half of proximal tubule has relatively high concentration of chloride (approximately 140 mEq/l) as compared with first part of it (105 mEq/l).
- **Creatinine:** It is a large molecule than urea. So the amount filtered by glomeruli is not reabsorbed and so excreted in urine.

THE PLASMA CLEARANCE: CONCEPT

- It is ability of kidneys to clear/clean, the plasma of various substances, e.g. if in plasma, a substance is having its concentration as 1 gm per cent and this quantity passes in urine, then plasma is said to be cleared of this substance.

So it can be calculated as:

$$\text{Plasma clearance (ml./minute)} = \frac{\text{Urine flow ml./minute} \times \text{concentration in urine}}{\text{concentration in plasma}}$$

UREA CLEARANCE: A MEASURE/CONCEPT

- Clearance means to clear or clean the plasma of various substances.
- For example—if the plasma passing through the kidneys contain 0.1 gm of substance in each decilitre, and 0.1 gm of this substance also passes in the urine per minute; then 1 decilitre of plasma is cleaned/cleared of this substance per minute.
- Now this rule is applied to urea. Suppose the normal concentration of urea in each ml of plasma and glomerular filtrate is 0.26 mg. Quantity of urea in

  = urine/mt. is 18.2 mgm. So $\frac{18.2}{0.26} = 70\ \frac{1820}{26}$ ml/mt.

  It means 70 ml of plasma is cleaned/cleared of urea each minute.

PLASMA CLEARANCES OF USUAL URINE CONSTITUENTS

Name	*Glomerular filtrate*	*Urine (1 ml/mt)*		*Plasma clearance per minute*	
	Qty/mt	*Con.*	*Qty /mt*	*Con.*	
Urea	33	26	18.2	1820	70
Inulin	—	—	—	—	125
PAH	—	—	—	—	585

Inulin clearance : A concept

- It is of small enough molecular weight (5200). It passes through glomerular membrane as freely as crystalloids and water of plasma. Since it is neither reabsorbed nor secreted, hence all the glomerular filtrate so formed is cleared of inulin. So plasma clearance of inulin per minute is equal to GFR.
- Inulin concentration in plasma is 0.001 gm in each decilitre and 0.125 gm of it passes into urine per minute. So by dividing $\frac{0.125}{0.001}$ = 125 ml/mt. So by

measuring plasma clearance of inulin normal GFR can be determined.

- **Tubular load** of a substance is the total amount of the substance that filters through glomerular membrane into the tubules each minute, e.g. 1.25 ml of glomerular filtrate is formed per minute with a glucose concentration of 100 mg per cent; then tubular load of glucose is 100 × 1.25 = 125 mg glucose per minute.
- For most actively reabsorbed substances there is a maximum rate at which each can be re-absorbed, this is called 'tubular transport maximum (Tm).

Tm for secretion

—Creatinine = 16 mg per minute

—PAH = 80 mg per minute

HORMONAL REGULATION OF REABSORPTION

i. ***ADH*** Is manufactured by cells of hypothalamus (paraventricular nucleus) and is released from posterior pituitary -
   - Its secretion is stimulated by (a) Increased osmolarity in extracellular fluid which is detected by osmoreceptors within the hypothalamus; (b) decreased circulating blood volume detected by cardiovascular volume receptors; (c) decreased arterial blood pressure as detected by baro-receptors.
   - It increases water permeability in the collecting ducts and the distal convoluted tubules. It promotes the reabsorption of water under the influence of high medullary osmolarity and so increases the extracellular fluid volume while reducing its osmolarity.
   - Through direct vasoconstriction it helps to elevate arterial blood pressure (so name - vasopressin).

ii. *Renin-angiotensin—aldosterone system*:
   - JG apparatus releases renin which is activated by decrease in afferent arteriolar pressure, reduction in filtered Na^+ load and stimulation of renal sympathetic nerves.
   - Renin catalyses the conversion of plasma precursor protein angiotensinogen into angiotensin I which is further converted into angiotensin II by converting enzyme on the surface of vascular endothelium.
   - Angiotensin II promotes the release of alodsterone from adrenal cortex, which in turn, stimulates reabsorption of Na^+ and water from distal convoluted tubule and cortical collecting ducts leading to increased extracellular fluid volume and arterial blood pressure.
   - Other actions of angiotensin II are:
     a. Stimulation of arteriolar vasoconstriction
     b. Promotes ADH release
     c. Promotes drinking so increasing ECF volume. Aldosterone also acts by stimulating sodium-potassium ATPase pump on basolateral side of cortical collecting tubule membrane. It also increases sodium permeability of luminal side of membrane.

iii. ***Some other hormones contributing***
   - Parathyroid hormone is an important calcium regulating hormone. It increases tubular reabsorption of calcium in thick ascending loop of Henle and distal tubule. It also inhibits phosphate reabsorption by proximal tubule; of course magnesium reabsorption is stimulated through loop of Henle.
   - Increased blood volume → distension of cardiac atria → secretion of atrial-natriuretic-peptide (ANP) → inhibition of reabsorption of sodium and water by renal tubules and collecting ducts → increased amount of urine → decreased/normal blood volume.
   - Activation of sympathetics → constriction of both afferent and efferent arterioles → decreased GFR → decrease in sodium and water excretion. On sympathetic stimulation renin-angiotensin system is activated which promotes tubular reabsorption and decrease renal excretion of sodium.
   - Angiotensin specialities:
     —It stimulates secretion
     —It constricts efferent arteriole → reduction in peritubular capillary hydrostatic pressure → increases in tubular reabsorption from proximal tubules.
     —Constriction of efferent arteriole → reduction in renal blood flow → rise in filtration fraction in glomerulus → increased colloid osmotic pressure in peritubular capillaries → rise in reabsorption of sodium and water.
     —It directly stimulates sodium reabsorption via sodium potassium ATPase pump and sodium hydrogen exchange.

SUMMARY AND HIGHLIGHTS

- The tubular load of a substance is the total amount of a substance that filters through the glomerular membrane into the tubules each minute.
- Glucose is reabsorbed almost exclusively in the proximal tube; (first half). It is an example of secondary active transport and the energy is provided by Na^+-K^+-ATPase that pumps the Na^+ out of the cell.
- The water reabsorbed in the proximal segment is obligatory water reabsorption. In the distal tubule Facultative water reabsorption occurs and is regulated by ADH, which increases the permeability of the distal tubule to water. The tubular fluid leaving the proximal tubule is isotonic, in the collecting ducts, the reabsorption of hyperosmotic fluid takes place.

BIBLIOGRAPHY

1. Aronson PS. "The renal proximal tubule : A model for diversity of anion exchangers and stilbene sensitive anion transporters." Ann Rev Phy 1989;51:419.
2. Aukland K, et al. "Renal cortical interstitium and fluid absorption by peritubular capillaries." Amer J Phy 1994;266:F175.
3. Berry CA. "Heterogenecity of tubular transport process in nephron." Ann Rev Phy 1982;44:181.
4. Blaustein MP, Hamlyn JM. Sodium transport Inhibition, cell Ca^{2+} and hypertension. The Natriuretic Hormone/Na^+-Ca^{2+} exchange hypertension hypothesis." Amer J Med 1984;77:45.
5. Brenner BM, Humes HD. "Mechanics of glomerular ultra filtration." New Eng J Med 1977;148:277.
6. Breyer MD, et al. "Hormonal signalling and regulation of salt and water transport in collecting duct." Ann Rev Phy 1994;56:711.
7. Davis JO, Freeman RH. "Mechanism regulating renin release." Phy Rev 1976;56:1.
8. Gregor R. "In transport mechanism in thick ascending limb of Henle's loop of mammalian nephron." Phy Rev 1985;65:760.
9. Hall JE. "Control of sodium excretion by angiotensin : Intra renal mechanism and BP regulation." Amer J Phy 1986;250:R 960.
10. Navar LG. "Renal auto regulation : Perspectives from whole kidney and single nephron studies." Amer J Phy 1978;234:F 357.

31 Formation of Urine-III

DILUTE URINE: BASIC RENAL MECHANISM

- The glomerular filtrate which is recently formed is having same osmolarity as plasma (i.e. 300 mOsm/L)
- In proximal tubule solutes and water are reabsorbed in equal proportion. It means that fluid of proximal tubule remains iso-osmotic to the plasma (i.e. 300 mOsm/L).
- Next, in descending loop of Henle, by the process of osmosis water is reabsorbed. This approaches tubular fluid in the same concentration as the interstitial fluid of renal medulla which is - hypertonic (4 times more osmolarity of original glomerular filtrate).
- In thick segment of loop of Henle solutes (Na, K, Cl) are actively reabsorbed but this portion of nephron is impermeable to water. This makes the tubular fluid more dilute (hypo-osmotic-osmolarity reduced to one-third of plasma).
- In distal/cortical/collecting duct further NaCl reabsorption occurs with impermeability towards water so tubular fluid becomes more dilute.

Hairpin Counter Current Multiplier System (Wirz et al), (Concentrating the Urine)

Necessity

Sometimes as in deserts, the body needs conservation of water because of inadequate supply of water.

Peculiarities/special anatomy: The loop of Henle of one-third to one-fifth of the nephronsdip deep into medulla and then return to the cortex; some dip to the tips of papillae that project into renal pelvis. This group of nephrons with long Henle loop is called juxtamedullary nephrons.

Loop of Henle

a. Thick descending segment- is direct continuation of proximal tubules having diameter of 55μ and length of 6 mm having brush border cuboidal epithelium.
b. Then is its thin descending segment → hairpin bend of the loop → followed by thin ascending segment which is continued as thick ascending segment. These cells are lined by flattened epithelial cells without brush border → this ascends to renal cortex to form distal convoluted tubule which is 9 mm long with a diameter of 30μ. It's lined by cuboidal epithelium without brush border.

Hairpin Counter Current Multiplier System—Hyperosmolarity of Medullary Fluid

- In order to manufacture concentrated urine, there is necessity to create a very high osmotic pressure (hyperosmolarity) of medullary interstitial fluid.
- Normal osmolarity of body fluid is 300 mOsm/litre. As one goes deeper into medulla, this osmolarity may increase as high as 1,200-1,400 mOsm/litre. This is achieved by
  i. Active transport of sodium ions along with co-transport of chloride, potassium, etc. from thick portion of ascending limb of loop of Henle into interstitium. These ions are carried downwards into inner medulla by downward flowing blood in descending limb of vasa recta + diffusion into descending thin limb.
  ii. From collecting duct, small quantity of ions are also transported into medullary interstitial fluid. It is because of active transport of sodium and passive absorption of chloride ions along with sodium ions (electrogenic).
  iii. Role of ADH: It increases permeability of inner medullary portion of collecting duct. It also makes inner medullary collecting duct highly permeable towards water. All this increases urea concentration in medullary interstitial fluid (400–500 mOsm/litre).

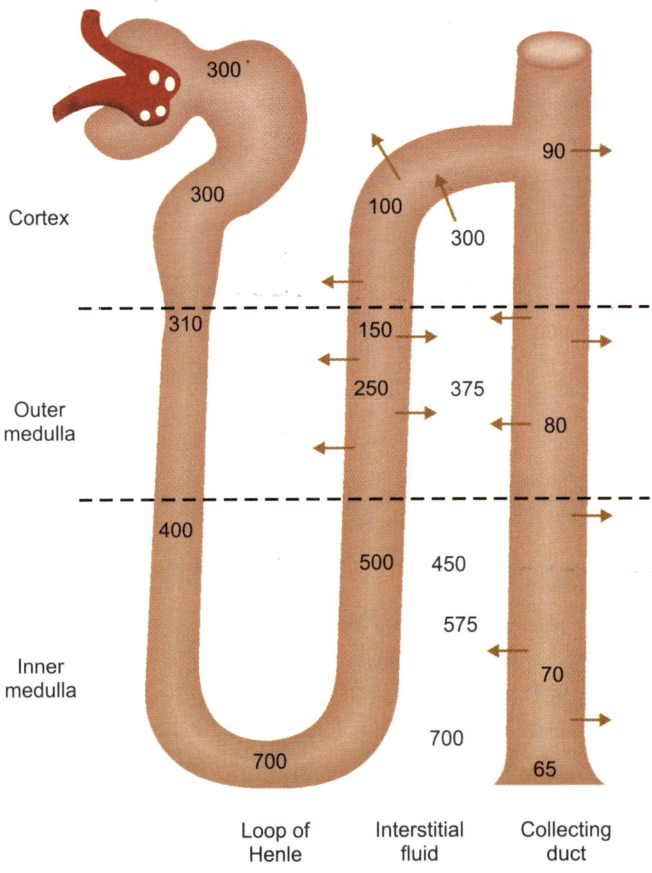

Fig. 31.1: Mechanism—Dilute urine

- ADH activation of adenylcyclase → cAMP in cell cytoplasm → this is diffused to luminal side of cell → formation of elongated vesicular structures in cytoplasm which fuse with luminal membrane, which becomes permeable for water. When no ADH these vesicles detach from this luminal membrane and return to internal position in cytoplasm making it again water impermeable.

Hairpin Counter Current Multiplier System—Justifying Name

- Sodium and other ions from thick ascending loop of Henle are transported into medullary interstitium. Its majority further diffuses into descending limb of vasa recta and descending thin Henle's loop. This NaCl is then carried to tip of papillae which further increases osmolarity.
- Remaining NaCl is carried back to ascending loop of Henle, where it is retransported by thick ascending segment to papillary interstitium.
- This repetitive reabsorption of NaCl by thick ascending loop of Henle (counter current) + continual inflow of new NaCl from proximal tubule into loop of Henle (multiplier) is the justification of name of the process.

Hairpin Counter Current Multiplier System—Vasa Recta: Counter Current Exchange Mechanism

- Inner medullary blood flow is very slight/sluggish (1-2% of total renal flow). This minimises removal of solutes.
- This is U shaped structure and both the arms of U are lying close to each other. This arrangement is done for easy exchange of fluid and solutes between two arms and both the arms are highly permeable to complete this function.
- All above arrangements have been made by the Nature to keep medullary fluid concentrated and for this, medullary solutes should not be removed. This is achieved by following illustration:
  - As blood flows in descending limb of vasa recta; certainly Na^+, Cl^- and urea diffuse from interstitial fluid into blood, and water diffuses into interstitium.
  - This raises the osmolar concentration of blood (up to 1200/1400 mOsm/litre)
  - Then as blood flows back in ascending limb, all extra molecules of Na^+, Cl^- and urea are diffused back into interstitial fluid from blood, while water diffuses back into the blood.
  - This concludes that blood flowing through vasa recta carries only minute amount of medullary interstitial solutes away form medulla.

Hairpin Counter Current Multiplier System—Overview

- Is the mechanism through which urine becomes hypertonic in relation to body fluids.
- Loop of Henle along with blood vessels passes from corticomedullary junction to the medulla and again return towards the cortex and thus stimulate this mechanism.
- Sodium and chloride from the fluid in ascending limb of loop of Henle are transferred into interstitial fluid. So tubular fluid is diluted causing rise in osmotic pressure of interstitial fluid.
- In distal tubule water is further reabsorbed due to ADH. This reduces the fluid volume and leads into collecting tubule in medulla and get same osmotic pressure as blood. The osmotic pressure of interstitial fluid is high. Due to ADH it becomes permeable to water and some part of water is reabsorbed. This

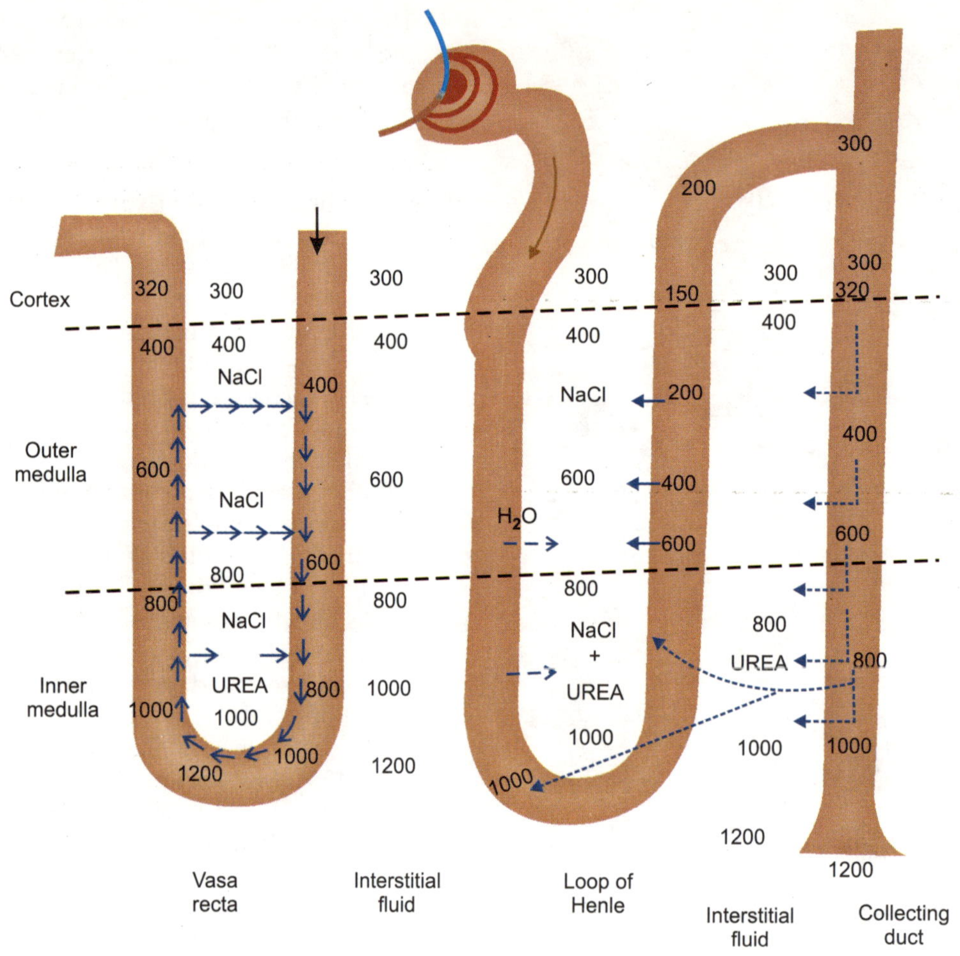

Fig. 31.2: Counter current mechanism (Urine concentration)

raises osmotic pressure of tubular fluid. It becomes same as interstitial fluid and urine becomes hypertonic.

- The excess of solute transferred from tubule is retained in medullary interstitial fluid for some time which is due to this mechanism. The outflowing blood loses the solute whereas inflowing blood takes up solute. Due to loop arrangement there is transfer of sodium salts from ascending limb although there is a low concentration gradient. There is high concentration gradient in interstitial fluid.
- This is called counter current multiplier system as low concentration gradient from tubule to interstitial fluid is multiplied in a longitudinal axis, i.e. from cortex to papillae.

Hairpin Counter Current Multiplier System—Highlights

- The nature of mechanism by which urine is rendered hypertonic to the body fluid is more complex part of renal physiology. Its essentials are more or less anatomical.
- The convoluted tubules are cortical structure; loop of Henle and collecting duct lie in medulla. The blood supply of medulla and papilla forms a loop like system derived from efferent. Vessels of juxtamedullary glomeruli running down into medulla and looping back to the cortex. Thus, both loop of Henle and blood supply of the medullary region form counter current system in which outflowing fluid flows counter to/ and in proximity to inflowing fluid.

PROCESS OF URINE FORMATION : AN OVERVIEW

Nature/Process	*Site*	*Activity*
Ultrafiltration	Renal/malpighian corpuscles	Nonselective filtration on the basis of hydrostatic pressure. A filtrate is formed. GFR is 125 ml/mt normally.
Re-absorption	Proximal convoluted tubule	Re-absorption of water, glucose, amino acid into blood
	Descending limb-loop of Henle	Passive process of water re-absorption
	Ascending limb- loop of Henle	Re-absorption of urea, Na^+, Cl^-
	Distal convoluted tubule	Re-absorption of water under influence of ADH; also of Na^+, Cl^-, HCO_3^-
	Collecting tubules	Water re-absorption under ADH effect
Tubular secretion	Distal tubules to a great extent	PAH, potassium NH_4^+, H^+, etc.

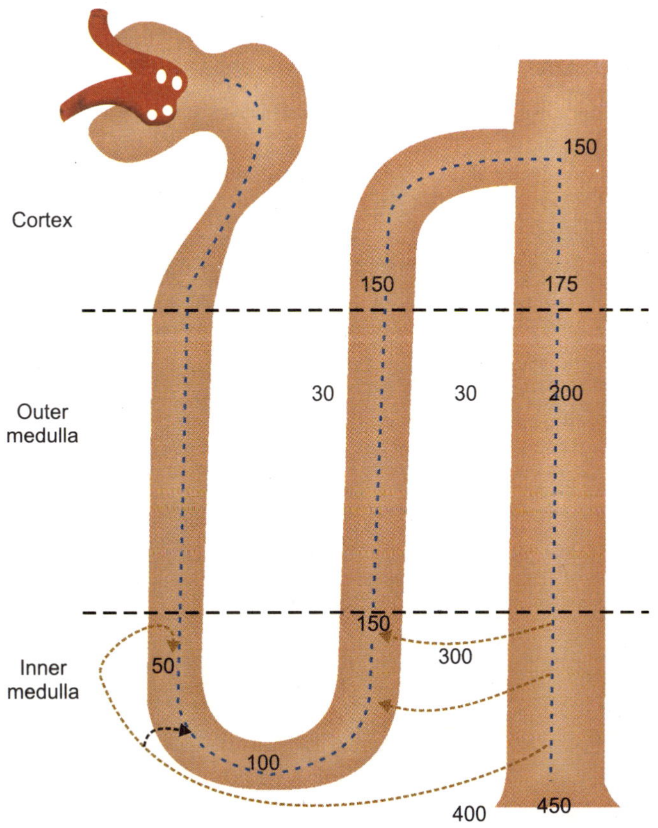

Fig. 31.3: Recirculation of urea

- A counter current system is a system in which the inflow runs parallel to, counter to and in close proximity to outflow for some distance. This occurs for both—the loop of Henle and vasa recta in the renal medulla.

BIBLIOGRAPHY

1. Woeff SD, et al. Regulation of predominant renal medullary organic solutes. Ann Rev Phy 1990;52:727.
2. Young DB, et al. Control of extra cellular calcium concentration by ADH thirst feedback mechanism. Amer J Phy 1977;232:R 145.
3. Young DB, et al. Effectiveness of aldosterone sodium and potassium feedback control system. Amer J Phy 1976;231:945.

THEME OF COUNTER CURRENT MULTIPLIER SYSTEM

1. The fluid entering the proximal tubule is iso-osmotic (300 mosmol). Fluid that enters the descending thin limb of Henle's loop is also hence iso-osmotic with rest of the plasma.
2. The descending thin limb is highly permeable to water and much less to NaCl and urea. As fluid flows deeper into hyperosmotic medulla, water is reabsorbed. So at hairpin turn its osmolality is equal to that of surrounding interstitial fluid (1,200 or 1,400 mosmol). The urea concentration of tubular fluid also increases because of two reasons; (a) Water is reabsorbed from tubular fluid; (b) Urea diffuses into descending thin limb from medullary interstitium (urea recycling).
3. The ascending thin limb is impermeable to water but highly permeable to NaCl. As NaCl rich tubular fluid moves up the ascending thin limb, NaCl diffuses passively into medullary interstitium (osmolality of NaCl of interstitial fluid is 600 mosmol while osmolality of NaCl in tubular fluid which enters ascending thin limb is 1000 mosmol).
4. Since ascending thin limb is permeable to urea, it diffuses from medullary interstitium into the tubular lumen (urea recycling).
5. The thick ascending limb of Henle's loop is impermeable to water. Tubular fluid is further diluted by active reabsorption of NaCl by this segment of nephron. Dilution occurs up to the extent that fluid leaving thick ascending limb is hypo-osmotic with respect to plasma (100 mosmol). ADH acts here.
6. So, fluid reaching the collecting duct is hypoosmotic with respect to surrounding interstitial fluid so in the presence of ADH water diffuses out of the tubular lumen— beginning of process of urine concentration. The maximum osmolality that the fluid in cortical collecting duct can attain is 300 mosmol.
7. As fluid in collecting duct continues through medulla, water is reabsorbed. This increases osmolality and mainly through urea. Permeability is increased by ADH. Because the urea concentration of the tubular fluid is increased by water reabsorption, some urea diffuses out of tubule lumen and into medullary interstitium.
8. The urine has an osmolality of 1,200 mosmol. It contains urea, and non-reabsorbed solutes. Because urea in tubular fluid tends to equilibrate with the interstitial urea, its concentration in urine does not exceed that of interstitium (600 mosmol). The high NaCl concentration of interstitium drives additional water reabsorption, concentrating the other non-reabsorbed solutes in tubular fluid.

Source:

1. Jamison RL, et al (1976). The urinary concentrating mechanism. New Eng J Med 295:1059.
2. Knepper MA, et al. The vasopressin regulated urea transporter in renal medullary collecting duct. (1990). Amer. J. Phy. 259: F393.

(1) and (2) quoted by Berne RM, Levy MN Physiology - Mosby year book, Third Edition.

32 Micturition

INTRODUCTION

a. Urine formed in the kidney passes out of the orifices of cribriform area into the renal calyces and pelvis. It then descends along the ureter to the bladder, where it accumulates. Periodically the bladder is emptied by the act of micturition.

b. The bladder is a muscular organ capable of changing its capacity tremendously by virtue of alteration in the tonus of its smooth muscle fibres. These are arranged in three layers. The external layer which runs longitudinally from fundus to the neck has been called detrusor-urinae but since expulsion of urine is accomplished by contraction of all layers, it is more applied to entire musculature. The urethral orifice is guarded by an internal sphincter of smooth muscle and is surrounded in urethra by striated muscle which functions as an external sphincter. Both of these sphincters are normally in a state of tonic contraction.
   - The bladder, prostatic and membranous segment of urethra are one functional unit, the object of which is (i) the accumulation in bladder of urine coming from the kidney and (ii), its periodic evacuation.

c. Urine collected in pelvis of kidney passes through the ureters to the bladder by virtue of contractions of its external and internal muscular layers. Contraction wave begin at the pelvic end and spread over the ureter with a velocity of about 20–30 mm per second thereby driving the urine ahead. The frequency of contractions varies with the rate of urine secretion into pelvis, but it is ordinarily given as occurring at intervals of ten to twenty seconds. Peristaltic waves are myogenic in origin. The upper portions of the ureter are innervated by the splanchnic nerves via the renal plexus; the lower structures via hypogastric plexus. These nerves apparently contain excitatory fibres which reflexly modify the irritability of ureters and so affect the rhythmicity and vigor of contraction. Inhibitory fibres have been described in the inferior mesenteric plexus, and sensory fibres are doubtless present, as evidenced by excruciating pain developed when calculi obstruct the free passage of urine. These peristaltic waves recur with a frequency of one to five per minute in man.

Table 32.1: During urination

1. Relaxation of sphincter which allows a few drops of urine to enter neck of urethra to create a powerful reflex.
2. Contraction of detrusor muscle at the same time.
3. Usually assistance by contraction of the abdominal muscle.
4. The striated (compressor urethrae) muscle expells last drops of urine from urethra.

BLADDER INNERVATION

- Double innervation, i.e. (a) Parasympathetic pelvic nerves, (b) sympathetic hypogastric nerves and (c) Pudic nerve.
- There are two important functions of hypogastric (sympathetic innervation), i.e. (i) they are important in maintaining the tone of internal sphincter during filling of bladder; (ii) they are solely concerned with vasomotor and sexual functions not with bladder function.
- Parasympathetic nerves coming from pelvic nerves (nervi-erigentes). Its stimulation causes contraction of bladder muscle (detrusor urinae) and relaxes internal sphincter. Both those actions serve to empty the bladder. Acetylcholine has the same effect.
- Afferent impulses from bladder are conducted almost exclusively by fibres in pelvic nerve. These fibres enter the spinal cord by the dorsal roots of S_2 and S_3. The fibres that conduct painful impulses enter the spinal cord in the dorsal roots of upper two or three lumbar nerves.

- The pudic nerves innervate the external sphincter. They come from the upper three sacral nerves. They also carry the afferent fibres from urethra.

FILLING OF BLADDER

i. The ureters enter the base of the bladder obliquely, forming a valvular flap which passively prevents reflux of urine. Urine is propelled into bladder by rhythmic peristaltic contractions of the ureters, gradually filling it. The bladder muscle in the same way as the muscular coat of other hollow viscera, can adapt its capacity to the contents without any considerable change in the intravesical pressure.

ii. A considerable amount of fluid 400 ml can be accommodated by stretching the bladder without significant rise of pressure, but as the volume progressively extends/exceeds this amount, the tension rises (up to 30 cm H_2O) due to tonic contraction of bladder musculature. In addition, detrusor muscles start contracting rhythmically, about 3 to 6 times per minute. When vesicular tension has reached a threshold level of about 18 cm. H_2O, stretch and tension receptors are excited, which create afferent impulses responsible for sensation of distension and desire to urinate. With filling to 600–800 ml powerful rhythmic contractions occur which are accompanied by painful sensation. These can be suppressed voluntarily until vesicular pressure has increased approximately to 100 cm of H_2O; above such pressure involuntary micturition follows.

MICTURITION: STRUCTURAL BEAUTY

1. Ureter penetrates the bladder obliquely through trigone. The ureter courses several centimetres under the bladder epithelium. When pressure rises in bladder due to any reason, ureter is compressed. This prevents backflow of urine whenever pressure is increased in the bladder.
2. When ureteric stone blocks it, reflex constriction is the result; of course it is associated with pain. This sympathetic reflex is reaching to the kidney which causes constriction of renal arterioles; which results into decrease in urinary output. This is named as "uretero-renal-reflex." Its purpose is to prevent excessive flow of fluid into renal pelvis when ureter is blocked.

THE MICTURITION

i. During micturition the detrusor contracts, the internal sphincter is relaxed and urine is evacuated with considerable force; the pressure within the bladder can rise up to 130 cm H_2O. Micturition is usually preceded by contraction of abdominal muscles and a slight expiratory effort with the glottis closed. Abdominal contraction can be sustained throughout the act to accelerate evacuation. In the male, the bulbocavernous muscle contracts rhythmically at the end of micturition, and thus the last drops of urine in the urethra are expelled (Piston stroke). In the female, micturition ends more abruptly.

ii. It is a reflex act, but normally it is commenced voluntarily. When its desire is felt, evacuation is prevented or performed voluntarily. In the first case, voluntary contraction of external sphincter reinforces the effect of internal sphincter and there is reciprocal relaxation of detrusor, the intravesicle pressure diminishes and desire to micturate ceases for the time being. The desire to evacuate the bladder can be voluntarily overcome as long as bladder contents are less than 700 c.c., there is then a painful sensation in hypogastrium and urgent need to evacuate. When desire to micturate is complied with, the voluntary contraction of external sphincter is inhibited, and a chain of reflexes commences which results in emptying of bladder.

iii. Before 18 months, the act is wholly automatic. Between 18 months and 3 years child develops bladder sensation and will signify desire to void but cannot control detrusor muscle. The bladder smooth muscles present two types of contractions waves - isotonic (bladder contents at constant pressure) and isometric (bladder contents at constant volume).

Table 32.2: Physiologic status of micturition

Condition	*Volume in bladder*
• First sensation of bladder filling at	100–150 ml
• First desire to void occurs at	150–250 ml
• The maximal intravesicle volume that can be tolerated without undue discomfort and at which micturition is effected normally.	250–450 ml

Table 32.3: Normal micturition

Sensation of bladder fullness → higher centre inhibition → pelvic floor, bladder neck or urethra relax → detrusor contracts to raise intravesicle pressure + contraction of anterior abdominal wall → bladder empties

Post voiding → if bladder empty → pelvic floor + intrinsic urethral sphincter contract to milk urine into bladder from proximal urethra → abdominal wall relaxes → inhibition of micturition returns.

EMOTIONS V/S MICTURITION

Due to anxiety or excitement, the ability of detrusor to relax is reduced and desire for micturition is developed even when the bladder contains only small quantities of urine. Therefore, frequency of urination develops.

PREGNANCY V/S MICTURITION

It causes loss of tone of detrusor muscle. So pressure in bladder remains low even when volume of urine within it is high. So during micturition act, bladder is not emptied completely and residual urine is always left which becomes the cause of urinary tract infection.

CLINICAL PHYSIOLOGY

a. ***Atonic bladder***: If sensory nerves fibres from bladder to spinal cord are destroyed; then transmission of stretch signals from bladder is inhibited and so prevents micturition reflex contractions. So bladder fills to its utmost capacity and overflows a few-drops through urethra. This is overflow dribbling—or outflow incontinence. It should be noted that this occurs inspite of presence/intact efferent connections between brain/spinal cord and bladder. It is seen in tabes dorsalis (tabetic bladder).
b. ***Automatic bladder***: If spinal cord is damaged above sacral region but sacral segments are still intact then typical micturition reflexes occur. The bladder loses tone and fails to response on spinal shock and no response of micturition reflex, so urine overflows by dribbling when bladder is full. During recovery stage of shock, when bladder is filled then it automatically evacuates since voluntary control is lost. This may be due to loss of control by higher centres.
c. ***Nocturnal micturition (enuresis, bed wetting)***: Commonly occurring in children below three years or in infants. Due to incomplete myelinisation of nerve fibres of bladder (motor) this lack of control occurs. Other causes include—psychogenic, lumbosacral vertebral defects—a neurological disorder, impairment of motor area of cerebral cortex.
d. ***Uninhibited-Neurogenic bladder***: It is due to lack of inhibitory signal from brain. That part of spinal cord or brainstem is damaged which interrupts most of the inhibitory signals. So "facilitatory signals" are continuously exciting the sacral centres so that even a small quantity of urine will elicit an uncontrolled micturition reflex. Spinal micturition centres are excited by higher centres because of lesion in some part of brainstem. This results into uncontrolled micturition. Frequency of micturition increases, i.e. small collection of urine collected in bladder will elicit micturition reflex.

Notes

Voluntary Urination

— Some muscular movements which are not essential for micturition, accompany the act. At the onset, the levator ani and perineal muscles are relaxed which decrease urethral resistance; glottis closed, diaphragm descends and abdominal wall muscles contracts, which accelerate the flow of urine by increasing intravesical pressure.

— Physiological capacity of bladder at birth—20 to 50 ml increasing four times during first year of life. In adult it can be as high as 600 ml specially in those persons who find lavatory facility difficult.

— Arrest of voiding stream, once initiated, is accomplished by powerful voluntary contraction of external sphincter and perineal muscle, and is associated with a sense of burning and urgency due to stimulation of somatic afferents in the region of membranous urethra. If contraction is sustained, urine is forced backwards into the bladder by collapse of posterior urethra, associated with gradual relaxation of the detrusor muscle.

CENTRES FOR MICTURITION

1. A spinal centre for micturition exists in 2nd, 3rd and 4th segments of spinal cord.
   Visceral afferent impulse from stretch receptors in bladder wall excited $\xrightarrow{\textit{pelvic nerves}}$ micturition centre $\xrightarrow{\textit{efferents via pelvic nerve}}$ contraction of detrusor muscle → urine is forced into posterior urethra → inhibitory signals to anterior horn cells of S_{2-4} → decreased frequency of impulse in pudendal nerve → relaxation of external sphincter.
2. Brainstem centre is located in pons. It exerts both facilitatory and inhibitory effects of spinal centre. It also inhibits spinal micturition reflex at an unconscious level, even when the bladder is filled. It is responsible for sustaining contraction of detrusor muscle and relaxation of external sphincter until the bladder is completely emptied.
3. In cerebral cortex, extreme medial aspect of sensory motor strip (para central lobule) is the area where intra vesicle changes are felt. By this centre one can feel degree of fullness of bladder, slight burning on

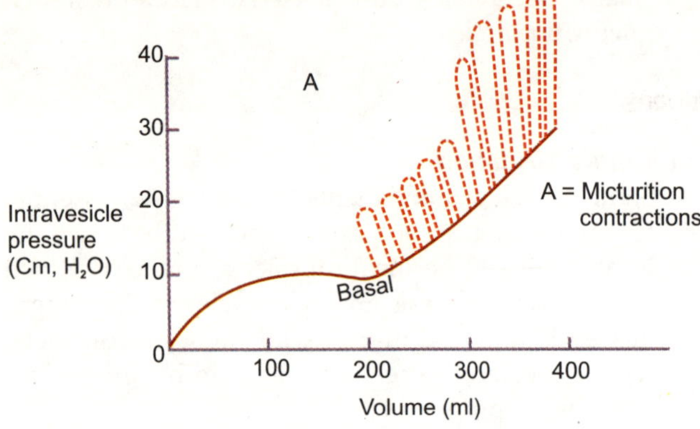

Fig. 32.1: Normal cystometrogram

initiation of voiding, pain of vesicle spasm, etc. It has following main functions.

- Cortex inhibits above mentioned lower centres until a suitable time and place is found for passing the urine.
- It can also induce a desire to void if it is interrupted once.

CYSTOMETROGRAM

It is the technique for demonstrating the relation between intravesical pressure and volume of urine in bladder. Pressure within the bladder is intravesical pressure. Graphical recording of pressure changes is cystometrogram.

Description

a. Segment/Presentation I
   Empty bladder, intravesical pressure is O, when 100 ml fluid is collected - 10 cm. H_2O pressure rises.
b. Segment/Presentation II
   Characterised by plateau. The amount of fluid collected in bladder is 300–400 ml, the pressure is 10 cms H_2O so no increase, which is because of adaptation by bladder through relaxation (Laplace law).
c. Segment/presentation III → Pressure increases with collection of 300–400 ml fluid, consciousness and urge for micturition begins due to detrusor muscle contraction. Voluntary control is possible up to 600–700 ml of urine and beyond which voluntary control lost (at 40 cm H_2O pressure with feeling of pain sensation).

33 Assessing Kidney-I: The Urine

PHYSICAL

i. ***Amount:*** Daily excretion for adult man on ordinary mixed diet is 1000–1800 ml.

Two-third to three-fourth is excreted during the day and the rest during the night. Children excrete three to four times more urine per kg of body weight than adults.

Factors affecting the amount are

a. Diet: A protein diet increases the amount of urea excreted and therefore the total volume of urine. In fasting less urine is excreted.

b. The environmental temperature: A high temperature that provokes sweating diminishes the amount of urine formed.

c. Body posture: The urinary volume increases in the horizontal position.

ii. ***Reaction***: pH of normal urine lies between 5.0 to 7.0, with a mean of 6.0 to 6.8. The extreme values of urinary pH are 4.8 and 8.2. This is due to the end products of protein metabolism, which give several acids on oxidation.

iii. ***Specific gravity***: Varies between 1.010 to 1.025 or 1.015 to 1.020, but can be 1.002 when large quantity of urine are excreted and 1.040 when volume is small. It is lowered in some forms of renal diseases, when excess of fluid being excreted and in diabetes-insipidus. In severe renal inefficiency it remains constant at 1.010.

Table 33.1: Urine—causes of increased amount (polyurea)

1. Increased intake of fluids
2. Nervous influences—emotions, excitement
3. Increased blood pressure due to increased force of heart beat
4. Presence of osmotically active substances within lumen of distal tubule, e.g. glucose, urea, mannitol, sodium chloride
5. Constriction of cutaneous arterioles (cold weather), leading to reflex dilatation of arterioles in splanchnic area and consequent rise of pressure in glomerular capillaries
6. Diabetes mellitus and insipidus, Hyperparathyroidism, Addison's disease, chronic glomerulonephritis.

Table 33.2: Urine—causes of diminished amount (Oligurea—Less than 500 ml)

1. Diminished intake of fluids
2. Low blood pressure, e.g. shock
3. Fevers and some type of renal diseases
4. Increased loss of fluids (Vomiting, diarrhoea, sweating)
5. Passive congestion of renal vessels by local compression, bilateral hydronephrosis
6. Diurnal variation—decreased during sleep, minimal values between 02.00–04.00 hours; maximal during first hour of rising and after meals. Findings reversed in night workers.

Table 33.3: Specific gravity variation

1. High specific gravity seen in excess sweating, glycosurea, acute nephritis, albuminurea and all cases of oligurea.
2. Low specific gravity is seen in excessive water intake, chronic nephritis, diabetes insipidus, etc. in all cases of polyurea except diabetes mellitus.
3. Low and fixed specific gravity (1.010–1.012) reflects failure of concentrating power of renal tubules or deficiency of ADH, e.g. chronic nephritis, arteriosclerotic kidney, diabetes insipidus, etc.

Table 33.4: Glycosurea—causes

1. Diabetes mellitus
2. Non-diabetic causes
   a. Glycosurea but no hyperglycaemia
   - Renal—low threshold; In advanced glomerulonephritis
   - Alimentary—after taking carbohydrates;

   b. Glycosurea with hyperglycaemia
   Hyperthyroidism, emotions, ether anaesthesia, infection or septic condition, increased intracranial pressure.

iv. *Others*
- Freezing point varies from 0.9 to 2.7°C (plasma is - 0.56°C).
- Colour is golden yellow, the intensity of which increases with the concentration.
- Odour is an aromatic one, and on standing it is ammoniacal. It is fruity/sweetish (ketone bodies), putrid (cystinurea, pus of cystitis), ammoniacal (bacterial action), faecal (recto-vesical-fistula).
- Urinometer is the instrument for determination of specific gravity.

CHEMICAL AS ORGANIC AND INORGANIC

1. ***Organic constituents:***
   a. *Urea:* Is the principal nitrogenous substance in urine. It is an end product of protein metabolism. Its normal values ranging between 25–40 gm daily. The greater part of urea excreted in urine is the result of metabolism of ingested proteins.
   b. *Uric acid:* Is a product of nucleo-protein metabolism. The exogenous uric acid varies with the diet while the endogenous comes from tissue destruction.
   c. *Creatinine:* Amount excreted is very constant in health and is roughly a measure of the muscle mass of an individual. Amount excreted is increased in fever and starvation owing to increased tissue breakdown.
   Creatine is a normal constituent of urine in children and of pregnant women. It is present in urine during involution of uterus, and not infrequently in normal adult urine. It is converted to creatinine on heating with acids. It is present as creatine phosphate in muscle. Creatinine is the anhydrous form of creatine. Ordinary muscular work does not increase the excretion of creatinine.
   d. *Hippuric acid:* Is formed in the body by the combination of benzoic acid (ingested with food) and glycine, which is split off from the proteins in food or synthesised in body. The daily excretion is 0.1 to 1 gm; it increases when the diet contains much fruits and vegetables.
   e. *Urinary indican (potassium - indoxysulphate):* Comes from the indole produced from tryptophane in the course of intestinal putrefaction.
2. ***Inorganic constituents:***
   a. *Chloride:* Chief source is NaCl of the food. Its normal daily excretion is 6 to 10 gm. Next to urea, chlorides are the most abundant urinary constituent, but in salt starvation and in pneumonia they may be absent.
   b. *Sulphates:* (Na, K, Ca, Mg) are produced exclusively by oxidation of sulphur containing amino acids - cysteine and methionene. A high protein diet will provoke an increase in urinary sulphate which is normally about 2 gm daily. Sulphur is present in urine in three forms—(a) Inorganic - 78–82 per cent (b) conjugated (ethereal) 4–7 per cent (c) Organic 15–20 per cent. As a result of putrefaction of tryptophane in large intestine - indole, skatole and phenol are formed. During absorption they combine with inorganic sulphates to form relatively harmless products which are excreted in the urine.
   c. *Phosphates (Na, K, Ca, Mg):* Total phosphates excreted daily in urine varies from 1 to 5 gm. This amount is dependent on the phosphorus containing substances ingested and on the elimination of Ca and Mg phosphates in the faeces. They have origin both as exogenous (phospho proteins of food) and endogenous (nucleoprotein).
   d. *Ammonia:* Its daily excretion is about 0.7 gm. Its amounts in urine is conditioned by the excess of acid over base excreted. An increase in acid formation (high protein diet, diabetic acidosis etc.) results in an increase in urinary ammonia.
   e. *Sodium - Potassium:* Their amount is dependent upon the diet. Normally 2 gm K and 4 gm. Na are eliminated daily. Small quantities of calcium (0.2 gm daily) and magnesium (0.15 gm daily) have been reported. Carbonates of food and vegetable acids (citric and tartaric acid) have been reported in urine of vegetarians.

ABNORMAL CONSTITUENTS OF URINE

a. *Proteins:* Chiefly albumin. Usually due to disease of cells of urinary tubule, so that proteins of plasma pass through them.
b. *Sugar:* Most frequently found is glucose or dextrose.
c. *Blood:* Urine is smoky red or black in colour. Identification of RBC under microscope may be done. In cases known as 'haemoglobin urea" as distinct from haematurea (blood in urine), corpuscles are not present. Benzidine test, spectroscopical examination and microscopical examination are available tests.
d. *Pus:* Pus cells may be seen under microscope.
e. *Bile:* Urine is dark green in colour. Tests for bile salt is Hay's sulphur test and for bile pigment is van den Bergh test.
f. *Acetone:* Acetone bodies consist of acetoacetic acid and β-hydroxybutyric acid and acetone; They are found in urine in condition of ketosis. Rother'a test is done for acetone.

Urinary Pigments

a. *Urochrome:* Principal pigment. It is a compound of urobilin or urobilinogen and a peptide.
b. *Urobilin:* Formed from haemoglobin. Of the 250 mg of bile pigment excreted daily, only 1–2 mg is excreted in urine. Its spectrum shows an absorption band in blue between E and F lines.
c. *Uro-Erythrin:* This gives a red colour to deposits of urates and uric acid.
d. *Coproporphyrin and Uroporphyrin:* Excreted in haematoporphyria. They are not normally derived from haemoglobin. Their increased excretion has been reported in fever, poisoning (sulphonal), rendering urine black.

Table 33.5: Colour of urine

Orange	Concentrated urine (restricted intake of fluid, fever, pyridium like drugs).
Red	Blood, anilin dyes, Pyridium
Dark brown	Altered blood (methaemoglobinurea, porphyrin, myoglobin)
Cloudy	Phosphates, urates, bacterial contamination.
Portwine	Porphyria
Brownish black	Alkaptonurea, melanin, methaemoglobin
Green	Carbolic acid, biliverdin.

MICROSCOPIC EXAMINATION OF URINE

A. *Sediments:*
   - Cells—WBC, RBC, epithelial cells
   - Casts—Hyaline, granular, fatty, waxy,
   - Mucus, spermatozoa, bacteria, yeast, parasites
   - Foreign bodies—starch granules from dusting powder
   - Crystals and amorphous chemical deposits
   - Acidic urine—Uric acid : urates
   - Alkaline urine—Urates and amorphous phosphates

B. Cells: WBC—Occasional leucocyte is of no significance. Increases in number seen in inflammatory diseases of urinary tract, contamination of urine from female genital tract.
   - Erythrocytes—Seen in fresh samples only
   - Epithelial cells—No diagnostic value. Cells are large with small nuclei.
   - Mucous threads—More ribbon like. Show faint longitudinal striations.
   - Small round cell—They arise from kidney and are slightly larger than pus cells. These are indicative of renal disease.
   - Transitional cells—They are more common when samples are obtained after ureteric catheterization or prostatic massage. Their presence is of no pathological significance.

C. *Casts:* These are produced by precipitation of proteins in renal tubules which are then pushed down by urinary flow. Red cell, leucocyte, epithelial, hyaline, granular, fatty and waxy casts are common. Their presence indicates renal origin of various cells.

D. *Crystals:* Common crystals are oxalate, phosphate, urates and uric acid. Exact typing of crystal is not of much clinical significance.

Table 33.6: Albuminurea—causes

1. Functional—Severe muscular exercise, pregnancy, prolonged exposure to cold, orthostatic.
2. Organic;
   a. Renal—Nephritis, nephrosis, carcinoma, tuberculosis
   b. Prerenal—Fever of toxaemia, ascites, drugs and chemical poisoning.
   c. Post renal—Pyelitis, cystitis, urethritis

Table 33.7: Haematurea—causes

1. Kidney—Acute glomerulonephritis, tuberculosis, neoplasm.
2. Lower urinary tract—Ureteritis, cystitis, neoplasm. Few RBC may present after strenuous exercise.

ASSESSING KIDNEY-II: RENAL FUNCTION TESTS

URINE EXAMINATION

For normal and abnormal constituents.

SPECIFIC GRAVITY TEST

Normal kidney gives urine with a specific gravity of 1.002-1.032 (maximum 1.040; corresponding to 1400 mOsm/l). In performing the test care should be taken to check the zero error on the hydrometer by immersing it in water and it should be measured at room temperature. No fluid/fruit is given after midday. Urine is obtained on waking and twice during following morning.

Administration of vasopressin or pituitrin may be used to achieve maximum concentration. In this test, deprivation of water is not needed. He is asked to empty his bladder and urine is saved as the first specimen. Pituitrin is given by subcutaneous route in a dose of 10 units (0.5 ml). Nothing is given orally until test is complete. Specimens are obtained at one and two hours interval after the injection.

The lowest concentration is 1.028. It is contraindicated in old age, heart diseases, renal failure, chronic illness, etc.

BLOOD UREA ESTIMATION

Normal range 20 to 40 mg per 100 ml of blood.

UREA CLEARANCE TEST

The concept of renal clearance can be applied to any substance that is present in the blood and is excreted in the urine. Urea clearance defined as least volume of blood (or plasma) containing an amount of urea equal to that excreted in one minute in urine. Thus, clearance is a ratio of the urinary excretion to the average blood level determine simultaneously. Normal urea clearance is 75 ml/minute when rate of excretion of urine was 2 ml or more per minute. Urea clearance gives an indication of the magnitude of GFR. The clearance is influenced by the rate of urine flow.

Since it is commonly used clinical test for kidney function, it is well to point out that urea retention does not occur until clearance has fallen to 30–55 per cent of the normal.

Thus: Give the patient 8 ml water/kg body weight at least one hour before the test begins, (water not more than 600 ml). At the beginning of the test the patient must empty his bladder and the time is recorded. In exactly one hour, the patient is asked to void again. Measure the quantity of urine in ml and divide by 60 to calculate (V), i.e. number of ml per minute. Near the midpoint of the test withdraw blood by venepuncture and determine the value of urea nitrogen in mg/100 ml. (B) Determine the urea nitrogen content of the urine and express as mg/100 ml (U).

Calculation as :

$$C_M = \frac{UV}{B} \text{ OR in per cent } C_M = \frac{100\ UV}{75\ B}$$

If quantity of urine excreted is less than 2 ml/minute the formula for standard clearance -

$$C_S = \frac{U\sqrt{V}}{B}$$

U = mg urea per ml urine
V = ml urine excreted per minute
B = mg urea/ml of blood

Interpretation - 75–125 per cent - normal; 40–60 per cent - moderate impairment; 20–40 per cent marked impairment; less than 20 per cent clearance severe impairment. Standard clearance averages 54 ml/minute.

INULIN CLEARANCE

It averages 125 c.c. per minute. A valuable feature of the knowledge that inulin clearance measures GFR is that it becomes a "Yard stick" for the evaluation of renal clearance of any other substance. Inulin is a polysaccharide obtained from "dahlia tubers." Since the concentration of Inulin in glomerular filtrate is equal to that in plasma (Pin) the factor UV/Pin; C_{IN} gives GFR. (Normal is 110–150 ml/minute). It is filtered by glomerulus but is neither excreted nor absorbed by tubules.

IVP

(Intravenous pyelography) may be performed.

PLASMA ALBUMIN CONCENTRATION

Plasma albumin concentration and 24 hours urinary protein excretion are the best methods of assessing the severity of nephrotic syndrome.

PLASMA ELECTROLYTES

concentration may be required for diffuse renal failure or specific tubular defects. The most important are Na, K, Ca, HCO_3 and PO_4 concentration.

PHENOL SULPHONEPHTHALEIN

(PSP, phenol red) is secreted by tubules at a high rate as well as being filtered at the glomerulus, there being a Tm for PSP as there is for PAH. After its I.V. injection of 6.0 mg 1.6 mg can be normally recovered in urine at the end of 15 minutes and 3.6 mg at 2 hours. The quantity of dye in urine is determined by alkalinizing the urine with NaOH and checking it against a colour standard.

Tm GLUCOSE

The maximum capacity of the tubules to reabsorb glucose is measured by infusing glucose I.V. at a rate sufficient to maintain the plasma concentration above the threshold value. Inulin clearance is determined simultaneously. The amount of glucose appearing in the urine each minute (UV) is then subtracted from the amount filtered (i.e. the plasma concentration multiplied by the Inulin clearance) and the difference gives the TmG in mg/minute.

CREATININE CLEARANCE TEST

Approaches the GFR but it is complicated by the fact that a portion of creatinine is secreted by the tubules. Of course, in renal diseases its portion rises because of failure of filtration. In addition, mannitol and sodium thiosulfate can be used for clearance.

RENAL BLOOD FLOW

It is determined with the help of substances like "diodrast" or "PAH" which at low blood concentration are almost removed completely by tubular excretion in a single circulation through the kidney. It is normally 1,000–1150 ml/minute OR expressed as plasma flow about 600–700 ml/minute.

PSP TEST

Procedure Breakfast is withheld. Patient is given 300–400 ml of water to promote urinary excretion. He is advised to empty the bladder. 1 ml of solution containing 6 mg. PSP is injected after half an hour intramuscularly/intravenously. Three urinary specimens are collected after 15 minutes, one hour and then two hours. The output of dye PSP is estimated in each sample.

Results Normally, 25 per cent or more of dye is excreted in first 15 minutes (after I.V. administration). Then 70 per cent will be excreted during the two hour period.

Inference

- Impairment of PSP excretion
- Slight—59–40 per cent excretion of injected dye
- Moderate—39–25 per cent excretion of injected dye
- Marked—24–11 per cent excretion of injected dye
- PSP excretion is increased in hypertension, hyperthyroidism, acute nephritis (early stage).
- It is decreased in glomerulonephritis, tubular diseases, interstitial diseases, drugs (like sulphonamide, salicylate, diuretic), liver diseases (cirrhosis, CHF, low serum albumin).

Advantages Easy to perform, can be done in a short time, function of individual kidney can be assessed, test is useful in surgical cases in connection with operative risk.

Principle The dye is eliminated only by kidneys and its amount can be easily estimated by colorimetric methods. The time of its first appearance in the urine and the quantity eliminated within a definite period are taken as a measure of the functional capacity of the kidneys.

Notes Amount of PSP must be 1 ml. Patient is asked to empty the bladder at schedule time. It is insensitive to advanced changes. Dye excretion varies directly with urine volume in severe renal diseases.

RENAL FUNCTION TEST: AN OVERVIEW

1. **PAH clearance test.** It is 90 per cent cleared from plasma. Therefore, its clearance can be used as an approximation of renal plasma flow.
   So out of 100 ml it is cleared 90 ml.

   $$\text{So 1 ml} = \frac{90}{100}$$

   $$\text{and 650 ml (plasma volume)} = \frac{90}{100} \times 650$$

   $$= 585 \text{ ml/minute}$$

   $$\text{so actual plasma flow} = \frac{585}{0.9}$$

   Since extraction ratio for PAH is 90 per cent = 650 ml/minute.
   'The percentage of a substance removed from the blood is known as extraction ratio of PAH and it averages about 90 per cent in normal kidney.'
2. $$\textbf{Renal blood flow (RBF)} = \frac{\text{Clearance of PAH}}{\text{Extraction ratio of PAH}}$$

$$\text{Extraction ratio} = \frac{\text{Renal arterial PAH-renal venous concentration}}{\text{Renal arterial PAH concentration}}$$

$$\text{Extraction ratio} = \frac{650 \text{ ml/minute}}{1\text{-}0.45 \text{ (Hematocrit)}} = 1182 \text{ ml/minute}$$

3. **Filtration Fraction.** 17–19 per cent since plasma flow is ranging between 600–700 ml/minute
4. **Inulin clearance**

$$\text{GFR} = \frac{U_s \times V}{P_s} = C_s = \frac{125 \text{ mg/ml} \times 1 \text{ ml/minute}}{1 \text{ mg/ml}}$$

= 125 ml/minute
Us = Urine concentration of the substance
Ps = Plasma concentration of the substance
V = Urine flow rate
Cs = Clearance rate of a substance

34 Homeostasis: Acid–Base Balance and Regulation

Acid–base balance is vitally important. It means maintenance of the homeostasis of the hydrogen ion concentration of body fluids. Even a slight deviation from normal causes pronounced changes in the rate of cellular chemical reactions. This in turn, threatens the survival.

THE TERM pH

It is a symbol used to mean the hydrogen ion concentration. It indicates the degree of acidity and alkalinity of a solution. A pH of 7 indicates neutrality, while greater than 7 indicates alkalinity and less than 7 is acidity.

THE TERM BUFFER

In terms of action, a buffer is a substance that prevents marked changes in a pH of a solution when an acid or base is added to it.

Buffer consists of two kinds of substances and are referred as buffer pairs. Most of the body fluid buffer pairs consists of a weak acid and a salt of the acid like

Bicarbonate pairs $\frac{NaHCO_3}{H_2CO_3}$; $\frac{KHCO_3}{H_2CO_3}$ etc.

Plasma protein pairs $\frac{\text{Na proteinate}}{\text{Proteins (weak acid)}}$

Haemoglobin pairs $\frac{KHb}{Hb}$ $\frac{KHbO_2}{HBO_2}$

Phosphate buffer pairs $\frac{Na_2HPO_4}{NaH_2PO_3}$

The proper ratio of hydrogen and hydroxyl ions in the blood and the body is spoken as acid–base balance. Since the only free acid in the blood is carbonic acid (H_2CO_3) formed by the union of CO_2+H_2O; and since sodium bicarbonate is the important alkali; the pH is determined by relative amount of each of these present; or by the ratio $\frac{H_2CO_3}{NaHCO_2}$. The carbonic acid of the blood is equivalent to 0.0015 molar solution, while the concentration of the bicarbonate is 0.03 m; the ratio of these two in blood is therefore 1/20. This ratio represents the acid–base balance and is equal to pH 7.4 (Range 7.3–7.5). A fall in pH much below 7.3 is called acidosis (grave situation resulting in coma and death) and pH beyond 7.5 constitutes alkalosis (convulsions and fatal results).

pH buffering depends on chemical reactions which reduce the effect of the addition or removal of H^+ on the final (H^+). Any weak acid and its conjugate base can act as a pH buffer system. If H^+ is added it can combine with the base to form more acid, as predicted by law of mass action. This removes H^+ from solution and so there is less of a reduction in pH than would otherwise have occurred. If H^+ removed from the system, this will favour dissociation of acid, releasing protons which limit increase in pH.

ROLE OF BUFFERS

Buffers react with a relatively strong acid (or base) to replace it by a relatively weak acid (or base). That is to say, an acid which highly dissociates to yield many H^+ ions is replaced by one which dissociates less highly to yield fewer H^+ ions. Thus by buffer reaction, instead of strong acid remaining in the solution and contributing many H^+ ions to drastically lower the pH of a solution, a weaker acid takes its place, contributes fewer additional H^+ ions to the solution and thereby lowers its pH only slightly. Because blood contains buffer pairs, its pH fluctuates much less widely than it would without them.

Examples ....

1. H_2CO_3 + KHb (buffer) ⟶ $KHCO_3$ + HHb.

↑↓ ↑↓

H^+ (*few*) + HCO_3^- H^+ (*few*) + Hb

The above state is buffering of carbonic acid inside RBC by potassium salt of haemoglobin. Each molecule of carbonic acid is replaced by a molecule of the acid, haemoglobin. Since haemoglobin is a weaker acid than carbonic acid, fewer of these haemoglobin molecules dissociate to form H^+ ions. Hence, fewer hydrogen ions are present in RBC intracellular fluid than would have been present without the buffering of carbonic acid by potassium salt of haemoglobin.

2. Lactic acid + $NaHCO_3$ ⟶ Na lactate + H_2CO_3

↑ ↑↓

H^+ (*few*) + Lactate H^+ (*few*) + HCO_3^-

Above is buffering of lactic acid (non-volatile acid) by basic carbonate salt which also buffers other non-volatile acids. Carbonic acid (a weaker acid than lactic acid) replaces lactic acid. So fewer hydrogen ions are added to blood than would be if lactic acid were not buffered.

BICARBONATE BUFFERS: AT A GLANCE

HCl (*strong acid*) + $NaHCO_3$ ⟶ H_2CO_3 (*weak acid*) + NaCl

and

NaOH (*strong base*) + H_2CO_3 ⟶ H_2O + N_aHCO_3 (*weak acid*)

It is not a very powerful buffer due to large difference between pH of extracellular fluid, i.e. 7.4, and pK of bicarbonate buffer, i.e. 6.1. Even then it is more important because concentration of its two constituents is regulated separately, i.e. bicarbonate is regulated by kidney while CO_2 is regulated by the respiratory system.

Phosphate buffer: Is more useful inside RBC and other cells. The weak acid is H_2PO_4 (unprotonated form); the base is HPO_4. The buffer system in plasma consists of NaH_2PO_4 (weak acid) and Na_2HPO_4. Within the RBC, the system consists of KH_2PO_4 and K_2HPO_4 since in RBC Na^+ concentration is low and K^+ concentration is high.

$H_3PO_4 \longleftrightarrow H^+ + H_2PO_4^-$

$H_2PO_4 \longleftrightarrow H^+ + HPO_4^{2-}$

$HPO_4^{2-} \longleftrightarrow H^+ + HPO_4^{3-}$

This system is more effective in ICF than ECF because (a). Total phosphate concentration is greater in ICF than ECF and (b) Intracellular pH is some what lower than extracellular pH.

PHOSPHATE BUFFER

- Phosphate buffer is effective in buffering tubular fluid in kidneys, because
  1. Phosphate becomes greatly concentrated in tubular fluid due to excess water reabsorption as compared with phosphate; and
  2. pH of tubular fluid becomes more acidic than pH of ECF.

PHOSPHATE BUFFER: AT A GLANCE

HCl (*strong acid*) + Na_2HPO_4 ⟶ NaH_2PO_4 (*weak acid*) + NaCl

So when strong acid, i.e. HCl is mixed with a fluid rich in phosphate buffer system, a weak acid (NaH_2PO_4) is produced which creats a very mild change in pH.

On another side

NaOH (*strong base*) + NaH_2PO_4 ⟶ Na_2HPO_4 (*weak base*) + H_2O

If a strong base (NaOH) is mixed with a fluid rich in phosphate buffer, a weak base (Na_2HPO_4) is formed which prevents changes in pH.

It is more powerful than bicarbonate buffer because it has pK of 6.8 which is near pH of body fluids, i.e. 7.4, but overall buffering capacity is less than the bicarbonate buffer because the concentration of phosphate in extra cellular fluid is only 1/6th that of bicarbonate.

Protein Buffer: Is of two types viz. plasma proteins and haemoglobin buffer and later is more important, because of (a) quantity of haemoglobin is more; (b) reduced haemoglobin is even superior; (c) CO_2 enters the capillary at the tissue level, there develops a threat of fall in pH in the venous blood, but pH does not fall appreciably as haemoglobin by now has become a stronger buffer (within the veins).

$HPr \longleftrightarrow H^+ + Pr^-$

RESPIRATORY MECHANISM FOR pH CONTROL

- Respiration plays vital role here. With every expiration CO_2 leaves the body in the expired air. This less CO_2 in extracellular fluid combines with water to form carbonic acid whose amount is also reduced hence forth. If the amount of carbonic acid in blood decreases, the concentration of hydrogen ion also decreases, and pH increases.

- An increase in CO_2 content of blood, decreases pH called *acidaemia*. It can be brought about in many ways viz. by decreasing the elimination of CO_2 by the lungs (as by voluntarily holding the breath) by breathing air rich in CO_2, by decrease in alkali reserve, and by inability of the heart adequately to supply O_2 to the tissues. In muscle the lactic acid acting upon $NaHCO_3$ forms sodium lactate and carbonic acid, and thus causes acidosis by increasing the acid and decreasing the alkali reserve. Whatever the cause, acidosis results in increased stimulation of the respiratory centre, since neurones of the respiratory centre are sensitive to changes in arterial blood CO_2 content and pH changes. This causes increased rate and depth of respiration causing much elimination of CO_2 and also reduces carbonic acid and hydrogen ions and increase pH back towards normal level.
- The carotid chemoreflex is another device by which respiration adjusts blood pH and in turn, adjusts pH.
- By voluntary forced ventilation of the lungs a larger volume of CO_2 is expelled from the blood. As a result H_2CO_3 is lowered and pH of blood is increased, a condition called *alkalaemia*. The resulting lack of stimulation of respiration induces apnoea until an amount of CO_2 has been formed and retained by the body sufficient to lower the pH to its normal value.

SOME PRINCIPLES - pH AND RESPIRATION

1. A decrease in blood pH below normal (acidosis) tends to cause increased respiration (hyperventilation) which tends to increase pH back towards normal. In other words, acidosis causes hyperventilation which acts as a compensating mechanism for acidosis.
2. Prolonged hyperventilation may increase blood pH enough to produce alkalosis.
3. An increase in blood pH above normal (alkalosis) causes hypoventilation which serves as a compensating mechanism for the alkalosis by decreasing blood pH back towards normal.
4. Prolonged hypoventilation may decrease blood pH enough to produce acidosis.

KIDNEY: pH CONTROL

Kidneys play a vital role in pH control. Kidney tubules by excreting many or few hydrogen ions, in exchange for reabsorbing many or few sodium ions control urine pH and thereby blood pH. If for example blood pH decreases below normal, kidney tubules remove more hydrogen ions from the blood to the urine and reabsorb more sodium ions from the urine back into the blood, thereby decreasing urine pH but increasing blood pH back towards normal. In nutshell, urinary mechanism of pH control is a device for actually eliminating more or fewer hydrogen ions from the body at a rate matching the number entering the blood.

When pH of body fluid decreases urine pH also decreases due to certain activities of distal tubule cells which acidify the urine. It is illustrated by :

Distal tubules secrete hydrogen ions into the urine in exchange for basic ions which they reabsorb. CO_2 diffuses from tubule capillaries into distal tubule cells where enzyme carbonic anhydrase accelerates the combining of $CO_2 + H_2O$ to form carbonic acid. The latter dissociates into hydrogen ions and bicarbonate ions. Hydrogen ion then diffuse into the tubular urine where they displace basic ions (Na oftenly) from a basic salt of a weak acid and thereby change the basic salt to an acid salt or to a weak acid which is eliminated in the urine. During this happening, the displaced sodium or other basic ion diffuses into a tubular cell. Here it combines with bicarbonate ion left over from carbonic acid dissociation to form sodium bicarbonate which then diffuses and reabsorbed into the blood.

So sodium bicarbonate is conserved for the body. Extra hydrogen ions are added to the urine and thereby eliminated from the body. Finally, this increases blood pH back upward toward normal and decreases urine pH. In nutshell, hydrogen ion secretion from distal tubule in exchange for sodium ions makes blood more alkaline by making urine more acid.

KIDNEY pH CONTROL

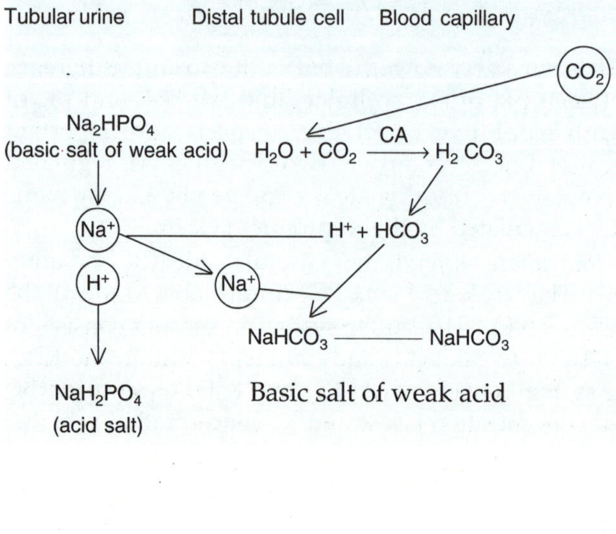

Tubular urine — Distal tubule cell — Blood capillary

CO_2

Na_2HPO_4 (basic salt of weak acid)

$H_2O + CO_2 \xrightarrow{CA} H_2CO_3$

Na^+ — $H^+ + HCO_3$

H^+ — Na^+

$NaHCO_3$ — $NaHCO_3$

NaH_2PO_4 (acid salt)

Basic salt of weak acid

Distal tubule cells synthesise ammonia which diffuses into tubular urine, there to combine with hydrogen to form an ammonium ion, which displaces sodium or some other basic ion from a salt of strong acid to form an ammonium salt. The basic ion then diffuses back into a tubule cell and combines with a bicarbonate ion to form a basic salt which in turn diffuses into tubular blood. Distal tubules secrete more hydrogen and ammonium ions, or in other words make the urine more acid when pH of body fluid decreases below its normal mean.

ACIDOSIS

i. *Diabetic ketosis*, starvation are such states when abnormally large amounts of non-volatile acids enter the blood.

ii. *Compensation*
   - Respiration becomes deep and fast removing more CO_2 and thereby decreasing carbonic acid and hydrogen ion content of blood towards normal (hyperventilation).
   - The kidneys increase their action of H^+ and NH^{4+} in exchange for reabsorbed Na^+. This removes some of the added acid ions and lessens the decrease in blood base carbonate.
   - Basic bicarbonate buffers immediately react with the acids. This decreases the ratio of base bicarbonate Carbonic acid of blood which decreases blood pH.

iii. *Manifestations*
   - It (acidosis) stimulates the respiratory centre which manifests into hyperventilation.
   - It depresses CNS and thus causing disorientation, coma, etc.
   - Renal tubules can excrete either hydrogen or potassium in exchange for sodium which they absorb. In general, the more hydrogen they excrete, less potassium is excreted. In acidosis therefore, in which tubule excretion of hydrogen increases, potassium excretion decreases. This may lead to hyperkalaemia a dangerous condition because it can cause heart block.

iv. *Acidaemia due to CO_2 Retention*
   - It should be remembered here that role of lungs in acid–base regulation consists in excretion of CO_2 at such a rate to maintain arterial CO_2 tension about 40 mmHg.
   - In some instances rate of CO_2 excretion is reduced, e.g. upper respiratory tract obstruction, certain lung diseases. So Pco_2 of arterial blood is raised or fall in pO_2 occurs. Patients with chronic pulmonary disease may not always have demonstrable abnormality of acid–base balance, but on mild exertion or increased tissue metabolism (fevers) acidaemia may be precipitated. Even when lungs are normal, respiratory acidaemia can occur if the sensitivity of respiratory centre is reduced, e.g. morphine or barbiturates administration. If the situation is not corrected by lungs, the situation is reversed by kidneys.

v. *Acidaemia due to excessive acid production:* Body metabolism produces acid substances, which if unbuffered in the cells and in the body fluids, would cause intolerable changes in pH. Among the end products of metabolism are carbonic, sulphuric and phosphoric acid. Lactic, propionic, citric and acetoacetic acid are also normally produced in small amounts in intermediate metabolism, but with the exception of lactic acid, they are not normally found in the extracellular fluid in amounts sufficient to influence acid–base balance. Lactic acid accumulates sufficiently during severe muscular exercise to require buffering in the body fluids as well as within muscle cells. If however, there is a metabolic block which results in accumulation of one or more of such acids, or in failure of utilisation, the buffering capacity may be exceeded and acidaemia appears; e.g. hypoxia of ventilatory failure or cardiac arrest.

   The commonest clinical cause of severe non-respiratory acidaemia is uncontrolled, diabetes mellitus with acidosis ketosis. Same thing but less severe may also occur in starvation because of increased utilisation of body fat for energy production.

   Kussmaul's breathing by lungs is the compensatory mechanism. Kidney greatly increases the excretion of hydrogen ions by the usual mechanisms, and retains bicarbonate.

vi. *Acidaemia due to drug ingestion:* Drugs taken orally like ammonium chloride cause acidaemia. Ammonia is largely converted into urea in the liver, produces large amount of HCl. There follows a reduction of plasma bicarbonate and secretion of acid urine. Barbiturates that depress ventilation are common cause of respiratory acidosis.

vii. *Acidaemia of renal origin:* Since in normal metabolism acids are continually being produced (e.g. 50 m equivalent H_2SO_4 are formed per day); failure of renal function must result in accumulation of acid in the body.

   The usual excretory mechanism (s) for H^+, namely the glutamine-ammonium ion and the hydrogen ion sodium ion exchange presumably decrease in efficiency approximately in proportion to the decrease in solute concentrating power of the kidney, so that as renal disease progresses acidaemia tends to increase. With accumulation of anions, e.g. sulphate and phosphate and the retention of hydrogen ions, the blood bicarbonate is lowered. The increase in CO_2 excretion via lungs affect the pH (Henderson-Hasselbalch equation) but does not effect a net excretion of H^+; thus restoration to normal can only occur if the kidneys recover their ability to secrete acid.

Acidaemia due to abnormal loss of base: Loss of intestinal secretions, either through prolonged diarrhoea, or from an intestinal fistula results in loss of HCO_3^- along with equivalent amount of Na^+ and K^+ and a certain amount of Cl^-. Although, such loses cause considerable water and electrolyte depletion, with reduction in extracellular fluid volume, it is in fact the loss of HCO_3^- which is responsible for acid–base disturbance. Excretion through the lungs reduces the (H_2CO_3) so that acid–base ratio is restored at a lower level of bicarbonate buffer concentration. The kidneys produce an acid urine with a high concentration of NH_4^+, and an increased excretion of H^+ in the form of $H_2PO_4^-$.

METABOLIC ACIDOSIS

Causes

- Lactic acidosis—due to accumulation of lactic acid during excess metabolism of Carbohydrates and in circulatory shock.
- Diabetic ketoacidosis.
- Uraemic Acidosis.
- Diarrhoea—Bicarbonates ion of pancreatic juice are excreted thus producing acidosis.

Metabolic alkalosis : Causes

- Vomiting—gastric contents (HCl) are expelled.
- Diuretics—large quantity of acidic urine excreted.

ALKALOSIS

Some situations like ingestion of an excessive amount of an alkaline drug, hyperventilation, or excessive vomiting can produce alkalosis. In compensated alkalosis carbonic acid also increases but the base bicarbonate - carbonic acid ratio and pH remain normal. In uncompensated case the ratio and pH increase.

i. *Alkalosis due to drug ingestion:* Ant acids are example. They neutralise gastric HCl. In consequence, HCO_3^- of intestinal secretion tends to be reabsorbed whereas normally much of it is converted to H_2CO_3 in the gut. If $NaHCO_3$ is taken in amounts greater than are required to neutralise the HCl secreted, there is in addition, absorption of HCO_3^- which leads to a high plasma bicarbonate and since the (H^+) is reduced, to alkalaemia.
ii. *Alkalaemia due to loss of gastric secretion:* Vomiting leads to this type of consequences. It is due to loss of hydrogen ion secreted by the stomach. Alkaline tide is the another situation responsible for this sort of consequences. In prolonged vomiting of pyloric stenosis—plasma chloride progressively diminishes and is replaced by bicarbonate which increases roughly in proportion to the loss of chloride, and since respiratory function is usually normal the (H_2CO_3) is little altered.

Patients suffering from prolonged vomiting are unable to take adequate food, and breakdown of tissue fat is increased with developing starvation-ketosis. This condition is itself a cause of acidaemia and its occurrence in association with severe vomiting may lead to confusing plasma anion pattern characterised by almost normal (HCO_3^-) but low (Cl^-). It is thus possible for a patient to be in alkalosis and ketosis simultaneously.

Besides vomiting, administration of diuretic drug also causes alkalosis since it results in excretion of large volume of acidic urine (e.g. thiazides etc.).

Metabolic alkalosis seldom develops acutely. The magnitude of respiratory compensation is normally quite small, since the response of the carotid body chemoreceptors to an increase in arterial pH is much less than their response to a fall in arterial pH.

Role of kidney in correcting alkalosis:

$H_2CO_3^-$ derived from H^+ secretion may be normal or elevated slight but because of slight increased filtered load of HCO_3^- even a somewhat increased rate of H^+ secretion is insufficient to recover all of the filtered HCO_3^-.

Kidneys can secrete HCO_3^- under the condition of chronic alkalosis. HCO_3^- excretion therefore increases, $(HCO_3)_p$ falls, and arterial pH decreases towards normal.

Tubular secretion of H^+ helps to maintain a normal pH despite the continuous production of acid metabolites, (other than CO_2) in the body. This normally results in an acid urine which excretes about 50–80 m moles of H^+ every 24 hours. Though small but it is vital to acid–base homeostasis. Kidney absorption of HCO_3^-, occurs in exchange for secreted acid. This maintains the physiological (HCO_3^-), (25 m mol/L) which is crucial for pH control since any reduction in HCO_3^- favours dissociation of carbonic acid and a fall in pH.

ACID–BASE BALANCE: OVERVIEW EFFECTS

Acidosis

- CNS depression—patient disorientates and then comatose.
- Increased rate and depth of respiration.

Alkalosis

- CNS over excited. Peripheral nerves are effected before CNS sometimes nerves start firing without stimulation. This leads to tetany.

TREATMENT

- *Acidosis*: To neutralise acid, large amounts of $NaHCO_3$ should be ingested by mouth. Sodium lactate/gluconate may also be used.
- *Alkalosis*: Ammonium chloride is often administered orally. Its ammonia portion is converted into urea by liver. This reaction liberates HCl which react with buffer of body fluids to shift pH towards acidic side.
- *Renal compensation*:
  a. *Acidosis*: In respiratory acidosis, kidney secretes an excess of hydrogen ion. It causes increased concentration of $NaHCO_3$ in extracellular fluid.
  b. *Alkalosis*: In respiratory alkalosis, large amount of $NaHCO_3$ are lost into urine.

THEME OF ACID–BASE REGULATION

1. Firstly, there exists secondary active transport of hydrogen ions in early tubular segments. The sodium ion is transported from lumen to tubular cell and thence to interstitium and ultimately to peritubular capillaries. The hydrogen ion is extruded from cell towards lumen by counter transport mechanism via Na^+ H^+ counter transport.
2. Besides this there exists Primary active transport of hydrogen ions in late distal tubules. This contributes only 5 per cent of total hydrogen ions secreted; but here they are concentrated many more times and energy for this process comes through hydrogen transporting ATPase (ATP → ADP). This whole is a function of intercalated cells located at distal and collecting tubule. The source of hydrogen ion is - $CO_2 + H_2O \rightarrow H_2CO_3 \rightarrow H^+ + HCO_3^-$. HCO_3^- extruded towards interstitium and thence to blood, while H^+ enters lumen.
3. The HCO_3^- filtered by glomerulus, combines with H^+ secreted to form H_2CO_3, which dissociates into H^+ and HCO_3. This HCO_3^- is then extruded from the cell towards interstitium and then to blood, so each time a hydrogen ion is formed, a bicarbonate ion is also formed; and another interesting thing is that the HCO_3^- that enter extracellular fluid are not the same HCO_3^- that are removed from tubular fluid.
4. Now think of acidosis, which means, the ratio of CO_2 increases than HCO_3 ions in extracellular fluid. So rate of hydrogen ion secretion increases than bicarbonate ion filtered by glomeruli, so there are only few HCO_3^- to react with H^+. To compensate it, buffers (phosphate and ammonia) are coming into action. Furthermore, as told earlier, with each H^+ secreted, a HCO_3^- is formed and extruded in extra cellular fluid to compensate.
5. The NH_3 secreted combines with H^+ to form Ammonium NH_4^+ which acts as a buffer system. This has got two specialities viz. (a) Most negative ions in tubular fluid are Cl^-, so $H^+ + Cl^- \rightarrow HCl$ may occur but since HCl is a very strong acid and fall of pH may be drastic so this does not become evident and only thing happens is $NH_4^+ + Cl \rightarrow NH_4Cl$ and it is a very weak acid; (b) When NH_3 combines with H^+ to form NH_4, the concentration of ammonia is decreased in tubular fluid → still more ammonia to diffuse from epithelial cells into tubular fluid. So rate of NH_3 secretion into tubular fluid is controlled by amount of excess hydrogen ions which are due to be transported. Of course the source of ammonia is glutamate (60%), and other amino acids/ amines (40%).
6. Now think of alkalosis, which means, ratio of HCO_3^- to dissolved CO_2 increases. This further means, low secretion of H^+; increased HCO_3^- concentration in ECF and increased filtration of HCO_3^- by glomeruli. Any way, since HCO_3^- first combines with H^+ before reabsorption, so excess HCO_3^- are passed into urine, of course, carrying with them Na^+ (loss of $NaHCO_3$).
7. Renal mechanism of adjusting pH, can keep on functioning for hours or days. It cannot work within seconds or minutes. The total amount of buffers in whole body is 1,000 m moles (pH 7–7.8). Kidneys can remove about 500 m moles of either acid or base/day.

BIBLIOGRAPHY

1. Aronson PS. Mechanism of active H^+ secretion in the proximal tubule. Amer J Phy 1983;245:F64.
2. Astrup P, et al. The acid–base metabolism a new approach. Lancet 1960;1035-1039.
3. Cogan MG. Fluid and Electrolytes: Physiology and pathophysiology: Appleton and Lange. 1991.
4. Cresef R. Terminology of acid–base regulation. Lancet 1962;i:419-424.
5. Davenport HW. (1961). The ABC of acid–base chemistry. 5th edn. Chicago University Press and 6th edn. (1974).
6. Frazer SC, Stewart CP. Acidosis and Alkalosis a modern view. J Clin Path 1959;12:195.
7. Knepper MA, et al. Ammonium transport in the kidney. Phy Rev 1989;69:179.
8. Morgan HG, et al. Acid–base monitoring of open heart surgery. J Clin Path 1963;16:545.
9. Roose A, Boron WF. Intraceullular pH. Phy Rev 1981;61:296.
10. Seldin DW, Giebisch G (Eds). Regulation of Acid–Base Balance. Raven Press. 1989.

35 Homeostasis: Body Temperature: Regulation

The maintenance of certain temperature is of vital importance to the organism because all biologic processes are conditioned by temperature.

- The average normal body temperature is generally considered to be 98.6°F (37°C) when measured orally and ranging between 97° to 99° (35.9 to 37.3°C).
- It is 1°F (0.6°C) higher when measured rectally.
- Temperature in the mouth is taken by placing thermometer under the tongue and keeping the mouth closed, for one complete minute.
- If it is to be recorded by axillary channel, the thermometer is placed in axilla and is left in place for 5 to 10 minutes, with the arm held tightly against the thorax. The axillary temperature is usually 0.2 to 0.4°C (0.36–0.72°F) below the temperature in the mouth and 0.5 to 1°C (0.9–1.8°F) below that of the rectum.
- Those animals which are able to maintain a relatively constant body temperature inspite of great variation of external temperature are homeothermic, whereas animals in which body temperature varies with that of environment are poikilothermic (cold blooded).

TEMPERATURE VARIATIONS

- The temperature of the viscera is 1 to 1.5°C (1.8–2.7°F) above the temperature in axilla; it is highest in the liver.
- The blood is cooled as it passes through lungs. Therefore, it is warmer in right ventricle than in left ventricle.
- The lower limit of body temperature compatible with life in man is 27 to 29°C (80.6° to 84.2°F). A rise of temperature to 44 or 45°C (111.2 or 113°F) produced fatal disturbances in central nervous system.
- Diurnal variation Temperature is maximum between 5 and 8 pm and minimum between 2 and 6 am This cycle may be reversed in night workers.

HEAT LOSS

Heat loss by conduction: Suppose a person is sitting on a chair or bed (or any object) then heat is lost from our body to that object and the process continues till an equilibrium state is reached between body and the object. The same thing occurs between our body and surrounded atmosphere, i.e. body loses heat to atmosphere till equilibrium state is reached. So this heat loss by conduction is considered as a self-limiting process, as well as, it represents only a small percent of the total heat loss from the body.

So this consists in the transmission of heat from one molecule to another in a solid, liquid or gaseous body. It depends on the conductivity of the body and the difference in temperature between the two points in contact.

Loss by convection: Heat is first lost by conduction and then carried away by convection currents. This consists in transmission of heat in currents of liquids or gases resulting from differences in density or other causes. The air surrounding a radiant body is heated and rises; colder air replaces it and thus currents are formed which carry away heat from the radiant body. This justifies the use of fans in summer since by fans more heat is lost by convection and loss by evaporation is also increased in this way. Convection increases with the speed of air current up to 125 km (78 miles) per hour but beyond this speed the convection does not increase.

The convection process is really a special case of transfer by conduction. When surrounding material is a fluid and when that fluid becomes lighter at a higher temperature, the layer of the fluid next to a warm object will rise when it is heated, and it will be replaced by another mass of the cool fluid.

So convection is promoted by movement of air across body surfaces.

Heat loss by Radiation: This is in the form of infrared rays (electromagnetic waves). This is dependent on temperature difference between temperature of body surface and average temperature of surroundings. If temperature of body is greater than surroundings then heat will be radiated from the body to atmosphere till equilibrium state is reached. Reverse can also occur, i.e. if temperature of surrounding is more than body surface than heat is lost from atmosphere to body till equilibrium state is reached.

Evaporation: In this situation when temperature of surroundings is more, then body gains heat from atmospheric surroundings. Then in this situation, body can get rid of this extra heat only by means of evaporation and nothing else. But in humid weather (hot-muggy summer days) one feels more uncomfortable because this evaporation is greatly reduced in such atmosphere and secreted sweat remains in a fluid state. One ml of water absorbs 0.58 kcal during evaporation.

An optimum sense of well being is felt with an environment temperature around 20°C (68°F) and a relative humidity of 50 to 60 per cent. Evaporation diminishes as atmospheric humidity increases. With a temperature of 37°C and 100 per cent humidity, it would be impossible for the organism to lose heat either by radiation or evaporation; in this case the temperature of the skin rises above that of environment and heat is thus eliminated by radiation but mainly by vaporisation. Heat is tolerated better in a dry weather than in a damp one, hot volleys, near rivers, workshops and badly ventilated mines etc.

Perspiration

i. Insensible perspiration consists in the evaporation of such a small amount of water that it vaporises as soon as it is excreted.
ii. This water passes through the skin by diffusion and osmosis and not as result of activity of sweat glands.
iii. For a man of 1.8 sq. meter surface area with BMR as 40 kcal./sq. meter/hour; the basal metabolism is 72 kcal/hour (1728 kcal/day). Thus about one quarter of heat is lost by the skin even when no sweating occurs.
iv. *Body too hot:* steps for decreasing temperature:- (a) Vasodilatation: possibly due to inhibition of vasoconstrictive centre located in posterior hypothalamus. (b) Sweating, (c) Phenomenon like shivering/chemical thermogenesis are inhibited and thus heat production is decreased.

SWEAT : A REVIEW

i. It is a dilute watery solution, with a specific gravity 1.002 to 1.003 and its pH varies between 5 to 7.5. Of course sweat due to exercise is less acidic than heat sweat.
ii. It is a fluid coming from sweat glands which are highly developed in man and horse while dogs and cats have these glands only on the pads of their paws.
iii. The sweat secretion is not a simple filtration of blood plasma through the glandular epithelium because, when glands are active then circulatory/histology/physical and chemical phenomenon typical of true secretion are observed.
iv.
   - Before the sweat secretion actually begins; there occurs "primary secretion" which is an active secretory product of epithelial cells lining the coiled portion of sweat gland. The cholinergic sympathetic fibres elicit the secretion. It does not contain protein (difference from plasma). As this secretion passes through the ducts, NaCl is reabsorbed here.
   - When these glands are stimulated slightly, this secretion passes slowly through the ducts so almost all NaCl is reabsorbed and hence their concentration is reduced; to say 5 mEq/liter → reduction in osmotic pressure → more water is reabsorbed → very much concentration of other constituents like urea, lactic acid, potassium ions etc.

Table 35.1: Composition of sweat

Density........	1.003 (1.001 – 1.006)
pH	5 – 7.5 (5.2 - heat) 5 – 7.5 (6.6 - exercise)
Water	99.2 – 99.6 per cent
Sodium	75 – 250 mg per cent (150 mg %)
Chlorine	70 – 346 (180) mg per cent
Potassium	17 mg per cent
NPN	23 – 94 mg per cent (42 mg %)
Ash	144 – 566 mg per cent
Sulphate	4 – 6 mg per cent (average 5)
Freezing point	0.13 – 0.54°C (0.24°C average)
Rate of secretion	1.5 to 4 litres per hour capable of losing 8 pounds body weight per hour.

Table 35.2: Factors causing sweat stimulation

- Increase in temperature of environment
- Physical exercise—due to discharge of impulses from nerve centres
- Psychic factors, e.g. emotions, fear etc.
- Stimulation of nerve centres by factors like asphyxia etc.
- Sleep
- Reflexes, e.g. local warming of a limb, certain gustatory stimuli, centrepetal stimulation of sciatic or splanchnic nerves, etc.

- Just opposite actions take place when it passes very fast through duct → very little NaCl is reabsorbed → concentration is increased to 60 mEq/litre → reduction in water reabsorption.

v. In acclimatised person, there is a decrease concentration of NaCl in sweat so there is better conservation of salt. This effect is also achieved by increased secretion of aldosterone hormone.

vi. In great secretion of sweat, electrolyte level of blood may decline particularly of sodium chloride and this may lead to dehydration. One of the preventive measures coming into action in this situation, is secretion of aldosterone hormone in excess which acts in similar way as it acts on renal tubules. Its ultimate aim is to minimise loss of sodium chloride in the sweat when its blood concentration becomes low.

vii. Besides this hormonal balance, another preventive measure is number of sweat glands. A person living in tropics from a much longer time is having increased number of sweat glands. If this man, then shifts to temperate zone then these glands may be inactivated; but if he continuously lives in tropics then these glands will be working permanently.

viii. About 50 per cent of the total sweat produced on a hot day comes from the skin of trunk, about 25 per cent from lower limbs, and the remaining 25 per cent from the head and upper limbs. Sweating of the hand and feet is due to emotion and anxiety.

ix. Sweat may be of many types depending upon stimulus which evokes it : After few minutes exposure to warm environment sweating begins on all skin areas, of course most noticeable in forehead, upper lip, neck, chest, trunk.

Mental states produce sweating on palm and sole, as well as in axilla. Its centre lies in cerebral cortex while above thermal stimulus produce sweating and centre of its lies in hypothalamus.

SWEAT GLANDS

a. *Eccrine glands*: Distributed over whole surface of body. 2,000,000–3,000,000 in number. Their aggregate mass is equal to half that of one kidney. Most abundantly found on palm of hand, sole of feet, neck and trunk. They occupy almost an area of 2.5 miles. Secrete dilute fluid.

b. *Apocrine glands*: Found in axilla, nipples, labia and mons veneris. Secretion is of characteristic odour.

c. *Innervation*: These are innervated by cholinergic fibres of sympathetic nervous system; but some adrenergic fibres have also been reported. Stimulation of sympathetic fibres causing sweat secretion liberates acetylcholine which passes into sweat, and that is stimulated. Atropine inhibits it.

The nerve centre controlling sweat secretion located in hypothalamus. Sweat secretion can be inhibited by local application of cold on the skin (by drinking iced water for a short time or by submerging a limb in cold bath).

The sympathetic system is of fundamental importance in regulation of heat loss by evaporation of sweat. If the temperature rises sweat is secreted by all sweat glands, except those in a denervated area.

REFERENCES

1. Human physiology by Bernardo A Houssay.
2. Kuno Y. "Physiology of human perspiration" J and A., Churchill London, 1935.

HEAT PRODUCTION

i. Practically all the heat in the human body is derived from the oxidation of organic foods. Oxidation and therefore heat production take place in tissues themselves. Every tissue contributes to this, but skeletal muscles, furnish the largest amount. The glands except the liver, are of minor importance. Increasing heat production is therefore achieved by increasing the activity of muscles.

ii. A fall in external temperature from 30°C to 25°C or 20°C does not increase heat production since at this level, one is able to maintain its body temperature by merely decreasing the amount of heat loss, i.e. by physical regulation. However, when atmospheric temperature is lowered to 15°C or 7.5°C this physical regulation does not work but at this point, it is necessary to step up heat production. This is the onset of chemical regulation which is accomplished by muscle tension, shivering, chattering of teeth. Shivering (involuntary exercise) begins when skin temperature has dropped to approximately 19°C (66°F) and may increase oxidation by as much as 400 per cent. Before shivering, there occurs irregular activity of muscle units contracting out of phase with one another known as thermal muscular tone and later on the activity becomes regular and phasic called shivering.

iii. Heat cannot be produced by muscles paralysed by disease, a relaxant drug (e.g. curare), or by an anaesthetic. The temperature of an anaesthetized patient thus tends to fall to that of environment and for this reason surgical operation theatres are kept warm.

iv. **So when body is too cold: the sequence of events**
   - Vasoconstriction (skin) throughout the body.
   - Piloerection:- due to sympathetic stimulation the muscle (arrector pili) attached to hair follicle, contracts. It leads to upright projection of hair. This is more important in animals than human being.
   - Heat production via shivering, sympathetic stimulation, secretion of thyroxine.
   - Primary motor centre for shivering is located in posterior hypothalamus near the wall of third ventricle. This centre is normally inhibited by centre located in pre-optic area of anterior hypothalamus, but when the temperature falls, this centre gets stimulation, leading to transmission of shivering signals into lateral column of spinal cord and thence to anterior motoneurons. Due to this there occurs increase in tone of skeletal muscle throughout the body which leads to shivering.
   - Sympathetic stimulation can also increase the body temperature by releasing epinephrine and norepinephrine—a process called chemical thermogenesis (this depends upon amount of brown fat present in animals but not in human beings). This acts by uncoupling of oxidative phosphorylation.

PHYSIOLOGY OF FEVER

Fever occurs when some condition like infection interfere with the normal regulation of body temperature. Due to infection, some toxic agents called pyrogens are produced by infective agents like bacteria, virus, foreign allergic proteins, etc.

Thus, because of fever, the temperature regulating centre is at higher temperature but the temperature of the blood reaching the temperature regulating centre is still low. To compensate, vasoconstriction, pale - shivering are produced which constitute so called *chills*. Due to these responses heat loss is reduced and heat production is increased and temperature of body rises which continues until newly indicated temperature is reached. In man, shivering can raise the metabolic rate only 2–5 times. Shivering serves as an unconscious, automatic function of temperature regulation, executed by the somatic division of the nervous system.

When pyrogens are removed by any means (drug administration, etc.) then blood temperature is still raised in comparison of thermostat. To compensate blood vessels of skin dilate and sweating occurs and temperature drops back to normal. This is *crisis*.

Because of the dependence of the rate of chemical reaction on temperature, the metabolism increases about 7 per cent for each 1°F rise in body temperature. A disproportionate amount of this increase is in protein metabolism. Therefore, when a person has fever, the diet should be protein rich.

High temperature would appear to aid in the destruction of some bacteria, so the temperature itself may be a part of defence mechanism. Of course, very high fevers (105° F or above) can be quite harmful if it is long and continued. The nervous system is specially prone to be damaged, and neuronal cells once destroyed can never be replaced.

Dehydration is another cause of fever, besides the infection. It is due to lack of available fluid for sweating as well as, the fact that this dehydration state is having a direct effect on temperature regulating centre located in hypothalamus.

The pyrogens: These are toxic substances secreted by the invading organisms which can raise the body temperature. Such pyrogens can also be released from damaged body tissues as well as from damaged or degenerated leucocytes which is called 'leucocyte pyrogen' which is released from buffy coat of WBC. These are polysaccharides toxins.

Role of Interleukin–I

a. When bacteria enters the body, they are attacked and destroyed by WBC, tissue macrophages and lymphocytes. On digesting the bacteria, interleukin–I is released (synonym-leucocyte pyrogen/endogenous pyrogen). It when reaches to hypothalamus produces fever. The maximum amount of interleukin–I needed to cause fever is only a few nanograms.

b. Many workers are of the opinion that these interleukins first form prostaglandins which increases body temperature. Now aspirin- an analgesic inhibits the formation of prostaglandin from arachidonic acid, so it reduces fever.

- If hypothalamus is compressed by brain tumours then fever is evident.
- Neurogenic fever when there is any injury to nervous structures like vicinity of third ventricle, internal capsule, medulla or upper part of spinal cord.
- Surgical fever—arising from extensive aseptic operation and due to toxic substances liberated by injured tissue.
- Antipyretic drugs
  - —Aspirin (salicylates) etc. lower the temperature in fever by increasing heat elimination. They act through drawing water from tissues into the vessels and thus increasing the volume of fluid in heat radiating system of body.
  - —Alcohol leads to cutaneous vasodilatation. This hastens heat loss, for skin is warm and moist. So it is a wrong belief that alcohol will warm a person. In fact it further lowers the body temperature since it increases heat loss.
  - —The morphine and other anaesthetic agents depress cerebral activity and produce sweating.

FEVER: CHANGES OCCURRING

- Increased metabolic rate in proportion to increase in temperature.
- Pulse rate and blood pressure increases which returns to normal as temperature is stable.
- Pulmonary ventilation increases.
- Blood: becomes concentrated, blood chloride decreases so little or no chloride is excreted in urine. Ingested chloride is retained in great part in tissue fluid. As temperature falls, retained chlorides are excreted causing polyurea.
- Metabolism: protein breakdown increases so great excretion of urea, nitrogen, creatinine. Great consumption of fats and carbohydrates. Ketosis/acidosis occur if adequate carbohydrates are not taken.
- Malaise, headache, depression, loss of appetite, constipation, delirium etc. are symptoms.

TEMPERATURE RECEPTORS

- In skin both cold and warm receptors are present.
- When skin is chilled:
  - — Shivering results which causes heat production.
  - — Skin vasoconstriction is promoted to diminish the transfer of body heat to the skin.
- Deep receptors are found in abdominal viscera, and spinal cord. These are sensitive towards body core temperature rather than body surface temperature. They mainly detect cold temperature rather than warmth.

NERVOUS CONTROL OF TEMPERATURE

a. ***Peripheral nerves:***
   - Motor nerves: There occurs rapid fall in temperature in animals in which spinal motor centres have been destroyed.
   - Vasomotor nerves: Which constrict and dilate cutaneous nerves.

b. ***Cerebral cortex*:** The decorticate dog maintains a normal temperature and responds normally to heat and cold. Of course on exposure to cold shivering occurs earlier and body temperature falls easily. Removal of cerebral cortex in dog and man does not seriously impair temperature regulation.

c. ***Spinal cord*:** If it is cut in the neck, above the sympathetic outflow, body temperature regulation becomes extremely poor.

d. ***Hypothalamus*:** The thermostatic control exercised by hypothalamus is two fold
   i. A nerve centre located in the anterior part controls the loss of heat and thereby prevents overheating of the body. On its destruction (pathologic or experimental) the animal or person behaves normally in a cold environment, but on exposure to heat the usual methods of losing heat are imperative and the body temperature rises. On the other hand, heating the anterior centre by electric means sets the mechanism for thermolysis into action - the animal pants and sweating of the pads of the feet and vasodilatation occurs; this results in a fall of body temperature of several degrees.
   ii. The posterior centre governs heat production and thereby prevents chilling of the body. After its destruction exposure of the animal to cold does not increase metabolism or heart rate; heat production lags and the body temperature falls. Its stimulation causes a fall in body temperature.
   iii. Hypothalamic injury can lead to temperature misregulation. Rostral lesion may lead to hyperthermia with fever leading to death. More caudal hypothalamic lesion, extending laterally lead to hypothermia, if the environment is cool.

TEMPERATURE REGULATION: ROLE OF ENDOCRINE GLANDS

a. ***Thyroid*:** Its hormone exerts calorigenic effect and raise BMR. Cold acts on hypothalamus and provokes a discharge of impulses that increase the secretion of TSH from adenohypophysis which stimulates thyroid gland. In hyperthyroidism the skin is usually warm and temperature is high but everything is within the normal range and hyperthermia is not observed. On the contrary, thyroidectomised animals have a cold skin and subnormal temperature.

Exposure to cold $\xrightarrow{TSH}$ raised secretion of thyroxin

b. ***Adrenals***: Adrenaline (either from parenteral route or by discharge from adrenal medulla) causes an increase in metabolic rate and a little rise in temperature. Adrenalectomised animal don't resist cold well.
Sudden exposure to cold → release of adrenaline → rise in blood pressure and constriction of minute vessels.

c. ***Pituitary***: Anterior pituitary exerts a continuous indirect action on heat production by maintaining a normal level of thyroid and adrenal functions.

d. ***Hypothalamus***: The peripheral receptors stimulate posterior hypothalamus at the level of mammary bodies. This area also receives signals from anterior hypothalamus. It provides heat conserving and heat producing reactions.

DISTURBANCES IN THERMO-REGULATION

a. ***Heat Cramps (Miner's cramp)***: The main cause is decrease in NaCl content of body. In this the body temperature is not elevated. The main disturbance lies in exceedingly painful and spasmodic contractions of muscles, specially of those which had been employed in work. The administration of 0.2 per cent NaCl to drinking water is a safeguard. The profuse sweating may dehydrate the body and loss of NaCl in sweat may induce such cramps. Hard work in a hot climate may require the intake to be increased by an extra 7–21 gm of Nacl.

b. ***Heat stroke (Sunstroke)***: A high degree of external temperature coupled with great humidity renders it difficult for the body to lose heat by any means (viz. conduction, convection, radiation etc.) and sunstroke may then happen. The outstanding features are cessation of sweating (dry, hot skin) and a very sharp rise in temperature. Pulse and blood pressure are above normal. The person is generally unconscious with reflexes lacking altogether; he may be delirious or in convulsions. The body temperature may rise to even 110°F and at this level brain cells are quickly and badly effected. The temperature may be reduced by ice packs and cold baths. Alcohol makes a man more susceptible along with heavy clothing and obesity. It seems likely but by no means proved, that sudden cessation of sweating and circulatory failure are the causes of fatal hyperpyrexia. Sunstroke is term applied to those cases of heat strokes which occur during exposure to tropical sun.

c. ***Heat exhaustion (prostration)***: Here body temperature may be normal or little below normal and skin may be cool and clamy (moist). Cardiovascular system is at fault as indicated by low blood pressure and very rapid, weak and soft pulse. Complete rest is generally sufficient for recovery.

   Upon sudden exposure to a high temperature there is a dilatation of peripheral vessels which greatly increase the vascular space. If more exertion is done then heat exhaustion may ensue because of more load on cardiovascular system. The patient is uncomfortable, dyspneic, confused, may be unconscious, skin is moist with profuse sweating.

d. ***Hyperpyrexia:***
   — 106°F or above (41.2°C) of temperature extremes is accompanied by weakness, mental confusion, headache, increase in respiratory rate and finally loss of consciousness. Such higher temperatures are incompatible with life.
   — Local haemorrhagic or parenchymatous degeneration of cells occur throughout the body, specially in brain, along with liver, kidney etc.
   — Many persons acclimatise to this exposure with high temperature, e.g. soldiers for tropical duty, miners in south Africa (humidity 100%). The main changes of this acclimatisation include- maximum rate of sweating, increase in plasma volume, diminished loss of salt in sweat and urine.

Exposure to Cold: Hypothermia

- Persons exposed to cold without adequate protection begin to shiver as the body temperature falls; the heart rate increases, skin vessels constrict and blood pressure rises. These compensating reactions fail if the body temperature falls below 32°C (90°F), and shivering is replaced by muscular rigidity; consciousness is impaired and reflexes are sluggish. Death usually occurs at about 26°C (77°F).
- *Artificial Hypothermia*: The body temperature can be reduced to 27°C (80°F) by packing the body with ice. At this temperature the oxidation of glucose ceases and metabolism is reduced by some 30 to 40 per cent. The cardiac and respiratory rates are reduced, arterial pressure is low, and patient passes into a state of suspended—animation from which he can completely recover if he is allowed to warm up slowly. In such situation the circulation can be interrupted for 10 to 15 minutes so that surgical operations on heart and

large blood vessels become practicable. At low temperatures there may be metabolic acidosis, (which can be compensated by $NaHCO_3$ administration) and, ventricular fibrillation (at 80°F or below 27°C) (which can be restored on re-warming by injection potassium citrate/OR application of electric shock to ventricles). In such situation the temperature in lower third of oesophagus is often measured since it is closely correlated with cerebral temperature.

FUNCTIONS OF SKIN

i. ***Regulation of body temperature***
ii. ***Excretion***: salt and metabolites are excreted in sweat.
iii. ***Water balance***: Through sweat secretion and temperature regulating mechanism, water balance of body is maintained.
iv. ***Acid–base balance***: Through sweat - which is acidic in reaction, it takes part in maintaining acid–base balance.
v. ***Sensation***: Through various receptors, sensation like touch, pain, temperature are felt through skin.
vi. ***Synthesis***: Ergosterol $\xrightarrow[\text{(present in skin)}]{\text{Sun ultraviolet rays}}$ Vitamin D
vii. ***Secretion***: Sebum, sweat, milk (from breast) are important substances secreted.
viii. ***Store house***: Substances like fats, salt, water, glucose are stored.
ix. In animals like frog etc., it is a means through which *gaseous exchange* occurs.
x. It *protects* body's internal structures
xi. *Absorption* also occurs through skin.

SUMMARY AND HIGHLIGHTS

Normal body temperature is 98.6°F. This is beautifully maintained by balance between heat loss and heat production. It is measured by putting thermometer under the tongue for one complete minute. Fever is caused by infection, dehydration etc. Artificial hypothermia is used for some cardiopulmonary surgery.

BIBLIOGRAPHY

1. Atkins E. Pathogenesis of fever. Phy Rev 1960;40:580-646.
2. Bard P. DMCK Rioch Amer J Phy 1934;109:515.
3. Cooper KE. Temperature regulation and hypothalamus. British Medical Bulletin 1966;22:238–42.
4. Cooper KE, Ross DN. Hypothermia in surgical practice, London: Cassell. 1960.
5. Cooper KE, et al. Observation on the site and mode of action of pyrogen in rabbit's brain. J Phy 1967;191:325–37.
6. Dinarello CA, SM Wolff. Pathogenesis of fever in man. New Eng J Med 1978;29:607–12.
7. Du Bois EF. Fever and regulation of body temperature. Springfield : Illinois : Thomas. 1949.
8. Hemingway A. Shivering. Phy Rev 1963;43:397–422.
9. Hillton SM, Lewis GP. Functional vasodilatation in submandibular salivary gland. British Medical Bulletin 1957;13:189–96.
10. H Johnson, JMK. Spalding. J Phy 1963;166:24.
11. Kuno Y. Human Perspiration. Oxford Blackwell, 1956
12. Moore DM, et al. Studies on pathogenesis of fever. XVII-activation of leucocyte for pyrogen production. J Exp Med 1970;131:179–88.
13. Parkes AS (Ed.). Hypothermia and effects of cold. Brit Med Bull 1961;17:1-73.
14. Robinson S, Robinson AH. Chemical composition of sweat. Phy Rev 1954;34:202–220.
15. Sawyer ME, T Schlossberg. Amer J Phy 1933;104:172.
16. Wolestenholme GEW, Birch J. Pyrogens and fever: Ciba foundation symposium : Edinburgh: Churchi Livingston. 1971.

36 Kidney in off Mood (Renal Diseases)

RENAL PATHOPHYSIOLOGY—HIGHLIGHTS

1. *Glomerular disease*: On glomerular inflammation, there occurs increased capillary permeability and occasionally acute discontinuity of capillary basement membranes. This leads to protein urea, haematurea and WBC also leaks into the urine. The protein may be precipitated in the tubules to form casts. So due to inflammation the glomeruli become swollen and hypercellular due to infiltration with neutrophils and monocytes and because of proliferation and hydropic swelling of mesangial and endothelial cells. This causes blockage of blood flow through most of the glomerular capillaries which causes decreased filtration fraction which results into decreased GFR which may terminate into oligurea or anurea (little and no urine formation respectively).

   The acute inflammation of glomeruli subsides within two weeks. Sometimes if many of the glomeruli are destroyed beyond repair; and in small percentage of patients progressive renal deterioration takes place leading to chronic renal failure.
2. *Tubular disease*: This is caused by ischaemia, toxic substances and it leads to oligurea or anurea if nephrons are damaged in great number. If oligurea persists azotemia (sharp rise in nitrogenous waste products in the blood) and acute renal failure results.

In any chronic renal disease, the tubules may be destroyed or may develop irregular atrophy with interstitial fibrosis and thickened peritubular basement membranes. Such chronic changes are associated with decreased ability to pump sodium, synthesise ammonium ion, exchange hydrogen ions.

Uraemia

- Is a systemic toxic state resulting from acute or chronic failure to eliminate urine. It may be caused by urinary tract obstruction as well as parenchymal renal disease. It may have some other complications like CNS toxicity (tremor, lethargy, twitching, convulsions, coma etc.), pericarditis, pulmonary oedema, pneumonitis, gastroenteritis, pancreatitis, anaemia, bleeding tendency, uraemic frost. The patient may progress into a state of uraemic coma and for which acidosis is the main contributing factor. Respiration is deep and rapid in coma with a fall in arterial blood pressure.
- Disturbances of acid–base balance and fluid electrolyte metabolism are also present.
- It means—advanced renal insufficiency—deriving its name from increased blood urea level.

Acute renal failure: Oligurea is suddenly developed. Previous water intake may lead to pulmonary oedema or cardiac failure and hyperkalaemia which results from lack of excretion of dietary potassium and endogenous potassium from the breakdown of blood, necrotic tissue and catabolism of negative nitrogen balance. It may result in cardiac arrhythmias and sudden death.

Chronic Renal Failure

- Here the big problem is acidosis since kidney fails to excrete hydrogen ions as ammonia and fails to reabsorb adequately all the filtered bicarbonate. Sulphates, phosphates and other anions accumulate leading to acidosis.
- Hypocalcaemia also exists due to defective absorption of calcium from GIT. It further results in secondary parathyroid hyperplasia with demineralisation and resorption of bone, osteomalacia. Renal-rickets are seen in children under such circumstances. In such long- standing states peripheral nerve degeneration may develop causing sensory and motor problems.

Major decrease in number of functioning nephrons → reduction in GFR → decrease in renal excretion of water and solutes. If their number falls to 5–10 per cent then death may result due to electrolyte and fluid retention. This is because of hypertrophy of blood vessels and glomeruli and functional changes which cause vasodilatation; that kidney continue to functions normally inspite of 70 per cent loss of nephrons.

FEW DISEASES AT LENGTH

Glomerulonephritis (A Cause of Acute Renal Shut-down):

a. He was Richard Bright (1827) who described this disease. He is not only the father of renal pathology but he has taught us many things in this aspect.
b. Diffuse glomerulonephritis primarily involves kidney glomeruli but secondarily damage reaches to other parts of the nephron as well as intestinal tissues.
c. It is classed into three stages—
acute—characterised by acute renal insufficiency, oedema and a varying degree of hypertension.
Subacute—oedema and albuminurea.
Chronic—hypertension and renal failure.
d. For a long time the disease may progress only in the mesangium, with no urinary changes if basement membrane is little involved. This is a period of silent nephritis—a latent phase preceding chronic glomerulonephritis, which may manifest itself clinically only decades after the initial episode of acute glomerulonephritis, if indeed there has been such an episode.
e. Streptococci bacteria (group A Haemolytic) is the cause. Its infection from throat, ear (otitis media) may damage the kidney. These organisms may initiate an autoimmune process in human glomerulonephritis. Sensitisation of kidney tissue is an essential feature and inflammation is allergic in character due to antigen-antibody reaction in the glomerulus. The structural element of glomerulus which is involved in antigen-antibody reaction is the basement membrane. Hypersensitivity is the another causative factor.
f. Acute glomerulonephritis is characterised by pain in the back (due to stretching of glomeruli capsule), fever, oedema, hypertension, urinary changes (high specific gravity, presence of albumin, blood, casts, low urea content with a corresponding non-protein retention in blood, oligurea, high coloration etc.).
g. The subacute stage is characterised by oedema, urinary findings (albumin urea), blood changes (high blood cholesterol, low serum albumin, reversal of albumin/globulin ratio, no retention of urea), low BMR etc.
h. Signs of renal failure appears in chronic stage. Filtration rate and renal plasma flow reduced, Tm reduction.

Pyelonephritis

a. Is a focal, suppurative inflammation of the interstitial tissue of the kidney and renal pelvis. The causative organism is *E. coli* while others include aerobacter-aerogenes, pseudomonas, staphylo and streptococci etc.
b. Acute state is characterised by pain and tenderness over the kidney, fever, leucocytosis and pyurea. In chronic cases there is contracted kidney, renal failure with or without hypertension.
c. Medulla is effected more as compared with the cortex. Since the primary function of medulla is to provide the counter current mechanism of concentrating the urine, such patients have normal renal function except for reduced ability to concentrate the urine.
d. The infection reach the kidney via blood or from lower urinary tract by way of ureters to the kidney.
e. Sequence of events/damage:
Inability of bladder to empty completely → bacteria multiply and bladder is inflamed-cystitis → It may be localised → may reach the renal pelvis due to vesico-ureteral reflex where urine is propelled up; so infection reaches to ureter and kidney.

Nephrotic Syndrome

a. Is a symptom complex of massive proteinurea, hypoproteinaemia, oedema (generalised anasarca), hyperlipaemia and lipiduria.
b. The various causes include—hypersensitivity, circulatory diseases (constrictive pericarditis), metabolic diseases (diabetic glomerulosclerosis), pregnancy (toxaemia), and hereditary.
c. Normally negative charge of basement membrane repel the negatively charged plasma proteins. Due to any reason if there is loss of this negative charge of basement membrane, glomerular capillaries allow protein (albumin) to pass through the glomerular membrane.
d. Conditions increasing the permeability of glomerular membrane include:
   — Chronic glomerulonephritis - amyloidosis - (due to accumulation of abnormal proteinoid substance in the blood vessel wall, thus damaging basement membrane of glomeruli.
   — Minimal change nephropathy - in children - 2 to 6 years, due to increased permeability of capillary membrane → 40 gm of plasma protein excreted

in urine → fall in plasma protein concentration below 2 gm/dl → fall in colloid osmotic pressure (from normal 25 to 6/8 mmHg) → leakage of fluid from capillaries causing oedema throughout the body.

OTHER ASSOCIATED CONDITIONS

Anaemia: chronic renal failure: Normally the erythropoietin is secreted by kidney tissues which stimulate the bone marrow to produce erythrocytes. In kidney diseases this substance is not secreted in adequate amount so it results into diminished number of erythrocytes and hence anaemia.

Osteomalacia in renal failure: Serious kidney damage reduces the availability of calcium to the bones. Vitamin D must be converted into 1, 25 dihydroxy cholecalciferol in liver and kidney before it promotes calcium absorption from the intestine.

Renal glycosurea (tubular disorder): Besides diabetes mellitus; the tubules may be at fault. Because of their diminished or Zero reabsorptive power, glucose may pass into urine each day; of course it is a benign condition.

Amino acid urea (tubular disorder): may lead to cystinurea - may terminate into renal stones; and simple glycinurea; beta amino isobutyric acid urea.

Renal hypophosphataemia (tubular disorder): Phosphates are failed to be reabsorbed → plasma phosphate concentration falls → diminished calcification of bones.

Acidosis in renal failure: Normally 50–80 millimoles/day more metabolic acid is produced than alkalis. So on renal failure acid accumulates in body and as pH falls below 6.8 death may result.

Increase in urea and other NPN: Renal failure : urea, uric acid, creatinine are end-products of protein metabolism to maintain homeostasis. In renal failure their concentration rises ten times from normal values.

Nephrogenic diabetes insipidus : Occasionally ADH is not affecting renal tubules so constantly dilute urine is excreted. When adequate quantity of water is not taken, dehydration becomes the main diagnostic point of the disease.

Fanconi syndrome : Characterised by failure to reabsorb sodium bicarbonate which causes metabolic acidosis, and increased excretion of potassium and calcium and so nephrogenic diabetes insipidus. So increased urinary excretion of amino acid, glucose, phosphate results.

Causes are hereditary, renotoxic drugs, renal ischaemia etc. affecting mainly tubular cells.

LITHOTRIPSY

- Is the use of ultrasonic or shock waves to pulverise kidney stones. The stones are either excreted or removed from body.
- Two types
  — ESWL (extra corporeal shock wave lithotripsy)
  — Percutaneous lithotripsy
- Former is used on smaller stone, breaks up the stone with external shock waves from a machine called lithotrip.
- For larger stone, a type of endoscope called nephroscope is inserted into kidney through a small incision. The ultrasonic waves from this instrument shatter the stones and fragments are removed through nephroscope.

DIURETICS

These are the substances that increase the rate of urine volume output. Their most important use is to reduce extra cellular fluid volume as required in oedema and hypertension.

- ***Osmotic diuretics***: When substances like urea, mannitol, Sucrose, glucose, etc. are injected, they increase the osmotic pressure in the tubular fluid. This then greatly reduces the water reabsorption. This leads to flushing of large amount of tubular fluid in urine, e.g. when blood glucose concentration in diabetes mellitus rises above transport maximum for glucose, then excess remains in tubules, acts as an osmotic diuretic causing polyurea. They act mainly on proximal tubule.
- ***Loop diuretics***: mechanism:- by decreasing active reabsorption of sodium-chloride potassium
  Site - Thick ascending loop of Henle
  Examples - Furosemide (lasix), ethacrynic acid (edicrin) bumetanide
  Steps:
  — The theme is decreasing active reabsorption by blocking Na, K, Cl cotransporters located in luminal membrane of epithelial cells.
  — By increasing the quantities of solute in distal part of nephron, they behave as osmotic agent
  — Inhibition of Na and Cl reabsorption in loop of Henle → more of these ions excreted along with water excretion → dilution is impaired.
  — Decreased reabsorption of Na, Cl, ions → decreased renal medullary interstitial fluid concentration of these ions → reduced renal

medullary osmolarity → urinary concentration impaired further due to decreased reabsorption of fluid from collecting duct which reduces maximal concentrating, ability of kidney → roughly 30 per cent of glomerular filtrate may be delivered into urine → great urine output for few minutes, under acute conditions.

— By above chain of events counter current multiplier system is disrupted.

- ***Thiazide diuretics***: e.g. chlorothiazide (diuril)
  Mechanism: Blocking Na-Cl-Co transporter in luminal membrane of tubular cell.
  Site - Early distal tubule
  Result :- 5 per cent of glomerular filtrate may pass into urine.
- *Carbonic Anhydrase Inhibitor*:- e.g. Acetazolamide (diamox)
  Mechanism: Blocking sodium-bicarbonate reabsorption
  Site: Proximal tubule
  Disadvantages: Acidosis (some degree) due to excessive loss of bicarbonate ions in urine.

Steps:

1. HCO_3 + H^+ (Secreted in tubular fluid → H_2CO_3 → CO_2 + H_2O → CO_2 diffuses into tubular cell and recombine with H_2O to form H_2CO_3 in presence of carbonic anhydrase → HCO_3^- released + H^+. This HCO_3^- can diffuse across basolateral membrane and can be absorbed into the blood. If thus carbonic anhydrase is blocked then bicarbonate ion cannot be reabsorbed from tubular fluid.
2. Since HCO_3^- reabsorption and H^+ secretion are coupled to Na^+ reabsorption through sodium-hydrogen-ion counter transport mechanism in luminal membrane. So decrease in HCO_3^- reabsorption also reduce sodium reabsorption. This further acts as osmotic diuretics.

- *Spironolactone as diuretic:*
  Example: Aldosterone inhibitors/competitive inhibitors also called potassium sparing diuretics.
  Site— Cortical collecting tubular epithelial cells
  Mechanism— competing with aldosterone for receptor sites in cortical collecting tubule epithelial cells → decreases sodium reabsorption and potassium secretion in this tubular segment → sodium retains which acts as osmotic diuretic. So potassium is secreted/less excreted/increase in extracellular potassium level.
- *Amiloride and triamterene*:
  Mechanism: Inhibition of sodium (Sodium channel blockers) reabsorption and potassium secretion in collecting tubules.
  Steps: By these drugs entry of sodium into sodium channels of the luminal membrane of collecting tubule epithelial cell is decreased → decreased sodium transport across basolateral membrane of cell → decreased activity of Na K ATPase pump → decreased secretion of potassium into tubular fluid.
- *Water and alcohol*: as diuretic mechanism- by inhibiting secretion of ADH
- *Vasopressor receptors inhibition*: Such antagonists by inhibiting its receptors, prevent the activity of ADH
- *Xanthines* (Caffeine—theophylline)
  Mechanism—by increasing GFR and decreasing sodium reabsorption.

READ AND DIGEST: DIURETICS

1. **What should be the quality of a diuretic?**

Ans. Along with the effect of diuresis (increased output of water), it should lead to natriuresis (more excretion of sodium). If sodium will not be excreted → retained in the body → fluids will become hypertonic → elicitation of osmoreceptor response → increased secretion of ADH → more reabsorption of water → effect of diuretic is nullified.

DIALYSIS

Dysfunctions of kidney are treated by dialysis of blood of patient and is carried out by a machine called 'artificial kidney.'

Principle of Functioning

- Because of impaired kidney functions, some toxic waste products which have been accumulating, need to be removed like urea etc.
- Dialysis means diffusion of solutes from an area of higher concentration to the area of lower concentration through a semi permeable membrane.
- Blood flows continuously between two thin membranes of cellophane, outside the membrane is dialysing fluid. Cellophane is porous to allow constituents of plasma to diffuse in both direction, i.e. from plasma to dialysing fluid and vice versa. This means if concentration of a substance is greater in plasma than dialysing fluid, then it will be transferred from plasma to dialysing fluid.
- As told earlier this diffusion depends upon many factors like concentration gradient of solute between two solutions, surface area of membrane, permeability of membrane, time during which this contact has been made.

Procedural Details

- To prevent coagulation, a small amount of heparin is infused into blood as it enters the artificial kidney.
- Normally:
  — Total amount of blood in artificial kidney is less than 500 ml.
  — Total diffusion area is ranging between 0.6–2.5 sq. meters while rate of flow may be many ml/minute.
  Dialysing fluid:This does not contain urea, ureate, sulphate, creatinine or phosphate.

Notes

- Artificial kidney can function more rapidly than two kidneys as far as urea clearance is concerned (Normal kidney = 70 ml/minute Artificial kidney = 225 ml/minute)
- It is used 4 to 6 hours/day thrice a week.
- But artificial kidney cannot be dominant over normal kidney because of other functions like erythropoietin production, etc.

BIBLIOGRAPHY

1. Adler S, et al. Diabetic nephropathy: Pathogenesis and treatment. Ann Rev Med 1993;44:303.
2. Brenner BM. Nephron adaptation to renal injury or ablation. Amer J Phy 1985;249:F 324.
3. Brezis M, Epstein FH. Cellular mechanism of acute ischaemic injury to kidney. Ann Rev Med 1993;44:27.
4. Co. FL, et al. Pathogenesis and treatment of kidney stones. New Eng J Med 1993;327:1141.
5. Gabow PA. Autosomal dominant polycystic kidney disease. New Eng J Med 1993;329: 332.
6. Savin V, et al. Circulating factor associated with increased permeability to albumin in recurrent focal segmental glomerulosclerosis. New Eng J Med 1996;334:878.

MULTIPLE CHOICE QUESTIONS : EXCRETION

1. Nephron was first experimentally demonstrated by:
   a. Ludwig
   b. Heidenhain
   c. William Bowman
   d. Malpighi [ ]
2. Structural and functional unit of kidney is:
   a. Glomerulus
   b. Nephron
   c. Peritubular capillary network
   d. Renal interstitial fluid [ ]
3. Hormone renin is secreted by:
   a. Tubular secretion
   b. Gastric mucosa
   c. Proximal part of intestinal mucosa
   d. Juxtaglomerular apparatus [ ]
4. The average glomerular pressure is said to be:
   a. 10 mmHg
   b. 100 mmHg
   c. 70 mmHg
   d. 50 mmHg [ ]
5. Average pressure in Bowman's capsule is:
   a. 50 mmHg
   b. 10 mmHg
   c. 14 mmHg
   d. 100 mmHg [ ]
6. Which of the following substance is neither reabsorbed nor secreted in any segment of tubules:
   a. Urate ion b. PAH
   c. Inulin d. Urea [ ]
7. Total amount of a substance in plasma which is passing through kidney per minute is called:
   a. Tubular load
   b. Plasma load
   c. Plasma clearance
   d. Counter current mechanism [ ]
8. Transport maximum of glucose is:
   a. 320 mg/min
   b. 125 mg/min
   c. 250 mg/min
   d. 100 mg/min [ ]
9. Water acts as a diuretic because:
   a. Inhibition of ADH
   b. Increases tubular osmotic load
   c. Increases GFR
   d. Idiopathic [ ]
10. The renal blood flow per minute is: (UPSC 1982, 83)
    a. 500 ml b. 750 ml
    c. 1000 ml d. 1300 ml [ ]

---

1 c 2 b 3 d 4 c 5 c 6 c 7 b 8 a 9 a 10 d

VIVA VOCE : EXCRETION

1. Enumerate the main functions served by kidney ?
   a. Excretion of waste products derived from metabolism, toxic substance, drugs etc.
   b. Maintenance of acid–base balance of body.
   c. Regulation of normal blood pressure.
   d. Maintenance of fluid and electrolyte balance.
   e. Plasma osmolarity is maintained.
   f. Detoxicating function (hippuric acid formation).
   g. Synthetic functions: Ammonia, renin, prostaglandin, erythropoietin.
2. What is juxtaglomerular apparatus?
   The epithelial cells of distal tubules where it lies in apposition to the afferent arterioles become condensed into collection of tall tightly packed cells called 'macula densa' which along with juxtaglomerular cells and few intervening granular cell is collectively known as 'J.G. apparatus'.
3. Enumerate the functions of J.G. apparatus ?
   a. Renin hormone production.
   b. Controlling renal blood flow.
   c. Lumen of glomerular arteriole is adjusted by macula densa.
4. What is glomerular filtrate and glomerular filtration rate (GFR)?
   The fluid that filters through glomerular membrane into Bowman's capsule is known as 'glomerular filtrate' and its quantity formed per minute in all nephrons of both kidneys is GFR.
5. How afferent arteriolar constriction is going to effect GFR?
   If afferent arteriolar constriction is there, it causes decreased blood flow into glomerulus which leads to decreased glomerular pressure and hence a decrease in GFR; certainly opposite effects will be noticed on their dilatation.
6. What is the effect of efferent arteriolar constriction on GFR?
   a. On its stimulation, outflow resistance from glomeruli is increased which tends to increase the glomerular pressure and finally terminating into increased GFR. If degree of efferent arteriolar constriction is severe blood flow through glomerulus becomes sluggish.
   b. Opposite manifestation is also possible but that is apparent on severe constriction. Since this leads to sluggish blood flow; which is capable of increasing plasma colloid osmotic pressure which terminates into fall in GFR.
7. Name substance which is neither reabsorbed nor secreted by kidney tubules?
   Inulin
8. What is the composition of glomerular filtrate ?
   Its composition is same as that of plasma except that it has no significant amount of proteins.
9. Define the term 'plasma clearance' ?
   It is defined as ability of kidneys to remove various substances from plasma

$$\text{Plasma clearance}\left(\frac{\text{ml}}{\text{min}}\right) = \frac{\text{Amount of urine}\left(\frac{\text{ml}}{\text{min}}\right) \times \text{concentration in urine}}{\text{Concentration in plasma}}$$

10. Define the term 'transport maximum' (Tm)?
    For every actively reabsorbed substance there exists a maximum rate at which it can be reabsorbed. This is Tm.
11. Mention the Tm of glucose, plasma protein, haemoglobin?
    Glucose = 320 mg per minute.
    Plasma protein = 30 mg per minute.
    Haemoglobin = 1 mg per minute.
12. Anaemia usually occurs in renal insufficiency ? Why
    Kidneys are producing 'erythropoietin' (ESF) normally. This in turn acts on bone marrow to increase the red blood cell production. But in renal insufficiencies there is not existing adequate quantity of this substance; owing to which diminished red cell population is there; terminating into anaemia. Besides this various other factors like urea, hydrogen ions, potassium in higher concentration contribute towards anaemia, also.
13. What do you understand by 'water intoxication'?
    16 ml/minute is maximum urine flow during water diuresis. If due to any reason water ingestion is more rapid, the problem of swelling of cells become worst terminating into convulsions and death. It is all due to hypo-osmolar intestinal fluid.
14. Enumerate classical features of micturition reflex ?
    a. Its onset is at 5th intrauterine life.
    b. Parasympathetics are motor nerves to bladder called 'nerve of emptying'.
    c. On emptying external sphincter closes, detrusor relax; bladder neck closes.
    d. It is 700 ml called 'optimum capacity', up to which the inhibition of emptying the bladder can be exerted by voluntary effort.
    e. Section of sympathetic nerves do not interfere in continence so they are no longer 'nerves of filling'.
    f. Bladder becomes automatic when any damage occurs to spinal micturition centre.
    g. Voluntary control of micturition does not appear until the age of 2 to 3 years upto which bladder is emptied reflexly.
    h. 100 to 150 ml of urine in bladder sensation of filling 150 to 250 ml of urine in bladder feeling of a desire to void.
15. What is nephrotic syndrome?
    It is characterised by massive proteinurea, marked reduction of plasma protein, marked increase in plasma lipids, oedema. Hypertension and haematurea are not prominent. The primary defect lies in capillary basement

membrane which allows protein to escape into glomerular filtrate. Among the causes are amyloidosis, lupus erythematosus, syphilis etc.

QUESTION BANK

1. Draw a labelled diagram of Nephron.
2. Explain
   a. The mechanism of concentration of urine,
   b. Mechanism of reabsorption of bicarbonate in the proximal nephron. (Raj Univ First MBBS, 2001)
3. Describe tubulo-glomerular feedback theory.
4. Write in brief about control of micturition.
5. Write short notes
   a. TmG
   b. Inulin clearance test
   c. Automatic bladder
   d. Hormones secreted by kidney.
   e. Renal blood flow and its regulation.
   f. GFR
   g. Diuretics
   h. Dialysis
   i. Counter current mechanism
   j. Acute kidney shut down (Raj Univ 1991, MD)
   k. Urea clearance tests (1982)
   l. Microanatomy of nephron (Raj Univ 1980, MD)
   m. Inulin clearance (Raj Univ First MBBS, 2001)
   n. Tubular Transport maximum (Raj Univ First MBBS, 2001)
6. Discuss the role of kidney in maintaining acid–base balance.
7. Draw a labelled diagram of juxtamedullary nephrone. Discuss mechanism of tubular reabsorption and secretion. (Raj Univ 1996, MD)
8. Write a note of pH maintenance by kidney (Raj Univ 1985, MD)
9. Describe the histology of renal tubules. How are various tubular functions carried out? (Raj Univ 1999, MD)
10. Describe the formation of urine in man and in desert animal. How do you account for differences (Raj Univ 1991, 1993 MD)
11. Discuss
    a. The structure and function of JG apparatus. (Raj Univ 1991, 1992, MD)
    b. Renal function tests (Raj Univ 1985, MD)
    c. Why is micturition reflex effected in spinal cord injuries.
    d. Pathophysiology of chronic renal failure and principles of treatment (Raj Univ 1989, MD)
    e. The physiology of normal and abnormal micturition (Raj Univ 1986, MD)
    f. Heatstrokes (Raj Univ First MBBS, 2001)
    g. Diurnal variation of core body temperature. (Raj Univ First MBBS, 2001)
12. How much is the normal osmolality of plasma. What is the greatest contributor to it. What are the factors maintaining osmotic gradient in medulla of kidney. What is its significance?
13. Differences (a) Osmotic and water diuresis.
14. Name the sites where Na^+ and glucose are co-transported. How is this principle used in clinical practice?
15. How does kidney produce concentrated urine. Describe counter current mechanism? (Raj Univ1983, 1992, MD)
16. How do you evaluate kidney efficiency in an individual? (Raj Univ 1979, MD)
17. How is the water distributed in body. Discuss its regulation? (Raj Univ 1990, 1996, MD)
18. a. Describe the major homeostatic mechanisms which maintain the tonicity and volume of E.C.F.
    b. Describe the mechanism of action of various buffers in blood. [BF/2003/08 (MD)]

UNIT 6

Boon of Nature

"Certainly we are able to see this wonderful world by our eyes and listen the melody of Nature by ears, but what to say about modern noise which is a pollution in this advancement of civilisation."

Special Senses

37 Sense of Vision: I, II, III, IV, V, VI

VISUAL OPTICS

Basic physical principles of optics are very important to be studied first before we call our eye as a camera.

- Light rays travel through air at a velocity of approximately 300,000 km/sec. but much slower through transparent solids and liquids. The refractive index of air itself is 1.00. If light travels through a particular type of glass at a velocity of 200,000 km/sec., the refractive index of this glass is 300,000 divided by 200,000 or 1.50.
- When light waves travelling forward in a beam strike an interface that is perpendicular to the beam the waves enter the second refractory medium without deviation, of course their velocity is decreased. On the other hand, if light waves strike an angulated interface, the light waves bend if refractive index of two media are different from one another. This bending of light rays at an angulated interface is called refraction and degree of refraction depends on (a) ratio of the two refractive indices of two transparent media and (b) degree of angulation between interface and wave entering:
- Concave lens diverge light rays while convex lens converge them.
- If lens is ground with exactly proper curvature parallel light rays passing through each part of the lens will be bent exactly enough so that all the rays will pass through a single point called *'focal point.'* The distance beyond a convex lens at which parallel rays converge to a common focal point is called *'focal length of a lens.'* The refractive power is measured in terms of *Diopter*.
- The lens system of eye is composed of four refractive interfaces : (a) The interface between air and anterior surface of cornea; (b) interface between posterior surface of cornea and aqueous humor, (c) interface between aqueous humor and anterior surface of crystalline lens of eye (d) interface between posterior Surface of lens and vitreous humor.
  Refractive index of air - 1; Cornea 1.38, aqueous humor 1.33, crystalline lens 1.40, vitreous humor 1.34.
- The lens system of an eye can focus image on retina. The image is inverted and reversed. However the mind perceives objects in upright position.

ERRORS OF REFRACTION

- Eye is considered to be normal (emmetropia) if parallel light rays from distant objects are in sharp focus on the retina when the ciliary muscle is completely relaxed.
- *Myopia (near sightedness)*: when ciliary muscle is completely relaxed the light rays coming from the distant objects are focussed in front of the retina. It is due to a long eyeball. Since concave lens diverges the rays, so it is corrected by placing concave lens in front of the eye. Person is unable to see distant objects clearly.

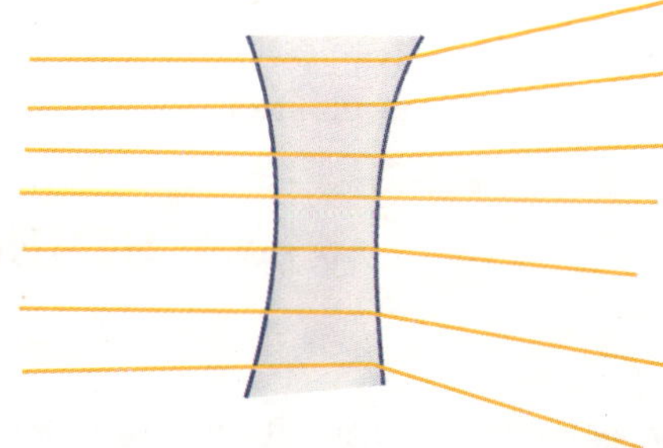

Fig. 37.1: Concave lens: divergence of rays

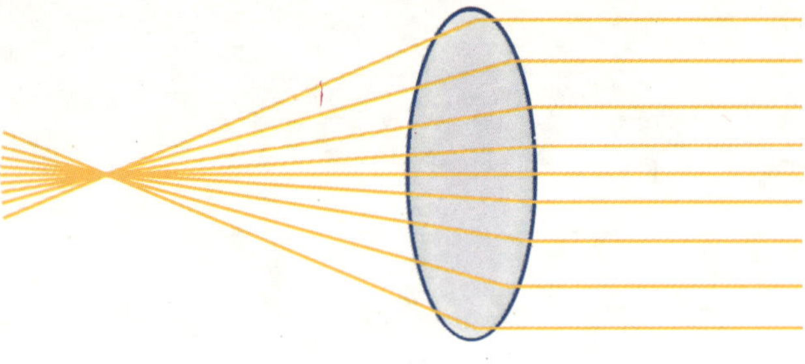

Fig. 37.2: Convex lens

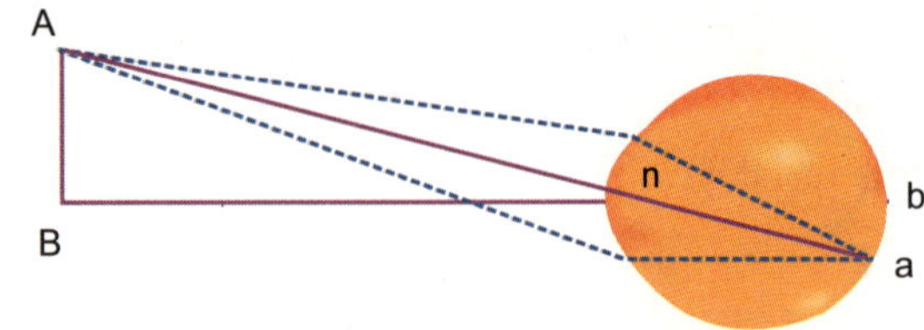

Fig. 37.3: Reduced eye

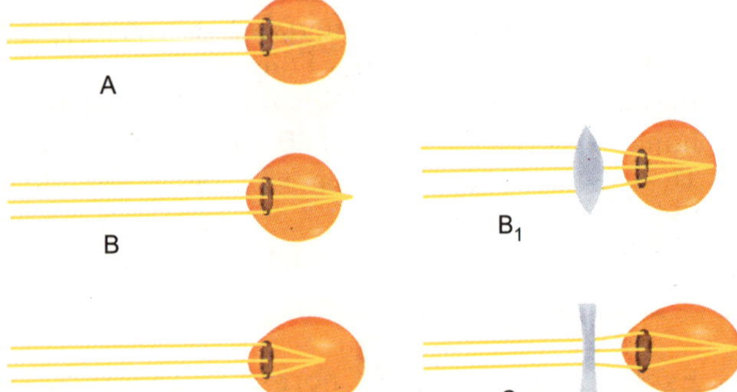

Fig. 37.4: Common errors of visions (A = Emmetropia (Normal eye, B = Hypermetropia, B1 = Corrected with convex lens, C = Myopia, C1 = Corrected with concave lens

- *Hypermetropia or hyperopia (far sightedness)*: Eyeball is too short, parallel light rays are not bent sufficiently by the lens system; they are focussed behind the retina. A convex lens in front of the eye corrects the error. Person is unable to see near objects clearly.
- *Presbyopia*: As age advances lens grows larger and thicker and loses its elasticity which is due to denaturation of lens proteins. Power of accommodation decreases. Eye remains focussed permanently at an almost constant distance which depends on physical characteristics of individual's eye. Eyes cannot accommodate for both near and far vision. So old persons must wear bifocal glasses with upper segment normally focussed for distant vision and lower segment for near vision.
- *Astigmatism:* This refractory error is caused by an oblong shape of cornea/lens. Because the curvature of astigmatic lens along one plane is less than curvature along other plane, light rays striking the peripheral portions of lens in one plane are not bent nearly so much as are rays striking the peripheral portions of other plane. It is obvious that all light rays passing through an astigmatic lens don't come to a common focal point because light rays passing through one plane focus far in front of those passing through the other plane. For its correction, usual procedure is to find a spherical lens by 'trial and error' that corrects the focus in one of the two planes of the astigmatic lens. Then an additional cylindrical lens is used to correct the error in remaining plane and for this both axis and strength of required cylindrical lens must be determined.
- *Cataract is an ageing process*: A cataract is a cloudy or opaque area in the lens. Proteins of lens fibres are denatured; later on some proteins coagulate to form opaque areas in place of normal transparent protein fibres. Surgical removal of entire lens is the remedy and is replaced by powerful convex lens of +20 diopter in place of removed lens.

INTERESTING FACTS

1. The rate of blinking is once every five seconds, or 17,000 times each day or $6^1/_2$ million times a year.
2. If eyes are shut tightly, the light apparently seen are phosphenes. This luminous appearance is due to excitation of retina caused by pressure on eyeball.
3. History:- The original bifocal lenses were invented by Benjamin Franklin (1706–1790)—He joined the two lenses in a metallic frame. In 1889, J. L. Borsch welded them together.

STRUCTURAL ASPECTS

Human eyeball is roughly spherical being little flat from above downwards.

EYEBROW

A thickened ridge of skin covered with short hairs. Protects the eye from vivid light.

EYELIDS (PALPEBRAE)

- Are two movable folds placed in front of the eye. The upper lid is attached to small muscle levator-palpebrae-superioris - an elevator of lid. Around both lids there is orbicularis oculi muscle which closes the eyelids. They are covered externally with skin and internally with conjunctiva—(mucous membrane).
- Eyelids protect the eye from bright light, foreign objects and it covers the eyes during sleep.
- Palpebral fissure is nothing but the slit between the edges of lids. Outer angle of this fissure is external canthus while inner angle is internal canthus. It is the size of this fissure which gives appearance to eye—large or small.

EYELASHES

- From the margin of each eyelid, a row of short thick hairs project called eyelashes. The follicle of eyelashes receive a lubricating fluid from the sebaceous glands which open into them. On getting infection *sty* results (pimple/furuncle).
- The tarsal/meibomian glands are lying between conjunctiva and tarsal cartilage of each eyelid. These are elongated sebaceous glands, the duct of which open on edge of eyelid. Their distension is called *chalazion*.

CONJUNCTIVA

Is a thin stratified mucous membrane which is reflected on to the inner surface of eyelid. It covers the exposed part of eyeball. It serves the purpose of lubrication and protection.

LACRIMAL APPARATUS

i. Consists of lacrimal gland, lacrimal duct, lacrimal sac and nasolacrimal duct.
ii. Lacrimal gland is a compound gland. It is about the size and shape of an almond. It is lodged in a depression of frontal bone at upper and outer angle of the orbit.
iii. Lacrimal ducts (6–12) lead from the gland to the surface of conjunctiva of upper lid. The secretion (tears) flows into two tiny lacrimal ducts and is conveyed into lacrimal sac at the inner angle of the eye.
iv. The lacrimal sac is the expanded upper end of naso-lacrimal duct, a small canal that opens into the nose. It is oval in shape measuring 12–15 mm in length.
v. It secretes tears.

Table 37.1: Composition of tears

Water	98.2%
solids	1.8%
Sodium, potassium, ammonia	0.79%
Urea	0.03%
NPN	0.05%
Sugar	0.6%
NaCl	0.66%
Albumin, globulin lysozyme	

vi. It keeps the surface of eye moist and help in removing the foreign bodies, bacteria, dust, etc.
vii. This gland does not develop sufficiently to secrete tears until about fourth month of the life.

MUSCLES OF THE EYE

i. Intrinsic muscles—are ciliary muscles and muscles of iris.
ii. The extrinsic muscles hold the eyeball in place and control its movements. They include four recti (straight) and two oblique.

Table 37.2: Control of eye movements

Muscle	*Action*	*Nerve supply (Cranial)*
Superior rectus	Up and In	III
Inferior rectus	Down and In	III
Medial rectus	Inwards	III
Lateral rectus	outwards	VI
Superior oblique	Down and out	IV
Inferior oblique	up and out	III

Table 37.3: Ocular movements

1. Eye axes move to the same side, e.g. right, left, up, down.
2. Eye axes move in opposite direction, e.g. convergence divergence.
3. Eyeball rotates round their axes clockwise or anti-clockwise.
4. Sometimes these muscles (specially recti—medial and lateral) are unequal in length or strength, the equilibrium of opposed muscles is upset and is then turned in direction of stronger muscle producing a squint (strabismus).

NERVES OF EYE

i. Optic nerve concerned with vision only
ii. Oculomotor nerve supplying medial/superior/inferior recti and inferior oblique muscle, ciliary muscle, circular muscle of iris
iii. Trochlear nerve controls superior oblique muscle
iv. Abducent controls lateral rectus

v. Ophthalmic—a branch of trigeminal nerve supplies general sensation, sending branches to cornea, ciliary body, iris, lacrimal gland and conjunctiva.

EYE ORBIT

Are bony cavities in which eyeballs are contained. Bones assisting are : frontal, malar, maxilla, palatine, sphenoid, ethmoid, lacrimal. During many forms of illness the body fat is oxidised at an unusual rate, during those situations the orbital fat diminishes and eyeballs sink in the orbit.

EYEBALL ... spherical shape.

Fibrous tunic ... sclera, cornea

Vascular tunic ... choroid, ciliary body, iris

Nervous tunic ... Retina

FIBROUS TUNIC

- *Sclera*: covers posterior five sixth of eyeball. It is supplied with few blood vessels. Its nerves are derived from ciliary nerve. It is opaque, white and smooth externally. It maintains the shape of eyeball and also protects the delicate structures contained within it. It is separated from choroid by lymph space.
- *Cornea (window of eye)*: Covers anterior sixth of eyeball and is directly continuous with sclera. It is well supplied with nerves, lymph vessels but is destitute of blood vessels.

CORNEAL REFLEX

Twist a cotton into fine hair like. Lightly touch the lateral edge of cornea at its conjunctival margin with this cotton wisp. Patient should see straight. Blinking occurs if reflex present. Two sides should be compared. Central part of cornea should not be touched because of risk of corneal ulceration. Doctor should keep his little finger on cheek of patient.

VASCULAR TUNIC

- *Choroid*: thin, dark brown membrane lining the inner surface of sclera. It consists of dense capillary plexus, small arteries and veins, carrying blood to and from plexus. Between these vessels are pigment cells which with other cells form a network - stroma : It is dark and opaque so that it darkens the chamber of eye by preventing reflection of light. It extends to the ciliary body.
- *Ciliary body*: includes orbicularis ciliaris, ciliary processes and the ciliaris muscle. The fibres of ciliary muscle arise from sclera near the cornea, and extending backward are inserted into outer surface of ciliary process and choroid. This muscle is chief agent in accommodation. When it contracts, it draws forwards the ciliary process, relaxes the suspensory ligament of lens and allows lens to become more convex.
- *Iris (rainbow):*
  - — Is a circular, coloured disc suspended in aqueous humor in front of lens and behind the cornea. It is attached at its circumference to the ciliary process with which it is practically continuous, and is also connected to sclera and cornea at the point where they join one another. It hangs free in interior of eyeball. The colour of the eye is related to number and size of pigment bearing cells in iris.
  - — If no pigment or very little ... blue eye
  - — If large amount of pigment ...black/brown/gray
  - — In the middle of iris there is a circular hole called pupil.
  - — Two sets of muscles - sphincter pupillae - fibres arranged like sphincter with its fibres encircling pupil.
  - — Dilator pupillae - fibres radiating from pupil to the outer circumference of iris. The action of these muscles is antagonistic.
  - — The iris regulate the amount of light entering the eye and thus assisting in obtaining clear images, which is accomplished by these muscles. When eye is accommodated for a near object or stimulated by a bright light the sphincter muscle contracts and diminishes the size of pupil. When eye is accommodated for a distant object or the light is dim, the dilator muscle contracts increasing size of pupil.
  - — Functions of Iris - (i) It adjusts the amount of light falling on retina. (ii) It helps to avoid errors of refraction by cutting off the peripheral rays. (iii) It increases the depth of focus. (iv) Surface is covered with epithelium which phagocyte proteins and small particles from aqueous humor to make it clean.
  - — Pupil diminishes the amount of light entering eye. It improves vision largely by reducing aberration as well as by increasing depth of focus. As distance between object and eye is decreased, the depth of focus also diminishes which is counteracted by decreasing the diameter of pupil.
  - — Pupillary reflexes: (size of pupil is 8 mm in diameter in weakest light intensity to 1 mm at maximum light intensity)
    - a. *Light reflex:*
      - i. When light falls on one eye the pupil constricts. This is the direct pupillary reflex. In such an instance, even the pupil of other eye constricts which constitute indirect

pupillary reflex. The degree of constriction depends upon intensity of light and state of adaptation.

ii. Visual receptors are stimulated when light falls on retina. The afferent impulse passes along afferent fibres running in optic nerve and tract to be terminated into pretectal nucleus. From here fibres are relayed to Edinger-Westphal nucleus of both sides. Efferent impulses are passed along third cranial nerve to sphincter pupillae which contracts to make the pupil constricted.

iii. By this reflex amount of light entering the eye is adjusted. It also improves the vision by decreasing aberration (spherical/chromatic).

b. *Accommodation reflex:* Afferent impulses from retina are carried to visual cortex along visual pathway. The fibres then reach to Edinger-Westphal nucleus and ventro median nucleus of oculomotor nerve nucleus through descending fibres/frontal eyefield.

c. *Near reflex:* When a person looks upon a near object three changes take place namely pupillary constriction + convergence + increased anterior curvature of lens. This is near reflex.

d. *Cilio-spinal reflex (Pupillary skin reflex):* If skin of the neck is pinched; dilatation of pupil results. The pathway is as - pain endings → middle cervical segments of spinal cord → spino-thalamic projection → thalamo-cortical projections. Post-ganglionic fibres from superior cervical ganglion to 'dilator pupillae' via long ciliary nerves.

NERVOUS TUNIC

Retina: Innermost coat of eyeball. A delicate nervous membrane, which receives the images of external objects and transfer the impression evoked by them to the visual centre in brain. It occupies the space between the choroid coat and the hyaloid membrane of the vitreous body and extends forwards almost to the posterior margin of ciliary body where it terminates in a ***jagged*** margin called ***ora serrata***.

The seventh layer is of rods and cones which act as end organ/receptor for optic nerve.

The blind spot: The optic nerve pierces the eyeball not exactly at its most posterior part but a little to inner side. This point is insensitive to light called blind spot. There are no rods and cones at this point and rays of light falling upon it produces no sensation.

Macula lutea (yellow spot): Is situated about 2.08 mm to the outer side of the exit of optic nerve and is the exact centre of retina. In its centre is a tiny pit *fovea centralis* which is the centre of direct vision. At this point there is an absence of rods but a great increase in cones. This is a region of greatest visual acuity. In reading, the eyes move so as to bring the rays of light from word after word into centre of fovea. Here each cone is connected to one ganglion cell from which one fibre leads to the brain. Else where in retina several cones or rods are connected to one ganglion cells and one fibre of optic nerve.

Functions of Retina

Vision: Due to cones, the fovea is responsible for visual acuity, bright/day light or photopic vision and colour vision. The peripheral retina due to rods is responsible for dim light (scotopic vision).

It is concerned with various reflexes like accommodation, fixation, visuospinal, etc.

It also helps to maintain tone/posture and body equilibrium.

Rods: Photoreceptors of retina. Sub-serves dim light. 110–125 million in number. 40–60 μ long and 2 μ in diameter : it is made up of outer segment - thin cylindrical part composed of myelin like substance and contains rhodopsin- inner part - broad

Cones: Concerned with bright light vision, colour vision and visual acuity. 6–7 million in number. 28–85 μ long and 2–5 μ in diameter.

In fovea - only cones; in periphery rods; intermediate part - contains both.

Consists of—outer part—smaller and transversely striated, inner part larger and longitudinally striated. Inner segment of rods contain cytoplasm + its organelles, along with mitochondria; these mitochondria supply energy for their proper functioning. Synaptic body is that part of rods and cones which connects them with subsequent neuronal cells/horizontal and bipolar cells.

REFRACTIVE MEDIA

- *Crystalline lens* enclosed in its capsule is a transparent refractory body with convex anterior and posterior surfaces. It is placed directly behind the pupil where it is retained in position by counter balancing pressure of the aqueous humor in front and vitreous body behind and by its own suspensory ligament. In infancy it is almost spherical, in adult of medium convexity and in the aged considerably flattened. The capsule surrounding lens is elastic.
- It is convex on all sides but its posterior surface is more curved than anterior surface. It is about 11 mm in diameter and thickness of central part is ranging between 3.6–3.9 mm. It is divided into two parts—

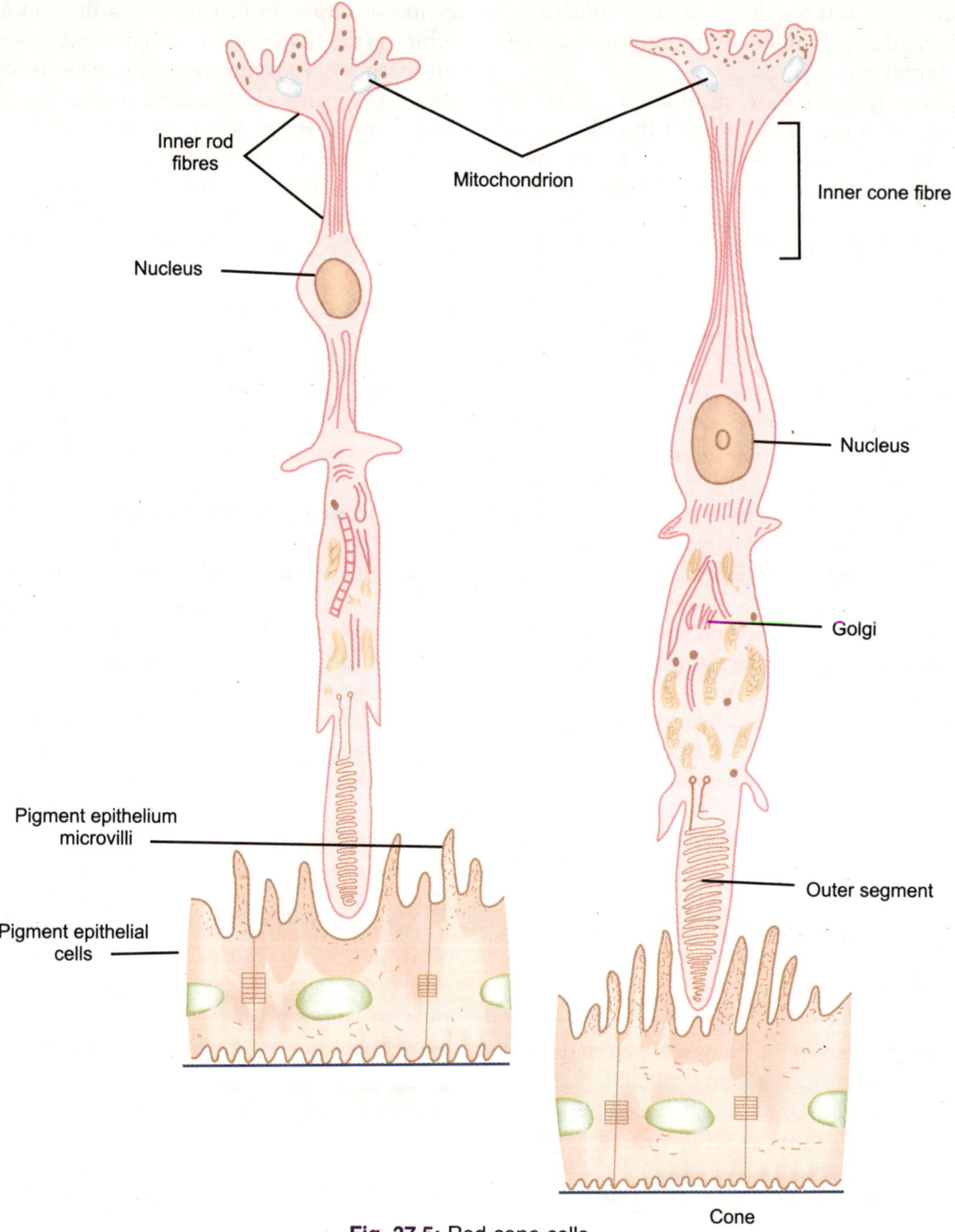

Fig. 37.5: Rod-cone cells

softer outer part cortex and hard central part the nucleus.

- The refractive index of whole lens is 1.42 (cortex - 1.38; nucleus 1.43).
- It is main refractory apparatus which focusses the light on retina and thus aids vision.
- It derives its nutrition entirely from aqueous humor and partly from vitreous humor. The process of active transport is said to occur between lens and aqueous humor because of subscapsular epithelium. R. Q. of lens is one (essential source of energy for lens is carbohydrate; metabolic activity is confined to cortex).

Intraocular Fluid

- Fills the eye which maintains sufficient pressure in the eyeball to keep it distended.
- The aqueous humor which lies in front and to the side of lens, and vitreous humor which lies between lens

and retina. Aqueous humor is freely flowing fluid while vitreous humor is a gelatinous mass held together by fine fibrillar network.

- Aqueous humor is formed at rate of 2 to 3 cubic mm per minute. It is secreted by ciliary process which are linear folds projecting from ciliary body into space behind the iris where the lens ligaments also attach to eyeball. It is formed as an active secretion of the epithelium lining the ciliary process.
- It flows between the ligaments of lens, then through pupil and finally into anterior chamber of eye. Here the fluid flows into angle between cornea and iris, then through a meshwork of trabeculae, finally entering the canal of Schlemm which empties into extraocular veins.
- Normally intraocular pressure ranges between 12–20 mmHg (average 15 mmHg)
- In conditions where large amount of debris is accumulated in aqueous humor (as seen in intraocular infection, haemorrhage etc.); then adequate reabsorption of fluid from anterior chamber is prevented. This raises the tension, i.e. glaucoma. This is because of the fact that this debris gets itself accumulated in trabecular spaces which leads to canal of Schlemm.

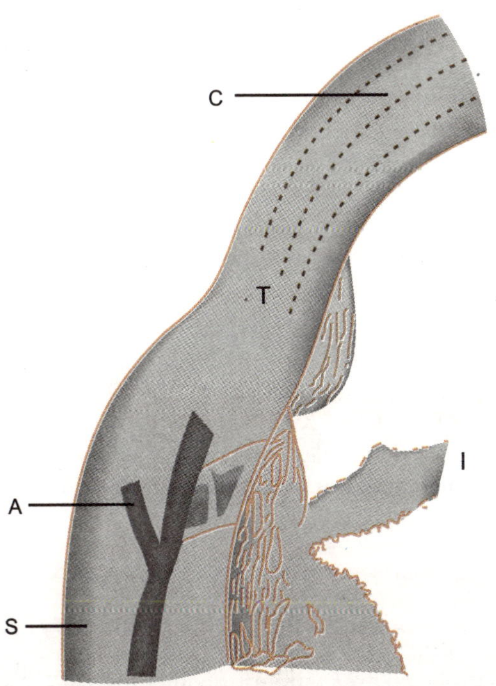

Fig. 37.6: Outflow of aqueous humor (A = Blood veins, S = Sclera, C = Cornea, I = Iris, T = Trabeculae

- It is worth remembering here that there exists larger number of RE cells which clean the trabeculae system by their phagocytic action.
- The secretion of aqueous humor starts with active transport of sodium ions into spaces between epithelial cells. To maintain electrical neutrality they attract Cl^- as well as HCO_3^-. They then cause water osmosis.
- The Schlemm canal is a thin walled vein extending all the way around eye. Its endothelial membrane is very much porous.

Glaucoma

- Is the name given to raised intraocular tension (from 20/30 to 70 mmHg). It is one of the common causes of blindness. As the pressure rises the axons of optic nerve are compressed where they leave the eyeball at the optic disc. This compression blocks axonal flow of cytoplasm from neuronal cell bodies in the retina to peripheral optic nerve fibres entering the brain. This results into inadequate nutrition which terminates into death of affected neurones. Compression of retinal artery also contributes to inadequacy of nutrition. Pilocarpine eye drops are used which reduces the secretion or enhances absorption.
- In acute eye inflammation, WBC + debris can block these trabecular spaces and may raise the tension. In old age fibrous occlusion of these trabeculae may raise the tension.
- Surgical treatment consists of opening the spaces of trabeculae or to make direct channels between fluid space of eyeball and subconjunctival space outside the eyeball.

VITREOUS HUMOR OR BODY

- Is a jelly like material covered by a homogenous membrane-the hyaloid membrane, occupying posterior compartment. It is made up of a series of lamellae arranged concentrically round hyaloid canal.
- Its refractive index—1.34
- Functions—(i) Maintains shape and pressure of eye ball. (ii) Acts as a refractive medium.
- It gets liquefied in cases of retinal detachment where retina floats in vitreous cavity.
- Differences from aqueous humor : (1) Its glucose content is less (2) Concentration of pyruvic and lactic acid is higher.
- It provides nutrition to lens; it prevents retinal detachment; as well as it gives support to lens posteriorly.
- It contains mucoproteins and residual proteins.

LIGHT THROWN ON EYE

BINOCULAR VISION

The value of two eyes instead of one is that true binocular vision is possible. Its components are:

a. *Convergence*
   - Is necessary to turn the eyes inwards, in order that two images of a given object may lie upon corresponding points of the two retinae. It is voluntary up to some extent and is brought about by innervation of medial rectus muscle.
   - Although two images are formed but observer sees only one. This is because of the fact that two images are physiologically fused giving impression of one single image. But it is possible only when two images are focussed at respective points on retina called corresponding points (two fovea). The opposite of corresponding point is disparate point; and when both images are focussed at these points diplopia is the result (single image will be doubled).

b. *Optic chiasma:* The optic fibres from each retina pass backward through the optic foramen and shortly after leaving the orbit the two nerves come together, and fibres from the inner portion of each nerve cross (outer fibres don't cross). This is optic chiasma.
   - On looking at a near object in a bright light → pupil constricts → entering rays are directed towards central part of lens where refractory power and convexity is greatest and to fovea centralis.
   - In a dim light → pupil dilated → rays are directed towards peripheral part of retina
   - Constriction of pupil is brought about by stimulation of circular muscle of iris by oculomotor nerve.
   - In stress (excitement, fear) autonomic nerves are stimulated causing its dilatation, (ophthalmic branch of trigeminal nerve).

c. *Accommodation*: Is the ability of the eye to adjust or focus objects at different distances because a sharply focused image must fall upon retina in order to produce clear vision.
   - Eyes are rest/fixed upon distant objects → suspensory ligament exerts a tension upon capsule of lens which keeps the lens flattened, particularly the anterior surface to which it is attached. It is a passive process.
   - Eyes fixed upon near objects (reading, sewing etc.) → ciliary muscle contract drawing forward choroid coat → releases tension of suspensory ligament upon lens capsule allowing anterior surface of lens to be more convex. It is an active process and is more or less fatiguing.
   - In emmetropic eye, parallel light rays are focused on retina. Rays from objects closer than 6 m from observer are focussing behind retina and so it appears blurred. This problem should be solved, i.e. rays should be focused on retina. This is made possible by increasing the distance between lens and retina or by increasing the curvature or refractive power of lens. So the process by which curvature of the lens is increased is accommodation.
   - At rest lens is held under tension by lens ligaments. It is pulled into flattened shape because of elasticity of lens capsule. When gaze is directed at or near the object there occurs contraction of ciliary muscles which decreases the distance between edges of ciliary body and so relaxes the lens ligament, so it appears more convex shaped. This shape-wise change increases its refractive power 10–12 times. The above mentioned contraction of ciliary muscle is due to contraction of longitudinal muscle fibres near corneo-scleral-junction.
   - Sphincter like action of circular muscle fibres. Due to this edges of ciliary body are brought closer.
   - Autonomic control... Ciliary muscles are controlled by ANS. Parasympathetic stimulation → contraction, of ciliary muscle → relaxation of lens ligament → increase in refractory power → eye is capable of focussing on objects nearer at hand.
   - Sympathetics are exerting a weak effect in relaxing the ciliary muscles but almost no role in accommodation.

PUPILLARY REFLEX (Two types)

a. *Pupillary light reflex*: It contracts when light falls on it, which starts after a latent period of 0.05 sec. and reaches to peak by 0.1 sec.

   Impulse arises in rods and cones $\xrightarrow{\text{retina}}$ optic nerve → optic chiasma $\xrightarrow{\text{decussation}}$ optic tract → pretectal area (superior colliculus) $\xrightarrow[\text{nuclear}]{\text{colliculo}}$ III nerve nucleus → ciliary ganglion → post ganglionic fibres arise which supply sphincter pupillae through short ciliary nerves.

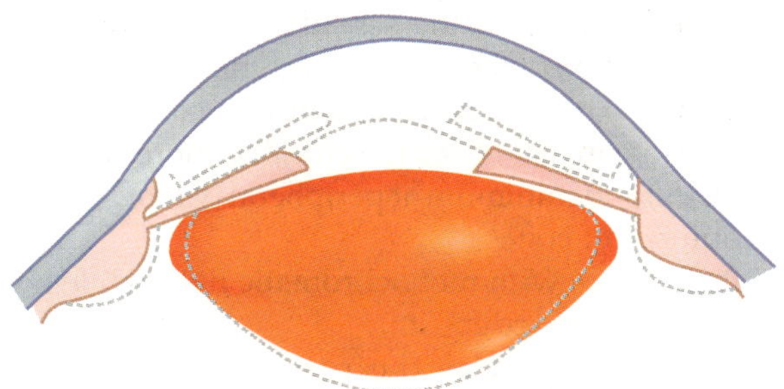

Fig. 37.7: Accommodation

b. *Accommodation reflex:*
- Adjustment of optical apparatus to make it suitable for near vision. It is not a pure reflex process but to some extent a willed movement.
- It includes visual path from retina to occipital cortex. From here the impulse is relayed in frontal eye field (Area 8) and then carried by corico-nuclear fibres passing through anterior limb of internal capsule to III cranial nerve nucleus of opposite side through which impulse reaches to muscles involved in accommodation.
- The stimulus for it is visual clue. The blurring of image and chromatic aberration are the two important factors affecting it.

Argyll Robertson pupil: Is an abnormal state where light reflex is lost but accommodation reflex persists. It is seen in cerebral syphilis and the lesion is in sylvian aqueduct. Its opposite is called Wernicke's hemianopic-pupillary reaction in which light falling on blind half of retina, elicits light reflex but not accommodation reflex.

Near reflex remains intact. The defect is bilateral. Painful stimulus are unable to dilate such pupil and they don't respond to atropine. The affected pupils are smaller and unequal in size. The site of lesion is pretectal/tectal area; or may be in posterior commissure, or in oculomotor nucleus (synapse between afferent and efferent neurones), or involvement of sympathetic and parasympathetic in iris itself (various views about site of lesion).

Myotonic/Adies pupil: Pupil reacts either not at all or very little to light. It shows near reflex. Pupillary constriction occurs very slow and delayed. Young women are main sufferers. Tendon reflexes are reduced. It is an unilateral benign disease. Affected pupil is larger comparatively. It dilates with atropine.

PHOTOCHEMISTRY OF VISION

- A light sensitive pigment *rhodopsin or visual purple* is contained in the outer segment of rod that projects into the pigment layer of the retina. It is actually a mixture of *scotopsin* (-a protein) and *retinene*—(a carotenoid pigment).

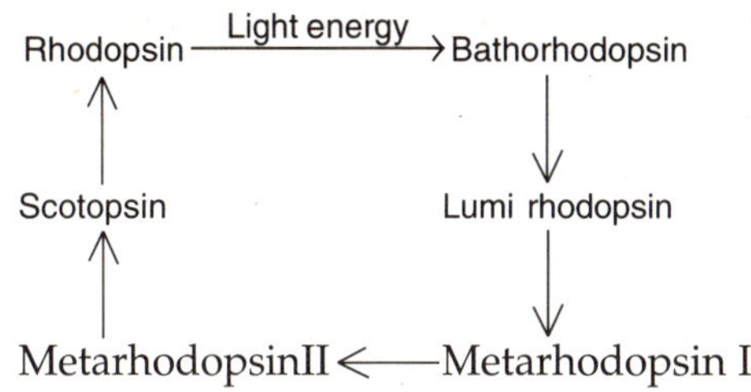

Photochemistry of Vision

- The degraded rhodopsin is reformed in the presence of enzyme 'retinal isomerase.' Once II-cis retinal is formed it recombines with scotopsin to reform rhodopsin.
- Vitamin A is present in both cytoplasm of rods and in pigment layer of retina. Night blindness occurs in severe vitamin A deficiency. The reason is clear that when enough vitamin A is not present then adequate amount of rhodopsin is not formed. In this condition the vision is not adequate in the night. This occurs when an individual remains on diet deficient in vitamin A
- Rod-receptor potential : Light thrown on retina → rhodopsin decomposes → decrease in membrane conductance for sodium in outer segment of rod → Hyperpolarisation of entire rod membrane (receptor potential).
- Qualities of receptor potential:
  i. A visual image impinged on retina for only a millionth of a second can cause the sensation of observing the image sometimes for longer than a second (Receptor potential reaches at peak in 0.3 sec. and lasting for more than a second; In cones these changes are more fast).
  ii. It allows the eye to discriminate light intensities through a range many thousand times greater than will be otherwise possible.
- Activated rhodopsin → activate many molecules of transducin (a protein present in inactive form in membranes of disc and cell membrane of rod) → It

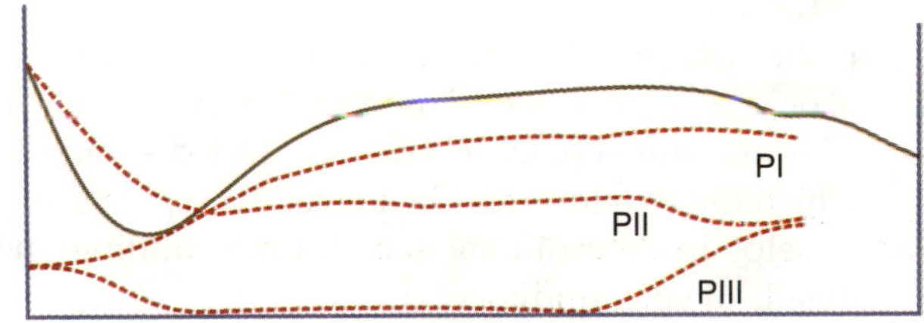

Fig. 37.8: Electroretinogram

activates many more molecules of phospho-di-esterase → hydrolyses molecules of cGMP → closure of sodium channels in light (but in dark continued influx of sodium ions) → This excites the rod → Rhodopsin kinase another enzyme present in rods, inactivates the activated rhodopsin and entire cycle reverses back.

- *Receptor potential*
  1. It is the first potential change occurring because of falling of light on photo receptors.
  2. Early phase: Zero latent period. It is dominated by cones. It is seen even in the presence of metabolic inhibitors. The potential generated by cones (single) is larger than rod (single). It is directly proportional with change in physical energy of stimulus.
  3. Late phase: Latent period 1 m sec. It is inhibited by metabolic inhibitors and cold. It is many-many times more sensitive than early phase.

Electro-retinogram (ERG)

1. The graphical record of gross electrical changes taking place in retina on exposure to light is ERG.
2. After a very brief latent period - a negative a wave is seen. It is followed by positive b wave. Then a slow rising 'c' wave and last d wave when light is turned off. a-b and c wave are due to activity of photo receptors, bipolar cells and pigment epithelium respectively; while d wave is due to interaction between receptor potential and dc component.
3. Its pattern depends on - nature of receptors dominating in retina, adaptation by eye, wavelength of stimulus and number of stimuli.
4. It is useful in studying retinal physiology + diagnosis of retinal disease. It is subnormal when retina fails in function. When rods and cones fail to perform their duties it is extinguished.
5. The receptive field of a cell is an area of retinal stimulation which alters the activity of that particular cell. It has a central and a peripheral part and response on both these parts is opposite.

VISUAL ACUITY

i. Is the sharpness to which the details and contours of objects are perceived. It is usually defined in terms of minimum separable—the shortest distance by which the two lines will be perceived separately.
ii. It helps in determining shape, form, outline and details of surroundings.
iii. It depends upon the sensitivity of retina to light illumination of the surface, the time of exposure, and ability to recognise the distance of parallel rays.
iv. It is maximum at fovea centralis (more number of cones) and minimum at peripheral part of retina (less number of cones).
v. It increases with monochromatic light while errors of refraction reduce it.
vi. It is expressed as the reciprocal of the angle subtended at the nodal point of the eye—visual angle which is generally one minute when retinal images are separated by 4.5μ.

DARK ADAPTATION

- It is a common experience that after entering from brightly illuminated area into a dark room, the vision at first is very poor but after sometime is improved. This is dark adaptation.
- It involves two separate processes - (i) Removal of after image from retina and (ii) Resynthesis of bleached rhodopsin in the rods.
- It is not possible in vitamin A deficiency. Time taken for dark adaptation is directly proportional to intensity of light and duration of exposure and inversely proportional to vitamin A content. It is completed within one hour.

LIGHT ADAPTATION

- Is nothing but disappearance of dark adaptation. If a person suddenly passes from a dim to brightly illuminated area, intense and uncomfortable light is felt by him but stage passes after a while.
- The decreased sensitivity of the eye or an increase in visual threshold in the light, is light adaptation.
- It is a very rapid process. The pupil constricts, vision changes from rods to cones, bleaching of photo pigment occurs which reduce their concentration in the receptors, inhibition type of functional changes occur in retina.

DARK AND LIGHT ADAPTATION: AT A GLANCE

- A person in bright light → large amounts of photo-chemicals are reduced to retinal and opsins + much of retinal is changed into vitamin A → concentration of photosensitive chemicals reduced → reduced sensitivity of eye towards light → light adaptation.
- If a man remains in a dark room for a longer time then the pigments (retinal + opsin in rodcones) are converted back into light sensitive pigments.

Vitamin A is also changed into retinal to provide more light-sensitive pigments.

- When light intensity is increased, then signals transmitted by different cells of retina viz. bipolar, horizontal, amacrine, ganglion cells increase their intensity of firing.
- Pupillary size also controls this phenomenon.
- When a person comes out from a film hall (cinema) in bright light, then entire visual image is bleached having little contrast between its different parts. Initially this is a poor vision: It remains poor until retina has adapted sufficiently or adequately for the fact that darker areas of object/image will no longer stimulate the receptors in excess.
- On the contrary, when a person enters the - darkness (say from bright light to a cinema hall) then initially sensitivity of retina is very slight and upto the extent that even light spot in the image are unable to excite the retina. Of course, after dark adaptation light spots are being registered.

DARK ADAPTATION

- The increased sensitivity of eye or a decrease in visual threshold in the dark is dark adaptation.
- Factors affecting: Time period is related to intensity and duration of previous exposure to light. Rate of adaptation is slow The persons who use to work in dim light like radiologists, aircraft pilots, etc. wear deep red goggles instead of waiting for few minutes in a dark room. It is decreased in hypoxia, vitamin A deficiency etc.
- Mechanism or physiological changes:- Dilatation of pupil. Regeneration of photo pigments. Change in functional re-organisation of retina leading to reduction in lateral inhibition. It is the property of retina. Spatial and temporal summation + responsiveness increased at retinal level. So more light enters the eye through dilated pupil and thus the sensitivity is increased.

VISUAL MECHANISM

To appreciate any object by the eyes is an interesting mechanism in which various steps are involved. This section consists of all those steps.

RECEPTOR POTENTIAL (STIMULATED ROD-CONES)

When light falls on retina, its photochemical substance is decomposed which causes a sustained 'receptor potential' which lasts as long as the light continues. This has got some unique characteristics :

(i) It is positive (ii) its intensity is proportional to the logarithm of light energy in contrast to the more linear response of many other receptors, (iii) Neither rods nor cones generate action potential. The receptor potential themselves acting at the ends of the axon, are believed to induce signals directly in successive neurones.

ROLE OF BIPOLAR; HORIZONTAL CELLS

- The axons of rods and cones make intimate contact with the dendrites of both bipolar and horizontal cells. These cells transmit no action potential but, transmits signals of the electrotonic variety. Horizontal cells transmit signals laterally in retina and bipolar cells transmit signals from rods and cones to the ganglion cells. These cells have more extensive fibre networks in the peripheral retina than in central retina and area of inhibition is great in periphery but circumscribed in the central retina. This explains that 'lateral inhibition' is caused by signals carried in horizontal cells which have extensive connections in outer plexiform layer of retina.
- There are two types—depolarising, and hyperpolarising. They provide opposing excitatory and inhibitory signals in visual cortex.
- One of such cells respond to neuro-transmitter glutamate released by rods and cones on depolarisation. Another variety of bipolar cells receive their signal from horizontal cells which are inhibitory; so they cause inhibition.
- This reciprocal relationship between two types of bipolar cells provides second mechanism for lateral inhibition. Secondly, both positive and negative signals are transmitting visual information to the brain.

GANGLION CELLS

i. Transmit continuous nerve impulses at a rate of about 5/second even when retina is in total darkness.
ii. These cells are famous for their 'ON', 'OFF' response. When light falls, there is an intense transient discharge which increases very weakly. This is 'ON' response of these cells. When light is turned off, opposite effect occur, which is OFF response.

Actually, when light falls on retina, there is existence of a minute spot of light shining on the very centre of the 'retinal field' of a peripheral ganglion cell (excited area). There also exists a concentric area surrounding the spot of light on retina which is called 'Inhibited area' and the phenomenon is named as *'Lateral inhibition.'* So when the light is turned off, this inhibited area (which exits adjacent to the excited area) transmits large number of impulses; or better to say that impulse rate from here increases at first to a level considerably greater than normal rate of discharge, and this effect lasts for a fraction of second until the cells re-adapt to their normal level of discharge. Of course, the intermediate zone (area between excited and inhibited area) possesses 'ON-OFF response' in which they fire both when light is turned on and when it is turned off.

iii. W Cells: 40 per cent of total population. Diameter less than ten micrometers. Transmit signals to their optic nerve fibres at rate of 8 m per second. They receive excitation from rods via bipolar + amacrine cells. Inner plexiform layer of retina is rich in dendrites of these cells. These are concerned with detection of directional movements.

iv. X cells: 55 per cent population, diameter 10–15 micrometer. Rate of transmitting impulse to optic nerve is 14 m/sec. In contrast to W cells, their dendrites are not richly distributed in inner plexiform layer of retina. They receive signals from one cone, so are responsible for colour vision. Their signals represent discrete retinal location.

v. Y cells: Largest (35 micrometer diameter), rate of transmission of nerve impulses is 50 m/sec (faster). Population 5 per cent. They respond to rapid changes in visual image. More clearly, when we see any exciting vision, these cells inform CNS instantaneously, so one feels it without accuracy in its place of location.

vi. Amacrine cells: One type of such cells is responding very strongly at the onset to a visual signal; but this response vanishes early also.

vii. Other types of such cells respond to movement of a spot in some specific direction.

So they are acting as analyser of visual signal in the beginning.

TRANSMISSION OF VISUAL SIGNAL: LATERAL INHIBITION

1. When flat light is applied to retina OR all photoreceptors are stimulated equally - then:- Signals passing through excitatory bipolar cell is stimulatory, while passing through hyper polarised bipolar cell is inhibitory, which is coming through horizontal cells, laterally.

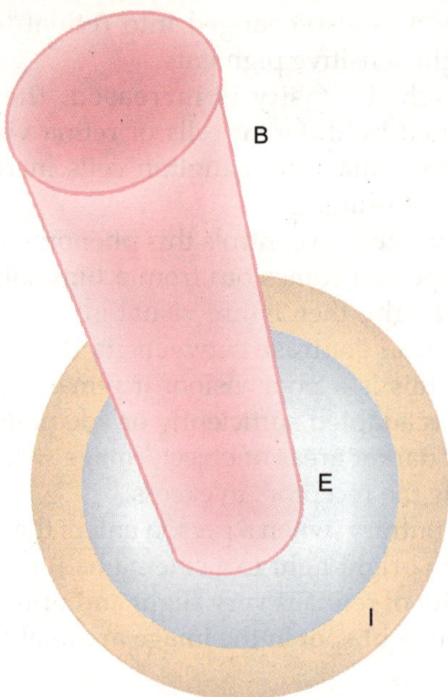

Fig. 37.9: Retinal area: Excitation inhibition (E = Excited area, I = Inhibited area, B = Light beam)

2. A contrast border is present in visual scene - i.e. a scene in maximally bright position but with dark borders - then - opposing effect.
3. Central photoreceptor is stimulated by bright light spot while two lateral receptors are in dark. The bright spot will excite directly bipolar cell. But because one of the lateral receptor is in the dark so it will inhibit horizontal cell. So it loses its inhibitory effect on bipolar cell, which causes intensification or more excitation of bipolar cells.

FUSION OF IMAGES (CONVERGENCE)

i. When an object is seen with two eyes, one image of the object fall on the retina of each eye. Although, two images are formed, one sees only one object and not two. This is because of the fact that two images are physiologically fused and give the impression of single image. Such fusion of images will occur only when the two images of a single object fall on specific points on the two retinae. These two points are called *'corresponding points'* (two fovea are corresponding points). Opposite of it is *'disparate points'* (retinal points which are not corresponding). When the two images fall on disparate points, a single object will be seen double called *'Diplopia.'* During near vision, the eyes converge to turn the retina in such a way that the two images of the object fall on corresponding retinal points which is essential for perfect vision.

ii. Crude fusion is inherent in the newborn baby due to inherited conjugate movements of the eyes. As visual system becomes more developed, the ability of the two eyes to fixate on the same object of attention reaches to great accuracy of fusion. Then, along with the development of persuit movement, the pathway for controlling the conjugate movements of the two eyes normally develop equally.

iii. Lateral geniculate body consists of successive nuclear layers. Corresponding points of two retinae transmit signals to these layers; therefore it is said to play a remarkable role in fusion of images. When the eyes are appropriately oriented, the retinal images will be appropriately superimposed upon each other, in the respective layers.

LACK OF FUSION : SQUINT (STRABISMUS; CROSS EYEDNESS)

1. It means a constant lack of parallelism of the visual axes of the eye. In this condition the two retinal images don't correspond with each other and there is a tendency for one of the retinal images to be suppressed so that it gives rise to no conscious perception, so the state of *Kahin-pe-nigahe-Kahin-pe-nishana appears. So it is a manifest deviation of visual axes in one or more position of gaze, or more simply the visual axes from both the eyes are not united upon the object or point looked at.*
2. A constant lack of parallelism of the visual axes of the eyes.
3. Causes include:
   — over convergence.
   — Paralysis of one extraocular muscle,
   — congenital
   — Mechanical (due to pressure on eye from within the orbit)
   — spasm of an extraocular muscle.
4. Types include:
   — Uniocular (one eye affected)
   — Dynamic (vigorous movements of eyeballs bring further lack of parallelism)
   — alternating (Either eye fixes; or both eyes remain steady or move alike when either eye is indifferently covered;
   — Concomitant (deviating eye follows the other in its movements, the angle between visual axes remain same).
   — Convergent (internal squint; visual axes converge).
5. The degree of squint can be detected by strabismometer.
6. In paralytic squint diplopia is common.
   - *Stereoscopic acuity:* It is the ability of an observer to detect the smallest difference in distances of two objects from him. It is expressed as least difference between angles formed by lines of sigh of two objects. The difference in angle is called stereoscopic parallax. It may be as little as two seconds. At maximum acuity a difference of 0.15 mm distance between two objects can be detected when objects are about 1 meter away, from observer.

FIXATION MOVEMENTS OF EYE

Are those movement that cause the eyes to fix on a discrete portion of the field of vision.

i. The eyes are said to be in a position of rest (primary position) when their direction is maintained simply by the tone of ocular muscles, i.e. when the gaze is straight ahead and far away and not directed to any particular point in the space. The visual axes are then parallel. When the eyes view some definite object they are turned by the contraction of the ocular muscles and converged so that the visual axes meet at the observed object and an image of the object falls upon a corresponding point on each fovea. The closer the object to the eye, the greater the degree of convergence. This movement of the eyes for the acute observation of an object is called *'fixation.'* The point where the visual axes meet is called *'fixation point,'* and the lines joining the latter to the fovea, i.e. the visual axes are sometimes called as fixation lines. The widest limits of vision in all directions within which eyes can fixate is called, *'field of fixation.'*

ii. Two types of fixation exist
   - *Voluntary:* The person moves his eyes to find the object on which he wants to fix his attention. The centre for it is located in frontal lobes (premotor cortical regions, bilaterally). If this area is destroyed then person is unable to unlock the eye from one fixed point and move it towards another point.
   - *Involuntary:* When one finds the object then he constantly keep, his eyes over it. This is controlled by secondary visual area of occipital cortex (Brodman area 19—anterior to area 17 and 18). Naturally on its destruction, one will not be able to fix his eyes on the desired object. When

superior colliculi are destroyed then this type of movement will not be possible.

iii. Suppose we are travelling in a train or in a car. Then through the window we observe many scenes by jumping from one scene to the next at an average rate of 2 to 3 jumps per seconds. This is called saccades. Brain does not fixate the attention, so we are not very much conscious of the scenes. This is opticokinetic movement.

iv. During reading, the situation is little difficult. Eyes here are trained to scan the scene. So one is able to extract the important informations.

v. Mechanism of fixing:
   - When an object is focussed or fixed on retina (specially on fovea), then this spot moves at a rapid rate across the cones. It is also drifted across the cones. Because of this the focussing of object tends to move towards the edges of fovea. But then it is reflexly brought on centre by a flickering movement. So this is an automatic response.
   - When an object is moving; then the cerebral cortex develops ability to fix it automatically. This is called pursuit movements. It is quite evident that when an object moves up and down (wave like) then initially eyes are unable to adjust themselves accordingly; but later on eyes also develop smoother movements according to the movement of object to fix it exactly.

vi. Superior colliculus: Important role
   - If there is a sudden visual disturbance, the eyes are turned in that direction.
   - The optic nerve from eyes to colliculi, divide into two branches - one going to visual cortex while other going to superior colliculi. The fibres are made up of Y type.
   - Signals are also going to other brainstem levels via medial longitudinal fasciculus, so that whole body is turned towards the direction of side of visual disturbance.

vii. Stereopsis: Or depth perception: There are two possible concepts:
   - It is a fact that right eye observes a little more of right hand side of the object. It is also true for left eye in the same way that left eye observes a little more towards left side of the object. This is a natural disparity. So images are not registered at the same time. This becomes more worse as the object is brought nearer to the eye. This gives space for mechanism of stereopsis.
   - Another interesting scientific fact is that few additional nerve fibres are running in addition to main trunk of fibres; but they run one to two degrees on either side of the main track. There are two to three or more such tracks which are running few degrees apart from the main trunk. So this may disturb the registration of the image. This is depth perception or stereopsis.
   - Monocular depth perception: Persons with one eye can also judge for length, breadth, thickness of any object with accuracy. It is dependent upon various factors like:
     —Distribution of light and shade in visual scene.
     —Relative apparent sizes of known objects. The size of an image of an object on the retina is inversely proportional to distance of the object from the observer. When the distance is more, the size of the image is smaller, and vice versa.
     —Apparent change of colour of an object at a distance; e.g. green trees appear blue from a distance which is because of the fact that atmosphere is not transparent.
     —Parallax is also important (means - when head moves in one direction then objects nearer to observer move to opposite direction while objects at a distance move in same direction.

LESIONS AT VARIOUS LEVELS: VISUAL PATH

1. *At optic nerve:* If one optic nerve is affected then there will be total blindness of corresponding eye.

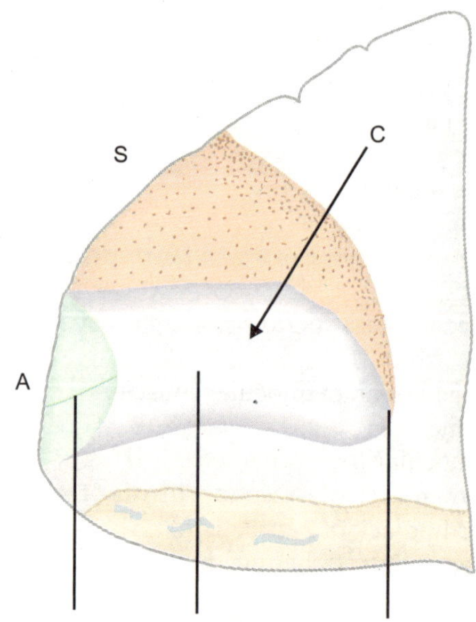

Fig. 37.10: The visual cortex (A = Primary visual cortex, C = Calcarine fissure, S = Secondary visual area)

2. *At optic chiasma:*
   - Unilateral lesion on outer angle leads to unilateral loss of vision involving temporal half of retina (loss of nasal vision on same side).
   - On involvement of both lateral angles the effect is binasal hemianopia.
3. *At optic tract:* Homonymous hemianopia
4. *At lateral geniculate body:* Homonymous hemianopia.
5. *At optic radiation:* Homonymous hemianopia
6. *At occipital cortex:* Bilateral destructive lesion of both visual cortex leads to total blindness.
7. When striate area of one hemisphere is damaged, it leads to homonymous hemianopia.

NEUROPHYSIOLOGY OF VISION

The image is the adequate stimulus which excites the sensory receptors in the retina which are capable of transforming the energy of the stimulus into a nerve impulse which is conducted by suitable nerve fibres to appropriate cell station in the brain.

SENSORY RECEPTORS: RODS-CONES

- Their outer segment is rod like so this name is derived. It is about 60 microns long and 2 microns thick, lying next to pigment epithelium. There are about 120 millions rods. It terminates in the so called ellipsoid. The cell nuclei of rods lie together with those of the cones, forming the external nuclear layer. The dendrites of rods and cones connecting with bipolar cells form the external plexiform layer.
- The cones resemble a flask with a narrow neck, corresponding to the outer segment, and a plump inner segment. They are 52 microns in length (slightly shorter than rods), but their thickness is in reverse proportion to their length. The transition between inner and outer segment is marked by an indentation or waistline, marking the place where the cone fits into neuroglial ring that surrounds the opening in the outer limiting membrane. This latter keeps the cone fixed in its place. The cell body and nucleus are found just inside the outer limiting membrane in the outer nuclear layer. From this structure the cone fibre runs inward to terminate in cone pedicle which are all placed in the middle zone of outer plexifrom layer. There are approximately 6 million cones in retina.

  After impulses leave the retinae, they pass backward through the 'optic nerves.' At the 'optic chiasm' all the fibres from nasal halves of retinae cross to the opposite side, where they join the fibres from opposite temporal retinae to form 'optic tracts.' The fibres of each optic tract synapse in 'lateral geniculate body' and from here 'geniculo-calcarine fibres' pass through 'optic radiation' (OR 'geniculo-calcarine tract' to the 'visual cortex' (occipital-lobe- calcarine area).

LATERAL GENICULATE BODY

i. Each lateral geniculate body is composed of six clearly demarcated nuclear layers, separated by intervening layers of the white matter. The layers have been numbered 1 to 6, from surface inward. Layers 1, 4, 6 receive signals from the nasal retina of opposite side, while layers 2, 3, 5 receive signals from temporal portion of ipsilateral retina.
ii. It projects entirely on the visual cortex. So it acts like a relay station which relay information from the optic nerve fibres into geniculo-calcarine-tract without altering it significantly.
iii. Neurons which are excited here; constitute 'excited area.' Immediately adjacent to this area, there is 'inhibited area' which is called 'lateral Inhibition' which enhance the degree of contrast in the visual pattern.
iv. It plays a major role in fusion of visual images because corresponding points of the two retinae transmit visual signals respectively to the successive nuclear layer of lateral geniculate body.
v. It differs from ganglion cells in the way that

   They respond less to diffuse light, They adapt more rapidly and completely Their activity is influenced by vestibular, reticular and cortical impulses, There is diffuse antagonistic surroundings, but effect on central receptive field is more marked.

THE VISUAL CORTEX

i. Detection of visual scene is the function of visual cortex lies mainly in calcarine fissure located bilaterally on the medial aspect of each occipital cortex. Brodmann area 17 is the primary visual cortex which lies almost entirely on the medial aspect of the cerebral hemisphere, but extends onto the outer surface of the occipital pole. So area 17 is the visuo-sensory area and forms an anatomic, functional entity. Outside area 17 are two other areas which are also concerned with visual reactions. These are 'area 18' (para striate area) and area 19. Area 18 has been considered the visuomotor field and area 19 the visuopsychic field. In man area 18 + area 19 (7,839 mm^2) is almost three times as large as area 17.

ii. The macula is represented at the occipital pole of the visual cortex and the peripheral regions of retina are represented in concentric circles farther and farther forward from the occipital pole. The upper portion of the retina is represented superiorly in visual cortex and the lower portion inferiorly.

iii. Fibres from the corresponding upper retinal quadrants end in cells above the calcarine fissure, and fibres from corresponding lower quadrants end in cells below the fissure. At the extreme anterior end of the calcarine fissure is the representation of the most peripheral nasal retina of the opposite side.

iv. Bars of light/lines/edges are stimulus for cells of layer IV of primary visual cortex.

v. The receptive fields are arranged in different directions like vertical, horizontal and oblique.

vi. Three types of cells are present namely simple cells which indicate location and orientation of a line or border in visual field; the complex cells indicate orientation of position, while hypercomplex cells indicate angles and orientation.

iv. *Anomalies*:

- Wide spread destruction of areas 18 and 19, lead to word blindness (alexia) which means that person cannot identify the meanings of words which he sees.
- Sometimes a person sees that scene which he has seen years back. Such type of happenings are there when 'lower border of temporal cortex is stimulated (complicated visual perception).
- A person sees very well the plate, fork and food; but he cannot use the fork to have the food from the plate. This means he is unable to correlate the visual images with the motor functions. This happens when angular gyrus (region where parietal, temporal and occipital lobes come together) is destructed.
- Optical auras (lines, stars, discs, triangles, etc.) are seen when area 17 + 18 + 19 are electrically stimulated.

EXAMINATION OF EYES

OPHTHALMOSCOPY

Principle: Whenever light is thrown in the eye of a patient through the pupil, some part of it is absorbed by pigments, while remaining part of light is reflected back into the eye of the observer. This reflected light follows the same path by which it has entered the eye, so if we have to see the inside structure of eyeball, we have to look through same path but it is not possible in ordinary circumstances. So pupil appears as a black spot from outside.

Discovery of ophthalmoscope has solved this problem. So "this is an instrument by which we can see and study the different structure lying inside the eyeball because same path is followed by this light rays. By this instrument we can examine retina and its blood vessels as well as refractive state of eye—hypermetropia, myopia, emmetropia.

Instrument : Ophthalmoscope is used, which is having a mirror with a central hole for observing called sight hole. Space for different lenses moving on a turrent ranging from +20 to -20 D.

Other requisites: are atropine or homatropine drop, dark room, source of light above and behind the patient's head.

Method

- From a distance of one metre
- Direct examination
- Indirect examination.

From a Distance of One Metre

- Throw the light by ophthalmoscope into patient's eye through pupil and try to see the red reflex also known as *fundus glow*. Once it is identified do not miss it.
- Look for any opacity which will be visible in the form of dark patches.
- Nothing more will be visible from one metre distance.

Direct Examination

- For detailed study of fundus doctor has to go as near to the patients eye as he can, just like looking directly in the eye of patient.
- In hypermetropia the divergent rays are focussed behind retina and a clear erect image is formed, while

in myopia convergent rays are focussed in front of retina so a clear inverted image is formed.

Observation

- *Optic disc*: It marks the entry of optic nerve. It is rounded or oval in shape. Pinkish or reddish in colour but not white. Its margins are clear. It has got a central depression called physiological cup from which blood vessels are arising.
- *Blood vessels*: Retinal blood vessels—arteries appear red, veins may be dull, arteries are not pulsatile.
- *Macula*: It is present on temporal side of optic disc. It is star shaped. It is devoid of blood vessels.

Abnormalities

- *Papilloedema*: swelling of optic disc
- *Papillitis:* infection to the disc.
- *Retinal haemorrhage*: dark patches suggestive of hypertension or internal injury.

Precautions

- Dilation of pupil is necessary which is done by atropine.
- This is to be done in a dark room.
- Before starting you must be familiar with the instrument.
- Throw the light and use the ophthalmoscope in horizontal and vertical direction for correct focussing of fundus glow.
- Relax your accommodation, as well as doctor's eye should be emmetropic.

Importance

The ophthalmoscopic examination have virtually made the eye a window of the brain, not only the local condition of eye but also the systemic condition of nervous, cardio-vascular and renal origin bring about changes in fundus of eye. Diabetes and hypertension also effect the retina.

RETINOSCOPY

It is a reliable and objective method for determining the state of refraction of the eye. It can be applied in case of children, illiterate, adults and where other subjective methods are not needful.

Principle: It is based on the fact that on tilting the reflecting mirror the emerging rays of light move in different direction according to the state of refraction. The plane minor is used to illuminate the fundus and the glow of the fundus through the pupil with the shadow of the iris are observed.

Method

- Patient is comfortably sitting on a chair and doctor stands at little distance.
- Light is thrown through pupil into eye of patient and red reflex or fundus glow is observed.
- Move the mirror in horizontal as well as in vertical direction and note the direction of movement of glow.

Observation

- If movement is in same direction it suggests emmetropic, hypermetropic or myopia of less than ID.
- If movement is in opposite direction it is suggestive of myopia of more than ID.
- If glow is suddenly disappearing and then suddenly re-appearing it is also suggestive of either emmetropia or myopia-less than ID.

Notes

1. Pupil should be dilated.
2. This experiment is done in dark room
3. This can also be done by concave mirror
4. A trial frame is put and appropriate lenses are put over it and retinoscopy is continued till refractive error is corrected, so that appropriate number of glasses can be given.

VISUAL ACUITY

- *Snellen's test type*: It is employed to measure the ability of the subject in discriminating different letters which are constructed so that their details subtend a known angle at a given distance from the eye. The basis is that two points or lines separated by a space having a visual angle of one minute can be resolved by the average normal eye.

  Nine rows of letters printed in black upon a white background are there. The rows of these letters are arranged in descending order of size from above down. The width of line forming the letters of first row subtends an angle of one minute at 60 metres from eye whereas letters from two to nine rows have a visual angle of one minute at 36, 24, 18, 12, 9, 6, 5 metres respectively. The subject stands at a distance of 6 meters (20 ft.) and reads these letters with one eye closed. If subject cannot read beyond '12 metre' line then his visual activity is 6/12 (numerator is 6 and denominator is the distance at which the smallest letters can be read by eye). Normal visual acuity is 6/6.
- The distance of 6 metre is selected to eliminate the possibility of accommodation.

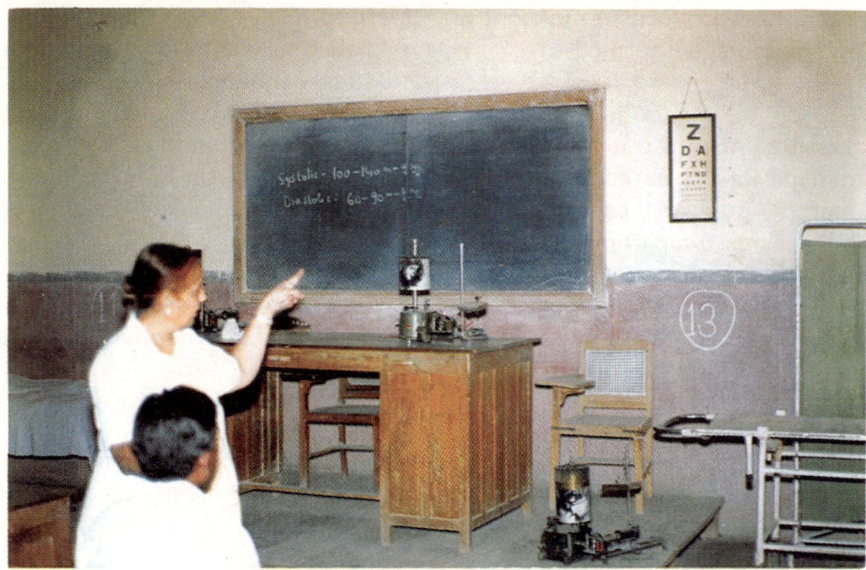

Fig. 37.11: Testing distant vision
(*Courtesy*: Dept. of Physiology, SP Medical College, Bikaner)

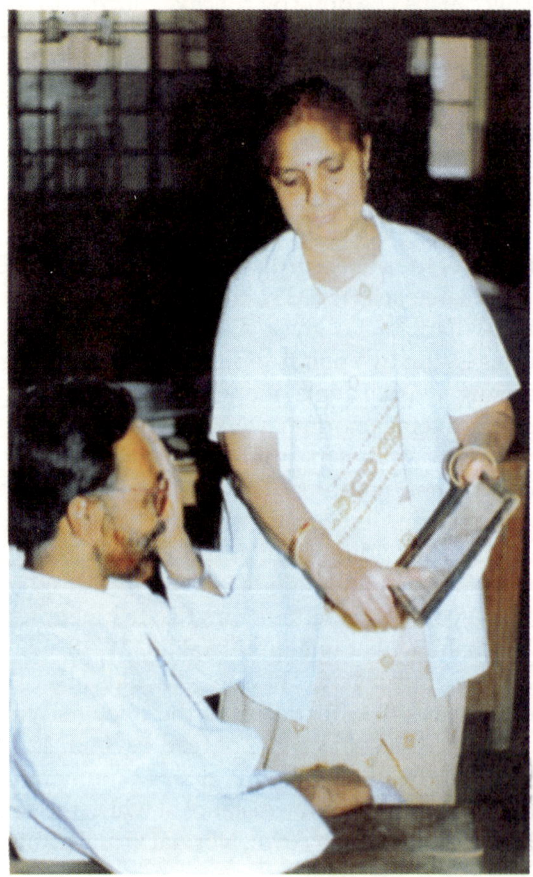

Fig. 37.12: Testing near vision
(*Courtesy*: Dept. of Physiology, SP Medical College, Bikaner)

- Suppose there are two separate lines which we see as two because they are separated from each other by a minimum distance which is called "minimum separable distance."
- Visual acuity (v) is recorded according to d/D.
  d = distance at which letters are read.
  D = distance at which they should be read.
- (d = 6 m from test types). If only top letter is visible than vision is 6/60. If it is less than this, then patient is moved towards the test types until they can read the top letter. If top letter is visible at 2 m distance then visual acuity is 2/60. If in any case, it is less than 1/60, then it is examined or told as counting fingers, hand movements, perception of light, or no perception of light.
- Glasses: Take the glass. Hold it and look at an object through it. Move the lens from side to side and watch the object. If it moves in opposite direction to lens, then the lens is convex. If in same direction then lens is concave.
- For spherical/cylindrical lens, look at a straight object through it, and then slowly twist it round. In case of a cylindrical lens the object will take an oblique position.
- To determine near vision Jaeger's chart is used. Vision is observed from a distance of 12 to 14 inches.
- Factors affecting visual acuity:
  — Refractory errors: myopia, hypermetropia and astigmatism decrease visual acuity because of out of focussing of image on retina. Chromatic and spherical aberration also decrease the visual acuity because of degradation of retinal image.

- Brightness: Proper illumination is the main factor in visual acuity. In high illumination visual acuity is increased while it is decreased in poor illumination.
- It increases also with background illumination.
- Visual acuity is maximum in central fovea while minimum in periphery.
- The object should be of proper size. Patient should also be given adequate/proper time to have a view of it.
- Technique of measurement is also an important factor.

• Physiological basis:
- Suppose we are viewing two lines (object) which are separated from each other by a definite distance. It means in order to view two such separate lines (i.e. duality of an object) they must be separated by a minimum space. The two images of these two lines will stimulate two cones equally and one cone lying between them is stimulated in somewhat a different way. This is because of diffraction or chromatic aberration which makes these images diffuse; but not sharp. Because of this the ganglion cells connected to these cones, discharge differently and this differential discharge is appreciated. If on the other hand these two lines are so close to each other that with less separable distance then adjacent cones are only stimulated, with impossible differential discharge of ganglion cells; and so duality cannot be reported and they appear as a single piece. Cones are having diameter between 1.5–4μ. The distance separating the two lines or images on retina is inversely related to visual acuity. It is 4.4μ when visual acuity is one, and it is 1µ when visual acuity is three (normal visual acuity is one; highest may be three). It means or is better to say that even at highest level of visual acuity the distance separating the two images may be equal to diameter of a single cone.
- Amacrine as well as horizontal cells are improving the visual acuity by the mechanism of lateral inhibition. The strongly stimulated cone will inhibit the poorly stimulated adjacent cone. It leads to magnification of neuronal discharge from the adjacent ganglion cells and thus visual acuity is increased. Here, the another factor which plays a role is receptive field of the ganglion cells, which is large for rods, less for cones in extra foveal region while is minimum at fovea centralis. This explains that visual acuity increases from peripheral part of retina towards the fovea. At fovea centralise, there is one to one relationship between cones—horizontal cells bipolar cells—ganglion cells—geniculate cell etc.
- These are the steady movement of eyeball which shift the image on retina. This also facilitates the activation of cones and visual acuity. In almost all cases, the image moves over 2 to 4 cones in the retina which further help visual acuity.
- The ability to detect a dark spot or a dark line on a uniformly bright background is minimum detectable visual acuity. Here the diameter of cone is not the limiting factor.

PERIMETRY

Perimetry: The marking out or mapping out of field of vision of an individual. It is measured by Perimeter.

Field of vision: Area of external world seen by fixing the eye at a point, that area is known as field of vision of that eye.

Factors on which field of vision depends :

1. Object
2. Eye itself

Object

a. *Size:* If bigger is the size of object more will be visual field.

b. *Illumination:* Better the illumination better the field.

c. *Colour of object:* For the white object field of vision best and for red and green it is less than 20°. Cones are responsible for perception of colour vision. At the periphery cones are less so the colour light has less field of vision.

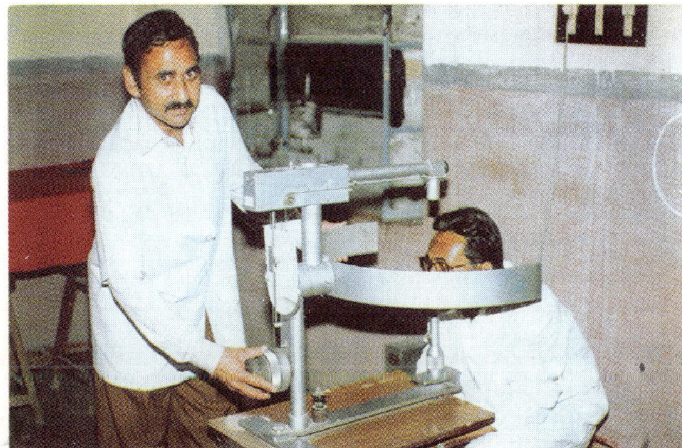

Fig. 37.13: Testing field of vision by perimeter (*Courtesy*: Dept. of Physiology, SP Medical College, Bikaner)

Terms to Denote Loss of Field of Vision

Visual field has been subdivided into four quadrants - Lateral half (temporal field) and medial half (nasal field) can be made by drawing an imaginary line through the fixation point. These two quadrants have been further subdivided into upper and lower quadrants by drawing an imaginary horizontal line through the point of fixation.

Confrontation Method: Field of vision determination

The doctor stands or sits facing the subject. One eye of the patient is covered, and he sees at the nose bridge of the examiner. As a test object—either extended finger or white headed pin is used. The doctor brings the test object forward behind the subject's head and notes the point when it is first seen by the patient. One eye is tested at one time and process is repeated from various directions.

In another method, the doctor stands/sits facing the subject at a distance of two feet. One eye is examined in one time. The doctor places a test object (e.g. extended finger) in between himself and the patient but outside his own visual field. The test object is then moved from periphery towards mid line. The patient is told to point out when he first observes the object. The doctor compares the position when he first sees the object with that it was first seen by the patient. This procedure is repeated in various directions.

Eye : The degree of field of vision is different in different sides. Let the field of vision from upper side is 60° for lower side 70°. For nasal side 60° temporal side 90°, so we can say field of vision is maximum on temporal side.

In case of protruding eye the field of vision is more than 120° e.g. in frog's eye.

This visual field is compared with a hemisphere, visual field subtends an angle of 160° in horizontal plane and an angle of 130–135° in vertical plane, and central point forms visual axis.

Binocular field is the combination of two uniocular fields. About 120° of each eye's field overlap, only a crescent shaped area is left where overlapping does not occur is known as temporal crescent

Perimeter : It is an instrument with which the visual field is recorded. It has following parts

ARC : This is made up of heavy metal. It is more than half of a circle. Its concavity faces the subject and it is pivoted on the vertical stand. It can be rotated on the axis. On its inner side in the centre there is a lighted cross fixation object. On the concavity test object moves, on its convexity there are marking.

Stand: It gives stability to the instrument. It has a vertical limb upon which the arc is pivoted. The vertical limb is broad and helps to screen the activity of examiner. It bears a circular scale to read the meridian on which the arc is brought.

Chin Rest : Two grooves present on it, one on right side and one on left side, you should keep your eye in a straight visual axis. For changing the position of visual axis we require two grooves. For right eye we use left chin rest and vice versa. We can move chin rest backward and forward and keep distance between eye and object 33 cm. We can also make it up and down.

Chart holder: This is made up of metal and soft rubber. There are two fixing points or needle on it. A punching needle is also present.

Arrangement of object: There are three plates for arrangement of object. By first plate one can make illumination. We can make bright faint or fainter. By second plate we can change colour, i.e. white, red and green and by third plate we can adjust the size of the object, i.e biggest, small, smallest by using these plates we can obtain 64 arrangement of object.

Arrangement for Movement of Object

Object is light which move on arc by very big adjust screw. This screw is very big because it makes the movement of object easy.

Perimeter chart: Ideally perimetry should be conducted on a concave spherical surface having three dimension, but in practice the picture is required to be drawn on a plane paper. The central point of map corresponds with the visual axis and concentric lines called isopters are drawn around the axis. Ten circles are present. First circle written as 10 and last circle is 100. If a substance is placed at 60° it subtends an angle of 60° on visual axis.

Procedure

- Exercise should be done in dark room.
- Chart should be in chart holder.
- White light must be selected.
- Ask the patient to put his chin on left side of chin rest.
- Ask the patient to fix his right eye on object and never allow to move the eye or head.
- Ask the patient to perceive the object and knock the table.
- Bring object from periphery to centre to find out blind spot. Bring object from opposite side of centre.
- Move the arc by 15° and again repeat the process.

Significance

- It is used in findings out the site of lesion in visual pathway.
- Any area of blindness in the visual field. (Scotoma) can be found.
- To locate and in finding dimensions of blind spot. Size of blind spot is increased in infection.

Clinical Aspect

- *Scotoma*— Area of blindness in visual field
- *Anopia*— Complete blindness
- *Hemianopia*— Loss of half the visual field. It is of two types (1) Bitemporal (2) Binasal hemianopia
- *Quadrentanopia*— Loss of ¼ field of vision.
- *Heteronymous hemi anopia*— Bilateral hemianopia in which similar, i.e. corresponding halves (e.g. temporal halves of both side) of the field of vision are lost.
- *Homonymous hemianopia*— Loss of opposite halves of vision, i.e. loss of temporal side of one eye and nasal side of other eye.
- Concentric dimensions of field of vision occurs during
  a. Hysthesia (2) Papilloedema
    - Central scotoma
    - Damage in optic disc or optic neuritis
- Some time vitamin A deficiency.
- Bilateral hemianopia - Both sides temporal vision goes away (a) tumours of pituitary gland which press optic chiasma
- *Binasal hemianopia*—due to pressing of the crossing fibre of optic chiasma
- Heteronymous hemi-anopia → damage in optic tract.

Stereoscopic vision: This is the perception of the solidity of the object or 3 dimensional view of the object. This perception is actually a test for diffusion of two eyes in a corresponding point image of single object formed at two sites of retina.

Amblyloscope: An instrument used for stereoscopic vision. It is a sort of binocular.

Method: Ask the subject to see through the two arms of ambyloscope with his two eyes. In one he will see the picture of a cage in other a picture of bird. Now ask him to reduce the angle between two arms until he sees a single object, i.e bird in the cage.

Blind spot: It represents projection of that area where the optic nerve enters the retina. It subtends an angle of 5.5° in width and 7.5° in height. Its centre lies about 15.5° to the lateral side of the fixation point and 1.5° below the horizontal meridian. Vision is absent.

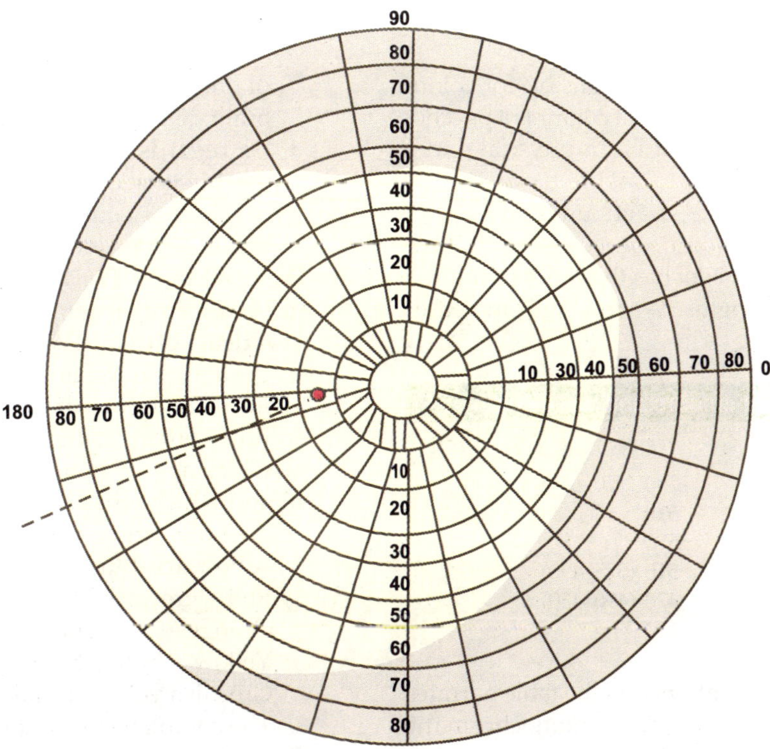

Fig. 37.14: Perimetry chart

Perimeter chart: This is a circular chart used to record the visual field. The central point of the map corresponds with visual axis and the concentric line circles are drawn called isopters around this axis. The isopters are measured in degrees. A point on a isotope in any given meridian is a measure of an angle subtended by that point with the visual axis at the nodal point of the eye. While constricting the chart. The radii (meridians) are marked in dotted lines at 10° interval.

TONOMETRY

Instrument used to measure intraocular tension is tonometer. The cornea of the eye is anaesthetised with a local anaesthetic and footplate of tonometer is placed on cornea. A small force is applied to a central plunger so portion of cornea is displaced inward. This displacement is recorded on its scale which is calibrated in terms of intraocular pressure.

Cornea: It is the window through which the light rays pass on their way to the retina. In order to fulfil this function, the tissue must be transparent. It must also possess the proper curvature and correct refractive index, so that light rays, coming form objects at infinity, are imaged on retina, for it is at the anterior corneal surface that major portion of refraction of light takes place.

i. It is the round, transparent convexity in anterior part of the eyeball.
ii. Corneal epithelium is stratified but non-cornified in order to preserve its translucency. It has remarkable regeneration power.
iii. Normally no blood vessels are present. It gets its oxygen supply from atmosphere and aqueous humor. Glucose diffuses through it. As the final consequence of metabolism lactic acid accumulates which diffuses into aqueous humor and CO_2 is going out in atmosphere.
iv. Its thickness is 0.5 - 1 mm.; diameter is 11 mm. (vertical) and 12 mm. (lateral). Non-medullated nerves are richly supplying it.

Blind spot: It represents the projection of that area where the optic nerve enters the retina. It subtends an angle of 5.5° in width and 7.5° in height. It's centre lies about 15.5° laterally to the fixation point and 1.5° below the horizontal meridian, vision is absent.

COLOUR VISION

i. These are the 'cones' that are responsible for colour vision. Although the sensation of colour is a psychological attribute of vision, it has a physical and a physiologic basis.
ii. The day light visible spectrum consists of *'VIBGYOR'* (violet, indigo, blue, green, yellow, orange and red). The violet has the shortest and red has longest wave lengths. Wave length increases from violet to red.

Table 37.4: Different colours and wavelength

Colour	*Wavelength (mμ or nm)*
1. Red.	700 (720–650)
2. Orange	610
3. Yellow	580
4. Green	510 (575–490)
5. Blue	470 (490–450)
6. Violet	420

- The wavelength mentioned in the table narrates that for example - an orange monochromatic light of wavelength of 610 nanometers stimulates almost hundred percent of red cones, fifty percent of green and forty percent of blue cones. So our brain detects it as orange.
- As regards white colour is concerned, it is a combination of all the wavelengths of spectra. It is said that equal stimulation of all red, green, and blue cones will give us sensation of white.

iii. There are three *'Primary colours'* namely red, green and blue. Proper admixture of these can produce all varieties of colour. When they are mixed in correct proportion, the mixture has a white colour, black colour really means absence of colours.
iv. Complementary colours are those
   a. which appear in negative after image,
   b. and which when blended in proper proportion give the 'grey impression' e.g. red and green, yellow and blue, black and white.
   Red + greenish blue = white
   Orange + cyan blue = white
   Yellow + indigo blue = greyish white
   Greenish yellow + violet = white
   The complementary colour for green is purple.
v. There are three fundamental qualities of the colour:
   - *Hue*: Colour itself like red, blue, green etc.

- *Intensity (luminosity)*: like 'bright red,' or 'pale blue' one red light can be brighter than another red light but have the same hue. A red pigment may be made darker by mixing some black pigment with it.
- *Saturation:* Whether purely primary colour or mixed with some other colour, e.g. pure blue, bluish green.

  Hue is defined as wavelength, however, saturation cannot be measured in terms of physical units but only in terms of sensation of brightness.

  Within visible spectrum, a normal human subject can recognise 150–200 hues, which means that human eye has remarkable 'hue discrimination power.' It can detect a difference of 1 nm in wavelengths in 'blue green' and 'yellow regions.' Number of factors may influence the perception of hue like contrast phenomenon, brightness (Hue changes with luminance - Bezold - Brucke - Phenomenon).

  Brightness or luminosity is a measure of reflection of light falling on an object. It is expressed like 'very dim,' 'dazzling' etc.

vi. *Colour Blindness:*

1. *Monochromates (Achromate):* No cones have been reported, only rods are responsible for vision. They cannot differentiate the hue and they match the different colours only by their luminosities.
2. *Dichromates*: Having only two types of cones. They are further classified as -
   a. *Protanopes*: The red sensitive cones are missing, so the person can differentiate between blue and green, but tend to read 'red' as 'green.'
   b. *Deuteranopes*: They have no green sensitive cones.
   c. *Trichromates*: They are persons having all the three types of cones, i.e. normal persons.
   d. *Blue weakness*: rare, blue cone missing, sometimes genetically inherited.

vii. *Theories of colour vision*:

a. *Young - Helmholtz–Theory (1801)*:

- This states that there are three types of cones with three fundamental sensation— red, green and violet. These cones contain three photochemical substances corresponding the three fundamental colour sensations.
- This also suggests the presence of specific nerve fibres and specific cortical cells, corresponding specifically to each photochemical substance for each colour sensation. The different photoreceptors after being stimulated, transmit different types of messages to visual cortex.
- It is assumed that each of photoreceptor is stimulated to some degree by all of the spectral frequencies but for a particular colour sensation, the specific photoreceptor is chiefly affected by the specific wavelength. The blue receptor will be stimulated maximally at the short end of the spectrum but minimally at strong (long) end of spectrum.
- Thomas Young (1773–1829) established this theory. Hermann Von - Hemholtz (1821–1894); a German scientist, working independently elaborated the details of the problem of colour vision made earlier by Thomas Young and he showed that he can match most colours by mixing wavelengths chosen from red, green and blue bands of the spectrum.
- The sensation of different colours is appreciated when different wavelengths in varying degree of amplitude strike the retina and are registered in visual area of the brain. The sensation of many colours are produced by combined stimulation of the three types of receptors of different intensities whereas white colour sensation arises when all the three receptors are equally stimulated.

b. *Granit's modulator and dominator theory* (1943):

- He investigated the sensitivity of light of different wavelengths in dark and light adapted eyes.
- Dominators: According to him there are some ganglion cells which are stimulated by whole of the visual spectrum. These ganglion cells are called dominators. They are of two types; i.e. dominator for rods and dominators for cones. According to him - dominator cone indicates about the intensity (brightness) of light only and not the colour.
- Dominator rod in dark adapted eye respond maximally to wavelength 500 mμ.
- Modulators: He also observed that some ganglion cells are only stimulated by a narrow wavelength band in light adapted eye. These cells are called modulators, which are of three types-

  —One group stimulated by blue light (wavelength 450–470 nm),

— another group stimulated by green light (wavelength 520–540 nm),

— still another group stimulated by red yellow light (wavelength 580–600 nm) According to him, in a light adapted eye, if green light falls on retina, the modulators for green colour will be stimulated maximally while others are not. So modulators are responsible for different colour sensations.

Neurological Basis: Colour Vision

i. When light falls on retina (of a particular wave length) there occurs 'coding process' not only in retina but in lateral geniculate body and visual cortex also. This neural coding of retina is involved in the perception of colour.
ii. The C-Horizontal cells are depolarised or hyperpolarised depending on wavelength of light. In this way, the colour is ultimately coded in terms of magnitude and polarity of horizontal cell potential.
iii. The R-G cells are depolarised by 'red' and hyperpolarised by 'green' whereas Y-B cells are depolarised by 'yellow' and hyperpolarised by blue.
iv. The colour opponent ganglion cells respond selectively to different wavelengths of light. There is an evidence of a coding process in the retina that converts colour information into ON and OFF, responses, individual ganglion cells; e.g.; red 'on' blue 'off', green 'on' blue 'off', red 'on' green 'off' or vice versa such type of on-OFF response is also seen in lateral geniculate body.
v. The differential responses of three types of cones and colour coding at different levels in the visual system leads to generation of a specific pattern or response for a particular wavelength of light. This is interpreted by the visual centre as a particular colour and thus the colour is perceived.

Polychromatic Theory

It is believed that there are seven types of receptors in man; six out of them have simple modulators like response while seventh one has twin responses; one in extreme red and another in extreme violet, and when stimulated produce a sensation of crimson light. All these receptors are arranged in three units;

a. A tricolour unit consisting of orange, the green and blue-violet or indigo receptors;
b. A dichromatic unit comprising the yellow and the blue receptors which are complementary in colour to one another.
c. Another dichromatic unit comprising the red and blue green receptors which are also complementary in colour to one another.
   At the normal fovea, at medium light intensities and average visual angle, the tricolour unit has the greatest activity but it is helped by both the other units.
d. *Cluster theory (Hartridge):* There are three retinal receptors almost similar in size (red, green, blue). They tend to form small clusters/aggregator of these three receptors. It can account for high acuity of eye using light of different wavelengths. Of course there is no proof of different colour receptors in retina.

Tests

a. *Holmgren's Worsted test*: Subject is given two skeins of wool, a pale pure green and a vivid red, and told to select from a bundle of skeins all those of same colour, whatever the depth of shade may be. It is not satisfactory one because -
   i. It requires a certain amount of intelligence and colour education and
   ii. People who are more or less colour blind can pass the test.
b. *Edridge - Green Lamp*: With the apparatus a small circle of colour can be shown for a short time. Test can be made more delicate by interposition of fog glasses.
c. *Ishihara's plates*
   Numerous coloured dots. Each plate used, is a card on which an irregularly array of coloured dots is printed, so that a letter or figure is formed by the dots of one colour, other colour forming the background. Some cards are designed to be read easily by normal subjects but not by colour blind, others to be read more easily by the colour blind than normal, others again to be interpreted differently by the normal and colour blind.
d. *Spectroscopic tests* : The subject in this test is to identify the spectral colours, their limit and position.

Simultaneous Contrast

- A colour or shade is influenced by its background, e.g. a blue against a yellow background is more vivid than if placed against any other colour. This is simultaneous contrast. Maximum effects are produced when complementary colours are used.
- More clearly, when an object of a particular colour (say of red) is observed against a background of its complementary colour like green then both colours appear to be brighter. This phenomenon is simultaneous contrast.

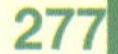

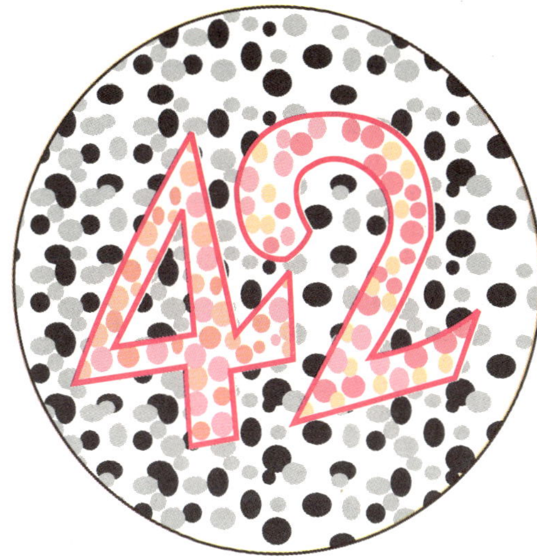

Fig. 37.15: Ishihara chart

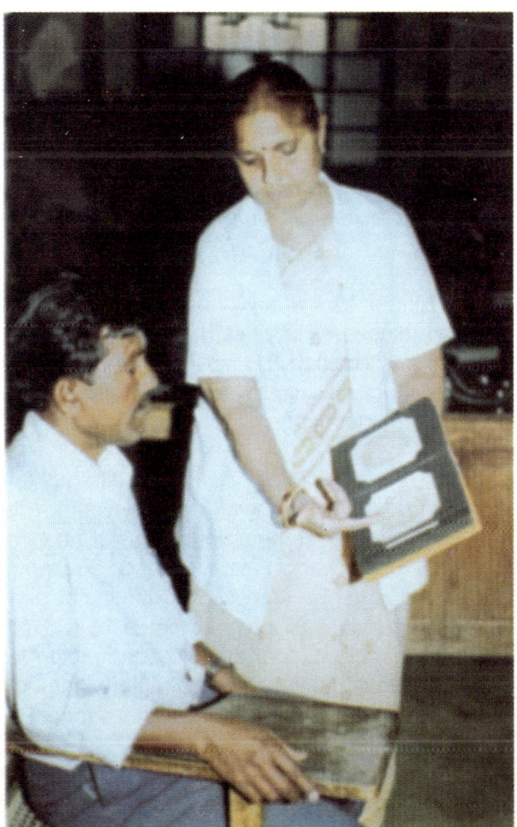

Fig. 37.16: Testing colour vision by Ishihara chart (*Courtesy*: Department of Physiology, SP Medical College, Bikaner)

Successive Contrast

On staring at a coloured figure until eye is fatigued and then transferring the gaze to a uniform white background, one sees a negative after image in its complementary colour, e.g. red object gives green after image. A positive after image is obtained on closing the eyes after gazing at a bright light; it is followed by a negative after image.

After image: Even after removal of an object, the visual impression persists, called after image.

a. *Positive:* When an object is removed, or person turns his head away from object, or even one closes his eyes, then impression of the object persists for a while. This is positive after image. This further means that photochemical changes which started in rods and cones, are still continuing.
b. *Negative:* Now if a person observes a coloured object, and then he suddenly turns to a white background; it means he is continuously observing the object in complementary colour. Now say, if the object is yellow, red/or white, then he sees it as blue/green/black. This is negative after image.

Photochemistry: Colour Vision

- Photochemicals in the cones have almost same chemical composition as that of rhodopsin in rods. Only differing is photopsin in cones is different from scotopsin of rods.
- Colour sensitive pigment of cones = retinal + photopsins

- The photochemicals present in cones are blue sensitive pigment, red sensitive pigment, green sensitive pigment.
- It is believed that cone pigments are also conjugated proteins. When fovea cones are bleached by strong light, addition of 11-cis retinal, can cause re-synthesis of the pigments.
- When light falls on cones, the pigments of cone are broken down in similar way like rhodopsin. They are regenerated also in similar way like rhodopsin synthesis, (of course regeneration of cone pigments is faster; and they don't breakdown as readily as rhodopsin breaks down).

SOME TERMS: SENSE OF VISION

Law of squint. False image is displaced towards the side of paralysed muscle. The false image is fainter than true one, since it falls on less sensitive part of retina of squinting eye.

Contraction of pupil. It is caused by sudden increase in light intensity (light reflex), accommodation for near vision (accommodation reflex), stimulation of ciliary ganglion/nerve/ third nerve, sleep, severe pain, loss of aqueous humor, paralysis of cervical sympathetic nerve.

Dilatation of pupil. It is caused by sudden decrease in light intensity, fear/excitement, late stages of asphyxia, accommodation for distant vision, third nerve paralysis, stimulation of cervical sympathetic.

Phakoscope.

- Shows following reflections:- a bright upright image at air-corneal junction, a faint upright image from anterior surface of lens, a faint inverted image from posterior surface of lens.
- On accommodation, middle image moves, coming nearer anterior one, other two remaining stationary.

Stereoscopic vision. In fact the separate retinal images are not absolutely identical, their fusion in brain produces a visual sensation which has depth and solidarity.

Rod receptor potential is not a depolarising one but is a hyperpolarising one?

- This is a common question asked to physiologists. The inner segment of the rod continuously pumps sodium from inside to outside of the rod. Due to more passage of Na^+, the inside becomes rich in electronegative potential. But outer membrane is also typical, i.e. in dark state, it is leakly to Na^+. Because of this passage of Na^+ from out to inside due to leakage, this inside negativity is neutralised or balanced. This is normally - 40 mV electronegativity under dark conditions when the rod is not excited.
- Now suppose rod is excited by light. This decreases the conductance of sodium of outer segment of rod. So this leakage of Na^+ from outer towards interior of rod is suppressed. This increases the negativity inside and if energy striking rod is more, then more will be the electronegativity inside which means hyperpolarisation.

Chromatic aberration. The shorter waves (397-492 mμ) are refracted to a greater extent on passing through a lens than the longer waves (e.g. 585-723 mμ - orange red). Hence the image formed by lens will have colour fringes - chromatic aberration. It is to be remembered that white light is composed of light waves whose wavelengths range between 723-397 mμ.

Example:- Examine the spectrum through spectroscope. It is not possible to focus red and violet bands simultaneously.

Amacrine cells. There are following types:

- One are part of direct pathway for rod vision (rod biopolar cells amacrine cells ganglion cell)
- Other type of such cells, respond strongly at onset of visual signal but respond dies out rapidly.
- Other type of cells respond strongly at offset of visual signal, but response again dies rapidly.
- Other type of such cells respond to movement of a spot across the retina in a specific direction.
- Other types of such cell responds at both the instances, i.e. at on and off.

So these cells are types of interneurones that help in beginning analysis of visual signals before they leave the retina.

Young-Helmholtz theory of colour vision

- Suppose there are there types of cones each having a specific photochemical substance, e.g. XYZ (X is acted principally, by red light) (Y acted by green light) (Z acted by violet light).
- Colour blind occurs when X absent in red blindness, Y in green blindness. But this happens to be fallacious because if Y substance is absent in green blindness, patient cannot distinguish between white and purple, but this does not happen.

Reduced eye

- Because refractory index of cornea is different from air more of the refractory power of the eye is provided by anterior surface of cornea, not by crystalline lens.
- The refractory power of lens within eye - 20 Diopter. If it is removed from eye; then it is surrounded by air. Then its refractory power will be many times more. This is so because refractory index of fluid surrounding lens is not significantly different from refractory index of lens itself. This little difference decreases the amount of light refraction at the lens interfaces.
- If all the refractory surfaces of eye are added together and then considered to be one single lens the optics of normal eye may be simplified and represented at reduced eye.
- In reduced eye the total refractory power is 59 Diopters when lens is accommodated for distance vision.

- If the light rays are parallel to the axis (line through the middle) of a lens/curved mirror, they come to the principal focus. If the lens has adequate convexity, these diverging light rays will bent and coverage on conjugate focus. So distance to conjugate focus is greater than to principal focus for lens.
- The power of a lens to bend light depends on (i) refractory index of lens, (ii) curvature of surfaces.
- Refractory power of a lens is expressed in Diopters and 'focal distance' is a distance between a biconvex lens and principal focus.
- The shorter the focal distance be, greater the refractory power of the lens will be.
  — When focal distance is 100 cm the lens is said to get a power of 100/100 = 1 Diopter
  — When focal distance is 20 cm then lens is said to get a power of 100/20 = 5 Diopters
- As the parallel rays are diverged by biconcave lens and there is no focal point. So the power of biconcave lens will be expressed in terms of its ability to counteract converging ability of biconvex lens so power of biconcave lens is expressed in terms of negative diopter, while power of biconvex lens is expressed in terms of plus Diopters.

Helmholtz theory of accommodation

- Radial fibres of ciliary muscle contract and pull choroid forwards.
- Thus, suspensory ligament is slackened and tension on lens capsule is relaxed.
- Lens in virtue of its own elasticity becomes more convex.
- Contraction of circular fibres of ciliary muscle reduces circumference of lens, making anterior surface bulge forwards.
- Atropine paralyses accommodation by interfering with third nerve which supplies ciliary muscle.

Astigmatism. Due to spoon shaped curvature of cornea, i.e. radius of curvature is different in different planes, causing inability to focus vertical and horizontal lines simultaneously.

Spherical aberration. Rays passing through the periphery of convex lens are strongly refracted. So they are focussed in front of those passing through the centre of the lens. So when centre of an image is focussed its edges are blurred and vice versa.

BIBLIOGRAPHY

1. Bill A. Blood Circulation and fluid dynamics in the eye. Phy Rev 1975;55:383.
2. De Valois RL, et al. Normal mechanism of colour vision: In Darian Smith I (Ed.) Hand book of physiology sec. I, Vol. IIII, Bethesda, Md American physiological society 1984;525. (Quoted by Guyton AC in Textbook of Physiology, WB Saunders).
3. Eckmiller R. Neural control of persuit eye movements. (Quoted by Guyton AC in Textbook of Physiology, WB Saunders). Phy Rev 1987;67:797.
4. Gurnery AM, et al. Light flash physiology with synthetic photosensitive compounds. Phy Rev 1987;67:583.
5. Hillman P, et al. Transduction: invertebrate photo receptors: Role of pigment bistability. Phy Rev, 1983.
6. Kanko A. Physiology of retina. (Quoted by Guyton AC in Textbook of Physiology, WB Saunders). Ann Rev neurosci 1979;2:169.
7. Koretz JF, et al. How the human eye focuses. Sci Am 1988;92.
8. Lam DM-K, Shatz CJ. (Ed.). Development of visual system MIT press. (Quoted by Ganong WF in Review of Medical Physiology, Lange Publications).1991.
9. Liebman PA, et al. The molecular mechanism of visual excitation and its relation to structure and composition of rod outer segment. (Quoted by Guyton AC in Textbook of Physiology, WB Saunders). Ann Rev Phy 1987;49:765.
10. Mac Nichol EF. (Jr.) Three pigment colour vision. (Quoted by Guyton AC in Textbook of Physiology, WB Saunders). Sci Amer 1964;211:48.
11. Marks WB, et al. Visual pigments of single primate cones. Science 1964;143:1181.
12. Owen WG. Ionic conductances in rod photo receptors. Ann Rev Phy 1987;49:743.
13. Rushton WAH. Visual pigments and colour blindness. (Quoted by Guyton AC in Textbook of Physiology, WB Saunders). Sci Amer 1975;232(2):64.
14. Sherman SM, et al. Organisation of visual pathway in normal and visually deprived rats. Phy Rev 1982;62:738.
15. Toates FM. Accommodation function of human eye. Phy Rev 1972;52:828.
16. Van Essent DC, et al. Information processing in primate visual system: An integrated systems perspective. (Quoted by Ganong WF in Review of Medical Physiology, Lange Publications). Science 1992;255:4'9.
17. Wolf G. Multiple functions of Vitamin A. (Quoted by Guyton AC in Textbook of Physiology, WB Saunders). Phy Rev 1982;64: 738.

38 Sense of Hearing: Ear (Auditory Apparatus)

It acts as a highly differentiated and specialised mechanoreceptor which extracts and transmits to the CNS-the information about the acoustic environment. It represents 'many-in-one' like "apne-rang-hazaar."

EXTERNAL EAR

It consists of Pinna and External auditory meatus.

Functions of Pinna

- Slight in man.
- To collect sound waves and reflect them into meatus.
- To locate sounds. We locate a sound by turning the head until the sound is equally loud in both ears.

External-Auditory-Meatus: 2.5 cm long. In its walls are hairs, sebaceous glands and ceruminous glands which secrete an oily fluid which keeps membrane tympani moist and hinders entry of insects or particles of dirt. It is first directed upwards and backwards, then forwards and inwards to end at tympanic membrane. It enables sound waves to impinge perpendicularly on tympanic membrane.

TYMPANIC MEMBRANE

It is an oval, stretched, semitransparent, fibroelastic membrane which separates the external auditory meatus from the middle ear. It is 0.1 mm thick.

MIDDLE EAR (TYMPANUM)

Boundaries

a. Inner wall - shows
   i. Fenestra ovalis a foramen covered in by a very thin layer of hyaline cartilage.
   ii. Fenestra rotunda ......
b. *Anteriorly:* Shows a canal 'Eustachian tube' which is lower canal; while upper canal contains tensor tympani muscle.
c. *Posteriorly:* shows
   Aditus—a passage leading from upper part of tympanum to mastoid antrum. On its inner wall there are two bulges—one for external semicircular canal and another for facial nerve—the 'Aqueductus—Fallopii.'

Contents - (i) Ossicles (ii) Muscles - tensor tympani and stapedius (iii) Air

Ossicles

- *Malleus (handle hammer)*: having large, rounded head articulating with incus. Muscle tensor tympani is inserted into neck.
- *Incus (anvil shaped)*: articulating with head of malleus. It is attached by a ligament to posterior wall of tympanic cavity.
- *Stapes (stirrup shaped)*: Its head articulates with long process of incus. Its neck serves for insertion of

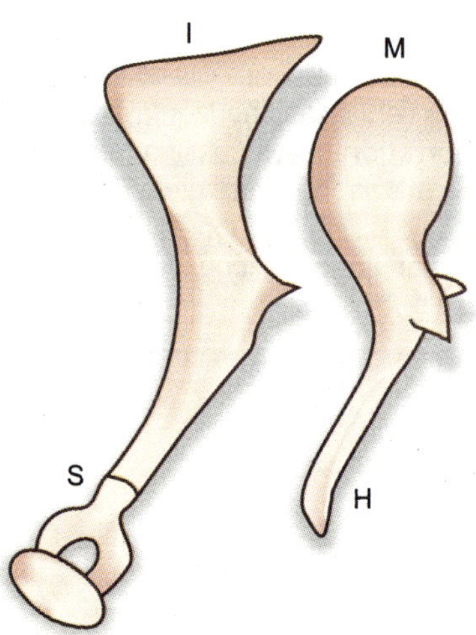

Fig. 38.1: Left ear ossicles (I = Incus (body), M = Malleus (head), H = Head, S = Stapes (head)

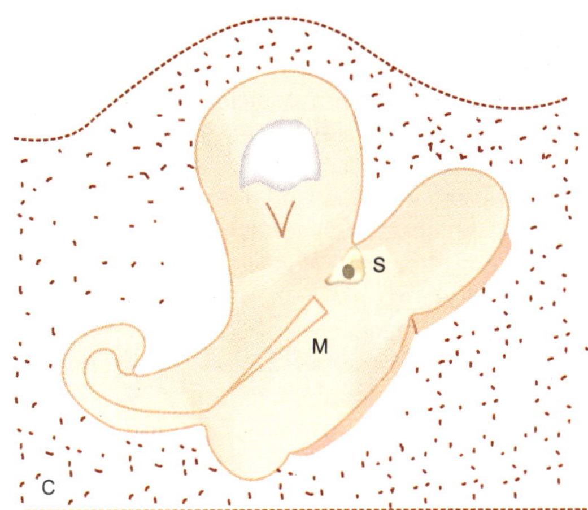

Fig. 38.2: Ear: An outlook (V = vestibule (internal ca, C = Cochlea, M = Middle ear, S = Stapes bone)

stapedius muscle. Its footplate or faceplate is attached to margins of fenestra ovalis by a membrane.

Functions of Ossicles

a. To transmit vibration from large tympanic membrane (60 sq. m.) to the small fanestra ovalis (3 sq. m.), thus increasing pressure or power.
b. To modify vibrations by diminishing their amplitude and thus increasing their force or power, aiding transference of vibrations from air to fluid. Combined effect increases pressure or force of vibrations 60 fold, thus overcoming inertia of labyrinth. It is the pressure which is more significant to overcome the inertia.

Peculiarities of Middle Ear

i. *Impedance matching*
   - The surface area of tympanic membrane is about 55–60 mm^2; whereas that of oval window is about 3–3.2 mm^2.
   - The force of sound on the tympanic membrane is transmitted through the three ossicles to the oval window and pressure of the sound is thus magnified by 15–20 times (Pressure = force per unit area).
   - The middle ear ossicles acting as a lever system allows all the energy of a sound wave impinging on the tympanic membrane to be applied to the small faceplate of stapes, causing approximately 20 times as much pressure on the fluid of cochlea as is exerted by the sound wave against the tympanic membrane. Since fluid has greater inertia than air, it is clear that increased amount of pressure are needed to cause vibrations in the fluid. In this way, the tympanic membrane and ossicular system provide "Impedance matching" between sound waves in air and sound vibrations in the fluid of cochlea. In the absence of this matching, more than 90 per cent of sound energy would have been reflected from tympanic membrane back into the air, and therefore would be lost and thus sensitivity of hearing would have been decreased. The medium on the medial side of the oval window is a liquid and matching system facilitates transfer of power from air (light-compliant) to the fluid (heavy-stiff).

ii. The tensor tympani muscle which is attached to the malleus, when contracts causes the tympanic membrane to become taut and so its contraction causes reduction of amplitude of vibration of eardrum; which is thus protected from injury when pressure of sound wave is too high. On the other hand, contraction of stapedius draws the stapes more outwards, thus reducing the impact on the end organ of hearing (organ of Corti) in the internal ear. When amplitude of sound is very high (loud noisy sounds; noise pollution) these two muscles contract reflexly, and thus protects the internal ear as well as eardrum from any possible damage which may terminate into deafness. Another function of this mechanism is partly to allow adaptation of the ear to sounds of different intensities. This has been also called as, *'attenuation reflex.'*

iii. For the eardrum to vibrate freely and thereby set in motion the other conduction mechanism, the air pressure on the two sides of the drum must be same. A gas enclosed in body cavity is speedily absorbed by the blood and surrounding tissues, hence the pressure of gas is gradually reduced. To prevent this from occurring in tympanic cavity, the eustachian tube permits air to flow from the pharynx into middle ear. Thus, an equality of pressure on the two sides of eardrum is assured. The tubes are open, however, only during yawning, swallowing and while blowing the nose.

iv. *Functions: Attenuation Reflex Impedance Matching*
   —Protection of cochlea from damaging vibrations caused by excessive loud sound.
   —In a noisy atmosphere; certain background sounds may mask the main sound vibrations so by these those sound is masked. In this way one is able to concentrate on main sounds, i.e. 1000 cycles per second.
   —Another function of these two muscle is to decrease a person's hearing sensitivity to his own speech.

— When loud sound waves are transmitted through ossicular system into CNS; there occurs reflex contraction of both these muscles. The tensor tympani pulls the handle of malleus inwards while stapdius muscle pulls the stapes outwards. These two opposing forces produce a high degree of rigidity, i.e. reducing ossicular conduction of low frequency sound. The opposing forces decrease the sound transmission. A reflex is initiated by loud sound which causes contraction of these muscles called tympanic reflex. It prevents auditory receptors from damage which may be due to loud sounds.

v. *Functions of middle ear: Few more points*

— Bekesy found that at all frequency of sound upto 2400 cycles per second, the central conical part of tympanic membrane moves in and out and handle of malleus move as a single unit.

— The malleus and incus are closely bound together and suspended by elastic ligaments. They move as a single unit. The axis of rotation is through anterior and lateral processes and transmits the vibrations to head of stapes. The ossicles function as a lever system converting mechanically the resonant vibrations of tympanic membrane into movements of stapes against posterior edge of oval window. The vibrations are then transmitted to perilymph in scala vestibuli.

— Three types of conduction

1. *Ossicular:* Conduction of sound waves from external ear $\xrightarrow[\text{membrane}]{\text{tympanic}}$ middle ear $\xrightarrow{\text{auditory ossicles}}$ cochlear fluid.
2. Air: Sound waves may be conducted in the cochlear fluid through membrane of round window (secondary tympanic membrane). Not normally required.
3. Third way is possible through transmission of vibrations of the bones of skull. Tuning fork may be directly applied to the skull. These vibrations which are generated by bones of skull are transmitted to cochlear fluid.

READ AND DIGEST

- Impedance means obstruction or opposition to the passage of sound waves, through any object.
- Because of the fact that solid objects have impedance; so usually when sound is passed to solid object then sound waves are not transmitted.
- Now, auditory ossicles are also solid objects; but sound impedance is comparatively less. So remaining more sound energy developed by tympanic membrane is transmitted to cochlear fluid by ossicles.
- This difference between ossicles and solid object is because ossicles act like a lever system; and, ossicles increase the sound pressure which arrive at oval window; All this is to set vibrations in fluid present in cochlea.
- The entire process by which tympanic membrane and lever system of ossicles convert the sound energy into mechanical vibrations in fluid of inner ear is called "Impedance matching."
- Role of tympanic membrane: Acts as a resonator which reproduces sound vibrations.
- Role of auditory ossicles: Vibrations in tympanic membrane are transmitted through malleus and incus to reach the stapes; thus causing to and fro movements of stapes against oval window as well as perilymph.
- Role of eustachian tube:
  — Not concerned with hearing.
  — It equalises the pressure on either side of tympanic membrane.
  — It connects middle ear with posterior part of nose and forms passage of air between middle ear and atmosphere.

INNER EAR

Like the middle ear, it is a cavity in the temporal bone of the skull. It consists of 'cochlea;' the 'saccule,' the 'utricle' and the 'semicircular canal.' Only 'cochlea' functions in the hearing process.

Cochlea: (Snail) is a tube that is coiled into a helix whose two and a half turns decrease in size as it progresses away from the middle ear. The shape of the cochlea resembles a snail shell. A cross-section of the cochlea shows that the coiled tube contains three tubular regions, namely *'scala vestibuli,' 'scala media'* and the *'scala tympani.'* The scala vestibuli and the scala media are separated from each other by the *'vestibular membrane'* which actually is designed to maintain a special fluid in the scala media that is required for normal function of the sound receptive hair cells. Therefore as far as sound transmission is concerned, scala vestibuli and scala media are considered as a single chamber. Similarly scala media and scala tympani are separated from each other by *'Basilar membrane.'* Distal ends of the scala vestibuli and scala tympani are continuous with each other by way of the *'Helicotrema.'*

Basilar Membrane : Peculiarities

a. The fibres near helicotrema vibrate at low; fibres at cochlear base vibrate at high frequency?
   i. It is containing almost 20,000 basilar fibres which are projecting from bony centres of the cochlea, towards the outer wall. Actually these fibres are

stiff/elastic/hair like structure which are free at one end, so they vibrate like reeds of harmonium. The length of these fibres is 0.04 mm at the base of cochlea, while it assumes the length as 0.5 mm at helicotrema; means almost 12–13 fold increase in length. This is the reason that shorter fibres near the base of cochlea vibrates at higher frequency, while fibres near helicotrema vibrate more easily at a low frequency.

ii. The volume and elasticity of the fibres near the helicotrema is almost hundred times great, as compared with the fibres near the stapes. This also explains the above fact that area near the base of cochlea vibrates at higher frequency while fibres near helicotrema vibrate more easily at low frequency.

iii. 'Fluid loading' is another fact. The fluid mass is comparatively less at base of cochlea as compared with the area near to helicotrema. This also explains the fact.

b. Travelling wave

i. A high frequency sound wave travels only a short distance along the basilar membrane before it reaches its resonant point and then it fades away; A sound wave with medium frequency travels upto midway only and then fades; while a sound wave with very low frequency travels completely or on entire basilar membrane, before it dies.

ii. Basilar fibres are having high coefficient of elasticity near the stapes, and comparatively decreasing coefficient farther along the membrane. This explains the fact that the sound wave travels fast along the initial portion of the basilar membrane but then it becomes slow and more slow as it goes farther and farther into cochlea.

c. Organ of Corti:

- This important organ seated on the basilar membrane is actually the apparatus that transduces mechanical energy into electric impulses. It is also the site of 'hair cells' which are the actual sensory receptors and are connected to fibres of statoacoustic nerve (VIII). The hair cells have projecting hairs or fibres that extend upwards and are embedded in a tongue like, stiff tissue *'tectorial membrane'* which lies above in scala media. It is an important anatomical feature that the tectorial membrane is hinged at a point not on the basilar membrane so that motion of the basilar membrane causes the hair cells to bend. Upper ends of hair cells are fixed tightly in a structure called *'reticular lamina'* which is a rigid structure and is continuous with a rigid triangular structure called *'rods of Corti'* which rests on each *basilar fibre.* So basilar fibre, rods of Corti and reticular lamina all move as a unit. The *hair cells* are said to be of two types—the *'internal and external'*—internal are 3500–4000 in number and having diameter of 12 µm while external cells are 20,000 in number but with a diameter of only 8 µm.
- The inner hair cells are sensory cells which generate action potential in auditory nerves. They are stimulated by movements of fluid.
- The outer cells are motile. They shorten on depolarisation, while lengthen on hyperpolarisation. The incoming sound is amplified by reduction in damping of basement membrane.

d. The fluid medium:

- The scala media is filled with a fluid *'Endolymph'* which contains potassium in very high concentration but sodium in a low concentration. This fluid is secreted by *'stria vascularis'* - an area located on outer wall of scala media and is said to be highly vascular.
- Perilymph is the fluid contained by scala vestibuli and scala tympani; and this fluid is quite identical with CSF (Cerebro-spinal-fluid).

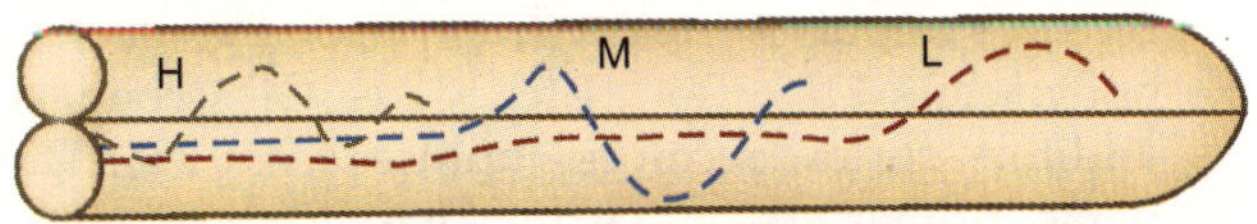

Fig. 38.3: Travelling waves (H = High frequency wave, M = Medium frequency wave, L = Low frequency wave)

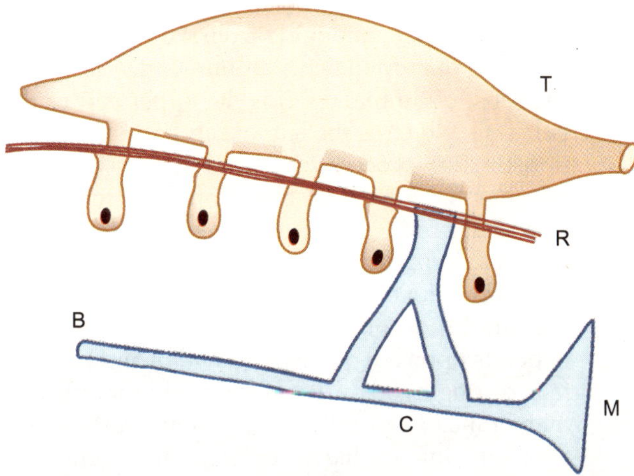

Fig. 38.4: Hair cells tectorial membrane (R = Reticular lamina, C = Rods of Corti, T = Tectorial membrane, B = Basilar membrane, M = Modiolus)

- An electric potential of 80 mV exist between endo- and perilymph with positivity inside and negativity outside the scala media and is named as *'endocochlear potential'* and is due to continued secretion of potassium ions into scala media by stria vascularis.

e. Action potential: Auditory nerve fibre:
When basilar fibres bend towards scala vestibuli, the hair cells depolarise; while hyperpolarisation occurs on opposite side. This generates 'hair cell receptor potential.' This is further because of opening of cation conducting channels; which cause rapid movement of positively charged potassium ions into the tips of stereocilia, which cause depolarisation. It has also been suggested by many workers that a transmitter preferably glutamate is released during depolarisation.

f. Loudness: Mechanism: Following are postulations
   i. As sound becomes louder → increase in amplitude of vibration of basilar membrane + hair cells → hair cells excite nerve ending at more rapid rates.
   ii. Increase in sound amplitude → more and more hair cells stimulated → spatial summation of impulses → loud sound.
   iii. Some hair cells are having high threshold value. It means that certain hair cells cannot be stimulated until vibrations on basilar membrane reaches to a certain intensity. So when such cells get stimulation, the loud sound is appreciated.

g. Potentials - Other than Endocochlear:
   i. Corti lymphatic: The hair cells as well as supporting cells of cochlea have a negative potential (intracellular) with respect to fluid bathing them. It is ranging from -20 to -80 mV.
   ii. Cochlear microphonic: Is an immediate response to acoustic stimulation. It is the upper end of the hair cells which is the site of mechano-electrical-transduction-process. It may be regarded as receptor potential having no true refractory/threshold period. It produces stimulus wave. Its amplitude is directly proportional to displacement of cochlear partition. With the increase in intensity of stimulus, the amplitude of response is also increased. It depends upon adequate oxygenation and hence it fails during hypoxia. It has been told that plasma membrane of hair cell furnishes abundant surface area for ionic exchange between hair cells and perilymph.
   iii. Summating potential
      — Positive one—is more sensitive towards hypoxia. It originates in outer hair cells-
      — Negative one—more resistant. It increases the amplitude after mild injury to organ of corti.

The Auditory pathway:

- The nerve cell bodies of dendrites that arise from hair cells, constitute 'spiral ganglion' situated within the internal ear, which sends axons to the cochlear nerve, (dorsal and ventral cochlear nuclei located in upper part of medulla). Organ of Corti is represented or 'unrolled' again and again in the brain. The pathway are both crossed and uncrossed so that each cochlea is represented in both sides of the brain.
- Second order neurons arise from cochlear nuclei, pass mainly to opposite side of the brainstem through 'trapezoid body' to terminate into 'superior olivary nucleus.' Some other fibres enter lateral lemniscus directly to terminate at 'nuclei of lateral lemniscus.'
- The third order neorons from superior olivary-nucleus ascend in lemniscus to the 'inferior colliculus,' whereas those from nuclei of lemniscus proceed to the medial geniculate body and from here auditory radiations pass on to internal capsule to the 'primary auditory area.'
- A cerebellar auditory centre has also been reported in 'tuber vermis' which receives fibres from dorsal cochlear nucleus.
- Descending pathway has been reported which has fibres which terminate on both the cells of origin of olivo cochlear bundles and on neurons of the ventral cochlear nucleus. These are called 'centrifugal extra - reticular - auditory control system.'

AUDITORY CORTEX

i. Lies on the supra-temporal-plane of the *superior temporal gyrus*, but also extends over lateral border of the *temporal lobe*, over much of the insular cortex and also to most lateral portion of the parietal operculum.
ii. It has been broadly divided into two parts—*A I* (or 'short latency area; OR *Primary Auditory cortex*) receives impulses mainly from medial geniculate body; while *A II* (or 'long latency area; OR secondary auditory cortex) receives impulses from A I. The name 'primary receptive area' has also been given

to AI since on electric stimulation, it makes an individual capable of listening all sorts of sounds e.g. tingling, roaring etc., while A II has been designated as *'Interpretive area'* since on electric stimulation, it makes an individual to listen whole sentences and then to interpret them also.

iii. Auditory cortex is not necessary, at least for learning responses to tones, or for discriminating between tones. It is required, however, for recognition of simple auditory pattern, such as differences between two different sequences of three tones each - 'high-low-high;' 'low-high-low.' This sort of discrimination depends upon integrity of insular and temporal areas.

iv. The direction of the sound can be judged by two mechanisms:
   - By time interval between entry of sound into one ear and then into opposite ear.
   - By the difference between intensities of the sounds in the two ears.

   If one is standing exactly in front of the sound source, the sound will reach to both ears exactly at the same time. If right ear is closer to the sound as compared with the left; then sound waves enter the right ear earlier than the left.

v.
   - Destruction of primary auditory cortex only on one side in human beings has little or no significant effect on hearing because of many other crossover connections.
   - If auditory association areas are destructed, then the poor sufferer will be unable to interpret the meaning of the words.

vi. Destruction of auditory cortex on both sides of brain, makes a person unable to detect the sound direction. This mechanism is located in superior olivary nuclei. Its lateral part first of all compares the intensity of sound and then it sends signals to auditory cortex to estimate the direction.

vii. When we listen to a symphony-orchestra then within the so called mixture of all instruments, we can concentrate on one single instrument, and can reject other sounds. This is possible by some fibres moving retrograde (from superior olivary nucleus to cochlea) which are inhibitory in nature. They can reduce sound intensity as much as 15–20 decibels (Centrifugal signals).

viii. A young man (before ageing) can hear between 20–20, 000 cycles per second (frequency of sound). In old age it falls to 50–8000 cycles per second.

HEARING MECHANISM

Sound wave-from air to tympanic membrane

↓ middle ear

Rocking movement of stapes

↓ Pressure changes in perilymph

Basilar membrane - moves up and down

↓

Hair cells - move side ways

↓ Receptor potential + Release of neurotransmitter?

Nerve impulse through VIII N

↓

Sound perception by brain

DEAFNESS (HEARING IMPAIRMENT)

Any abnormal condition or disease process which interferes with the conduction of sound to the inner ear; with the transduction to nerve impulse in the cochlea; or with their transmission to the appropriate levels of the nervous system, can cause impairment of hearing or deafness.

a. *Conductive deafness*: Sound wave energy does not reach the internal ear satisfactorily. Its causes include:
   - Accumulation of dry and hard wax' in external canal. It can be easily corrected.
   - Otosclerosis is a localised disease of bony capsule of the labyrinth and a common cause of this sort of deafness. It involves destruction of bone in neighbourhood of window and replacement by new bone which may be deposited around the stapes footplate in such a way so as to interfere with its motion and ultimately to fix it in the oval window. The loss of hearing is due to increasing stiffness and because of it, stapes and oval window become firmly adherent and therefore it fails to move properly when the eardrum vibrates.
   - Perforation of eardrum—which may result from the inequality of the air pressure between middle and the external ear cavities. The effect of perfora-

tion upon hearing depends upon its position and size but it usually involves the low frequencies.

- A temporary conductive impairment can occur when eardrum membrane is strongly retracted by a negative pressure in middle ear and it also increases its stiffness. This condition is experienced in air craft during descents from altitude.

b. *Nerve: OR Sensory neural Deafness*: Is caused by damage to cochlear mechanism or to the auditory nerve. Its leading cause is the increasing *'noise pollution.'* In its earliest form it appears as TTS (temporary - threshold shift) when noise exists which is of more intensity than normal. If it is of very high intensity and appears continuously, i.e. day by day, it can turn into permanent impairment named as 'Permanent - threshold - shift' (PTS).

This type of deafness may be congenital also, or may occur as a result of some infection like meningitis or mumps.

- Meniere's syndrome is a form of such type of deafness, accompanied by violent attacks of vertigo. Hearing for low frequencies is affected and tinitus is often present. All this is because of increased hydrostatic pressure of the endolymph, causing bulging of the walls of the cochlear duct. Auditory nerve is also affected due to such changes. Lastly a progressive nerve deafness occurs with advancing age called 'Presbycusis.'

DEAFNESS: CAUSES

— Noise induced
— Drugs: Quinine, streptomycin, gentamycin, chloramphenicol, frusemide, NSAID-Aspirin
— Infection: Otitis media
— Genetic: Otosclerosis, sensory-neural deafness
— Sudden: Viral infection, acoustic neuroma

HEARING TESTS

a. *Rinne's Test*: Is performed by using tuning fork. The vibrating fork is first placed on the mastoid process. When the patient reports that he can no longer hear its tone by bone conduction, it is removed from the bone and vibrating prongs are held up to the open ear canal. The normal ear should then hear the fork by air conduction and continue to hear it for about 45 seconds. This positive Rinne's test is also characteristic of sensori-neural impairment. If the fork is heard longer by bone conduction, the test is negative and a conductive loss is present.

b. *Weber test*: It consists simply in placing the vibrating fork on the patient's head and asking him to report in which ear he hears it. If one ear has a sensori-neural lesion the sound will be heard in the opposite, i.e. the better ear. If however, one has a fixed stapes, the sound will be heard in the same, i.e. worse ear.

c. *Schwabach test*: In this, patient's bone conduction hearing is tested against the presumably normal hearing of the examiner. If there is a conductive lesion, the patient will be able to hear the tuning fork longer than the examiner, because the presence of the lesion excludes masking noise. If a neural lesion is present, the patient will hear tuning fork for a shorter time than the examiner.

TESTS OF HEARING

Rinne's: Base of vibrating tuning fork is placed on mastoid process till person stops hearing. Then it is held in air. A normal man hears vibrations in air after completion of bone conduction. In conduction deafness, vibrations in air not heard after completion of bone conduction. In nerve deafness, vibrations are heard in air after bone conduction is over.

Webers: Vibrating tuning fork is put on skull vertex. Normally one hears equally on both sides. In conduction deafness, sound is louder in diseased ear because here masking effect of environmental noise is absent. In nerve deafness, sound is louder in normal ear.

Schwabach: Here, bone conduction of patient is compared with normal person. In conduction deafness, bone conduction is better than normal. In nerve deafness, bone conduction worse than normal.

THEORIES OF HEARING

1. *Helmholtz Resonance Theory (1863):* A series of resonators were presumed by him in cochlea, each capable of tuning to a different frequency. Rods of Corti may also act as resonators. Short fibres of basilar membrane near the oval window respond to higher frequency and longer fibres near the apex respond to lower frequency.
2. *Rutherford Telephone Theory (1880):* Cochlea is working as a telephone transmitter. It transfers sounds into nerve impulses of the same frequency, which is then analysed by CNS.
3. *Place Theory:* Entire cochlea is a tuned structure. Basilar membrane and organ of Corti respond to sound of different frequency. This report is reaching to the brain that which part of organ of Corti has been stimulated.
4. *Wever—Resonance Volley Theory (1949):* It is a combina–tion of two—(a) Telephone theory .... Response of whole cochlea to low frequency and, (b) Place theory—Cochlear analysis of higher frequency.

EFFICIENT HEARING - DEPENDS ON

i. Proper transmission of the sound waves by conducting mechanism to the inner ear.
ii. The generation of nerve impulses by the receptor (organ of Corti)
iii. The conduction of impulses by the auditory nerve to the cerebral cortex.
iv. The setting up of sensation in auditory area of the brain.

SOME INTERESTING COMMENTS

Von Bekesy (1951–60)

a. Basilar membrane may be regarded as a gelatinous sheet, enveloped by thin homogenous layer of fibres, forming a continuous structure with the organ of Corti. Graded stiffness is its another characteristic, which is greatest at the stapes and decreases towards the apex. So the stiffness of cochlear partition is one hundred times greater at the stapes as at apex.

Engstrom (1962): The stereocilia (hairs) are as stiff micro levers which transmit the vibrations of tectorial membrane to the cuticular plate and thus to the interior of hair cell.

Weiner and Ross: External ear is protective in function. It helps to shield the drum membrane from damage by blows. It also helps to maintain a favourable temperature and humidity for membrane.

Zwislocki (1962): Part of the sound energy reaching the drum is reflected back, while rest is absorbed by the drum. The amount of reflected and absorbed energy depends upon mechanical impedance of ear. If drum acts like a rigid plug which presents infinite impedance then all energy will be reflected. If it matches impedance to that of air in external canal all energy will be absorbed. So the impedance depends upon frequency of sound being transmitted by ear.

MASKING

i. Inspite of the ability of the ear to analyze complex tones and separate out individual frequencies weak sounds may be completely inaudible in the presence of sounds of greater intensity. This phenomenon is called masking.
ii. The common example is—In a railway journey unless the voice is louder, one cannot hear it. The loudness of the voice can be revealed when the train stops. So weaker sounds may be completely inaudible in presence of louder sounds and this is masking.
iii. The degree of masking to which one component is masked by the other is measured by finding the threshold. The sounds of almost same frequency cause fluctuations in loudness.
iv. Since low tones affect the whole length of the basilar membrane, whereas high tones affect only a limited region near the stapes (Bekesy). According to this pattern of excitation of the basilar membrane, it is said that, 'low tones are much more effective in masking high tones than vice versa.'
v. Masking by noise is used in clinical audiometry to 'block' the better ear so that it will not respond to loud sounds or to bone conducted sounds used in testing the worse ear and thus give a false result.
vi. Noise—Is described in psychological terms as a sound which causes annoyance or disturbance. If it is a long-term exposure, it may lead to deafness, of course, loss of hearing depends upon frequency value of noise.

AUDIOMETRY

It is an important investigation for auditory dysfunction. It is a valuable method for diagnosing ear disease, degree of deafness.

Pure Tone Audiotmetry

Introduction

— It is an electronic device that consists of pure tone generator, an amplifier and an attenuator.
— The frequency can be selected from pure tone generator by frequency selector switch. Intensity of stimulus is controlled by hearing level dial/ attenuator.

Method

— In a sound proof room the ability of patient to hear tones in frequency range of 125, 250, 500, 1000, 2000, 4000, 6000, 8000 Hz. Pure tone sensitivity can be measured by air and bone conduction.
— The operator increases the intensity of stimulus till it is heard by the patient. Then he slowly decreases the intensity until patient no longer listens the notes/ tones. The process is repeated several times.

Audiogram

— Is a graph showing the hearing sensitivity for air and bone conducted sound.

Principle

— Inner ear, i.e. cochlea is lying in bony cavity, i.e. temporal bone called bony labyrinth.

— Hence if skull is vibrating; it can produce vibrations in cochlea itself.
— Therefore, if a tuning fork is placed on any bony protuberance of the skull (specially on mastoid process) will cause a person to listen the sound.
— This device provides pure tones of various frequencies through earphones. At each frequency the threshold intensity is determined and plotted on a graph as a percentage of normal hearing.

Nerve Deafness: Audiogram

i. Deafness occurs due to loud sound. Low frequency sounds are louder as well as more damaging to organ of Corti.
ii. Certain drugs are also damaging like streptomycin, kanamycin, chloramphenicol etc.
iii. It means damage to cochlea/auditory nerve/CNS pathway.
iv. It means total loss of ability to listen sound tested by both, air and bone conduction.

Conduction Deafness: Audiogram

i. Due to middle ear infection, otosclerosis (hereditary disease causing fibrosis).
ii. Face plate of stapes become ankylosed by bony overgrowth to the edges of oval window.
iii. If stapes is removed and replaced with metal prosthesis then the person will be able to hear again
iv. In such circumstances, the sound wave cannot be transmitted easily through the ossicles from tympanic membrane to oval window.

Advantages

— Any type of hearing loss can be evaluated.
— It gives a measure of degree of hearing loss.
— It makes basis for treatment like hearing aid, tympanoplasty etc.
— Useful for medicolegal purposes.

SOUND AT A GLANCE

It, in its objective sense, consists of air vibrations. When a violin string is plucked, it vibrates forwards and backwards. In doing so, it condenses the air in front of it and rarifies the air behind it. These condensation and rarefactions travel through the air at a rate of 1,090 feet per second. The vibrations of a shorter string produce a greater number of waves per second and the pitch of the sound is higher, but whether the string be plucked gently or violently does not affect the number of vibrations per second, and consequently the pitch will remain the same.

i. *Pitch:* Depends on the frequency of vibrations. Human ear can appreciate a range in frequency from 16,000–20,000 per second. Within these limits we can distinguish about 11,000 different pitches. It is determined by the number of vibrations per second. The sensitivity of the ear varies with pitch.
ii. *Loudness (Intensity)*: of sound depends on the amplitude of the waves. It is more or less, a psychological concept which refers to the auditory sensation. The unit of measurement is called 'Bel,' (named after Alexander Graham Bell who developed telephone), which indicates 'differences of intensity. The reference intensity is that of the faintest audible sound in a quiet room of the same pitch as that of the sound with which it is to be compared. It is recorded on a logarithmic scale : or "It is a logarithm of the ratio of the intensities of that sound and a standard sound."

$$1\text{bel} = \log \frac{\text{intensity of sound}}{\text{intensity of standard sound}}$$

Bel is a large unit so decibel (1/10th of bel) is generally used.

Examples

Conversational voice at 12 ft. = 5 bel.
Loud motor horn at 25 ft. = 10 bel
Limit of ear's endurance = 13 bel.
Quiet street = 30 decibel
Noisy street = 60-80 decibel
Faintest audible sound = 0 decibel
Average office = 40 decibel

When decibels are plotted against the frequencies, an audibility curve (audiogram) is obtained. The threshold for hearing in man is least between 1000 and 3000 vibrations per second.
iii. *Timbre (Quality)*: Musical notes of same amplitude and pitch, produced by different instruments, vary in quality because the sound waves produced are peculiar to the instrument. The compound waves are produced by the fusion of sine waves whose wave lengths are $^1/_2$, $^1/_3$, $^1/_4$ etc., those of fundamental note, i.e. the compound wave is the algebraic sum of the fundamental note and its overtones which are a characteristic of the instrument.

When a string vibrates, it vibrates as a whole forward and backward; the waves thus formed constitutes the fundamental sound and determine its pitch. But the string, at the same time, vibrates in its parts, i.e. each half, third and fourth of the string vibrates independently of the whole string. This causes other waves and other sounds, the overtones, to accompany, and to fuse with the fundamental wave. These overtones vary with different sorts of instruments; in consequence, each distinct source of sound impresses its overtones upon the fundamental tone and enables us to recognise the source. So, "A violin string having 2,000 vibrations per second is set into vibrations; a similar string in piano is also caused to vibrate with the same force as the violin string; the two sounds have the same pitch and the same intensity, but no body mistakes one for the other. This is colour or timbre.

vi. *Resonance*: When a sound wave falls upon an object like a windowpane, it causes this to vibrate. When a person sings a certain note near a piano, the piano continues for a short time to send out the same note after the singer has stopped because the string which corresponds in number of vibrations to that of the note sung is thrown into sympathetic vibrations, or resonance.

SUMMARY AND HIGHLIGHTS—THE EAR WORKS

- As a Detector: It is capable of recording minute amounts of mechanical energy in the form of vibrations of the air molecules.
- As an analyzer: It gives detailed information of intensity and frequency spectrum of these air-borne vibration and about pitch-loudness, etc. also.
- As finder of direction—of sound in close collaboration with brain.
- As a transducer: Is capable of converting mechanical energy of sound into the form of electro-chemical energy which activates the concerning nerve fibres.

BIBLIOGRAPHY

1. Borg E, et al. The middle ear muscles. Sci Amer August-1989;PP74.
2. Davis HA. Model for transducer action in cochlea. Cold spring harbor symp. quant. Biol XXX, sensory receptors, 1966. (Quoted by Best and Taylor in Physiological basis of Medical Practice 1967—Williams and Wilkins Co.).
3. Davis H, et al (Ed.). Hearing and deafness. Revised ed. Holt. Rhinebart and winston Inc. 1960. (Quoted by Best and Taylor in Physiological basis of Medical Practice, 1967—Williams and Wilkins Co.).
4. Engstrom H, et al. Structure and function of sensory hairs of inner ear. (Quoted by Best and Taylor in Physiological basis of Medical Practice, 1967—Williams and Wilkins Co.). J. Acoust Soc. Am 1962;34:1356.
5. Guth PS, et al. Neurotransmission in auditory system : A primer for pharmacologist. Ann Rev Pharma Toxi 1982;22:383.
6. Hudspeth AJ. The cellular basis of hearing : The biophysics of hair cells. Science 1985;230:745.
7. Kay RH. Hearing of modulation in sounds. Phy Rev 1983;62:187.
8. Masterton RB, et al. Neural mechanisms of sound localisation. Ann Rev Phy 1984;46:275.
9. Nadol JB (Jr.). Hearing loss. (Quoted by Ganong WF in Review of Medical Physiolog—Lange Publications). New Eng J Med 1993;329:1092.
10. Patuzzi R, et al. Tuning in mammalian cochlea. Phy Rev 1988;68:1009.
11. Rhode WS. Cochlear mechanism. Ann Rev Phy 1984;46:231.
12. Rubel EW. Ontogeny of auditory system function. Ann Rev Phy 1984;46:213.
13. Sachs MB. Neural coding of complex sounds. Ann Rev Phy 1984;46:261.
14. Von Bekesy G, et al. The mechanical properties of ear: In Handbook of experimental psychology (ed. SS Stevans) John Wiley & Sons. Inc. New York 1951. (Quoted by Best and Taylor in Physiological basis of Medical Practice, 1967—Williams and Wilkins Co.).
15. Von Bekesy G. Experiments in hearing; McGrew Hill Co. Inc. New York 1960 (editor & translator EG Weaver). (Quoted by Best and Taylor in Physiological basis of Medical Practice, 1967—Williams and Wilkins Co.).
16. Weiss TF. Relation of receptor potential of cochlear hair cells to spike discharges of cochlear neurons. Ann Rev Phy 1984;46:247.
17. Zwislocki J. Analysis of some auditory characteristics: In Handbook of Mathematical psychology, Vol. III. John Wiley & Sons Inc. New York 1965. (Quoted by Best and Taylor in Physiological basis of Medical Practice, 1967—Williams and Wilkins Co.).

39 Chemical Senses: Sense of Taste

Tongue is the organ of taste.

TASTE SENSATION AND THEIR DISTRIBUTION

Sweet taste at tip, salt on dorsum, sour at sides and bitter at the back of tongue. Metallic and alkaline tastes have also been reported.

TASTE BUDS—THE END ORGAN OF TASTE SENSATION

a. *Distribution*: Mainly on tongue, but also found in soft palate, pharynx, epiglottis, arytenoid process (inner surface), fauces (anterior pillars).
b. *Functional anatomy*:
   i. Taste (neuro-epithelial) cells—fine hair like processes are projecting at the outer end through an epithelial depression called 'inner gustatory pore.' These sensory nerves are taste end organs.
   ii. Supporting cells: Peripheral and central; former are spindle shaped while later lies in between the taste cells. They encircle the small opening called inner taste pore; which is connected with outer taste pore situated upon the tongue surface through a small canal.

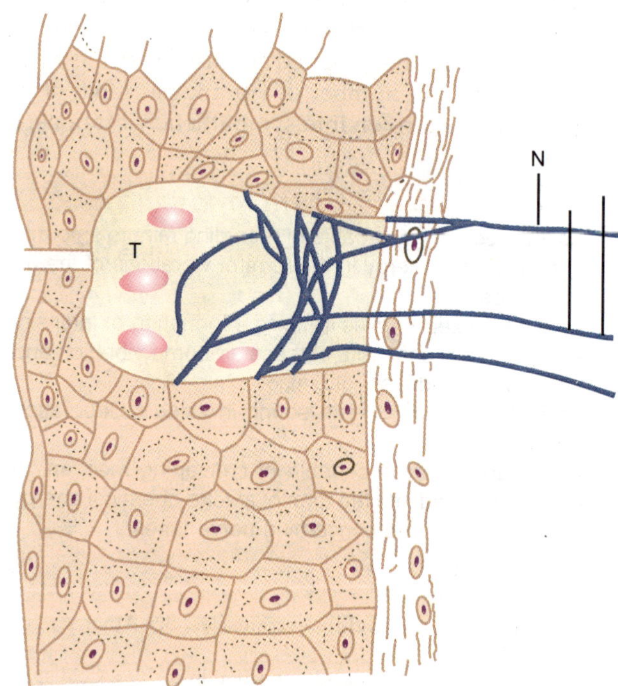

Fig. 39.1: Taste bud (N = Nerve fibre, T = Taste cell)

PATH OF TASTE SENSATION

1. *First order neurone* :
   a. From anterior two-third of tongue : Taste fibres first enters the lingual nerve, then chorda tympani and finally join the trunk of facial nerve (VII cranial). Cell station situated in upper part of *tractus solitarius*.
   b. From posterior one-third—fibres pass along glossopharyngeal nerve and entering cell station in the petreous ganglia. The axons of these cells pass along IX cranial nerve to end in lower part of *tractus solitarius*.
2. *Second order neurone*: from the nucleus of *tractus solitarius* second order neurone arise, cross in mid line, pass through medial lemniscus to end in thalamus.
3. *Third order neurone*: arises from thalamus, pass through posterior limb of internal capsule and ending in inferior part of post central gyrus of cerebral cortex. Its lesion therefore causes loss of taste and general sensation of opposite half of tongue.

PAPILLAE OF TONGUE

- *Circumvallate*: Largest, circular, containing taste buds, form a V shaped row near root of tongue.

- *Fungiform:* Resemble fungi, found on tip and side of tongue.
- *Filiform*: Bear delicate brush like processes highly developed on tip, found on anterior third of tongue.

TASTE BLINDNESS

For certain substances many of us are taste blind. "Phenylthiocarbamide" is a substance commonly used by psychologists to demonstrate taste blindness.

TASTE THRESHOLD

1. Sour taste by HCl..... 0.0009 N
2. Salty taste by NaCl ..... 0.01 M
3. Sweet taste by sucrose .... 0.01 M
4. Bitter taste by quinine ...... 0.000008 M

TASTE PREFERENCE

1. An adrenalectomized animal will certainly prefer drinking water with a high concentration of sodium chloride in preference to pure water.
2. The animal who has been given a high dose of insulin; will have a low blood sugar level. So sweetest food will be selected by it among many samples.
3. The animal from which parathyroid gland has been removed, will select an eatable rich in calcium chloride.
4. If a person becomes sick after taking a particular eatable, then he develops taste aversion for it (negative taste preference).

STIMULATION: TASTE BUDS

1. Membrane of taste cell is negatively charged inside with respect to outside.
2. Taste substance when attaches itself to taste cell's hairs → loss of negative potential → depolarization of cell.
3. Substance → reacts with taste villi → receptor potential is initiated. This means opening of ion channel; which is entry of sodium ions for depolarization. As the substance is taken away by saliva, the whole process comes to an end.
4. A weak signal is transmitted through nerve fibre as long as the stimulus is in contact with the taste bud, while a strong signal is immediately transmitted by the nerve.

BIBLIOGRAPHY

1. Oakley B, et al. Neural mechanism of taste. Phy Rev 1966;46:173.

40 Chemical Senses: Sense of Smell (Olfaction)

It is also a chemical sensation. For smell a substance must be in gaseous form. It is most primitive of all sensation. Smell sensation is often blended with taste sensation viz. Sweet smell (chloroform) pungent smell (ammonia).

OLFACTORY AREA

- Olfactory epithelium is that part of nasal epithelium which is sensitive to smell and confined to nasal mucosa of olfactory area, yellow coloured. Olfactory area is formed by superior nasal concha, upper part of septum and roof of nose.
- Olfactory cells—Are receptor cells for smell sensations. They are bipolar cells derived from CNS. They are 100 million in number interspersed among subtentacular cells. The mucosal end of olfactory cell forms a knob from which 'olfactory hairs/cilia (0.3 micrometer diameter; 200 micrometer length) project into mucus which coats the inner surface of nasal cavity. These cilia react to odour in the air and then stimulate the olfactory cells. Glands of Bowman are present among olfactory cells in the olfactory membrane which secrete mucus/watery/oily substance.

MECHANISM OF OLFACTION

- The membrane of cilia contain large number of protein molecules which binds itself with different substances whose smell is to be felt (odorant substances). These proteins are called 'odorant binding-proteins,' and this binding is the adequate stimulus for olfaction.
- By such type of binding, ionic channels are opened up which allows large number of positively charged sodium ions to flow to the interior of the olfactory cell and depolarise it.
- Another possibility is that receptor binding protein becomes activated (adenyl cyclase) and then protrudes to interior of the cell. It in turn catalyses the formation of cAMP; which act on many other membrane proteins to open ion channel through them.
- Qualities of substance to be smelled -
  1. Only volatile substance that can be sniffed into nostrils can be smelled,
  2. Stimulating substance should be slightly water soluble
  3. It must be slightly lipid soluble.
- The membrane potential of resting olfactory membrane is—55mV. Then on stimulation/depolarisation there is generation of action potential from once every twenty seconds upto two/three per seconds. Most of the substance cause membrane depolarisation. A few substances may cause hyperpolarisation of membrane which decrease the firing rate of nerves.

OLFACTORY PATHWAY

- Bipolar nerve cells of olfactory epithelium are first order neurone. Each receptor cell give rise to only one axon which joins with those derived from other receptors forming collectively olfactory nerves; which are non medullated having neurilemmal sheath.
- This nerve enters 'olfactory bulb' by piercing the cribrifom plate. Here, the axon makes synapses with dendrites of mitral cells and tufted cells to form olfactory glomeruli—a globular structure.
- These mitral and tufted cells are second order neurones and their axons constitute the olfactory tract which proceeds towards anterior perforated substance and divides in olfactory trigone into olfactory striae—medial, intermediate and lateral.
- The axons of tufted cells leave the tract for ending in opposite bulb through medial olfactory striae. This tract after entering the anterior commissure passes bilaterally to nucleus of striai terminalis, olfactory tubercle and to amygdaloid nucleus complex.

- The axons of mitral cells pass through lateral olfactory striae, and, end in anterior olfactory nucleus, pre pyriform cortex and peri amygdaloid cortex and these two are primary olfactory cortex. While Entorhinal cortex is the secondary olfactory cortex.

OLFACTORY SYSTEM: HISTORICAL VIEW

- Group of nuclei located in mid-basal part of brain. It is anterior and superior to hypothalamus. It is medial olfactory area—the very old olfactory system.
- Prepyriform and pyriform cortex along with cortical portion of amygdaloid nuclei constitute lateral olfactory area—the old olfactory system.
- The latest olfactory pathway is:- It passes through thalamus; and then to dorsomedial nuclei of thalamus and then to orbito-frontal cortex (latero-posterior-quadrant).

NOTES

- Loss of sense of smell is called *Anosmia* while *hyperosmia* means sensitiveness to odours, which is seen in hysteria, raised intracranial pressure.
- The olfactory receptors become insensitive to a particular substance after exposure to a specific period of time. This is *olfactory adaptation*.
- *Threshold of olfactory sensation* is the minimum concentration of different odorous substances to arouse olfactory sensation.
- Substances having strong odour *mask* the odour of weaker substances. If the odorous substances are of equal strength then the odours of both are perceived.
- One can distinguish between 2,000–4,000 different odours.
- An instrument *'olfactometer'* is used to determine maximum—identifiable—odour (MIO) of a substance.
- Methyl mercaptan can be smelled in least quantity, or it is a substance of low threshold value. So it is usually mixed with the gases so that whenever any gas leakage occurs, it would be identified.
- Centrifugal fibres have been reported. These are the fibres running backwards from olfactory part of cerebral cortex to olfactory bulb. From here inhibitory fibres are running to mitral and tufted cells. These fibres make the olfactory capacity of one individual very sharp to distinguish one odour from other. This is also responsible for adaptation of olfactory receptors.
- There are various olfactory stimulants like pippermentary, ethereal, pungent, putrid etc. etc. Some one may be odour blind for one substance which means lack of appropriate receptor protein in olfactory cell for that substance.

BIBLIOGRAPHY

1. Duck E. The sense of smell and its abnormalities New York, Churchill Livingstone. 1974.
2. Getchell TV. Functional properties of vertebrate olfactory receptor neurones. Phy Rev 1986;66:772.
3. Lat J. Self selection of dietary components. In code CF and Heidel W. (Eds.) Handbook of Physiology, Sec. 6, Vol. I, Balti more, Md. Williams and Wilkins 1967, 367.
4. Moulton DG, et al. Structure and function in peripheral olfactory system. Phy Rev 1967;47:1.

MULTIPLE CHOICE QUESTIONS : SPECIAL SENSES

1. The sweet taste is felt at following part of tongue:
   a. Tip
   b. Sides
   c. Back
   d. Mid dorsal region [ ]
2. Bitterness is felt at following part of tongue:
   a. Tip
   b. Sides
   c. Mid dorsal region
   d. Back of tongue [ ]
3. Aqueous humor is secreted mainly by:
   a. Cornea
   b. Lacrymal gland
   c. Epithelial cells lining ciliary process
   d. Iris [ ]
4. The refractive index of whole lens is:
   a. 1.42
   b. 1.38
   c. 0.5
   d. 2.5 [ ]
5. The lens free eye is called:
   a. Aphakic
   b. Myopic
   c. Presbyopic
   d. Cataract [ ]
6. The dioptric condition of eye in which with accommodation at rest parallel rays are focused mainly in front of retina is:
   a. Hypermetropia
   b. Astigmatism
   c. Anisometropia
   d. Myopia [ ]
7. Structure in retina concerned with bright light vision and colour vision is:
   a. Rods
   b. Bipolar cells
   c. Cones
   d. Horizontal cells [ ]
8. In which of following part of retina visual acuity is maximum:
   a. Region N of ora serrata
   b. Peripheral
   c. Fovea centralis
   d. All of above [ ]

9. The surface area of tympanic membrane is:
   a. 55 sq. mm.
   b. 3.2 sq. mm.
   c. 1.3 sq. mm.
   d. 100 sq. mm. [ ]
10. Primary auditory cortex is:
   a. Brodmann's area 41 in superior portion of temporal lobe
   b. Broca's area
   c. Prefrontal lobe
   d. Limbic lobe [ ]
11. Presence of one sound decreases an individual's ability to hear other sounds; phenomenon is:
   a. Deafness
   b. Nystagmus
   c. Sound localisation
   d. Masking [ ]
12. Range of sound frequencies audible in human being is:
   a. 20–20,000 cycles per second
   b. 50 cycles per second
   c. 1000–4000 Hz. [ ]
13. The pitch of average male voice in conversation is:
   a. 250 Hz
   b. 1000 Hz
   c. 120 Hz
   d. 0 Hz [ ]
14. Refractive index of cornea is:
   a. 1.38
   b. 1.40
   c. 1
   d. 1.33 [ ]

---

1 a **2** d **3** c **4** a **5** a **6** d **7** c **8** c **9** a **10** a **11** d **12** a **13** c **14** a

VIVA VOCE : SPECIAL SENSES

1. Enumerate the functions of tear ?
   i. Moistening and lubrication of eyeball.
   ii. Minimising the unevenness of cornea and thus improving vision.
   iii. Supply O_2 and nutrients to cornea.
   iv. Cleansing and protective action.
   v. Its oily secretion seals the inner margin of moving lids to surface of eyeballs.
2. What is necessary stimulus for smell ?
   i. The substances must be volatile.
   ii. It must be water soluble.
   iii. It must be lipid soluble.
3. Define protanope and deuteranope ?
   i. Protanope means lack of insensibility to red light.
   ii. Colour blind person lacking green cones is deuteranope. Both confuse red with green and so they are called redgreen blind.
4. Enumerate functions of cornea ?
   i. Light transmission.
   ii. Convergence of light.
   iii. Focusing the light on retina, being, a refractory medium.
5. What is Argyll-Robertson pupil ?
   Here loss of light reflex occurs with intact near reflex. It is a bilateral defect commonly seen in neuro-syphilis. They do not give good response to atropine. It suggests a neurological disease. They do not dilate by painful stimuli. The usual site of lesion is in pretectal or tectal area but destruction of small afferent fibres in optic nerve can produce it.
6. What is the function of cones ?
   They are concerned with bright light vision, visual acuity and colour vision.
7. What is the function of rods ?
   They are concerned with dim light vision. No part is taken in colour vision and visual acuity.
8. What is Hemianopia ?
   When loss of vision affects one half of retina of each side, state or condition is Hemianopia.
9. What is field of vision ?
   It is the part of external space that can be seen by one eye when gaze is fixed in one direction. It is subdivided into nasal and temporal field of vision.
10. What is Perimetry?
   It is mapping the visual field and the instrument is called Perimeter. It is used to find out limitations of a peripheral field of vision which is important among aeroplane drivers or pilots respectively.
11. What is accommodation?
   It is defined as adjustment of eye whereby the image of both distant and near objects are accurately focussed on the retina. It depends on state of refraction of eye.
12. Name the instrument used to project light into subject's pupil along the light of observer's eye?
   Ophthalmoscope. Fundus is usually examined and along with its condition of refractive media of eyeball, degree of refractive error as well as its state can be known.
13. What is nystagmus ?
   It is actually a reflex maintaining visual fixation on stationary points while body rotates. It is nothing but characteristic Jerky movement of eye observed at beginning and end of a period of rotation. It is not initiated by visual impulses and present in blinds.
14. How much is the pitch of male and female voice?
   Male: 120 Hz.
   Female: 250 Hz.

QUESTION BANK

1. What is decibel. How much is the loudness level of normal conversation. How is the loudness of different sounds detected by ear.
2. Short notes
   a. Dark and light adaptation (Raj. Univ. First M.B.B.S. 1995)
   b. Organ of Corti (Raj. Univ. 1991, M.D.)
   c. Taste buds (Raj. Univ. 1992, M.D.)
   d. Presbyopia
   e. Accommodation reflex (Raj. Univ. First M.B.B.S. 1995)
   f. Tests of hearing (Raj. Univ. 1986, M.D.)
   g. Binocular vision (Raj. Univ. 1980, M.D.)
   h. Colour blindness (Raj. Univ. 1985, M.D.)
   i. Photo chemistry of vision (Raj. Univ. 1980, M.D.)
   j. Mechanism of hearing
   k. Deafness (Raj. Univ. 1992, M.D.)
   l. Hemianopia (Raj. Univ. 1992, M.D.)
   m. Role of cornea in normal vision (Raj. Univ. 1976, M.D.)
   n. Mechanism of image formation in retina [Raj. Univ. 2000, M.Sc. (Med. I)]
   o. Cochlear microphonic potentials (Raj. Univ. 2000, M.D.)
   p. Electroretinogram (Raj. Univ. 2000, M.D.)
3. Describe
   a. Neural pathway of vision (Raj. Univ. 1995)
   b. Impedance matching device of middle ear (Raj. Univ. 1995)
   c. The mechanism of pitch perception of sound? (Raj. Univ., 1986 M.D.)
   d. Photochemistry of vision (Raj. Univ., 1985 M.D.)
   e. Physiology of accommodation in different animals (Raj. Univ. 1985, M.D.)
   f. Briefly histology of retina and discuss its receptor function with special reference to theories of colour vision (Raj. Univ. 1988, 1990 M.D.)
4. What is visual acuity? Discuss its physiological basis. How will you test it in a patient? (Raj. Univ. 1994, M.D.)
5. Discuss
   a. Physiology of colour vision (Raj. Univ. 1996, M.D.)
   b. Visual pathway with special reference to histology of visual cortex (Raj. Univ. 1996, M.D.)
   c. The mechanism of pitch perception of sound (Raj. Univ. 1980, 1986, M.D.)
   d. The mechanism of vision (Raj. Univ. 1995, M.D.)
6. Give electrophysiology of hearing (Raj. Univ. 1985, M.D.)
7. Give an account of ocular movement and their control. Write a note on strabismus (Raj. Univ. 1986, M.D.)

UNIT 7

Communication and Control

"The hormonal system acts as a mediator between psyche and soma. It is controlling the entire body mechanics in association with central nervous system."

Endocrines

41 Introduction
(Ductless Glands Producing Hormones)

(Endon = within; krino—to separate; hormone = hormao = to arouse, to stimulate)
These glands include a number of diverse tissues and organs which are distributed throughout the body.

STRUCTURAL PECULIARITIES

1. Glands are composed of clumps of secretory cells arranged in columns lining the sinusoids (exception—thyroid and neurohypophysis)
2. No duct found.
3. Profuse blood supply.
4. Structural alteration may occur to pour hormone in blood circulation.
5. Blood vessels supply the gland by forming thin walled sinusoids.

HORMONE

It is a chemical messenger elaborated by endocrine gland, poured directly into blood stream and affect the activities of the selective target cells, at distant places within the body.

MECHANISM OF HORMONE ACTION

- Because of their large molecules they are unable to enter the cells. So they bind themselves with specific receptors present in cell membrane of target cells.
- Bound hormone → changes permeability of cell → ion and substrates pass into the cell.
- Bound hormone trigger off production of second messenger within cell which enhances ion permeability cyclic {adenosine monophosphate (AMP)}.
- Steroids initially bind to a specific high affinity receptor protein in cytosol. The complex is then transported to the nucleus of the cell where it reacts with nuclear chromatin. This combination influences the synthesis of mRNA which directs the synthesis of specific protein enzyme in endoplasmic reticulum; thus acting as a template.
- The enzyme may also be synthesised at ribosome level, i.e. activity is at level of translation of information carried by mRNA on ribosomes.
- The receptor may be present at a membrane level. So it is also possible that initiating hormonal event is activation of a membrane receptor.
- Level of cyclic nucleotides:
  - Cyclic AMP—a nucleotide playing a leading role in hormone synthesis.
  - Glucagon—Cause large increase in cAMP in liver but smaller in muscle.
  - Epinephrine—Cause great increase in cAMP in muscle than in liver.
  - Insulin can decrease hepatic cAMP.
  - There are specific receptor sites in different cell membranes where hormone combines which causes activation of adenylate cyclase.
  - In adipose tissues cAMP may activate lipolysis by stimulating 'protein kinase' which enhances lipase activity.
  - The kinases also phosphorylate other proteins like nucleoprotein.
  - cAMP may affect regulatory systems at chromatin level of transcription and possibly at ribosomal protein level of translation.
- In absence of calcium, the action of protein hormones may be inhibited. Ionised calcium of cytosol is important signal (sources are extracellular fluid, tissue bound calcium mobilisation of intracellular calcium, etc.).

SECOND MESSENGERS

1. cAMP
2. *Calcium ion and calmoduline*: (or Troponin C)

Hormones → increases Ca^{2+} + another protein calmodulin called calcium calmodulin complex → activates various enzymes in the cell. Examples are myosin kinase in smooth muscles, in skeletal muscle calcium ion + troponin C.

3. *IP_3* (Inositol triphosphate)
   Hormone receptor complex → activation of enzymes PIP_2 (phospholipase) → PIP_3 $\xrightarrow{\text{protein kinase C}}$ release of Ca^{2+} into cytoplasm of target cell → physiological actions.
4. cGMP (Cyclic guanosine monophosphate)—Similar with cAMP by acting on protein kinase A.
5. DAG (Diacylglycerol)—It's produced from PIP_2. Rest of mechanism is the same.

LOCATION OF HORMONE RECEPTORS

a. *Cell membrane*: Receptors of catecholamines, protein hormones (pituitary, pancreas, parathyroid, etc.).
b. *Cytoplasm*: Receptors of steroid hormones (of target organs).
c. *Nucleus*: Receptor of thyroid hormone in nucleus of cell.

REGULATION—HORMONE RECEPTORS

- If hormone secreted in excess $\xrightarrow{\text{Down regulation}}$ No. of receptors decrease
- If hormone secreted less $\xrightarrow{\text{Up regulation}}$ No. of receptors increase
- Hormone receptor complex $\xrightarrow{\text{endocytosis internalization}}$ enters the cell

THYROID HORMONE: ACTION

- The thyroid hormones cause increased transcription by certain genes present in nucleus.
- Hormone first bind directly with receptor protein in the nucleus. They activate the genetic mechanism on binding to intranuclear receptor, the thyroid hormone remains active and exert its full effects.

ALDOSTERONE: ACTION

- Enters the cytoplasm of renal tubular cell which contains the receptor protein. This complex is transported into nucleus. This binds at specific point to DNA strands which stimulate the process of transcription to form mRNA. It then diffuses into cytoplasm and at ribosome level new proteins are formed by the process of translation. In this case, proteins which promote sodium reabsorption appear in renal tubular cells after 30-45 minutes. This explains the delay in onset of action of steroid hormones.

HORMONE MECHANISM: AN OVERVIEW

1. All neurotransmitters combine with receptor. This causes a conformational changes in protein structure of receptor. This either opens or closes different ionic movement like Na^+, K^+, Ca^{++}, etc. As an example catecholamines are quoted which are capable of changing membrane potential of smooth muscle cell causing either excitation or inhibition which depends upon type of receptor.
2. ACTH, TSH, LH, FSH, parathormone, glucagon, catecholamine, vasopressin, secretin act via cAMP. The stimulating hormone first binds with specific receptor—on the membrane surface of target cell. The protruding portion of receptor is activated to become adenyl cyclase which causes conversion of cATP to cAMP. This activates a cascade of enzymes, i.e. only a few molecules of activated adenyl cyclase in cell membrane can activate many molecules of next enzyme.
3. Insulin binds with that part of receptor which is protruding. This leads to structural change in receptor molecule. This leads to formation of activated kinase, which then promotes phosphorylation of substances inside the cell.

CRITERION FOR ENDOCRINE GLAND

1. A typical syndrome is induced by its destruction by disease/experimental removal (e.g. castration, tubercular destruction of adrenal glands, removal of thyroid etc.).

Table 41.1: Differences

Hormones	*Enzymes*
1. Produced by endocrine glands.	Produced by duct bearing glands.
2. They may be steroids, modified amino acid, peptides, amines or protein.	Always protein in nature.
3. They are carried by blood.	Carried by ducts. They act at their site of secretion.
4. May be excitatory or inhibitory.	They act as biocatalysts.
5. Consumed during metabolism may influence synthesis, activation or inhibition of some enzymes in their target organs.	Produced in same quantity at end of reaction.

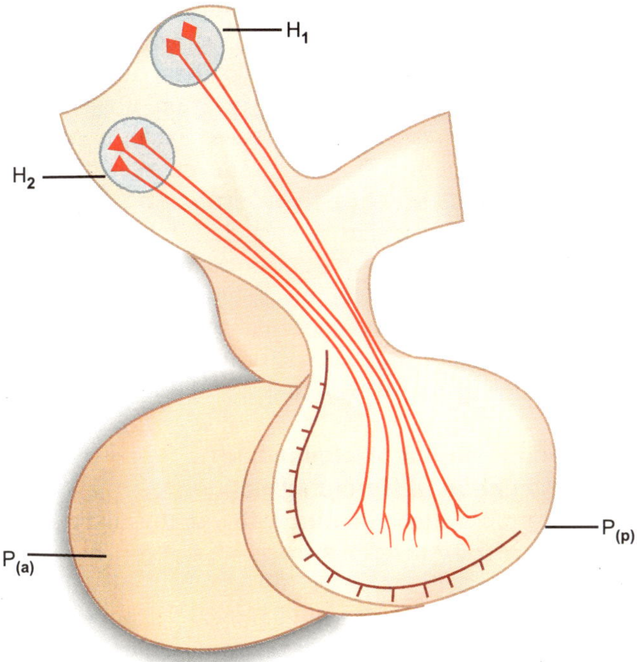

Fig. 41.1: Hypothalamo-hypophyseal-perital vessel-A faithful neuro-endocrine relation (H_1 = Hypothalamus (Paraventricular nucleus) H_2 = Hypothalamus (Supraoptic nucleus) $P_{(p)}$ = Pituitary (posterior), $P_{(a)}$ = Pituitary (anterior)

2. The deficiency state induced by removal or destruction of gland should be repairable by administration of suitable extracts of the gland or by grafting the removed gland into a distant site in the body.
3. Administration of large doses of glandular extract should produce signs of over dosage.

MECHANISM OF HORMONE ACTION: ELABORATION

Some common terms

i. *Paracrines:* At some instances, chemical signal producing cells produce some chemical which diffuses into target cells situated close to the cells which is producing this chemical; e.g. enterochromaffin cells (ECL) secreting histamine which encourages HCI production by oxyntic cells. Insulin hormone also diffuses to stimulate glucagon secretion.

ii. *Autocrines:* Here the producer cell manufacture chemical signal which instead of diffusing stimulate the producer cell itself; e.g. growth substance of cancer cells.

iii. *Eicosanoids:* These are derivative of saturated fatty acid - archidonic acid, and famous types are—prostaglandins and leucotrienes.

iv. *Receptor:* It is a big protein molecule. They are synthesised by cells where they are present. They are naturally degraded and degraded receptors are replaced by newly synthesised receptors. Large number of receptors are regulatory proteins; which are special big sized molecules of protein which have been created for catching the ligand. These regulatory proteins may be cytosolic, or nuclear or membrane bound.

v. *Different types of regulation*
   a. *Down* → no or few receptors are available to bind with fresh molecules of hormones. So addition of fresh doses of hormone at this stage will either produce no effect or a very little effect.
   b. *Up* → opposite of down. All the receptors are free; no ligand is available to bind with receptor. So addition of little amount of hormone will lead to profound action.
   c. *Internalization* → It is a variety of down regulation. It means entire receptor ligand complex enters within the cytoplasm, e.g. insulin.

vi. *G-proteins* → (Internal switch board of body) They are present in the cell membrane between the receptor and catalytic unit. Their participation is necessary in most of the classical protein-peptide-hormones, eicosanoids, and some biogenic amines. It is not required for insulin, epidermal growth factor and insulin-like growth factor (ILGF, EGF).

vii. *Ligand* → It is a chemical substance which can combine with its specific receptor in the target cell to produce RLC (receptor-ligand complex). Hence forth, the hormone or a drug molecule whose chemical structure is closely similar to the hormone, is a ligand.

viii. *Grade A hormones:* Ligands like ACTH, noradrenaline adrenalin LH, FSH, GnRH, TSH, hCG etc. Here catalytic agent is adenyl cyclase and second messenger is cAMP.

ix. *Grade B hormones:* Examples are Angiotensin II, Vasopressin etc. Catalytic unit is Phospholipase C, and second messenger are inositol triphosphate (IP), diacyl glycerol-DAG, and Ca^{++} ions.

x. *Protein Kinase:* The second messenger stimulates the respective protein kinase. This activated protein kinase now acts upon a specific enzyme which leads to biological effects.
   - cAMP is formed from ATP in the cytosol
   - IP3 (inositol-triphosphate) is formed from phospholipid of cell membrane.

- Varieties of protein kinase: (a) Protein kinase A stimulated by second messenger cAMP (b) Protein kinase C stimulated by IP_3, DAG, Ca^{++} (c) MLCK

Receptors: An Overview

A. *Membrane bound receptor*

- The membrane of target cell contains receptor. It has two regions— one for binding with ligand, and other is to identify it whether it is agonist or antagonist.
- If ligand is antagonist then nothing happens, if it is agonist then series of action ensues.

The receptor ligand complex stimulates G protein lying within the cell membrane. This actives G protein which in turn stimulates the catalytic unit for respective hormones, i.e. of grade A and grade B. This stimulated catalytic unit in turn activates/stimulates the production of second messenger (of respective hormones, i.e. grade A and B). This in turn activates the protein kinase which in turn now activates specific enzymes within the cell and this produces biological effects of hormone. It is to be remembered that for the actions of some hormones like insulin, epidermal growth factor (EGF), insulin like growth factor (IGF), the G protein is not required.

B. *Cytosolic receptor*

- A part of these receptor is covered by a protein called HSP (heat shock protein) (Examples are adrenal cortical steroids, androgens, progesteron).
- Cell membrane is easily crossed by steroid hormones which leads to formation of receptor-ligand-complex. This removes HSP (heat shock protein) from receptor so it is now uncovered. This facilitates the movement of receptor ligand complex towards nucleus and it attaches itself on highly specific area of DNA which is made up of genes. This leads to formation of mRNA (from DNA-through process of transcription). This leads to the formation of highly selective variety of protein. All this is called expression of genes.

C. *Nuclear receptors:* Examples are estrogen, thyroxine, tri-iodothyronene. The hormone crosses the cell membrane and reaches to receptor straight. Rest procedure is same as that of cytosol receptors.

D. *Signal transduction.* The hormone-neurotransmitter-autacoid etc. so called chemical signal forms receptor-ligand-complex as received by target cell. This initiates post-receptor-binding events which terminates into biologic effects. All this is called signal transduction.

Hormone Receptor Mechanism in Implementation of Hormonal Action

All neurotransmitters combine with receptors in the post-synaptic membrane. This leads to a conformational change in protein structure of receptor. This leads to altered movement of ions, which means channels open for some ions, while closing for some other ions (e.g. adrenaline and noradrenaline).

Calcium-calmodulin-transducting System

- The hormone first binds with membrane bound receptor.
- This leads to formation of receptor ligand complex.
- This makes G protein activation.
- This facilitates the entry of Ca^{++} from extracellular fluid to intracellular region.
- This causes increase in concentration of free Ca^{++} in cytosol.
- This free Ca^{++} binds with calmodulin in cytosol to form calcium-calmodulin complex.
- This causes the biological action.

42 Master Gland: Pituitary

> Here in this well concealed spot, almost to be covered by a thumb nail, lies the very important structure which controls emotions, reproduction and entire human behaviour. It is one of the smallest of endocrines but the master gland of the body—the pituitary.
>
> —Harvey Cushing

The pituitary consists of anterior lobe (Adeno-hypophysis); and a posterior lobe (Neuro-hypophysis). The adult pituitary gland only weighs between 0.4–0.6 gm; and up to 0.8 gm in women who have been pregnant. Of the total weight 75–80 per cent is adenohypophysis.

The anterior lobe is epithelial in structure, and is derived from Rathkey's pouch—an upgrowth from the pharynx. The posterior lobe of nervous structure, is developed from the floor of the third ventricle, and remains attached to the hypothalamic region of the brain by a stalk or infundibulum, in which a very narrow channel of communication with the ventricle remain open.

The posterior lobe consists of pars nervosa, and a pars intermedia. Former consists of non-medullary nerve fibres, which connect the pituitary with hypothalamus, and a varying amount of nerve cells, and neuroglia; while the later is an epithelial investment of the pars nervosa, derived from Rathke's pouch, and is composed of basophil cells.

Table 42.1: Lobes and parts

Lobes	*Parts*
Anterior	Pars anterior Pars tuberalis
Posterior	Pars intermedia Pars nervosa Median eminence Infundibulum

Table 42.2: Hormones form anterior lobe

- Growth hormone
- Thyroid stimulating hormone (TSH) or thyrotropin
- Adreno-cortico-tropin (ACTH)
- Gonadotropin (FSH, LH, prolactin)
- β-Lipotoropin (β-LPH)
- γ-Melanocyte stimulating hormone (γ-MSH)

HISTOLOGY

Pars anterior consists of columns or masses of epithelioid cells and cells found are :

Eosinophil (acidophil) cells: They are granular alpha cells. They secrete "growth and lactogenic hormone." They are 35 per cent in number.

Basophil (Beta) cells: Their granules take basic stain. 15 per cent in number. They produce TSH, ACTH, FSH, LH.

Chromophobe cells (inactive cells): They don't secrete any hormone. They are called chief or reserve cells. 50 per cent is the number. They are non-granular and not staining.

GROWTH HORMONE

(Somatotropic SH; Somatotropin)

Its molecular weight is 22005. It is a small protein molecule having 191 amino acids.

Actions : Growth

It stimulates the multiplication of the epiphyseal cartilage and thus increases the length of cartilage bones.

It increases muscular, visceral growth. It stimulates growth of thymus and also increases the secretion of milk during lactation.

It does these functions by increasing amino acid uptake and protein synthesis. It also reduces the breakdown of proteins?

Table 42.3: Hormones and growth

Hormone	*Mode of action*
Growth Hormone	a. *Anabolic effect:* Retention of protein. RNA synthesis and protein in liver + peripheral tissues is stimulated. Transfer of amino acid from ECF to interior of cell is promoted. b. *Lipid mobilisation:* Turn over of depot lipids. So initial fall of NEFA followed by increase in liver lipids, ketonaemia and ketonurea. c. *Pancreotropic effect:* Increase blood glucose level. Release of insulin as well as glucagon.
Thyroxine	It potentiates the effect of growth hormone as well as protein synthesis. Brain suffers most in its deficiency. It helps the cell differentiation. It potentiates action of somatomedins.
Insulin	Anabolic effect. Helping amino acid uptake and so protein synthesis. Diabetic animal fails to grow. It causes growth in hypophysectomised animals.
Androgens and oestrogen	Androgens by anabolic effect. Adrenal-androgen secretion + bone growth in females.

Phases of Growth (After Birth)

1. Rapid growth in first year (net weight gain from 8–20 lbs approximately).
2. Slow but progressive growth (from 3–12 years).
3. Accelerated growth during puberty (during 12–15 years).
4. Slow phase may be terminal (after 30 years).

Main Types of Growth

- *Neural:* Immediate growth of brain, spinal cord, eyes, ear. They attain their optimum size.
- *Lymphoid:* Tonsils, thymus, adenoid reach their peak on attaining puberty.
- *Reproductive:* Rapid growth at puberty.

***Carbohydrate Metabolism*:** Decreased use of glucose for energy, enhancement of glycogen deposition in the cells, diminished uptake of glucose by cells, increased insulin secretion along with decreased sensitivity to insulin. So it is said to produce diabetes mellitus—a *diabetogenic hormone*.

***Fat Metabolism*:** Release of fatty acids from adipose tissues so their concentration in body fluid is increased. Fatty acids are also converted to acetyl CoA. In its excessive production, sometimes the quantity is so large to produce keto acids (acetoacetic acid) thus causing ketosis.

***Protein Metabolism*:** It enhances all facets of amino acid uptake and protein synthesis by cells. It also reduces the breakdown of proteins.

***Bones*:** Increased deposition of protein by osteogenic cells which cause bone growth; these cells are produced in great quantity; converts chondrocytes into osteogenic cells.

Growth effects of growth hormone are mediated through somatomedin C. It has got insulin like effects, i.e. it promotes glucose transport across the cell (its molecular weight 4500).

Growth Hormone v/s Somatomedin

- These are small proteins (polypeptides) produced by liver; they have very potent effect on bone growth. In some races, this somatomedin is congenitally absent; which explains the small stature of those persons, in spite of normal concentration of growth hormone in plasma.
- Growth hormone does not act on bones directly but acts through somatomedin which is secreted by liver on stimulation by growth hormone.
- It is of two types:
  a. Somatomedin C (IGF-1-insulin like growth factor)—acts on bones.
  b. Insulin like growth factor II.
- Generally, growth hormone binds with plasma protein loosely so it is released quickly. But somatomedin binds with plasma protein very strongly so they are released slowly from plasma proteins and so its action also lasts for many hours as compared with growth hormone. It acts via cAMP.

READ AND DIGEST: GROWTH HORMONE

Q. How does growth hormone influence protein metabolism?

Ans.

- GH enhances transport of most of amino acids to interior of cell through cell membrane. This increased concentration of amino acid in cell causes protein synthesis (similarity with insulin).
- It excites increased RNA translation which promotes protein synthesis.
  It stimulates transcription of DNA in nucleus; so that more RNA is formed.
- Breakdown of cell protein is also decreased. This is because of the fact that it mobilises large quantity of free fatty acid from adipose tissues; which is used for supplying the energy.

Q. Growth hormone influences carbohydrate metabolism. How?

Ans.

- Glucose utilisation by cell is decreased. It causes increased mobilisation of fatty acids for energy which leads to more formation of acetyl CoA, which inhibits the glycolytic breakdown of glucose.
- Even then, any quantity of glucose which enters the cell, is polymerised into glycogen and accumulates in the cell. This leads to early saturation of cell with glycogen.
- All this leads to pituitary diabetes which is insensitive with insulin. This diabetogenic effect of GH, further stimulates pancreatic islets to produce more insulin. As a result "burning out" of islet cells occur which aids in diabetes mellitus.
- For complete action of growth hormone, carbohydrates as well as adequate availability of insulin is necessary.

Q. What are the mechanism of bone growth?

Ans.

- Long bones grow in length at the point where epiphysis is separated from shaft. The shaft becomes elongated because of growth of new cartilage which changes into new bone. This further separates shaft with epiphysis.
- Osteoblasts cause deposition of new bone on the surface of old; while osteoclasts remove old bone. When construction (i.e. deposition) is greater than destruction (i.e. resorption), then bone increases in thickness. GH stimulates osteoblasts, i.e. construction.

Q. It enhances fat utilisation. How?

Ans.

- It causes release of fatty acids from adipose tissues; so their concentration in body fluids is increased. They are then converted into acetyl CoA. This effect is sometimes so great that accumulation of acetoacetic acid takes place which leads to ketosis — a fatal state.

REGULATION

Its normal concentration in blood plasma is 1.5–3 ng/ml. It is chiefly regulated by nutritional status/stress of body, e.g. hypoglycaemia or low concentration of fatty acids, exercise, excitement, trauma, etc. In chronic conditions; its secretion correlate more with degree of cellular protein depletion than with the degree of glucose insufficiency.

- The secretion of growth hormone is decreased in REM sleep. Glucose, cortisol, FFA, growth hormone itself are other stimuli which decrease its secretion (negative feedback mechanism).
- Hypoglycaemia, exercise, protein meal, glucagon, stress oestrogen/androgens are some of the stimuli which increase its secretion.
- It is controlled by hypothalamus. GRH (growth hormone releasing hormone) as well as growth hormone inhibiting hormone (somatostatin) have been reported to be secreted from hypothalamus. The secretion of somatostatin is more tonic while of GRH is episodic.
- Under the hypothalamic effect, anterior pituitary produces growth hormone—which causes an increase in IGF-I (insulin like growth factor-somatomedin); which in turn exerts a direct inhibitory action on secretion of growth hormone from anterior pituitary. It also stimulates somatostatin secretion. Hypothalamic lesion or section of pituitary stalk inhibits growth hormone secretion.

	IGF-I	IGF-II
1.	70 amino acid	67 amino acid
2.	Liver and other tissues are its source	Diverse tissues are source
3.	Plasma binding protein	Plasma binding protein
4.	Skeletal + cartilage growth	Growth during foetal development

ACTH—AT A GLANCE

- It is a straight chain polypeptide containing 39 amino acids with a molecular weight 4,500.
- Its main actions include:
  - — Synthesis and release of cortico steroids from adrenal gland.
  - — Enhances synthesis of steroids from cholesterol.
  - — Mild stimulation in dispersing melanin granules on skin.
  - — It can cause lipolysis and stimulate insulin secretion from pancreas through cAMP.
  - — Its administration leads to retention of Na, Cl, H_2O, hyperglycaemia, increase in level of circulating free fatty acids, increased excretion of uric acid, decrease in eosinophil and lymphocytes.
- It is controlled by CRH from hypothalamus. High levels of ACTH inhibits further synthesis of ACTH.

TSH—AT A GLANCE

- It is a glycoprotein of molecular weight 30,000. Two polypeptide chains TSH a and TSH b. It is very rich in sulphur containing amino acid consisting of 11 disulphide residues and contains fucose, mannose, galactose, glucosamine and galactosamine.
- Functions:
  - — It increases the release of thyroxin from thyroid gland into circulation.
  - — It binds to specific membrane receptors, thus activating thyroidal adenylate cyclase causing increased cellular cAMP and increases the rate of removal of inorganic iodide from blood by thyroid and incorporation of iodide in thyroid hormone.

- cAMP acts as a second messenger and activate protein kinase which causes phosphorylation which results into immediate increase in secretion of thyroid hormones along with prolonged growth of thyroid tissue.
- Controlled by TRH from hypothalamus whose release is dependent on calcium ions and the process is non-ribosomal.

PANHYPOPITUITARISM

(Decreased secretion of all pituitary hormones)

Dwarfism

- Rate of development is greatly decreased. A child of 10 years appears as 4–5 years. He does not pass through puberty; never secreting sufficient quantity of gonadotropic hormones to develop adult sexual functions.
- In adults the effects are : hypothyroidism, decreased secretion of glucocorticoids by adrenals, decreased secretion of gonadotropins. So the patient is a lethargic person - gaining weight.
- *Lorain Levy type* (Infantilism): Stunted but proportionate growth, due to arrest of skeletal growth, intelligence is normal and proportionate to age, underdeveloped gonads and sexual secondary characters do not develop, adiposity is seen, low BMR, intractable polyurea.
- *Brissaud type*: Excessive fatty deposition, clubby face, lack of initiative and dynamicity, low intelligence.
- *Mixed type*: Both types of features seen.
- *Short features*: Due to gonadal dysgenesis having XO chromosomal pattern, instead of XX or XY pattern.
- *Sexual ateliotic dwarf*: Sexually mature but is a dwarf.
- *Laron type*: Dwarfism because of deficiency of somatomedins; otherwise growth hormone level is normal or tissue fails to respond to circulatory somatomedin, e.g. African pygmies.
- *Acromicria*: Due to hypofunctions of eosinophil cells. Is characterised by emaciation, retarded development of bone, hand, feet and face, loss of hair and sexual functions.

Simmond's disease: It is due to atrophy of anterior lobe, together with extreme depression of adrenal cortical activity along with its target sites like thyroid and gonads. It is characterised by some general symptoms like loss of axillary and pubic hair, dry and wrinkled face, smallness of hands and feet; anaemia, atrophy of gonads, hypoglycaemia and low metabolic rate (due to associated thyroid hypofunctioning), mental deterioration, amenorrhoea or impotence, adrenal insufficiency, diminished urinary excretion of gonadotropins.

Sheehan's syndrome: Sheehan described milder variety of above symptoms of Simmond's disease after child birth; which is characterised by haemorrhage along with peripheral circulatory failure. According to him hypothalamo-hypophyseal portal vessels are being obstructed. All this is known after him.

Fröhlich's syndrome: It is also known as "dystrophia-adiposo genitalis" and of prepubertal or infantile variety occurring as a result of inherent defect of pituitary. It is characterised by striking features combined with dwarfism and obesity. Subjects are lethargic or somnolent and are of subnormal intelligence. They are craving for sweets having voracious appetite usually called "fat boy." Children become idiotic and stupid. In Fröhlich's syndrome of adult type there is excess deposition of fat in males occurring in such a way that it is having feminine distribution. Skin of face and body is smooth, soft and without hair and hips are broad. Extreme obesity is seen in females. Degeneration of sex is there. The picture is reverse as that of acromegaly, i.e., small pretty hands and feet slender and tapering finger tips with narrow pointed terminal phalanges, subnormal BMR with increased sugar tolerance, diabetes insipidus is common.

HYPERPITUITARISM

Giantism or Gigantism

- Hyperpituitarism depend on the age of the patient at which hormonal hyperfunction becomes apparent. In early age the result is giantism while at a later date, the result is acromegaly, and it depends on whether ossification has been completed or not.
- So before completion of ossification (epiphysis of bone has not fused with shaft); the growth in length is favoured so person looks like a giant. It is always due to pituitary hyperplasia. A definite tumour is usually present with enlargement of sella turcica, but in milder forms there may be merely hyperplasia of the anterior lobe.
- Associated with skeletal overgrowth there may be later development of symptoms of pituitary insufficiency, specially impotence in men, and amenorrhoea in women. The pituitary activity may inhibit the action of insulin so that glycosurea develops and it is common for giants to die with symptoms of diabetes.
- The skeletal overgrowth is caused by hyperplasia of the eosinophil cells of the anterior lobe, while subsequent sexual insufficiency is due to pressure on the cells of that lobe which are concerned with sexual stimulation.

Acromegaly: It is a result of hyperpituitarism after completion of ossification. Great enlargement of hands and feet (akors = extremity; megaly = enlargement), large face with prominent frontal sinuses, forward protrusion of lower jaw, excess development of supraorbital ridges causing forward slanting of forehead, nose increases as much as twice of its size, foot needs a shoe of large size. Kyphoses may be marked, huge hands reaching to knees. Patient with his bent back, "gorilla like" picture is attained due to protruding lower jaw, skin becomes coarse thick and furrowed which is more marked in scalp which is corrugated like "Bull dog" thick coarse hair, profuse sweating, increased sexual excitement.

MIDDLE LOBE OF PITUITARY

- It produces MSH (melanocyte-stimulating hormone).
- α MSH is smaller containing 13 amino acids and is identical to the first 13 amino acids of ACTH. It has some corticotropic activity.
- Functions : It increases deposition of melanin by the melanocytes of skin.
- Its action is inhibited by cortisone, hydrocortisone, epinephrine and norepinephrine.
- β and γ MSH have also been reported.

HOUSSAY DOG/ANIMAL

- Anterior pituitary gland is related to carbohydrate metabolism.
- Houssay made dogs diabetic by doing pancreatectomy. Those dogs when subjected to hypophysectomy (removal of pituitary), showed amelioration of the diabetes. Such a preparation called Houssay dog after him and they lived for a longer period without insulin.
- Young (1937, 53) showed that administration of anterior pituitary extract to adult dogs and cats for a period of several weeks might result in a permanent state of diabetes mellitus. Severe damage to permanent islet cells was found.

POSTERIOR PITUITARY (Neurohypophysis)

- It is composed of pituicytes (glial like cells) - they don't secrete any hormone but act as a supporting structure. Two hormones - ADH (antidiuretic hormone vasopressin) and oxytocin.

Antidiuretic Hormone (ADH)

- It is formed primarily in supraoptic nuclei of hypothalamus and then transported to posterior pituitary. It is chemically a polypeptide.
- In its presence, permeability of collecting ducts and tubules to water increases very much so water is conserved in the body.
- It is a cyclic polypeptide having 8 amino acids : structures here isoleucine replaced by phenylalanine and leucine replaced by lysin - (distinction from oxytocin).
- Alcohol inhibits its secretion.
- It is having molecular weight of 1000.
- It also stimulates the contraction of gallbladder, intestine and urinary bladder.
- ***Regulation***: It is regulated osmotically. On administration of concentrated electrolyte solution; more ADH is secreted; while its secretion is reduced or inhibited on administration of dilute solution.
- Decreased blood volume leads to increased production of this hormone.

Osmotic regulation: Modified neurone receptors are present in or near hypothalamus called osmoreceptors. Now when extracellular fluid becomes concentrated, fluid is pulled by osmosis out of these osmoreceptors, which is a signal to release ADH. Reverse is true when extracellular fluid becomes dilute.

Feedback control: Body fluids concentrated → hypothalamus produces ADH → kidney → permeability of tubules increased → most of the water is reabsorbed from tubular fluid → so electrolytes are continuously lost in urine → extracellular fluid is diluted or normal osmotic composition.

- Their higher concentration is having very potent effect of constricting the arterioles everywhere in the body and so increase the blood pressure. So the name vasopressin has been given.
- In its deficiency, water and electrolytes are not reabsorbed so they are excreting in plenty giving rise to a state *diabetes insipidus* in which urine volume is increased and patient may develop dehydration.

Diabetes insipidus: The disease occur when ADH secretion is inhibited. The urine is not concentrated; specific gravity remains constant (1.002, 1.006) the urine output may go as high as from 4–6 litres daily to 12–15 litres daily; this creates a constant thirst. Patient may be dehydrated. So the disease can be treated by insufflating powdered posterior pituitary extract into nose (0.1 microgram only).

It may be due to tumour of hypothalamus or pituitary, or injury to hypophyseal stalk.

The other actions of ADH includes: contraction of smooth muscle of body (intestinal, bile duct, uterus). Both ADH and oxytocin are adsorbed to a carrier protein whose molecular weight is 30,000.

Oxytocin Hormone

- It stimulates the pregnant uterus towards the end of gestation.
- It is also playing a leading role in the process of lactation. It causes milk to be expressed from alveoli into ducts which can be obtained by baby through suckling mechanism. It causes contraction of myo-epithelial cells (Let down reflex).

FORMATION AND FATE OF NEUROHYPOPHYSEAL HORMONES

For a long time, it was believed that the cells of pars intermedia migrated posteriorly into neurohypophysis and liberated posterior pituitary hormones. It is now suggested that certain specialised cells (pituicytes of Bucy, or parenchymatous glandulnar cells of Gersh) secrete these hormones. Hypothalamo-neuro-hypophyseal unit act as a neurosecretory mechanism.

These are secreted as polypeptides and become linked to plasma proteins. Major part of inactivation occurs in liver and kidney and excreted in urine.

Control of neural lobe : Its functional activity is entirely dependent on its nerve supply from hypothalamus. The innervation is constituted by 100,000 unmyelinated fibres arising from supraoptic and paraventricular hypothalamic nuclei. These fibres converge to the pituitary stalk and end in all three parts of neurohypophysis—the median eminence, the infundibular stem and infundibular process.

The basis of belief are: A lesion placed in supra-optico-hypophyseal tract in the hypothalamus results in loss of posterior pituitary functions, atrophy of all three parts of gland, loss of extractable activity from the gland, disappearance of neurones from supra-optic and paraventricular nuclei. Electrical stimulation of supra-optico-hypophyseal tract results in rapid discharge of posterior pituitary hormones as milk ejection, antidiuresis, increase in intestinal peristalsis, increased uterine activity, and slight increase in blood pressure.

FUNCTIONS OF POSTERIOR LOBE (NEURAL LOBE)

a. ***Anti-diuretic action*:** Very small doses of posterior pituitary extract (or purified vasopressin) are effective in inhibiting a water diuresis. Emotional stress produced in variety of ways is found to be associated with antidiuresis, (Verney, 1947).

b. ***Pressor action*:** Larger doses of vasopressin are required to elicit a pressor than an antidiuretic response. Electrical stimulation of supra-optico-hypophysial tract in conscious animal excites a slight increase in blood pressure of the same type as that of following injection of vasopressin.

c. ***Intestinal peristalsis*:** As told by Cushing, "A patient with tumours that have destroyed neurohypophysis ... are notably victimised by chronic constipation." But at the same time it is also true that large doses of vasopressin are required to elicit an observable increase in intestinal peristalsis.

d. ***Hyperglycemic action*:** Both posterior pituitary hormones lead to hyperglycaemia. In rabbits vasopressin has greater effect while in dogs, oxytocin is more effective. It is unlikely that posterior pituitary plays a physiological role in regulating the blood sugar.

e. ***Oxytocin on uterus*:** Elaboration and discharge of a principle by pituitary constitutes an important factor in the birth mechanism. It forms part of mechanism controlling uterine activity during normal labor. The ascent of sperms in the genital tract, increase in uterine activity following mating or mechanical stimulation of genitalia or uterine cervix, etc., are all mediated by oxytocin release.

f. ***Milk ejecting action*:** It is well known that stress may inhibit the flow of milk and this inhibition may, however, be overcome by injection of oxytocin. It is of interest that after a single injection of oxytocin, lactation proceed normally without the need of further injection in majority of cases.

BIBLIOGRAPHY

1. Boumann G. Growth hormone binding proteins. Proc Soc Exp Biol Med 1993;202:392.
2. Houssay BA. New Eng J Med 1936; 214.
3. Houssay BA. Endocrinol 1942;30:884.
4. Houssay BA, et al. Endocrin 1931;15:511.
5. Houssay BA, et al. JH Phy 1932;77:81.
6. Hughes JP, et al. The nature and regulation of the receptors for pituitary growth hormones. Ann Rev Phy 1985;47:469.
7. Isaksson, OGP, et al. Mode of action of pituitary growth hormone on target cells. Ann Rev Phy 1985;47:483.
8. Kelly PA, et al. The prolactin/growth hormone receptor family. End Rev 1991.
9. Klabiniski A, et al. Diagnosis and treatment of hormone secreting pituitary adenomas. New Eng J Med 1991;324:822.
10. Kolata G. New growth industry in human growth hormone. Science 1986;234:22.
11. Melned S. Acromegaly. New Eng J Med 1990; 322:966.
12. Menninger RP. Current concepts of volume regulation of vasopressin release. Fed Proc 1985;4:55.
13. Muller EE. Neural control of somatotropic function. Phy Rev 1987;67:962.
14. Sklar AH, et al. Central nervous system mediators of vasopressin release. Phy Rev 1983;63:1243.
15. Vance ML. Hypopituitarism. New Eng J Med 1994;330:1651.
16. Young FG. Rec Prog Horm Res 1953;8:471.

43 Iodine Homeostasis: Thyroid

The thyroid gland is one of the most labile organs in the body. It maintains metabolism by means of its iodine containing hormone—the thyroxin.

This gland is situated at the root of the throat, having two lobes, one on either side of trachea, joined by thin tissue called "isthmus." Its weight is 20–25 gm, and is a highly vascular gland, (3.5–6 ml/gm/minute is blood flow).

HISTOLOGY (MICROSCOPICAL STRUCTURE)

- It is found to consist of follicles lined by low/tall cuboidal epithelium;
- The follicles are 15–150 µm in diameter having spherical or oval shape;
- The follicles are filled with a protein material consists of thyroglobulin which constitutes 75 per cent of soluble proteins and is the main storage form of thyroid hormone;
- The follicles are surrounded by vascular stroma which also contain lymphatics;
- The border of the thyroid epithelial cell is having microvilli;
- Within the cell; cytoplasmic vesicles are seen. They have absorbed the colloid from follicles through a process of pinocytosis. Vesicles are filled up with a colloid material secreted by epithelium;
- In between follicular cells "para follicular cells" are found (rich in mitochondria) which synthesise hormone called "*thyrocalcitonin*" which reduces calcium level of blood,
- This gland produces three hormones—*thyroxin, triiodothyronine and calcitonin.*

Thyroid cartilage of larynx is also called Adam's apple.

FUNCTIONS OF THYROID GLAND (THYROXINE)

Metabolism

- General BMR is increased so it is a calorigenic hormone. It stimulates O_2 consumption of all tissues except brain, spleen, testis.
- In O_2 consumption; great role is played by mitochondria. In hypothyroidism O_2 consumption of mitochondria of cell is decreased while it is increased in hyperthyroid states.
- ***Carbohydrate***: Absorption of monosaccharides by intestine is stimulated. It stimulates glycogenolysis and thus produces hyperglycaemia. It reduces sugar tolerance. Insulin breakdown is also enhanced.
- ***Protein***: In its small doses protein synthesis is stimulated while in large doses; breakdown of proteins takes place. Excessive protein breakdown elevates nitrogen elimination which may lead to wasting of tissues.
- ***Fat***: In hypothyroid states blood cholesterol level is raised. Lipids are mobilised from their stores so their level is increased in blood. Thyroid hormone accelerates oxidation of free fatty acids by β oxidation.
- Thyroid hormone causes increased need for vitamin. So little vitamin deficiency may occur on excess secretion of thyroid hormone.
- Increased amount of thyroid hormone decreases the body weight and decreased production of thyroid hormone increases body weight.
- Thyroid hormone directly excites the heart which in turn increases heart rate. This may increase the strength of the heart. But when quantity of thyroid hormone is markedly increased → increased protein catabolism → decreased strength of heart muscle.

THYROID AND THE HEART

- These hormones increase the number and affinity of β-adrenergic receptors in heart and thus increases its sensitivity to ionotropic and chronotropic effects of catecholamines.
- Heart has got two MHC (myosin heavy chains) isoforms-α-and β-MHC. They are encoded by two homologous genes located on short arm of chromosomes 17. β MHC is having less ATP-ase activity than αMHC. αMHC are predominating in adult-ventricle and their level is increased by administering thyroid hormones.

- In hypothyroidism, expression of α MHC gene is depressed and, β MHC is enhanced.

- Thyroxin → vasodilatation → increased blood volume.
- Thyroxin → increased metabolism → more utilisation of O_2 and formation of CO_2 → increased rate and depth of respiration.
- Thyroid hormones → increased motility and rate of secretion of digestive juices → increased appetite and diarrhoea.

THYROID: CELLULAR METABOLISM

1. On its administration, number and activity of mitochondria is increased. This results into formation of ATP which supplies energy to cell, for its proper functioning.
2. But on its extreme high doses, mitochondria actually swell → uncoupling of oxidative phosphorylation → more production of heat + less production of ATP.
3. Activity of enzyme Na-K-ATP-ase is increased. So metabolic rate of body is increased; because of more heat production by this enzyme. Under the effect of thyroid hormones, the cellular membrane becomes leaky to sodium ions which activate the sodium pump which further increases heat production.

- Excess thyroid hormones → increased protein catabolism → muscle becomes weak.
- Excess thyroid hormone → increased reactivity of the neuronal synapses in the cord areas which control muscle tone → tremors (fine muscular 10-15/sec different from tremor of Parkinson's diseases).

THYROID AND TISSUE

1. It causes nuclear transcription of large number of genes.
2. Before doing this, all thyroxine is de-iodinated by one iodine ion, forming T_3 which has got a high affinity to cellular thyroid hormone receptors.
3. Any way on binding with receptor, transcription process is initiated. It leads to formation of large number of mRNA and it forms new proteins.

- Thyroid hormone → exhausting effect on CNS and muscles → feeling of constant tiredness and inability to sleep in patient of hyperthyroidism.

THYROID V/S NERVOUS SYSTEM

- Its large doses leads to rapid mentation, irritability and restlessness.
- In adult brain, thyroid hormone enters and so found in grey matter.
- They exert a marked effect on brain's development. In hypothyroid infants there occurs abnormal development of synapses, defective myelination and retarded mental development.

- Lack of thyroid hormone → menorrhagia → complete loss of libido
- Great excess of thyroid hormone → impotency.
- Excess thyroxin → increased stroke volume → increased pulse pressure → increased blood flow through tissue between heart beats (systolic increased, diastolic decreased).

CHOLESTEROL METABOLISM V/S THYROID

- It lowers cholesterol level.
- It is independent of stimulation of O_2 consumption.
- It is due to increased formation of LDL receptors in the liver which causes increased removal of circulating cholesterols.

SYNTHESIS

- Iodine is one of the necessities of life, for without iodine the thyroid hormone cannot be built and without that hormone, normal life is impossible although, one may still survive. Iodine, of course, does not exist in free form either in the blood or in the tissues.
- Iodine metabolism has been described as a grand cycle in which iodine in the form of iodide ions is extracted from the blood by thyroid, converted into thyroxin and possibly other hormones, discharged as such into the blood, and carried to every cell in the body, where it exerts a profound effect on metabolic and enzymatic activities.
- Iodide consumed in food and water are absorbed and carried to the iodide pool in the extracellular fluid.
- The first stage is the accumulation of inorganic iodide from the blood, in which it is present at very low concentration of about 0.24 μg/100 ml plasma in man. This accumulation is an active transport process, occurring against concentration gradient, is energy dependent, and competitive inhibition occurs by other anions like perchlorate and thiocyanate. Thiocyanate was used once upon a time in treatment of hypertension and it was then proved that it is goitrogenic compound. It is found in plants of the cabbage family and is formed by the breakdown of inactive mustard oil glycoside precursor.
- Iodine is found in the blood in two forms:
  i. Inorganic iodide, and
  ii. Organic or protein bound iodine (PBI)—its level is a reliable index of thyroid secretory activity (normal level—4-8 μg %).
- The salivary glands as well as thyroid seem to be concerned with the iodine cycle. These glands concentrate iodide ions into the saliva, the concentration

being 30 times that of plasma. The salivary glands are responsible, at least in part, for the degrading of thyroxine in the body and the recycling of the iodine to the thyroid as iodide ion. The saliva test for radio iodine secreted by the glands is of marked diagnostic value in thyroid disease.

- Iodides ingested orally are absorbed by GIT and 1/5th of their amount used by thyroid gland.
- The basal membrane of thyroid cell has ability to pump the iodide actively to the interior of the cell so-called iodide trapping.
- Endoplasmic reticulum and Golgi apparatus synthesise and secrete glycoprotein molecule called thyroglobulin into the follicles.
- The major substrates are tyrosine amino acid which combines with iodine to form thyroid hormones.
- These hormones are formed within the thyroglobulin molecules.
- The first essential step in formation of thyroid hormone is conversion of iodide into oxidized form of iodine and this oxidation is promoted by enzyme peroxidase and its accompanying hydrogen peroxide. When this enzyme is blocked or it is genetically absent, formation of thyroid hormone falls to low level.
- Oxidized iodine will bind directly with amino acid tyrosine. Iodinase enzyme activates or accelerates this action. Tyrosine is first iodized to MIT and then to DIT. Then more DIT are coupled with each other to form thyroxine.
- 1 mol. MIT + 1 mol. DIT → Tri-iodo-thyronine (MIT = mono-iodo-thyrosine; DIT = di-iodo-thyrosine)
- Each thyroglobulin molecule contains thyroxine (1-3 molecules). The ratio between tri-iodo-thyronine and thryoxine is 1:10—(for every one molecule of tri-iodo-thyronine there are ten molecules of thyroxine). In this form thyroid hormones are stored in follicles.
- The thyroxine and tri-iodo-thyronine are first cleaved from the thyroglobulin-molecule and then these hormones are released. About 90 per cent of released material is thyroxine and rest is tri-iodo-thyronine.
- After releasing in the blood, it combines with:
  - globulin to form TBG (thyroid binding globulin) normal value 1-1.5 mg/dl.
  - Thyroxine binding pre-albumin and albumin.
- As these hormones come in contact with their target tissue, most of thyroxine is de-iodinated to form additional tri-iodo-thyronine. So its amount is increased - (35 µg/day + 35 µg/day by this reverse T_3).
- A latent period of 2-3 days has been reported with thyroid injection. Then its activity is increased, reaching at peak level in 10-12 days and then decreases. Tri-iodo-thyronine (T_3) acts more rapidly than thyroxine (T_4) (latent period 6–12 hours).

DIFFERENCES BETWEEN T_4 AND T_3

	T_4	T_3
1. Total serum level	8 µgm%	0.15 µgm%
2. Secretion into plasma	80 µg/day	8 µg/day
3. Binding	99.9% binds to TBG, very small amount to TBPA and albumin	Mainly bound to TBG and albumin, little to TBPA
4. Action	Onset is slow but duration is long	Rapid onset of action. More potent and more active
5. Others	• Extracellular hormone • Stable precursor of T_3 since it is converted to T_3	Penetrates tissue fluid rapidly so is an intracellular hormone

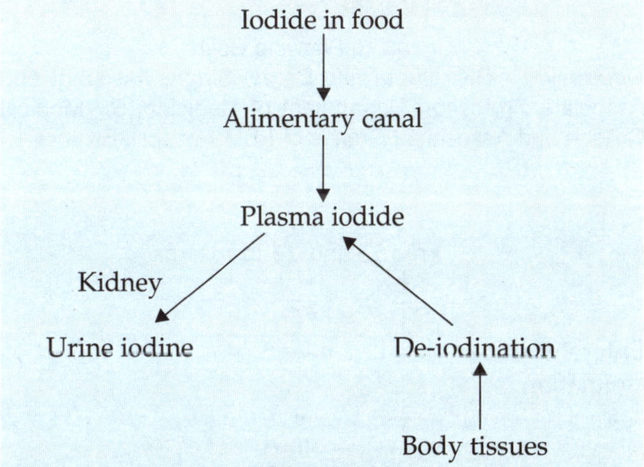

Diagram I

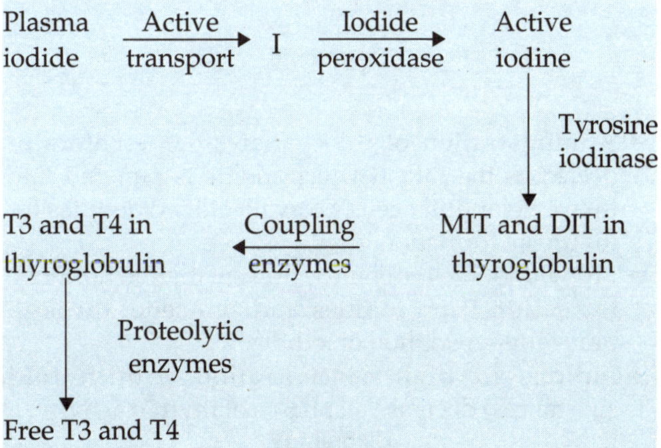

Diagram II

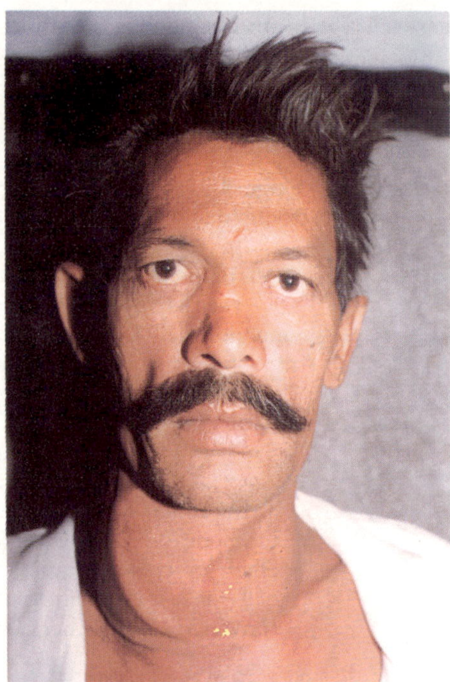

Fig. 43.1: Showing Goitre
Courtesy: Dr BK. Gupta and Dr VB Singh, Assistant and Associate Professor, Department of Medicine, SP Medical College and Associated Groups of PBM Hospital, Bikaner

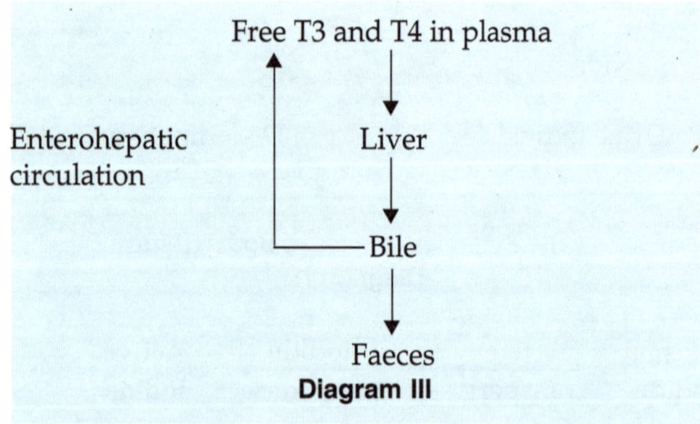

Diagram III

- Administration of thiocyanates or perchlorates decreases the rate at which iodide is pumped into thyroid glandular cells. So availability of iodides for thyroxine formation is reduced.
- Propylthiouracil/thioureas prevent thyroid hormone formation from iodides and tyrosene, through preventing oxidation of iodides.
- Iodides in high concentration (Antithyroid substances) decrease all phases of thyroid activity.

Diagram IV

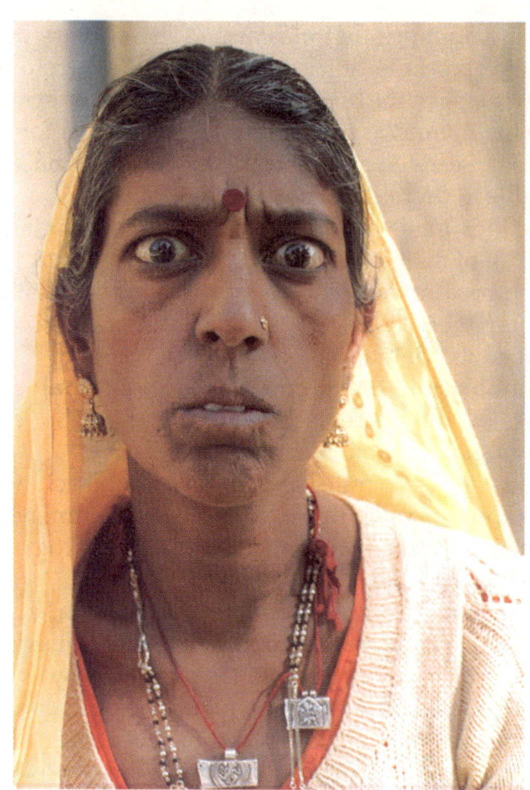

Fig. 43.2: Showing exophthalmos
Courtesy: Dr BK. Gupta and Dr VB Singh, Assistant and Associate Professor, Department of Medicine, SP Medical College and Associated Groups of PBM Hospital, Bikaner

HYPERTHYROIDISM (GRAVES' DISEASE, EXOPHTHALMIC GOITRE)

- Clinically, it is marked by classical triad of—hyperthyroidism because of excess production of thyroid hormone; exophthalmos (protrusion of eye balls) and goitre. Pathologically it is diffuse hyperplastic enlargement of the thyroid.
- It is an example of an entire organ starting and continuing to hyperfunction without any regard to the needs of the body. It bears no apparent relation to iodine deficiency. There is often a very definite history of nervous or psychic shock, not infrequently sexual in character. It is much commoner in women than in men in the proportion of 5 to 1. It usually begins in early adult life and onset is often sudden and acute.
- The four cardinal signs are: enlargement of thyroid gland, exophthalmos, tachycardia and tremors.
- Exophthalmos is a major problem in Graves' disease. It consists of—lid lag—the inability of upper lid to follow the movement of lid together with retraction

of the upper lid, giving the eyes a staring appearance; and proptosis.

- The eye displacement is due to oedema of the orbit, which may be so marked as to produce an extreme degree of proptosis. There is a deposition of mucopolysaccharides rich in hyaluronic acid in fat tissues of the orbit. It is due to EPS (exophthalmos - producing substance).

HYPERTHYROID CRISIS

- Increased severity of hyperthyroid symptoms.
- Thyrotoxic crisis is most commonly because of infection and previously untreated or undertreated hyperthyroidism.
- It may also develop after subtotal thyroidectomy, or, within a few days of ^{131}I therapy when acute irradiation damage may lead to transient rise in serum thyroid hormone levels.
- Patient should be treated with broad spectrum antibiotic and rehydration therapy.

HYPERTHYROIDISM: IODINE INDUCED

- On administration of iodine, hyperthyroidism may result.
- It may be administered as - antiarrhythmic agent, radiographic contrast media, prophylactic iodination programme, etc.
- The disease is mild and self-limiting.

- *Diagnostic tests (Hyperthyroidism)*: Increased basal metabolic rate, decreased plasma TSH level because of negative feedback mechanism, (it is measured by radio-immuno-assay).
- *Treatment:*
  — Consists of surgical removal of gland.
  — Administration of high concentration of iodides and thiouracils.

HYPERTHYROIDISM: CLINICAL FEATURES

A. *Cardiorespiratory:* Tachycardia, palpitation, increased pulse pressure, dyspnoea on exertion, exacerbation of asthma, angina, ankle oedema.
B. Neuromuscular: Nervousness, irritability, tremor, muscle weakness.
C. Ocular: Lid lag, lid retraction, exophthalmos, corneal ulcer, diplopia, papilloedema, ophthalmoplegia, loss of visual acuity.
D. Goitre: Diffuse/nodular
E. General: Fatigue, thirst, anorexia, nausea vomiting, amenorrhoea, loss of libido, apathy, heat intolerance.

Thyroid Storm

- Causes a fulminating increase in sign and symptom of thyrotoxicosis. In past years it was a postoperative complication, but nowadays medical storm is common because of various drugs available with us. The syndrome is characterised by extreme irritability, delirium or coma, fever (41°C + or more), tachycardia, restlessness, vomiting, diarrhoea, hypotension, etc. The condition may be worst by super added symptoms like apathy, coma. Postoperative complications may be there like sepsis, haemorrhage, etc.
- It does not appear to be an acute increase in severity of thyroid hyperfunction.
- *Treatment basis:* Put patient in cool and humidified O_2 tent, cooling blanket if hyperpyrexia, digitalisation to check fibrillation. If shock—I.V. pressor agents, large doses of antithyroid agent (100 mg propyl thiouracil every 2 hour), beta adrenergic blocking agents (propranolol), regular ECG monitoring, large doses of dexamethasone.

GOITRE

- This is an indefinite term applied to enlargement of thyroid gland. This may be an evidence of: (i) primary hyperplasia, (ii) compensatory hyperplasia to meet the increased demand of tissues for hormones, (iii) increased storage of colloid.
- *Types:* (i) Diffuse colloid goitre, (ii) Exophthalmic goitre (Graves' disease), (iii) nodular or adenomatous goitre. The macrofollicles respond to iodine therapy indicating that they are related to iodine deficiency.
- *Diffuse colloid goitre:* (simple, endemic, adolescent goitre) Most physiological form of thyroid disease since is an example of compensatory hypertrophy. The main cause is the deficiency of iodine. It is much more commoner in women than in men; in girls at time of puberty. This enlargement is also seen at the time of pregnancy and lactation.
- *Nodular goitre:* As the time passes goitre tends to become nodular, sometimes new tissues are formed called adenoma. The ^{131}I is a reliable index of the rate of secretory activity of uptake by thyroid gland.
- *Hashimoto's disease (Lymphodenoid goitre):* Common in women at the time of menopause. Thyroid is enlarged, moderately firm, with prominent hypothyroidism. Lymphoid tissues are abundant.
- Graves' disease is an autoimmune disease in which antigen activates T lymphocytes which stimulate B lymphocyte to produce circulating antibodies against antigen. In Hashimoto's disease, antibodies damage thyroid cells.
- Other antibodies are formed against components of TSH receptors. These are TSI (Thyroid-stimulating immunoglobulins)—which activate the receptors producing hyperthyroidism.

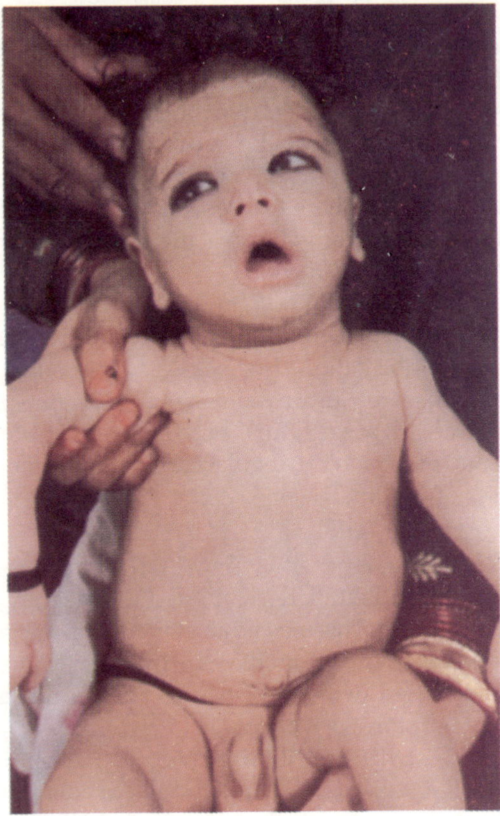

Fig. 43.3: Cretinism
Courtesy: Dr PC Khatri, Associate Professor, Department of Paediatrics, SP Medical College and Associated Groups of PBM Hospital, Bikaner

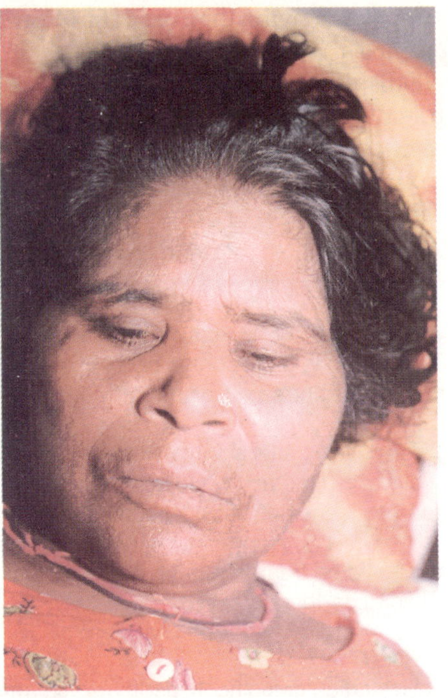

A

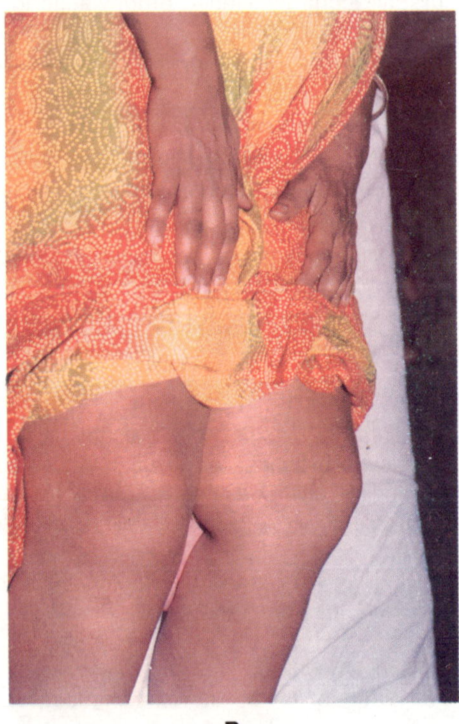

B

Figs. 43.4A and B: Hypothyroidism with polyarthritis
Courtesy: Dr LA Gauri, Associate Professor, Department of Medicine, SP Medical College and Associated Groups of PBM Hospital, Bikaner

Cabbage and turnips contain progoitrin and a substance which converts it into goitrin—an active antithyroid agent. Thiocyanates are also occasionally ingested with food.

GRAVES' DISEASE — A VIEW

- There occurs a defect in suppressor T lymphocyte which permits helper T lymphocyte to stimulate b lymphocyte to produce thyroid auto-antibodies. So high circulating level of T_4 and T_3 inhibit TSH secretion so TSH level is decreased.
- Increasing level of thyroid hormone leads to increased formation of antibodies; while decreased level of thyroid hormones (due to treatment of condition) leads to lowering the formation of antibodies (but not completely preventing their formation).
- Other substances which are similar to TSH may be found in such patients. These are actually immunoglobulin antibodies; which bind with same receptor to which TSH

binds. So it also induces cAMP formation which leads to hyperthyroidism. These antibodies are called TSAb. Their stimulating effect on thyroid gland is long. This TSAb leads to increased secretion of thyroxine which may suppress TSH formation by anterior pituitary.

CRETINISM (HYPOTHYROIDISM IN CHILDREN)

- If the thyroid does not develop properly during foetal life, or if it is acted on during that period by goitrogenous influences, the child is born a cretin.
- The cretin child is a dwarf physically and mentally. The mind, skeleton, sexual organs are having delayed growth.
- The abdomen is pot bellied with protruding umbilicus. The child is deaf, dumb and idiot.
- Skin is rough, dry, wrinkled.
- Low blood sugar and iodine and body resistance is low.
- Face is typically presented—thick parted lips, large protruding tongue with dribbling of saliva and broad nose. Skin is yellow because of deposition of carotene.

CRETINISM — A VIEW

- Most common cause is maternal iodine deficiency.
- Congenital anomalies of hypothalamo-hypophyseal-thyroid axis that cause goitre can lead to congenital hypothyroidism.
- T_4 crosses the placenta.

MYXOEDEMA (GULL'S DISEASE)—HYPOTHYROIDISM IN ADULTS

- This is a condition of thyroid deficiency in the adult which usually appears at the age of forty years.
- Two classes of cases are seen : (a) Thyroid deficiency—which may be due to thyroidectomy, neoplasm, chronic thyroiditis, or radio iodine therapy, (b) Pituitary deficiency of TSH which may be due to tumours, etc.
- The clinical picture in advance case is so characteristic that the disease can be diagnosed at a glance. The woman is heavy and intensely phlegmatic; the face is broad and devoid of all expressions. The basal metabolic rate is characteristically low.
- The face is swollen, puffy having oedematous look. The deposited material myxomatous tissue consists of a semifluid substance rich in protein and mucopolysaccharides. Hoarseness in voice because of swelling of tongue and larynx. Hair fall out from axilla, pubic, head and outer third of eyebrow.

MYXOEDEMA—ANOTHER VIEW

Normally skin contains a variety of proteins mixed with polysaccharides, hyaluronic acid and chondroitin sulphuric acid. In hypothyroidism these substances accumulate → water retention is promoted → characteristic puffiness of skin. When thyroxine given → mobilisation of proteins → diuresis → myxoedema goes off.

- Mental conditions are impaired (loss of memory), sex degenerates leading to amenorrhoea/impotency, low blood sugar and iodine. Blood cholesterol level is raised so chances of high blood pressure are bright. Lethargy and apathy are other symptoms.
- The disease derives its name to a solid pseudo-edema of the skin and mucous membranes caused by infiltration with an acid mucopolysaccharide (hyaluronic acid) so that the tissue appears to be myxomatous. It is this infiltration which serves to iron out the expressive wrinkles and folds of the face so that all the patients have a strong family resemblance to one another. The change is most marked in the face, neck, supraclavicular fossae, and backs of hands which are fat and clumsy. The mucous membranes are also infiltered so that the tongue is thick and there is swelling of mucous membrane in nose, mouth, larynx, bronchi and alimentary canal. Cardiac edema is not associated with increased capillary permeability. There is advanced atrophy of the interstitial cells of the testis, accounting for such gonadal symptoms like impotency and loss of desire.
- *Diagnostic tests*: Low free thyroxine in blood (T_4) reduced BMR, increased level of TSH, blood cholesterol level is increased because of its diminished excretion by liver in bile.

SUBCLINICAL HYPOTHYROIDISM

- It is described as low level of thyroid hormones but raised level of TSH.
- Patients are clinically euthyroid and asymptomatic.
- Thyroxine should be given since such patients are mildly hypothyroid.

SECONDARY HYPOTHYROIDISM

- There is atrophy of inherently normal thyroid gland caused by failure of TSH secretion.
- It is seen in hypothalamic or anterior pituitary disease, autoimmune lymphoid - hypophysitis.

REGULATION OF SECRETION

a. *Role of anterior pituitary*:
   - Hormone TSH (thyroid stimulating hormone—thyrotropin) is secreted from anterior pituitary;

which increases the production of thyroid hormones. Both these control each other by negative feedback mechanism, i.e.

— Increased thyroxine in body fluids → decreases secretion of TSH by anterior pituitary → excess thyroxine production is checked.
— Decreased thyroxine in body fluids → increased secretion of TSH by anterior pituitary → more production of thyroxine.
— Thyroid hormone reduces the number of TRH receptors on cells which secrete TSH.

TSH—AN OVERVIEW

- The thyroidal changes resulting from removal of pituitary are as reduction in size, vascularity and weight, histologically reduction in height of epithelial cells of acini and increased amount of acinar colloid; reduction in all chemical process of iodine metabolism.
- All these changes are reversible on administration of TSH.
- Injection of excessive doses of TSH results in hyperplastic thyroid gland and signs of hyperthyroidism. The acinar cells show hypertrophy and hyperplasia with a reversal in polarity of mitochondria and Golgi apparatus. The colloid undergoes a peripheral vacuolisation so that it appears basophilic rather than eosinophilic and becomes reduced in amount as stored hormone is liberated into the blood in increased amounts.
- Under the effect of TSH there occurs - increased proteolysis of thyroglobulin with release of thyroid hormone into circulating blood, increased activity of iodide pump which increases iodide trapping, increased iodination of tyrosine and increased coupling to form thyroid hormones, increased size and secretory activity of gland, increased number of thyroid cells, epithelium changes from cuboidal to columnar or activity of thyroid cells increases under TSH effect.
- Pituitary is related to exophthalmos. The EPS (exophthalmos-producing substance) is liberated in association with TSH. Recently LATS (long active thyroid stimulator) has been found in blood of thyrotoxic and exophthalmic patients and which may not be of pituitary origin.
- Its regulation is influenced by two factors:
  a. Blood concentration of thyroid hormone: Rise in thyroid hormones in blood depresses TSH secretion and fall in thyroid hormone in blood activates TSH release (negative feedback).
  b. Nervous influences from hypothalamus through hypothalamo-hypophyseal-portal vessels. If pituitary stalk is cut or pituitary gland is transplanted to a distant site in body, the activity of thyroid is decreased. The hypothalamus exerts a tonic influence in maintaining the basal level of thyrotrophic secretion and by means of nervous reflexes, to modify TSH release in accordance with requirement of the environment. Lesions in anterior hypothalamus result in reduced thyroid function while its stimulation leads to increased thyroid activity.
  In many of hyperthyroid patients, many substances are found in their blood. They are named as 'immunoglobulin - antibodies.' They bind with the same membrane receptors which bind. TSH. They lead to the development of 'thyroid stimulating antibodies (TSAb). Excessive stimulation of thyroid gland under its effect can lead to depression of production of TSH by anterior pituitary. They exert a prolonged stimulating effect on thyroid gland.

b. *Role of hypothalamus:*
- It secretes TRH (thyrotropin - releasing hormone) in hypothalamo-hypophyseal-portal vessels. This in turn stimulates TSH from anterior pituitary which stimulates thyroid to produce more thyroxin. If this area of hypothalamus (median eminence) is stimulated electrically, it produces increased amount of thyroxine and on the contrary, if this area is destructed, thyroxine secretion is inhibited.
- TRH is a tripeptide amide. It first binds to TRH receptors in pituitary cell membrane.
  — It then activates second messenger system (phospholipid) to produce phospholipid C which ultimately leads to release of TSH.
  — It is present at various places of hypothalamus like anterior, paraventricular nucleus, suprachiasmatic nucleus, ventromedial nucleus, dorsomedial nucleus, etc.

c. *External temperature*
- Cold climate stimulates and hot depresses thyroid functions through hypothalamus by releasing hormones and partly through reflex mechanism (vasomotor reflex).

d. Through vasomotor reflexes, this gland is also controlled by autonomic nerves (sympathetic and para sympathetic nerves).

THYROCALCITONIN

(Blood calcium lowering hormone from parafollicular cells of thyroid)

- Polypeptide in nature, structurally identical with parathormone. It lowers the blood calcium level.
- More blood calcium level will depress while less blood calcium level stimulates its secretion (negative feed back).
- Polypeptide having 32 amino acids, molecular weight 3,400.
- *Actions*
  - — Facilitates deposition of calcium on bones. It depresses activity of osteoclasts (counteracting parathormone). Decreasing bone resorption.
  - — Increases excretion of calcium in urine by kidney via inhibiting reabsorption of calcium from renal tubules.
  - — Calcium absorption is prevented by intestine into blood. It decreases the formation of new osteoclasts.

DIFFERENCES BETWEEN CALCITONIN AND PARATHYROID FEEDBACK

Calcitonin	*Parathyroid feedback*
It operates more rapidly.	It takes comparatively a longer time to reach to peak activity.
It is a short term regulator of calcium ion concentration.	it sets the long term level of calcium ions in extra cellular fluid
——	This system of control is having overriding effect.
Its effect is weak because: a. Parathyroid hormone overrides it. b. The daily rates of absorption and deposition of calcium are very small.	——

ASSESSING THE GLAND: THYROID FUNCTION TESTS

Direct Tests

i. *RAIU* means radioactive iodine uptake which is most common. The ^{131}I is used but ^{123}I is preferred because it delivers lower radiation dose. It is usually measured 24 hours after administration of isotope. It varies inversely with plasma iodide concentration and directly with functional status of thyroid gland. Normally it is 5 to 30 per cent of administered dose of isotope. Higher values are suggestive of hyperfunctioning states.

Normal thyroid can concentrate iodine 10,000 times more than other tissues.

RADIOACTIVE IODINE UPTAKE—AT A GLANCE

- This can be measured by using tracer doses of radioactive iodine isotope which is without any deleterious effect on thyroid gland.
- The tracer is given orally and gamma ray counter is placed over the neck. Another site is over the thigh and in that case the values are subtracted from neck counts.
- Isotope commonly used is ^{123}I: half life 0.55 day—(half life of ^{131}I is 8.1 days; ^{125}I of 60 days).
- In patients of hyperthyroidism, iodide is rapidly incorporated into T_4 and T_3 which are released rapidly - this leads to rise in amount of radioactivity, which later on levels off and may start to decline within 24 hours while it still rises in normal subjects. In hypothyroid patients uptake is low.
- Since radiation kills the cells; so large amounts of radioactive iodine destroy thyroid tissue. So this therapy is sometimes useful in treating some benign thyroid cancer.
- Chances of radiation-carcinogenesis and germ cell mutation should be kept in mind.

ii. *Protein bound Iodine (PBI)*: Normal 3.5–7.5 µgm per cent. Its level decreases in hypothyroidism, pregnancy and thyroiditis; while increases in hyperthyroidism and on oral administration of oral contraceptives. It is a reliable test. It reflects the index of circulating level of T_4 and T_3.

iii. *Serum Thyroid Hormone levels*:
Normal Total serum T_4—3-8 µgm per cent, Free T_4 .. 2 ng per cent.
Normal Total serum T_3—0.15 µgm per cent, Free T_3 .. 1.5 ng per cent. All these values are increased in hyperthyroid while decreased in hypothyroid states.

iv. *Blood sugar*: This rises in hyperthyroid while decreases in hypothyroid states. (Normal 80-120 mg%).

v. *BMR:* Means O_2 consumption of the subject under mental and physical rest. Normally ± 20 per cent. It is increased in hyperthyroid and decreased in hypothyroid states.

vi. *Serum cholesterol*: Increases in hypothyroid and decreases in hyperthyroid states (normal value 150-250 mg%).

vii. *Serum creatinine*: Normal 0.6 mg per cent. Increases in hyperthyroid and decreases in hypothyroid states.

viii. *Thyroid binding globulin (TBG)*: Its level is increased in pregnancy, liver diseases, myxoedema; while decreased in administration of androgens/ oestrogens/cortisone, acromegaly, severe prolonged illness.

ix. Thyroid imaging (scintiscanning) This helps to detect retrosternal-prolongation of thyroid.

Test for Controlling Mechanism

Measurement of basal serum TSH concentration is useful.

Other Aspects

- Myxoedema is a disease which can be diagnosed on telephone since voice becomes slow and husky. Memory also becomes poor.
- In some patients, exophthalmos is made worst by thyroidectomy. It is due to an autoimmune attack on extraocular muscle and orbital connective tissue by cytotoxic antibodies. Steroids may lead to immuno-suppression.
- The reaction time of stretch reflex is shortened in hyperthyroidism while it is prolonged in hypothyroidism. So measurement of reaction time of ankle jerk (Achilles reflex) is an important way of evaluating thyroid functions.
- In hypothyroidism hair is coarse and sparse, skin dry and yellowish (carotenaemia), cold is poorly tolerated, poor memory, slow mentation and in some patients severe mental symptoms - "myxoedema madness."
- Thyroxine → increases BMR → increased need for vitamins → precipitation of vitamin deficiency syndromes.
- Carotene $\xrightarrow[\text{Thyroxine}]{\text{Liver}}$ vitamin A. So in its deficiency this conversion is not possible so carotene accumulates which gives yellowish tint to skin (sclera not yellow difference from jaundice).
- Muscle weakness is common with hyperthyroidism so named "thyrotoxic myopathy" which runs parallel with the advancement of the disease. It may be due to accelerated catabolism of proteins. It affects the expression of MHC genes in skeletal and cardiac muscle.

BIBLIOGRAPHY

1. Chopra IJ, Solomon DH. Pathogenesis of hyperthyroidism. Ann Rev Med 1983;34:267.
2. Dumont JE, et al. Physiological and pathological regulation of thyroid cells proliferation and differentiation by thyrotropin and other factors. Phy Rev 1992;72:667.
3. Dussault JH, et al. Thyroid hormones and brain development. Ann Rev Phy 1987;49:321.
4. Gershengorn MC. Mechanism of thyrotropin releasing hormone stimulation of pituitary hormone secretion. Ann Rev Phy 1986;48:515.
5. Kouridos IA, et al. The regulation and organisation of thyroid stimulating hormone genes. Rec Prog Horm Res 1984;40:79.
6. Lenzen S, et al. Thyroid hormones, gonadal and adrenocortical steroids and function of Islet of Langerhans. Endocrin Rev 1984;5:411.
7. McClung MR, et al. Treatment of hyperthyrodism. Ann Rev Med 1980;31:385.
8. Refetoff S, et al. The syndromes of resistance to thyroid hormones. Endocrin Rev 1993;14:348.
9. Samuels HH, et al. Regulation of gene expression by thyroid hormone. Ann Rev Phy 1989;51:623.
10. Woeber KA. Thyrotoxicosis and the heart. New Eng J Med 1992;327:94.

44 Protective Envelope: Adrenals

Human adrenal is an organ with dual character. The adrenals are more essential to life than is the pituitary. They play leading role in determining whether any person is sick or well. Patients with adrenal insufficiency often die from minor infections and stresses.

It consists of cortex and medulla. The cortex is developed from the mesoderm of the wolffian ridge in conjunction with the sex glands. The medulla is ectodermal in origin and arises from neural crest together with sympathetic nerve cells. The cortex is yellow coloured because of its high lipid content. It is made up of three zones:

i. *Zona glomerulosa*: It is rich in lipids specially cholesterol, raw sterol material from which the corticoids are formed. It is so named because the cells are arranged in clusters bearing a feeble resemblance to glomeruli. This zone is the source of hormone *"Aldosterone"* which is famous for its property of retaining salt and water and increasing the loss of potassium. This zone is not under the control of ACTH from adenohypophysis, but it works autonomously.

ii. *Zona fasciculata*: The clear cells are there with a low RNA and a high lipid content. It secretes steroids which are mainly concerned with carbohydrate (mainly), fat and protein metabolism. Examples are—corticosterone (with an OH at position II and more correctly called hydroxycorticosterone, cortisone; with an O at position 11 and OH at position 17-11-dehydro-17-hydroxycorticosterone).

iii. *Zona reticularis*: Cells here are compact cells having high RNA and a high lipid content. It secretes sex hormones or androgens (androsterone). A small amount of oestrogen may be produced in addition to androgen, so that a tumour of adrenal cortex may on rare occasions be associated with feminising rather than masculinising effects.

All these hormones may be mentioned as salt, sugar and sex hormones.

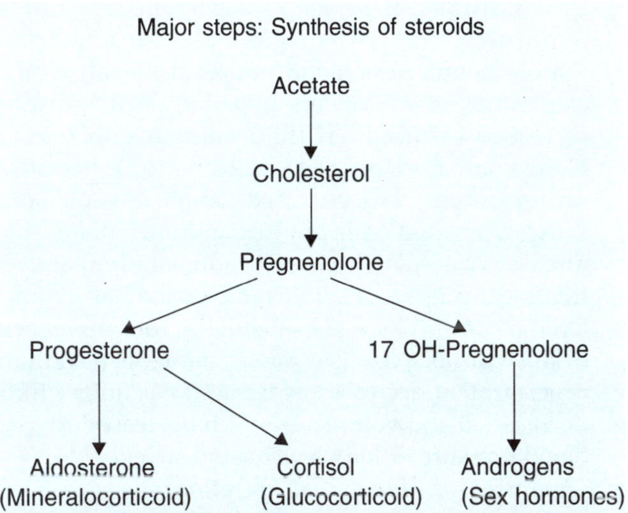

- All steroid hormones have a parent ring of cyclo-pentano-perhydro-phenanthrene.
- Most naturally occurring steroids contain alcohol side chain called sterols.
- A and B rings of nucleus are joined in a trans or cis configuration. Oestrogen does not show such isomerism since their A ring is aromatic.

DIFFERENT STEROIDS

Mineralocorticoids	*Glucocorticoids*
• Aldosterone (very potent)	• Cortisol (very potent)
• Desoxycorticosterone	• Corticosterone
• Corticosterone	• Cortisone
• 9 α flurocortisol (synthetic slightly more potent than aldosteron)	• Prednisone
• Cortisol	• Methylprednisone
• Cortisone	• Dexamethasone

MINERALOCORTICOIDS (ALDOSTERONES)

- It causes increased reabsorption of sodium by tubular epithelial cells. This causes increased level of sodium in extracellular fluid. There occurs simultaneous osmotic absorption of water in equal quantity approximately. This limits the concentration of sodium in extracellular fluid. This increased extracellular fluid volume increases the venous return and hence cardiac output and finally arterial blood pressure is increased.
- Because of increased level of sodium in extracellular fluid, much of the potassium is lost in urine which decreases level of potassium in blood (from normal 4-5 mEq/l. to 1-2 mEq/l); this is called hypokalaemia responsible for muscular weakness, because of preventing the transmission of action potential.
- In conditions of *primary aldosteronism* 'Conn's Syndrome' the patient generally suffers from hypokalaemia (less blood potassium level) which causes muscular weakness, hypertension (because of increased extracellular fluid volume + increased blood volume + increased venous return + increased cardiac output). This increased sodium level of blood causes decreased renin production from kidney. This disease is caused by tumour of adrenal gland and so treatment consists of surgical removal of the gland.
- On the contrary, if a person suffers from deficiency of this hormone, i.e. *hypoaldosteronism*; then sodium concentration decreases in extracellular fluid which decreases blood volume → which decreases arterial blood pressure → hypotension and shock.
- ***Regulation of aldosterone secretion:***
  - — So by above discussion it is clear that it is regulated by sodium and potassium ion concentration in extracellular fluid, renin-angiotensin system, ACTH of anterior pituitary.
  - — A very low concentration of potassium can cause manifold increase in secretion of aldosterone.
  - — Renin-angiotensin system is activated in response to decreased blood flow to kidney, which may alter the concentration of aldosterone.
  - — Likewise decreased sodium concentration in ECF can increase the secretion of aldosterone.

CELLULAR MECHANISM : ALDOSTERONE SECRETION

- Since it is lipid soluble, so it readily diffuses to interior of tubular epithelial cells.
- There, in cytoplasm, it combines with receptor protein which is highly specific.
- This complex enters the nucleus, where it induces DNA to produce mRNA related to the process of sodium and potassium transport.
- The mRNA diffuses back into the cytoplasm, where with ribosomes it causes protein formation.
- The proteins so formed is a mixture of receptor protein, enzymes, membrane transport proteins, etc.
- One of the enzymes increased is Na-K-ATPase which is the principle part of the pump for Na-K exchange at basolateral membrane of tubular cells.
- Approximately 30 minutes are required before new RNA appears in the cells; + 45 minutes are required before rate of sodium transport begins to increase. So effect of aldosterone is significant after a few hours.

STRANGE BUT TRUE: ALDOSTERONE V/S OEDEMA

- At one glance, it appears true that under the effect of aldosterone hormone, there is reabsorption of sodium, chloride, bicarbonate. This in turn promotes increased water reabsorption from tubules by stimulating ADH secretion + by creating osmotic gradient across the tubular membrane. All this leads to increased extracellular fluid volume. It may be sometimes enough to cause generalised extracellular oedema.
- But moderate quantity of this hormone does not cause oedema. Increased electrolyte concentration → polydypsia (more thirst) → polyurea (increased urinary output). Of course this urine may contain little quantity of electrolytes but its increased volume keeps washing more and more electrolytes from body fluids. This nullifies the chances of oedema.

GLUCOCORTICOIDS

Actions

Carbohydrate metabolism: Gluconeogenesis is stimulated (new production of glucose).

They also cause mobilisation of amino acids from extrahepatic tissues, mainly from muscles; so these amino acids now become available to promote the formation of glucose. They also cause decreased utilisation of glucose by the cells.

All these above mentioned mechanisms cause an elevation in blood glucose level, i.e. hyperglycaemia (diabetes mellitus) - so called *adrenal diabetes.*

Protein metabolism: Corticosteroids cause reduction in protein stores of the body (except liver). It is due to increased destruction as well as reduced synthesis of proteins. In excessive production of steroids; muscles become excessively weak.

Everywhere protein deficiency occurs, but their level is elevated in liver and plasma.

Fat metabolism: They also promote mobilisation of fatty acids from adipose tissues. This increases the concentration of free fatty acids in the plasma which is used for energy. They also cause increased oxidation of fatty acids in the cells. This makes a man obese (excess deposition of fat in chest and head—moon face, buffalo like torso) and also creates ketogenic effects.

During *stress*, excessive corticosteroids are liberated which causes fright, fight or flight attitude. This is all achieved by mobilisation of amino acid, fatty acids and neoglucogenesis.

When the infection occurs, this is proceeded by inflammation which may be sometimes more fatal/ injurious than even infection. This inflammation is blocked by steroids. So they are anti-inflammatory in action. They act by blocking early stages of inflammation and if it has begun, it causes rapid resolution of inflammation.

ANTI-INFLAMMATORY ACTION : AN OVERVIEW

- Mainly the stages of inflammation are:
  (i) Release of chemicals from damaged tissue cells. Like histamine, bradykinin, prostaglandins, leukotrienes, etc.; (ii) Blood supply of inflamed area is increased - the effect called erythema; (iii) Because of increased capillary permeability, there is leakage of large quantities of pure plasma out of capillaries into damaged area leading to clotting of tissue fluid - non-pitting oedema; (iv) Infiltration of inflamed area by leukocytes; (v) Growth of fibrous tissue helping in healing process.
- The steroids are anti-inflammatory in action through: (i) Blocking early stages of inflammation before it actually begins, (ii) Rapid resolution of inflammation.
- Cortisol decreases the capillary permeability which prevents loss of plasma into the tissues.
- Cortisol suppresses the immune system. T lymphocytes are specifically decreased which decrease tissue reaction which would otherwise promote further inflammatory process.
- Cortisol decreases the formation of prostaglandins and leukotrienes. It prevents emigration of leukocytes into inflamed area.
- Lysosome contains some proteolytic enzymes which are released by damaged cells.
- Cortisol increases production of erythrocytes. Anaemia has been reported in their less production while polycythaemia in their excessive production.

Steroids leads to *eosinopenia* and *lymphopenia*.

STEROIDS AND ALLERGY

- The basic allergic reaction between antigen and antibody is not affected by cortisol.
- It blocks the inflammatory response to allergic reactions as it blocks in other types of inflammatory responses.
- They are capable of preventing shock or death in anaphylaxis.

CIRCADIAN RHYTHM—STEROIDS

- The secretory rate of CRF, ACTH, and cortisol are high in early morning but low in late evening.
- Plasma cortisol ranges between 5 mμ/dl (around mid-night) and 20 μg/dl an hour before arising in the morning.
- Maximum daily production of cortisol occurs between 4 and 10 a.m. Bursts are frequent in early morning; least frequent in evening.
  Reference: Moller J D. (1993). Amer J Phy 264: R 821. "On the nature of circadian clock in mammals.
  Source: Review of medical physiology by W. F. Ganong. Lange medical book.

STEROIDS AS ANTI-INFLAMMATORY AGENTS: SOME NEW PERSPECTIVES

1. Phospholipase A_2 is inhibited which in turn, reduces the release of arachidonic acid from tissue phospholipids. All this reduces the formation of leucotrienes, thromboxanes, prostaglandins.
2. The movement of NF - $_{K}$B to the nucleus is inhibited, which, in turn exerts inhibitory effect on release of cytokines.

HYPERADRENALISM

a. *Cushing's syndrome*

1. It was first described by Harvey Cushing (1932). It is characterised by:
   - i. Painful adiposity (obesity) confined to face, neck and trunk but spares the limbs. "Moon face" and "buffalo neck";
   - ii. Hirsutism in females and preadolescent males;
   - iii. A dusky plethoric appearance;
   - iv. Peculiar striations of the skin of abdominal wall;
   - v. Muscular weakness and atrophy;
   - vi. Vascular hypertension (systolic);
   - vii. A tendency to diabetes;
   - viii. Kyphosis of upper thoracic spine;
   - ix. Sexual dystrophy (amenorrhoea in females and impotency in males). The most characteristic is deep red, round, full moon face (atrophy of testes and ovaries + hypertrophy of adrenal cortex).
   - x. Polycythaemia with cyanosis of face, feet and hands.
   - xi. Loss of minerals from bones leading to osteoporosis, softening or brittleness.
   - xii. Eosinopenia, lymphopenia, NaCl retention leading to oedema with low blood potassium. It may arise either as a result of pituitary tumour (excess ACTH) or from primary hyperplasia or tumour of adrenal cortex. Cushing's disease is restricted to cases associated with pituitary

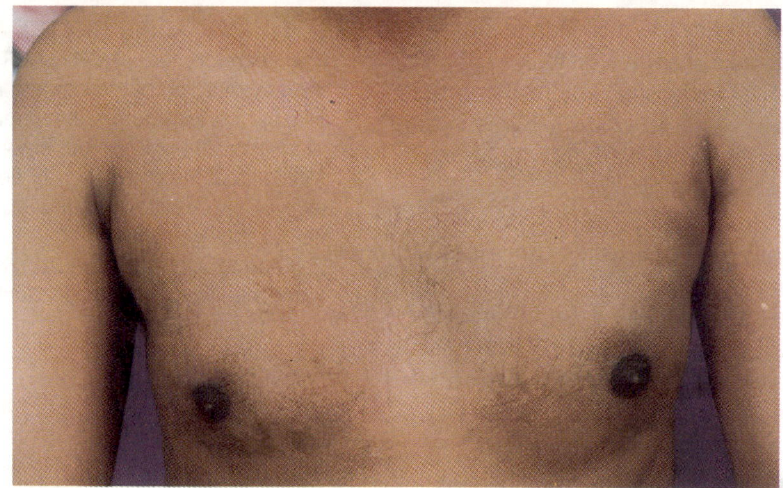

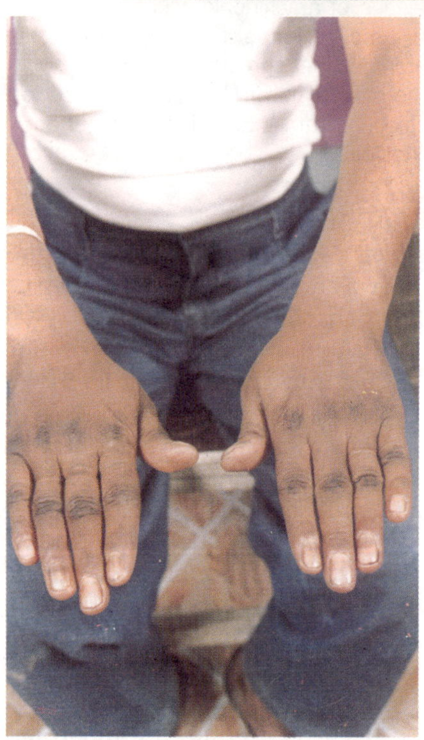

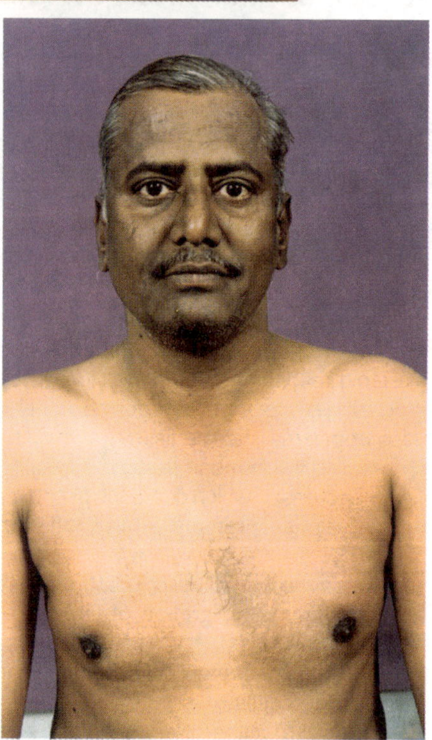

Fig. 44.1: Patient of Addison's disease—Note site of pigmentation
Courtesy: Dr Harish Badjatya, Assistant Professor, Department of Medicine, SP Medical College and Associated Groups of PBM Hospital, Bikaner

tumour while Cushing's syndrome is referred to condition due to primary adrenal tumour.

b. ***Adreno-genital syndrome***:

i. In this, presence of an excess of masculinising hormones (androgens) produces a striking variety of clinical changes, depending on age and sex. In girls, if abnormality is present in the first few weeks of intrauterine life, the result is female pseudo-hermaphroditism; if late in intrauterine life or in boys, the result is precocious puberty.

ii. The clinical picture is characterised by hirsutism, virilism and great muscularity so that a boy presents picture of Hercules with premature development of sex organs. In girls, there is a development of both primary and secondary male characters the clitoris become enlarged and hair develops on the face and body (hirsutism). In women, the sex organs atrophy, amenorrhoea and obesity, the voice is deep and hirsutism is marked on the face and body. Adult males show no sexual change except in rare cases where there is a feminising effect. Urinary 17-keto-steroids are elevated, serum sodium and blood sugar levels are low and serum potassium is high.

CHRONIC ADRENAL INSUFFICIENCY—ADDISON'S DISEASE

1. Thomas Addison (1855) has first of all attracted attention towards this disease. In his words the principal features are, general languor and debility, remarkable feebleness of the action of heart, irritability of stomach, and a peculiar change of colour in the skin, occurring in connection with a diseased condition of the suprarenal gland. The colour of the skin presents a smoky or dingy appearance, or various shades or tints of deep ambour or chestnut brown. This skin discolouration usually increases with the advancement of the disease. The anaemia, languor, loss of appetite and feebleness of the heart become aggravated. A darkish streak usually appears on the commissure of the lips, the body wastes. Pulse becomes smaller and weaker, hypotension develops. The patient gradually sinks and expires.
2. Loss of salt and water balance includes depletion of sodium and chloride together with a rise in plasma potassium. This involves a flow of water from extracellular into intracellular compartments, with an accompanying decrease in plasma volume. These changes in turn lead to circulatory failure with a fall in blood pressure and decreased blood flow to organs. In kidney, a fall in blood flow is accompanied by a decrease in glomerular filtration rate resulting in renal failure which finally may prove fatal.
3. The pigmentation (as described above) ranges from light yellow to deep brown is most marked on exposed parts and regions like areola of nipple, genitals, etc. The mucous membranes of the mouth and vagina are often pigmented. There is loss of hair over the body and axilla.
4. Changes in general metabolism affecting principally carbohydrates, but also protein and fat, are due to insufficiency of 17-hydroxycortico steroids, produced by zona fasciculata. The hypoglycaemia may be attributed to failure of gluconeogenesis, owing to the proteins not being broken down in the liver to amino acids from which sugar can be formed. The muscular weakness and hypotension also may be due to interference with protein metabolism. The loss of body and axillary hair as well as loss of weight may be associated with lack of anabolic hormones from zona reticularis.
5. There may be remissions and exacerbations of symptoms called *crisis*; marked by extreme arterial hypotension, decrease in blood volume, GIT symptoms (nausea, vomiting, diarrhoea, loss of appetite) shock and sometimes terminating in death; which is partly due to hypoglycaemic shock.

   Acute crisis is usually because of :
   i. Bilateral adrenalectomy;
   ii. Massive adrenal haemorrhage destroying glands or widespread thrombosis,
   iii. Sudden stress (trauma, surgical operation, acute illness) superimposed on adrenals gravely damaged by chronic disease or atrophied as a result of prolonged administration of cortisone with consequent suppression of normal ACTH response of pituitary-adrenal-axis to the stress. The abrupt withdrawal of oral cortisone under these conditions will precipitate a crisis of insufficiency.

In fully developed acute crisis, the features are pain abdomen, headache, lassitude, which may be accompanied by nausea, vomiting, diarrhoea. The temperature may shoot to hyperpyrexic levels. If disease is still uncontrolled the patient becomes confused, restless and circulatory collapse develop which may terminate into coma and death. It represents two distinct syndromes namely. Sodium loss, and deficiency of 17-hydroxycorticosteroids.

ADDISON'S DISEASE: CLINICAL FEATURES

1. Insufficiency of glucocorticiods: weight loss, weakness, nausea, vomiting, anorexia, diarrhoea/constipation, hypoglycaemia, postural hypotension.
2. Insufficiency of mineralo-corticoids: hypotension.
3. Increased ACTH secretion: pigmentation.
4. Loss of adrenal androgen: decreased body hair specially in females.

NELSON'S SYNDROME

It is the association of locally invasive pituitary tumour with very high levels of ACTH and hyperpigmentation which may occur in some patients with Cushing's disease following bilateral adrenalectomy.

REGULATION OF GLUCOCORTICOID SECRETION

It is controlled entirely by ACTH from anterior pituitary. It is further controlled by releasing hormones from hypothalamus (ACTH-RF/CRF corticotropin releasing factor), through negative feedback mechanism.

CRF is a peptide composed of 41 amino acids. Cell bodies are located in its paraventricular nuclei.

- More cortisol in blood → inhibitory signal from hypothalamus → diminished production of ACTH → less cortisol.
- Less cortisol in blood → stimulatory signal from hypothalamus (more CRF) → increased production of ACTH → more cortisol. This increased ACTH production also enhances the secretion of melanin-producing hormone (MSH) which is responsible for pigmentation (Addison's disease). This MSH causes the melanocytes to form pigment melanin and these cells are found in between dermis and epidermis of the skin.
- Hypothalamus also receive many nervous connections from limbic system and lower brainstem.
- In ACTH stimulated steps:
  i. Enzyme "Protein Kinase A" is activated which causes conversion of cholesterol to pregnenolone. This explains the fact that ACTH is necessary for the formation of adrenocortical hormone.
  ii. Adenyl cyclase in the cell membrane is activated; which then induces the formation of cAMP in cell cytoplasm. This cAMP then activates the intracellular enzymes which causes formation of adreno-cortical hormones. (Example of cAMP as second messenger).
- ACTH chemically is a large polypeptide having a chain of 39 amino acids.

ACTH: AN OVERVIEW

- It was found that atrophy of adrenal cortex occurred in hypophysectomised rats and repair took place under the influence of pituitary implants (Smith 1913–1930).
- Adrenal cortical overactivity was associated with basophil adenoma of pituitary. In acute states of stress when ACTH is secreted in increased amount, basophil degranulation occurs (Harvey Cushing 1910–1927).
- Out of 39 amino acids, the first 13 amino acids of ACTH show a similar sequence to that of MSH which accounts for melanocyte stimulating activity on the part of ACTH.
- Its inactivation occurs very rapidly. It is not excreted in the urine though appreciable amounts of administered dose may be recovered from kidney tissues. Its half-life in rat is about one minute.
- Its extra-adrenal activities are : fat mobilisation, ketogenic effect, melanocyte stimulation, etc.
- Adrenal activities: Administration of ACTH induces: Increased size of adrenal, depletion of ascorbic acid content of adrenal within half an hour, a fall in adrenal cortical cholesterol concentration, increased release of adrenal steroids.
- Regulation: Release of hormone at increased rate is one of the body's defence reactions towards stress/trauma and ACTH given in pharmacological doses in conditions like rheumatoid arthritis, etc. is of use.
- It is mainly controlled first by feedback of its target gland hormones (adrenal steroids) and second, by an influence from CNS via hypothalamus.

A THOUGHT ON STEROIDS

Steroids: life saving	*Steroids: life threatening*
• Relief from allergic manifestation viz bronchial asthma, anaphylaxis, etc.	• Hyperglycaemia
• Anti-inflammatory action	• Hypertension
• Prepares the individual against stress	• Mobilisation of fats from adipose tissue + more oxidation of fatty acids • Obesity • Eosinopenia + Lymphopenia, i.e. diminished resistance.

- So steroid therapy should be advised to patients when it is really necessary. Once started they should not be withdrawn suddenly but their withdrawal should be gradual (tapering doses).
- Adrenal diabetes is moderately insulin sensitive.

ANABOLIC STEROIDS—A VIEW

Anabolic = protein building drugs. They mimic the effects of testosterone and other male sex hormones. They can build up muscle tissue, strengthen the bones and speed muscle recovery following exercise or injury. They are also used to treat osteoporosis in postmenopausal women and some types of anaemia. Weightlifters, body builders and athletes, use them to build muscle strength and bulk and to undergo vigorous muscular training. They are banned because of their adverse effects.

HIRSUTISM

A perplexing problem:

- Is the growth of terminal hair "in a male pattern" in a female. It is often racial as well as familial. It is very common after menopause. The main cause is excess production of androgens by ovary/adrenal.
- Investigations required:- diurnal cortisol levels, ACTH, testosterone, sex hormone binding globulins, 17-OH progesterone, luteinising; FSH ratio; ovarian ultrasound, dexamethasone suppression test.
- Management:
  — Electrolysis, shaving,
  — Waxing and depilatory creams,
  — Oral anti-androgen (e.g. cyproterone acetate),
  — Removal of any endocrinal cause,

— Spironolactone has a dual action of blocking the androgen receptor and of inhibiting androgen production. So is an alternative therapy. Cimetidine is also performing the same role, but is of not much benefit in this case.

CAUSES IN FEMALES

1. Genetic
2. Idiopathic
3. Adrenal (Cushing's disease, tumour, congenital hyper-functioning)
4. Ovary—tumour, polycystic ovaries
5. Drugs—phenothiazines, minoxidil, phenytoin.

Virilization: Means enlargement of clitoris, deepening of the voice, temporal recession, breast atrophy, acne, increased size of shoulder girdle muscles, frontal balding.

SYMPATHIN

During sympathetic stimulation, a chemical substance resembling adrenaline in its action, is liberated from sympathetic endings supplying the smooth muscles of skin. This is sympathin and in most mammals this and nor-adrenaline are identical.

ADRENAL CORTICAL FUNCTION: CLINICAL TESTS

1. If a test dose of corticotrophin is administered, fifty per cent reduction in eosinophil number is seen. This observation is absent in adreno-cortical-insufficiency.
2. Normally, diuresis occurs within 30–45 minutes of drinking water. But in adrenal insufficiency this excretion of excess water is much delayed.
3. Other tests include—tendency to hypoglycaemia during fasting, sensitivity to insulin, and uric acid creatinine ratio which is normally increased during cortical stimulation.

BIBLIOGRAPHY

1. Burnstein KL, et al. Regulation of gene expression by gluco-corticoids. Ann Rev Phy 1989;51:683.
2. Funder JW. Adrenocortical steroids and brain. Ann Rev Phy 1987;49:397.
3. Keller Wood ME, et al. Corticosteroid inhibition of ACTH secretion. End Rev 1984;5:1.
4. McEwen BS, et al. Adrenal steroids receptors and actions in nervous system. Phy Rev 1986;66:1121.
5. Meyer JS. Biochemical effects of cotricosteroids on neural tissues. Phy Rev 1985;65:946.
6. Ozawa S, et al. Electrophysiology of excitable endocrine cells. Phy Rev 1986;66:887.
7. Quinn SJ, et al. Regulation of aldosterone secretion. Ann Rev Phy 1988;50:40.
8. Revier CL, et al. Mediation by corticotropin releasing factor (CRF) of adenohypophyseal hormone secretion. Ann Rev Phy 1986;48:475.
9. Schneider EG, et al. Effect of osmolality on aldosterone secretion. Endocrinology 1981;116:1621.
10. Schneider EG, et al. Effect of sodium concentration on aldosterone secretion by isolated perfuse canine adrenal glands. Endocrinology 1984;115:2195.
11. White PC, et al. Congenital adrenal hyperplasia. New Eng J Med 1987;316:1519.

45 Homeostasis: Blood Sugar Regulation—Diabetes Mellitus

WHY IS BLOOD SUGAR REGULATION NECESSARY?

This is a question which may be asked to physiologists. Explanations are:

- The glucose is the only nutrient which can be utilised by (as well as necessary) brain, retina and germinal epithelium of many tissues to meet their demands, so it becomes necessary to regulate glucose metabolism in a beautiful way.
- Excess glucose collection → increased osmotic pressure in extracellular fluid → cellular dehydration → loss of glucose in urine → fatal termination.
- Above sequence must be checked so its regulation becomes essential.

LIVER AND INSULIN

- Insulin leads to diffusion of glucose from extracellular fluid to cells by simple mechanism of facilitated diffusion.
- But liver cells are highly permeable to glucose so insulin will have a little effect on transport of glucose through the liver cell membrane.
- An enzyme glucose-6-phosphatase is abundant in liver cells which causes de-phosphorylation of glucose which has already been phosphorylated. This does not cause trapping of glucose inside the liver cells, but leads to release of glucose from liver into the blood and therefore, liver glycogen level is decreased and blood glucose level is increased.
- A special enzyme glucokinase is also present in liver cells which causes phosphorylation of glucose. Its level increases following 6 to 12 hours after administration of insulin.

All these above facts explain the following circumstances :

i. The action of insulin on muscle and other peripheral tissues of the body causes rapid transport of glucose into peripheral cells and thus reduces blood sugar level.
ii. At this moment, dephosphorylating action of glucose-6-phosphatase enzyme dominates, which leads to decreased level of liver glycogen.
iii. A number of hours later, there occurs slow build up of enzyme 'glucokinase' which enhances glucose phosphorylation and in this way, it promotes increased use of glucose as well as increased storage of glycogen, by the liver cells.

- From above paragraphs it becomes reasonable to say that liver acts as a glucose-buffer-system. Glucose can readily penetrate hepatic cells in either direction, passing from extracellular spaces into hepatic cells to be stored as glycogen, or the glycogen being split to glucose that then passes rapidly into extracellular fluid.
- Besides the above buffering action, the liver also is capable of producing new glucose—so-called "*Neoglucogenesis*" and by this means also it regulates blood sugar level. It manufactures glucose from amino acids and glycerol derived from fats.

DIABETIC SYMPTOMATOLOGY: ACTIONS OF INSULIN

- Glucose probably combines with a carrier substance in the cell membrane and then is transported to the inside of the membrane, where it is released to the interior of the cell. The carrier then returns to the outer surface of the membrane to transport additional quantities of glucose. This is simple "facilitated diffusion" which does not occur against concentration gradient. The main thing or fact is that for better operation of this facilitated diffusion insulin is essential.
- One fact is that this transport of glucose does not occur in brain since that occurs through blood-brain barrier

and so also is true through intestinal mucosa as well as through tubular epithelium of the kidney. But on the contrary this glucose transport by insulin is most effective in skeletal muscle, adipose tissue, into heart, uterus, etc.

- So in insulin deficiency the sugar absorbed from bowel is not utilised and it accumulates in the blood. So sugar is not utilised to satisfy the needs of the body the cell actually starves in spite of presence of abundant sugar outside. This leads to symptoms *'Polyphagia'* (excessive eating/sense of hunger), weakness, loss of weight. *Pruritus* also may be a prominent symptom which is apparently due to the accumulation of unused sugar in the tissues.
- The large amount of sugar in the blood causes withdrawal of fluid from the tissues by reason of osmosis so that there is great thirst - so called *Polydipsia* (excessive drinking of water). This effect is also responsible for cellular dehydration. Elevation of blood sugar level from normal levels to higher or highest/fatal side can cause considerable *dehydration of cells* which constitutes important cause of diabetic coma.
- Whenever the quantity of glucose entering the kidney tubules in glomerular filtrate rises above 225 mg per minute, a significant amount of sugar begins to spill into the urine, and when this quantity rises above the tubular maximum (325 mg per minute), then all the excess sugar will be lost in the urine. This sugar is followed by loss of water so that marked *'Polyurea'* results. This polyurea is further due to osmotic diuretic effect of glucose in the kidney tubules. This water loss may also accompany an obligatory loss of electrolytes with it which may aid to further dehydration which is a cause of diabetic coma.
- Insulin influences hepatic neoglucogenesis through FFA (free fatty acids) mobilisation. When low insulin level is there, then FFA are taken up by liver and gluconeogenesis is stimulated by acetyl CoA derived from fatty acid oxidation.
- ***Fat metabolism: role of insulin*:** The adequate insulin causes proper transport of glucose into cells so that cell is full of energy. On the contrary, if glucose is not available to the cells (due to deficiency of insulin or diabetes mellitus), then the major share of the energy required by the body is then supplied by fats. Due to deficiency of insulin, the activity of lipase is increased in fat depots resulting in excess production of free fatty acids which pass into circulation raising its level in plasma. This leads to overall increase in quantity of lipoproteins and their constituents like triglycerides—cholesterol and phospholipids. Excess cholesterol synthesis is further due to increased production of acetyl CoA. This excess lipid content is responsible for atherosclerotic changes which may precipitate myocardial attacks, angiopathy in retinal and renal arteries.
- In diabetes mellitus (deficiency of insulin) catabolism of fat is increased with production of ketone bodies and free fatty acids along with decreased synthesis of fatty acids and triglycerides.
- Increased production of acetyl CoA is a feature of diabetes mellitus; some of it is converted into aceto-acetyl CoA and then in liver into acetoacetic acid and its derivative β hydroxybutyric acid and acetone passes into circulation in greater amount to produce ketonaemia and ketosis. This liberates H^+ and lowering of blood pH stimulates respiratory centre, thus producing rapid and deep respiration—*Kussmaul breathing (air hunger).*
- ***So dehydration + acidosis + polyurea + hypovolaemia + hypotension leads to unconsciousness in a diabetic patient which we may call diabetic coma.***
- ***Insulin and protein metabolism*:** Just like insulin promotes transport of glucose across the cell membrane; here too, protein transport across the cell membrane is also promoted under the effect of insulin, but of course, intensity is less.
- Deficiency of insulin leads to diabetes mellitus which means carbohydrates are not metabolised. This causes mobilisation of both proteins and fats from tissues and, they are used for energy. So it is better to say that under the influence of insulin (better utilisation of carbohydrates), catabolism of tissue proteins is decreased but protein anabolism is proceeding successfully.
- By the above paragraph it is also told that insulin is essential for growth of an animal. The growth promoting action of insulin is, of course, due to: (a) direct effect of insulin on protein anabolism; (b) protein sparing effect of increased carbohydrate metabolism; (c) Growth hormone also promotes body growth by increasing the rate of insulin production, (d) formation of mRNA.

PHYSIOLOGICALLY IMPORTANT POINTS—INSULIN

i. It is produced by β-cells of islets of Langerhans. These cells contain coarse, round granules which are precursor of insulin. Any stimulus which causes insulin secretion is often associated with degranulation of β-cells. These granules are insulin containing covered packets in the cytoplasm, which are having rectangular/round shape. The number of granules determine the insulin content of the gland.

ii. Insulin is inactivated by digestive enzymes, so it is not suitable for oral administration.

iii. It combines with a globulin and is carried in blood with them. In circulation its half-life is 5 minutes only.

iv. Eighty per cent of its is metabolised in kidney and liver through many ways.

v. The normal value of insulin in plasma is 25–50 units or 1–2 mg. The normal basal rate of insulin secretion in man is 0.5 to 1 U/hour. After each meal rate of insulin secretion increases. During the overnight fast it is 10–20 μU/ml by morning and after meals it may reach to peak values as high as 100 μU/ml.

CHEMISTRY OF INSULIN

- It consists of two polypeptide chains (A and B).
- These two chains are interlinked by disulphide bridges.
- 21 amino acids in chain A; and 30 amino acids in chain B are present.
- Its molecular weight - 5734. Iso electric pH 5.4.
- It is soluble in dilute alcohol, stable in acid but not in alkaline solution. It is destroyed by proteolytic enzymes, so inactive by mouth.
- Normal pancreatic tissue is rich in zinc. This means, insulin remains stored in it as zinc salt.
- It is rich in cystine, leucine, glutamic acid. Tryptophane, methionene and hydroxypronaline are absent.

PREPARATION OF INSULIN

- Soluble: Watery solution, 6 hours is duration of action but acts quickly.
- Lente: Insuline zinc suspension. Slow absorption. Injection effective for 24 hours. Prolonged action.
- Protamine: (extracted from nuclei but containing arginine or lysine). Slow absorption. Prolonged action.
- Zinc + Protamine: Remains soluble for months. Action starts within 6–8 hours but lasting for 48–72 hours.
- Globin: (obtained from Hb. + $ZnCl_2$) delayed action.
- Regular insulin + retard insulin - Quick and prolonged action.

MECHANISM OF ACTION: INSULIN

- Insulin first binds with and activates membrane receptor protein having molecular weight 3,00,000.
- This insulin receptor is a combination product of two alpha subunits lying outside the cell membrane and two beta subunits protruding into cell cytoplasm. This leads to formation of a proteinkinase—an activated enzyme which causes phosphorylation of other cytosol enzymes.
- Any way:
  - — As insulin binds with membrane receptor, the cell membrane becomes highly permeable to glucose. The increased glucose transport is because of opening of gates in a glucose transport protein—which is a membrane protein with a molecular weight of 55,000.
  - — Cell membrane at the same time becomes impermeable for amino acids, potassium-magnesium and phosphate ions.
  - — Many other intracellular metabolic enzymes show changed state of phosphorylation.
  - — Other slower effects are: altered role of translation of mRNA at ribosome to form new protein, changed rate of DNA transcription.

INSULIN EXCESS

Is producing hypoglycaemia. It is characterised by anxiety, hunger, cold sweat, tremulousness, etc. If this fall of glucose continues and remains untreated, then patient may be comatosed with resulting fatal end. Irreversible brain damage is a serious manifestation which is characterised by confusion, slurring of speech, coma, etc. Of course, body itself meets with the hypoglycaemic situation by releasing glucagon and catecholamines. Administration of glucose corrects the situation, or glucose like drinks, e.g. orange juice are equally effective.

- It may also exist when insulin level is excess due to insulin secreting tumour (insulinoma); or due to hyperplasia of β cells. All such symptoms are severe in morning because of depleted hepatic glycogen reserve after an overnight fast. Hypoglycaemia may be confused with epilepsy or psychosis.
- ***Macrosomia*** means high birth weight and large organs in infants of diabetic mother. This is because of the fact that foetal pancreas is stimulated by glucose and amino acid from the blood of the mother. Of course, it is protease of placenta which can destroy free insulin of maternal blood, but it is antibody bound insulin which is protected and reaches the foetus.

***Coma in diabetes*:** As told earlier, acidosis and dehydration together cause the state of unconsciousness in a diabetic patient. Lactic acidosis may complicate the stage. Acetone breath and Kussmaul's breathing are diagnostic points in such states. Brain oedema has also been noticed in many patients with diabetic acidosis.

DIFFERENCES BETWEEN TWO STATES

Hyperglycaemic coma	*Hypoglycaemic coma*
Due to high blood glucose level	Due to fall in blood glucose level
Cause - insulin - under dose, infection	Due to over dosages of insulin
Breathing- deep + rapid (Kussmaul's breathing)	Laboured breathing
Diminished CNS reflex	Often bilateral extensor plantar response
Marked glycosuria and ketonuria	No. specific characteristic feature
Marked dehydration	Hydration normal

CAUSES OF DIABETES MELLITUS

a. ***Heredity*: *It is the basis of diabetes.*** It is probable that there is a specific gene for every specific enzyme within a cell. When that gene is lost or altered, the corresponding enzyme is also lost or altered.
Diabetes is present from birth in the form of an inherently defective carbohydrate mechanism which can be triggered in a variety of ways. The defect may remain in a latent form for many years which is called *'latent diabetes.'* The disease is transmitted as a recessive genetic characteristic.

b. ***Obesity*: *Is open door for diabetes.*** The glycosuria of middle-aged persons often disappears when body weight is reduced to a sufficient degree.
Furthermore, the diabetic effect of obesity is believed to be caused by the depression of glucose metabolism in the presence of excess fatty acids in the blood.

c. ***Role of hormones*:** Pituitary hormone specially growth hormone is able to influence the course of diabetes mellitus. Growth hormone is a diabetogenic one. Diabetes may be associated with acromegaly. Administration of this hormone (GH) leads to hydropic changes in the beta cells associated with an early reversible phase of diabetes, followed later by an irreversible phase with complete destruction of beta cells.
Adrenal cortical hormones are also diabetogenic. The administration of hydrocortisone causes marked hyperglycaemia.

d. ***Pancreas*:**
   - The most obvious and immediate cause of diabetes is insulin deficiency which may be actual (through lessened production) or relative (through increased demand on the part of the tissues).
   - Ratio of alpha to beta cells is responsible for the diabetic state.
   - Prolonged overactivity of the islets, as in continued hyperglycaemia from any cause may lead to work-exhaustion of the beta cells (or burning out of cells).
   - Certain cytotoxic agents (Alloxan and streptozotocin) destroy β cells and hence are used experimentally to produce diabetes in animals (Alloxan-Diabetes).

DIFFERENCE BETWEEN TWO TYPES OF DIABETES

Insulin dependent (Juvenile onset)	*Insulin insensitive (Maturity onset)*
1. Seen before fourteen years of age	Seen after forty years
2. Family history of diabetes uncommon	Commonly there is family history of diabetes
3. Patients are insulin sensitive	Patients are insulin resistant
4. Low or no insulin secretion	Initially low or increased insulin secretion followed by decrease
5. Ketosis seen, if kept untreated	Ketosis - often not seen
6. Patients are underweight	Patients are normal or over-weight

REGULATION OF INSULIN SECRETION

Following are the factors taking part in its regulation :

i. ***Blood glucose level*:** Blood glucose level and insulin secretion exert a negative feedback control on one another. It has been observed that when glucose level of blood perfusing the pancreas is increased to higher values (or towards higher side), the insulin concentration of pancreatic venous flow shows a marked increase. On the contrary, when glucose level of perfusing blood is normal or low, the insulin level in pancreatic venous flow is also low. β cells of islets express specific receptor that recognise glucose and respond by synthesis and secretion of insulin via second messenger. Another view holds that β cells are directly stimulated to produce insulin by glucose or other metabolites.

ii. ***Diet:*** Insulin secretion is stimulated by administration of certain amino acids (like arginine, leucine, etc.) as well as by fatty acids (β-hydroxy-butyric acid, acetoacetic acid).

iii. ***GIT hormones*:** If glucose is fed orally, it will cause profound secretion of insulin; as compared with parenteral administration of glucose. The same is also true with administration of above mentioned amino acids and fatty acids. This confirms that GIT hormones (gastrin, secretin, pancreozymin, cholecystokinin, etc.) tend to stimulate insulin secretion. This action is mediated through gut factor (GIP); which is now recognised as enteroglucagon which is secreted from gut on a carbohydrate diet.

iv. ***Autonomic nerves***:
- When blood sugar level decreases, sympathetic nuclei of hypothalamus is stimulated, which in turn releases adrenaline from adrenal medulla as well as from sympathetic nerve endings. This adrenaline activates adenylcylase enzyme, which converts much of ATP into cyclic adenylic acid; which activates glucose-6-phosphatase and under its effect glycogenolysis in liver cells is stimulated. All this chain of reaction results into conversion of glycogen into glucose which then diffuses into blood to raise blood glucose concentration.
- Right vagus supplies the pancreas, so its stimulation leads to increased insulin release. This effect is increased by acetylcholine/cholinergic agents while it is inhibited by atropine.
- Controversy is that administration of epinephrine inhibits insulin release via interaction with a receptors.

v. ***Oral hypoglycaemic agents***:
- Tolbutamide and sulfonylurea are orally effective agents which exert their effects of increasing insulin release, through; closing ATP sensitive K^+ channels on β cells as well as by increasing tissue sensitivity to insulin. These agents are said to be ineffective in IDDM and after pancreatectomy.
- While phenformin, biguanides, etc. (oral hypoglycaemic agents) cause glucose utilisation. Their mechanism of action includes inhibition of oxidative metabolism of glucose and increasing anaerobic glycolysis within cells, decreasing glucose absorption from GIT Their side effect includes lacto-acidosis.

vi. ***Potassium depletion***: Decreases insulin secretion. This is the reason that thiazide group of diuretics which on their administration cause loss of K^+ and Na^+ in urine, decreases glucose tolerance and therefore diabetes is worsened. Besides K^+ depleting effects, pancreatic islet cell damage is also responsible for it. Insulin causes hyper-polarisation of plasma membrane. In vivo, it alters distribution of Na^+ and K^+ between extra- and intracellular spaces. It may directly act on membrane bound Na^+/K^+ ATPase. It increases cytosolic Ca^{2+} level by releasing Ca^{2+} from bound form within the cell.

vii. ***Cyclic AMP***: Increases insulin secretion by increasing intracellular Ca^{2+}.

viii. ***Exercise:*** Does the same effect as of insulin. The persons who are regularly doing exercise, they should take either extra calories or reduce their insulin dosage. This is a treatment of diabetes. Entry of glucose is enhanced into cell by exercise, under anaerobic conditions.

GLUCAGON

i. It is a small protein, having a molecular weight of 3482 and is composed of 29 amino acids. It is produced by A (alpha) cells of islets of Langerhans of pancreas and also from upper gastrointestinal tract. In A cells human pre-proglucagon is found (other sites are brain and lower GIT) and is said to be a product of mRNA.

ii. ***Metabolism***: It enters the portal circulation and is first presented to the liver. About 5-10 minutes is its half-life in circulation. Portal : systemic ratio of it is 1.5 : 1. Its basal rate of secretion is 100-150 µg/day. It is mainly degraded by the liver tissue. This explains its rise in blood level in the diseases like liver cirrhosis in which decreased hepatic degradation takes place.

iii. ***Actions***
- Its main effect is glycogenolysis in the liver which in turn increases blood sugar concentration. It is therefore called hyperglycaemic factor.
- Glucagon increases hepatic gluconeogenesis.
- It does not cause glycogenolysis in extrahepatic tissues - a distinction from catecholamines.
- It enhances lipolysis in adipose tissue. On glucagon administration there is a sharp increase in blood glucose level and consequent rise in insulin levels. These override any tendency of glucagon to mobilise free fatty acids. Any way, its lipolytic activity leads to increased ketogenesis.
- Its large exogenous doses leads to exert positive ionotropic action on heart, but it does not alter myocardial excitability; of course, it is mediated through myocardial cyclic AMP. It should be remembered that it plays no role in regulating cardiac function. Due to increased hepatic deamination of amino acid performed by glucagon, it also exerts calorigenic action. It also stimulates the secretion of growth hormone, pancreatic somatostatin.

iv. ***Regulation of secretion***:
- Hypoglycaemia stimulates and hyperglycaemia suppresses glucagon release.

- Glucagon secretion is stimulated by amino acids, since these are the amino acids that are converted to glucose in the liver under the influence of glucagon.
- Its secretion is increased during starvation—perhaps it is an attempt to maintain a normal blood glucose concentration. It reaches at its climax on third day of fast—at the time of maximum neoglucogenesis.
- A glucagon stimulatory factor is released from mucosa of GIT Gastrin and CCK stimulates while secretin inhibits release of glucagon.
- On stimulating sympathetic nerves, glucagon secretion is stimulated. This effect is mediated via β-adrenergic receptors and cyclic AMP. Vagal stimulation also increases glucagon secretion.

INSULIN AND LIPIDS

- It stimulates fatty acids biosynthesis.
- It is the key hormone monitoring the availability of glucose - suppressing release of FFA when glucose is available and permitting rapid mobilisation when glucose level falls and lipids are needed to provide energy.
- It increases activity of enzyme lipase through cyclic AMP (by inhibiting its conversion from lipase b to lipase a). By this, it favours the uptake and deposition of triglycerides from VLDL and chylomicrons into adipose tissue.

FACTORS INFLUENCING INSULIN RELEASE

- *Stimulators:* Glucose, amino acids, GIP, ketone bodies, glucagon, parasympathetic stimulation, cyclic AMP, salicylates, β-adrenergic stimulation.
- *Inhibitors:* Somatostatin, α-adrenergic stimulation, diazoxide, prostaglandins, alloxan, diphenylhydantoin, sympathetic stimulation.

GLUCAGON SECRETION

- *Stimulators:* Amino acid, gastrin + CCK, cortisol, exercise, infection, acetylcholine, stresses, β-adrenergic stimulators, growth hormone, glucocorticoid.
- *Inhibitors:* Glucose, somatostatin, secretin, insulin, ketones, FFA, α-adrenergic stimulators.

INSULIN ACTIONS

- *Liver:* Decreased glucose output due to decreased neo-glucogenesis and increased glycogen synthesis, increased protein and increased lipid synthesis, decreased ketogenesis.
- *Muscle:* Increased glucose entry, increased amino acid uptake, increased protein synthesis in ribosomes, decreased protein catabolism increased ketone uptake, increased glycogen synthesis
- *Adipose tissue:* Increased fatty acid synthesis, increased glucose entry, increased triglyceride deposition, activation of lipase, increased K^+ uptake, inhibition of hormone sensitive lipase.
- *Others:* Increased cellular growth.

OTHER ISLET CELL HORMONES

a. *Somatostatin:*

i. It is a tetradecapeptide hormone and is a 14-amino acid peptide with a carboxy terminal cysteine residue in disulphide linkage to another cysteine residue at position 3.

ii. It is found in D cells of pancreatic islets.

iii. It inhibits the secretion of insulin, glucagon and pancreatic polypeptide. It, however, inhibits to the intestinal absorption of glucose. Since it tends to inhibit secretions of two antagonistic hormones; its clear-cut action on metabolism cannot be predicted.

iv. It inhibits release of growth hormone and TSH, ACTH and prolactine from anterior pituitary. It also tends to inhibit the gastric acid and pepsin secretion, secretion of pancreatic enzymes, intestinal motility and absorption, secretion of GIT hormones like VIP/pancreozymin/secretine, etc. It can therefore develop gallstones and dyspepsia.

v. It is first isolated from hypothalamus. It is widely distributed throughout central and peripheral nervous system. It acts as a spinal transmitter, i.e. it plays a role in neurotransmission. It can also be traced from mucous membrane of GI tract.

vi. It is regulated by many factors. Glucose, amino acids (arginine/leucine) when infused stimulate its secretion. Glucagon also stimulates its production. Epinephrine (via α-adrenergic mechanism) inhibits while acetylcholine stimulates its secretion. GIT hormones like cholecystokinin-P pancreozymin increase its secretion. Due to inhibition of CCK secretion contraction of gallbladder diminished which aids in precipitation of gallstones.

b. *Pancreatic polypeptide (PP):*

i. It is a linear polypeptide containing 36 amino acid residue and is produced by F cells in the islets.

ii. Its stimulants include protein meal, muscular exercise, hypoglycaemia. Arginine and leucine when given orally stimulate its secretion but their intravenous administration is ineffective which suggests the interference of GIT hormones as mediator. Its secretion is decreased by somatostatin and intravenous glucose.

iii. It mainly causes glycogenolysis in liver without altering blood glucose level; of course, level of plasma glycerol and free fatty acids decline.
iv. Its plasma level is 60-100 pg/ml.
v. Its secretion is said to be controlled by cholinergic nerves. Atropine decreases its plasma level.

TYPES OF DIABETES MELLITUS

i. *Maturity onset type (Non-insulin dependent diabetes NIDDM, ketosis resistant diabetes)*
It is having its onset generally over the age of 40 years. It is having insidious onset, and is rarely associated with ketosis. There is impaired insulin secretion as well as insulin resistance specially in skeletal muscles. Patient being of stocky built and overweight if not actually obese. It is not associated with total loss of the ability to secrete insulin. There is a strong genetic component in this type. Patients with this type of disorder also have a deficiency of GLUT 4 glucose transporters in insulin sensitive tissues.
ii. *Early onset (Juvenile type, insulin dependent IDDM)*: It is seen before the age of 25 years and is with the deficiency of circulating insulin due to failure of pancreas to produce enough insulin in thin patient and a proneness to ketoacidosis. It is an autoimmune disease, with the fact that anti B cell antibodies causing destruction of B cells. Of course, a genetic factor predisposes to the development of antibodies.

GLUCOSE-TOLERANCE TEST (GTT)

a. **Preparing the patient** He should be taking carbohydrate rich diet for three days prior to the test. All drugs affecting carbohydrate metabolism should be discontinued for at least two days. He should not do any strenuous exercise on previous day of the test. He should observe an overnight fast and avoid smoking.
b. **Procedure** Call the patient in the morning. A fasting sample of blood is drawn and also urine is collected. Then person is given 75 gm glucose dissolved in 300 ml water, orally to drink, in about five minutes. Blood and urine samples are collected at 30 minutes interval for at least 2 hours. Blood samples are estimated for glucose while urine samples are qualitatively tested for glucose.
c. **Interpretation** (i) Normally fasting level is 75–110 mg per cent; with oral glucose load, concentration increases to <140 mg/dl in less than one hour, which returns to normal by 2 hours. No sugar detected in urine. (ii) 140–200 mg/dl impaired glucose tolerance (2 hours glucose level).

DIABETES MELLITUS—ANOTHER SILENT KILLER

The complications other than acidosis + coma include:

a. Micro-vascular abnormalities → Proliferative scarring of retine - diabetic retinopathy and of kidney diabetic nephropathy. It is due to overgrowth of blood vessels.
b. Micro-vascular abnormalities → It is because of accelerated atherosclerosis which is due to increased LDL in plasma. It finally terminates fatally in myocardial infarction and strokes.
c. Neuropathic abnormalities → Named as diabetic neuropathy which involves ANS and peripheral nerves. It along with above changes reduces body resistance towards infection which terminate into ulceration and gangrene specially in feet.
   i. Intracellular hyperglycaemia $\xrightarrow[\text{reductase}]{\text{Aldose}}$ increased sorbitol formation in cell → reduced Na^+K^+ ATPase.
   ii. Intracellular hyperglycaemia → formation of AGEs (advanced glycosylation end products) → Blood vessels are damaged + response of WBC towards infection is impaired.

BIBLIOGRAPHY

1. Arimura A. Recent progress in somatostatin research. Biomed, Res 1981;2:233-37.
2. Foster DW, MC, Garry JD. The metabolic derangements and treatment of diabetic ketoacidosis. New Eng J Med 1983;309:159.
3. Gerich JE. Oral hypoglycaemic agents. New Eng J Med 1989;321: 1231.
4. Hazel Wood. Synthesis, storage and significance of pancreatic polypeptide in vertebrates. In islets of Langerhans edited by S. J. Coopsstein and D. Watkins : New York Academic Press. 1981
5. Hers HG. The control of glycogen metabolism in the liver. Annu Rev Biochem 1976;45;167-89.
6. Horwitz DL, et al. Circulating serum C peptide. New Eng J Med 1976;295:207.
7. Hougen TJ, et al. Insulin effects on monovalent cation transport Na^+/K^+ ATPase activity. Amer J Phy 1978;234:C 59.
8. Koerker DJ, et al. Somatostatin: hypothalamic inhibitor of endocrine pancreas. Science 1974;184:482-84.
9. La Raia PJ, et al. Glucagon effect on adenosine 3′-5′ monophosphate in rat heart. Amer J Phy 1968;215:968.
10. Morglian HE. Identification of mobile carrier mediated sugar transport system in muscle. J Biol Chem 1964;239:369.
11. Park CR, et al. Mediated transport of glucose in mammals and its regulation. J Gen Physiol 1968;52:286.
12. Philips LS, et al. Somatomedins. New Eng J Med 1980;302:371-38.
13. Pilkis SJ, et al. Hormonal regulation of hepatic gluconeogenesis and glycolysis. Ann Rev Biochem 1988;57:755-83.
14. Unger RH L. Orci. Glucagon and A cell. New Eng J Med 1981;304: 1581.
15. Yen SS, et al. Effect of somatostatin in patients with acromegaly suppression of GH - prolactin insulin and glucose levels. New Eng J Med 1974;290:933-938.

46 Calcium-Phosphorus Control: Parathyroid

They are most difficult organs to be traced on account of their small size, as well as resemblance to the lobules of fat.

These glands are minute structures, not more than 5 mm in diameter, four or more in number; inferior group may be embedded in the substance of thyroid. Three main sets of cells are found:

a. ***Chief cells***: Are the only cells until puberty, have scanty cytoplasm and a relatively large and deeply stained nucleus.
b. ***Oxyphil cells***: Appear after puberty and increase in number with age. They are rich in phospholipids. It contains acidophilic granules. They are much more numerous in women. They don't appear to elaborate the parathyroid hormone.
c. ***Water clear cells*** *(Wasserhelle cells = German)*: Appear in very small number after puberty. They appear to be derived from chief cells. They are rich in glycogen which is soluble in water.

ACTIONS

- It helps to maintain normal blood calcium level.
- If this gland is removed, blood Ca^{2+} level falls.
- It regulates the excretion of inorganic phosphate in the urine.
- It mobilises calcium from the bones, so it raises blood calcium level.
- This hormone was discovered in 1925 by Collip and is polypeptide in nature.
- It elevates serum alkaline phosphatase activity.
- It affects renal tubular reabsorption of Ca and P.
- It increases absorption of Ca and P from intestine and lowers serum phosphate.

CALCIUM METABOLISM

- It is an indispensable mineral and is a constituent of all animal fluids and solid tissues.
- *Distribution:* It constitutes 2 per cent of the weight of adult body. In skeleton (90%), muscles 8 mg/100 gm of net weight, plasma (9-10.5 mg/100 ml), blood (4.5-6 mg per 100 ml), CSF (5 mg/100 ml). Negligible amounts are deposited in skeleton before fifth month of intra-uterine life.
- The concentration of plasma in the blood gives the total concentration in the blood, which is 9–11 mg per 100 ml (4.5–5.2 mEq/l). It is present in the plasma in three forms - ionised, complexed, and protein bound. The protein bound is non-diffusible and attached to albumin and globulin fractions of plasma proteins (mainly albumin) in the proportion of 0.84 mg/gm of protein. The other two states, i.e. ionised and complexed are diffusible.
- Although the three fractions of calcium in the plasma are believed to be in equilibrium with one another, the level of ionised calcium is regarded as most immediately related to the activity of parathyroid gland. The ionised calcium in plasma is raised in hyperparathyroidism, and in this condition, there is a reduced ability for plasma proteins to bind calcium.
- A raised ionised calcium is more significant than a raised total calcium, and is the cause of hypercalcaemia. The complexed calcium fraction is combined with citrate and phosphate, and level will be raised in renal failure.
- The non-diffusible calcium, varies with protein concentration of the plasma. Lymph, which has a lower concentration of protein than plasma, has also a lower calcium content. The CSF calcium, which is practically protein free, is entirely in diffusible form and has a concentration approximately equal to that of diffusible fraction in the plasma. Therefore, the CSF calcium is taken as an index of diffusible fraction of plasma calcium because the CSF is an ultrafiltrate.

- The function of the parathyroids is to regulate the metabolism of calcium, phosphorus and bone. At a given pH, there is a strong tendency for the solubility product of calcium and phosphorus to remain constant—the one rises and the other falls and this constancy depends upon the parathyroid hormone—***the Parathormone***.
- Normally it is poorly absorbed by GIT However, vitamin D promotes an active transport system. Normal intake is 1 gm/day. Absorption of phosphate ion is easy.
- About 9/10 part of calcium is excreted in faeces, 1/10th part in urine. About 90 per cent of calcium is reabsorbed in tubules.
- Phosphate is a renal threshold substance, i.e. when its concentration in plasma is below the critical value of about 1 mmol/litre, no phosphate is lost into urine because all in glomerular filtration is reabsorbed. Thus, the kidney regulates phosphate concentration in extracellular fluid by altering the rate of phosphate excretion in accordance with plasma phosphate concentration. Phosphate excretion by kidney is greatly increased by parathyroid hormone.

FACTORS AFFECTING CALCIUM METABOLISM

1. *Increased:* Acidity in stomach, bile and bile salts, hypocalcaemia (low intake of calcium, pregnancy, lactation), parathormone, growth hormone, high protein diet.
2. *Decreased:* Presence of alkalies, reduced secretion of bile and bile salts, hypercalcaemia (high Ca intake), excess of inorganic phosphate.

MAGNESIUM METABOLISM

- Human body contains about 20 gm of it; majority of it is found in muscle and bone.
- Its normal concentration is 1.8–2.4 mg per cent of which some is protein bound.
- Hypomagnesaemia also leads to tetany. Besides its symptoms, it is characterised by mental confusion. It is seen in hyperparathyroidism.
- A low calcium intake will increase magnesium absorption from ileum and vice versa. Both these minerals are absorbed by a common pathway (involving a common carrier system). Vitamin D does not play any role in its absorption.
- Parathormone increases the absorption of it from the intestine and calcitonin has reverse effect (Care and Keynes, 1964).

PARATHORMONE—CHEMISTRY

- It is a single chain polypeptide consisting of 84 amino acids.
- Its molecular weight is 9,500.
- Initially synthesised in chief cells as pre pro-hormone.
- Degradation is rapid. Half-life is 18 minutes.
- Oxidation of the hormone by hydrogen per oxide mainly destroys its biological activity, but this may be restored by reduction with cysteine in acid at elevated temperatures (Teshjian, et al. 1963).

HYPERCALCAEMIA—AN OVERVIEW

- Lassitude, fatigue, backache, weakness, difficulty in walking, waddling gait, constipation, poor appetite, nausea, vomiting, slow pulse rate with shortening of QT interval of ECG are vague symptoms. Many of these are due to decreased muscular excitability. Increases in ionised calcium raises the electrical resistance of the cell membrane and increases end plate potential. It may be due to hyperparathyroidism.
- The other causes are: faulty technique in collecting blood, osteolytic bone tumours, myeloma, malignant tumours of bone which secrete a substance like parathormone, overdoses of vitamin D, sensitivity to vitamin D, bed rest in Paget's disease, peptic ulcers. Emergency parathyroidectomy is useful. Parathyroid crisis may occur with calcium level up to 17 mg per cent.

VITAMIN D: CALCIUM METABOLISM: AN OVERVIEW

- Most important is vitamin D_3 (cholecalciferol) which is formed in the skin as a result of irradiation of 7-dehydrocholesterol (a substance normally found in the skin) by ultraviolet rays from the sun. So the sun is said to be the richest source of vitamin D.
  7-dehydrocholesterol $\rightarrow$ vitamin D_3 (cholecalciferol)
- This cholecalciferol is converted into 25-hydroxycholecalciferol which occurs in the liver. This process is self-limiting by feedback mechanism. By this feedback, conservation of vitamin D becomes possible in liver for future use.

  Vitamin $D_3 \xrightarrow{\text{Liver}}$ 25-hydroxycholecalciferol
- This, 25-hydroxycholecalciferol is converted into 1, 25-dihydroxycholecalciferol which is the most active form of vitamin D. This conversion takes place in proximal tubules of kidney which explains the importance of kidneys in effectiveness of vitamin D. Furthermore, this conversion needs parathormone without which this conversion does not take place. So parathyroid hormone exerts a potent effect on functional aspect of vitamin D.

  25-hydroxy-cholecalciferol $\xrightarrow{\text{Parathormone-kidney}}$ 1, 25 Dihydroxy-cholecalciferol

- This 25-hydroxycholecalciferol forms calcium binding protein in intestine epithelial cells. This facilitates calcium transport into cell cytoplasm. So rate of calcium absorption is directly varying with quantity of this binding protein.
- This 1, 25-dihydroxycholecalciferol also leads to the formation of alkaline phosphatase in epithelial cells; and calcium stimulated ATPase in brush border of epithelial cells.
- 1, 25-dihydroxycholecalciferol → calcium binding protein + alkaline phosphatase + calcium stimulated ATPase binding protein → increased absorption of calcium binding protein → plasma calcium ion concentration (controlled by parathyroid).

RICKETS

Occurring in children due to deficiency of vitamin D which affects reabsorption of Ca and P from renal tubules which leads to inadequate mineralization of growing bones. Its manifestations are: collapse of chest wall, kyphosis (forward bending, excessive curvature of spine with convexity backwards), lordosis (excessive curvature of lumbar spines), hepato-splenomegaly. In advanced states tetany may result, bowing of hands and legs, Harrison's sulcus due to pulling of diaphragm inwards a groove in rib formed.

OSTEMOALACIA (RICKETS IN ADULT)

Causes

a. *Deficiency of vitamin D:* Low intake, inadequate synthesis in skin, reduced absorption in intestine.
b. *Renal causes:* Renal failure (chronic), renal tubular acidosis.

Characterised by pain, bone and muscle tenderness, waddling gait + myopathy; hypoglycaemia (feet are wide apart; duck walk) may lead to tetany.

OSTEOPOROSIS

- Loss of bone matrix and minerals and due to disturbed homeostasis, i.e. decreased bone formation and increased bone resorption.
- Due to these high risk of fracture.
- Hips, vertebra are commonly affected.
- Common in women at the age of 60 years.
- Risk factors include: heredity, excess intake of alcohol/caffeine/protein/steroids/smoking, early menopause/ovariectomy, sedentary life, endocrine disorders like hypothyroidism/Cushing's disease/hypogonadism/acromegaly.

HYPERPARATHYROIDISM

- Primary hyperparathyroidism may be caused by adenoma, carcinoma, etc. Usually, water clear cells are involved but chief cells are also influenced.
- Secondary hyperparathyroidism is associated with secondary hyperplasia which results from calcium deprivation, and in turn may produce an excess of hormone causing further decalcification. The chief organs affected due to excess production of this hormone are:

i. ***Bones***: Decalcification is the main effect. This is followed by osteoporosis, i.e. removal of decalcified organic material by osteoclasts—the phagocytes of the bone.

ii. ***Gastrointestinal tract***: Hypercalcaemia is responsible for abdominal symptoms. Increased Ca^{2+} concentration in the sympathetic ganglia impedes the transmission of afferent stimuli and diminish their efferent discharge which result in constipation. It is associated with gastric atony, dyspepsia, nausea and vomiting. Peptic ulcer usually develops in some cases which is duodenal. Indigestion may be due to pancreatitis which may be acute, recurrent or relapsing.

iii. ***Renal changes***: When disease proves fatal, death is due to renal failure. Renal insufficiency itself gives rise to secondary hyperparathyroidism, which in turn may be responsible for further renal damage. A fine deposit of calcium occurs in the renal tubules and the interstitial tissue of pyramids. Renal calculi may develop with accompanying pyelonephritis and renal insufficiency. There may be calcification of tubular epithelium and the tubular basement membrane.

iv. ***Biochemical changes***: The calcium extracted from the bones appears in the blood in large amount, and this may elevate blood calcium level (from 10 mg% normal to even 20 mg%). The blood phosphorus (normal 1.3 mg) is below normal (1.1 mg) because the renal threshold for phosphorus is lowered by excess of parathyroid hormone. The urinary excretion of calcium is greatly increased so that there is a negative calcium balance. Metastatic calcification is a natural accompaniment of the extensive decalcification of the skeleton.

HYPOPARATHYROIDISM

The clinical manifestation is *Tetany*. It can be produced in variety of ways, all of which are connected directly or indirectly with low calcium up to 6 mg per cent from normal 9 to 11 mg per cent. Pure parathyroid tetany is best seen when parathyroids have been removed. There is a marked drop in blood calcium and a decreased excretion of calcium in the urine. The blood phosphorus is normal or raised. The tissues are depleted of calcium and tetany develops owing to increased neuromuscular irritability and this hyperexcitability is shown by twitching of the muscles, convulsions. The low calcium is the key to the clinical picture, for it facilitates the transmission of nervous impulses across the myoneural junction, as a result a great increase in neuromuscular excitability.

Its main cause is lowered level of calcium in blood and tissue fluid. This increases the proportion of neuro-excitatory factors like Na, K, etc. which causes tetany.

Features

- General convulsions.
- Slight pressure on limb may cause—flexion of elbow and wrist; flexion of fingers at metacarpophalangeal but extension at interphalangeal joint. Thumb in the palm and finger tips drawn together; feet extended and plantar flexed ***(Corpo pedal spasm or Trousseau's sign)***.
- Spasm of glottis with inspiratory stridor ***(Laryngismus-stridulus)***.
- Taping of facial nerve near styloid process may cause facial spasm ***(Chvostek's sign)***.
- Increased excitability of motor nerves to electric current ***(Erb's sign)***.
- When kidney functions are failed → reabsorption of calcium by tubules is diminished → more excretion or less blood level of calcium → tetany.
- Deficiency of vitamin D (Rickets) → diminished absorption of calcium by GIT → tetany.
- Malabsorption syndrome of intestine → diminished absorption of calcium by intestine → tetany.
- Alkalaemia (Vomiting/excess intake of alkali) → alters ionic balance → decreasing ionic Ca^{2+} → tetany.

PHYSIO-PATHOGENESIS: TETANY

- As ancient as 1909, Maccallum pointed out that plasma calcium was depressed in tetany and condition was immediately relieved by intravenous administration of calcium. At that time, it was believed to be due to some endogenous toxic metabolite (guanidine) which was destroyed by parathyroids but after parathyroidectory this substance accumulates.
- Calcium deficiency is the direct cause of this neuromuscular hyperexcitability in such conditions. It is generally accepted that determining factor in the tetany production is the concentration of ionised calcium in the plasma and extracellular fluids of the body rather than total calcium concentration. The increased neuromuscular excitability appears to be due to a change in cell membrane potential with decrease in ionised calcium level, lowering the electrical resistance of the membrane and reducing end plate potential.
- A reciprocal relationship exists between phosphate and calcium concentration in plasma. Hyperphosphataemia therefore undoubtedly increase the severity of tetany, but it does not play primary role in its development.
- It is rapidly abolished by IV injection of Ca, gluconate. Parathormone relieves tetany but only for a few hours and should be administered parenterally. But patient develops adaptation from it so it is of not much use. So vitamin D by mouth with calcium supplementation will control neuromuscular symptoms. But this regime is not safe since it may cause hypercalciuria and thus kidney stones as well as vitamin D toxicity may also develop.
- ***Idiopathic and infantile tetany***: Causes are—defective parathyroid functions, hypocalcaemia. It may occur in the first week of life specially in premature infants and those born by diabetic mothers. It is characterised by paroxysms of generalised hyperactivity rather than by spasms of muscles; the first symptom is laryngeal stridor. Tetany of infant is generally an accompaniment of rickets.
- By citrate, the EDTA and phosphate administration tetany may be produced since they reduce the level of ionised calcium as this happens with very large transfusion of citrated blood. The EDTA is a chelating agent.
- ***Milk fever***: In cows, sometimes tetany (hypocal caemia) develops after calving as a result of loss of calcium in the milk. Condition is treated by intravenous injection of calcium.
- ***Accouncheur's hand of tetany***: The feet are extended at ankles and toes are plantar flexed. Spasm of eyes muscles may be seen and occasional retention of urine occurs.
- ***Tetany in dogs*** (extensively studied) characterised by—fall in plasma calcium (from 10 to 6 mg%) a rise in plasma inorganic phosphate (from 5 to 9 mg%), increased excitability of skeletal muscles to galvanic stimulus, reduced urinary excretion of calcium and phosphate, fibrillary twitching of muscles followed by tonic or clonic muscular contraction, head is dorsiflexed. Jaws are clenched; limbs are either stuffy

extended or jerk violently, rapid noisy breathing, muscle phosphocreatine is reduced, death is because of asphyxia through spasm of laryngeal/thoracic muscles.

CONTROL OF PARATHYROID SECRETION

- It is the blood calcium level which controls.
- Low blood calcium level → stimulates parathyroid secretion and hypertrophy of gland.
- High blood calcium level → decreases parathyroid secretion.

BONE PHYSIOLOGY

- It is composed of organic matrix (30%) and bone salts (70%). Former is made up of collagen fibres (95%) + ground substance; which is made up of ECF + proteoglycans specially hyaluronic acid and chondriotin sulphate.
- Collagen fibres have great tensile strength.
- ***Bone salts***: Made up of calcium and phosphate (hydroxyapatite) - $Ca_{10}(PO_4)_6(OH)_2$. Each crystal measuring 400 (Long) × 10-30 (thick) × 100 (wide) Angstroms in dimensions. The Ca/p ratio varies between 1.3 and 2.0 (2.2:1).
- ***Concrete bony structure***: Tensile strength by collagen fibres while calcium salts provide great compressional strength to bone. Hydroxyapatite crystal lies adjacent to each segment of fibre, bound tightly to it.
- Hydroxyapetite crystals fail to precipitate in spite of supersaturation of ions because of presence of pyrophosphate in plasma which acts as inhibitor.
- ***Bone calcification:*** Osteoblasts → secretion of collagen molecules and ground substance $\xrightarrow{\text{Polymerisation}}$ Collagen fibres → osteoid (a cartilage-like material in which calcium salt will soon precipitate) → osteocytes → calcium salts begin to precipitate on the surface of collagen fibres which is at first appearing at interval along each collagen fibre thus forming nidi (nest-like structures) which rapidly grow and multiply into finally hydroxyapatite crystals.
- ***Osteoblasts***: Bone is continuously being deposited by these cells. They are found on outer surface of bones and in bone cavities.
- ***Osteoclasts***: Bone is continuously absorbed by these cells, which are large phagocytic multinucleated cells. They project villi-like process which secretes proteolytic enzymes from their lysosomes as well as acids like lactic and citric from their mitochondria and secretory vesicles. These either digest or dissolve the bone matrix. They also induce phagocytosis of minute bone matrix particles and release them in the blood.
- ***Osteocytes***: Main cells of developed bone derived from matured osteoblasts, small flat and rounded cells embedded in bone lacunae. Neighbouring cells form tight junctions. These run into canaliculi and ramify throughout bone matrix, they maintain the exchange of calcium between bone and extracellular fluid, they maintain the bone as living tissue.
- ***Homeostasis***: Bone deposition and absorption process is well maintained to keep total mass of bone constant.
- Once osteoclast begins to develop, it eats the bone within 2 to 3 weeks making a tunnel having diameter of 0.2 to 1 mm. By this time, osteoblast appears which continues the formation of bone, forming the concentric layers to fill that tunnel back. This is essential because it has to withstand stress and old bone requires new matrix.
- ***Laboratory finding***: Osteoblasts secrete large quantities of alkaline phosphatase which may diffuse into blood. So blood alkaline phosphatase level is increased which is an indicator of osteoblastic activity. ***Role of vitamin D***: In smaller quantities it promotes bone calcification by increasing absorption of Ca and P from intestine. Sometimes it enhances mineralisation of bone. In large doses, it causes absorption of bone. In absence of vitamin D, the effect of parathyroid hormone in causing bone absorption is greatly reduced or prevented.

BIBLIOGRAPHY

1. Barnes DM. Close encounters with an osteoclast. Science 1987;236:914.
2. Blaustein MP. Physiological effects of endogenous ouabain: Control of intracellular Ca^{2+} stores and cell responsiveness. Amer J Phy 1993;242:C 1367.
3. Garel JM. Hormonal control of calcium metabolism during reproductive cycles in mammals. Phy Rev 1987;67:1.
4. Gross M, et al. Physiology and biochemistry of Vitamin D dependent calcium binding proteins. Amer J Phy 1990;259:F 195.
5. Habener JF, et al. Parathyroid hormone : Biochemical aspect of biosynthesis, secretion, action and metabolism. Phy Rev 1984;64:985.
6. Inesi G. Mechanism of calcium transport. Ann Rev Phy 1985;47:573.
7. Nijweide PJ, et al. Cells of bone: Proliferation, differentiation and hormonal regulation. Phy Rev 1986;66:855.
8. Riggs BL, et al. The prevention and treatment of osteoporosis. New Eng J Med 1992;327:620.
9. Wasserman RH, et al. Calcium transport proteins, calcium absorption and vitamin D. Ann Rev Phy 1983;45:375.
10. Wozney JM, et al. Novel regulators of bone formation: Molecular clones and activities. Science 1988;242:1528.

$\xrightarrow{\text{Polymerisation}}$

Local Hormones

Apart from endocrine glands there are number of tissues in the body, which liberate chemical substances, which act in strictly localised way. They are local hormones. They are active near their site of origin. They are never transmitted distally.

HISTAMINE

a. It is liberated when tissues are damaged.
b. Functions:
   - Dilatation of capillaries while arterioles are also dilated. It increases capillary permeability which results into leakage of fluid causing oedema. It causes flushing of face, fall in systolic blood pressure, tachycardia. Meningeal vessels are also dilated leading to headache.
   - It stimulates secretion of gastric acid and pepsin mainly and to a lesser extent of pancreatic/salivary/sucus entericus, etc.
   - It increases tone of smooth muscles (intestinal, uterine, bronchiolar). It precipitates attack of bronchial spasm in asthma.
   - It is responsible for anaphylactic shock.
   - Its release is associated with itching and pain.
   - It may be concerned in maintenance of sustained growth of embryonic tissues and rapid wound healing by tissue regeneration.

c. It is destroyed (oxidised) by enzyme histaminase.
d. ***Stimulators for release are***: Injection of foreign protein, physical stimuli (injury, cold, pressure), chemicals (morphine, pathedene, tubocurine, etc.).
e. ***Antihistaminics:*** These are agents which antagonise the actions of histamine. They act by the mechanism of competitive inhibition. Here the drugs compete for the receptor sites where histamine is normally bound. In this way, the actions of histamine is blocked on blood vessels, smooth muscles, itch receptor, capillary permeability, etc. By these antihistaminics, only histamine is inhibited; not SRS-A (slow-reacting substance of anophylaxis).
f. ***Anaphylactic shock:*** When antigens react with antibodies, histamine is released and a shock-like condition develops. These antibodies pass into circulation. If second intravenous injection of the same substance is given, then it produces severe reactions which differs from species to species. In bronchial asthma, along with histamine, SRS-A is also released (slow-reacting substance of anophylaxis) which gives rise to bronchospasm in bronchial asthma.

SEROTONIN (5-hydroxytryptamine; Enteramine)

- Majority is found in platelets, intestinal mucosa, brain, mast cells, etc.
- Blood normally contains 0.1 µg/ml during coagulation only a part is excreted in urine.
- *Actions—Heart*—Stimulation of heart constricting blood vessels. On I.V. administration → hypertension + tachycardia- followed by hypotension and bradycardia through baro-and chemoreceptors.
- This (5-HT) is released in serotoninergic nerve endings in brain. It does not cross blood-brain barrier (BBB), so rarely have action on brain. If it is injected into cerebral ventricles, it may produce a lethargic state.
- Its precursor 5-hydroxytryptophane can cross blood-brain barrier, which is then converted into 5-HT by action of enzyme 5-hydroxytryptophane-decarboxylase present in brain and that is associated with induction of sleep.

Respiration

Produces hyperpnoea—(reflex apnoea also). Produces bronchospasm and so can precipitate an attack of bronchial asthma.

Kidney

Antidiuretic action. Ureteric spasm → stoppage of urinary flow.

Smooth Muscles

Tone increases. Stimulates intestinal peristalsis leading to evacuation of intestines.

Nervous system: Produces pain through stimulating free nerve endings. It does not cross blood-brain barrier. It plays role in maintenance of mood and normal behaviour.

BRADYKININ

- These are polypeptides containing 9–11 amino acid residues.
- They are formed in lymph, plasma, extracellular fluid.

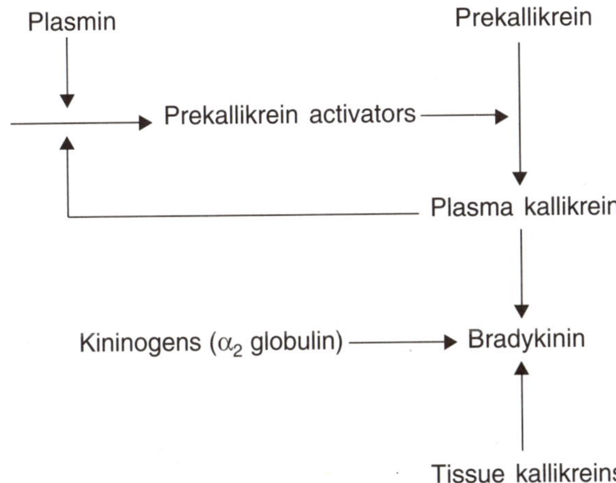

Mechanism of formation of bradykinin

- Bradykinin is inhibited by tissue carboxypeptidase as well as by kallikrein inhibitors present in body. There are two kininases (enzymes destroying the kinins):
  - — Kininase I—carboxypeptidase.
  - — Kininase II—is a converting enzyme which converts angiotensin I into angiotensin II—found in lungs.
- This is the substance responsible for vasodilatation during secretion of sweat, salivary, exocrine pancreas secretion.
- Actions:
  - — Increase motility and dilatation of vascular smooth muscle, which result in hypotension, flushing, increased capillary permeability, tachycardia, increased cardiac output, etc. (similarity with histamine).
  - — They stimulate the movement of WBC towards injured area.
  - — They increase salivation and lacrymation.
  - — They cause local oedema, allergic manifestation, inflammatory response.
  - — Through vasodilatation they increase blood flow in active tissues.
  - — They adjust the vascular tone by relaxing it during rise of local temperature.
  - — Glucocorticoids inhibit release of kinin. Aspirin antagonises its peripheral action on bronchial muscle and nerve endings.

PROSTAGLANDINS

Introduction

Prostaglandins are generic names for a group of structurally related biological active compounds. The term was coined by Von Euler and Goldblatt to the lipid found in seminal plasma but manufactured in prostatic tissues.

Physiological Effects

i. They lower the blood pressure by reducing the tone of smooth muscles of blood vessels. Medullin is anti-hypertensive substance of kidney which is a prostaglandin isolated from renal medulla. They increase heart rate via sympathetic stimulation.
ii. Following administration of pentagastrin and histamine, they inhibit gastric secretion.
iii. They are stimulant to smooth muscle activities.
iv. They possibly increase intestinal motility.
v. They have some oxytocic functions during labour.
vi. They counteract permeability response of toad's bladder to vasopressin.
vii. It inhibits aggregation of platelets in lower doses.
viii. They are affecting smooth muscle tone of genital passage and fallopian tubes.
ix. In CNS, they modulate the actions of chemical transmitters released at nerve endings. They also modulate the actions of hormones.
x. They inhibit release of glycerol and free fatty acids from adipose tissues.

Therapeutic Uses

i. Prevention of conception
ii. Initiation of labour
iii. Termination of pregnancy
iv. As bronchodilator in asthma
v. Control of blood pressure
vi. Prevention of lipolysis
vii. Prevention and cure of peptic ulcer.

Chemistry

These are a group of unsaturated twenty carbon fatty acids that contain a five-membered ring within its molecule. Same basic structure termed prostanoic acid is contained by each. Four groups (PGA, PGB, PGE and PGF) are constituted according to their variation in double bonds and hydroxyl and ketone groups within its structure. E and F are again subdivided into six primary prostaglandins—PGE_1, PGE_2, PGE_3, PGF_{1a}, PGF_{2a}, PGF_{3a}. E series is ether soluble having keto group at 9 carbon atom while F series is phosphate soluble having hydroxyl group in position 9.

Synthesis

They are synthesised in cell membrane and the enzyme responsible for its synthesis is prostaglandin endoperoxide synthase. Aspirin inhibits this synthesis.

Metabolism

They are quickly metabolised by enzyme 15-hydroxyprostaglandin dehydrogenase present in mammalian tissue.

Notes

i. Human seminal vesicles, prostate, umbilical cord vessels, menstrual fluid, kidney, pancreas, lungs, brain, amniotic fluid, iris of sheep, calf thymus, bovine brain are some of tissues which produce prostaglandins.
ii. They can be assayed by gas-liquid chromatography.
iii. Lipid materials of unknown chemical nature like darmstoff, menstrual stimulant, vesiglandin, medullin, irin are now believed as prostaglandin.
iv. Thromboxanes are those prostaglandins which cause aggregation of platelets; while prostacyclin are those which inhibit such platelet aggregation.

BIBLIOGRAPHY

1. Beaven MA. Histamine. New Eng J Med 1976;294:80.
2. Haigler HJ. Serotonin receptors in brain. Fed Proc 1977;36:2159.

48 Hormonal Function: Other Organs

These are the hormones and central nervous system structures which are regulating the body machinery as a whole. It is quite interesting that some other structures are also acting as endocrine organs.

RENIN-ANGIOTENSIN SYSTEM

- Renin is an acid protease secreted by the kidney. Angiotensinogens are circulating in combination of plasma protein-globulin.

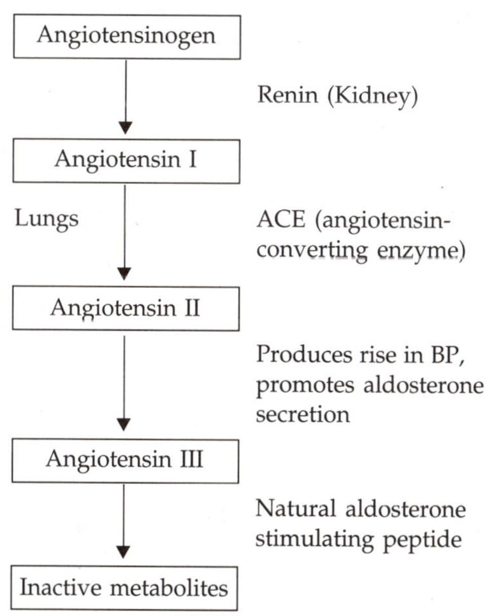

- ***Functions of angiotensin II:***
  - — Secretion of aldosterone stimulation.
  - — Rise in blood pressure.
  - — It acts on hypothalamus to increase vasopressin secretion + water intake.
  - — Constriction of arterioles → increases peripheral resistance and thus raises blood pressure. It is 4 to 8 times more potent than nor-adrenaline. It requires sodium to exert its full activities.
- ***Angiotensin I***: It acts as a precursor of angiotensin II. Besides renin; these are peptidases which can produce it from angiotensinogen. Renin is secreted from kidney JG cells.
- ***Stimuli for renin secretion***:
  - — Fall of arteriolar pressure at JG cell level → stimulation of intrarenal baroreceptors → stimulation of renin secretion.
  - — It varies inversely with plasma potassium level which indirectly affects Na^+ and Cl^- transport across macula densa cells.
  - — There exists a feedback inhibition of renin secretion via angiotensin II.
  - — Increased sympathetic discharge increases renin secretion.

ERYTHROPOIETIN

- It is a circulating glycoprotein. It is mainly secreted by the kidney but approximately 10 per cent role is played by liver also. When one is exposed to hypoxia, its secretion is stimulated. This in turn stimulates bone marrow to produce more red blood cells.
- It converts erythropoietin sensitive cells (stem cells) to pro-erythroblast through stimulation of synthesis of mRNA. It has been seen that anti-erythropoietin antibodies block its action and produce anaemia.
- Removal of pituitary produces anaemia which is cured by administration of pituitary extract. Erythropoietic effect of pituitary extract is due to ACTH, TSH and LH. Oestrogen inhibits erythropoiesis.
- Its half-life is five hours. Destroyed by liver. Its molecular weight is 23,000. Its stimulants are: hypoxia, anaemia, administration of cobalt salts and androgens. Alkalosis developed at high altitude favours its release.
- It is the liver which manufacture the globulin and that is converted into erythropoietin by renal factor. Hypoxia stimulates liver to produce this globulin.

PINEAL GLAND (Seat of the soul, third eye of lower vertebrates)

- It arises from roof of third ventricle.
- Melatonin is its active principal. It sometimes depresses and sometimes facilitates the gonadal functions. It may inhibit the onset of puberty. It is rapidly metabolised in liver and excreted by kidney. Its secretion is increased during dark period of the day and maintained during daylight hours.
- It is cone shaped. 8-12 mm long, 5-8 mm wide.
- Two types of cells found are:
  - Parenchymal cells—irregular slender process with club-shaped termination. It is like a secretory granule.
  - Glial cells - (supporting cell).
- Highly vascular. No nerve fibre seen.
- Functions:
  - Secretes growth inhibiting hormone.
  - Secretes a factor which inhibit ACTH.
  - Secretes a factor responsible for lightening of skin complexion.
  - Secretes a substance, which cures a mental disease named schizophrenia.
  - It influences the secretion of aldosterone.

MELATONIN

- Chemically - N-acetyl-5 methoxytryptamine.
- It acts on melanophores of toads and lightens the skin.
- Its synthesis is decreased in light and increased in dark.
- Its concentration in minute amount found in peripheral nerves.
- It is metabolised in liver.

ANP (ATRIAL-NATRIURETIC-PEPTIDE)

- Secreted by the heart. Muscle cells in atria contains necessary granules. It causes natriuresis by increasing glomerular filtration rate and sodium excretion by tubules. It also lowers blood pressure.
- In brain its effects are opposite of angiotensin II. The neurons containing ANP are involved in lowering blood pressure and promoting natriuresis.

MULTIPLE CHOICE QUESTIONS : ENDOCRINES

1. Fibres originating in hypothalamic nuclei descend in neural stalk. This tract of fibres serves important functions by connecting posterior pituitary with hypothalamus. What is the name of this connections?
   a. Tract of Goll
   b. Hypothalamo hypophyseal tract
   c. Spinotectal tract
   d. Tract of Burdach [ ]
2. Loss of axillary and pubic hair, dry and wrinkled facial skin, anaemia, mental deterioration, atrophy of gonads acute adrenal insufficiency, low metabolic rate, loss of teeth, smallness of hand and feet, shrunken appearance of facial features are characteristics presented by your patient. What is your diagnosis?
   a. Hypothyroidism
   b. Addison's disease
   c. Simmond's disease (Pituitary cachexia)
   d. Cushing's syndrome [ ]
3. Following is the quantity of ingested iodine required for synthesis of thyroxine:
   a. 30 mg per week
   b. 100 mg per week
   c. 50 mg per week
   d. 1 mg per week [ ]
4. Thyroxine increases the metabolic activities of following tissues *except*:
   a. Muscles
   b. Liver
   c. Kidney
   d. Brain [ ]
5. The hyperthyroid person feels difficulty in sleep in spite of muscular and CNS exhaustion because:
   a. Production of hypnotoxin
   b. Release of amphetamine
   c. Depressing the synapses
   d. Exciting effects on synapses [ ]
6. Growth hormone is chiefly regulated by:
   a. Presence of any disease
   b. Sex
   c. Age of person
   d. Nutritional status of body [ ]
7. Following are hormones of anterior pituitary *except*:
   a. Growth hormone
   b. Thyrotropine
   c. Follicle-stimulating hormone
   d. Oxytocin [ ]
8. The yellowish tint of skin in hyperthyroid state is due to:
   a. Carotenemia
   b. Increased blood cholesterol
   c. Less haemoglobin
   d. Less RBC [ ]
9. Clinical test for evaluation of thyroid function in connection with peripheral nervous system is:
   a. Knee jerk
   b. Reaction time of ankle jerk (Achilles reflex)
   c. Babiniski's sign
   d. Corneal reflex [ ]
10. Adrenal cortex secretes following hormones *except*:
    a. Glucocorticoids
    b. Aldosterone
    c. Epinephrine
    d. Sex hormones [ ]
11. The pigmentation in Addison's disease is due to:
    a. ACTH
    b. Thyroxine

c. MSH
d. ACTH and MSH [ ]

12. Which of the following cells is responsible for bone formation?
a. Fibroblasts
b. Osteoblasts
c. Macrophages
d. Osteoclasts [ ]

13. Which of the following form of calcium is more important as regards its functions?
a. Ionic
b. Non-ionic
c. Diffusible
d. Combined with other substances [ ]

14. The lethal level of blood calcium to cause tetany is:
a. 20 mg per cent
b. 100 mg per cent
c. 7 mg per cent
d. 10 mg per cent [ ]

15. Which of the following glands is considered to be the seat of soul by philosophers?
a. Pineal body
b. Thyroid
c. Pituitary
d. Adrenals [ ]

16. Following are actions of vasopressin *except*:
a. Antidiuretic
b. It lowers blood pressure
c. Increase in intestinal peristalsis
d. Raising blood pressure [ ]

17. Antidiuretic hormone:
a. Secreted by pituicytes
b. Increases water reabsorption
c. Stimulates body growth
d. Reduced GFR [ ]

---

1 b **2** c **3** d **4** d **5** d **6** d **7** d **8** a **9** b **10** c **11** d **12** b **13** a **14** c **15** a **16** b **17** b

VIVA VOCE : ENDOCRINES

1. Define a hormone.
It is a chemical substance produced by a group of specialised cells and regulates the activities of distant parts through entering the blood stream. The term hormone refers to a chemical messenger in the blood stream (hormone = to arouse).

2. What is hypothalamo-hypophyseal portal system ?
It appears to act as a vascular link between nervous system and adenohypophysis arising in one set of capillaries and ending in another so-called portal system. Hypothalamic hormone which are trophic for anterior pituitary are transmitted as neurosecretory material to the portal capillaries in neurohypophysis and then to adenohypophysis.

3. What are the main metabolic effects of growth hormone?
a. Rate of protein synthesis is increased.
b. Rate of carbohydrate utilisation is decreased.
c. Mobilisation of fats is increased.

4. Skin becomes considerably darkened in Addison's disease. Why?
In Addison's disease, inadequate adrenocortical hormones are produced. To compensate them, corticotrophin secretion from adenohypophysis is augmented and along with it probably MSH secretion (melanocyte-stimulating hormone) from 'pars intermedia' is also produced in excess which is responsible for skin darkening effect.

5. What is Houssay animal?
Growth hormone is diabetogenic. On removing pituitary gland (hypophysectomy) hypoglycaemia results. So if pituitary gland is removed in pancreatectomized animals, the symptoms of diabetes (hyperglycaemia, glycosuria, ketone bodies) disappear. This type of experiment was first done by Houssay in dogs so it is named after him. Such an animal may live for long periods without insulin.

6. Describe the characteristic features of a patient of acromegaly.
It is a result of hyperpituitarism after completion of ossification. Great enlargement of hands and feet (akors = extremity; megaly = enlargement), large face with prominent frontal sinuses, forward protrusion of lower jaw, excess development of supraorbital ridges causing forward slanting of forehead, nose increases as much as twice of its size, foot needs a shoe of large size. Kyphoses may be marked, huge hands reaching to knees. Patient with his bent back, 'gorilla-like' picture is attained due to protruding lower jaw, skin becomes coarse thick and furrowed, which is more marked in scalp, which is corrugated like 'bull dog' thick coarse hair, profuse sweating, increased sexual excitement.

7. Comment on condition 'Fröhlich's syndrome'.
It is also known as 'dystrophia-adiposo genitalis' and of prepubertal or infantile variety occurring as a result of inherent defect of pituitary. It is characterised by striking features combined with 'dwarfism and obesity', subjects are lethargic or somnolent and are of subnormal intelligence. They are craving for sweets having voracious appetite usually called 'fat boy'. Children becomes idiotic and stupid. In Frohlich's syndrome of adult type, there is excess deposition of fat in males occurring in such a way that it is having feminine distribution. Skin of face and body is smooth, soft and without hair and hips are broad. Extreme obesity is seen in females. Degeneration of sex is there. The picture is reverse as that of 'acromegaly', i.e. small pretty 'hands and feet', slender and tapering finger

tips with narrow-pointed terminal phalanges, subnormal BMR with increased sugar tolerance, diabetes insipidus is common.

8. Hypocalcaemia leads to tetany. How?
   Hypocalcaemia leads to increased excitability of central nervous system as well as peripheral nerves due to more neuronal permeability. This results into tremendous discharge from nerves to peripheral skeletal muscles terminating into tetanic contractions.
9. What is the lethal calcium level where tetany starts?
   It is 7 mg or so per cent (usually 30% below normal level).
10. How much is normal calcium phosphate ratio?
    Ca/P ratio varies between 1.3 and 2.0 on a weight basis.
11. Hyperparathyroidism leads to formation of kidney stone. How?
    Hypersecretion of parathyroid hormone causes excess mobilisation of calcium and phosphate and these are excreted by kidney where they are deposited or precipitated leading to formation of calcium phosphate, calcium oxalate stones.
12. What is parathyroid poisoning ?
    Due to more secretion of parathyroid hormone, the calcium and phosphorus level rises exceedingly in body fluids. This excess amount is unable to be excreted by kidney and so they form crystals ($CaHPO_4$; calcium phosphate crystals) which are now tending to be deposited elsewhere like lung alveoli; kidney tubules, gastric mucosa, walls of entire arteries, thyroid, etc. All this terminates into fatal results. The lethal level of calcium for such changes is said to be 17 mg per cent. Kidney stones are also formed (described earlier).
13. Enumerate functions of Thymus.
    a. During foetal and postnatal life, it forms small lymphocytes.
    b. It is believed that 'thymus hormone' is produced by it, which induces antibody formation, which are immunologicaly active.
    c. It is involved in autoimmune disease where it undergoes hyperplastic changes.
    d. Before birth, small lymphocytes migrate from here and settle at their usual sites for multiplication.
    e. Removing this gland; 'myaesthenia gravis' is reversed and ameliorated.
14. What is glucagon? Mention few of its action.
    a. It is formed from a large precursor molecule inside cells of islets of Langerhans of pancreas.
    b. It stimulates neoglucogenesis as well as breakdown of glycogen in liver.
    c. It causes breakdown of glycogen into glucose causing rise in blood sugar level.
    d. It raises metabolic rate (BMR; Calorigenic action).
    e. It promotes secretion of insulin, growth hormone and pancreatic somatostatin.
    f. In its large doses positive ionotropic effects on heart is exerted but no alteration on heart excitability.
    g. It is not promoting glycogenolysis in muscles.

QUESTION BANK

1. Name diabetogenic hormones and describe mechanism of their regulation.
2. Short notes:
   a. Tetany
   b. Diabetes insipidus
   c. Glucagon
   d. Adreno-genital syndrome (Raj. Univ. 1989, M.D.)
   e. Addison's disease
   f. Structure and function of thymus gland (Raj. Univ. 1981, M.D.)
   g. Thyroid function tests with their significance (Raj. Univ. 2000, M.D.)
   h. Calcitonin
   i. Hormone-receptor mechanism (Raj. Univ. 2000, M.D.)
   j. Releasing factors
   k. Somatostatin
3. Discuss at length about the role of adrenal steroid hormones as life savers as well as life threateners.
4. Describe the role of second messengers in mediation of hormonal action (Raj. Univ. 1995).
5. What are secretions of posterior pituitary hormones? How are they regulated and what are their physiological actions? (Raj. Univ. 1997, M.D.).
6. Discuss the comparative physiology of endocrine pancreas.
7. How do you evaluate thyroid function test in an individual? (Raj. Univ. 1995, M.D.)
8. Describe the role of mineralocorticoid and add a note on adrenocortical function test (Raj. Univ. 1985, 1994, M.D.).
9. Describe structure and mechanism of action of growth hormone.
10. Discuss patho-physiological effects of glucocorticoids. (Raj. Univ. 1995, M.D.)
11. Describe hypothalamic regulation of pituitary gland. (Raj. Univ. 1990, M.D.)
12. Explain how growth hormone produces its effects. List the major factors that affect the secretion of growth hormone. Explain the cause of pituitary dwarfism and gigantism. (Raj. Univ. 1990, 1994, M.D.)
13. Enumerate the hormones of thyroid gland and list the general functions of each. Distinguish between hypo and hyperthyroidism and describe consequences of each. (Raj. Univ. 1993, M.D.)
14. Discuss hypothalamus as neuro-endocrine system. (Raj. Univ. 1992, M.D.)
15. Describe hormones acting on mammary gland. (Raj. Univ. 1992, M.D.)
16. Discuss the role of thyroid gland in body. Describe pathophysiology of Graves' disease. (Raj. Univ. 1986, 1991, MD)
17. Discuss the mechanism of calcium homeostasis in body. Briefly discuss disorders. (Raj. Univ. 1983, 1986, 1988, M.D.)
18. Describe the various mechanisms by which chemical messengers act. (Raj. Univ. 2000, M.D.)

19. Explain:
    1. Skin becomes considerably darkened in Addison's disease. Why?
    2. Hyperparathyroidism leads to kidney stones. How?
    3. Dose of corticoids should be tapered off after long term use. Why?
    4. Excess production of aldosterone can cause hypertension. How?
    5. A patient of diabetes mellitus complains of polyphagia—polydipsia and polyurea. Why?
    6. Exophthalmos is not cured completely after thyroxine attains normal level. Why?
    7. Blood glucose level is needed to be maintained or regulated. Why?
20. Discuss:
    a. Anti-inflammatory action of steroids.
    b. Mechanism of COMA in patient of diabetes mellitus.
    c. Mechanism of action of hormones in general.
    d. Formation and secretion of thyroid hormone.

BIBLIOGRAPHY

1. Hackenthal E, et al. Morphology, physiology and molecular biology of renin secretion. Phy Rev 1990;70:1067.
2. Krantz SB. Erythropoietin. Blood 1991;77:419.
3. Maack T. Receptors for ANF. Ann Rev Phy 1992;54:11.

UNIT 8

Perpetuation of Race

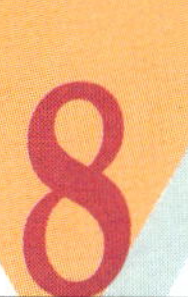

- "**Menopause:** Oh! my teaming date has drunken up with time.
- **Puberty:** A happy go lucky tomboy changes into full adult, often moody and imaginative, like Romeo and Juliet.
- **Menstruation:** It is funeral of unfertilised ovum."

Reproduction

49

Sexual Status: Female Partner: Becoming Familiar

FEMALE SEXUAL ORGANS

Vulva or external genitalia: Its components are:

- ***Mons pubis*** is a mount of fat situated in front of the symphysis pubis and covered by skin and hair.
- ***Labium majus*** is a fold of fat and skin lying below mons pubis. It is having hair on outer surface while is smooth internally. It contains sweat and sebaceous glands.
- ***Labium minus*** is a smaller fold of skin under the labium majus containing both sweat and sebaceous glands.
- ***Clitoris*** is highly vascular organ made up of erectile tissue and is counterpart of the male penis in the female.
- Area between labia minora is *vestibule*. Above it there is urethral orifice and below is the vaginal orifice.
- ***The external urethral meatus*** lies an inch below the clitoris, looking like a slit.
- ***The vaginal orifice*** (introitus vaginae) occupies the lowest third of vestibule and in virgin, it is covered by hymen—an incomplete membrane and is torn after coitus and childbirth.
- On either side of vaginal orifice are ***Bertholin's glands*** which secrete mucus during coitus for the purpose of lubrication.

VAGINA

It is a muscular tube extending from vulva to cervix. It is always warm and moist. Secretion is coming from cervical glands, in smaller amount, and exudate from vaginal wall. Due to presence of Doderlein's bacilli the reaction is acidic which prevents the growth of pathogenic organisms. During pregnancy this acidity is increased. Before puberty and in elderly life this reaction is less acidic—which explains the infection of this place the vulvovaginitis.

UTERUS (WOMB)

It is a thick-walled, pear-shaped hollow muscular organ which receives fertilised ovum, which develops here until birth. Its tapering end is cervix which projects into upper vagina. The area of insertion of fallopian tube into uterus is *cornu*. The opening of cervix into vagina is external os which is round until the birth of first child; after which it becomes a transverse slit. The constriction marking the junction of the cervical canal and uterine cavity proper is anatomical internal os of the cervix.

FALLOPIAN TUBES

These are two tubes extending from the cornua of the uterus to the ovaries. It has a small lumen which communicates with the uterine cavity medially and opens into peritoneal cavity laterally. The broad ligament of the uterus and ovaries are below the tubes.

OVARY

These are two in number and classed as female sex glands and located one on either side of pelvic wall. It projects freely into the peritoneal cavity and is the only abdominal organ not covered by peritoneum. It is suspended from cornu of uterus by the ovarian ligament. It is very closely related to fallopian tube. It lies behind the fallopian tube and the broad ligament. It performs two main functions:

a. The production of ova for the purpose of procreation; and
b. The production of sex hormones.

PUBERTY AND ADOLESCENCE (Adolescence-to grow; Latin)

Modern description of adolescence is "*teenager." It is the period of life during which carefree child becomes responsible adult.* Puberty (pubertas - adulthood; Latin) is the state of becoming functionally capable of procreation; and is the first part of adolescence, remainder being concerned with mental and emotional adaptation to sex functions which develop to their full maturity *"Menarche"* — the onset of menstruation, which is a manifestation of puberty.

PSYCHOPHYSIOLOGICAL CHANGES

Happy go lucky tomboy changes into a self-conscious girl better to call "Juliet/Laila" who is interested in her appearance, may be moody and is often imaginative and curious. Her confidence becomes another girl rather than mother. She begins to feel that she is grown up and finds it more difficult to obey orders and looks for independence. The sex hunger becomes manifest. The phase of active physical growth makes girl temporarily awkward and lanky in her movement; thereafter figure becomes full feminine and shrill voice of child changes to slightly deeper and more melodious (musical) tone of the adult. Menstrual flow itself if preceded by mucoid vaginal discharge and periodic hypogastric pain possibly due to uterine contraction. Acne of face and back is often a nuisance for 1-2 years after menarche possibly due to increased adrenal activity (androgen secretion and 17-ketosteroid in urine). Temporary enlargement of thyroid is also noticed. Body contour changes by deposition of fat, skin pigmentation notably on vulva, sometimes around the eyes, mouth and nipples, and on abdominal wall in the form of linea nigra. Some development of breast and pubic hair usually precedes onset of menstruation, average interval being 2 years. Axillary hairs appear later.

During childhood anterior pituitary is concerned with physical growth. It is capable of gonadotrophic activity but inhibited by hypothalamus. At puberty, as a result of secretions of releasing factors by hypothalamus, all the activities of glands are increased and this is manifested by sudden change in stature just before or after menarche (growth hormone effect), increased adrenal cortical activity (adrenocorticotrophic effect), skin pigmentation (MSH), onset of ovarian activity (gonadotrophin effect). Cyclic production of gonadotrophines and oestrogen in amount approaching those found in adult is often demonstrable by 10 years of age. Oestrogen secretion by ovaries and of androgen by adrenals induces epiphyses closure. Skeletal growth then ceases, girl is more curious and anxious about her genitalia.

HERO HORMONE OF FEMALE SEX—PROGESTERONE

Active Principle of Corpus luteum:

a. *Sources*: Corpus luteum, adrenal cortex and placenta.

b. *Functions*:

1. • Essential to maintain pregnancy hence therapeutically used in "threatened abortion" for embedding of ovum (causes hypertrophy of endometrium).
   • For formation of placenta so pregnancy proceeds up to full term, inhibits uterine muscle so prevents expulsion of ovum.
   • Promotes secretory changes in mucosal lining of fallopian tubes and these secretions are important for nutrition of fertilised dividing ovum as it traverse fallopian tube before implantation.
2. Inhibits menstrual cycle and ovulation.
3. Responsible for pre-menstrual changes in uterine mucosa.
4. Enlargement of birth canal, due to growth of vagina and relaxation of pelvic ligament.
5. It acts synergistic as well as antagonist with oestrogen.
6. Development of breast: Lobular development is promoted as well of alveoli to enlarge as well as secretory. It does not allow milk to be secreted. Also causes swelling of breast due to increased fluid in subcutaneous tissues.
7. Exerts mild catabolic effect on proteins similar to glucocorticoids.
   Progesterone has been called as nature's contraceptive for it serves to prevent the ripening of another ovum until the next cycle starts.
8. Protein catabolic effect (only significant during pregnancy, since proteins are required by foetus).
9. It is synthesised from cholesterol.

PROGESTERONE AND ELECTROLYTE BALANCE

- It like aldosterone causes sodium and water retention by kidney tubules (distal). But strangely it may cause increased excretion of sodium and water. When progesterone combines with the receptor, then no place is left for aldosterone and progesterone exerts many times less potent action than aldosterone. So the cause is competition between it and aldosterone.

Indication for Treatment (use in gynaecological practice)

1. Inhibition of ovulation and suppression of ovulation pain.
2. Spasmodic dysmannorrhoea (corrects painful ovulatory cycles into painless anovulatory bleeding).
3. Pre-menstrual tension.
4. Pregnancy test (oestrogen progesterone mixture is used which will induce uterine bleeding in non-pregnant while it will fail to do so in pregnant state).
5. Amenorrhoea.
6. Abortion (threatened or habitual).
7. Carcinoma of body of uterus.
8. Endometriosis.

9. Metropathica hemorrhagica.
10. Infertility (given in second half of menstrual cycle to get good secretory endometrial response.
11. Control of MC: Women occasionally request help from a doctor because their menstrual period is to occur on a date which may cause them some frustration more particularly from young girls who have some theatrical or alternative appointments, a tiring long journey, as well as wedding which has to be arranged at an inappropriate time for reason beyond control. By using synthetic oestrogen progesterone combination it is easy to postpone menstruation indefinitely. Its main disadvantages are—it may take one or two months for monthly cycle to return back to its normal rhythm, and a patient may also feel certain side effects since "no drug is safe in therapeutic, each and every drug has got its own side effects."

PROGESTERONE: MECHANISM OF ACTION

- It is lipid in nature, so it easily crosses the membrane of target cell. There it combines with its receptors in cytosol. It forms receptor hormone complex which moves to specific part of DNA. Then transcription of mRNA results which leads to synthesis of new proteins which leads to its biological effects.
- It was discovered by Corner and Allen (1930, Americans) and was named progestin by them. It was named as progesterone by Sir Henry Dale.

HERO HORMONE OF FEMALE SEX—OESTROGEN

- These are compounds which can produce oestrus in ovariectomised animals.
- *Types*:
  a. Natural—Sterol derivative, not effective orally.
  b. Synthetic—Not sterols but benzanthracene compounds. Effective by mouth, e.g. Ethinyl oestradiol, diethylstilboestrol.
- Oestradiol—natural hormone secreted by ovary. Oestrone—less potent. Found in adult female urine and increasing during pregnancy.
- *Source*: (1) Ovary is chief source—from its Graafian follicle (liquor folliculi and follicular epithelium) and interstitial cells (2) Adrenal cortex (3) Placenta (4) Testes.
- *Chemistry:* The oestrogens are C-18 steroids and differs from androgen in lacking the methyl group C_{10}.
- *Functions:*
  1. Responsible for all puberty changes.
  2. Responsible for proliferative stage of menstrual cycle.
  3. Causes growth of uterus during pregnancy.
  4. Synergistic action with oxytocin and thus helps in parturition (delivery of child).
  5. Inhibits thymus.
  6. Like aldosterone, it increases reabsorption of water and electrolytes from renal tubules thus increasing blood volume, of course, action is comparatively milder than aldosterone.
  7. It increases total body protein which is indicative by positive nitrogen balance.
  8. It causes increased deposition of fats in subcutaneous tissue and in other regions to give a feminine structure.
  9. It increases skeletal growth. Retention of calcium and phosphate is also increased after its administration.
  10. Stimulates oestrus in young animals.
  11. Stimulates secretion of ACTH from anterior pituitary.
  12. Maintains negative feedback relation with FSH from anterior pituitary.
  13. Synergistic action with progesterone, e.g. menstrual cycle, breast growth.
  14. It is also essential for maintenance of corpus luteum.
  15. It has a significant plasma cholesterol lowering action and thus helps in prevention of atherosclerosis.
  16. Vaginal epithelium is changed from cuboidal to stratified which is comparatively more resistant to trauma and infection.
  17. It causes increased osteoblastic activity. It also causes an early union of epiphyses with shaft of the bone. So growth of the female ceases earlier as compared with the male.

OESTROGEN ACTION: INTRACELLULAR MECHANISM

On entry into target cells oestrogen combines with receptor protein molecules in the cytoplasm within a few seconds. This combination interacts with specific portions of chromosomal DNA. This leads to formation of mRNA within a few minutes through the process of transcription. The RNA diffuses to the cytoplasm where it leads to increased formation of proteins.

METABOLISM: SEX HORMONES

- Both these two hormones are transported in blood, bound mainly with albumin and specific oestrogen progesterone binding globulins.
- The liver conjugates oestrogen to form glucoronides and sulphates, 1/5th of them excreted in bile while the remainder is excreted in the urine. Liver, further converts potent oestrogen into least potent or impotent oestrogen.

Because of these two reasons in patients suffering from liver diseases; there is increased activity of oestrogen (hyperoestrinism).

- Progesterone is also degraded by liver and major product is pregnanediol.

Metabolism

1. From its source, it is widely distributed in blood, muscles, urine, etc.
2. Oestradiol → oestrone and oestriol → metabolised in liver; made inactivated by conjugating with glucoronic acid and then excreted in urine.

THE OVARIAN CYCLE

i. *Hormonal basis:*

It has got three basic components—the arcuate nucleus of hypothalamus, the gonadotrophs of pituitary gland and the ovary. The arcuate nucleus (hypothalamus) generates a signal once per hour or two, that eventuates in the release of a bolus of GnRH (gonadotropin-releasing hormone) into pituitary-portal circulation, to which the gonadotrophs respond by releasing a pulse of LH and FSH. Immature ovarian follicles respond to these pulses of gonadotropic hormones by increasing in size and secreting increasing quantities of estradiol, which achieve peak levels in the circulation near midcycle. This process occupies approximately 14 days. When estradiol exceeds a threshold of 200 pg./ml. for at least two days the negative feedback action of steroid is interrupted and its level comes down to almost zero. Then graafian follicle undergoes full maturation → massive estradiol formation → follicular rupture → ovulation → corpus luteum formation → progesterone secretion. The life of corpus luteum is 14 days after which it undergoes luteolysis a new follicle is selected for development and the cycle is repeated. The ovary, therefore, times the events of the menstrual cycle. Its characteristic 28 days duration simply represents the sum of durations of follicular development and of the functional life span of corpus luteum.

ii. *Stages of development of follicle*:

- *Formation of primordial follicle*: The primitive precursor of the ovum is oogonia. It is estimated that there are about 5 lakh primary oogonia (oocyte) at birth. By puberty this number is considerably reduced to 1.5 to 2 lakh. From fifth month of intrauterine life, their multiplication by mitosis is coming to an end, but meiosis starts within oogonia, and it converts oogonia into oocyte, and this meiosis stops at the stage of prophase. Those oocyte that don't mature undergo some form of degeneration.
- The ovaries are enveloped by a single layer of cubical epithelium called 'germinal epithelium' and few of this epithelial cells are spindle cells which form ring around the oocyte. This spindle cell layer is further enveloped by a thin layer of stroma called basal lamina.
- This entire structure (spindle cells + basal lamina + ovum) is called primordial follicle.
- *Primordial to primary follicle*: As told above, the oocyte is surrounded by a layer of granulosa and is referred as primordial follicle. It is called primary follicle when spindle cells are converted into a single layer of cuboidal epithelium.
- *Primary to mature follicle*: The above mentioned cuboidal cells multiply and thus produce several layers of itself; so-called *granulosa cells*. Meanwhile, *zona pallucida*—a mucopolysaccharide layer—is formed round oocyte. This mucopolysaccharide gives it a glistening appearance, and is produced by granulosa cells. These granulosa cells now produce fluid called liquor folliculi which occupies its central cavity called *Antrum*. Ovarian stroma starts condensing round the maturing follicle. *Theca interna* is the name given to the layer just outside the basal lamina while the layer external to it is *theca externa*. A mature follicle is called graafian follicle.
- *Graafian follicle*: Large vesicles which protrude on free surface of ovary, and is having diameter up to 10 mm. It is a thin-walled structure holding follicular fluid under pressure. The ovum is enclosed in a thick membrane zona pellucida which is covered with a layer of follicular cells *"Corona radiata."*
- Basement membrane of intact follicle provides a barrier to the passage of essential nutrients into the follicular fluid, which in turn stops the ovum and granulosa cells from developing. So what suggested is that one of the actions of LH is to increase the permeability of the blood-follicle barrier.
- Lumen of the graafian follicle is a pretty sleepy place. The ovum resides there in an arrested state of meiotic division from soon after birth until shortly before ovulation. Then presumably under the action of LH, meiosis is resumed and the first polar body is extruded. Granulosa cells appear to be relatively inactive in intact follicle. They are

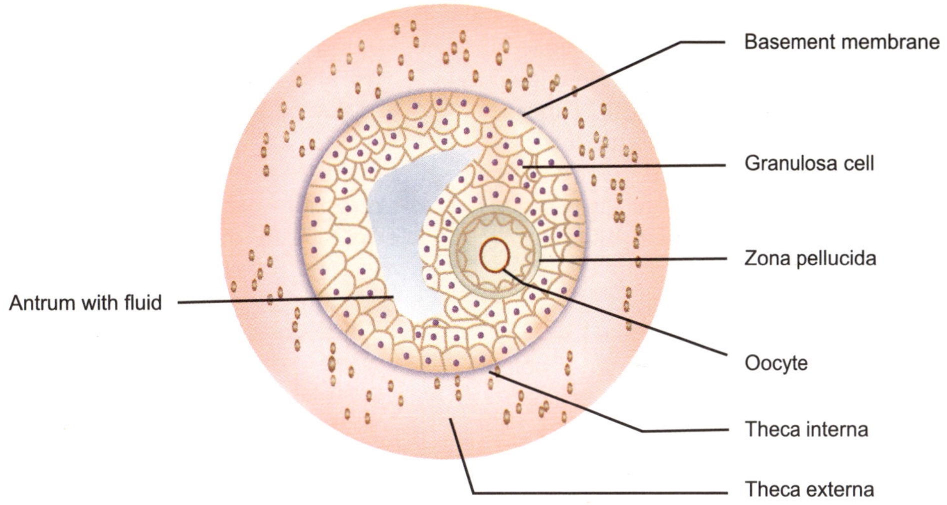

Fig. 49.1: Graafian follicle

small, half-starved looking creatures with comparatively little cytoplasm, but they blossom forth into luteal cells, after ovulation.

iii. *Ovulation*

A. The matured graafian follicle rupture and ovum is discharged, at about middle of menstrual cycle. This is ovulation; which means a process by which an ovum is discharged from a mature graafian follicle to form a gamete (secondary oocyte). Ovulation usually continues until the age of 45-50 years. Before puberty and during childhood the ovary grows in size. The connective tissue stroma increases. There is, however, no ripening of primordial follicle and no ovulation until the time of menarche. Ovulation may, however, be delayed until the age of 15, 16 or 17 years.

B. *Its causes include:* Necrosis or weakening of cells of stigma or of the cement substance between them, degeneration of theca and granulosa cells in the region of stigma.

C. *Role of LH:* Inhibits the growth of granulosa cell and cement substance between granulosa cells, disintegrates in presence of it.

D. *Mechanism:* Enzyme theory—It proposes that active enzymatic or vascular processes result in deterioration and disruption of the follicle wall. Hyaluronidase is secreted into follicle causing decomposition of mucopolysaccharides in the follicular fluid → swelling of follicle due to more osmotic pressure.

- *Endosmosis theory*—It relates ovulation to change in follicular pressure or volume.
- If we mix up both the above theories, the following facts are exposed:

—Fall of intrafollicular hydrostatic pressure occurs prior to ovulation.

—There occurs increased dispensability of large mature follicles.

—Inherent elasticity of wall decreases prior to ovulation.

—The enzymes degrade the follicle wall and contents and increase the osmotic pressure with decrease in maximal tensile strength and all these contribute to rupture of follicle.

E. *Accepted steps of ovulation:*

1. Growth and maturity of the follicle occur without an increase in hydrostatic pressure.
2. A rapid increase in size of follicle immediately prior to rupture is accompanied by a fall in intrafollicular pressure.
3. Stigma formation and localised rupture occur despite generalised distribution of enzymes throughout follicular fluid (and wall).

F. *Endocrine regulation:*

1. FSH results in growth of the unstressed radius of ovarian follicle.
2. Oestrogen also results in growth of follicle but mainly affects its mass and volume of follicle wall. The lumen of antrum remains relatively small.

3. The LH might act to increase the number of osmotically active particles. An enzyme identical with testicular hyaluronidase is said to be present in liquor folliculi of mature follicles which decrease the elastic limit and increase the number of osmotically active particles. The LH acts synergistically with FSH to cause rapid swelling of follicle before ovulation.

G. *Tests:*

— Basal body temperature is raised in post-ovulatory phase by 0.5°C. It is recorded before leaving the bed in early morning.

— On measurement, urinary metabolites of progesterone are on higher side as compared with anovulatory woman.

— Uterine mucosa on examination, indicates of the secretion of progesterone (secretory phase).

— Electrical changes in pelvis.

iv. *Corpus luteum:* After expulsion of ovum from the follicle, the granulosa and theca cells of the follicle undergo luteinisation and mass of cell becomes corpus luteum which secretes mainly progesterone. These cells become greatly enlarged and develop lipid inclusion which gives them a yellow colour. The change of follicular cells into lutein cells is completely dependent on LH by adenohypophysis, hence the name luteinising hormone is given.

After seven to eight days of ovulation, it attains a size of 1.5 cm. After this time it involutes, loses its secretory function as well as lipid constituents. After a period of 10 to 15 days, this is replaced by connective tissue (corpus albicans). So the life span of corpus luteum in case of non-fertilisation appears to be 14 days while if fertilisation occurs, it is maintained. Its degeneration is characterised by decreased vascularity.

On the other hand, in general, one ovum is expelled from the ovaries during each monthly sexual cycle. All developing follicles that do not ovulate, start degenerating called atretic follicles. The phenomenon of atresia is characterised by degeneration of ovum contained within it, disappearance of follicular cells and in growth of connective tissue.

v. *Monthly ovarian cycle :* A summary—The adult ovary undergoes a cycle of activity which usually lasts 28 days. The cycle starts on the first day of menstruation and can be divided into two phases. The first phase is follicular phase which lasts for 14 days during which ripening of ovum takes place. The secretion of FSH by anterior pituitary causes graafian follicle to ripen and level of oestrogen to rise also. Other actions of FSH includes—stimulation of mitotic division of the granulosa cells, conversion of stroma into theca, helping theca interna to produce oestrogen, appearance of FSH and LH receptors on the granulosa cells. High levels of oestrogen thus produced depresses the FSH secretion by negative feedback mechanism and thus encourages the secretion of LH by adenohypophysis. When correct ratio of LH to FSH is attained, LH brings out its specific actions which include—stimulation of ovulation, formation and proper functioning of corpus luteum which secretes progesterone hormone in large quantities and development of atresia in atretic follicles.

If pregnancy does not occur, the level of LH falls by negative feedback mechanism and corpus luteum begins to degenerate. This causes a fall in level of both oestrogen and progesterone and releases FSH again, which in turn brings about the ripening of a graafian follicle and so the cycle continues.

It is GnRH (gonadotropin-releasing hormone) secreted by hypothalamus, which brings about the secretion of FSH and LH from adenohypophysis. Chemically, it is a 10-amino acid peptide. Once secreted into circulation; it is rapidly degraded with half-life of 2-4 minutes. Its secretion is not continuous but its release is episodic (short bursts) due to depolarisation of arcuate neurons. The average frequency of its release has been measured as 60 minutes to 4 hours. Its secretion is stimulated by norepinephrine neurons while decreased by opioidergic system through secretion of β-endorphin.

FSH; LH; ICSH; AN OVERVIEW

- Some observers indicated that ovarian functions were humorally controlled by some substance external to the ovary. This hypothetic substance was termed "generative ferment" and "X substance" by others. The gradual atrophy and suppression of sex functions because of pituitary disorders (acromegaly, Frohlich's syndrome) and atrophy of gonads indicated clearly the pituitary as a source of this substance. So:
- FSH = Concerned with ripening of ovarian follicles or spermatogenesis.
- ICSH/LH = Concerned with ovulation, luteinisation and maintenance of interstitial tissue of gonads.
- LTH = Maintain luteal activity.
- Their source within the pituitary is basophil cells.
- FSH is a glycoprotein, rich in carbohydrate. Its hormonal activity is destroyed by ptyalin. So its

activity is dependent upon integrity of carbohydrate fraction. It is not destroyed by trypsin.

- LH is also a glycoprotein. Its biological activity is not destroyed by ptyalin.
- The inactivation of pituitary gonadotropins in the blood stream proceeds more slowly as compared with other pituitary hormones. Their small amount excreted in urine. Ovarian tissue inactivates gonadotropins.
- If FSH and LH are administered together, then follicular ripening, ovulation, corpus luteum formation follows. The optimum doses for ovulation is FSH:LH (10:1).
- This synergism is best seen as far as ovarian weight is concerned. FSH given alone increases weight of ovary.

FEW MORE FACTS : MONTHLY OVARIAN CYCLE

1. *Initiation of ovulation*:
   a. Proteolytic enzymes are released from thecaexterna from lysosomes → dissolution of capsular wall → weakening of wall → swelling of entire follicle + degeneration at stigma.
   b. Secretion of prostaglandins in the follicular tissues (local hormones causing vasodilatation) → plasma transudation into follicle → follicular swelling → degeneration at stigma with follicular rupture.
2. *Atresia*: One follicle which becomes highly developed secreting more oestrogen than others which causes vicious cycle as follows: (a) FSH enhances both granulosa cells and theca cells to proliferate which leads to further oestrogen production and in this way a new cycle of proliferation begins; (b) FSH + oestrogen increase the number of FSH and LH receptors on granulosa and theca cells; thus another such vicious cycle is promoted; (c) Large amount of this oestrogen from follicle depress further enhancement of secretion of FSH and LH by adenohypophysis and so further growth of less well-developed follicle is arrested.
3. Throughout childhood (before puberty), the granulosa cells provide nourishment to ovum and secrete oocyte maturation-inhibiting factor which keeps the ovum in its primordial state, suspended during this entire time in prophase stage of meiotic division.

SEXUAL ACT (THE COITUS)

Sex is an emotional as well as a physical experience.

a. *Male act*: It is completed in three different stages:
   i. ***Erection of penis***: Any psychic stimulation/gentle massage of glans penis will cause erection penis and initiation of sex drive. Stimulation of anal epithelium, perineal structures, scrotum, kissing, gently massaging the breast of female partner, even thinking of sexual thoughts or dreaming can all initiate sex drive. These impulses pass through pudendal nerve-sacral plexus and thence to sacral part of spinal cord and then finally to highest—the cerebrum. Erection is the first effect of sexual act. It is caused by parasympathetic impulses passing from sacral part of spinal cord to penis through nervi-erigentes. Due to this parasympathetic stimulation arteries of penis are dilated which leads to flow of arterial blood under high pressure into erectile tissue of penis (cavernous venous sinusoids) which are normally empty. This leads to ballooning of erectile tissue which converts the flaccid penis into hard and elongated one.
   ii. ***Ejaculation:*** It means emission of semen from the penis. This act is completed by: (a) peristaltic contraction (in ducts of testis, epididymis, vas deferens—to cause expulsion of sperm into internal urethra), (b) rhythmic contraction (in prostate and seminal vesicles). Sympathetic stimulation causes rhythmic contraction of muscles lining the male genital tract. Rhythmic impulses are sent through S_1 and S_2 from cord and then to skeletal muscles through pundendal nerve.
   iii. ***Lubrication***: Lubrication is important because without it the sexual act becomes rather painful which may inhibit the sexual drive. "Bulbourethral glands" and "glands of Littre" secrete mucus in males while bilaterally located 'Bertholin glands in female' produce mucus. Lubrication establishes a satisfactory massaging action during coitus.

b. *Female act*: Sex drive is developed in the same way like psychic and physical stimuli (massaging perineal and anal structure, kissing, breast massaging). These sensations are mediated through sacral plexus in spinal cord, which are taken to cerebrum and is partly responsible for orgasm. Located around the introitus and extending into the clitoris is erectile tissue. All these stimuli lead to rapid inflow of blood into this erectile tissue so that introitus tightens around penis which is a sufficient stimulation for males to ejaculate.

Now, let us be familiar with some sexual terms:

i. *Libido*—Sexual impulse.
ii. *Potentia*—Erection of penis.
iii. *Orgasm*—Climax of sexual pleasure feeling followed by immediate relief of nervous and physical tension, with pleasurable lethargy and sleepiness. In man it is accompanied by emission of semen

while in females is by rhythmic contraction of muscles around vagina.

iv. ***Priapism***—State of sustained erection of penis not accompanied by sexual desire, but accompanied by pain and venous thrombosis. Usually occurs in fourth decade of life.

v. ***Masturbation***—Young children of both sexes tend to handle their external genitalia and feel it pleasurable. It creates sensation of shame, guilt otherwise it is harmless.

vi.

- On intercourse, sperms are deposited in upper regions of vagina, while fertilisation takes place in fallopian tube. On reaching the fallopian tube; they undergo some changes which are collectively called capacitation, which includes: (i) increased entry of Ca^{++} inside spermatozoan; (ii) activated motility; (iii) loss of acrosomal membrane. Similarly, ovum after releasing from graafian follicle is surrounded by three layers of germinal epithelium called 'cumulus oophorus' as well as coating of zona pallucida.
- Sperms can exist in female genital tract for 24–72 hours but remain active and highly fertile for only 24 hours. Similarly, a mature ovum is also fertilisable for 12–24 hours. Only one sperm, out of millions is required or able for fertilisation, for the reasons that zona pallucida of the ovum has a lattice type of structure, and once the ovum is punctured, some substance diffuses out of ovum into the lattice to prevent penetration by other sperms, of course, many sperms try to penetrate the ovum.

HYPOTHALAMIC - HYPOPHYSEAL-PORTAL SYSTEM

i. Hypothalamic nuclei (supraoptic and paraventricular) are connected with posterior pituitary through unmyelinated 'hypothalamico-hypophyseal-tract.'

ii. Neurones originating in various parts of hypothalamus send nerve fibres into median eminence and into tuber cinereum which is the hypothalamic tissue that surrounds the hyophyseal stalk. These neurones are not meant for passage of nerve signals; but they secrete hormones called 'hypothalamic neurosecretory substances' which are immediately absorbed into hypothalamic-hypophyseal-portal capillaries and carried directly to the sinuses of adenohypo-

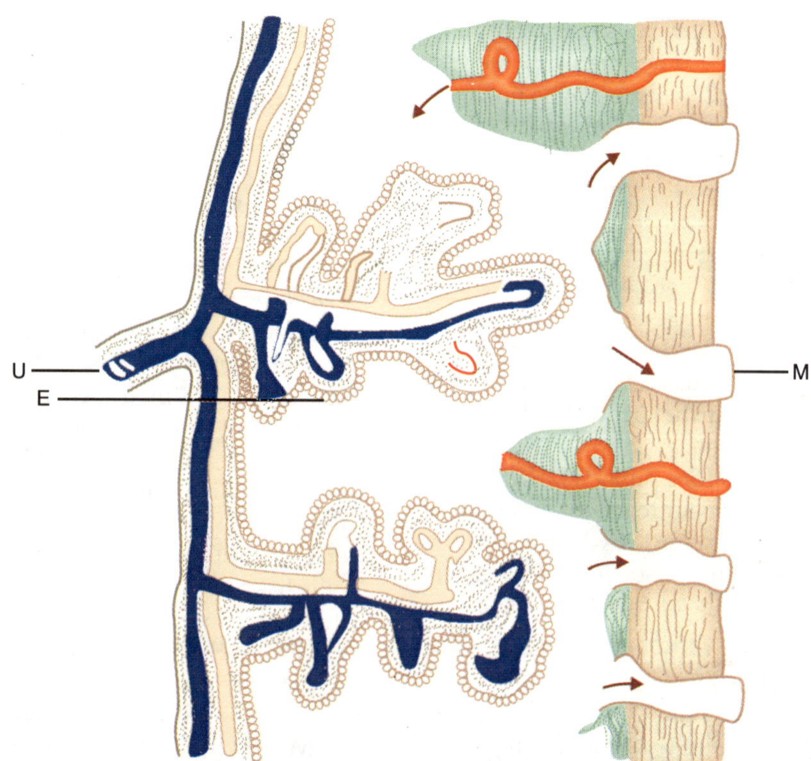

Fig. 49.2: Placental and maternal portions together with physiological process in progress M = Maternal portion, U = Umbilical cord, E = Embryonic portion

physis. They are also called Releasing Hormones (RH).

iii. The fibres of hypothalamico-hypophyseal tract synthesises hormones—ADH and oxytocin in paraventricular and supraoptic group of nuclei and it contains 1,00,000 nerve fibres, and it proceeds through stalk hypothalamus. These hormones reach the neurohypophysis via the same tract, where they are stored in the form of granules.

iv. Evidences indicate that human hypothalamicpituitary system forms a well-differentiated functional unit by midgestation. Dopamine, serotonin, noradrenaline are all present in foetal hypothalamus by 12 weeks of gestation and all of hypothalamic nuclei and tubulo-infundibular dopaminergic system are well differentiated by 15 weeks. An intact hypothalamico-hypophyseal-portal system is established as early as 11.5 weeks of gestation and GnRH containing neurones in MBH (medio-basal-hypothalamus) with axon terminal in contact with portal capillaries of median eminence are present by 16 weeks of gestation. Hypothalamic control of foetal gonadotropic activity appears to be operative as evidenced by parallel increase in hypothalamic GnRH content and foetal pituitary gonadotropin secretion.

v. This unit maintains the endocrinal function at a normal level. In the absence of neural control the activity of some glands is depressed either or falls completely.

vi. It is responsible for maintaining rhythmic activity, e.g. ovary during normal sexual cycles.

vii. It acts as an intermediary between varying external environment and endocrine system.

viii. It possibly acts as a part of central mechanism involved in feedback action of target gland hormones.

ix. Halsted's principle of deficiency, e.g. ovarian transplants survive better in an ovariectomised animal than in a normal animal; because ovariectomised animal has a higher level of circulating gonadotrophic hormone than a normal animal possesses.

x. All vertebrates possess a system of vessels passing from median eminence to the anterior lobe of pituitary. These vessels are portal that they start as capillaries in, form vascular trunks and break up into sinusoids of anterior pituitary.

xi. The direction is from median eminence to anterior pituitary.

xii. The effects of pituitary stalk section are conditioned by subsequent state of portal vessels, i.e. if vessels regenerate across site of cut, the pituitary functions may be regained or if regeneration is prevented. The pituitary functions may be greatly reduced.

BIBLIOGRAPHY

1. David Rodbard. Mechanics of ovulation. J Clin Endcrin 1968;28:849.
2. Espey LL, Lipner H. Enzyme induced rupture of rabbit Graafian follicle. Amer J Phy 1965;208:208.
3. Espey LL, H Lipner Amer J Phy 1963;205:1067.
4. Espey LL. Amer J Phy 1967;21:1397.
5. Goodmand AL, Hodgen GD. J Clin Endorinol Metab 1977;45:837-40.
6. Greenblatt RB. Ovulation: stimulation, suppression, detection. 1966. Philadelphia J.B. Lippincott Co.
7. Keyes PL, Wiltbank MC. Endocrine regulation of corpus luteum. Ann Rev Phy 1988;50:465.
8. McCann. Effect of progesterone plasma LH activity. Amer J Phy 1962;202:601.
9. Phol and E. Knobil. The role of CNS in the control of ovarian function in higher primates. Ann Rev Phy 1982;44:583-593.
10. Rasmussen DD, et al. Endogenous opioid regulation of GnRH release from human MBH in vitro. J Clin Endocrinol Metab 1983;57:881-84.
11. Reiter ED, et al. Neuroendocrine control mechanism and onset of puberty. Ann Rev Phy 1982;44:595.

50 Sign of Womanhood: Menstruation

Synonyms : menses, monthly period, being unwell, the curse, funeral of unfertilised ovum, weeping of uterus.

INTRODUCTION

- Cyclic discharge of blood, mucus and certain other substances from the uterus in the reproductive life of female at an average interval of 28 days (24–34 days) is called 'menstruation' and is occurring every month from puberty to menopause.
- Its duration is 4 to 6 days without pain. It begins as a pink discharge consisting of cervical mucus and blood rich in leukocytes. It is heavier on second and third day when it is dark red in colour consisting of blood, endometrial and cervical secretions, endometrial debris and bacteria.
- 30-40 c.c. of blood along with 30-40 c.c. serous fluid is discharged in total, which is composed of blood, striped off endometrium, mucus, leukocytes and unfertilised ovum. During each cycle uterine mucosa hypertrophies.
- The first menstruation in a girl's life is called 'menarche' and after it a girl should menstruate every month if her periods are regular.
- Menstrual blood is predominantly arterial, with only 25 per cent of the blood being of venous origin.
- The above mentioned amount discharged depends on various factors like thickness of endometrium, medication, and disease affecting clotting mechanism.
- Along with the blood and necrotic material tremendous number of leukocytes are released in menstrual blood. This explains the resistance of uterus towards infection during these days.
- A substance 'fibrinolysin' is released along with menstrual flow which prevents clotting. It should be remembered that presence of clots in menstrual blood indicates towards any pathology.

PHYSIOLOGY OF MENSTRUATION

The endometrial changes are divided into :

i. *Resting/Postmenstrual Phase*

ii. *Proliferative/Reparative Phase*

These two phases are described together. This is characterised by increasing amount of 'oestrogen' secreted from ovary. This is further controlled by 'FSH' principal from adenohypophysis. Under its effects first of all the menstruated endometrium heals and becomes normal. Then slow proliferative changes start appearing; e.g. mucosa thickens (from 1 to 2-3 mm), vascular supply increases, endometrial glands become longer and tortuous, vasodilatation, etc. This stage lasts for Ist to 14th day of menstruation (1st-5th day resting phase; 6th-14th day proliferative phase). Oestrogen secretion rises under the effect of FSH which leads to maturation of follicles. In urine, maximum excretion of oestrogen (inactive estriol) may be observed.

On 14th day ovulation takes place with the formation of corpus luteum. Secretion of hormone 'progesterone' begins. Due to high oestrogen level and beginning of progesterone secretion; the oestrogen secretion and FSH are inhibited and their level declines to almost zero (negative feedback mechanism).

iii. *Premenstrual/Secretory Phase*

Now, under the effect of hormone progesterone mucosa further thickens (from 1-3 mm to 5-6 mm), glands are much more enlarged and tortuous and distended with mucus, capillaries are dilated like sinus, stroma cells proliferate, secretory vacuoles containing glycogen appear above nuclei. This uterine secretion/milk can provide nutrition to fertilised ovum and this is the reason that this phase is also named as 'secretory phase'. Then once the ovum implants in the endometrium, the

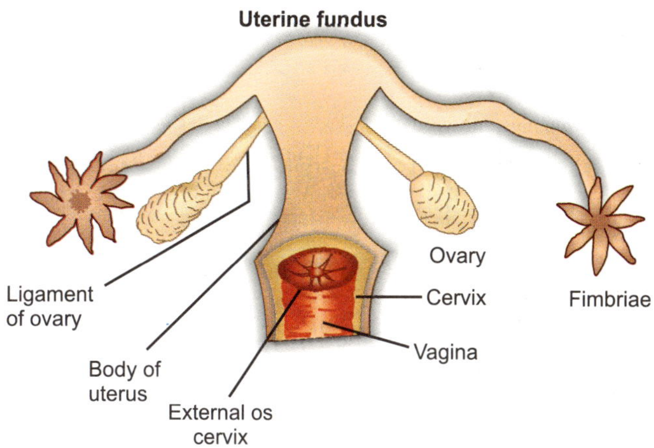

Fig. 50.1: Female reproduction

trophoblastic cells on the surface of blastocyst begin to digest the endometrium and to absorb endometrial stored substances, thus making still far greater quantities of nutrients available to early embryo. The secretion of progesterone is under the control of LH principal of adenohypophysis so it is also named as progestational phase. Corpus luteum attains maximal size on 19th-27th day of menstrual cycle. In urine pregnanediol appears 2 to 3 days after ovulation, rises to maximum about one week before the period and falls 2–3 days before the onset of menstruation.

- Mediobasal hypothalamus causes pulsatile release of GnRH (Gonadotropin-releasing hormone) which controls most of the female sexual activity.
- Hormone 'inhibin' is important in causing decreased secretion of FSH and LH towards the end of female sexual month. It is secreted by corpus luteum (female) and sertoli cells (male).
- Norepinephrine and epinephrine increase GnRH pulse frequencies. Conversely, opioid peptides, e.g. enkephalins, β endorphin reduce the frequency of GnRH pulse.
- It is also controlled by the highest centres (limbic cortex). So any sort of stress alter menstrual cycle in some or other way.

iv. *Menstrual/Destructive Phase.*

- Approximately two days before menstruation, the level of progesterone also declines to zero because of negative feedback mechanism. So menstruation is caused by this sudden reduction of both oestrogen and progesterone hormone at the end of monthly ovarian cycle. If a course of progesterone is given after a course of oestrogen, typical endometrial pre-menstrual changes occur; and if then progesterone is suddenly withheld, bleeding takes place which is identical with menstrual discharge (withdrawal bleeding).
- The spiral arteries continue to lengthen disproportionately to the growth of endometrium. Some time before menstruation there is a reduction in blood supply to the endometrium which shrinks and compresses the spiral arteries. The blood is then further slowed until there is a state of stasis. Finally, the spiral arteries constrict and set themselves for menstruation. After a period of ischaemia of the endometrium, individual spiral arteries relax and haemorrhage occurs through rupture of the wall of an arteriole or capillary. The blood may escape through epithelium or may collect in underlying tissue to form a haematoma which discharges into lumen of the uterus. But constriction and relaxation of these vessels don't occur synchronously so that some bleeding continues. This explains the normal duration of menstruation (4–6 days). Gradually the vessels close permanently and an intact circulation begins through the basal arteries. This marks the end of menstruation and also commencement of a new follicular phase.
- Another theory of menstruation holds an additional spasm and then necrosis of the walls of spiral arteries, leading to spotty haemorrhages that become confluent and produce the menstrual flow. This vasospasm is probably produced by

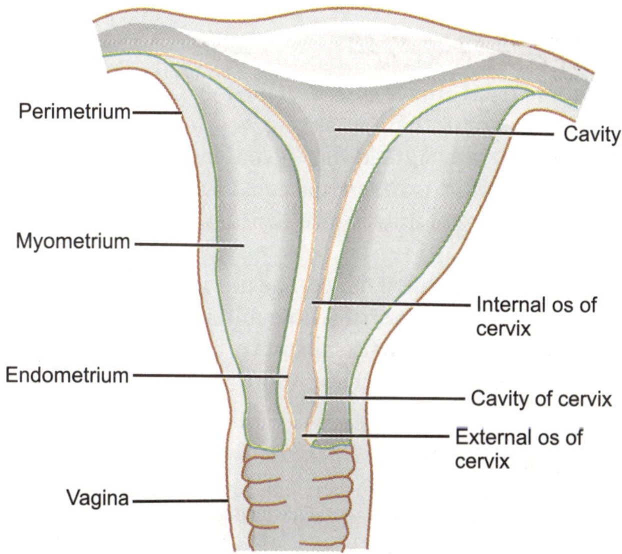

Fig. 50.2: Uterine section

locally released prostaglandins. There are large quantities of prostaglandins in the secretory endometrium and in menstrual blood and infusion of PGF_2 produce endometrial necrosis and bleeding.

- One theory of onset of menstruation holds that in necrotic endometrial cell, lysosomal membrane breakdown, with the release of enzymes, that foster the formation of prostaglandins from cellular phospholipids.

SURGE: A VIEW

1. Very high level of oestrogen (which persists for 36 hours) along with little level of progesterone $\xrightarrow[\text{(vicious cycles)}]{\text{positive feedback}}$ massive production of LH and vigorous production of FSH → known as LH and FSH surge respectively.
2. LH surge causes ovulation + formation, maintenance of corpus luteum which produces both these sex hormones.
3. LH has got specific effects on granulosa and theca cells. They are converted to more progesterone secreting cells, and less oestrogen secreting cells. So rate of secretion of oestrogen falls about one day before to ovulation while small amounts of progesterone are secreted so all this leads to rapid growth of follicle, diminished oestrogen secretion and beginning of secretion of progesterone.
4. A 'luteinization inhibiting factor' has been mentioned which acts like a local hormone. It checks luteinization process until after ovulation.
5. Graafian follicle is named after De Graaf — a Dutch Naturalist (1672).

NO SEXUAL CONTACT

The menstrual phase is a part of the safe period and some women are having strong sex desire at that time but it is generally agreed that sexual intercourse (coitus) is prohibited during menstrual cycle. Medical arguments against practice of intercourse (coitus) during menstrual cycle

i. Sexual excitement may cause uterine congestion and increase the menstrual flow and that more vascular and friable vaginal walls may be injured but these are theoretical considerations with little practical significance.

Hormonal interactions—a summary: Oestrogen content of blood rises when ovary is stimulated by FSH (from anterior pituitary) and when concentration of this hormone (ovarian) reaches a certain level, it in turn acts to suppress the output of FSH and excite LH principal of anterior pituitary so concentration of oestrogen upon which proliferative stage of menstruation, depends is thus reduced and this LH principle stimulates development of corpus luteum, but as the concentration of progesterone rises in blood, LH production suppressed with the result that integrity of luteal tissue cannot be maintained. With the fall in concentration of oestrogen and progesterone, menstrual bleeding occurs and FSH secretion is then resumed with commencement of another cycle.

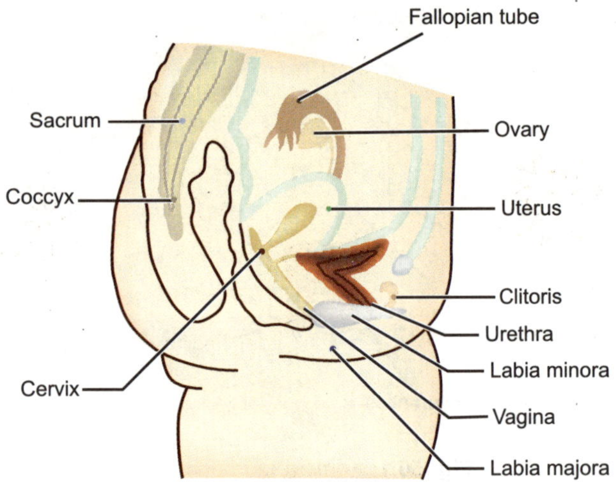

Fig. 50.3: Female reproduction

ii. If there is chronic or latent infection in the genital tract of either male or female, there is danger of 'salpingitis' if coitus is practised during menstrual cycle.

SAFE PERIOD

Sexual intercourse must be restricted to those times in menstrual cycle when there is very little chance that an ovum will be available for fertilisation. When there is normal cycle of 28 days safe period comprises 4 days of menstrual cycle itself, 3 days postmenstrually and 9 days premenstrually. In all women, the safest of all periods is 7 days preceding menstruation. The only disadvantage is that this simple calculation is not safely applicable to any one except that lady who is having regular menstrual cycle. Many couples use contraceptives during the fertile period but take a chance to enjoy sexual pleasure during the safe period. If ovulation is occurring normal in a woman, i.e. on 14th day of menstrual cycle, then the best chances of pregnancy on intercourse (coitus) occurs on 12, 13, 14, 15 days of menstrual cycle so-called 'fertile period' (opposite of safe period).

MENSTRUAL CYCLE IN RELATION TO LACTATION

Popular belief that return of menstrual cycle results in deterioration in supply and quality of milk is WRONG. In women who do not lactate menstruation usually reappears 6–8 weeks after delivery and is regular within 3 month. After abortion the 1st menstrual cycle generally appears in 4–6 weeks and ovular in 75 per cent.

PREMENSTRUAL TENSION SYNDROME

It occurs in the late luteal phase and is characterised by emotional upset, headache, oedema, changes in appetite or craving for certain foods, breast swelling and tenderness, constipation, decreased ability to concentrate, a sensation of abdominal bloating, acniform eruptions, depression/irritability/tension/fatigue.

There are many hypothesis to explain this syndrome like oestrogen excess or progesterone deficiency, vitamin deficiency, altered aldosterone production, altered neurotransmitter, modulation of salt and water balance, hypoglycaemia, altered endogenous opiates or endorphin modulation of gonadotropin secretion, etc. but no one is perfect in explaining the pathophysiology of this syndrome. Oral contraceptives are widely believed to afford relief from premenstrual tension symptoms. Some workers suggest that this syndrome is of less intensity in users of oral contraceptives than in non-users. In general oral contraceptive therapy is not a suitable treatment for this syndrome.

MENOPAUSE

It is natural cessation of menstruation and is counterpart of menarche. It is attained between 42–52 years depending upon environment, racial factor, number of pregnancy which a woman had, age of menarche, socio-economic factors, etc.

Physical Changes

Breast shrivel and becomes flat except in obese (fatty) woman in whom they remain large and pendulous. Anterior pituitary responds by functional changes and thyroid, adrenal are also altered. The shoulders become flat, waist line is lost, there may be slight growth of hair on face. Plasma and urinary levels of calcium and potassium tend to rise having relationship with osteoporosis. Increase in weight is common but not generally believed.

GIT

Universal tendency of flatulence so constipation, dyspepsia, abdominal discomfort while appetite may be increased or decreased.

Endocrine

Obesity, slight virilisation, low BMR, dryness skin, reduction in mental power and concentration, raised cholesterol.

Genital Tract

a. Vulvular skin becomes thin and pale with progressive atrophy.
b. Vagina is dry with low glycogen with senile vaginitis.
c. Uterus diminishes in size shrinks but does not disappear.
d. Atrophy of cervix with diminution in its mucous secretion.
e. Ovulation finally stops in ovary with gradual decrease in oestrogen production.

Menstrual Changes

Three classical changes during which period ceases:

1. Sudden stoppage.
2. Gradual diminution in amount of loss with each regular period until they disappear.
3. Gradual increase in spacing of period until they finally stop for an interval of six months. Any woman who menstruates after a gap of 6 months must be considered to be suffering from postmenopausal bleeding.

CVS

The commonest change is 'hot flushing and sweating' which are occurring in daytime but are worse at night in bed and this night sweating disturbs patient's rest. Functional derangement of cardiac action with palpitation are common and angina pains of effort are complained of at this time. Vasodilatation is followed by vasoconstriction so after a flush comes 'cold shiver'.

HORMONE REPLACEMENT THERAPY

1. **Actions.** It improves physical/mental and sexual well being. By it atrophic changes are diminished. It reduces the risk of coronary artery diseases. It restores calcium balance, so further loss of bone is checked; of course, bone loss again starts on cessation of hormone replacement therapy.
2. **Doses.** Conjugated estrogens are used (0.625-1.25 mg/day).
   - It is equivalent to ethynylestradial (5-10 μg) - three weeks treatment and then one week gap.
   - A progestin is added for 10 to 12 days each month (medroxy-progesterone acetate/norethisterone; 2.5 mg daily).
   - Oestrogen alone is used in hysterectomised women and also when progestin is not tolerated or is contra-indicated.

3. **Mechanism.** It reduces the risk of ischaemic heart diseases through favourable changes in lipid profile (raised HDL: LDL ratio), inhibition of LDL oxidation, reduced arterial impedance, increased production of PGI_2 etc.
4. **Risk.** Predisposition of breast cancer, gallstones, migraine etc.

Psycho-Physiological Changes

'Pin and needle sensation' with headache and noises in ear, with increase in sexual feeling. Fundamental reason for emotional upset is menopause represents end of reproductive era. She is worried unnecessarily about the fact that her husband will not give that love and affection and out of physical tiredness she will be unable to perform routine household activities. This age is also a time of STRESS in home since children at this age cause more worries to parents (often needless). All these things give menopause a bad name so it is the main reason why so many women approach it with fear.

Physiologic Basis of Treatment

'A woman will not like to listen menopause since to stay young desire is there;' so it is the primary duty of a doctor to convince her patient and to tell exact physiological basis of her hormonal state. Intelligent ladies must start this new phase of life with a great confidence, tolerance and scientific knowledge given by doctor. *If this will not be practised, she will be continuously looking for shadow of a shadow.*

Other Menstrual Problems

- This includes 'menstrual migraine' which is characterised by headache which is localised to one side of head. This headache is severe and accompanied by nausea and vomiting. Since it is associated with menstruation, they are relieved temporarily by pregnancy.
- Premenstrual tension is a symptom complex characterised by headache, emotional upset and disturbed mood, enlargement—congestion and pain in breast, oedema of feet and ankles.

  It all occurs seven to ten days before the onset of the period. Symptoms are relieved by the onset of menstrual flow. The symptoms may be aggravated by undue anxiety, unhappy life, psychoneurosis, etc. Retained body fluid must be eliminated with diuretics, if necessary.
- Amenorrhoea—Absence of menstrual periods
  Dysmenorrhoea—Painful menstruation
  Metrorrhagia—Bleeding from uterus more than once in a month
  Menorrhagia—Scanty, abnormal profuse flow during regular periods.

MANAGEMENT OF MENSTRUATION (Menstrual Hygiene)

i. All the superstitions/folklore above mentioned should be resisted and corrected before society on clear physiological/scientific grounds and it should be told to social authorities that a menstruating woman must visit temples as well as kitchen of house.
ii. Menstrual discharge is usually controlled by means of an absorbent "sanitary pad" or diaper which has to be changed regularly.

WITHDRAWAL BLEEDING

In any case, if ovary is removed and then oestrogen and progesterone therapy is continuing, then bleeding will not occur naturally. But as soon as these hormones are suddenly withdrawn/discontinued, then bleeding will occur identical with menstruation. This is called "withdrawal bleeding."

HIGHLIGHTS AND SUMMARY

This cycle consists of two parts—the follicular and luteal phases. During the follicular phase approximately the first half of menstrual cycle, several follicles are stimulated with FSH secreted by adenohypophysis. From that group of follicles one usually emerges in mid follicular phase as the dominant (or graafian follicle) and the major source of estradiol in the late follicular phase. After the mid cycle, ovulation occurs, marking the onset of second part of menstrual cycle the luteal phase. The remainder of graafian follicle, now lacking an egg and some of its surrounding cells is transformed into corpus luteum which secretes progesterone. The functional lifespan of corpus luteum is 14 days, after which it undergoes luteolysis. On 27th day progesterone level comes to zero because of negative feedback mechanism. So zero level of both these hormones constitute the basis of menstruation as shown in Table 50.1.

BIBLIOGRAPHY

1. Di. Zerege GS, GD Hodgen. Folliculogenesis in the primate ovarian cycle. Endo Rev 1981;2:27-49.
2. Ferin MD, et al. The hypothalamic control of the menstrual cycle and the role of endogenous opioid peptides. Rec Prog Horm Res 1984;40:441-85.
3. Frommer DJ. BMJ. Changing age of menopause. 1964;ii 349-351.
4. Gruhn JG, Kozer RR. Hormonal regulation of menstrual cycle. New York, Planum Publishing Corporation. 1989.
5. Hammond CB, Maxson WS. Physiology of menopause : Current concepts. Upjohn. 1983.

Table 50.1: Highlighting the physiology

Phase uterine changes	*Ovarian changes*	*Control and comments*
	Resting Phase	
1-5th day Endometrium heals becoming normal	Corpus luteum degenerated. Inhibitory action of progesterone absent so rising oestrogen level and follicles maturing.	Oestrogen controlled by FSH (anterior pituitary) which is controlled by GnRH from hypothalamus.
	Proliferative Phase	
6th-14th day Mucosa thickens (1-2 mm) Glands become larger, tortuous, vessels dilate.	Follicles maturing releasing oestrogen. On 14th day ovulation takes place.	Positive feedback mechanism between oestrogen — FSH and GnRH.
	Premenstrual Phase (Luteal)	
15th-27th day Glands more enlarged. Secretory vacuoles appear. Mucosa further thickens.	Corpus luteum grows. Progesterone secretion.	LH principal. Negative feedback between oestrogen and FSH.
	Menstrual Phase	
28th day	Corpus luteum degenerates.	Lack of progesterone negative feedback.

6. Herzberg BN, et al. Depressive symptoms and oral contraceptives. BMJ 1970;4:142.
7. Hsueh AJW, et al. Direct inhibitory effect of oestrogen on Leydig cell function in hypophysectomised rats. Endocrinology 1978;103:1096-1102.
8. Hsueh AJW, et al. Extrapituitary action of GnRh. Endocrinol Rev 1981;2:437-61.
9. Judith L. Vaitukaitis. Premenstrual syndrome. New Eng J of Med 1984;311:1371 : 21.
10. Ken N Muse, et al. The pre-menstrual syndrome: Effects of medical ovariectomy. New Eng J Med 1984;311: 1345 : 21.
11. Lai JH, SSC Yen. Induction of a mid cycle gonadotropin surge by ovarian steroids in woman : a critical evaluation. J Clin Endocrinol Metab 1983;57:797-802.
12. Loraine JA, Bell ET. Hormone excretion during normal menstrual cycle. Lancet 1963;i:1340-42.
13. Mason AJ, et al. Complementary DNA sequence of ovarian follicular fluid inhibin show precursor structure and homology with transforming growth factor -beta. Nature 1985;318:659-63.
14. Means E, Grant ECG. Anoular as an oral contraceptive. BMJ 1962;75.
15. Robert L. Reid, S.S.C. Yen. Pre menstrual syndrome. Amer J Obst and Gynae 1981;139: 85.
16. Ryan KJ, et al. Steroid formation by isolated and recombined granulosa and thecal cells. J Clin Endocrinol Metab 1968;28: 355-58.
17. Yen SS, A Lein. The apparent paradox of negative and positive feedback control system on gonadotropin secretion. Amer J Obst Gynae 1976;126:942-54.

51 Most Delicate Period: Pregnancy

Pregnancy is delicate of all delicate period in the life of woman. It gives a sense of pleasure—a state of motherhood which marks this success of life of a lady. In first trimester the lady is in trouble because of nausea—vomiting : in second trimester she forms a nest of thoughts regarding the development and future of her child : While in last trimester she is again worried about the delivery process which is most exaggerated by other women of the society. In these bunches of thoughts this period passes and the lady attains and enjoy—the motherhood.

FERTILISATION

This is the union of an ovum and a spermatozoon, occurring usually at ampulla of the fallopian tube, 36–48 hours after ovulation. A ***zygote*** is formed from this union containing 46 chromosomes in its nucleus; which are contributed by sperm and ovum (23 from each).

The new cell (zygote) travels towards the uterus aided by ciliary and peristaltic movements of the fallopian tube. It is nourished by the secretions in the tube and food previously stored around the ovum. During this journey it takes the zygote three days to divide and subdivide to form a mass of cells ***'Morula'***. Later on, a cavity develops at one end of morula which contains some fluid and whole structure is called ***Blastocyst***. It arrives at uterus by fourth or fifth day. Its outer layer of cells is called ***'Trophoblast'*** and collection of cells at one pole inside the 'blastocyst' is called ***'Inner cell mass'***. The layer of cells connecting the inner cell mass and the trophoblast will form ***'Body stalk'***.

As a result of conception, the corpus luteum continues to grow and more progesterone is produced, which promotes the growth and development of the secretory endometrium into the *'Decidua.'* Due to these secretory changes the glands of endometrium become dilated, more tortuous, more secretory, more vascular, more thick. Therefore, in this way, it provides a rosy, nourishing bed for the developing foetus.

The 'blastocyst' usually rests on 'decidua' of 'fundus-uteri.' The trophoblast secretes an enzyme which erodes the decidua and some blood vessels. So the blastocyst becomes embedded in decidua. When fully embedded the 'blastocyst' is surrounded by a pool of maternal blood. The trophoblast develops into the *'placenta and chorion'* while inner cell mass forms the *'foetus, umbilical cord and amnion.'*

DEVELOPMENT OF PLACENTA AND CHORION

There are three distinct layers of cells of trophoblast—outerlayer—syncytium; middle semi permeable layer Langhan's layer—inner layer—primitive mesenchyme.

These above three layers arrange themselves into finger like projections (these are primitive chorionic villi and trophoblast now called primitive chorion) which multiply or proliferate invading decidua and maternal blood vessels. Foetal capillaries appear in mesenchymal core of each villus. One portion of primitive chorion next to decidua basalis outgrows the other portion, (almost three weeks after fertilisation) which eventually atrophies. The portion that outgrows is called 'chorion frundosum' while the portion which atrophies is called 'chorion laeve'.

The collection of villi of chorion frundosum form the 'placenta' while remaining of 'chorion laeve' forms the 'chorion'. The placenta is completely developed at about 12th week of pregnancy.

The cells of the body stalk elongate and later on become 'umbilical cord'. The differentiation of cells of inner cell mass results in formation of two cavities—amniotic cavity and yolk sac.' The amniotic cavity contains fluid called 'liquor—amnii'. This amniotic cavity rapidly outgrows the yolk sac and fills the cavity of blastocyst. Its lining called amnion becomes adherent to the chorion and also lines the foetal surface of placenta and umbilical cord.

FERTILISATION—FEW FACTS

- Foetus and the mother are two genetically distinct individual and foetus may be regarded as a transplant of foreign tissue in the mother. But it is not rejected and hence tolerated. The reason being that the placental trophoblast which separates maternal and foetal tissues does not express the polymorphic class I and II MHC genes, but it expresses HLA-G-a non-polymorphic gene. So antibodies against foetal proteins don't develop.
- The blastocyst becomes surrounded by an outer layer of syncytio-trophoblast (multinucleated mass) and an inner layer of cytotrophoblast (individual cells). The former erodes the endometrium and blastocyst burrows into it, so called implantation—the usual site of it is dorsal wall of the uterus.
- Fertilisation usually occurs in mid portion of fallopian tube. Human ovum secretes a chemotectic factor which attracts sperm towards egg. Many sperms contact zona pellucida—a membranous structure that surrounds ovum. Then occurs acrosomal reaction, i.e. the breakdown of acrosome—the lysozyme like on the head of sperm. Various enzymes are released including trypsin like protease—the acrosin which facilitates the penetration of sperm through zona pollucida. The one sperm fuses to the membrane of the ovum. This fusion sets off a reduction in the membrane potential of the ovum that prevents polyspermy, i.e. entry of more than one sperm. This fusion causes structural change in zona pellucida which further prevents entry of other sperms.

PLACENTA (means = a cake; mini endocrine gland) Is a flat circular organ with a diameter of 20–25 cm, weighing 450 gm (1/6th of baby's weight) and is attached with umbilical cord and its membranes. It is having two surfaces—'maternal' (dark, red, irregular) and 'foetal' (grey with blood vessels running in different directions).

Its Functions

a. It acts as a *'connecting link'* between foetus and mother.

b. *Nutritive:* Food substances in their simplest forms like amino acid, glucose, fatty acids, mineral salts and vitamin are carried in maternal blood and are transmitted to the foetus through placenta. The rate of transfer from mother to foetus increases with advancement of pregnancy. Substances with molecular weight less than 1,000 can easily cross placenta. In emergency it converts glycogen into glucose stored in decidua (*glucogenic function*). The sources of foetal fat are—transfer of fatty acids and cholesterol across the placenta, synthesis of fat from carbohydrates.

c *Excretion:* Waste products of metabolism like urea, NPN, creatinine etc. are excreted by foetus into placenta through arteries.

d. *Gas exchange across placenta*: Because of its respiratory functions, it has been named as *'uterine lung'*. The placenta contains two separate moving blood streams—maternal and foetal separated from one another by one or more layers of foetal and maternal tissues which we call the placental membrane. The partial pressure of oxygen is higher on maternal side than on foetal side of membrane and only process involved in transfer of oxygen from maternal to foetal blood across placental membrane is diffusion.

   CO_2 diffuses 20 times as rapidly as O_2 by pressure gradient. The Pco_2 in foetal blood is 40–46 mm Hg while in maternal blood it is 40–45 mm Hg. This is the development of low pressure gradient across the placental membrane.

e. *Storage*: It is storehouse of glycogen, fats and proteins. Thus it can control the foetal blood glucose level. Iron and calcium are also stored. In early days of pregnancy it therefore acts in the same way as liver acts in adults.

f. *Protection*: It allows protective antibodies to pass to the foetus.

g. *Enzymatic capabilities*: The enzymes present in placenta include—'Glycerophosphate dehydrogenase', 'Lactate-dehydrogenase', 'Glucose-6-phosphate-dehydrogenase,' 'Mono-amine-oxidase,' 'Ribonuclease,' 'glucoronidase,' 'Maltase,' 'Arginase,' 'ATPase,' 'Acid and Alkaline phosphatase,' 'Deoxy ribonuclease,' 'Lysozyme,' 'Inulase cathepsin(s),' 'Cholin esterase,' 'Adenylate kinase,' 'cytochrome oxidase,' 'catalase,' 'Lipase,' 'succinate-dehydrogenase,' 'Glutamic-pyruvic-transaminase,' 'NADP,' 'Inorganic pyro phosphatase.'

STORY OF PREGNANCY BEHIND CURTAIL

a. *Maturation of Ovum*: Shortly before ovum is released from G. follicle, by meiosis its nucleus divides and first polar body is expelled from nucleus of ovum this becoming secondary oocyte. Each of 23 pairs of chromosomes loses one of the partners to the polar body so 23 unpaired chromosomes remain in the secondary oocyte, at this point fertilisation occurs.

b. *Fertilisation of Ovum*: Only one sperm is required for fertilisation of ovum. After coitus (sexual intercourse) sperms are deposited in vagina (almost half billion) but only 1000–3000 succeed in traversing the fallopian tubes to reach ovum. Sperms can remain fertile in female genital tract for 24–72 hr (highly fertile for 12–24 hr). Again on another side ovum after ovulation is fertilisable for upto 24 hr (8–12 hr maximum fertilisable period). Due to own motility of sperms,

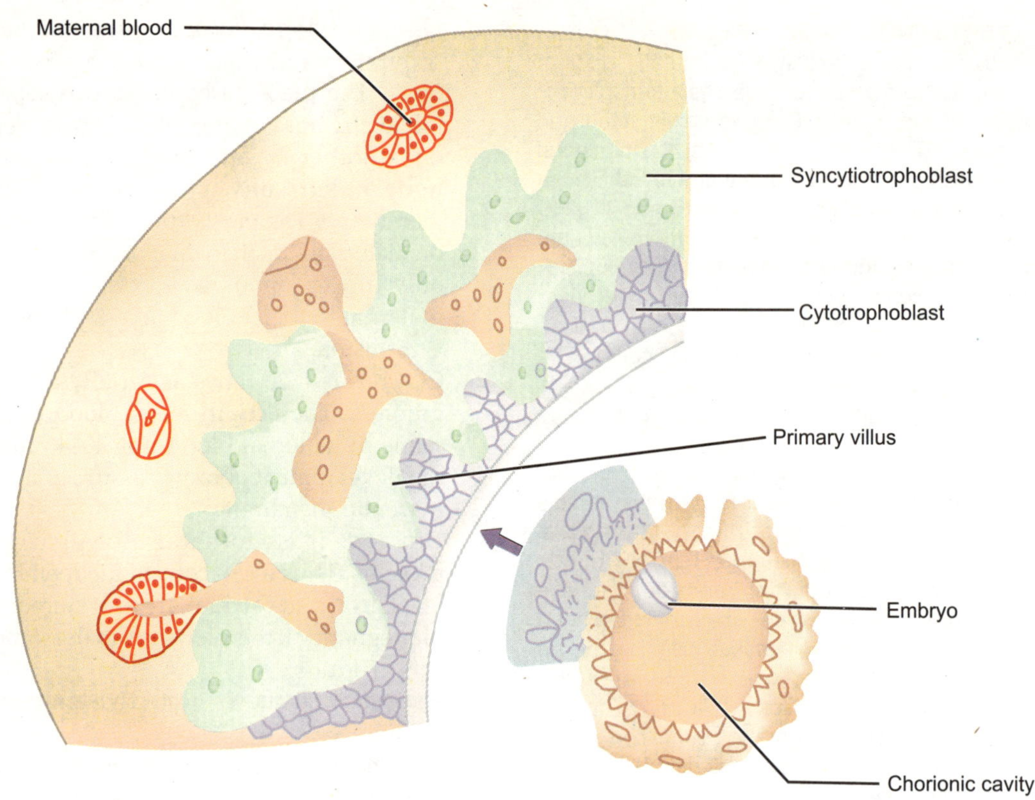

Fig. 51.1: Section through a human conceptus

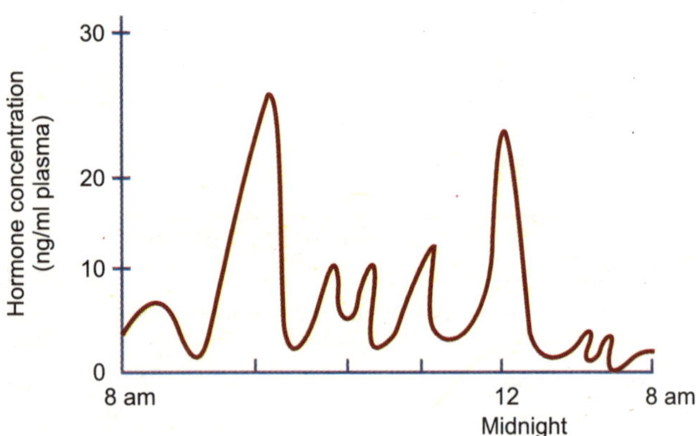

Fig. 51.2: Growth hormone variation: throughout day

propulsive movements of uterus and fallopian tubes, oxytocin secretion by posterior pituitary sperms are transported through uterus to the ovarian end of fallopian tubes within 5 minutes. Once sperm enters the ovum, its head forms 'male pronucleus' by swelling and later on complete complement of 46 chromosomes (23 pairs) is reformed in fertilised ovum (remaining 23 chromosomes coming from female pronucleus).

c. *Entry of ovum in fallopian tube*: We already know ovum is discharged in peritoneal cavity by a process called ovulation The fimbricated ends of each fallopian tube fall naturally around ovaries and inner surface of fimbriated tentacles are lined with ciliated epithelium and cilia continuously beat towards abdominal ostium of fallopian tube. By this ovum enters either fallopian tube. Ova can even enter opposite fallopian tube.

d. *Transport of ovum through fallopian tube*: After fertilisation additional three days are normally required for transport of ovum through tube into cavity of uterus. Fertilisation of ovum normally takes place soon after ovum enters fallopian tube but this process cannot occur until 'cumulus oophorus' (granulosa cells attached to outside of ovum) are dispersed from ovum. Transport mechanism is completed by

i. Feeble fluid current caused by ciliated epithelium lining tube since cilia are beating towards uterus.
ii. Isthmus of fallopian tube remains contracted for first three days following ovulation and after 3 days

time due to rapidly increasing progesterone, this region loses spasm, allowing thus entry of ovum in uterus.

e. *Implantation of ovum in Uterus:*
   i. Implantation means 'living in endometrium' in addition fertilised ovum remains in uterine cavity, so implantation occurs on 7th–8th days following ovulation. During this period ovum gets nutrition from fallopian tube secretion and 'uterine milk'. This is blastocyst stage.
   ii. Then trophoblast cells appears over surface of blastocyst which secrete proteolytic enzyme which liquefies cells of endometrium thus releasing much fluid and nutrients and their absorption through phagocytosis process, also additional trophoblast cells form cords of cell that extend into deeper layer of endometrium and attach them. Thus blastocyst eats a hole in endometrium and attaches to it at the same time. After this implantation trophoblasts and sublying cells proliferate rapidly forming placenta and membranes if fertilised ovum is implanted in endometrium. Continued secretion of progesterone cause stromal cells to swell still more and to contain more nutrients, these cells called 'decidual cells' and whole mass is decidua.

ESTIMATION OF PROBABLE DATE OF DELIVERY (CONFINEMENT) (NEAGELE'S METHOD)

The first day of last menstruating period (LMP) is taken. The actual date is calculated by adding roughly 7 days and then counting forwards 9 calendar months. Suppose LMP is 3rd Sep. adding 7 days, comes 10th Sep. and then 9 calendar months, this comes to 10th June, but this is approximate figure, plus-minus of fortnight period may be there.

HORMONAL REGULATION OF PREGNANCY

Placental Hormones

i. ***Oestrogen:*** Major amount of 'estriol' (E_3) is formed, then comes 'estrone' (E_1), and 'estradiol' (E_2).
   The major androgenic precursor to placental oestrogen is DHEAS (dehydroepiandrosterone sulphate).
   Estriol is weak excepting that it increases utero placental blood flow. It also stimulates liver enzymes to increase binding proteins.

ii. ***Progesterone:*** Its majority is formed by circulating maternal cholesterol. It is metabolised to pregnanediol and excreted in maternal urine.

iii. ***hCS (Human-chorionic somatomammotropin):***
   - Source—syncytiotrophoblast
   - molecular weight 38,000.
   - Functions as 'maternal growth hormone of pregnancy; which means—retention of nitrogen, calcium, potassium; lipolysis, decreased glucose utilisation.
   - Large quantities are present in maternal blood but very little reaches to foetus. Its peak level is achieved during last four weeks of gestation.
   - It has no luteotropic and prolactin like activity.
   - Synonyms : Human placental lactogen (hPL), chorionic growth hormone—Prolactin (CGP).
   - Functions as prolactin and in some instances causes lactation.
   - Protein deposition like growth hormone.
   - Decreased utilisation of glucose by cells so increasing blood sugar level + release of fatty acid from their stores and thus provides energy to foetus.

iv. ***hCG (Human chorionic–gonadotropin):***
   - It is a glycoprotein, containing galactose and hexosamine.
   - molecular weight 38,000.
   - Produced by syncytiotrophoblast.
   - It is primarily luteinizing and luteotropic having little FSH activity.
   - It acts on same receptor as LH.
   - Its small amounts also produced by foetal liver and kidney.
   - Its presence in urine is the index of pregnancy tests.
   - It exists in two forms—hCG A (molecular weight 18,000), and hCG B (molecular weight 28,000).
   - Other actions are: intrinsic thyroid stimulating activity, regulation of steroid production in the foetus during early pregnancy.
   - It prevents involution of corpus luteum. So it continues to secrete progesterone so large quantity of nutrients are available.
   - Also exerts interstitial cell stimulating effect' on testes resulting in production of testosterone which causes growth of male sex organs in male foetus.

v. ***Neuropeptides in placenta:***
   - GnRH (Gonadotropin-releasing hormone) related with regulation of hCG. Synthesised in cytotrophoblast.
   - Somatostatin : It is involved with inhibition of hCS release. Synthesised by cytotrophoblast in first trimester.

- TRH, CRH, ACTH< β-endorphin, β-lipoprotein etc.
- Their presence suggests that foetoplacental unit functions like—hypothalamo-pituitary target unit.

vi. ***Other peptides (Pregnancy specific)***
- β_1 glycoprotein (SP_1)—synthesised by syncytiotrophoblast, with a molecular weight of 90,000.
- Relaxin secreted and synthesised by corpus luteum of pregnancy.
- Other peptide growth factors, e.g. epidermal growth factor, inhibin, activin.

Other hormones

i. ***Thyroid***: Pregnancy → increased GFR → increased urinary excretion of iodine → depletion of iodine pool → to compensate gland enlarges with increase in iodine uptake. High levels of circulating oestrogen stimulate TBG.

ii. ***Parathyroid:*** Enlarged → Ca^{2+} absorption from bones of mother → normal Ca^{2+} concentration is maintained as foetus removes Ca^{2+} for ossifying its own bones.

iii. ***Pituitary:*** Anterior lobe increases so increasing secretion of growth hormone, TSH, ACTH, etc. Decrease in FSH and LH.

iv. ***Adrenal***: Increase in gluco and mineral corticoids. So tendency to retain fluid leading to hypertension.

SIGNS OF PREGNANCY

1. ***Suppression of Menstruation (Amenorrhoea):*** This is the first sign of pregnancy which leads a woman to think herself pregnant. But other cause of amenorrhoea may be kept in mind.
2. ***Morning sickness:*** Nausea and vomiting in early morning in first trimester particularly when a woman first rises from her bed. Normally it has got no side effect on health but it should not be in too much excess. Sometimes this sensation is also felt in afternoon or even in the evening.
3. ***Irritability of bladder:*** This is felt in early weeks and in the last two weeks. This frequency of micturition is due to pressure on bladder by growing uterus. As uterus become an abdominal organ, pressure on bladder is relieved. At the end of pregnancy the frequency is caused by the descent of presenting part into the pelvis.
4. ***Quickening:*** It is the first conscious feeling by mother of foetus in uterus. This feeling is just like 'fluttering of a bird in closed hand.' Most commonly occurs at 18–20 weeks or just above midterm. Uterus comes to lie closely in contact with abdominal wall and so uterine movements are transmitted to abdominal walls hence mother is made conscious of them.
5. ***Abdominal changes:*** Progressive enlargement of abdomen is of great significance with appearance of pigmentation called striae—gravidarum. In primi gravid woman the abdominal muscles are more strong and taut so enlargement of uterus is not so noticeable. State of umbilicus is also important. In first three months it is deepened and retracted, in second trimester it becomes shallower, in last two months it becomes everted and protruded above skin.

Positive Signs

1. Radiological X-ray evidence.
2. Foetal heart—It is a faint double sound like 'tickling of watch under pillow heard from 20–24 weeks. Rate is 120-140 per minute. Best heard by putting stethoscope in midline above symphysis.

Probable Signs

1. Shape of uterus—Globular shape of uterine body in early weeks the asymmetry of growth
2. Intermittent uterine contraction 'Brixton Hicks contraction
3. Changes in cervix—Softening of cervix as well as increase in its secretion are important evidence in favour of pregnancy.
4. Vaginal changes—Bluish cyanosed colour due to congestion seen in 2nd and 3rd months is characteristic of pregnancy 'Jacqemier's-sign.
5. Vaginal pulsation (osianader's sign) Pulsation in lateral fornices in 2nd or 3rd month of pregnancy due to increased size of uterine arteries. Increase in vaginal secretion occurs.

THE PHYSIOLOGICAL CHANGES DURING PREGNANCY

If ovum is fertilised by spermatozoa, pregnancy begins lasting for 280 days (about ten menstrual cycles). The changes are -

a. ***Vagina***: Increased vascularity and so increased secretion. Bulging of lower anterior wall at vulva. Pelvic joint also becomes loosened.

b. ***Cervix***: Light hypertrophy of its tissues. Increased vascularity. Increased glandular secretion so 'softening of cervix'. The cervix of a non pregnant uterus is of same consistency as tip of nose while during pregnancy it softens like consistency of lip.

c. ***Breast:***
   i. As early as second or third week of pregnancy woman may be conscious of prickling and tingling sensation in breast.
   ii. From second month there is a sense of fullness followed by visible increase in size, mammary tissues become firmer and nodular.
   iii. Nipples share in size, become darker in colour and more erectile.
   iv. From about fourth month a few drops of thin oily fluid *COLOSTRUM* (a poor emulsified fatty secretion and precursor of true milk which is secreted after delivery) can be expressed.
   v. During third month a deposit of pigment in areola around the nipple appears, the depth of colour varies from deep pink to dark brown or even black. (In the late months a faint secondary areola may be seen outside the primary areola but this is marked only in very dark woman).
   vi. Veins of the breast become more distended and prominent, may be seen as dark blue lines coursing over the breast just under the skin. This enlargement is due to hypertrophy of parenchyma stimulated by high oestrogen content of the blood. The actual elaboration of secretory cells is believed to be due to progesterone.

d. ***Ovary and Tubes:*** Increased vascularity. Ovary on one side will be found enlarged owing to the presence of corpus luteum of pregnancy. As the uterus rises up in to abdomen, tubes and ovary come to lie almost vertically by the sides of the uterus, By the third trimester ovaries are flattened.

e. ***Blood:***
   i. Increase in total blood volume which on full term increases upto 25%. Red cell volume is either maintained or increases, this is due to introduction of a new and enormously vascular organ the pregnant uterus and chorio-decidual space.
   ii. Also slight leucocytosis rapidly rising before labor persisting during first three or four days of post-delivery period (puerperium).
   iii. ESR is greatly increased but is not of a great diagnostic value, purely physiological fact.
   iv. Fibrinogen content of blood is increased and at term is between 325–400 mg per cent—a point which may be linked with blood clotting after delivery. "Globulin fraction of plasma proteins (both alpha and beta) also increases while albumin fraction falls. Since haemoglobin falls so pregnant woman if given iron from the beginning will not develop "physiologic anaemia."

f. ***Urinary system:***
   i. Rate of urine formation by pregnant lady is slightly increased due to increased load of excretory products.
   ii. GFR increases as much as 50%, thus increasing rate of water and electrolyte loss in urine. Renal plasma flow is also markedly increased proving that "kidneys are under some special strain during pregnancy".
   iii. Ureters show hypertrophy of their walls specially in lowest portion while upper portion is dilated, because of compression by enlarged uterus as ureter pass over pelvic rim thus increasing intra-ureteral pressure. Progesterone and relaxin also play a role in relaxing ureters. This ureteral and pelvic distension facilitates the renal infection.

g. ***Weight gain by mother:*** In first-three and four months pregnant lady loses weight due to nausea but during remaining two trimesters the average weight gain is 24 pounds.

h. ***Uterus and Birth canal:***
   i. Uterus enlarges due to hypertrophy and hyperplasia of its muscles, which are 10 times more longer and 6 time more wider than non-pregnant state.
   ii. Its weight increases upto 1000 gm at full term.
   iii. The lymphatic tract of the uterus enormously increases during pregnancy. The collecting channels in broad ligament, share in this growth.
   iv. Uterine nerves also increase in size and functionally are more active that is why uterus during pregnancy is more susceptible to reflex simulation better to say emotional stimuli.
   v. It also alters in shape, in the first three months, it loses its pyriform shape and become more and more globular while from fourth month it again becomes more oval as it grows up in the abdomen.
   vi. Both arteries and veins supplying, share in growth by becoming more angular and tortuous, growth is such that pregnant uterus become in sense part of blood vascular system and react as such to vasomotor influences such as nervous shock and certain drugs.
   vii. Size: "Its size is taken as a rough index of period of pregnancy attained"
   8th week: size of a egg.
   12th week: about the size of large orange (upper border palpable above pubic-symphysis)
   16th week: It has risen above brim of pelvis, its fundus is 4" above pubic symphysis.
   20th week: finger breadth below umbilicus

24th week: Just above the umbilicus
28th week: It has reached above one-third distance between umbilicus and xiphisternum.
36th week fundus of uterus approximately at ensiform cartilage. During last three or four weeks of pregnancy its sinks again, comes to lie one or two finger breadth below xiphisternum.

i. *Average gain in extracellular fluid during pregnancy (water retention)*

Product of conception	1.5–2 litres
Uterus and breast	0.7 litres
Blood plasma	0.5 litres
Extragenital interstitial fluid	2.5 litres
Total	5.2 to 5.7 litres

PREGNANCY: SOME MORE FACTS

1. *Respiration:* Total amount of oxygen used by mother shortly before delivery is more. This is due to increased BMR during pregnancy + increased size. This also causes increased minute ventilation. Progesterone increases the sensitivity of respiratory centre to CO_2. Furthermore, the growing uterus presses upwards against abdominal contents;which presses upwards against diaphragm; which decreases total excursion of diaphragm. This causes increased respiratory rate to maintain extraventilation.
2. *Nutrition:* 375 mg of iron is required by foetus to form its own blood; while extra 600 mg is needed by mother for her own. Normal store of iron is 100 mg so chances of anaemia is bright in these days. Because calcium is poorly absorbed by GIT in absence of vitamin D so adequate vitamin D is also necessary.

ABNORMALITIES OF PREGNANCY

a. *Hyperemesis gravidarum*: Condition characteristically begins as slowly progressive exaggeration of morning sickness. It is happening of first trimester of pregnancy. This is of course serious when vomiting occur very frequently at all times of the day or if it persists in spite of treatment. Vomiting is induced by even sight, smell thought of food. "Patient is unable to retain any food or fluid." Two cause can be mentioned on clear physiological grounds, one is 'neurotic' (psychosomatic) and other is toxic. Neurotic or psychosomatic—At the level of subconscious mind there is manifestation of psychological mind. In many instances baby is not wanted due to socio-economic factors while sometimes woman is anxious for baby better to say "wishful thinking" and sometimes there is disharmony between husband and wife. Another factor claimed to cause this is, diminution of glycogen reserve of liver and such deficiency is known to be associated with hyperexcitability of sympathetic nervous system which leads to reverse peristalsis of stomach. Glycogen deficiency is result rather than cause of vomiting but when vomiting is established, this will maintain it.

b. *Toxaemia of Pregnancy—Eclampsia:* Toxaemia constitutes a group of disease frequent during pregnancy having common features hypertension, oedema and albuminurea B.P. above 140/90 is abnormal called pre-eclampsia and when it is accompanied by convulsions, eclampsia is name given. This is the reason that blood pressure of pregnant lady should be checked fortnightly/ monthly. Oedema is more common during pregnancy. This is also due to obesity (longer the belt shorter the life). Lady will note that her face particularly eyelids are puffy on rising in morning, abdominal skin is thickened. She will also note that "her wedding ring is getting tight—very delicate test for hand oedema. Oedema of vulva marks severity of pre-eclampsia. This disorder is more common in primigravid woman with a history of familial hypertension, eclampsia is further characterised by disturbance of vision, headache, vomiting and epigastric pain.
Convulsion preceded by twitching and rolling of eyeballs, bitten tongue with foaming at mouth with violent contraction of limbs, and face become distorted. During fit the lady is unconscious and it lasts usually for one minute and faeces-urine may also be passed with a rise in pulse rate and temperature. During fit pupils don't react to light.

Terms Used in Pregnancy

i. Primi gravida: One who is pregnant for the first time.
ii. Primipara: Woman at the end of her first labor and thereafter.
iii. Multigravida: Woman during her second or subsequent pregnancies.
iv. Multipara: Woman who has had more than one child.
v. Nullipara: Woman who has not any children.

PREGNANCY TESTS

The term 'pregnancy test' is a misnomer. These procedures measure human chorionic gonadotropin and not the presence of a foetus. Its level is abnormally raised in pregnancy, hydatidiform mole, chorion epithelioma, malignant teratoma; while its level is decreased in incomplete abortion.

Biological Methods

These detect HCG in blood or urine of a pregnant women. First morning sample of urine is collected in a clean and sterile container.

At least 100 ml. of urine should be taken. No water or liquid diet after 8 pm previous night. Before collection of urine drugs like aspirin, salicylates, sedative should not be given. Within two hours of collection the sample should be tested. Urine should be clear, if not, filter it. Various such types of tests are listed:-

Immunologic Methods

The various tests employed are 'gel diffusion method,' 'complement fixation technique,' 'radioimmunoassay,' 'haem agglutination inhibition test' (HAI), 'precipitation test,' 'latex agglutination inhibition technique' (LAI).

PREGNANCY TESTS

First morning sample of urine is used.

1. *Ascheim-Zondek (1927) test (Mouse test)*: 0.4–0.5 ml of morning urine from a lady thought to be pregnant is injected by subcutaneous route twice daily for 3 days into 3–4 immature mice. On 4th-5th day animal is sacrificed and ovaries are extracted, Test is positive if blood filled follicles/corpora lutea found in ovaries.
2. *Friedman test (Rabbit test)*: 2 Rabbits (mature female isolated from males for 6 weeks) are injected with 10–15 ml of test urine by intravenous route. One is examined after 24 hours while second after 2 days. Test is positive if fresh corpora lutea appear in ovaries.
3. *Hegben Test (South African female clawed toad)*: 20–30 ml urine injected into dorsal lymph sac of animal. Test is said to be positive when appearance of large number of ova within 6–12 hours is there.
4. *Sperm shedding test (Galli-Mainini test)*: 5 ml urine injected into dorsal lymph sac of South African female clawed toad. Its urine after 1–2 hours examined for spermatozoa whose presence marks the positivity of the test.
5. *Kuperman test (ovarian hyperaemic/rat test)*: 2 ml of urine to be tested is injected by intraperitoneal route twice with an interval of one hour into prepuberal rats: Animals are examined for hyperaemia or blushing of ovaries at 2, 6, 12, and 24 hours.

Pseudo Pregnancy

Prolonged secretion of prolactin with corpus luteum retention together with delay in return of normal cycle for some time occurs in rats, mice and other species. This is pseudo pregnancy. Best stimulants are stimulation of cervix with glass rod, sterile coitus. So it is a neuro-endocrinal reflex. Sometimes due to strong emotional effects many women thinks themselves to be pregnant (pseudocyesis).

SUMMARY AND HIGHLIGHTS

Either as a result of the normal act or by artificial insemination, a tremendous number of sperm are introduced into the vaginal vault. The sperm, by their own motility, enter the uterus and travel up the fallopian tubes. Fertilisation usually takes place there. The fertilised egg is then carried down the fallopian tube to the uterus. Approximately 7 or 8 days after fertilisation it becomes implanted in the uterine wall.

Placenta marks a beautiful connection between mother and child. It is classed as a mini endocrine gland secreting various important hormones.

All other hormones are increased in amount so their activities is also increased. Pregnancy period is diagnosed by its typical sign and symptoms.

There are various pregnancy test available in literature.

BIBLIOGRAPHY

1. Diczfalusy E and Troen. Endocrine function of human placenta. Vitamin and Hormones 1961;19:229-311.
2. Dwain D. Hagerman. Enzymatic capabilities of placenta. Fed Proc 1964;23:785.
3. Jaffe LA. Electrical regulation of sperm egg fusion. Ann Phy Rev 1986;48:191.
4. James, Metcalfe, et al. Gas exchange across the placenta. Fed Proc 1964;23:774.
5. Lotgening FK et al. Maternal and foetal responses to exercise during pregnancy. Phy Rev 1985;65:1-29.
6. Nisula BC, et al. Evidence that chorionic gonadotropin is increasing thyro tropic activity. Biochem Biosphys Res Commun 1974;59:86-91.
7. Pekonen FH, et al. HCG and thyroid function in early human pregnancy. Circadian variation and evidence for intrinsic thyrotropic activity. J Clin Endocrinol Metab 1988;66:853-56.
8. Seron-Ferre M, et al. Role of HCG in regulation of foetal zone of human foetal adrenal gland. J Clin Endocrinol Metab 1978;46: 834-37.
9. Symposium on placenta. Amer J Obst Gynae 1962;84:1541-1798.
10. Walker WH, et al. The human placental lactogen genes : structure, function, evolution and transcriptional regulation. Endocr Rev 1991;12:316.
11. Wassarman PM. The biology and chemistry of fertilisation. Science 1987;235:553.
12. Wassarman PM. Fertilisation in mammals. Sc Amer 1988;78.
13. Wolf DP, et al. (Eds.) In vitro fertilisation and Embryo transfer. New York. Plenum publishing corporation. 1988.

52 Labour: Parturition

Labour or parturition, is the process by which the products of conception—the foetus, liquor amnii, placenta and membranes—are separated and expelled from the uterus.

INTRODUCTION

- Obstetrically, normal labour is that in which the child presents normal vertex of head, and which is having no complication and which is completed by natural unaided efforts of the mother within 24 hours.
- The word 'eutocia' is reserved for normal, while the word 'dystocia' is used for abnormal or pathological labor.

STAGES OF LABOR

The entire process is divided into three stages—namely:

First Stage or Stage of Dilatation

- The hallmark of this stage is periodic pains; due to uterine contractions. This can also be felt as hardness of uterus. At the onset the pain is weak, but along with the time it goes severe, beginning in the back and passing round to the front of abdomen and thighs. These contractions lead to dilatation of cervix which is accompanied by a slight discharge of blood stained mucus which is called 'show.' This is due to separation of foetal membranes and minute laceration of cervical mucosa. This stage lasts from 12–18 hours. At the end of it there is commonly a sudden gush of fluid, indicating that foetal membranes have ruptured and liquor amnii has escaped.

Second Stage or Stage of Expulsion

- After completion of first stage, the pains usually stop for few minutes but then re-start with greater frequency and now they are of down bearing nature. Abdominal muscles also contribute to uterine contractions. The effect of these pains is to drive the head through the cavity of the pelvis. As it descends, it presses upon the rectum and because of it, the lady feels a desire to defecate and the faeces are squeezed out during each contraction. As head comes further down, it presses on perineum which also bulges during each pain; the vulva also gaps more and more and with further descending of the head, the opening changes from slit to an oval shape and ultimately a circular opening. The perineum is so pressed that it appears thin and stretched. Behind it, the anus is also stretched that it appears as a 'D shaped opening' through which bulging of rectum may be seen. The alternate advance and recession of the head during and between the pains go on until the largest diameter of the head is forced through the vulva by a strong pain. Head is rapidly born by a movement of extension of the neck-brow and face of the child sweeping in succession over the perineum. This stage is further characterised by excruciating pain.
- This second stage lasts for two to three hours; at the end of which the uterus may be felt as a firm ovoid tumour extending upto just below the umbilicus.

Third Stage or Stage of Delivery

- This gives little relief to the lady because there is short cessation of pains. Of course, uterus starts contracting once again. Frequently there are little gushes of blood during the pains, indicating the separation of the placenta. In the end, the placenta is expelled by a strong pain into the vagina and then to exterior. This stage lasts from few minutes to an hour (average 20 minutes). Here the woman may have a shivering fit called ***'physiological chill of labour'*** which is due to cooling of body surface by perspiration, combined with the effects of severe muscular exertion.

THE PHYSIOLOGY OF PARTURITION

It very simply means, 'the process by which baby is born.' Following physiological factors contribute the entire process.

a. *Hormonal factors*: Following is the role played by various hormones -
   i. *Oestrogen: Progesterone*—Of course during the entire pregnancy period both these hormones are secreted in greater quantities; but in third trimester (7th to last month); the level of oestrogen is increased tremendously than progesterone. This is in fact a natural adjustment since progesterone inhibits uterine contractility so it is helping to prevent expulsion of the foetus; and on the other hand oestrogen increases the degree of uterine contractility; so it is a natural aid to the process of parturition.
   ii. *Oxytocin*: This hormone secreted from neurohypophysis increases the uterine contraction, and thus expulsion of child is facilitated. It has been observed that rate of oxytocin secretion is increased at the time of labor. Further, it has been seen that on hypophysectomy the labor process is prolonged.
b. *Mechanical factors*:
   - As the name suggests that irritation of uterine cervix is important in eliciting uterine contractions.
   - Uterus, during last few months of pregnancy undergoes periodic episodes of slow/weak but rhythmic contractions named as, *'Braxton Hicks contraction.'* At the end of pregnancy they become stronger enough to stretch the cervix which facilitates parturition.
   - Above series of contractions are caused by positive feedback mechanism. According to this concept, stretch of the cervix by head of the foetus becomes finally great enough to elicit a reflex increase in contraction of uterine body. This pushes the baby forward which further stretches the cervix and thus initiating a new cycle. This process continues again and again until the baby is expelled.
   - An initial contraction of the uterine body can force the foetal head or the fluid in amniotic cavity against the cervix to irritate it up to the extent of tear/stretch etc. This acts as an additional contraction of uterine body.
   - This cervical irritation by foetal head also stimulates posterior pituitary to release 'oxytocin' which further augments uterine contraction.
   - On this stretch mechanism, we can explain early delivery of twins, probably because of double irritation.
   - These labor contractions then also involve abdominal muscles which are also then thrown into contractions. This further adds to positive feedback mechanism; described above.
   - Above delivery of placenta the bleeding is limited to only 350 ml.

PARTURITION : FEW MORE INTERESTING FACTS

- The pituitary gland of foetus secretes oxytocin which further stimulates uterine contraction. In addition cortisol from foetal adrenal gland and prostaglandins from foetal membranes also stimulates uterine contraction.
- The uterine contraction during labor begins at the top of fundus and spread downward over the body. Furthermore, intensity of uterine contraction is more at top and body of uterus but weak in lower segment, near the cervix. This explains that each uterine contraction tends to force the baby downwards towards the cervix.
- The head of the baby is the first part to be delivered (normal vertex presentation). The head acts as a wedge to open the structures of birth canal to facilitate the delivery process.
- During each uterine contraction, 25 pounds force is exerted on foetus from uterine muscle and abdominal muscles.
- Initially uterine contractions occur every half hourly. Later on they occur every 1 to 3 minutes, with a very short period of relaxation. This is fortunacy provided by the Nature that these contractions are intermittent otherwise strong uterine contractions may cause stoppage of blood flow through placenta.

SUMMARY AND HIGHLIGHTS

- A decline in progesterone synthesis and release by placenta is necessary in order to permit forceful uterine contraction to occur at the end of term. Decline in progesterone is necessary a part of labor initiation. Oestradiol and esterone are elevated during last month of pregnancy in peripheral plasma. A rise in oestrogen just before parturition may be important in initiation of labor only in the presence of declining progesterone concentration.
- Mechanical irritation of uterus by foetus which is a positive feedback mechanism is another important physiological mechanism of delivery of child.

BIBLIOGRAPHY

1. Stabenfeldt GH, et al. Peripheral plasma progesterone levels in cow during pregnancy and parturition. Amer J Phy 1970;218:571.
2. Thorburn GD, Chalis JRG. Endocrine control of parturition. Phy Rev 1979;59:863.

53 Climax of Motherhood: Lactation

Suckling at breast is not going to spoil body figure but it is going to establish a heavenly relation between mother and child

- Reproductive behaviour can be divided into two broad phases sexual and parental. Both phases are programmed and under hormonal control. The sexual phase consisting of courtship and mating, is predominantly controlled by gonadotropins. The second or parental, phase is concerned with the care and feeding of the young. It begins after ovulation and has its peak after parturition. At this time secretion of sex steroids and gonadotropins has fallen to low levels, whereas that of '*Prolactin*' has risen to peak. The hormone prolactin acts as a releaser of parental behaviour.
- The period immediately following labor is called puerperium during which maternal organs return to their normal condition and lactation is striking phenomenon of this period.

BREAST AND HORMONES

i. Ductile system of the breast is developing and branching under the effect of oestrogen which is produced by placenta in tremendous quantity. It also increases the stroma of the breast and hence large quantities of fat are laid down in stroma.

ii. Under the effect of progesterone, growth of lobules, budding of alveoli and development of secretory character in cells of alveoli takes place.

iii. Prolactin

   a. *History*: it was discovered in 1928, as a lactogenic substance present in extracts of pituitary gland of the cow. In 1960–70 this has been identified, measured in human blood.

   b. *Source: chemistry*—Prolactin, presumably of pituitary origin is also found in relatively high concentration in human amniotic fluid. It probably has 18 amino acid. The amino acid sequence indicate that both prolactin and growth hormone arose from a common ancestral precursor molecule early in vertebrate evolution.

   c. *Actions*:

      i. Prolactin and STH together can induce full lobulo-alveolar- mammary growth in the rat. The ovarian hormones are believed to promote mammary growth mainly by stimulating secretions of prolactin and STH by adenohypophysis, and, by synergizing with these adenohypophyseal hormones, and, by sensitising the mammary gland to these hormones. Specific prolactin receptors have been detected in breast tissues of animals and these receptors increase in number with oestrogen treatment.

      ii. *Lactogenic*: It has long been established that adrenal cortical hormones as well as prolactin are essential for initiation and maintenance of lactation. If it is suddenly reduced (by hypophysectomy or administration of prolactin lowering drug), lactation ceases. After parturition lactation continues in an environment in which circulating oestrogens are low but prolactin is high. The act of suckling provides an important stimulus for the continued production of prolactin.

      iii. *Others*:

      - Hyper—prolactinaemia may be associated with amenorrhoea in women and reduced potency in males. Its metabolic actions are similar with growth hormone but to a less extent.
      - It orients the birds to care and protection as well as nutrition of its offspring. So it is designated as 'parental hormone.'

CONTROL OF SECRETION

1. It is under inhibitory control from hypothalamus. This inhibition is mediated by 'prolactin-inhibitory-factor (PIF) liberated by hypothalamus into portal vessels as a result of afferent dopaminergic impulses. It is a small molecule. The suckling stimulus, estradiol, reserpine, epinephrine, and acetylcholine are found to reduce hypothalamic PIF content in rats.

   Similarly 'prolactin releasing factor' also exist. 'Thyrotropin releasing hormone' is an important physiologic regulator of prolactin. Evidence for a prolactin releasing factor besides TRH has been obtained but its physiologic role is not certain.
2. Nursing appears to be most powerful and specific of all physiologic stimuli for prolactin release. It is mediated by cutaneous sensation arising from breast and nipple.

THE PROLACTIN

Inhibitors	*Stimulators*
1. Dopamine and its agonists	1. Dopamine antagonists
2. PIH	2. Catecholamine depletors (reserpine; alphamethyl dopa)
3. Glucocorticoid	3. TRH
4. Thyroid Hormone	4. Sleep
	5. Suckling
	6. Hypoglycaemia
	7. H_2 antagonist
	8. Exercise
	9. Pregnancy
	10. Opiate agonists
	11. Oestrogen

3. Stresses of all kind can cause prolactin release. This is seen most markedly after major operations with general anaesthesia. This explains galactorrhoea after major operations. The events like sleep, sexual intercourse with orgasm, tranquillising drugs are causing a rise in serum prolactin level.
4. The mean serum prolactin level is raised by oestrogen which also enhance responsiveness to prolactin-releasing-stimuli. These effects are apparent after several days of administration of oestrogen.
5. L-dopa (an anti-Parkinsonism drug) reduce serum-prolactin. With this drug the level goes to minimum two hours after its administration which comes to normal within 2–3 hours. This is initially decarboxylised to dopamine which then acts on hypothalamus and pituitary. Another such drug 'bromocriptine' also reduces serum-prolactin level.

   Serum-prolactin level is raised by 'Chlorpromazine and antipsychotic drugs' which inhibit dopaminergic transmission by blockade of dopamine receptors. Morphine raises its level in blood.

PHYSIOLOGY OF LACTATION

Milk is obtained from mammary glands of most species principally as a result of neuro-endocrine reflex. When baby suckles the breast, sensory impulses are transmitted through somatic nerves to the spinal cord and then to the hypothalamus. The afferent neural impulses are generated following stimulation of receptors in teat or overlying skin of mammary gland and results in rapid discharge of oxytocin (and vasopressin to a lesser extent) from neuro-hypophysis into blood. Oxytocin in turn causes contraction of myo-epithelial cells surrounding the alveoli and small ducts, thereby forcibly ejecting the milk into larger ducts, sinuses or cisterns, from where it can be passively withdrawn.

The myoepithelium of mammary glands also contracts in most of the species (mice, goats, rabbits) when mechanical stimulus is applied to skin overlying the mammary gland or directly to exposed mammary tissue. Direct activation of myo-epithelial cells is causing this action. So it has been suggested that suckling may mechanically stimulate myo-epithelium of mammary gland to contract for ejection of milk. All this constitute *'Let down reflex of milk ejection/draught.'*

The stimulus of suckling is followed by a depletion of prolactin in pituitary of rat (upto 90%). Physical or emotional stimuli associated with suckling may remove the hypothalamic inhibition over prolactin release. This prolactin releasing reflex may become conditioned.

Lactation: Hypothalamus and Adenohypophysis

Adenohypophysis is essential for lactation; without anterior lobe hormones lactation terminates and mammary glands regress. The secretion of possibly all adenohypophyseal hormones is thought to be influenced by hypothalamic neurohumours which reach the adenohypophysis by way of the hypophyseal portal vessels arising in median eminence of hypothalamus and traversing the infundibulum.

Prolactin from acidophil cells of anterior lobe is essential for both initiation and maintenance of lactation, being necessary for DNA synthesis and for milk secretion in mammary glands. Pituitary prolactin content rises in late pregnancy, continue in early lactation and declines with declining lactation, while decline is seen in non-suckled females, administration of large quantities of oestrogen and progesterone; while it is said to be more sensitive towards altered blood levels of thyroxine.

Presence of PIF has been demonstrated (prolactin—inhibiting factors). It is always present, possibly stored in hypothalamus and hypothalamic response to suckling stimulus is one of temporary inhibition of tonic release of this substance. It inhibits release of prolactin from pituitary.

Besides prolactin; ACTH and STH, thyroxin and insulin are also essential for lactation and hence they are also classed as 'galactopoietic hormones'. Both ACTH and STH have prolactin sparing effects in restoration of lactation in the hypophysectomized animal. Thyroxine has definite galactopoietic activity and increases in the rate of thyroxine excretion or utilisation in lactation may themselves induce increased TSH secretion by negative feedback. Thyroid secretion rates are greater in lactating than in non-lactating females. Thus, the pituitary content of each of the 'galactopoietic triad' necessary for lactation—namely 'Prolactin ACTH and STH can be depleted in response to suckling.

Food-intake increases in lactation to meet the demand for raw materials in milk, at the direction of appetite-controlling-mechanism in hypothalamus. Raised levels of lactogenic hormone increase food-intake and this action may account for increased appetite in pregnancy. The food consumption is also increased by suckling, while weaning is followed by diminished food-intake. Premature weaning results in cessation of milk synthesis and rapid involution of the secretory epithelium of the mammary glands. Stimuli associated with suckling or milling are essential for the maintenance of lactation.

Secretion of lactation maintaining hormones (Prolactin, STH, ACTH) and their level in blood. Occur in response to stimuli of both neural and systemic origin, operating at hypothalamic level. Their lowered level in blood may increase their rates of secretion from pituitary by negative feedback mechanism and for this to occur, releasing hormones from hypothalamus are playing a leading role.

LACTATION AT A GLANCE

A. *Two hormones from pituitary, for breast growth—preparing for lactation*:
   Mammogen I—stimulate duct system under the influence of oestrogen.
   Mammogen II—Growth of lobular alveolar system under the influence of progesterone.
   Prolactin is the main hero hormone of lactation.

B. *Initiation of lactation*
   High ovarian hormone levels during pregnancy would promote glandular development whereas sharp fall in concentration at parturition would permit lactation to begin. Oestrogen and progesterone exert an antagonistic effect towards prolactin at mammary gland level.

C. Maintenance of lactation
   Stimulus by suckling causes a nervous reflex release of lactogenic hormone from pituitary (prolactin) which maintains lactation. This establishes role of nervous/psychic factor.
   ACTH + Prolactin—best combination
   Thyroxin also maintains.

D. *Milk ejection*—Let down reflex/draught.

E. The milk secretion occasionally occurs in a child shortly after birth is '*witches milk*' which is explained on the basis, that foetus is exposed to ovarian hormones and elimination of these after birth might result in liberation of prolactin from infant's pituitary.

BREAST IN PUERPERIUM

During first few days of puerperium there is little change in breast. They become full and markedly congested making the lady very much sensitive. Early milk is called '*colostrum*' which is sticky yellow fluid containing leukocytes engorged and bloated with fat droplets. It is then replaced by true milk. It contains numerous globules and cell fragments together with free fat droplets, lymphocytes, monocytes, histiocytes, desquamated epithelial cells and colostrum corpuscles. It contains little fat but larger amount of antibodies.

INHIBITION OF MILK EJECTION

Psychogenic factors (stress, emotions, frustrations, excitement) are creating problem for nursing the baby. Generalised sympathetic stimulation can inhibit milk ejection by inhibiting oxytocin release from posterior pituitary. '*Stress during this nursing period is just like a double edged sword or two fold threat, since on one side it is harming the mother, while on another side it is damaging to the baby.*'

SEXUAL CYCLE AND LACTATION

Since lactation act is occurring due to hormone 'prolactin' from adenohypophysis which reduces the other gonadotropins from here and hence oestrogen and progesterone too. So sexual cycles are prevented during lactation. On the contrary during pregnancy hormone prolactin is inhibited due to oestrogen and progesterone. So lactation is prevented during pregnancy.

THE MILK EJECTION REFLEX

Stimulators	*Inhibitors*
1. Emptying of breast	1. Delayed breastfeeding
2. Suckling	2. Keeping baby awaiting for feeding
3. Night feeds.	3. Bottles
4. Prolactin in blood	4. Medication
5. Sensory Impulses	5. Stress, pain, doubt
6. Expression of milk	

COMPOSITION OF COW'S MILK (%)

Water	87.1
Proteins	3.2
Fat	3.9
Salts	0.9
Lactose	4.9
pH	6.6–6.8 (slightly acid)

HUMAN MILK

Amount 600–800 ml/day, 2500 ml have been noted

1. Water		87.5 gm per 100 ml
2. Protein	Total	0.7–1.5 gm/100 ml
	Caseinogen	0.14–0.74 gm/100 ml
	lactalbumin	0.43–0.97 gm/100 ml
3. Lactose		6–7.8 gm/100 ml
4. Fat		2–7 gm/100 ml
5. Cholesterol		0.01 gm/100 ml
Lecithin		0.04 gm/100 ml
6. pH		7–7.6
7. Vitamin A		200–500 I.U./100 ml
Vitamin B_1		2–4 I.U./100 ml
Vitamin C		1–12 mg/100 ml
Phosphorus		15–25 mg %
Calcium		7–72 mg %
Magnesium		4–6 mg %
Iron		0.12–0.72 mg %

Human milk is sterile, containing antibodies and antibacterial substances that are present in the mother's blood.

INVOLUTION OF MAMMARY GLANDS

After completion of lactation, mammary glands return to pre-pregnancy state. This is a regressive change. Secretion and secretory cells disappear as they are removed by macrophages. Lack of suckling causes retention of milk in breast which depresses secretion with resultant involutionary changes, during which glandular tissues are replaced by fats and connective tissue.

GYNAECOMASTIA

Breast development in male. Commonly bilateral but may be unilateral. Causes are many like—prolonged administration of oestrogen, testicular disorder, thyroid disorders (hypo and hyper), liver cirrhosis etc.

SUMMARY AND HIGHLIGHTS

Lactation is hallmark of puerperium. Prolactin is the main leading hero hormone of the process, secreted from anterior pituitary. It is further controlled by releasing hormone from hypothalamus. When child suckles at mother's breast an emotional set-up exist causing milk ejection by 'let down reflex.' Hormone oestrogen and progesterone continuously secreted by placenta during pregnancy have inhibitory control over prolactin. As placenta delivers this inhibition is removed and prolactin acts unopposed. Prolactin reduces other gonadotropins so sexual cycle is prevented during lactation. Early milk is 'colostrum' which differs from true milk in that it contains very little or no caseinogen, about 3 per cent protein (lactalbumin and lactoglobulin). Salts and lactose are present in the same concentrations as in true milk.

BIBLIOGRAPHY

1. Andrew G. Frantz: Prolactin. New Eng J Medicine 1978;298:201 (4).
2. Boyar RM, et al. Twenty four hour prolactin secretory pattern during pregnancy. J Clin Endocrine Metab 1975;40:1117-20.
3. Clark E. Grosvener. Contraction of lactating rat mammary gland in response to direct mechanical stimulation. Amer J Phy 1965;208:214.
4. Cowie AT. J Endocr. 1957;16:135.
5. CW Lloyd, Judith Weisz. Some aspects of reproductive physiology. Ann Rev Phy 1966;28:267.

54 Small but Important: Premature-Neonate (Foetal and Neonatal physiology)

ADJUSTMENT OF RESPIRATION: AFTER BIRTH

- A child starts normal respiratory rhythm within seconds after birth. When a child comes out from mother's body (asphyxiated state) to this external world which is comparatively cooler for him which creates sensory impulses originating in suddenly cooled skin.
- These two stimuli (asphyxiated state + cooler external atmosphere) stimulate respiratory centre and first inspiration starts in the form of a well known CRY.
- Before birth and at the time of birth alveoli are kept collapsed by surface tension of viscid fluid which fills them. Approximately a negative pressure of 25 mmHg is required to oppose this pressure and to begin the respiration by opening up the alveoli. Fortunately the first cry is so powerful to create a pressure of 60 mmHg, i.e. more than double of that is required. Of course second breath is much easier than first and within 40–60 minutes of birth the respiration becomes regular.
- Causes of hypoxia during delivery are:
  — Compression of umbilical cord
  — Premature separation of placenta
  — Excessive uterine contraction
  — Excessive anaesthesia given to mother.
- Failure to breath for 4 minutes lead to death in adult while infant often survives as long as 10–15 minutes. Permanent brain damage may result if breathing is delayed for 8–10 minutes.

PROBLEMS OF PRE-MATURITY

If a child is delivered before time certain problems should be kept in mind.

a. *Immature liver*: Up to first two weeks of life liver is still immature; so problems are:-
   - Bilirubin formed by destruction of RBC; does not form bilirubin glucoronide in liver so blood bilirubin level rises, i.e. Jaundice—also called physiological Jaundice of newborn which automatically subside in due course of time as liver gets maturity. Such newborn babies are kept under light (phototherapy).
   - Because of immature liver, plasma proteins concentration falls since it is the site of formation. This causes hypoproteinaemic-oedema.
   - Neoglucogenesis does not occur because of immature liver, so blood glucose level falls to 30–40 mg/dl and infant depends on stored fats for energy.
   - Blood clotting factors are formed normally in liver so they are not formed in adequate concentration so bleeding may result.

b. *Respiration*: Vital capacity and functional residual capacity is smaller in relation to infant's size. This may cause periodic breathing.

c. *Kidneys*: May also be immature. This may lead to severe disturbances in maintaining acid-base balance as well as fluid and electrolyte balance.

d. *GIT:* Absorption of fats is very poor, so it is advisable to give him a low fat diet. Absorption of calcium is also poor so it may lead to rickets which needs calcium and vitamin D therapy.

e. *Stability of body temperature*: Body temperature maintained below 96°F (35.5°C) may lead to serious consequences. This is the reason that incubators are used for premature child for stability of body temperature.

f. *Blindness in premature child*: If high oxygen concentration of pure O_2 is used to combat the respiratory distress → growth of blood vessels in vitreous humour of eye when this therapy is withdrawn → fibrosis → permanent blindness called retrolental fibroplasia. Upto 40 per cent O_2 is safe treatment.

PROBLEMS WITH NEONATE (NEWBORN)

a. *Respiration*: Tidal air per breath is 16 ml and respiratory rate is 40/minute. So minute respiratory volume is 40 × 16 = 640 ml/minute which is two times great as compared to adult in relation to body weight. This may lead to slow respiration because it is the residual air in lungs which controls the blood gas variation.

b. *Blood pressure*: On first day after birth it is 70/50 mmHg; then during next coming months it goes to 90/60 mmHg. Then rise is slow till it reaches to adult level.

c. *Immunity*: Antibodies diffuse from mother's blood to foetus through placenta.
The gamma globulin level of foetus decrease continuously after birth. But it is capable to protect infant from infectious diseases for about six months. So immunisation schedule starts after six month of age.

d. *Food and Digestion*:
   - Fat absorption by GIT is less.
   - Pancreatic amylase is also deficient.
   - Rich supply of calcium is needed. But vitamin D is also required for its absorption. Iron in adequate amount is also needed.
   - Vitamin C is also needed for proper development of bones, cartilage, intercellular structures, etc.

e. *Others:*
   - If a child is born of a mother having diabetes mellitus then Islets of newborn will be hypertrophied and hyper-functioning so more insulin will be produced which reduces blood sugar. This child may have stunted growth.
   - Similarly if a child is born of a mother having hyperthyroidism then the thyroid gland of newborn will be hypo-functioning because mother is taking treatment of hyperthyroidism. Another cause of reduced blood sugar level is immaturity of liver.
   - During first few days of life liver functions are quite deficient. It may lead to hypoproteinaemic oedema (due to less formation of plasma proteins), bleeding tendencies (because of too little formation of clotting factors).
   - Because of immaturity of kidney; the other problems of neonate include—acidosis, dehydration.
   - The newborn is rarely having allergic manifestation. But in initial days/months when antibodies first start developing in body of neonate then severe allergic manifestations are expected which in times to come may disappear.

BIBLIOGRAPHY

1. Battaglia FC, et al. Principal substrates of foetal metabolism. Phy Rev 1978;58:449.
2. Dallman PR. The anaemia of prematurity. Ann Rev Med 1981;32:143.
3. Heymann MA, et al. Factors affecting changes in neonatal systemic circulation. Ann Rev Phy 1981;43: 371.
4. Mortola JP. Dynamics of breathing in newborn mammals. Phy Rev 1987;67:187.

55 Reproduction

MALE PARTNER—I

- The substance of the testis consists of a mass of colloid tubules called convoluted seminiferous tubules bound together by a stroma of connective tissue. These tubules are lined by several layers of cells called *spermatogenic cells* which produce the spermatozoa and they undergo well defined changes in the course of transformation into spermatozoa. Initially, the germ cells are large round cells at the periphery of the tubule and are called *spermatogonia*, which alone are present in the immature testis. They multiply mitotically giving rise to *primary spermatocytes* which are larger than spermatogonia. Each divides into two smaller *secondary spermatocytes* and each of them in turn divides to produce two *spermatids*. The spermatids found near the lumen of the tubule are transformed directly into free spermatozoa. About half the number of spermatids or spermatozoa contain a Y chromosome and half X chromosome.

DIFFERENCES

Spermatogenesis	*Oogenesis*
1. Occur in seminiferous tubules of testes.	Occurs in ovarian follicles.
2. Meiosis produce four equal sized spermatids.	It produces one large ootid and three small polar bodies.
3. Spermatids are required to undergo transformation to become functional sperm.	Ootid is functional ovum.
4. Four functional sperms are produced from each primary spermatocyte.	One functional ovum is produced from each primary oocyte: Polar bodies are non-functional.
5. Differentiation of sperm occurs after completion of meiosis.	Differentiation occurs even before meiosis is complete.
6. Stages of spermatogenesis are closely associated with Sertoli cells.	Growing oocyte associated with follicle or granular cells.

- The sperms so released by seminiferous tubules are still immature. They cannot fertilise an ovum. They must attain motility for this purpose. It is the "*epididymis*" where non-motile sperm is changed into motile state and is considered as simply an ageing process; since they attain motility in almost 18 hours.
- The *Vas deferens* is considered a "store" of sperms. As long as they are stored they become dormant. They release CO_2 by their own metabolism which creates an acidic medium which inhibits the activity of sperm. During their storage, their fertility can be maintained for at least 42 days.
- *Seminal vesicles* are secretory glands rather than store houses. They secrete mucoid material which is rich in fructose and also have ascorbic acid, inositol, certain amino acids, phosphorylcholine etc. All this acts as nutrition for sperms and they also increase the bulk of semen. Its fructose content is directly controlled by circulating androgen and provides a sensitive index of androgenic activity.
- The contribution of *prostate* is in the form of an alkaline fluid containing citric acid, calcium, acid phosphate, fibrinolysin etc. It also adds to the bulk of semen. Its alkaline reaction is a boon by two-fold reasons : firstly acidic vaginal secretions are neutralised by its alkalinity and secondly—acidic reaction of secretion of vas deferens is also neutralised by its alkalinity and all this favours the fertilisation.
- Excessive temperature shortens the life of sperms and it also inhibits spermatogenesis. Increasing the temperature probably increases the rate of meta-

bolism of tubular epithelium and thereby causes the regenerative cells to burn out. This explains the descent of testes in scrotum and is to maintain the temperature of these glands below the body temperature. Scrotum is supplied with sweat glands which further adds in cooling testes. On cold days scrotal reflexes cause musculature of scrotum to contract, pulling testicles close to the body, whereas on warm days the scrotal musculature becomes totally relaxed so testicle hang far from the body.

- *"Cryptorchidism"* means failure of a testes to descend from abdomen into scrotum. A testicle remaining in abdomen throughout the life is incapable of forming sperm.

Fractions of Semen

- The process of ejaculation results in mixing of three distinct fractions of semen, which enter the urethra individually in rapid succession. The first fraction is coming from urethral and bulbo urethral glands and is clear viscid fluid in relatively slight amount. It mainly cleans and lubricates the urethra.
- The second fraction is from prostate along with most of spermatozoa and relatively small amounts of secretions from epididymis and vas deferens.
- The last fraction consists of mucoid secretion resulting from emptying of the seminal vesicles.

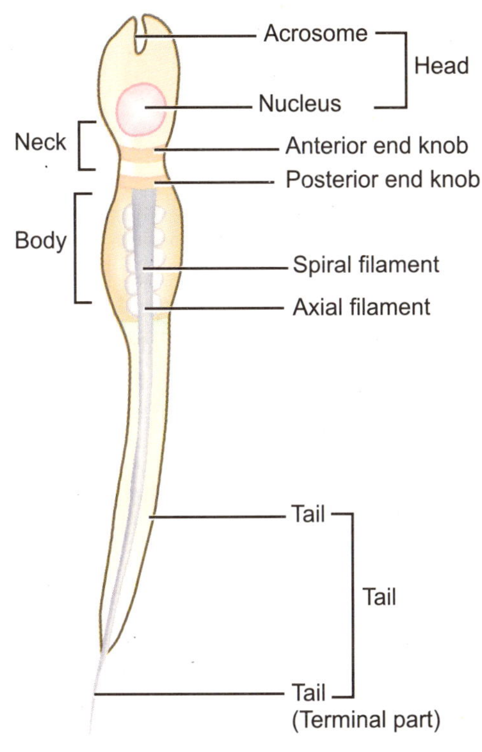

Fig. 55.1: Sperm (Human)

DIFFERENCE

	Sperm	*Ovum*
1.	Produced in testes	Produced in ovary
2.	Minute	Large
3.	Motile and active	Non-motile + inactive
4.	Made up of head, middle piece and tail	No different parts
5.	Has acrosome	No acrosome
6.	Very little cytoplasm	Large quantity cytoplasm
7.	Has an axial filament	No axial filament

MALE PARTNER—II (ANDROGENS)

The term androgen is used synonymously with the term male sex hormone, but it also includes male sex hormones produced elsewhere in the body besides the testes.

TESTOSTERONE : AN OVERVIEW

- Of the steroids isolated from testes, it is the most important and therefore regarded as male sex hormone. Another hormone is 44 androstene-3, 17-dione; but quantity of testosterone is greater.
- Chemically all androgens are steroid compounds; so can be synthesised either from cholesterol or directly from acetylcoenzyme A.
- After secretion, its some portion is fixed to the tissues and is converted within cell to dihydrotestosterone

which is the form in which testosterone exhibits its actions. The portion which is not fixed to the tissues is changed into androsterone and dehydroepiandrosterone which are then conjugated as glucoronides or sulphates and which is then excreted either in bile or in urine.

CELLS OF SERTOLI

These cells occur regularly at intervals around the tubules. They are having a large nucleus and are also possessing spindle shaped crystalloid near the nucleus. They are highly resistant towards many noxious agents. They also serve nutritive and supporting function towards developing spermatozoa. Due to their protective and nutritive support, spermatids undergo appropriate changes and are then transformed into spermatozoa. The spermatids attach themselves to Sertoli cells.

THE INTERSTITIAL CELLS (LEYDIG)

These are clumps of irregular polyhedral cells lying in connective tissue found in stroma of tubules of testes. They are known to secrete androgen. In foetus and newborn they are remarkably prominent due to stimulation by chorionic gonadotrophin; after birth they are atrophied; but, again become conspicuous at puberty.

TESTOSTERONE : FUNCTIONS

- It promotes the growth of many tissues like muscles, bone, kidneys, accessory sex organs, etc. Because of its effect on muscular growth it has been classed as ***"Youth hormone."*** This action is marked by increased blood supply of these organs.
- It causes development of primary and secondary sex characters viz. enlargement of penis, scrotum and testes to full size. Hair growth is also promoted, e.g. over pubis, upwards along linea alba, on the chest and face, etc. It decreases the growth of hair on the top of the head and this explains the fact that a man without functional testes does not become bald.
- Androgens are remarkably anabolic and cause nitrogen retention. Since it promotes growth so it is associated with deposition of proteins.
- It is essential for normal erythropoiesis. When its normal quantities are injected into a castrated adult the number of red cells increases.
- It increases basal metabolic rate which may be a manifestation of protein anabolism caused by testosterone.
- It also acts like hormone aldosterone, i.e. it increases the reabsorption of sodium in distal kidney tubules.
- On skin, it increases its thickness, raggedness of subcutaneous tissue, increased quantity of melanin to be deposited in skin. It is also said to increase the secretion of sebaceous glands. This explains acne on adolescence in many individuals.
- Typical male (masculine) voice is due to this hormone testosterone. In fact on injecting it leads to hypertrophy of laryngeal mucosa and enlargement of larynx.
- As mentioned earlier, it leads to bony growth—specially in thickness. Under its effect bony matrix is also increased with calcium retention. This explains its use in old age in osteoporosis.
- Stimulus for descending of testes in scrotum is certainly testosterone. They usually descend during last two months of gestation when the testes are secreting reasonable quantities of testosterone. Testosterone begins to be elaborated by the male at about second month of embryonic life.

CONTROL OF MALE SEXUAL FUNCTION

- Testes and pituitary gland interact with one another. It is well known that removal of testes results in the enlargement of the hypophysis and appearance of characteristic signet ring cells or castration cells.
- It is believed that FSH of hypophysis is mainly concerned with spermatogenesis. An injection of purified FSH into hypophysectomised animals (rats) prevents atrophy of seminiferous tubules and will restore gametogenic activity. There are FSH receptors attached to Sertoli cells in the seminiferous tubules, which binds FSH, which causes these cells to grow and secret various spermatogenic substances. Similarly testosterone is also having a tropic effect on spermatogenesis; or in other words, to initiate spermatogenesis, both FSH and testosterone are essential.
- It is said that activity of seminiferous tubule is controlled by negative feedback mechanism. It means that when seminiferous tubules fail to produce sperms, the secretion of FSH by anterior pituitary gland increases remarkably; and; conversely; when spermatogenesis proceeds rapidly, the secretion of FSH diminishes. This is possibly due to release of a hormone ***inhibin*** from Sertoli cells, which is exerting an inhibitory action on secretion of FSH by adenohypophysis as well as on hypothalamus on secretion of releasing hormone (GnRH).
- LH from adenohypophysis also exerts influence on spermatogenesis. The action is initially on Leydig cells to promote androgen secretion which in turn stimulates sperm formation. Quantity of testosterone secretion varies in proportion to the amount of available LH.

MALE PARTNER—III (SEMEN EXAMINATION)

Semen is collected in clean-dry condom or in a wide mouth test tube after abstinence for 4–5 days. Routine seminal fluid examination is advised in sterility/male infertility.

MICROSCOPICAL EXAMINATION

a. ***Volume***: Is measured in small graduated cylinder. It varies from few drops to 10 ml. (average 3–4 ml.; less than 1.5 ml. considered below normal).
b. ***Colour:*** odour—Whitish normally with typical seminal smell. If infective yellow colour and foul smell is imparted (musty or acrid odour).
c. ***Reaction***: Slightly alkaline, pH 7.2–8.0 (average 7.7).
d. ***Viscosity:*** Fresh semen is highly viscous. Self-liquefaction is completed in 15–30 minutes. Absence of liquefaction may inhibit the movement of spermatozoa.
e. Sperm ***motility*** can be studied by placing a drop of semen on a slide and then putting a cover slip over it. It is then examined under low and high power of microscope.

Azoospermia: Complete absence of spermatozoa.
Oligozoospermia: Only a few motile spermatozoa.
Necrozoospermia: Sperms present but immobile.

The proportion of motile to immobile sperms should be noted. If motility is very low repeat examination. Count at least 500 spermatozoa and put average percentage.

Motility duration should also be studied. For this a thick smear covered with coverglass is prepared and this preparation is sealed with vaseline and it should be examined hourly. A normal specimen shows little cessation of motility at the third hour after emission and cellular activity is noted at fifth or sixth hour.

Total Sperm Count

Its procedure is the same as that of TLC by haemocytometry except the *'Diluting fluid'* which is :

— Sodium bicarbonate .... 5 gm.
— Formalin ...... 1 ml.
— Distilled water ... to make volume 100 ml.
— Normally semen contains ... 100 million sperms/ml. of semen.

Morphological Examination of Sperms

Sperms can be examined for abnormalities like:

a. *Heads:* Too large or too small, pointed ragged edges atypical distribution of chromatin, presence of acidophilic vacuoles, double heads.
b. *Middle pieces:* Absent, swollen or bifurcated.
c. *Tails:* Double, curled, rudimentary or absent semen containing upto 20 per cent abnormal spermatozoa is still considered fertile.

Coagulation—Liquefaction (Seminal Fluid)

i. Coagulation results from action of prostatic clotting enzyme on a fibrinogen like precursor formed by seminal vesicles.
ii. Liquefaction is initiated by enzymes of prostatic origin.
iii. The protein fragments are degraded further to free amino acids and ammonia by the action of several polypeptides (proteolytic enzymes, aminopeptidase and pepsin.
iv. Liquefaction should be completed within 30 minutes.

BIBLIOGRAPHY

1. Berger FG, Watson G. Androgen regulated gene expression. Ann Rev Phy 1989;51:51.
2. Brooks DE. Metabolic activity in epididymis and its regulation by androgen. Phy Rev 1981;61:515.
3. De Jong FH. Inhibin. Phy Rev 1988;68:555.
4. Dufau ML. Endocrine regulation and communicating function of Leydig cell. Ann Rev Phy 1988;50:483.
5. Janne OA, Bardin CW. Androgen and anti-androgen receptor binding. Ann Rev Phy 1984;46:107.
6. McCann SM. Phy. and Pharm. of LHRH and somatostatin. Ann Rev Pharm and Toxico. 1982;22:491.
7. Means AR, et al. Regulation of testis Sertoli cell by FSH. Ann Rev Phy 1980;42:59.

56 Birth Control (Family Welfare)

BARRIER METHOD

Physical

1. *Condoms (Nirodh)*: Used by male, fitted over erect penis. Dry, deluxe (lubricated), super deluxe (thin, lubricated and coloured) are varieties. It prevents the semen from being deposited in vagina.

Advantages: Easily available, don't require super vision, provides prevention against sexually transmitted diseases and AIDS etc., safe and cheaper.

Disadvantages: May slip off or tear during coitus, interfere with sex sensation.

The condom was named after its inventor (English) who was personal physician to Charles II (1630–1685) who used a sheath of stretched, oiled sheep intestine to protect the king from Syphilis. Previously Italian anatomist Gabriel Fallopius (1523–1562) has designed penile sheaths (Lenin).

2. *Diaphragm (Dutch cap)*: Vaginal barrier made up of synthetic rubber or plastic material.

Inserted before intercourse and must remain there up to 6–8 hours after the sexual act. A spermicidal jelly is also used with it.

Advantages: No risk and contraindications.

Disadvantages: A trained person is needed for its application, if remained for a longer time toxic shock syndrome results.

Chemical

- Foam—Tablets/aerosols
- Cream—Jellies—Pastes—squeezed from a tube
- Suppositories—inserted manually
- Soluble films—C-film inserted manually.

INTRAUTERINE-CONTRACEPTIVE DEVICE (IUCD)

Introduction of a foreign body into uterus

- *Lippe's loop*: Double S shaped device. Made of nontoxic/noninvasive/durable plastic material made of polyethylene.
- *Copper T*: Metallic copper has got strong anti-fertility effect.
  - — *Advantages:* Low expulsion rate, no side effects, easy to fit, better tolerated.
  - — *Side effects:* Bleeding, pelvic infection, uterine perforation, pain, expulsion, cancerous changes etc.
  - — *Mechanism:*
    1. It causes a foreign body reaction which leads to cellular biochemical changes in endometrium which impair the viability of gamete and thus reduces chances of fertilisation.
    2. Copper seems to enhance cellular response in endometrium. It also affects enzymes in uterus. By altering biochemical composition of cervical mucus, copper ions may affect sperm motility capacitation and survival.

Oral Pills

1. *Combined*: Given orally for 21 consecutive days beginning on 5th day of MC followed by a break of 7 days during which menstruation occurs which is not a normal menstruation called withdrawal bleeding. It should be taken before going to bed. It contains 30–35 mg of synthetic oestrogen and 0.5 - 1 mg of synthetic progesterone. Synthetic preparations are used because natural preparations are destroyed by liver within a short time after their absorption from GIT.

   By government of India Ministry of Health

Mala-N	Mala-D
Norethisterone - 1mg	D-norgestrol 0.50 mg
Ethynyl oestradiol 0.03 mg	Ethynyl oestradiol 0.04 mg

Only Progesterone pill (mini/micro pill): They should be given in older woman who cannot take combined pill (contraindication/CVS risks)

Mode of action:

1. Combined pill prevent ovulation which is achieved by blocking the release of pituitary gonadotropins (2)

Only progesterone pills make cervical mucus thick and scanty which prevents sperm penetration (3) They also inhibit tubal motility so delaying transport of sperm and ovum to uterine cavity.

Once a month pill: Long acting oestrogen (Quine strol) + Short acting progesterone tried but disappointing results.

Male pill: Made of gossypol - a derivative of cotton seed oil is in news. It produces azoospermia/ oligospermia. Persons became permanently azoospermic and further it is toxic so research is continued.

Side effects of pills: Thrombophlebitis, ischaemic heart diseases, hypertension, hepatocellular adenoma, carcinogenic, breast tenderness, headache and migraine alteration in serum lipids etc.

Contraindication: Cancer breast/genitalia, liver disease, thrombo-embolism cardiac disorders, smokers, migraine, diabetes mellitus, gallbladder diseases, epilepsy.

Injectable Contraceptives

1. DMPA (Depot medroxy progesterone acetate)
2. NET-EN (Norethisterone—enantate)

   DMPA by suppressing ovulation and producing cervical mucus.

   Dose is: 1M injection 150 mg every 3 months. Require no motivation and does not affect lactation.

   NET EN—1M—doses of 200 mg every 60 days. Disruption of normal menstrual cycle is the main side effect.

Miscellaneous

1. *Abstinence*: Means no sexual contact. This is not practically possible since it will give birth to other complications like nervous breakdown/temperamental changes, etc. since it is inhibition of natural hunger.
2. *Coitus-interruptus* (Voluntary fertility control): The male partner withdraws before ejaculation and so deposition of semen in vaginal canal is prevented. It's difficult to be managed. The disadvantage is:- only a drop of semen is sufficient to cause fertilisation and precoital secretion of male may have sperms.
3. *Safe period* (Rhythm period, calendar sex, programmed sex)
   - 4 days of menstrual bleeding, seven days before and seven days after are safe period, i.e. least chances of conception.
   - This is all based on ovulation which occurs on 14th day (12–16 days range) of menstrual cycle. Since in this period ovum will be available for fertilisation.
   - The opposite of it is "fertile period" since many couples may wish for conception so not the "dangerous period."
   - Disadvantages:
     - —This holds true for those women who are having regular cycles; not for all because the post ovulatory period is fixed not the preovulatory period.
     - —This method is to be used only by educated and responsible couples with good co-operation/ motivation.
     - —Compulsory no sex programme for nearly half month or more.
     - —On regular menstrual cycle with periodicity of 28 days = ovulation within one day of 14th day of cycle.
     - —Periodicity of cycle is 40 days = ovulation occur within one day of 26th day of cycle.
     - —If periodicity of cycle is 21 days = ovulation occur within one day of 7th day of cycle.
   - For fertilisation, intercourse must take place between one day before ovulation upto one day after ovulation.
   - For calendar sex:- obtain the period of abstinence from calculations based on previous twelve menstrual cycle records. The first unsafe day is obtained by subtracting 20 days from length of shortest cycle and last unsafe day by deducting 10 days from the longest cycle.
   - For temperature rhythm—require abstinence until third day of rise of temperature.
   - For mucus rhythm—Require abstinence on all days of noticeable mucus and three days afterwards.
   - High failure rate.

Natural Methods

These are based on proper understanding of sexual science. They are not for everybody; but only for educated/motivated couples

1. *Basal body temperature* → It rises at the time of ovulation due to increased progesterone production. This rise is of course, very small, i.e. 0.3 to 0.5°C. It should be measured in early morning before getting out of bed. If it is high—means ovulation has taken place.
2. *Cervical mucus method:* At the time of ovulation cervical mucosa becomes clear watery resembling raw egg white, smooth, slippery and profuse. But after it under the effect of progesterone it becomes thick and less in quantity. So a woman uses a paper to wipe interior of her vagina to assess the characteristic of mucus. This will decide ovulation.

3. Mixture of both above method + Calendar Sex = Symptothermic approach.
4. Till a mother is performing breastfeeding actively ovulation does not occur so it is a safe period.
5. *Birth control vaccine*: Vaccine has been prepared from beta subunit of human chorionic gonadotropins (hCG). It will block continuation of pregnancy. Antibodies develop 4–6 weeks; reaches to maximum after 5 months and slowly decline reaching to zero level after 6–12 months. It requires more research.
6. The regular cycles are "anovulatory" in the absence of progesteronic effects. So simply analysing the urine for a surge in pregnanediol—the end product of progesterone metabolism during later half of sexual cycle, will tell us about ovulation. Its lack indicates failure of ovulation.
7. Common cause is endometriosis. It simply causes fibrosis throughout pelvis. This fibrosis sometimes so envelopes ovary which prevents the release of ovum into abdominal cavity.
8. Fallopian tubes are occluded by process of fibrosis. This constitutes salpingitis, i.e. inflammation of fallopian tube. So it is a common cause of female infertility.

Terminal/surgical (sterilisation)

1. *Male (Vasectomy):* Comparatively simple. It is customary to remove a piece of Vas (1 cm) after clamping. The ends are ligated and then folded back on themselves and sutured into position so that cut ends face away from each other. Person does not become immediately sterile but after at least thirty ejaculations. Here sperm production and hormone output not affected. Sperms produced are destroyed intraluminally by phagocytosis; and the rate of destruction is greatly increased.
2. *Female (tubectomy, Laparoscopy):* Through abdominal approach by using instrument called laparoscope.
3. *Abortion (MTP, medical termination of pregnancy):* Termination of pregnancy before foetus becomes viable (capable of living independently), which is administratively at 20 weeks. Early complications are:- haemorrhage, shock, sepsis, uterine perforation psychic complication, cervical injury, thromboembolism etc. while late complications are :- infertility, ectopic gestation, reduced birth weight, spontaneous abortion etc. Termination is permitted upto 20 weeks of pregnancy. When the pregnancy exceeds 12 weeks, opinion of two medical practitioners is required.

57 Unfortunacy Sterility: In/Sub-fertility

A woman is more conscious to become mother than in beauty and figure. Childlessness is really a tragedy in the career of a lady, which can cause a marital upset as well as personal unhappiness. The children are cementing substance for a married life. In western countries, large number of divorced couples are having no children.

Infertility implies apparent failure of a couple to conceive, Sterility indicates absolute inability to conceive for one or more reasons. Physiological sterility is present before puberty and after menopause. Infertility is termed primary if conception has never occurred, and secondary if patient fails to conceive after having produced a child or had an undoubted miscarriage (abortion). After menopause pregnancy is very rare/impossible because menopausal ovary contain no graafian follicle. It should be kept in mind that a girl may conceive before menstruation develops, if first ovum to be shed is fertilised, but this is rare because initial cycles are anovulatory.

FEW TERMS

Aspermia: Failure of formation or emission of semen.
Oligospermia: When count is less than 20 million sperms/ml.
Azoospermia: No spermatozoa in semen.
Asthenospermia: Reduction in vitality of spermatozoa.
Necrospermia: Spermatozoa are dead or motionless.
Teratospermia: Presence of high number of malformed spermatozoa in the semen.

INVESTIGATION/CAUSES

If a couple fails to achieve pregnancy after one year of regular unprotected intercourse, then they should be investigated.

Male Partner

a. *Azoospermia/oligospermia* "Failure to produce spermatozoa in sufficient number and with the capacity to fertilise."
   - Incomplete development of testes.
   - Late or non-descent of testes (the tissue temperature of scrotal testes is 2°C lower than rest of the body).
   - Previous orchitis due to previous mumps or infectious fevers.
   - Damage to testes (operation, accidents, X-rays main interference is with its blood supply).
   - Exposure of testes to heat (by wearing non-porous nylon underwears, varicocele).
   - Depression of testicular activity by diseases of other endocrine glands (hypothalamic-pituitary system).
   - Drugs. Sulfonamides may lower fertility temporarily, nicotine, deficiency of vitamin B_{12} and folate etc.
   - Male fertility falls after the age of 40 years.

b. *Epididymis/vas etc. at fault*
   - Accident/operation
   - Infection (most common gonorrhoea)
   - Congenital absence
   - Congenital/developmental obstruction.

c. *Defective/failure in deposition of sperm in vagina*
   - Premature ejaculation
   - Impotence
   - Penile abnormalities, e.g. phimosis, hypospadias
   - Retrograde ejaculation in bladder.

Female Partner

a. *Failure in ova production*: Rare
b. *Interference in passage of ovum*: Pelvic peritonitis, appendicitis, puerperal infection.
c. *Tubal obstruction*: Previous salpingitis, spasm of uterotubal junction, congenital hypoplasia.
d. *Absence/atrophy/hypoplasia of uterus*, tubercular endometritis.
e. *Cervix at fault*: Anatomical distorsion, faulty direction of cervix, polyp or other tumour.

f. *Vagina at fault*: Excessive acidity, purulent discharge, tumours.
g. *Secretion of abnormal mucus by uterine cervix.* This is produced in response of low grade infection or inflammation, or abnormal hormonal stimulation of cervix. This viscous mucous plug will prevent fertilisation.
h. *Human chorionic gonadotrophins*—a hormone extracted from human placenta—is having identical effects with LH; so is a stimulator of ovulation. So it is clear, that excessive use of this hormone → simultaneous ovulation from many follicles → multiple births

Process (coitus) at Fault

a. Apareunia and dyspareunia
b. Dry vagina because of lack of lubricants

Other Factors

a. Extreme anxiety
b. Genetic defect
c. Diet should not be very much deficient in nutritional values.

INVESTIGATION

Male Partner

- *Semen analysis*

	Fertility		
	Good	*Moderate*	*Low*
Volume (ml)	2-5	1-2	0.5-1
No. of sperms/ml	> 60 million	> 30 million	< 30 million
Motility at 6-8 hours	> 40	> 30	< 30
Normal morphology of head, body, tail (%)	80	50	< 50

- The practical importance of its chemical analysis is doubtful except in regards to fructose. If azoospermia is the result of obstructive lesion, the absence of fructose + sperms indicates the block at or below the level of ejaculatory ducts. High level of prostaglandins is disadvantageous. Urine may contain spermatozoa if ejaculation is done retrograde.
- *Testicular biopsy*: This helps to distinguish between a failure in spermatogenesis and an obstruction to their outflow.
- *Other tests*: Chromosomal studies, radiographs of sella turcica, sex hormone assays.

Female Partner

- *Tubal patency tests*:
  — Insufflation (Rubin 1970).
  — Hystero-salpingography, D and C (dilatation and curettage) hormone assays, cervical mucus studies, estimation of time and frequency of ovulation, laparoscopy: culdoscopy.

SEMEN NORMAL
(Examined within 2 hours of production)

- Total volume: 3–5 ml
- Sperm count: 60–120 million/ml
- Motility: 80–90 per cent
- Pus cells should be absent
- Counts below 20 million/ml are associated with infertility. Specimen obtained by masturbation in vicinity of laboratory.
- pH-alkaline (7-9): Liquefaction well in ½ hour.

MANAGEMENT OF MALE INFERTILITY

1. Education: sexual counselling
2. Avoidance of tobacco, alcohol, drug abuse
3. Reduce heat around scrotum—(avoid hot baths, wear loose cotton underwears, cotton clothing to encourage ventilation, control obesity)
4. Treat diabetes/thyroid diseases
5. Treat infection of sex organs by antibiotics
6. Hormones: testosterone, GnRH, pituitary hormones

Sperm penetration test: Is done by using zona free hamster egg which resembles the human ovum. A normal sperm is capable of penetrating the zona free hamster egg showing its fertilising capacity.

ARTIFICIAL INSEMINATION

The collection of semen by an emission occurring other than during coitus (usually by masturbation) and its transfer into upper vagina or cervical canal within two hours, is artificial insemination.

A. Insemination with husband's semen (AIH)
- Only indicates when any deformity of cervix makes it difficult for spermatozoa to enter is intracervical.
- It can also be put intravaginally with a pipette. It is indicated only when coitus is contraindicated + in retrograde ejaculation.

B. *Insemination with Donated Semen (AID):* When the woman is normal but man sterile then installation of semen (intravaginal/intracervix) which is donated will result in pregnancy. When donated semen is mixed with husband's semen, it is called A.I.H.D.

TEST TUBE BABY

- First such baby was Louis brown.
- Born on July 25, 1978.
- Fertilisation done in vitro (IVF).

- It occurred in a glass dish (not in a test tube) where eggs from mother's ovary are combined with father's sperm (in a salt solution). Fertilisation should occur within 24 hours and when cell division begins these fertilised eggs are placed in mother's womb.
- In our country, first such baby born on 6th August 1986.
- Another method is GIFT (Gamete-intra-fallopian-transfer). In this technique, sperm and ovum are made to fuse inside the body rather than fertilised outside. The difference is that sperms, after being treated is artificially placed at the ampicilliary end of fallopian tube of the mother where the fertilisation takes place. This method is more natural, simpler and successful.

INDICATIONS OF AIH

- Presence of persistent cervical mucus hostility with absence of sperm penetration.
- Oligospermia
- Retrograde ejaculation
- Impotency.

INDICATIONS OF IVF

- Irreparable uterine tubes
- Unexplained infertility
- Immunological infertility.

BIBLIOGRAPHY

1. Carr. BRGriffin ID. Fertility control and its complications. In William's Textbook of Endocrinology, J. D. Wilson D.W. Foster (Eds), 7th Ed. Philadelphia, Saunders. 1985.
2. Speroff L, et al. Clinical gynaecologic endocrinology and infertility, 4th ed., Baltimore, William and Wilkins. 1985.
3. The handy Science Answer Book—complied by Science and Technology department of Carnogie library of Pittsburgh 1994.
4. Wallach EE, et al. Modern trends in infertility and contraception control, vol. 3, Baltimore, Wiliams and Wilkins. 1985
5. Wenz AC, et al. Gynaecological endocrinology and infertility, Baltimore, William and Wilkins. 1988.

QUESTION BANK

1. **Explain:**
   a. Lactation remains inhibited during pregnancy. Why?
   b. Sexual cycle is prevented during lactation. How?
   c. Twins take birth earlier than single child. Why?
   d. Uterus is resistant to infection during menstruation. Why?
   e. Urinary tract infections are common during pregnancy. Why?
   f. How the newborn baby is protected against many diseases during initial month of birth?
   g. Testes are located in scrotum. Why?
   h. A newborn sometimes develops "hypoprotein aemic oedema" and low blood glucose. Why?
   i. Breathing starts at birth. How?
   j. Sexual act is usually not painful. Why?
   k. A premature infant is not treated with high concentration of oxygen. Why?
2. **Discuss:**
   a. Give an account of hormonal control of menstruation. How do oral contraceptives prevent ovulation (Raj. Univ. 1982 M.D.)
   b. Physiological forces for parturition.
   c. Measures for birth control and their physiological basis. Classify chemical contraceptives and relevance to safe period (Raj. Univ. 1988, M.D.)
   d. Maternal changes during pregnancy.
3. **Write short notes on:**
   a. Foetoplacental barrier (Raj. Univ. 1989, M.D.)
   b. Safe period
   c. Puberty
   d. Let down reflex
   e. Corpus luteum
   f. Menopause
   g. Placenta
   h. Toxaemia of pregnancy
   i. Pseudopregnancy
   j. Physiological effects of placental hormones (Raj. Univ. First M.B.B.S. 1995)
   k. Biological effects of ovarian steroids (Raj. Univ. First M.B.B.S. 1995)
   l. Control of secretion of prolactin (Raj. Univ. First M.B.B.S. 1995)
   m. Physiological basis of surgical contraceptive methods (Raj. Univ. First M.B.B.S. 1995)
4. **Describe:**
   a. The role of seminal vesicles, epididymis, prostate Sertoli cells in male reproductive system. State normal composition of semen.
   b. The various functions of oestrogen, progesterone, and testosterone with major differences among them?
   c. Hormonal regulation of pregnancy.
5. **Describe the mechanism of ovulation. Explain physiological basis of different methods of birth control (Raj. Univ. M.D. 1980, 1981, 1992). Describe modification of ovulation process by administration of hormones (Raj. Univ. 1982, M.D.)**
6. **Describe oestrous cycle. Correlate it with menstrual cycle (Raj. Univ. 1992, M.D.)**
7. **Write an essay on normal and aberrant sex differentiation (Raj. Univ. 1980, M.D.)**
8. **Describe testicular functions. How they are regulated. Discuss current researches on contraception in male (Raj. Univ. 1979, M.D.)**

MULTIPLE CHOICE QUESTIONS: REPRODUCTION

1. **Earliest changes to occur at puberty in boy is: (PGI 1989, Delhi, 1982)**
   a. Increase in size of testis
   b. Axillary hair

c. Pubic hair
d. Moustache ( )

2. **FSH and ICSH are secreted by: (AMC 1986, Delhi 1989)**
   a. Adenohypophysis
   b. Hypothalamus
   c. Ovaries
   d. Placenta ( )
3. **Important effects of Testosterone include all of the following *except*: (AIIMS, 1988)**
   a. Formation of foetal penis
   b. Descent of testis into scrotum
   c. Increased muscle development
   d. Initiation of ejaculation
   e. Increased thickness of skin ( )
4. **Penile erection is caused primarily by: (AIIMS 1982, 84, 89)**
   a. Reflex sympathetic constriction of arterioles
   b. Parasympathetically induced dilatation of arterioles
   c. Contraction of bulbocavernosus muscle
   d. Reflex parasympathetic constriction of venules
   e. Sympathetic induced constriction of veins ( )
5. **The onset of puberty in male is caused by: (AIIMS 1983)**
   a. Sudden ripening of testicles with secretion of large quantities of testosterone.
   b. Spontaneous secretion of FSH and LH by anterior pituitary gland at age of 12.
   c. An ageing process of hypothalamic sexual control centres.
   d. A sudden sharp decrease in hypothalamic sensitivity to testosterone. ( )
6. **The maximum production of hCG occurs during: (AIIMS 1983, AI 1989)**
   a. First trimester
   b. Second trimester
   c. Third trimester
   d. Implantation ( )
7. **The viability of spermatozoa within female genital tract is upto hours: (AIIMS, 1985, 88)**
   a. 6
   b. 12
   c. 24
   d. 48 ( )
8. **Semen contains all *except*: (AIIMS, 1983)**
   a. Fructose
   b. Thromboplastin
   c. Fibrinogen
   d. Prothrombin ( )
9. **Testis does not produce: (AI, 1989)**
   a. Estradiole
   b. Testosterone
   c. Fructose
   d. Inhibin ( )
10. **Function of luteinizing hormone is: (Delhi, 1988)**
    a. Follicle maturation and ovulation
    b. Milk secretion
    c. Progesterone secretion during ovulation
    d. Maintain placenta ( )

---

1 a 2 a 3 d 4 b 5 d 6 a 7 c 8 d 9 c 10 a

VIVA VOCE : REPRODUCTION

1. **What is ovulation ?**
   Discharge of ovum from ovaries into peritoneal cavity is called ovulation. It usually occurs on fourteenth day (14th) of menstrual cycle. Along with ovum a mass of granulosa and theca cell is also extruded. Ovary's graafian follicles are ruptured. Time range 13–17th day of last menstrual cycle.
2. **Mention cause responsible for ovulation ?**
   a. Weakening of stigma cells
   b. Degeneration of granulosa and theca cells in stigma region
   c. Secretion of 'hyaluronidase' into follicles leading to decomposition of mucopolysaccharides in follicular fluid
   d. Synergistic action of FSH and LH of adenohypophysis
3. **What is corpus luteum and mention its functions?**
   After ovulation, the follicles undergo luteinizing effect and mass of cells turn into so called 'corpus *luteum*' (*luteum* means yellow). Since these cells become enlarged and get lipids also and in this way they are constituted by columns of large conical cell with yellow pigment and distinct nucleus. Its main function is to secrete progesterone hormone.
4. **What is menstruation ?**
   It is cyclic discharge of blood, mucus, stripped off endometrium, unfertilised ovum, leukocytes, etc. from uterus at an average interval of 28 days and its duration is 4-6 days and also it is a painless cycle.
5. **What is female 'climacteric' ?**
   It is total time having duration of many months to many years during which sexual cycles are first becoming irregular terminating into final stoppage. Hot flashes, irritability, anxiety and other psychic states are chief characteristics of this period.
6. **What are an-ovulatory cycle ?**
   Cycles are said to be an-ovulatory when ovulation fails to occur. This may also lead to failure of development of corpus luteum, so enhanced progesterone secretion is not found.

7. **What is puberty ?**
   It is the onset of adult sexual reproductive life. 'Carefree child becomes a responsible adult'. It chiefly concerns with mental and emotional adaptation to sex function. 'Menarche' is the onset of menstruation. 'Happy go lucky tomboy changes into girl (self-conscious) often moody, imaginative and curious better called 'Juliet'. Obeying order is a difficult task.

8. **How it is possible that only one sperm enters the ovum for fertilisation while other's entry is prevented ?**
   It is well known fact that zonapellucida of ovum is having a lattice type of structure. A substance is said to be diffused into this lattice, as ovum is penetrated by one sperm. This substance is responsible for preventing the entry of other sperms.

9. **Why a pregnant lady gains weight ?**

a. Foetus	7 pounds
b. Amniotic fluid	4 pounds
c. Breast increase	3 pounds
d. Uterus increase	2 pounds
e. Protein increase	3 pounds
f. Fats increase	2 pounds
g. Fluids increase	3 pounds

10. **Enumerate function of placenta ?**
    Placenta is said as a 'cake' and a 'mini endocrine gland'.
    a. Nutritive : Water passes quite readily, concentration of sodium and potassium in both maternal and foetal blood is same; concentration of calcium in foetal blood is higher than maternal side. Blood sugar is higher in mother than foetus.
    b. Excretory : Anabolic waste products of foetal metabolism are carried to the placenta and then to maternal blood.
    c. Enzyme functions : Oxytocinase, histaminase, tissue thromboplastin.
    d. Endocrinal : Chorionic gonadotropins, progesterone, oestrogen, human placental lactogen, human chorionic somatotropins.
    e. Respiratory : High coefficient of oxygen utilisation.

11. **What are the physiological forces coming into action for process of parturition (labour; delivery) ?**
    a. Increase in oestrogen and decrease in progesterone level towards the end of pregnancy. Owing to decreased progesterone uterine contractions loss their inhibition facilitating delivery process.
    b. Secretion of oxytocin hormone from neurohypophysis which in turn increases uterine contractility.
    c. Vicious cycle is established by irritation of cervix-uteri leading to increased uterine contraction which again will cause more mechanical irritation by foetal head and so on.
    d. Contraction of uterus is joined by muscles of abdomen thus augmenting above vicious circle.

12. **What is 'lochia' ?**
    The place where placenta was attached previously undergoes autolysis which results into a vaginal discharge named as 'lochia'. At onset it is blood red but then afterwards it turns to serous in nature. It naturally stops within a week or so.

13. **Why lactation process remains inhibited during pregnancy ?**
    The two female sex hormones namely oestrogen and progesterone are continuously produced by placenta during entire time of pregnancy. Both of them are having inhibitory control over the production of 'prolactin hormone' from adenohypophysis. It is to be remembered that hormone 'prolactin' is responsible for milk secretion from breast along with the fact that it finally prepares the breast for milk secretion.

14. **The milk is ejected from breast as the baby sucks. How?**
    As the baby sucks it creates sensory impulse which reaches to head ganglion of autonomic system the 'hypothalamus' via somatic nerves; which on the other hand stimulates the secretion of hormone 'oxytocin' from neurohypophysis which causes myoepithelial cells of breast to contract causing milk ejection. Whole phenomenon is called 'ejection or let down reflex'.

15. **Sexual cycle is prevented during lactation? How?**
    Since lactation act is occurring due to hormone 'prolactin' from adenohypophysis which inhibits the action of oestrogen and progesterone- the hormones responsible for sexual cycle.

16. **Why immunisation schedule starts in a newborn after attaining age of six months ?**
    Antibodies (gamma globulins) from maternal side reaches to foetus through placenta by process of diffusion. Though it is true that there occurs a decrease in gamma globulin level of foetus after birth and the peak level of antibodies reaches at age of six years so there is decrease in immunity standard. But antibodies inherited from mother are still capable of protecting baby up to six month age. So immunisation starts after this age.

17. **What is the safe period ?**
    Coitus must be restricted when ovum is available for fertilisation. Four days of cycle itself, 9 days premestrually and 3 days postmenstrually are considered to be 'safe period' provided that cycle occurs at regular interval of 28 days. If many couples are using contraceptives during 'fertile period' they can just have a change to enjoy sexual pleasure during safe period. In all cases safe period is 7 days preceding menstruation.

18. **What is 'orgasm' ?**
    It is climax of sexual pleasure followed by immediate relief of nervous and physical tension with pleasurable lethargy. In males it is accompanied by emission of semen while in females by rhythmic contraction of muscles around vagina. It is said to be essential for ovum fertilisation as well as for transport of sperm towards ovum.

UNIT 9

The Fluid of Life

"Surgeons must be very careful when they take the knife! Underneath their fine incisions-stirs the culprit-blood-the fluid of life."

Blood

Introductory Outlines

The only connective tissue in body with liquid matrix (plasma) is the BLOOD in which formed elements (red and white cells and platelets) are suspended. Liquid part, i.e. 'Plasma' constitutes 55 per cent and is yellow coloured while remaining 45 per cent are formed elements (blood cells).

DETAILED COMPOSITION

Blood is red coloured in all vertebrates which is due to erythrocytes (RBC) as well as pigment haemoglobin contained within them. Due to its inorganic constituents it is 'salty in taste'. It is of characteristic 'smell' when drawn fresh.

In 'Plasma' 92 per cent is 'water' while remaining 8 per cent are 'solids' (In organic 0.9 or 1%, organic 7% or so). Inorganic constituents include 'sodium,' potassium, calcium, phosphates, copper, bicarbonates, chlorides, iodine, fluorine, iron etc. N. P. N. substances (urea, uric acid, creatinine, creatine, amino acid, xanthine etc.), neutral fats, phospholipids cholesterol, lecithin are also contained, as organic constituents. Proteins include albumin, globulin, fibrinogen and prothrombin. O_2, CO_2, N_2 are gases dissolved in plasma. Other organic constituents include antibodies, hormones, enzymes like carbonic anhydrase, phosphatases, transaminases, amylases, proteoses etc.

SPECIFIC GRAVITY

The specific gravity of whole blood 1055–1060, plasma 1025–1030, erythrocytes 1090.

Increased In

i. Loss of water and fluid from body, e.g. diarrhoea, vomiting (hyperemesis gravidarum, gastroenteritis, food poisoning).
ii. Inadequate intake of water.
iii. Burns, injuries, operation, i.e. passage of fluid into tissue spaces.

Decreased In

i. Excessive hydration (large quantity of water ingested, glucose or saline infusion,

REACTION

Average pH of blood is considered as 7.4 (7.3 to 7.45, i.e. alkaline). The erythrocyte's pH is lower than plasma. Lowest pH is 6.8 while highest is said to be 7.8. It is also evident that H^+ plasma (CO_2) is nicely balanced by OH^- ions.

FUNCTIONS IN GENERAL

Following are its chief functions:

i. *Nutritive function*: Various nutrients are carried through blood to various tissues for their growth and repair. Certainly nutrients are in form of amino acid, glucose, vitamins, lipids and are derived from digested food material.
ii. *Excretory function*: Waste products are removed through excretory organs by blood.
iii. *Respiratory*: It transports oxygen from air in lungs to tissues as well as CO_2 from tissues to lungs.
iv. *Blood as a protective medium*: It acts as a protective medium through carriage of antibodies. Its leucocytes are possessing famous property of phagocytosis.
v. *Participation in regulatory process*: It acts as a vehicle for carriage of hormones from ductless glands to different cells or tissues where they act.
vi. *Storage function*: Water and some essential electrolytes viz. sodium, potassium, glucose etc. are stored here and are supplied on demand.
vii. *Blood as a helper for clotting process*: Platelets which are one of the formed elements of blood are famous to assist clotting process in the following way through.

a. Sealing the damaged vessel.
b. Liberating thromboplastic material.
c. Liberation of serotonin which causes vasoconstriction.

VISCOSITY

a. The relative viscosity of water, plasma and whole blood is 1, 3 and 5 respectively.
b. It can be measured by an instrument called 'viscosimeter.'
c. Increased in: (i) Low temperature (ii) Increased number of cells (iii) High blood sugar level (iv) Low CO_2 tension 'acidosis', (v) high blood calcium level, (vi) decreased pressure gradient, (vii) decreased capillary lumen.

PLASMA PROTEINS

a. *Introduction:* Proteins of plasma includes - 'Albumin' (3.5–4.5%), 'Globulin' (1.5–3.5%), 'Fibrinogen' (0.2–0.4%), Prothrombin' (0.02–0.04%). Out of these, globulin fraction is divided further into – 'a' (alpha$_1$ globulin 0.2–0.4 gm%, alpha$_2$ globulin 0.4–0.8 gm%, beta globulin 0.4–0.8 gm%, gamma globulin 0.6–1.2 gm%). The famous albumin/globulin ratio is 2:1 (4.8/2.3). It is worth calling here in this reference that Arginine/Lysine ratio is 10/18.
b. *Description*:
   i. *Albumin:*
      1. It constitutes major part of plasma proteins.
      2. It is chiefly synthesised in liver.
      3. It can be coagulated by heat readily.
      4. Its molecular weight is said to be 69,000.
      5. Though it is insoluble in water but can be precipitated by full saturation of ammonium sulphate.
      6. It is said to exert almost 80 per cent of total osmotic pressure of plasma because of two reasons—firstly due to smaller size of its molecules and secondly due to its abundance (plenty).
      7. Many substances are carried by it as plasma bound specially hormones, bilirubin, antibiotics, sulphonamides, barbiturates, lipids etc.
      8. The albumin turnover:
         - Plasma albumin level in adult .... 3.5–4.5 or 5.0 g/dl.
         - Total exchangeable albumin pool .... 4–5 gm/kg body weight.
         - 35–45 per cent of this is intravascular and rest is in the skin.
         - 6–10 per cent of exchangeable pool is degraded per day; which is replaced by hepatic synthesis of 200–400 mg/kg/day.
         - Its synthesis is decreased during fasting but increased in nephrosis where excessive loss of albumin occurs.
   ii. *Globulin:*
      1. Though they are less in amount but are of high molecular weight as 90,000 to 1,300,000,
      2. Gamma globulins (γ) is the variety by which the antibodies are bound hence these are related with immunity.
   iii. *Fibrinogen:*
      1. It is to be recalled here that by uniting with thrombin, it forms fibrin which is the clot.
      2. Its molecular weight is 4,00,000.
      3. It is said to be precipitated by one-fifth saturation of ammonium sulphate.
      4. It is much more viscous than albumin owing to its large molecules.
      5. It can coagulate at 56°C temperature.
   iv. *Prothrombin:* It is famous in forming thrombin in presence of thromboplastin and calcium ions.
c. *Functions:*
   1. Fibrinogen and Prothrombin are main requisites for blood coagulation.
   2. When protein intake is not proper or adequate or during starvation, these act like 'protein reserve' probably through amino acid pool. Since their interchange to tissue protein is not proved so this is doubtful.
   3. It is a factor in maintaining blood pressure by providing 'viscosity' to the blood which maintains peripheral resistance.
   4. All plasma proteins contribute in 'maintenance of colloid osmotic pressure'. In this regard albumin contributes maximum owing to its smaller molecular weight. On the whole osmotic pressure created by plasma proteins is said to be between 25–30 mmHg.
   5. Plasma proteins after combining with leukocytes forms substances called 'trephones' which are essential for nourishment of body tissues.
   6. Many important substances are carried by plasma proteins specially hormones, enzymes, clotting factors.
   7. Acid-base balance of blood is regulated by them.
   8. The 'rouleaux formation' property of erythrocytes is facilitated by their globulin and fibrinogen fractions. In this way they assist in blood stability.

9. Immune substances so called 'antibodies' belong to gamma globulin group.
10. Metal binding proteins, e.g. ceruloplasmin, transferrin are provided to body mainly by alpha and beta globulins.

e. *Characteristics:*
   1. By various physical, chemical, electric and other methodology they can be separated into their respective constituents.
   2. The plasma proteins exert 25 mm mercury osmotic pressure (80% contribution from albumin; 20% contribution from globulin).
   3. It is capable of neutralising H^+ ions due to its ionising property so they assist in buffering action though their contribution is only one-sixth, as compared with whole blood.
   4. Viscosity of blood is due to plasma proteins which further is responsible for maintaining peripheral resistance as well as blood pressure. Less is the symmetry of the protein molecules, greater will be the viscosity. So shape of protein molecules is the causative factor for viscosity. On the whole, total blood viscosity is almost twice as compared with plasma, since corpuscles and proteins have equal viscosity.

f. *Origin or formation:*
   i. In embryo—they are produced by mesenchymal cells with first appearance of albumin and then others.
   ii. In adults the sources are—Liver is the chief source of albumin, majority of globulin, fibrinogen, prothrombin, lipoproteins.
   - Gamma globulins are coming from lymphoid tissue and plasma cells of reticulo endothelial system.
   - Food proteins also participate in their formation which is according to their amino acid constituents and pattern.
   - Disintegrated erythro and leukocytes are other sources.
   - Protein manufacturing process is said to be reduced in infectious diseases, starvation, liver diseases etc. ACTH as well as some vaccines (typhoid) is said to stimulate globulin formation.
   - About 150 mg of albumin per kg body weight is daily synthesised by liver.

g. *Serum:* It is a yellow straw coloured fluid having same composition of plasma without prothrombin and fibrinogen. When blood clot retracts, it releases this fluid so more clearly it is a residue of plasma after removing clot.

h. *Other proteins:*
   1. 'Glycoproteins' are constituted by hexosamine, sialic acid, hexoses, etc.
   2. Lipoproteins' which are said to be increased in liver diseases and obesity. Those such proteins having high percentage of glycerides are 'low density proteins' while those having reduced glycerides but increased cholesterol are 'high density proteins'.
   3. 'Ceruloplasmin' is copper containing protein (copper 0.34%). It is said to play role in transport of copper metal in plasma. Wilson disease is a famous example of low ceruloplasmin level. Actually it is α_2 glycoprotein capable of binding 90 per cent copper.
   4. Transferrin is responsible for absorption and transport of iron. It is a iron binding glycoprotein.
   5. 'Haptoglobulin' is that α_2 globulin which unites with pigment haemoglobin when it is released after erythrocytes destruction. It also controls renal threshold for haemoglobin. When there is severe haemolysis due to some abnormality, the released haemoglobin combine with haptoglobin. The resultant complex cannot pass through the kidney filter whereas free (unbound with haptoglobin) haemoglobin can pass. In this way haptoglobin saves the body from undue loss of haemoglobin in condition of hoemolysis as well as prevent blocking of renal tubules by haemoglobin.

Measurement of Specific Gravity (Copper sulphate method)

i. It is the ratio of the weight of blood to the weight of equal volume of water at 4°C. It is based on the principle that the drop of blood is delivered from a height of one cm above the fluid. On releasing the drop it breaks, loses momentum and then it behaves according to its gravity relative to the solution. It remains steady if its sp. gravity is same, if its sp. gravity is less, it rises up, it can sink to bottom if its sp. gravity is more. This above mentioned behaviour continues for 10–15 seconds.
ii. Solutions of different specific gravity are prepared covering the expected range (1049–1066) and containers are labelled, accordingly. Blood can be obtained by finger puncture or venepuncture and used before it clots. A pipette is filled with blood. Add one drop of blood from 1 cm above solution and watch its behaviour. Repeat it in all containers. Note down the specific gravity of the test solution

in which drop remains steady. It is the specific gravity of blood.

iii. Other solutions which can be used are—Glycerine and water (not recommended because of its hygroscopic nature).
   - Chloroform and Benzene (not recommended because of its volatile and inflammable nature).

BLOOD FILM

a. *Stain used* for staining film—it is 'Leishman's stain' which is eosinated methylene blue dissolved in acetone free methyl-alcohol. Its nature is 'neutral' since it is combination of both acidic and basic components. 0.15 gm of eosinated methylene blue is dissolved in 100 ml of acetone free methyl-alcohol.

b. *Qualities of good film*
   - It should be homogenous and thin covering at least three fourth portion of glass slide.
   - Neither longitudinal nor transverse striations should be present.
   - No gaps should be present.

   Longitudinal striations are due to uneven edges of spreader slide while transverse striations are due to stoppage at intervals while spreading the blood. Gaps are due to presence of greasy material, dust or fat on slide. Adequate size of blood drop should be taken since large drop may lead to formation of a thick film, while short films are formed with tiny drops.

c. *Preparation*: Two clean glass slides of uniform edges are taken. Get a prick with all aseptic precaution and put a drop of blood on the slide roughly one cm away from edges. Then take second slide (called spreader) and bring it near blood drop. By keeping the angle of 30–40° the spreader slide is moved towards another end of slide but movement should be gentle, uniform, neither fast nor slow. Wave it in air to make it dry. It will appear reddish yellow coloured if it is thin and one cell thick.

d. *Staining:* Blood film so prepared is put on a horizontal surface. Leishman's stain is poured over it drop by drop till it covers whole of the slide. It is put for two minutes. Stain should not be dried up in any case and to achieve this blowing of air through glass pipette is done. After this, equal quantity of distilled water is added and kept for eight minutes. After this wash the slide with tap water and dry it by waving it in air. Blood film is then examined under 'oil immersion lens of microscope' after putting one drop of 'cedar wood oil' in centre of the film.
   - The first two minutes of stain is 'fixation period'. Methyl-alcohol precipitates the protein component of the cell and hence the cells are fixed and it acts as a fixative.
   - Next eight minutes period is 'staining period' where distilled water dissociates conjugated dye since stain and distilled water are remaining in contact with each other. Distilled water is also said to maintain isoelectric pH since pH of Leishman's stain and water is 7 while that of blood is 7.4.
   - 'Cedar wood oil' is used because its refractive index is same as that of glass. This prevents double refraction.

SUSPENSION STABILITY: BLOOD

1. Haemolysis:
   If normal blood is centrifuged the corpuscles settle at bottom of the tube whereas supernatant plasma is clear or faint straw coloured. Under some conditions the haemoglobin may escape into the surrounding fluid which then becomes coloured. This is hemolysis.
2. Membrane permeability:
   The membrane of human erythrocyte is normally impermeable to haemoglobin, plasma proteins, Ca^{++}, Mg^{++}, K^+, organic phosphate ions. It of course, permits the passage of water, NH_4^+, H^+, Cl^-, HCO_3^-. On injury to cell membrane, potassium escapes freely. RBC membrane is not absolutely impermeable to sodium ions. So in absence of hemolysis minute amounts of sodium ion may pass from plasma into erythrocytes. The cell membrane is freely permeable to amino acid, urea, uric acid. Osmotic changes occur when CO_2 enters the blood and diffuses into the cell.
3. Chemical substances:
   - Ether/chloroform/benzene/alcohol act by dissolving lipid constituent of stroma of the cell.
   - Bile salts act by combining with protein constituents and saponin with cholesterol.
   - Acids act by penetrating the cell and increasing the osmotic concentration inside. It leads to swelling and liberation of haemoglobin.
   - Alkalies also cause haemolysis through stromatolysis. Certain chemical poisons, e.g. carbolic acid, nitrobenzene, arsenical preparations etc. are also famous to cause red cell destruction.
4. Substances of bacterial origin:
   a. *Bacterial or parasitic toxins:* Toxins of strepto/staphylo coccus, tetanus bacillus may cause RBC destruction. In extensive burns, infectious fevers (diphtheria, smallpox) intense haemolysis has been observed sometimes it may lead to haemolytic jaundice.

b. *Poisonous snake's venom:* Cobra, stringing insects, spiders are causing destruction of RBC. Snake venom is said to contain a principle which is capable of removing unsaturated fatty acids from lecithin molecule. The resulting product is lysolecithin and is haemolytic agent. Kephalin is also acted upon by snake venom in the same way. Since lecithin is present both in RBC and plasma and in all cells, the entry of snake venom into body leads to production of a haemolytic substance.

c. *Haemolysins from normal tissues:* Generally, they remain inhibited in normal way, but are liberated actively by disease/injury.

In pernicious anaemia, RBC are less fragile while in conditions like acholuric jaundice/purpura, their fragility is increased.

BIBLIOGRAPHY

1. Bing DH (Ed.). The chemistry and physiology of human plasma proteins. Pergamon, New York 1979.
2. Mcfarlane RG, Robb Smith AH. Functions of blood, Oxford Blackwell. 1961
3. Putnam FW. The plasma proteins. Academic Press, New York London Vol. I. 1960.
4. Rapaport SI. Introduction to Haematology 2nd ed. Philadelphia JB Lippincott. 1987.
5. Thompson RB. A short textbook of Haematology, Baltimore Urban and Schwarzenberg 1984.

59 Erythrocytes (Red Blood Corpuscles, RBC)

It is a unique and extraordinary structure which is the only cell without a nucleus in the body with a peculiarity of having life of numbered days. In the past it was regarded as a dead cell owing to its diminished consumption of oxygen and absence of nucleus but now it is said to carry out some metabolic functions; so it is better to call it as a specialised type of living cell.

INTRODUCTION

The normal erythrocytes in human body are biconcave disc shaped without nucleus. Their mean diameter is 7.2μ (ranging between 6–9 μ) and their average thickness is reported as 2.2 μ (ranging between 2–2.4 μ); their thickest part is lying near the periphery. So their central portion appears thinner and this get up of it gives them biconcave contour or dumbbell shaped when observed from edges or sidewise. The average volume of these cells is studied as 87 cubic microns (μ^3) and average area is 120 μ^2 to 135 μ^2. The red pigment "haemoglobin" is confined within these cells instead of being present as "free" in the plasma.

NUMBER AND VARIATION

In a healthy male, 50,00,000 cells per cubic mm is the normal number while healthy female is having 45,00,000 cells per cubic mm in their blood. Newborn child may have 70,00,000–80,00,000 cells per cubic mm in their blood.

Physiological Variation

Lowest count during sleep, increasing further after awakening and continuously rising throughout active working hours constitute what is called "diurnal variation."

During muscular exercise, spleen releases red cells in the general blood stream and thus increasing their population. Same event is repeated during emotions and high external environmental temperature." Owing to same reasons. "injection adrenaline" is also responsible for increasing their population.

"High altitude" is the chief culprit for increasing their population. This is the reason that inhabitants of mountain region (10,000 feet elevation from sea) have permanent high red cell count in comparison of those living at sea level. Travellers should not worry about this statement since trip to such places will cause immediate increase in the cell number for short duration. It is due to the fact that hypoxia develops at high altitude which acts as a stimulus for liberating a ESF (erythrocyte—stimulating factor, erythropoietin) substance from kidney tissues and which is chemically considered as glycoprotein with a molecular weight of 25,000 to 45,000. Lesser or say negligible amount of it is also said to be produced from liver. This erythropoietin then in turn acts on bone marrow to increase the rate of formation of erythrocytes. In first two three days very few erythrocytes appear but in consequent time the number is gradually increased as long as the subject remains in hypoxic state. It is to be remembered that if bone marrow is manufacturing erythrocytes very rapidly then the cells will be poured within circulation before their maturity, this sometimes may increase reticulocyte number so called reticulocytosis or even number of normoblasts may also be increased. If the subject is removed from hypoxic state then liberation of this substance will also be inhibited owing to lack of hypoxia as a stimulatory factor which will result finally into zero production of red cells. In fact, both these activities regulate each other through "negative feedback mechanism" meaning hereby hypoxia stimulates formation of erythropoietin which through bone marrow increases red cell population which alleviates hypoxia. On this ground the high red cell count among athletes can also be explained since severe muscular exercise leads to hypoxia which results into increased erythrocyte population, in comparison to a dull man lying in bed.

Factors increasing number	
Physiological	*Pathological*
1. Diurnal variations	1. Emphysema, pulmonary tuberculosis
2. Hypoxia (high altitude)	2. Congenital heart diseases
3. Muscular exercise	3. Chronic carbon monoxide poisoning
4. Emotion/excitement	4. Repeated small haemorrhages (rare)
5. Injections adrenaline	5. Chemical poisoning, e.g. arsenic, phosphorus, aniline dyes etc.
6. High external temperature	

Pathological Variations

- An increase in general erythrocyte population constitutes "Polycythemia" which may occur in following states :
- Conditions interfering with oxygenation of blood in lungs, e.g. emphysema, tracheal stenosis, pneumothorax, pulmonary tuberculosis, lung tumour etc.
- Congenital heart diseases.
- Chronic carbon monoxide poisoning.
- Repeated small haemorrhages (rare).
- Chemical poisoning, e.g. arsenic, phosphorus, aniline dyes etc.

On the contrary reduction in number of erythrocytes is called "Anaemia."

LIFE AND FATE

Since erythrocytes are devoid of nucleus, incapable of repair and reproduction so their days are numbered and it is suggested that lifespan of red cells in the circulating blood is 120 days, which further means that one hundred and twentieth of the mass of circulating red cell (25 gm approximately) must be removed daily from circulation by reticulo-endothelial cells. Ageing of cells is accompanied by gradual lipid loss together with diminished glycolytic enzyme activity. Of course ageing does not affect their morphological get up.

As far as their destruction is concerned almost 7–8 gm of haemoglobin is taken out from circulation daily. The first step in this breakdown is opening of the porphyrin ring system with the formation of compound "Verdo-haemoglobin" (Choleglobin) containing iron and protein with the formation of a chain by four pyrrole nuclei instead of a ring. In the next successive stage both protein and iron are lost but iron is stored in reticulo-endothelial cells in the form of haemosiderin and ferritin. This explains the fact that when excessive blood destruction results due to any reason, the hemosiderin gets deposited at its respective sites viz. spleen, bone marrow, liver. biliverdin is the next pigment, which remains after losing iron and protein from haemoglobin molecule and this is having structural similarity with protoporphyrin and is green coloured one. This pigment is present in abundance in herbivore animals and newborn infants. The pigment which is present in abundance in human being is bilirubin, a water insoluble lipophilic substance which flows in blood stream in association with α-globulin as bilirubin globulin (according to many workers it is albumin also which combines with bilirubin) and then transported to the liver. This pigment by passing through smooth endoplasmic reticulum of liver cells react with uridine—diphosphate glucuronate and forms bilirubin glucuronides. These pass to intestine by excreting in bile where they are acted upon by bacterial enzymes (the hydrolysis and reduction) and they are changed into so called bilinogens, which afterwards undergo auto-oxidation to be changed into stercobilin, the chief brown pigment of the faeces. Its small amount reaches the systemic circulation and excreted by kidney as urobilinogen and when urine is exposed to air it undergoes auto-oxidation and changed to urobilin. In routine faeces contain 100–200 mg per day of stercobilinogen and stercobilin, while urobilinogen is 0.5–2 mg per day is excreted.

The conjugation of bilirubin in liver is catalysed by enzyme glucuronyl transferase. Its activity is increased by drug "phenobaribitone." So hyperbilirubinaemia (Kernicterus) can be successfully treated by this drug.

About 10 per cent of daily red cell breakdown occurs intravascularly (and not within mononuclear phagocytes). It leads to release of 0.6 gm of haemoglobin each day into the plasma.

On the contrary drugs "Dianabol" (Methandrostenolonea-compound with androgenic activity)—competes with bilirubin for conjugating with glucuronides. As without conjugation the bilirubin cannot be excreted so this will cause "hyperbilirubinemia" (Jaundice).

Severe jaundice develops in "Crigler-Najjar disease" since this enzyme is absent.

Enzymes involved in glycolysis present in RBC.
Hexokinase
Phospho-hexo-isomerase
Aldolase
Phospho-hexokinase

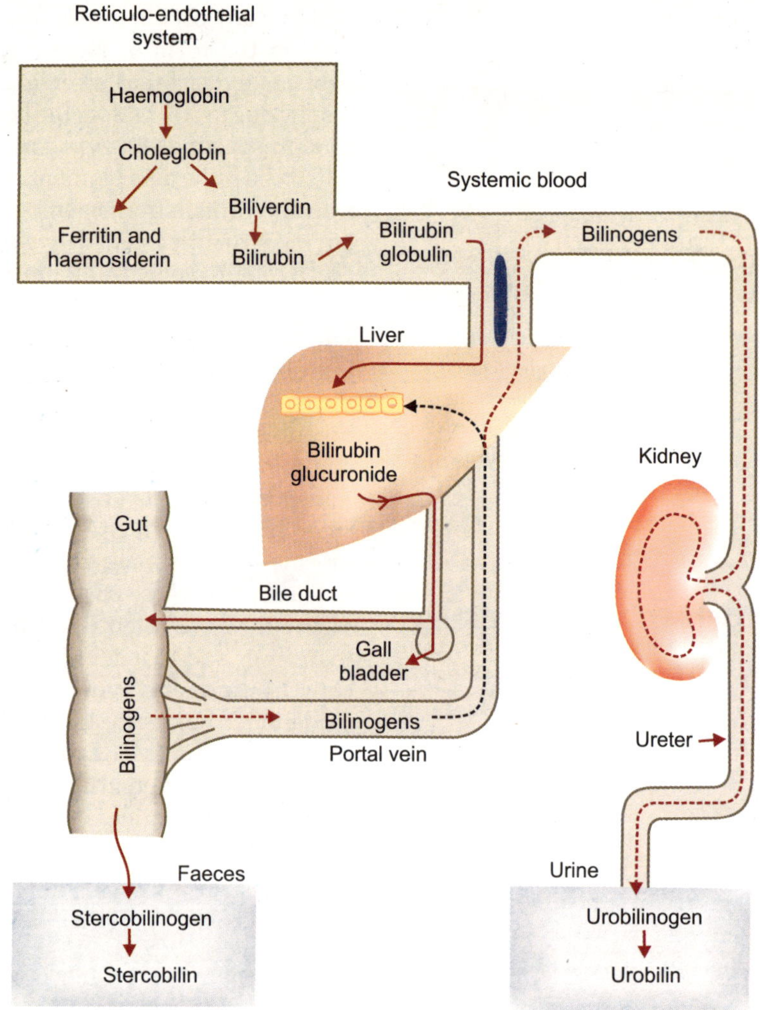

Fig. 59.1: Fate of RBC

Enolase
Glyceraldehyde dehydrogenase
Fumarase
Lactic acid dehydrogenase
Glucose-6-phosphate dehydrogenase

STRESSFUL LIFE OF RED CELL—A TRAGEDY

- It is destroyed by spleen macrophages, action of haemolytic substance in blood, simple wear and tear in blood stream.
- The cells are flung from the heart, into the arteries at high velocity. In their circulation, they are exposed to innumerable collisions not only with one another but with the arterial walls too. Some times the channel or passage is too narrow to give them space without marked distortion in their shape. Their membranes are always undergoing tension as a result of osmotic changes. In the last they cannot tolerate all these abuses and undergo so called fragmentation.
- According to one data, about 3,000,000 cells are destroyed in this way every second—so same number should be formed to maintain homeostasis. In a normal adult, between 5.6–6.7 gm of haemoglobin are removed and replaced daily. So a balance between blood formation and wastage is to be maintained.

(Rous, P; 1923) (Source—Physiological basis of Medical Practice by Best and Taylor Williams and Wilkins.

JAUNDICE

A. It is the symptom complex characterised by increased concentration of pigment bilirubin in the blood; which is easily recognised—first in the sclera of the eye and then in the skin and body fluids. It is produced in three different ways as:

B.

a. If for example, bile duct is obstructed by a gall-stone or tumour, then bile pigment cannot pass into the intestine and the faeces are pale. The bile pigments dammed back by obstruction are reabsorbed into the blood and the high concentration of this water soluble bile pigment leads to its excretion by kidney. The urine thus becomes dark greenish yellow in colour, giving positive tests for bile pigment. This is called "obstructive or post-hepatic jaundice."

b. Now when there occurs an excessive destruction of red cells, (and so haemoglobin too), the excess bile pigments are produced, and having passed through the liver is excreted into intestine. The amount of stercobilin is increased in faeces and they become dark brown (sometimes black). More bilinogen than normal is reabsorbed from the gut and the concentration of the urobilinogen in the urine is increased from a barely detective level to an amount which gives strong positive tests. This type of jaundice is called "haemolytic or pre-hepatic Jaundice."

c. Finally, if liver is diseased; then swelling of liver cells interfere with the flow of bile through the small bile canaliculi and re-absorption of water soluble bilirubin into the blood follows, just as in obstructive jaundice. Since in this condition many of the liver cells are in capable of functioning normally, water soluble bile pigments from breakdown of haemoglobin also accumulate. This is hepatic or toxic jaundice.

C. Laboratory test (Van-den Bergh's Test—1916)

Two forms of bilirubin exist, the one being converted into another in liver. On passage through the liver cells bilirubin—a water insoluble substance, is conjugated with glucuronic acid to form water soluble glucuronides (mono and di). These compounds are the main bile pigments found in obstructive jaundice in the blood, and by virtue of their water solubility, in the urine. They are responsible for "direct van-den Bergh" reaction seen in obstructive jaundice.

- On the contrary, in haemolytic jaundice, bilirubin itself appears in the blood, being held in solution by linkage to serum protein. The presence of alcohol allows it to pass into true solution to give indirect reaction.

D. *Normal Values:*

- Ranges between 0.2 to 0.8 mg per 100 ml. A patient does not appear to be jaundiced until serum bilirubin is above 2 mg. per 100 ml.
- In haemolytic diseases of newborn, the serum bilirubin may be over 30 mg per 100 ml and pigment is deposited in the basal nuclei which suffer permanent structural damage (Kernicterus).

E. *Symptomatology:*

- A patient of jaundice develops symptoms like itching/pruritus/urticaria (skin manifestations) because of increased serum bilirubin level.
- Because of liver damage, prothrombin—the main factor of blood coagulation is formed in either deficient amount or not at all. This blocks clotting mechanisms which explains bleeding tendencies in jaundice.
- Infants suffering from jaundice are treated by phototherapy (exposure to light). By exposure under white light, bilirubin $\rightarrow$ lumirubin which has a shorter half-life than bilirubin.

DETERMINATION OF LIFESPAN

1. Selective/differential agglutination technique: (Ashby—1928) It consists of transfusing the compatible red cells and then examining the recipient's blood from time to time for presence of foreign corpuscles which are counted in haemocytometer.
2. An isotope of nitrogen is used (N^{15}) to tag the red cell in the bone marrow. This is done by feeding glycine into which isotope has been incorporated. The disadvantage is that the uptake time is long and occurring in vivo; the tagged cells are not all of the same age and therefore, it is difficult to obtain precise determination of survival time.
3. Radioactive chromium (Cr^{51}) and iron technique is employed. Tagging takes place in vitro. The tagged cells are injected and their rate of disappearance from the peripheral blood is followed by means of serial samples. It has an advantage that external scanning over organs (liver, spleen) may be carried out at the same time to detect the sites of deposition of labelled cells.

ERYTHROCYTE SEDIMENTATION RATE

If a sample of blood taken out, mixed with anticoagulant and is allowed to stand in a tube, then owing to their

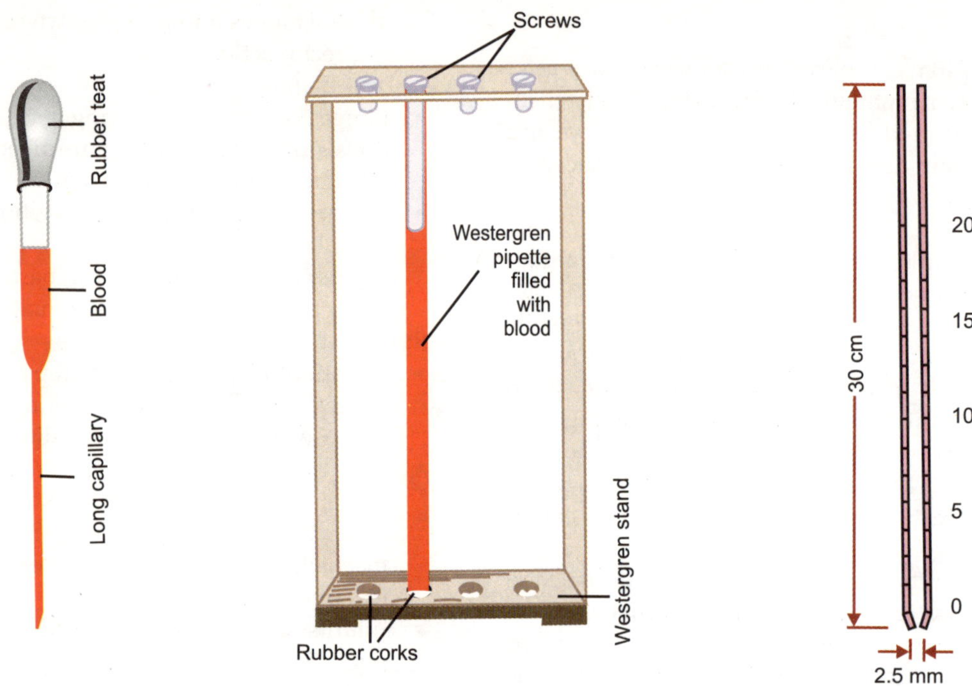

Fig. 59.2: Westergren's pipette in stand and long nozzled capillary pipette

high specific gravity, corpuscle settle at bottom and thus leaving clear plasma above. The rate at which this phenomenon takes place designated as erythrocyte sedimentation rate (ESR).

Importance

This test is much of prognostic value than the diagnostic one. This rate is increased in inflammatory conditions usually of chronic variety, e.g. tuberculosis, rheumatic fever, arthritis malignancies etc. An increased sedimentation rate is the index of worsening of a disease as well as presence of any organic lesion in the body. It is also said to increase in nephrosis, while reduction in sedimentation rate has been reported in allergic states, peptone shock, acholuric jaundice and sickle cell anaemia. Physiologically this rate is found to be increased in menstruation, pregnancy.

Factors Affecting

i. *Specific gravity:* Corpuscles of high specific gravity will certainly settle more quickly in normal plasma and of course if plasma is of low specific gravity then also normal corpuscles will settle quickly (RBC—1090, plasma 1030).
ii. *Clumping:* This indirectly means aggregation of corpuscles and aggregate mass will face rapid settling, owing to increased size.
iii. *Lowered viscosity:* If plasma viscosity is lowered, this settling rate will be increased.
iv. *Temperature:* A rise in temperature will accelerate the sedimentation rate while low temperature will slow down process.
v. *Shape of cell:* Rouleaux formation, discussed elsewhere.
vi. *Lecithin—cholesterol ratio:* Lecithin has got inverse while cholesterol has got direct relation with this phenomenon.
vii. *Erythrocyte concentration:* High population decrease ESR while decreased number increases the rate of settling.
viii. *Other factors:*
   - Rate is found to be faster when plasma fibrinogen level is increased.
   - Albumin decreases its level. This explains increased rate in state of nephrosis where serum albumin is reduced.
   - Dextran increases settling rate.

Determination

A. *Westergren's method*

i. The apparatus consists of Westergren pipette (uniform bore of 3 mm, marked with graduations from 0 to 200, 300 mm long, open at both the ends),

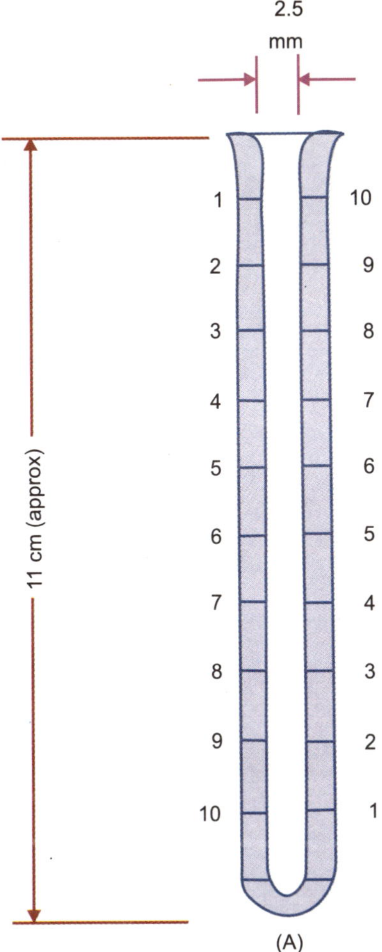

Fig. 59.3: Wintrobe's tube

and Westergren stand (can accommodate six pipettes, at upper end there is a screw cap which fits upon the pipette, it allows the pipette to remain in vertical position, at base there is a rubber cushion where lower end of pipette rests).

ii. The blood to be tested is collected intravenously. It is mixed with 3.8 per cent sodium citrate solution (4 parts of blood to 1 part of citrate solution; 1.6 ml blood mixed with 0.4 ml citrate minimum), which acts as an anticoagulant, dilutes the plasma and is isotonic with blood.

iii. The tube with this sample is filled with mark "O" and put exactly in vertical position for exactly one hour. At the end of one hour reading is taken by observing the upper level of red column above which there is a clear plasma. Unit is mm at the end of first hour.

iv. The main precautions are: There should be no clot in blood sample, tube should be clean and dry, blood should be filled with "O" mark, pipette should be fitted exactly in vertical position, room temperature must be recorded.

v. Normal values are:
- 3–5 mm at end of first hour (males)
- 4–7 mm at end of first hour (females)

B. *Wintrobe's Technique:*

i. The apparatus consists of Wintrobe tube (heavy cylindrical tube of uniform bore, graduated on the left hand from top of tube, each main division represents one cm and each smaller one mm), long capillary pipette (110 mm long and can reach upto bottom of Wintrobe's tube, can hold about 2 ml blood).

ii. Anticoagulant used here is double oxalate (potassium and ammonium). Sodium oxalate can cause crenation of cells and reduction in cell volume.

iii. Normal values:
- 0–7 mm in first hour (males)
- 0–15 mm in first hour (females)
- Rest of description is same

C. *Technical errors capable of modification*

Any clot, variations in room temperature, wrong position of tube, anticoagulants etc.

D. *Factors affecting rouleaux formation*

i. When number of RBC is more, more is rouleaux formation.

ii. Larger molecules usually increase the rate. Fibrinogen is better than gloublin which is better than albumin. In various diseases globulin concentration and its pattern changes which affects rate of rouleaux formation.

iii. Increase in MCV, decrease in MCH and spherocytosis all retard the rate of rouleaux formation.

ESR—Factors increasing	*ESR—Factors decreasing*
1. Increase in O_2	1. Increase in CO_2
2. Increase in cholesterol	2. Increase in albumin
3. Increase in globulin	3. Increase in lecithin
4. Increase in fibrinogen	4. Increase in nucleo protein
5. Dextran	5. Spherical RBC
6. Temperature above 20°C	

Rouleaux Formation

When a drop of blood is put in centre of a clean glass slide and examined under microscope after putting cover slip on it, erythrocytes will attach themselves like "pile of coins" or more clearly with their broad surfaces in

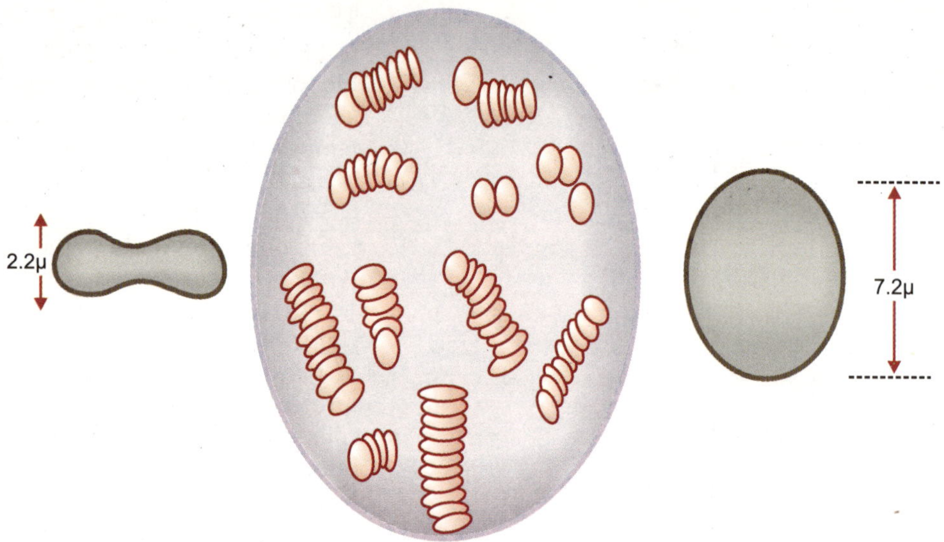

Fig. 59.4: Erythrocytes: Rouleaux formation

contact. This property is termed as rouleaux formation. With this property cellular mass increases so it will certainly increase the sedimentation rate so it is better to say that rate of sedimentation varies with the speed of rouleaux formation. This phenomenon should be distinguished from agglutination in which cells are clumped together and are not separable. It should be further noticed that this phenomenon does not exist inside the body since in actively circulating blood erythrocytes will not adhere with each other. Furthermore, routine biconcave shape is the main culprit for this phenomenon and as this shape is lost by any cause this property will also vanish, e.g. congenital haemolytic-jaundice. Each rouleau is consisting of 8–12 cells and on collecting more cells the repelling forces cause the rouleau to break. So it is a self limiting phenomenon as regards the size is concerned. When a rouleau is formed, its density is increased causing its sinking down. Red cells are negatively charged as they are suspending in plasma so they are separated in circulation, i.e. without rouleaux formation.

STRUCTURAL PECULIARITIES : A BOON

Since nature is the fountain head of all our problems and solutions, closer we keep to it better we realise it, so the non nucleated and biconcave shape of erythrocytes is really a boon for us in the following aspects:

i. For more efficiency the erythrocyte must absorb and release gases more quickly and this is a surface phenomenon, occurring at interface. So to meet this demand interface between each red cell and plasma should be great per unit of pigment haemoglobin, and this demand is fulfilled by its biconcave shape since this shape gives surface area 20 times more than sphere shaped structure. So this shape is fruitful for this purpose.
ii. Non-nucleated pattern provides maximum room for haemoglobin.
iii. Rounded edges protect the cells from injuries etc.
iv. One is the mechanical advantage, i.e. when the cell passes through narrow spaces like capillary bifurcation then due to this shape it will face minimal tension meaning by it will bend instead of breaking at those sites.

RED CELL FRAGILITY

1. A 0.9 per cent sodium chloride solution is isotonic with plasma.
2. When osmotic fragility is normal, RBC begin to haemolyse when suspended in 0.5 per cent saline, 50 per cent lysis occurs in 0.40–0.42 per cent saline, and lysis is complete in 0.35 per cent saline.
3. RBC shrink in solution with an osmotic pressure greater than that of normal plasma. In a solution with low osmotic pressure RBC swell—become spherical and burst, so loose hemoglobin (hemolysis) which colours the plasma.
4. Drugs and infection cause lysis of RBC. This is increased by deficiency of glucose-6-phosphate-dehydrogenase.

5. In hereditary spherocytosis the cells are spherocytic and haemolyse more readily than normal cells in hypotonic sodium chloride solution. The spherocytosis is caused by various abnormalities of protein network which maintains the shape and flexibility of red cell membrane.

FUNCTIONS

i. They are capable of absorbing as well as giving up of oxygen due to their peculiar shape, size and elasticity.
ii. They also carry carbon-dioxide from tissues and giving to pulmonary alveoli.
iii. As mentioned above they can easily pass through narrow spaces and by this property gaseous exchange take place at every cell level of the body.
iv. Because of containing haemoglobin it becomes store house of almost 2/3rd of body protein and furthermore bilirubin and biliverdin like pigments are derived out of it.
v. As blood group substances are contained herewith so they seem to be involved in blood group reactions.

Polycythaemia

Increase in number of red cells is the name given to this state polycythaemia.

Polycythaemia vera (Synonyms—polycythaemia rubra, Vaquez-Osler's disease).

Increase in red cell number irrespective of needs of body and count may go as higher as 7 or even 10 millions per cubic mm. Blood volume is also increased and due to more population of cells blood becomes more viscid. Haemoglobin is also increased and thereby raising colour index about 1. Moderate leucocytosis specially increase in polymorphonuclear cells. Hyperplastic bone marrow, moderate splenomegaly, distension of blood occurs in splanchnic vessels.

The skin and mucous membrane of mouth is red with blood shot conjunctiva due to increased red cell number. Due to more distension of cerebral vessels patient complains of vertigo and fullness in head and this vascular fullness may lead to some fatal results like peptic duodenal ulcer, retinal haemorrhage.

Erythrocytosis (Secondary polycythaemia)

This is actually an arrangement against insufficient oxygenation states like congenital heart diseases, CHF, emphysema, pulmonary arteriosclerosis. There exists no leucocytosis.

Relative polycythaemia

Marked loss of body fluids by vomiting and diarrhoea, low fluid intake etc. cause loss of plasma and hence causing apparent increase in red and white cells.

TOTAL ERYTHROCYTE COUNT

- It is done by haemocytometry techniques. Special diluting fluid called "Hayem's fluid" is used. It is composed of sodium chloride (0.5 gm) responsible for maintaining isotonicity of blood, "sodium sulphate" (2.5 gm) responsible for maintaining size and shape of red cells as well as maintaining blood isotonicity along with its fixative action, $HgCl_2$ (0.25 gm) acting as preservative and prevents growth of bacteria and fungus in solution and distilled water of course acts as solvent and to make total volume 100 cc. There is no need to destroy white cells since they are comparatively very less in number (700 : 1 ratio) so no trouble in counting. It is really an ideal fluid since on mixing with blood it neither causes haemolysis nor crenation.
- Counting is done in 5 small squares of red cell counting area of chamber under high power of microscope with low position of its condenser since it is an unstained preparation. Maximum light is required since excessive light makes them refractile. Prick is given with all aseptic precautions and blood is taken upto 0.5 mark of RBC pipette and is then filled with diluting fluid upto 101 mark. Contents are then mixed by rotating pipette in between palms of hand for 2–5 minutes. After discharging one or two drops chamber is charged as usual and then erythrocytes are observed and counted.

Calculation

Volume of one square = Length × Breadth × Depth

$$= \frac{1}{5} \times \frac{1}{5} \times \frac{1}{10} = \frac{1}{250} \text{ cubic mm.}$$

Since erythrocytes are counted in five squares so,

Total volume $= \frac{1}{250} \times 5 = \frac{1}{50}$ cubic mm.

Suppose $\frac{1}{50}$ cubic mm volume contains x no. of red cells

1 cubic mm. volume will have 50 ×

dilution is 200 times

So total number of cells comes as 200 × 50 ×

or 10,000 ×

STRUCTURE AND METABOLISM

- The stroma or framework of the cell actually is a lipoprotein complex arranged in three layers. Outer layer is of sialic acid determining the electric charge. This layer is crossed by pores responsible for ionic passage. Lipid constituent is mainly the phospholipid constituting 10 per cent and protein fraction constitutes 50 per cent. This lipoprotein complex has been designated as "elenin" which is also said to have A, B and Rh antigen.
- In spite of the fact of absence of nuclei and glycogen they are said to be metabolically active by utilising 1.5–2.2 milimoles of glucose per litre per hour which is almost equivalent to production of 25 calories of heat. Certainly this much energy is used for exit of sodium and influx of potassium against electro-chemical gradient. Potassium is said to be present in higher concentration than sodium. Carbonic anhydrase, catalase etc.—the enzymes of glycolytic system are also present within this cell. Due to inheritance of a sex linked recessive characteristics, glucose-6-phosphate-dehydrogenase is found also in very small amounts. Diminished quantity of glutathione making these cells readily haemolysed, is also reported.
- During metabolic processes "hydrogen peroxide" is formed within the cells but if it is not destroyed it may oxidise haemoglobin to methaemoglobin and furthermore it may harm to other those substances essential for maintaining integrity of these cells otherwise haemolysis may ensue. Glutathione per oxidase and catalase are the two substances performing role of protection; former acts by using hydrogen per oxide in oxidising reduced glutathione while later decomposes it into water and oxygen.
- On the whole it contains 60–70 per cent water and rest 30–40 per cent are solids including haemoglobin (29%), lipids (1%), other proteins (1%), above mentioned enzymes, organic substances (urea, amino acid, adenyl phosphate, creatinine), and inorganic substances (sodium chloride, potassium phosphate - 0.7%).

Red Cell Membrane

i. Erythrocytes possess a plasma membrane but it does not have internal membranes which enclose nucleus etc.
ii. The lipids constituting the membrane are—phospholipids, cholesterol and glycolipids. The phospholipids constitute a bimolecular sheet (hydrophilic + hydrophobic moieties). Cholesterol exists in its free—non-esterified form. The glycolipids are called ceramide (sphingosine + long chain fatty acid to which hexose molecules are attached. 55 per cent is phospholipid and remaining 45 per cent portion is cholesterol.
iii. Membrane proteins are of two types namely—peripheral proteins (quite easily separable from lipid bilayer, located at cytoplasmic face of membrane); and, "integral protein" (separation requires organic solvents or detergents).
iv. The membrane also possesses enzymes like G3 PD, ATPase, protein kinases etc. "ATPase" is a part of Na^++K^+ pump as well as of Ca^{2+} pump. Other enzymes present include "acetyl-choline esterase, lysosomal enzymes etc. (glycosidases, phosphatase etc.).

ERYTHROPOIESIS (PRODUCTION OF RED CELLS)

Site: It is area vasculosa of mesoderm of yolksac in early embryonic stage which forms erythrocytes and this constitutes "mesoblastic stage." Production takes place intravascularly. After third month of the foetal life spleen and liver becomes the main site for erythropoiesis so called "hepatic stage" where nucleated red cells are developing between blood vessel and tissue cells from mesenchyma. Nearly middle of foetal life this function is taken over by bone marrow and it is once again the bone marrow which acts as a sole region for erythropoiesis even after birth but this function continues upto approximately twenty years of age since after this time bone marrow of long bones become fatty; so after this crucial age, marrow of membranous bones, e.g. vertebrae, sternum, ribs produce these cells. But as the age advances further this marrow also becomes less productive and this explains the development of anaemia in old age.

Stages

Stage I: *Haemocytoblast*—18–23 μ diameter, large nucleus, thin rim of cytoplasm.

Stage II: *Pro-erythroblast* 15–29 μ diameter. No haemoglobin, appearance—Large nucleus with chromatin forming fine reticulum having several nucleoli. Deep violet blue cytoplasm.

Stage III: *Early Normoblast.* Comparatively small (Early erythroblast) sized cell but showing active mitosis. Fine chromatin network with disappearance of nucleoli, 11–17 μ size.

Stage IV: *Intermediate Normoblast.* Appearance of haemoglobin is hallmark though in initial phase. Resting nucleus shows further condensation of chromatin. Of course cell goes still smaller in dimension (10–14μ), but showing active mitosis.

Stage V: **Late Normoblast.** Cell diameter ceased to 7–10μ. Mitosis of course ceased and stage represents maturation. Haemoglobin of course increased giving cytoplasm an eosinophilic reaction. Degeneration of nucleus (pyknosis) which breaks and ultimately disappears through lysis or extrusion.

Stage VI: **Reticulocyte.** A network of reticulum is evident in cytoplasm. Chemically reticulum is composed of RNA. Their number is 1 per cent or even less than it remaining as it is throughout the life, of course, the reticulocyte population is increased when erythrocytes are being formed rapidly.

Stage VII: **Normal Erythrocytes.** Non-nucleated biconcave disc.

Maturation and Multiplication. Maturation comprises decreased cell size, condensation, and finally disappearance of nucleus, initiation of haemoglobin accumulation. Both maturation and multiplication do not proceed together.

A reticulocyte normally matures for 1–2 days in the marrow before entering the circulation, during which time haemoglobin synthesis continues and cell's size decrease.

Requisites

i. Tissue oxygenation is the chief regulator already discussed.
ii. Maturation factor. Vitamin B_{12}-cyanocobalamine. Growth of almost all cells of the body is notably depressed without vitamin B_{12} commonly called extrinsic factor since it is essential for DNA synthesis and without this vitamin nuclear maturation as well as division comes to an end and more specially rate of erythrocyte production is inversely affected if it is lacking. In brief it can be stated that in erythropoiesis maturation failure results in its deficiency. So for its proper absorption 'intrinsic factor' is required which is secreted from parietal cells of gastric glands. Its deficiency will certainly lead to either diminished or no absorption of extrinsic factor which finally terminate into a fatal state pernicious-anaemia. Along with it dietary deficiency of vitamin C can lead to anaemia.
iii. ***Folic acid:*** This is also required for DNA synthesis through formation of deoxythymidylate (a nucleotide essential for DNA formation).
iv. ***Hormones:*** Erythropoiesis is affected by various hormones at the same time. Insufficiency of thyroid, adrenal and anterior pituitary hormone terminates into anaemia. Inversely polycythemia results with hyperfunctioning of adrenal glands.
v. ***Metals:*** Copper though itself does not participate in haemoglobin molecule structure but it certainly stimulates or promotes haemoglobin synthesis. Liver is the storehouse of this metal. Manganese is also helping erythropoiesis on the same line but less effective than copper in comparison. Cobalt is said to have comparatively a more powerful effect here upto the extent that in higher quantities it may precipitate polycythemia. It is also a constituent of vitamin B_{12}.

SUMMARY AND HIGHLIGHTS

It is the simplest cell in the body; formed as a nucleated cell in bone marrow. It loses nucleus before it is released into circulation (at late normoblast stage of erythropoiesis). Its another characteristic content 'haemoglobin' appears at intermediate normoblast stage. On entering the circulation, it still possesses residual ribosomes, mitochondria and Golgi apparatus. These cytoplasmic organelles are lost after a day or so and RBC assumes the shape of flattened, or biconcave disc.

The advantage of biconcave shape and without nucleus—is exhibition of remarkable plasticity, being able repeatedly to squeeze through capillaries only one half of the diameter of the cell and then to return, undistorted, to its original biconcave shape. The high surface to volume ratio facilitate respiratory gas transfer which is the main function of erythrocytes.

Its diameter 7.2μ (7.8μm; 6-9μ); thickness 2.2μ (0.081 μm in thin part—2.6μm in thick part), volume 87 cubic μ.

Their lifespan is 120 days. On their fate, bilirubin is excreted in urine and faeces in the form of sterco and urobilin. Pathophysiology of Jaundice is deeply related to its destruction.

Their number in a normal healthy male 5–5.5 millions per cubic mm; in females 4–4.5 millions per cubic millimetre blood. Hypoxia (high attitude) is the main factor which increases their number through liberation of ESF (Erythropoietin) from renal tissues.

Rouleaux formation means arrangement of RBC like pile of coins. The rate of their settlement in a long tube is called ESR (sedimentation rate). This investigation is important more as a prognostic and then as diagnostic.

Their increased number leads to a pathologic state named polycythaemia, and decreased number of course is anaemia. They serve main functions viz. oxygen carriage, carbon dioxide carriage, maintenance of ionic, acid-base balance as well as blood viscosity and of course various pigments are derived from it.

BIBLIOGRAPHY

1. Bishop C, Surgenor DM (Ed). The Red Bood Cell. A comprehensive treatise—London Academic Press. 1964.
2. Berlin NI, et al. Life Span of Red Blood Cell. Phy Rev 1959;39:577.
3. Grewalt TJ, Jamesm GA (Ed). Formation and Destruction of Blood Cell. Leppincort, Philadelphia. 1970.
4. Harris JW, et al. The Red Cells. Cambridge—Harvard University Press. 1970.
5. Symposium on Disorders of Red Cell. Amer J Med 1966;41:657-830.

60 Haemoglobin (Red Pigment of Blood)

"In order to function as primary medium of exchange of oxygen and carbon dioxide, haemoglobin must fulfil four requirements viz. capable of transporting large quantities of oxygen, high solubility, good buffering action and releasing oxygen at appropriate pressure and normal haemoglobin fulfils all these eligibilities."

INTRODUCTION

It is a chromoprotein having non-specific simple protein 'globin' and a specific prosthetic group 'haem' which is an iron containing pigment. Iron remains in ferrous form and iron content of haemoglobin is 0.34 per cent. The proportion of globin and haem is 96 and 4 per cent respectively. It is having 400 times more affinity with CO_2 as compared with oxygen.

CHEMISTRY

It is a conjugated protein with a molecular weight 64,500.

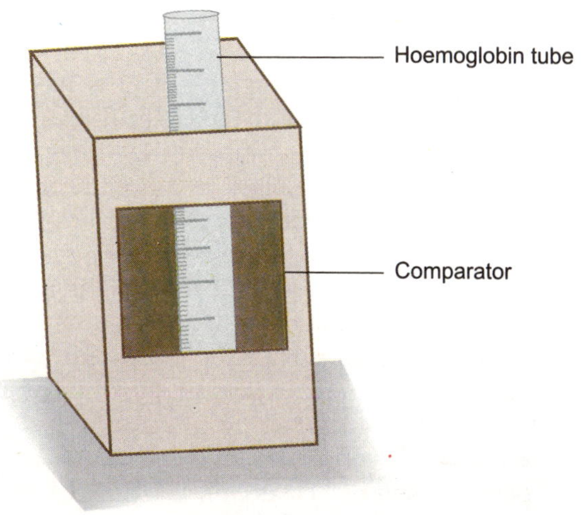

Fig. 60.1: Haemoglobinometer: Haemoglobin estimation (Sahli's method)

HEME

It is the prosthetic group of haemoglobin, and is an iron containing porphyrin derivative found not only in haemoglobin but also in cytochromes, peroxidase and myoglobin.

FUNCTIONS

1. Carriage of oxygen. It forms a compound called 'oxy-haemoglobin' which gives up oxygen when exposed to reduced pressure in tissues. 1 gm of haemoglobin can combine with 1.34 ml of oxygen at normal temperature and pressure.
2. Carriage of carbon dioxide—from tissues to lungs.
3. It helps in regulation of acid-base balance, so it is an essential buffer.
4. Various pigments are derived from it like bilirubin, stercobilin, urobilin etc.
5. Combination of heme and globin keeps the iron in ferrous state and also helps to combine molecular oxygen loosely with reversible potentiality.

FACTORS ESSENTIAL FOR BIOSYNTHESIS

Following is the list

i. First class proteins. Phenylalanine, leucine, histidine etc. are really needed for protein part of it.
ii. Vitamins—Specially C, B_{12}, folic acid, riboflavin, nicotinic acid.
iii. Metals—Iron, copper, cobalt, manganese are essential.
iv. Endocrines—Indirectly involved are thyroid, adrenal cortex and pituitary.
v. Overall control by gene located on autosomal chromosomes.

PORPHYRIA

It is a disorder of porphyrin metabolism in which abnormal porphyrins or large quantities of normal porphyrins are formed and excreted. 'Porphyrinuria' refers to increased excretion of porphyrins in urine which is coloured a 'wine red'. Condition is characterised by abdominal, mental and nervous symptoms.

FOETAL HAEMOGLOBIN (HbF)

1. It is present in foetal stage.
2. It compensates anoxia readily as compared to adult haemoglobin as it releases and combines with O_2 with great ease and releases CO_2 easily.
3. Foetal haemoglobin is resistant to alkali while HbA forms alkaline haematine.
4. It persists in congenital anaemia and thalassemia.
5. HbA and HbF are different chemically and spectroscopically.

NORMAL LEVELS

The haemoglobin level in healthy blood must be

- Male 14–17 gm per cent
- Female 12–15.5 gm per cent
- 14.8 or 15 gm per cent is considered as 100 per cent.

Types

a. *Adult Haemoglobin (HbA):* In adult red cells HbA makes up 90 per cent of the total. It contains two alpha chains and two beta chains (146 amino acids).

b. *Foetal Haemoglobin (HbF):*

   i. It is main component during foetal state.

   ii. Foetal red cells have considerably higher affinity for oxygen than do the adult red cells, e.g. at 20 mm of O_2 foetal haemoglobin can absorb 70 per cent oxygen while at same pressure the adult haemoglobin can only be saturated with 20 per cent oxygen. In the human, this discrepancy in relative oxygen affinities is due to the diminished interactions of HbF with red cell organic phosphates.

   iii. It releases oxygen more easily as compared to adult haemoglobin.

   iv. It does not release its oxygen load unless pressure is extremely reduced.

c. *Others*: Abnormals - S, C, D, G, M, I

HAEMOGLOBIN COMPOUNDS

a. *Additive Unstable*

   i. *Oxy haemoglobin*: Total oxygen carrying capacity is 15 × 1.34 = 20 ml. This is combination of haemoglobin with oxygen. When it gives up oxygen it is called reduced haemoglobin.

   ii. *Carbon dioxy haemoglobin*: Combination of Hb. With CO_2. Roughly (Carbo-haemoglobin) 10–30 per cent CO_2 is carried in this form.

   iii. *Methaemoglobin:* Iron of haemoglobin is in form (ferri-haemoglobin). Drugs like nitrites, chlorates, phenacetin, sulphonamides, methylene blue can produce it.

CO_2 AND HAEMOGLOBIN: A VIEW

1. One way: Oxygenation of haemoglobin molecule releases a proton, which in turn acts on bicarbonate to cause liberation of CO_2-, as
   $HHb + O_2 \rightarrow HbO_2 + H^+ + HCO_3^- \rightarrow H_2CO_3 \rightarrow H_2O + CO_2$
   This occurs in lungs. Reverse reaction occurs in peripheral tissues allowing CO_2 to be carried on venous side.
2. Second way: by formation of carbamino compounds as:
   $RNH_2 + CO_2 \rightarrow RNHCOOH$
   This binding is more stronger than oxyhaemoglobin.

OXYGEN AND HAEMOGLOBIN: AN OVERVIEW

- Its combination with O_2 is by virtue of its iron content. It readily combines as well as dissociate with O_2. Iron in haemoglobin is in ferrous state (divalent).
- Heme readily reacts with O_2 (trivalent).
- Each haemoglobin molecule contain four iron atoms. The oxygenation of one of the four hemes enhances the oxygen binding capacity of partly oxidised molecule so this molecule becomes fully oxygenated in preference to other haemoglobin molecules. The effect of this interaction of oxygenation of one heme upon the ease of oxygenation of other hemes results in peculiar sigmoid shaped curve. In absence of this interaction, the curve will get the shape of rectangular hyperbola.

b. *Additive stable*

   i. *Carbon monoxy haemoglobin:* CO is having 400 times more affinity with Hb molecule than oxygen. It is more stable as compared with oxy Hb. It is cherry pink coloured and its concentration is high in smokers. CO is slowly dissociated from heme.

   ii. *Nitro-haemoglobin:* Fumes of nitric oxide are having strong affinity for haemoglobin and forms stable compound.

   iii. *Sulfo-haemoglobin:* Haemoglobin with hydrogen sulfide. Green coloured.

c. *Degradation iron containing:*

   i. *Haem and Haematin*: Haem is formed when globin part is taken off. Haematin is oxidation product. Iron remains in ferric form.

   ii. *Haemin*: On further oxidation of haematin, it is formed.

iii. *Cytochromes*: Found in all animals and vegetable cells. These can be readily oxidised and oxidation product can be easily reduced.

iv. *Haemochromogen*: When haemoglobin is treated with acids (ferro haemochrome) or alkalies, globin part is denatured to form acid or alkali metaprotein which still links itself with haem. It is haemochromogen. If it is treated with oxidising agent, iron is converted into ferric form forming so called, 'ferri haemochrome'.

v. *Haem:* Combined with nitrogenous substances like denatured proteins, glycine, ammonia, pyridine are called ferrochrome.

OTHER HEME COMPOUNDS: A VIEW

1. Cytochrome: Widely distributed in plants and animal cells. They play a role in oxidation systems of cells. It acts by series of coupled reactions in which one of the cytochromes by molecular O_2 ultimately results in oxidation of a substrate, thus making energy available to the organism; haemoglobin here functions as a oxygen delivering agent.
2. Myoglobin: Is pigment of red muscle. Its molecular weight is 17,000. Iron content is 0.32 per cent. It is having higher oxygen binding capacity than haemoglobin. It can easily associate or dissociate than blood pigment. Molecule consists of one polypeptide chain and one heme group.

METHEMOGLOBIN: A VIEW

- It is dark coloured. When its large quantities are present, it gives a dusky discolouration to skin which resemble cyanosis.
- An enzyme system called NADH—methemoglobin-reductase system present in RBC converts it back, to haemoglobin.

d. *Degradation non-iron containing*:

i. *Porphyrin*: When haemoglobin is treated with strong acids or alkalies iron can be split from molecule and porphyrin may be set free which is in ring form. These porphyrins are proto or haematoporphyrins.

ii. *Bilirubin*: Biliverdin - urobilin and stercobilin.

DETERMINATION

i. *Requisites:* Includes haemoglobinometer or haemometer (Sahli's method) which contains a rack with standards fixed in front of a ground glass, a glass rod to stir, a specially graduated tube, a pipette with 20 cubic mm mark, a bottle containing distilled water, a bottle having N/10 HCl, a brush.

ii. To determine, graduated tube is placed between the standards in the rack. It is filled with N/10 HCl upto its lowest mark. Obtain blood and suck it in pipette upto 20 cubic mm mark. Dip its tip in acid. Blood and acid are then mixed. Wait for sometime. Add a drop of distilled water and mix again and match the colour with standard. Continue till colour is matched. Lowest point of meniscus, is to be read. To confirm the reading, add one more drop of distilled water and mix it. If in this second reading the colour is lighter then previous reading was correct. The reading what so ever is haemoglobin in gm per cent. Oxygen carrying capacity per 100 ml can also be calculated by remembering that 1 gm haemoglobin combines with 1.34 ml of O_2.

HAEMOGLOBIN UREA

- Due to haemolysis; the pigment haemoglobin passes into urine; so it is not converted into bilirubin. The urine—therefore is turned into portwine colour/dark brown/black coloured. This colouration is due to the action of urinary acid in converting pigment into acid hematin and methemoglobin.
- It should be remembered that haemoglobin cannot be retained within capillaries because of reasons like
  - — Environment of plasma is unsuitable for its action.
  - — Small size of its molecule
  - — So haemoglobin once escaped out from erythrocyte is useless.
- Paroxysmal cold haemoglobin urea: It occurs on exposure to cold. Persons are syphilitic in majority. Haemoglobin is liberated from erythrocytes by the action of an endogenous haemolysin which in presence of complement become fixed to red cells when the blood is chilled. This is in continuation of the fact that blood of such patient if cooled to 5°C outside the body and then subsequently warmed—then it undergoes haemolysis. It was studied by "Donath" so named "Donath phenomenon" after him.
- The disease is also seen after strenuous exercise—as in soldiers after long marches, i.e. March haemoglobinurea. The free pigment is oxyhaemoglobin not myoglobin. The fragility of erythrocytes is not increased.
- Nocturnal haemoglobinurea—is passage of haemoglobin/hemosiderin in urine specially in night. It is associated with haemolytic anaemia. Its cause is said to be susceptibility of red cells to acid metabolites and night destruction is attributed to accumulation of CO_2 during sleep. Some abnormality in stroma protein has also been blamed for haemolysis.

BIBLIOGRAPHY

1. Antonini E, Brunori M. Ann Rev Biochem 1970;39:977.
2. Astrup P. Red cell pH and Oxygen affinity of haemoglobin. New Eng J Med 1970;283:202.
3. Bunn HF, Jandle JH. Control of haemoglobin function within red cell. New Eng J Med 1970;282:1414.
4. Huchns ER, et al. Human embryonic haemoglobins. Nature 1964;201:1095.
5. Lehman H. Variation in human haemoglobin synthesis and factors governing their inheritance. Brit Med Bull 1959;15:40-46.
6. Lehman H, Carrell RW. Variations in structure of haemoglobin. Br Med Bull 1969;25:14.
7. Maclean N. Haemoglobin. Arnold, London. 1978.
8. Perutz MF, et al. The Structure of haemoglobin. Nature (London) 1960;185:416-22.
9. Perutz MF, et al. The haemoglobin molecule. Nature 1968;219: 29 and 131.
10. Perutz MF, et al. The haemoglobin molecule. Nature 1970;228: 551.
11. Riggs A. Functional properties of haemoglobin. Physiol Rev 1965;45:619.
12. Rimington C. The biosynthesis of Hb. Brit Med Bull. 1959;15:19-26.
13. White JC, Beaven GH. Foetal Hb. Brit Med Bull 1959;15:33-39.

61

Anaemia

In health the population of red cells and haemoglobin concentration are kept at normal levels by a nice balance between new formation and loss of red cells. Anaemia results when this balance is tipped one way or the other, that is—by a defect of blood formation or an increase in blood loss. Broad basically it is a condition in which blood haemoglobin level is reduced below normal limits.

IRON—DEFICIENCY ANAEMIA (HYPOCHROMIC—MICROCYTIC)

Anaemia which responds to proper adequate doses of iron is categorised as iron deficiency type.

Causes

a. Blood loss (gastric and uterine bleeding, post-menopause period).
b. Deficient intake (stomach and other digestive diseases, poverty, faulty dietary habits).
c. Excessive demand (menstruation, pregnancy, lactation, first two years of life).
d. Defective use (siderosis, defective intracellular iron containing enzyme).

Blood Picture

a. The total amount of haemoglobin is low but erythrocytes are not diminished in same proportion and hence colour index is low and anaemia is hypochromic.
b. Erythrocytes are smaller than normal (microcytic anaemia) or may be of normal size, so small pale cells are hallmark of this condition.
c. There exists leukopenia with relative lymphocytosis.
d. Thrombocytopenia is also said to exist.
e. Because of diminished size of erythrocyte MCV is also low.
f. MCH is also low as a result of smaller size of erythrocytes but also due to reduced pigment concentration throughout red cell substance.

Clinical Picture

a. The triad is the characteristic of disease viz. anaemia, atrophy of tongue's mucous membrane and brittle spoon shaped deformity of nails.
b. Bald and glazed tongue or 'angry red'.
c. Gastritis, poor appetite as well stomach mucosa may show superficial inflammation or even atrophy.
d. Paresthesia like numbness and tingling specially in arms or legs is evident too.
e. Spleen is never enlarged but palpable.
f. The condition is more common in middle aged women, as well as woman of child bearing period where deficient iron intake is there.

PERNICIOUS (ADDISON) ANAEMIA

The disease first described by Addison, so known after his name.

Blood Picture

a. All the formed elements of blood are reduced in number viz. erythrocytes, leukocytes and platelets;
b. Haemoglobin is also diminished but not in proportion so colour index is high and may be above one or even 1.5
c. The large sized cells 'macrocytes' can be readily seen in a stained film, but 'above normal size' of red cell is more valuable here as compared with presence of occasional macrocyte, i.e. the size here may vary from 4–12 μ (normal range 6–9 μ); of course many small cells 'microcytes' may also be present and this variation is collectively called 'anisocytosis.'
d. The red cells are hyperchromic with remarkable contrast to hypochromic or even achromic states, so this anaemia is 'macrocytic hyperchromic' type,
e. The cells varying remarkably in shape may be tailed or 'cocked hat shaped' called 'Poikilocytosis' (Poikilo = many fold),

f. The presence of 'reticulocytes' up to even 5 per cent is certainly a sign of immaturity (normal count 1%) so there is an increase in the reticulocyte count,
g. 'Nucleated red cells' may also be present which is again a sign of immaturity, which may be of normo or megaloblastic type. Nucleus may show even mitosis.
h. MCV and MCH are raised above normal, (high MCH is due to greater size of cell), MCHC is said to be normal.
i. There occurs decrease in number of white cells constituting 'leukopenia' which mainly affects polymorphonuclear cells so there occurs relative lymphocytosis. Furthermore polymorphonuclears are much more lobed in this type of anaemia than any other type of anaemia,
j. The platelets are much diminished in number called 'thrombocytopenia;'
k. Owing to increased blood destruction, bilirubin level is raised which is capable for making 'yellowish tinge of plasma' together with 'positive' indirect van den Bergh reaction' as well as increased urobilinogen in the urine;
l. Due to red cell diminishing the blood volume may be reduced but plasma volume may remain in normal range.

Clinical Picture

"The disease is so slow and insidious that the patient cannot fix up the exact date of his illness which all of a sudden becomes serious." Achlorhydria' and spinal cord symptoms are hallmark of the disease together with general anaemic symptoms like pallor, shortness of breath, headache, vertigo, palpitation etc. spinal cord symptoms like ataxia, spasticity, sensory disturbances.

As far as digestive disturbances are concerned 'soreshiny tongue (glossitis) together with atrophy of mucosa of fundus and body of stomach exists.

Treatment: Anti-anaemic Principle

For normal erythropoiesis two required factors are there. One is 'extrinsic factor' present in dietary food rich in Vitamin B complex, and is identified as vitamin B_{12} or cyanocobalamine. Its sources are liver, beef, rice polishing, yeast etc.

The other factor is secreted in gastric juice, called as 'intrinsic factor' and is fully essential for adequate absorption of extrinsic factor.

All the characteristic symptoms of disease mentioned above suggest lack of intrinsic factor.

HAEMOLYTIC ANAEMIA

Premature destruction and death of erythrocytes or in another way shortened lifespan of erythrocytes is the basis of this disorder.

Hereditary or intrinsic or intracorpuscular causes—defect here is residing within the cell and is transmitted by a gene.

Abnormal erythrocytes due to enzyme deficiency. Hereditary spherocytic anaemia.

Abnormal haemoglobin due to defect in haemoglobin protein synthesis—Haemoglobinopathies. (Thalassemia, sickle cell anaemia, drug-induced haemolytic anaemia).

Congenital spherocytic anaemia: "Red cells in this disease pass very slowly forwards and remains stagnant in splenic pulp, supply of glucose is reduced and cells become incapable of normal glycolysis can no longer maintain their normal energy stores and thus ensuing hemolysis." The spheroid shape of erythrocyte instead of normal biconcave shape is the main culprit here.

Due to this spheroid shape increased fragility ensues and excessive destruction of red cells lead to haemolytic jaundice (acholuric jaundice) because no bile appears in urine and jaundice is due to increased bilirubin production owing to increased erythrocyte destruction. Blood gives indirect van den Bergh reaction. Average lifespan of red cells is reduced to only 15 days (as compared with normal 120 days) so acute 'crisis' is expected.

CLASSIFICATION OF ANAEMIA

A. Anaemia caused by Blood Loss or Increased Blood Destruction

1. Post-haemorrhage—Acute and chronic (peptic ulcer, uterine bleeding, hookworm disease, purpura etc.
2. Haemolytic anaemia—Red cell destruction due to
   a. Intracorpuscular defect, i.e. abnormal red cell structure (hereditary spherocytosis, thalassemia, haemoglobinopathies, paroxysmal nocturnal haemoglobinurea; abnormal shapes render red cells more susceptible to phagocytosis).
   b. Extracorpuscular causes (i) Infective agents (malaria, virus etc.) (ii) Chemical agents (phenacetin, coal tar, quinine, sulphonamides), (iii) Physical agents (heat), (iv) Vegetable and animal poisons (snake venom), (v) Isoagglutinins (anti Rh, anti A and B, transfusion reactions, haemolytic diseases in newborn), (vi) Symptomatic haemolytic anaemia (chronic lymphatic leukaemia, malignancies) (vii) Paroxysmal cold haemoglobinurea, and (viii) Idiopathic acquired haemolytic anaemia.

B. Anaemia due to Defective Blood Formation

1. Nutritional anaemia (a) Iron deficiency (hypochromic microcytic) (b) Protein deficiency (c) Lack of folic acid (d) Vitamin C deficiency and riboflavin, nicotinic acid, pantothenic acid.
2. Lack or failure in absorption or in utilisation of specific anti-anaemic factor (vitamin B_{12}, cyanocobalamine)
3. Macrocytic anaemia (hypo or hyperchromic) with normoblastic bone marrow.
4. Anaemia due to interference with marrow functions either by depression or replacement (a) Infection (b) Toxic agents (X-rays, gold salts, benzol) (c) Renal diseases (d) Malignancy (e) Primary bone marrow failure (f) Replacement of marrow tissue by fibrous tissue.

Classification of Megaloblastic Anaemia

a. Pernicious anaemia
b. Macrocytic anaemia of pregnancy
c. Megaloblastic anaemia of infancy
d. Tropical nutritional macrocytic anaemia
e. Following total gastrectomy
f. Anti-metabolites and some drugs
g. Sprue—idiopathic steatorrhea

Blood film is characterised by 'micro spherulocytes and reticulocytes.' A spherocyte is smaller and thicker and spherical shaped. Reticulocytes may be even 20 per cent (instead of normal 1%). Leucocyte count may go as high as 12,000–15000/cu mm. and in state of crisis up to 80,000 even. There exists increased fragility of red cells.

"Chief symptoms are anaemia and jaundice and pathological lesions are splenomegaly and haemosiderosis."

Sickle cell anaemia: Disease is again hereditary characterised by haemolytic anaemia, acholuric jaundice, haemosiderosis with large number of reticulocytes. This disorder is greatly found in negro race and it was first described by Herrick (1910). As far blood picture is concerned there is marked anaemia and leucocytosis with prominent reticulocytes. Due to increase in bilirubin serum is deep yellow. Abnormal cells are phagocytosed by macrophages. In 'sickle cell trait' haemoglobin A (adult) and S (sickle cell) are present while in 'sickle cell anaemia' S and F (foetal) are present, bulk of course constituted by S.

As far as symptoms are concerned it is better to state, 'Before opening the abdomen of a coloured patient for any cause, it is better to observe blood film' At times patient may feel well but many times he presents symptoms. 'crisis' may occur periodically. Anaemia, painful muscles and joints, fever, leucocytosis, abdominal pain, general disability are symptoms in general.

Enlarged heart with thrill and systolic murmur, bone deformities, under weight—short trunk—long slender limbs—high domed skull (tower skull), neurological deformities are other peculiar features.

HAEMOGLOBIN "S"

- The α chains are normal but β chains are abnormal, because among 146 amino acid residues in each β-polypeptide chain, one glutamic acid residue is replaced by a valine residue.
- It is very insoluble at low O_2 tension and this causes the red cell to become sickle shaped.
- Heterozygous individuals have sickle cell trait and rarely suffer from severe symptoms. Homozygous individuals develop full blown disease. Sickle cell gene originated in black population of Africa but is resistant to one type of malaria.

Acquired haemolytic anaemia: (a) Idiopathic (unknown cause) (b) Extraneous agents

Protozoa .... Malaria
Virus ..... Primary atypical pneumonia
Bacteria ... Streptococci haemolytic and B. welchii
Chemicals ..... Toxic, e.g. trinitrotoluene
Animal and vegetable poisons ..... Snake venoms.

BONE MARROW HYPOFUNCTION: APLASTIC ANAEMIA

Primary aplastic anaemia generally appear in young individuals (15–35 years) and anaemia is capable of fatal results within weeks to months. Red, white and platelet cells all are reduced in number. Due to thrombocytopenia, purpuric bleeding as well as fever is common. Aplastic red bone marrow contain few cells and little more fats. Colour index is below normal but not significantly low. No evidence of haemolysis found. Though cause is unknown but the causative factor depresses bone marrow activity so no more blood is formed but destruction of blood continues so normal equilibrium upsets and anaemia ensues. None of the abnormality viz. polychromatophilia, reticulocytes, nucleated cells, macrocytes is found in film on the whole it is not a qualitative change but quantitative one.

Secondary aplastic anaemia may be due to some extraneous agents. Industrial poisons—(Benzol).

Drugs—(organic arsenicals, chloramphenicol, gold) Ionizing radiations.

SECONDARY ANAEMIA

Is a convenient term comprising a miscellaneous collection of anaemias which form one feature of a group of states or diseases of health.

Anaemia of infection is mild and normocytic normochromic type. There is decreased production of haemoglobin together with diminished iron absorption as well as diminished plasma iron level. Striking example is of subacute bacterial endocarditis.

Anaemia of pregnancy. In many cases there is some degree of iron deficiency leading to hypochromic microcytic type of anaemia.

Anaemia of renal disease seen in kidney diseases like chronic nephritis. It is possibly due to failure of elaborating erythropoietin–a marrow stimulating hormone.

Anaemia of malignancy as seen in leukaemia, lymphomas and due mainly to chronic blood loss from GIT interfering with production of intrinsic factor in cancer stomach.

Anaemia of nutrient deficiency like folic acid, iron, vitamin C, protein etc.

ANAEMIA : SIGNS AND SYMPTOMS

i. *Integumentary*: Pallor is most reliably discerned in mucous membranes, nail beds and lines of palm.
ii. *Respiratory and cardiovascular*: Increased rate and depth of respiration, tachycardia, angina of effort, night cramps, orthopnoea, cough, air hunger, exertional dyspnoea, palpitation, cardiac enlargement, ankle oedema, urinary frequency.
iii. *Gastrointestinal*: Anorexia, nausea, flatulence, constipation or diarrhoea.
iv. *Neuromuscular*: Headache, vertigo, faintness, roaring in ears, tinnitus, lack of power of mental concentration.
v. *Genitourinary*: Menstrual irregularity, cessation or profuse flow, urinary frequency, loss of libido.
vi. *Metabolic*: Low grade sustained fever, increased BMR.

BLOOD INDICES

These values are used to express the characters (absolute values) of individual cells in different types of anaemia.

a. *Colour index:* It is expressed as a ratio of haemoglobin to cells; i.e. it is obtained by dividing the haemoglobin value in gm /100 cc. by the red cell count, both values being expressed as percentages of normal. So

$$CI = \frac{\text{Percentage of Hb.}}{\text{Percentage of RBC}}$$

(14.5 gm/100 c.c. Hb. is said to be 100%) and (5 millions cell/cub. mm. red cells said to be 100%).

$$\text{So } \frac{100\% \text{ Hb}}{100\% \text{ RBC}} = 1$$

Normal colour index varies between 0.8 to 1.2. Increased value indicates towards hyperchromic state.

b. *Mean corpuscular volume (MCV):* This expresses the volume of individual red cell in cubic microns (μ^3). It is obtained by dividing the volume of packed cells expressed in ml per litre by the red cell count in millions per cubic mm.

Average MCV varies between 82–92 cubic microns. When it is raised the cell is macrocyte and cell is 'microcyte' on its decrease. Deficiency of some maturation factor induce macrocytosis, e.g. deficiency of B_{12} vitamin and folic acid leads to pernicious anaemia and nutritional anaemia respectively.

$$MCV = \frac{0.45 \text{ mm}^3}{5 \text{ millions}} = \left[1 \text{ mm}^3 = 1 \text{ mm} \times 1 \text{ mm} \times 1 \text{ mm}\right]$$

$$\text{or} = \frac{0.45 \times 1 \text{ mm} \times 1 \text{ mm} \times 1\text{mm}}{5{,}000{,}000} = \left[1 \text{ mm} = 1000 \text{ microns}\right]$$

$$= \frac{0.45 \times 1000\,\mu \times 1000\,\mu \times 1000\,\mu}{5{,}000{,}000} = \frac{0.45 \times 1000}{5}\mu^3$$

$$= \frac{45 \times 10}{5} = 90 \text{ microns}^3$$

$$\text{So MCV} = \frac{\text{Figure for packed cell volume in \%}}{\text{Figure for number of cells in millions}} \times 10$$

c. *Mean corpuscular Haemoglobin (MCH)*: It indicates the amount or weight of Hb present in a single cell. It is expressed in microgram. It may be obtained by dividing the haemoglobin in gm per hundred cc of blood by red cell count in millions per cubic mm.

1 gram = 1000 mg
= 1000 × 1000 micro gm
= 1000 × 1000 × 1000 milli micrograms (nanogram)
= 1000 × 1000 × 1000 × 1000 micro micro gm. (pico-gm.)
1 mg = 1000 microgram
1 microgram = 1000 milli microgram
1 milli microgram = 1000 micro-microgram or pico-gram

$$\text{So MCH} = \frac{15 \times 1000,000,000,000}{5000,000,000,00} \times \text{micro-microgram}$$

$$= \frac{15}{5} \times 10 = 30 \text{ picogram.}$$

So MCH $\frac{\text{Figure for gms of Hb. in 100 ml. of blood}}{\text{Figure for number of cells in millions}} \times 10$

Normally it varies between 27–31 micro-microgram. Its value increased in hyperchromic state, if decreased 'hypochromic state.' It is varying with the concentration of haemoglobin within the cell and with the number of the cell.

d. *Mean corpuscular haemoglobin concentration (MCHC)*: It is expressed in terms of percentage, and is the haemoglobin in gm. per 100 ml of blood divided by packed cell volume per 100 ml of blood.

1. $\frac{15}{45} \times 100 = 33.3$ per cent (45 = PCV of 100 ml of blood, 15 = haemoglobin in gm per 100 ml of blood)
2. $\frac{MCH}{MCV} \times 100 = \frac{30}{90} \times 100 = 33.33\%$

Smaller value (reduced saturation of haemoglobin in cells) seen in both hypo and hyperchromic states. The values are not increased unless blood is haemolysed. It is the index which indicates the degree of saturation of haemoglobin in red cell

IRON METABOLISM

1. As regards *'source'* is concerned green vegetables and some fruits are rich while milk contains only trace of it. Cereals are said to contain iron.
2. *Absorption*:
   i. It is better absorbed as 'ferrous' than 'ferric' state, and usual site is upper small bowel (duodenum and jejunum).
   ii. Factors affecting are:
   - Stomach acidity—favours absorption by reducing ferric form.
   - High concentration in diet—facilitates absorption.
   - Form—inorganic form is readily absorbed as well as ionizable form.
   - Reserve quota—if iron reserve is depleted, absorption increases while on its intactness only very small amount is absorbed.
   - Substances—Excess phosphate hampers absorption while it is hastened by low phosphate levels.

   iii. Feedback regulation:
   a. Liver secretes apotransferrin into the bile that flows through the bile duct into duodenum. Here it binds with free or conjugated iron (e.g. myoglobin, haemoglobin etc.) and this combination is called transferrin. This is attracted by intestinal epithelial cells. Then this transferrin molecule along with iron store, is absorbed by process of pinocytosis into epithelial cells and released on the blood side of these cells in the form of plasma transferrin.
   b. Excess stores of iron in body → formation of apotransferrin is decreased by liver → reduced concentration of this iron transporting molecule in the plasma and bile → less absorption of iron by intestinal apotransferrin mechanism → situation is balanced.
   c. Transferrin normally one-third saturated with iron; if fully saturated with iron; then → it does not accept no more new iron from mucosal cells → it also becomes difficult for transferrin to release iron to the tissues.
   d. Although, these feedback mechanisms do exist, but even then on taking large quantities of iron, it will be entering the blood; but will lead to massive deposition of hemosiderin in RE cells throughout the body and of course, it may be damaging.

   iv. Another representation (Granick—1943–46)
   - Ferrous iron passes from intestinal lumen into the mucosal cell where it is oxidised to ferric form, [ferric-hydroxide-phosphate-Fe(OH)]. It combines with a protein apoferritin—to form ferritin which is a iron-phosphorus-protein complex, and is a conjugate protein containing 23 per cent iron.
   - At the vascular surface of mucosal cell the iron of ferritin is reduced to ferrous form which is facilitated by Vitamin C. In blood stream it is oxidised and combines with B_2-iron binding globulin called "transferrin" (Siderophilin). This ferric iron diffuse across the capillary wall into tissue fluid but iron enters the cell in the ferrous form. In circumstances like hypoxia ferrous iron passes directly into the plasma without going to ferritin stage.
   - While iron is passing in considerable amount in blood, its concentration in plasma shows only little or no rise. This is due to the fact that it is taken up for manufacture of haemoglobin by red bone marrow; and after this utilisation, it is taken up by R.E. and parenchymal cells of other tissues where it is stored (liver, spleen, respiratory enzymes, muscle haemoglobin etc.).
   - The endogenous iron amounts to be 24 mg daily. The little amount which is excreted in urine, faeces etc. is available for re-use.

- Its excretion plays a negligible part in stabilisation of plasma iron level.
- The level of plasma iron represents the balance struck at any moment between iron from such sources, together with that absorbed from intestine and the iron taken up by the bone marrow and other tissues.

3. Dietary requirement—20 mg daily for adult male and 30 mg daily for adult female is dose recommended. In pregnancy and lactation period this may increase to 40 mg daily. Growing children requires 15-20 mg daily.
4. Blood iron:
   i. As haemoglobin in red cells. 15 gm of Hb per 100 ml of blood contains 50 mg of iron.
   ii. Transferrin is name given to its combination with plasma β globulin present in concentration of 2.5 gm per litre.
   Total iron biding capacity of plasma is 250–400 μg per 100 ml. The plasma iron concentration is 70–175 μg per 100 ml.
   Plasma iron increased—administration of iron salts, where red cell formation is depressed (aplastic-pernicious anaemia)
   Plasma iron decreased—on decrease of iron absorption, rapid red cell formation. With normal diet the level is constant.
   iii. As ferritin—serum ferritin is the best indicator of iron stores in the body.
   iv. Iron content of haemoglobin is 0.33 per cent, thus 100 ml of blood containing 15 gm Hb, contains 50 mg iron. As life of red cells is 120 days, 0.8 per cent of total blood haemoglobin, i.e. that contained in 50 ml of blood is daily destroyed releasing about 25 mg iron.
5. *Excretion:*
   i. Adult man on an adequate iron intake excretes about 0.4 mg in urine and 0.8 mg in bile daily (so it ranges from 0.5–1 mg daily).
   ii. Adult women—monthly menstrual loss—50 ml.
   Child bearing—iron content of foetus at term—400 mg.
   iron content of placenta and uterus—150 mg.
   iron content of blood loss at delivery—170 mg.
   iron content of milk during lactation—180 mg. (6 months)
   Total iron loss in 15 months—900 mg.
   Average daily iron loss—2 mg.
6. Significance:
   i. *Haemosiderosis:* In this condition iron is deposited in tissues in the form of hemosiderin. Malaria, hemolytic anaemia, blackwater fever are responsible for it since they are causing increased breakdown of red cells and that liberated iron is then being stored.
   ii. *Hemochromatosis*: This is an abnormal state when such haemosiderin deposits occurs in liver, spleen, kidney and other tissues.
   Hemochromatosis
   - Extensive deposits of colloid iron containing pigments called hemosiderin found in cells of liver, spleen and other tissues.
   - This haemosiderin contains 55 per cent iron which is made up of ferritin.
   - Total iron content of body is increased.
   - Other symptoms include—bronzing of skin, pancreatic sclerosis, liver cirrhosis, diabetes, testicular atrophy, etc.
   - It is a matter of debate to say this condition as inherited inborn error of metabolism.
7. *Transport and Storage*
   a. When plasma iron falls very low, iron can be removed from ferritin quite easily, but less easily comparatively from haemosiderin. The iron is then transported by plasma transferrin to those body parts where it is needed.
   b. Receptors are present in cell membranes of erythroblasts in bone marrow. Transferrin molecule combines with these receptors. Then it is ingested into erythroblast through process of endocytosis. On reaching there, this transferrin delivers the iron directly into mitochondria, where heme-synthesis takes place. So one who is not having an adequate quantity of transferrin, often suffers from anaemia.
8. *Summary*
   1. Body of healthy adult contains 4-5 gm (75–90 mmol) of iron in following forms:
      a. Blood Hb contains 2.5 gm (45 mmol)
      b. Storage iron (2/3 as ferritin, 1/3 as haemosiderin) amounts to 1–1.5 gm (18–27 mmol).
      c. Myoglobin, in red muscle contains 0.2 gm (3.5 mmol) of iron.
      d. Intracellular enzymes, accounts less than 0.1 gm of iron.
   2. Storage forms are—Ferritin—is water soluble consisting of a protein 'apoferritin' (mol. wt. 450,000). Haemosiderin—granular, water insoluble. Gives blue colour when ferricyanide is added to it.
   It is the essential element information of haemoglobin molecule, and is an essential constituent of myoglobin and respiratory enzymes while its deficiency may lead to iron deficiency anaemia.

3. A blood donation for transfusion (450 ml) depletes stores of 225 mg of iron. During lactation, a woman loses on additional 0.5–1 mg daily. About 20 mg of iron is needed daily to make new haemoglobin to replace the haemoglobin catabolized in breakdown of senescent RBC in mononuclear phagocytes.
4. A normal 70 kg man has—(iron)
   — 2.5 gm. iron in haemoglobin
   — 150 mg in muscle myoglobin
   — 15 mg in trace heme tissue enzyme
   — 1 gm in stores
   — 3 mg in plasma bound to transferrin on its way to cells.

ANAEMIA AND CIRCULATION

Because of anaemia, there exists less number of red cells. It leads to decrease in blood viscosity (as low as 1.5 times that of water as compared with normal 3); which decreases the resistance to blood flow in the peripheral vessels. All this increases the venous return to the heart. Furthermore, because of less number of erythrocytes, hypoxia ensues which causes the vessels of peripheral tissues to dilate which further increases the cardiac output to more higher levels. This increases the workload on the heart. This explains bright chances of myocardial infarction or cardiomegaly in anaemia.

Still anaemic patients can do better during 'rest' since even though each unit quantity of blood carries small quantities of oxygen which can meet the demand. But when an anaemic patient begins to exercise then the demand of tissue increases which cannot be met and cardiac failure often ensues.

BIBLIOGRAPHY

1. Charalton RW, Bothwel TH. Iron absorption. Ann Rev Med 1983;34:55.
2. Cook JD, et al. Evaluation of the iron status of a population. Blood 1976;48:449-55.
3. Finch CA, G Lenfent. O_2 transport in man. New Eng J Med 1973;206:407.
4. Huebers AA, Fuich CA. The physiology of transferrin and transferrin receptors. Phy Rev 1978;67:520.
5. Propper R, Nathan D. Clinical removal of iron. Ann Rev Med 1982;33:509.

The Leucocytes (White Blood Corpuscles: WBC)

When the call for help is heard, the bone marrow pours these cells in tremendous number into the circulating blood and when these cells reach to site of action, they reach to the tissues by migrating from blood so it is better to name these cells as loyal soldiers of the body.

INTRODUCTION

These cells differ from red cells in containing nucleus but at the same time they are devoid of haemoglobin. They are also comparatively less in number than erythrocytes. Their number in healthy blood varies between 4–11,000 cells per cubic millimetre of blood while erythrocytes are in millions; their proportion in blood is 700 : 1. They are not white as the name given but actually they are colourless appearing transparent in circulation.

MORPHOLOGY

As for as morphology is concerned, they fall into two categories—(a) Granulocyte and (b) A- or non-granulocytes.

a. *Granulocytes:* They are so named because of presence of granules in cytoplasm. They are further subdivided into three groups according to their staining reaction with 'Leishman's stain' which is a combination of eosinated methylene blue dissolved in acetone free methyl alcohol and since this stain is a mixture of both acidic (eosin) and basic (methylene blue) dyes so its nature is neutral. The cells having affinity with neutral part are called neutrophil, cells taking acid part eosinophil while basic part takers are basophil.

   i. *Eosinophils:* They are present in 2–4 per cent (1–5% also) in differential counts, with absolute number amounting between 150–450 cells per cubic millimetre of blood. This number increases in all allergic states (bronchial asthma, anaphylactic shock etc.), parasitic worm infestation, skin diseases and also tropical eosinophilia (Wein-Garton syndrome); all this increase in number named as eosinophilia. The reverse case eosinopenia meaning decrease in eosinophil population is under the endocrinal control depending upon release and amount of adrenocortical hormone and hence degree of their decreased number is taken as indication of severity of stress. ACTH administration is also a causative factor of this state. On break down these cells release histamine which on the other hand increases capillary permeability together with increased pouring of antibodies and thus inactivating the antigens. The nucleus appears bilobed (occasionally trilobed also) taking 'spectacle shape, while

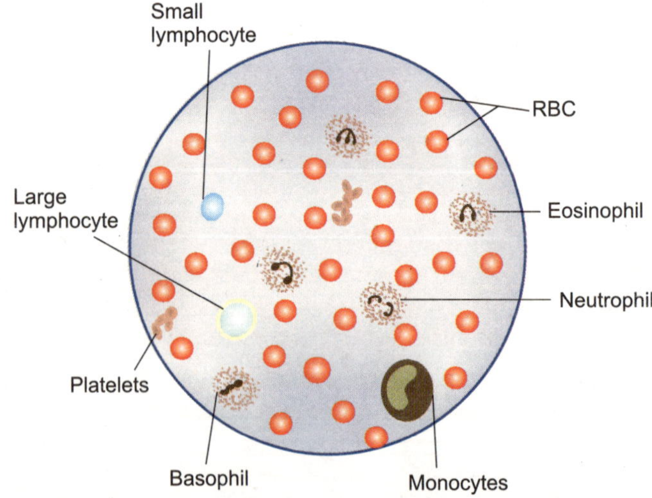

Fig. 62.1: Peripheral blood film (PBF) (Leishman's stain)

cytoplasm is packed with coarse, red refractile granules which may envelope cell wall even making it indistinct. They are also considered as mild phagocytic together with exhibition of chemotaxis but in comparison of neutrophils this property is insignificant. These cells are also said to contribute to dissolute the blood clots, by releasing pro-fibrinolysin substance which become activated to form fibrinolysin—an enzyme digesting the fibrin. Their usual size varies between 10–14μ. Comparative aspect. In horse 4 per cent, cow 5 per cent, dog 10 per cent, cat 5 per cent, goat 2 per cent, pig 3 per cent normally.

The granules contain EPO (Eosinophilic peroxidase enzyme having antibacterial activity and is also required for activities of mast cells during allergic inflammation), MBP (Major basic protein—rich in arginine and histaminase), and ECP (eosinophilic cationic protein).

ii. *Neutrophils (Thal-sainik)*: They appear in 50–70 per cent in differential count in healthy blood. Size/ diameter varies between 10–14μ. Nucleus may be many lobed (uni for one, bi for two, tri-tetra and penta for three, four and five lobes and multi for still many more) so this lobed pattern gives them another name of polymorph, while cytoplasm is characterised by fine granules, and these granules represent lysosomes containing à variety of digestive enzymes which makes the cell capable to remove ingested material. They are also rich in enzymes of glycolytic, respiratory and hydrolytic system including amylase, lipase, nucleotidase, protease, phosphatase etc. These cells are actively amoeboid showing phagocytic activities constituting what is called first line of defence, by quickly reaching to the site of infection. They are also supposed to show aerobic glycolysis. Besides the pathologic conditions of infection, there are certain physiological conditions which are capable of increasing their number—a condition named 'neutrophilia' and the factors include exercise, emotions, adrenaline or nor-adrenaline administration, menstruation, pregnancy, lactation etc. The granules are of two types—primary and secondary. Primary granules contain various proteolytic and amylolytic granules MPO (myeloper-oxidase enzyme granules), lysozyme enzyme granules—all cause bacterial disintegration. Secondary granules contain lactoferin, alkaline phosphatase, vitamin B_{12} binding protein, which inhibits bacterial growth.

Neutrophils are having various receptors on their surface membrane, which can bind substances like, prostaglandins, complement, immunoglobulin Ig etc.

iii. *Basophil:* Characterised by large coarse violet granules in cytoplasm, obscuring the nucleus and they amount between 0–1 per cent in differential counts. These cells are supposed to liberate heparin—a substance which prevents clotting so in this way these cells are very much similar to mast cells. Their granules are containing heparin, hyaluronic acid, histamine and serotonin (vasoactive agents). Whenever there is excessive bone marrow activity, e.g. chronic myelocytic leukaemia, polycythemia vera their number is increased; so also with chronic inflammation, number of basophils is increased (basophilia). Their size is 8–10μ and nucleus is lobed.

b. *Agranulocytes*: absence of granules from cytoplasm means agranular cell.

i. *Large lymphocyte*: These cells are classed as younger form of small lymphocytes. Their usual size is varying between 10–14μ with the percentage (%) between 20–40 (or 15–35% even) in differential counts. Nucleus almost covers ¾ part of the cell leaving remaining ¼ area for cytoplasm and is centrally located.

ii. *Small lymphocyte*: These cells are slightly bigger than erythrocytes varying between 7–10μ in diameter. Nucleus stains more deeply than surrounding narrow rim of cytoplasm which intervenes between it and cell wall and nucleus is relatively large and centrally placed.

Lymphocytes are mainly functioning as manufacturer of antibodies and physiologically are more plentiful in the blood of young children.

Pathologically lymphocytes are increasing their population in all chronic infection states while reverse case (means decrease in number-lymphocytopenia) is observed in response to adrenocortical hormones and ACTH administration (just like eosinopenia) and hence adrenalectomised animals show lymphocytosis—increase in their number.

Lymphocyte: Circulation and lifespan. Lymphocytes are now known to circulate through lymph nodes; entering by the blood stream and leaving by efferent lymph channels, to re-enter the blood stream by way of thoracic duct.

Lymphocyte: Control of blood levels.

i. Adrenal cortex controls lymphopoiesis. Adrenocortical hormones cause a rapid involution of thymus, lymph nodes and other lymphoid structures. Changes are reversed on adrenalectomy.

ii. Hypophysectomy causes a decrease in weight of thymus and spleen.
iii. Mild atrophy of lymphoid structures is seen on thyroidectomy.
iv. Increase in weight of thymus is observed on removal of gonads.
v. Marked atrophy of thymus in rats is observed on administration of testosterone.

Monocytes: (Transitional leucocyte as told by Ehrilich) biggest or largest cell with diameter ranging between 10–18 or 21μ. Nucleus having deep indentation and eccentrically placed with horseshoe kidney or even oval shape occupying only 2/3 part of cell while remaining part of the cell is occupied by cytoplasm. They are actively motile and phagocytic and considered as derivative of fixed histiocytes behaving as macrophages. They constitute 2–5 per cent of entire leucocyte population. They appear in 4–8 per cent or even 10 per cent in differential counts. An increase in their number so called monocytosis is observed in tuberculosis (advance stage), malaria, syphilis, bacterial endocarditis, monocytic leukaemia, glandular fever, brucellosis, infectious mononucleosus, etc. Arrest of tuberculosis is marked by increase in monocyte and decrease in lymphocyte counts. Fine chromatin threads are reported in this cell while coarse threads are seen in lymphocytes. Nuclear chromatin material is loose and network like while in lymphocytes lumpy chromatin is observed so its nucleus stains darker than monocyte's nucleus. MPO enzyme is absent.

PROPERTIES/FUNCTIONS

i. *Phagocytosis:* (phagein = to eat) The cytoplasm of the cell is projecting out its projections known as pseudo podia which engulf the foreign particle and finally draws it into cell itself, terminating in digesting that particle indicated by vacuole formation around it containing digestive enzymes; hence after digestion the foreign particle either disappears gradually or if not digested it is discharged from the cell.

Since natural substances found in the body are having electronegative charge like the phagocyte cells so they are naturally repelled by each other but foreign substances are having positive surface charge so they are attracted and ultimately phagocytosis occurs. 'More rough surface of foreign particle is—more will be the intensity of this process.' To promote this defensive process, body has some globin molecules termed as opsonins which first combines with the foreign material which facilitate the phagocytic cell to adhere to this combination.

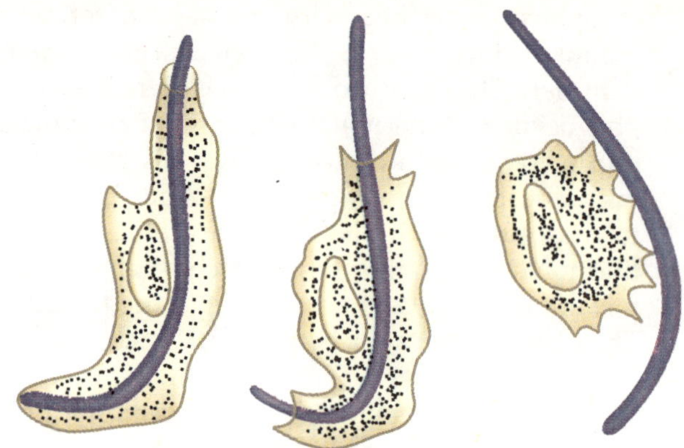

Fig. 62.2: Phagocytosis in stages

EVENTS OF PHAGOCYTOSIS

1. Binding of antibody coated antigen to receptors on membrane of phagocytic cell.
2. Hyperpolarisation of cell membrane followed by depolarisation and slow re-polarisation, increased free Ca^{2+} in cytoplasm.
3. Endocytosis of antigen-antibody complex with release of superoxide ions.
4. Fusion of phagocytic vacuole with lysosome.
5. Release of thromboxanes, prostaglandins, and leucotrienes.

The phagocytic cell is rich in lysosome filled with proteolytic enzymes (used for digesting foreign matter), lipase (used for digesting lipid membrane of foreign agents), bactericidal agents (used for killing bacteria, common are lysozyme and phagocytin). In this war, when foreign particles are killed, some breakdown substances are also formed by dead matter which is capable of destroying even phagocytes themselves; as per this property the neutrophil can destroy upto 30 bacterias or any other foreign matter before its own destruction while macrophage can destroy upto 100 such foreign particles.

So macrophages which are derived chiefly from monocytes are capable enough to digest bigger particles viz. senile erythrocytes, malaria parasite, tubercle bacilli etc., while neutrophils are capable for only an average sized bacteria. Sometimes when the notorious foreign particle is of much larger size like cholesterol crystals or bone pieces then many macrophages unite together to from so called 'giant cells' which is told as a cytoplasmic syncytium with large number of nuclei having greater phagocytic power. The term phagocytosis was first coined by Metchnikoff.

ii. *Diapedesis*: When WBC pass out of blood vessels, it is diapedesis. This passage is facilitated by pores of blood vessels through which white cells are squeezed. If the pore size is smaller than leucocyte then protein of white cell coming in contact with pore first will be temporarily constricted to allow passage for remainder of the cell (diapedesis = leaking through).

iii. *Chemotaxis:* The different chemical substances attract the white cells and the phenomenon is labelled as chemotaxis. Neutrophils and monocytes are attracted towards inflammation site which is called positive chemotaxis while reverse situation is classed as negative chemotaxis in which white cells are repelled. This property is certainly dependent upon concentration gradient which is maximum around the toxin or inflammatory foci and as we go away from this source this gradient decreases.

To summarise neutrophils and monocytes are the two free lances cells since they freely swim in search of foreign matter or bacteria. They project a processes pseudopodium from their cytoplasm and after it they pass out through process of diapedesis and after this escape they rush to the threatened area and destroy the invaders.

ANTIBACTERIAL ROLE OF NEUTROPHILS

1. During inflammation (i) Vaso dilatation of local fine blood vessels. (ii) Margination (adherence of WBC to vascular endothelium and emigration (going out of vessels by projecting pseudopodia); (iii) Chemotaxis (attraction of neutrophil by inflamed area/bacteria; (iv) digestion (by phagocytosis).
2. Margination is due to the fact that normally blood flows with a great velocity so it is axial or central stream. Because of any inflammation vasodilatation occurs which makes the blood flow sluggish so now blood occupies peripheral part of the vessel and then marginate.
3. Leucocytes specially neutrophils stick to vascular endothelium by complements and arachidonic acid metabolites (prostaglandins and leucotrienes—Synonym-eicosanoids).
4. Neutrophils have receptors on their surface, which can bind 'immunoglobulin (Ig), complement, arachidonic acid metabolites. Because of this binding the Ca^{++} moves to neutrophils from extracellular fluid which leads to contraction of actomyosin filaments which results into pseudopodial projection and emigration.
5. The chemotaxis is achieved by C5a' activated complement, PF_4 (platelet factor 4), leucotrienes.
6. Now after positive chemotaxis, phagocytosis begins, for which the bacterium has to be coated with opsonin (Ig, complement), which makes the bacteria sweeter in taste for neutrophils.
7. After phagocytosis, digestion begins due to primary and secondary granules of neutrophils as described earlier. As a result of metabolism, neutrophil produces H_2O_2 and superoxide (O_2) both are lethal to bacteria. This combination produces hypochloric acid and chlorine (HOCl) which are again lethal to bacteria. The lactic acid also accumulates because of metabolic activity of neutrophil; which is poured within phagocytic vacuole; which causes lowering of pH; resulting into death of bacterium.

LIFESPAN

Since from bone marrow they are poured in general circulation to fight against the invaders whenever they are existing (loyal soldiers) so naturally it appears evident that lifespan of white cells must be short. Granulocytes are said to live for 12–15 hours but if infection is marked this period may be still reduced. DNA labelled isotopes studies have revealed that lymphocytes live for 100–200 days but sometimes this period may be reduced to 3–4 days only. But in circulation stream total number of lymphocytes present is always less than amount discharged from thoracic duct. The reason being the lymphocytes pass out of the blood vessel through the process of diapedesis to tissue spaces from where they return to lymph nodes so in general circulation they appear less. Since monocytes live longer in threatened areas so they are having comparatively a longer life than other leucocytes. Whatever the presumptions may be but nothing can be told about correct life time of leucocytes.

After completing their lives, granulocytes are destroyed by RE cells (bone marrow, liver and spleen) while lymphocytes are destroyed by macrophages located in germinal centres of lymphoid tissue.

The life of lymphocytes may be months or years but this depends on body's need for these cells. The platelets are replaced once every ten days (about 30,00 platelets are formed each day per microlitre of blood).

PRODUCTION (LEUCOPOIESIS)

Granulopoiesis

Site—Red bone marrow is the usual place and reticular cell gives rise to stem cells which produce granulocytes. They develop extravascularly.

Stages: Primitive Leucocyte (Haemocytoblast).

Proliferation of stem cells. Large sized cells. Large nucleus covering cell cytoplasm. No mitochondria, no lobed nuclei, basophilic cytoplasm.

Stage I: *Myeloblast.* 12–18μ size. No granules in cytoplasm. Single large nucleus with fine chromatin and many nucleoli.

Stage II: *Pre myelocyte.* Granules in cytoplasm appear, majority is of neutrophilic type, less eosinophilic but basophilic granules are least. Large nucleus without nucleoli. Almost same size 12–18μ.

Stage III: *Myelocyte.* Greater amount of cytoplasm with more granules and clear staining reactions. Small nucleus without nucleoli but with coarse chromatin. Multiplication is active.

Stage IV: *Metamyelocyte.* More and conspicuous granular cytoplasm with indented nucleus. No more multiplication, but maturation. Amoeboid movements appear and they appear in circulation.

Stage V: *Mature white cell.* Indented nucleus change into lobed one. Distinct granular cytoplasm with staining characters. Start showing amoeboid movements. Individual lobes are connected with fine strand.

Lymphopoiesis (Development of lymphocyte)

Site–in embryonic stage mesoderm while in adult germ centre of lymphoid tissue.

Stages: The reticular cell of lymphoid tissue gives origin to stem cell which produces "lymphoblasts" which give rise to lymphocyte large as well as small.

Development of Monocytes

These cells develop from bone marrow histiocytes. They arise within the bone marrow from a common granulocyte macrophage progenitor cell. Monoblasts—promonocyte and monocyte make up from 1–3 per cent of marrow nucleated cells. A monoblast divides to give rise to two promonocytes, and each promonocyte divides once to give rise to two monocytes. Mature monocyte does not divide. Marrow transit time is six days.

Regulation of Leucopoiesis

The process of leucopoiesis govern is not still certain in scientific world but various hypothesis are there regarding its regulation. Some of them are listed below:

i. It is proposed that since they fight against foreign particles, bacteria or other invaders, many of leucocytes are killed in this war. A substance is liberated from dead or destructed white cells which is capable of promoting their own production. In this way we can presume that they regulate themselves.
ii. A hormone (Just like erythropoietin) is liberated which controls the whole process. Nothing reliable is known about it.
iii. Vitamin B complexes, folic acid, nucleotides are essentially required for their production and in their absence their production is inhibited.
iv. Role of thymus gland. Poor growth, failure in thriving, atrophy of lymphoid organs, small non-distinct lymph nodes, undeveloped lymph follicles of spleen, loss of normal immunological response of the body., reduction in number of lymphoid cells are few of some notable changes when thymus gland is removed (thymectomized animals) and in this way certainly the lifespan is reduced. Above are the changes only when thymus gland is removed shortly before birth or better called 'neonatal thymectomy.' Dramatically no such changes are noticed when the same gland is removed at an adult age. So by this experimental observation it is clearly evident that thymus is certainly playing a leading role in development of normal lymphoid system (but upto birth), after birth its role is over.

   Regarding explanation of this role, it can be understood that for proper differentiation, maturation of lymphoid cells, a suitable environment is produced or created by this gland and hence spleen, lymph nodes are such areas where these cells are populated and proliferated too. Secondly thymus gland is

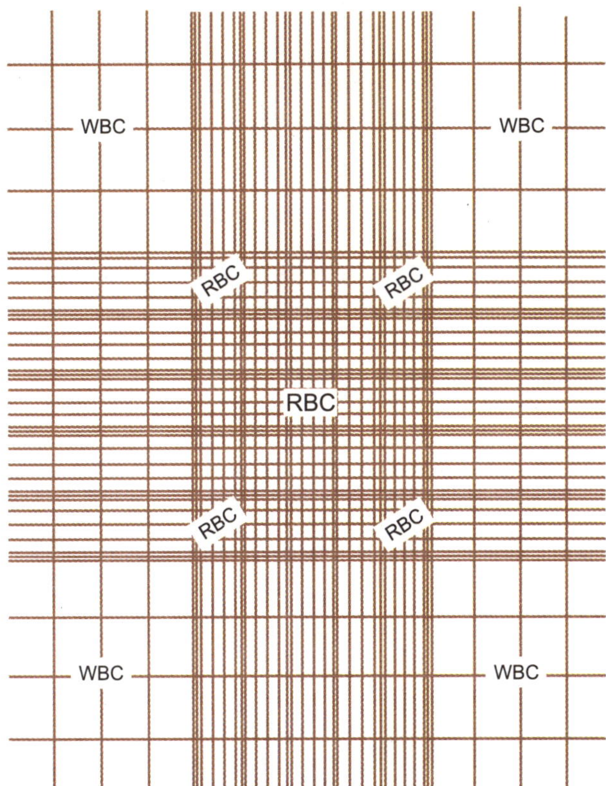

Fig. 62.3: Counting area of improved neubauer double counting chamber

supposed to produce a hormone thymosin which stimulates lymphocyte production as well development.

To sum up, "Thymus appears to play a major role in early life in maintaining the immunological integrity of the body, being the principal source of small lymphocyte which pass into the blood at the time of birth and are seeded to spleen and lymph nodes where they multiply for full immunological competence.

ABSOLUTE COUNTING

A special diluting fluid (WBC diluting fluid) is used for such counting which is composed of glacial acetic acid (0.2 ml) and gentian violet (0.1 ml. of 1% solution) together with distilled water to make volume 100 ml. Gentian violet stains the nuclei which are fixed by glacial acetic acid. Erythrocytes are destroyed by gentian violet.

WBC pipette is filled with blood to be tested up to mark 0.5 and rest part, i.e. upto mark II diluting fluid is filled. Both contents are mixed by rotating pipette between palms of hand for 2–3 minutes. First one or two drops are then discarded and chamber is charged as usual. Leucocytes appear as small rounded bluish violet dots spread homogeneously; of course they are counted in four corner squares of chamber. Dilution factor is 20.

Calculation. Area of one big square = Length × Breadth; So 1 × 1 = 1 sq mm.

Volume of one big square = Area × depth; So 1 × 0.1 = 0.1 cubic mm.

Counting is done in four squares so total volume = 0.4 cubic mm.

Suppose no. of cells counted in four squares = x

0.4 cubic mm. volume contains x no. of cells

So 1 such volume will have $\frac{x}{4} \times 10$ or $\frac{10x}{4}$

Dilution factor is 20.

So total number of cells comes to be $\frac{10x}{4} \times 20$ or 50 x

ARNETH COUNT

By this technique lobes of neutrophil nucleus are given importance and they are counted in percentage. In a healthy blood unilobed—12 per cent bilobed 25 per cent,

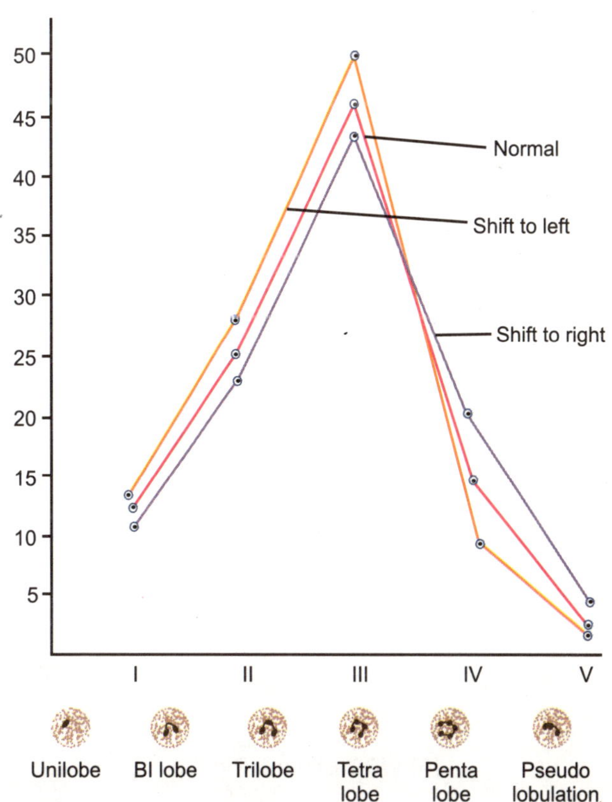

Fig. 62.4: Arneth count

Cellular Elements—Normal values			
Cell	*Average (Per cubic mm)*	*Normal range (Per cubic mm)*	*Percentage*
Total WBC	9,000	4–11,000	—
Neutrophil	5,400	3–6,000	50–70
Eosinophil	275	150–450	1–5 (2–4)
Basophil	35	0–100	0–1
Lymphocyte	2750	1,500–4,000	20–40
Monocyte	540	300–600	4–8–10
RBC	males	5.5–5 millions/cubic blood	mm
		females	4.5
Platelets	3,00,000	2,50,000–5,00,000	

trilobed 46 per cent, tetralobed 15 per cent, pentalobed 2 per cent are considered as normal. A relation has been established within lobes of nucleus and activity of bone marrow. So unilobed cells are youngest while multilobed are oldest. If unilobed cells are more (as normally seen in blood film of newborn) this means bone marrow is producing cells rapidly or its activity is increased (hyperactive bone marrow) and this is called shift to left which is commonly seen in acute infections, leukaemia, haemorrhages, high altitude, thyroid extract administrations, specific diet etc.

On the contrary if bone marrow activity is decreased, i.e. hypoactive marrow then pentalobed neutrophils will be more marked commonly called 'shift to right' generally met with pregnancy, pernicious anaemia, radiation therapy, toxic drug effects like sulphonamides, chloromycetine etc.

On looking through the microscope true and pseudolobulation should be differentiated. True lobulation of the nucleus is that in which lobes are well separated from each other or they may be connected with each other by a fine thin band of chromatin material, while pseudolobulation means lobes are not well separated but merged into each other or may be connected through a clear thick band of chromatin.

Generally in health trilobed cells are more because they are more mature hence their working efficiency is maximum in comparison.

SUMMARY AND HIGHLIGHTS (WBC—LOYAL SOLDIERS; NEUTROPHIL—THAL SAINIK)

Broadly of two types—Granulocytes and agranulocytes Phagocytosis (engulfing foreign particles), chemotaxis (attraction towards inflamed area), diapedesis (passing or squeezing out of blood vessels) are main properties or characteristics of WBC.

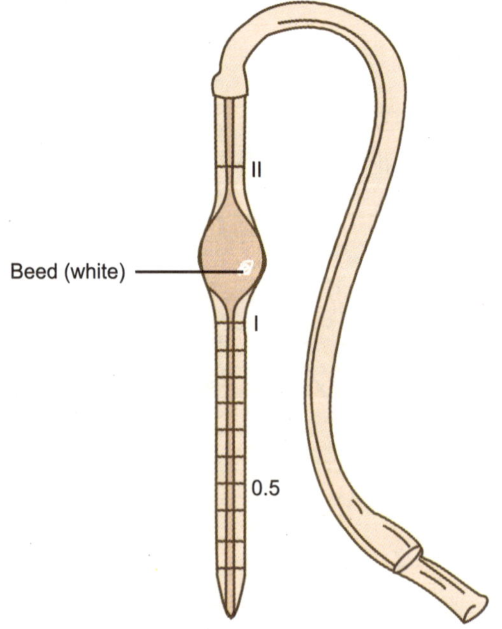

(A) WBC Diluting Pipette

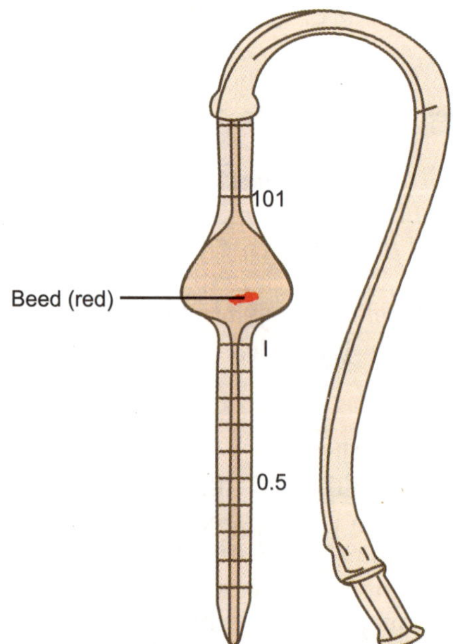

(B) RBC Diluting Pipette

Fig. 62.5: (A) WBC Diluting pipette (B) Pipette for absolute RBC counting (Note the difference of (A) marking 11 and 101 respectively and colour of beed)

During inflammation, following is the sequence—vasodilatation of local fine blood vessels, Margination, emigration, chemotaxis, phagocytosis and digestion of invader is there.

During leucopoiesis, multiplication occurs during myelocyte stage (granules also appear), while maturation takes place during metamyelocyte stage during which they project pseudopodia and appear in circulation.

In Arneth count number of lobes of neutrophils are counted in percentage and bone marrow's activity is decided (whether hyper or hypoactive).

Their total number varies between 4–11,000 cells per cubic mm. blood.

BIBLIOGRAPHY

1. Archer RK. The eosinophil leucocyte. Oxford : Balckwell. 1963.
2. Cline MJ. Metabolism of circulating leucocytes. Phy Rev 1965;45:674-720.
3. Metcalf D. Control of granulocyte and macrophages. Science 1991;254:529.

63

Immunity

Resistance of Body against Infection; Natural Immune or Defence System

It is better a sign of functional as well as structural integrity, of the body under which title, body learns to deal with infections more efficiently than in the past and one form of defence is rejection of those factors which are not part of body's own cellular structure.

NON-SPECIFIC IMMUNE SYSTEM (NATURAL IMMUNITY OR DEFENCE)

The members of the group include:

a. Surface epithelium of intact skin,
b. Mucus in alimentary as well as respiratory tract,
c. Gastric hydrochloric acid acting as an antiseptic,
d. Normal intestinal bacterial flora acting symbiotically,
e. Enzyme lysozyme present in sweat, sebum, tears, saliva, lacrymal gland's secretion,
f. Sneezing, coughing, vomiting reflexes,
g. Cilia of respiratory tube,
h. Basic polypeptides inactivating some gram positive bacteria
i. The effector cells are all leucocytes. Neutrophils are in first line of defence while monocytes can be transformed into macrophages whenever needed. Eosinophils are having doubtful phagocytic activity.
j. *Protection from virus:* By DNA-RNA mechanism a protein called interferon is synthesised against viral invasion which is capable to suppress the virus growth which is not checked by antibiotics.
k. Even then if any infective agent enters the body the inflammation and repair process immediately comes into action.
l. A very large protein properdin capable of direct destruction of gram negative bacteria. It is a serum macroglobulin having 8–10 times more molecular weight than gamma-globulins. Besides bacterial destruction it is also acting in virus neutralisation, erythrolysis. Its serum level is said to decrease in viraemia, bacteraemia, total body radiation, surgical trauma etc.

SPECIFIC IMMUNE SYSTEM

Before a detailed discussion is taken into consideration let us familiar with some concerning terms.

Antigens

In more simpler way it is defined as a substance foreign in character, protein in nature (sometimes may be polysaccharide too) which when gets entry in body will stimulate the formation of neutralising substances called antibodies. Generally the antigenic substances are possessing high molecular weight approximately 10,000 or more even. But this rule is not strictly implied since immune response can develop with a substance of even low molecular weight called 'hapten,' which will combine first with an antigenic substance to increase its molecular weight and this combination will then be capable of eliciting immune response; the examples in this series are chemical constituents of drugs and dust, industrial chemicals etc. Bacterial body proteins or liberated toxins are most potent antigenic substances.

Antibodies

These are key substance in this defensive part meaning that when body identifies a substance as foreign or not own or self the defensive antibodies are formed. These are protein in nature (gamma globulin of plasma proteins) consisted by polypeptide chains. By now following types of antibodies are known—*IgG* and *IgM* ... antibodies against microbes. IgA .... responsible for allergic reactions and formed in lymphoid tissue of, GI and respiratory tube.

IgD: Unclear function commonest immuno globulin. Mol. wt. 150,000. It may denote antigen taping capacity of B lymphocyte.

IgE: Not much known about it (Ig means immune globulines).

The antibody (gamma globulin) is formed by endoplasmic reticulum of plasma cells (which sometimes known as unicellular gland) which is rich in RNA constituting chief intermediary in protein synthesis process.

It may be surprising that cell may retain its ability to produce antibody long after infective organism has disappeared and further more persisting antibody may react in its full performance even with the new antigen.

Cellular or Lymphocyte or Cell Mediated Immunity

The chief type of cell designed for immunity is lymphocyte, meant that specific lymphocyte is sensitised against specific antigens. From immunity point of view lymphocytes are again divided into two

i. *T-Lymphocyte:* These are so named because they pass through 'thymus gland' and in fact approximately 80 per cent circulating lymphocyte are of this type and are not secreting any sort of antibody. Moreover, these are the cells responsible for above mentioned cellular immunity. These cells are said to fight against parasites, fungi, virus and few bacteria by direct fight. These are also capable of rejecting tissue transplant. After passing through thymus they reside in lymph nodes and lymphoid tissues. Irradiation, steroids and synthetic drugs (like azothioprine) are found to create inhibitory effect upon these cells. If any antigen enters second or more time, hypersensitive reactions are seen by producing a protein lymphokinase which is said to attract phagocytes and macrophages towards the area effected.

ii. *Main features of cellular immunity:* This type of immunity continues for years together or better to say for a much longer time as compared with humoral immunity. This is because of the fact that on exposure to antigen they continue to circulate in body blood and tissues for much longer time. Secondly it is better because only minute quantity of antigen can evoke lymphocyte release establishing this immunity. The famous examples in this series are tubercular infection, grafting tissues and even cancer cells.

iii. *Cells versus antigen : minutes of war:* On finding antigen the lymphocytes take the same characteristics as that of monocytes by swelling and thus increasing size. Then the sides of both (lymphocyte as well as invading agent) are attached with each other. Due to these proceedings the membrane of antigen undergoes autolysis, swelling and rupturing.

iv. *Manufacturing of lymphocytes:* Actually lymphocytes are lying in lymph nodes in their inactive state called 'lymphoblast.' On getting stimulation by the presence of antigen, this inactive form proliferate and release lymphocytes which are now called 'committed lymphocytes.' They are released because antibodies cannot be released by sensitised cells.

Humoral Immunity

i. This type of immunity depends upon antibody which are chiefly formed by plasma cells, which are present in lymph node, spleen and GI tract. Certainly the plasma cells are lying inactively at these respected sites in the form of plasmablasts. On getting stimulation in the form of any antigen they divide rapidly (500 cells within 4 days approximately). Due to this division process these cells develop granular endoplasmic reticulum which is the producer of gamma globulin antibodies at a rapid rate of 100 molecules per second.

ii. *B-Lymphocytes:* These lymphocytes after their release from bone marrow pass through 'bursa of Fabricius' (this structure is found in chickens as a mass of lymphoid tissue near cloaca in its GI tract but in humans this structure is not present but suspected in tonsil, intestine or appendix). Any way, from this structure the lymphocytes again reach lymph nodes and lymphoid tissue making these sites as their permanent residence. So these cells don't pass through thymus as T cells. These are providing humoral immunity but they amount to be only 20 per cent in circulation. They are capable to resist specific bacteria through antibody formation. They are said to possess finger like projections. They are having no capability of resisting abnormal mutant cells or intracellular bacteria.

Antigen Antibody Reaction

On the whole, it is an established fact that antibodies which are formed to suppress antigen is functioning as either to destroy or to inactivate the antigen. This aim is achieved in many ways -

i. *Neutralization of antigen*: The antibodies neutralise the toxic antigen after combining with it and this antigen antibody complex is then engulfed and destroyed by reticulo-endothelial cells (macrophages). Viruses are also exposed for phagocytosis by antibodies,

ii. *Bacterial agglutination:* Here instead of antigens many bacteria are linked together by antibodies in the form of chains or clumps better called agglutination. In this way bacteria are then easily phagocytosed.

iii. *Precipitation:* The antibodies when combine with antigen forming antigen antibody complex which then precipitates. It consists of large solid insoluble mass which is very easily destroyed by macrophages,

iv. *Complement fixation:* Complement is a complex lipoprotein substance normally present in circulating body fluids. The beauty in its way of acting that it waits for antibody to attach to antigen and then it will be attached to antigen and it is capable of penetrating cell wall and rupturing and destroying it. It is also capable of attracting white blood cells by chemotaxis process towards the site of antigen-antibody reaction. Its nine components are known till date from C^{-1} to C^{-9}.

v. *Opsonization:* Specific opsonizing antibodies (opsonins) and complement together destroy the invader sometimes. Since complement easily mixes with phagocyte's membrane, the opsonized bacteria is easily engulfed by phagocytes.

Differences between B and T cells

B Cells	*T Cells*
1. They don't pass through thymus but enter into bursa of fabricius.	They pass through thymus.
2. They are responsible for humoral immunity.	They are responsible for cellular immunity.
3. 20% of circulatory lymphocytes are of this variety.	80 per cent are of this type.
4. They are responsible for solid tissue grafts.	They are responsible for rejecting any transplants.
5. They fight against specific bacteria through their secreted antibodies.	They offer specific resistance to virus, fungi, parasites and only few bacteria.

CLONE

i. Suppose there are four brothers A, B, C and D. From each brother their progeny will develop and will form a distinct line or clone. So here, there will be four clone (A, B, C, D). Lymphocytes of our body are divided into numerous clones. Each clone has only one job and that is to tackle a highly specific antigen.

ii. When a multitude of cells arises from a single cell (e.g. when a single stem cell give rise to a spleen colony) that multitude of cell is called a clone. In normal hemopoiesis, mature blood cells originate from multiple stem cells, which means, normal hemopoiesis is polyclonal. Clone aggregates is termed as colonies.

INTERFERON

i. Is a polypeptide produced by cells invaded by viruses that passes to other cells and stimulates their resistance to infection.

ii. It is produced by fibroblasts, leucocytes, and T lymphocytes.

iii. It activates the immune system, possesses antitumour activity and has other cell regulating effects.

iv. It is of α, β and γ varieties. Lymphocytes produce alpha, while fibroblasts give rise to beta variety.

v. Interferons which were discovered and characterised by their antiviral activity, inhibit growth of variety of cells. Interferon β_2 may also limit TNF stimulated growth by its growth inhibitory effects.

Several monokines have been described like PAF (platelet activating factor), interleukin I. They activate helper T cell and acts as pyrogen.

Human immunoglobulins

Immunoglobulins	*Functions*	*Plasma concentration (μg/ml)*
1. Ig G	Complement fixation	12,100
2. Ig A	Localised protection in external secretion (tears, intestinal secretion)	2600
3. Ig M	Complement fixation	930
4. Ig D	Antigen recognition by B cells	23
5. Ig E	Releases histamine from mast, basophil cells	0.5

DEVELOPMENT OF IMMUNE SYSTEM

Passive Immunity

Temporarily immunity can be induced in a person without injecting any antigen. This task is achieved by injecting activated T cells, or by infusing antibodies. It lasts for only 2–3 weeks.

Allergy

Non-ordinary response of immune system. This allergic tendency is passed from parent to child, which is characterised by the presence of large quantities of Ig E antibodies, which are called reagins or sensitizing antibodies. Allergen is defined as an antigen that reacts specifically with a specific type of Ig E reagin antibody. When allergen enters the body allergen reagin reaction takes place which leads to subsequent allergic reaction.

Ig E antibodies are characterised by their strong affinity with mast cells and basophils. A single mast cell or basophil can bind as many as half a million molecules of Ig E antibodies. By the union of antigen (allergen)—antibody; immediate change in membrane of the cell occurs which is pulled. Many cells rupture releasing substances like histamine, leucotriens (slow reacting substances of anaphylaxis). Anaphylaxis, urticaria, asthma, hay fever are some of the different types of allergic reactions.

Immunosuppression

Drugs like cortisol (in heavy doses), 'cyclosporine cause immunosuppression.

Regulation of Immune Mechanism

- Immune mechanism should be neither less nor more. It should be just adequate.
- If it is more than sufficient, there will be death of too many innocent cells as well as damage to healthy tissues.
- If it is less than required, then antigens will be dominant and disease process will be facilitated.
- In order to regulate it to maintain an equilibrium there are regulatory T cells and helper T cells.

IMPORTANCE OF IMMUNE MECHANISM

- Through the lymphocyte mediated immunity, the body removes various antigen.
- Killer cells and natural killer cells kill the cancer cells. They also destroy virus infected cells.
- Tissues when transplanted to our body from foreign persons, are usually rejected called tissue rejecting.
- When any specific antigen comes in contact with T and B lymphocytes; the former form T cells while the latter forms antibodies.
- They are specific in their action; i.e. only specific type of antigen with which it can react can activate it.
- All the different lymphocytes that are capable of forming one specificity of antibody or T cell are called a clone of lymphocyte. All lymphocytes in each clone are alike.
- The macrophages in millions are present lining the sinusoids of lymph nodes, spleen and other lymphoid tissue. Most of the foreign antigens are first digested by these cells and antigenic products are liberated into the macrophage, which is then passed to the lymphocytes by these macrophages. This leads to activation of specified clones. Interleukin I is a substance secreted by macrophages which promotes the growth and reproduction of the specific lymphocytes.

Lymphocyte system—Humoral Immunity: The clones of B lymphocyte remain inactive (dormant) in hymphoid tissue prior to exposure to a specific antigen. On entry of antigen, B lymphocytes are also activated (by T cells; macrophages phagocyte antigen and present it to lymphocyte). These B lymphocytes enlarge immediately and take the appearance of lymphoblast; some of them then differentiate to form 'plasmablast which are precursor of plasma cells.

A sensitised lymphocyte produces many offsprings. Most of them remain ordinarily sensitised lymphocytes designed to fight against the specific antigen and die after sometime. Some of offspring become memory cells. A memory cell lives within a lymph node without any activity for many years. When a fresh invasion of that antigen occurs after a long time, the memory cell springs into life and repeatedly divides to produce a large number of lymphocytes of particular clone again.

VACCINATION

This can be done by various means like:

i. By injecting dead organisms which are unable to cause any disease but still have chemical antigenicity, e.g. whooping cough, diphtheria, typhoid fever etc.
ii. By injecting toxins which are treated with chemicals so that their toxic nature has been destroyed but antigenicity is still retained, e.g. tetanus, botulism, etc.
iii. By living organisms which are attenuated. It means that either the organisms have been grown in special culture media to destroy their toxic power; or they have been passed through a series of animals until they have been mutated enough that they will not cause any disease; but in all means they carry antigenic powers, e.g. poliomyelitis, yellow fever, measles, smallpox etc. (viral diseases).

T CELL

i. A cell surface T cell antigen receptor has been mentioned. It has following characteristics : (synonym—T cell marker)
   - It is clonotypic, i.e. recognition of single specific immunogenic determinant of an antigen. It is capable to differentiate between foreign MHC protein and self MHC protein (Major-histo compatibility complex).
   - Self MHC protein is tolerated and not at all reacted/rejected.
ii. The T cell antigen receptor is a multisubunit complex. On majority of T cells, the receptor complex

contains two disulphide linked polypeptide chains called α and β chains that mediate antigen recognition.

iii. *Helper T cells:* Are most numerous of T cells. They are supposed to secrete a series of protein mediator called 'lymphokine' which help in immune system. These include Interleukin 2, 3, 4, 5, 6, Interferon γ, Granulocyte—monocyte colony stimulating factor. HIV (AIDS) destroys or paralyse these cells. These cells also stimulate growth, proliferation, secretion of B cells. Due to these reasons these cells (or their interleukin) are sometimes referred as B cells stimulatory factors.
   The macrophages are also influenced by T cells in following ways :
   - Macrophages are activated much to perform 'phagocytosis' more efficiently.
   - Macrophages are chemotactically attracted towards the inflamed tissues and then their movement is slowed down.
   - Interleukin-2 further stimulates helper T cells and this vicious cycle goes on.

iv. *Cytotoxic T cells*: They are also named as 'killer cells' since they are capable of killing not only the microorganisms, but also body's own cells. They bind themselves to the attacking organisms, through receptor proteins present on surfaces of cytotoxic cells. On binding they secrete special proteins which make a hole in the membrane of attacked cell and through this hole cytotoxic substance is poured to destroy the respective cell.

v. *Suppressor T cells:* As the name suggests, they suppress the functions of both cytotoxic and helper T cells. Thus producing a braking effect on both types of T cells. So it is better to name these cells as 'regulatory cells.' Thus they exert a negative feedback control.

AIDS (ACQUIRED IMMUNODEFICIENCY SYNDROME)

Introduction

In the modern advancing scientific age certainly old diseases are controlled but it is also evident that they are replaced by new disorders and in this series it is the latest challenge to scientist. The main causative agent of this disorder is HIV (human-immuno deficiency virus), a human retro virus of lenti virus group. This virus further is subdivided into two distinct categories namely HTLV-I and HTLV-II (Human T lymphotropic-retro virus I and II respectively) and among these two HTLV-I is the commonest causative agent.

The disease is now coming up in the form of global epidemic. It was 1981 summer when the disease was first found out when pneumonia patients of unknown cause were found and all of them were having homosexuality in common, at New York and Los Angeles. Besides it, large number of cases have been reported at Western Europe, Central Africa, South America and Canada. It is epidemic in Central and East Africa and is becoming commoner in West Africa, where disease has got its another name 'slim disease' since severe weight loss is a common symptom there.

Disease classification system		
Group I	Acute infection	
Group II	Asymptomatic infection	
Group III	Generalised lymphadenopathy	
Group IV	Other diseases	Constitutional diseases Neurological diseases Secondary infection Secondary neoplasm Other conditions

The common denominator of AIDS is a profound immuno-suppression preferably of cell mediated immunity which switches to variety of opportunistic diseases which include certain infections and neoplasms. The main cause of this immune defect is quantitative as well as qualitative deficiency in subset of T lymphocyte.

Clinical symptoms: The infection starts from acute phase (group I) characterised by routine symptoms like myalgia, fever, rigor, diarrhoea, urticaria, abdominal cramps. This starts appearing 3–6 weeks after primary infection and it lasts for 2–3 weeks. The disease takes its full peak form after 7 years of initial infection (range 7–10 years), of course deterioration of immune system starts after 3 years of infection. Neurological involvement is also common in the form of HIV encephalopathy, dementia, meningitis, primary CNS lymphoma, peripheral neuropathy.

Diagnosis: Laboratory detection of HIV infection is accomplished by number of diagnostic tests. Most widely used test for HIV antibody is ELISA (Enzyme linked immuno-sorbent-assay). Non-specific laboratory findings with HIV infection includes anaemia, leukopenia (particularly lymphopenia), thrombocytopenia, hypocholesterolemia, hypergammaglobulinaemia (see Table).

Epidemiology: The risk of sexual transmission varies with particular sexual practices, anal intercourse is the most risky.

The risk of sustaining HIV infection from a needle stick with infected blood is approximately 1 : 250.

The HIV virus has not been shown to be transmitted by respiratory droplet spread, by vectors (mosquito) or by casual non-sexual contact.

Intravenous drug use and heterosexual contact with an infected partner are the two major risk factors for women who are at risk for gynaecological complications including candidal vaginitis, pelvic inflammatory disease and cervical dysplasia. With the rapid increase of HIV infection among women, there has been a corresponding rise in the number of perinatally infected children. The reason for greater risk for transmission with heterosexual intercourse in Africa and Asia than in United States may relate to cofactors like general health, presence of genital ulcers and number of sexual partners.

LABORATORY FINDINGS WITH HIV INFECTION

Test	Significance
1. ELISA	Screening test for HIV infection. Sensitivity 99.5 per cent.
2. Western blot	Confirmatory test for HIV. Specificity 99.9 per cent when combined with Elisa.
3. CBC	Anaemia, neutropenia, thrombocytopenia. Common with HIV infection
4. Absolute CD^4 lymphocyte count	Most widely used predictor of HIV progression
5. CD^4 lymphocyte percentage	It is more reliable than count
6. β_2 - Microglobulin	Not useful for intravenous drug users.
7. P^{24} antigen	Indicates active HIV replication

A-OR HYPOGAMMAGLOBULINAEMIA

(Deficiency of gamma globulin fraction of plasma proteins)

It is congenital, familial and sexlinked, present only in males. Symptoms are due to sexlinked recessive gene. The main events are inability to synthesise gamma globulin antibodies, atrophy of lymphoid tissue, failure of plasma and lymphoid cell differentiation, leading to absolute lymphopenia or generalised lymphocytic hypoplasia or thymus alymphoplasia.

HYPERGAMMAGLOBULINAEMIA

Gamma globulins are present more than their normal level, e.g. collagen or connective tissue disease, chronic liver diseases like cirrhosis, chronic granulomas etc.

THYMUS GLAND AND IMMUNITY

It plays a major role in early life in maintaining immunological integrity of the body because of acting as a main leading supplier of small lymphocytes which at the time of birth are seeded to spleen and lymph nodes which are their sites of multiplication and in this way develop immunological competence in full. In case of its removal in early foetal life the immune system fails to develop and also its removal shortly before or first few days after birth greatly impairs immune system. A hormone (thymic hormone) has been demonstrated which releases from this gland, diffuses throughout the body and activate growth of lymphoid tissue. This gland is said to play a leading role in immunologic tolerance in the way that on formation of early lymphocytes at rapid rate, innumerable lympho and plasmablasts seed the lymphoid tissues and each type of such cell is capable for immune reactions while some of these cells are capable of creating immunity against body's own proteins but such cells are rapidly bound with body's own proteins and are either destroyed or inactivated before they seed the lymphoid tissues. To sum up (1) It is a major site of lymphopoiesis in embryo as well in newborn, (2) It produces a hormone immunotropic in action. *On the whole 'In natal and early postnatal life it is main leading organ of immunologically competent cells.*

AUTOIMMUNITY

It literary means—protection against self; while actually it may be classed as 'injury to self' —so is criticised. Hence, it is a condition in which structural or functional damage is produced by the action of immunologically competent cells, or antibodies against normal components of the body.

Historical Background

- Metalnikoff (1900): noted that guinea pigs when injected with their own spermatozoa produced sperm immobilising antibodies.
- Ehrlich (1901): noted the production of antibodies against erythrocytes from other goats.
- Landsteiner (1904): Identified circulating auto-antibodies in paroxysmal cold haemoglobinurea.
- Dameshek (1938): Establishment of autoimmune basis of acute haemolytic anaemia.

Autoimmune Diseases: Characteristics

- Elevated level of immunoglobulins

- Autoantibodies can be demonstrable.
- At the site of lesion, there occurs accumulation of plasma cells and lymphocytes.
- Benefit occurs from steroid therapy (immunosuppression).
- Genetic predisposition of disease
- More than one autoimmune lesion occurs in one individual.

Autoimmune Diseases

A. *Haemolytic:* Haemolytic anaemias, thrombocytopenia, leucopenia,
B. *Organ specific/localised:* Graves' diseases and Hashimoto's diseases of thyroid gland, Addison's disease, orchitis, myasthenia-gravis, eye diseases, pernicious anaemia, Guillain-Barre syndrome.
C. *Systemic diseases:* (Non-organ specific), systemic lupus erythematosus, rheumatoid arthritis, polyarteritis nodosa, Sjögren's syndrome.

Pathophysiology, Autoimmunity

- Autoantibodies are easily detectable than cellular auto-sensitisation.
- Autoantibody formation may be a result of tissue injury and antibody may help in promoting immune elimination of damaged cell.
- Antibodies may cause damage by cytotoxic/cytolytic and toxic complex reaction (type 3)
- T lymphocytes when sensitised cause such reaction.

Once initiated this remains a continuous process until it is suppressed by immunosuppressive therapy.

Autoimmunity Mechanism

- Hidden antigens may not be recognised by body when they are released in circulation; immune process is induced.
- Cells may undergo antigenic alterations by any stimulus like physical/chemical/biological etc.
- Gross reacting foreign antigens may induce such immune response.
- T and B cell defect may lead to such reactions.

AUTOIMMUNE REACTIONS

Story is similar to famous proverb, 'Is Ghar ko aag lug gayi, ghar ke chirag se, or Ghar ka bhedi lanka dhaye. More clearly further we may sum up this process as, 'physiological remoteness and special nature of metabolism are the main preceding factors which prevent the standard blood levels of these body's own proteins which in future become strangers for body's immune system terminating into fatal results. For autoimmune reactions, (i) Circulating antibodies should be present in patient's serum, (ii) antigen should be known. The diseases under this heading are falling into following groups (i) Organ specific (The particular organ is attacked by inflammatory antibody leading to destruction of epithelial tissues, e.g. haemolytic anemias, Hashimoto's diseases of thyroid, Addison's disease, toxic adrenal atrophy etc.), (ii) Non-organ specific (many organs are involved with wide spectrum of autoantibodies and antigens circulate in body in excess, e.g. collagen diseases, rheumatic diseases etc.) so to conclude with, 'body can develop immunity against some of its own tissues, and this may be due to either escaping of body's own antigenic substance, or similarity in structure of body protein and antigen or due to exposure of body to certain haptens etc.

IMMUNOLOGICAL TOLERANCE

As above mentioned case of autoimmunity if we continue the story we can imagine that spoiling effects can occur due to this reaction and terminate even in death, but sometimes body's immune system learns to recognise the own antigenic substance and it does not form antibodies against its own protein but certainly remain capable against foreign material. This is immunological tolerance and certainly it appears quite theoretical or hypothetical. But unfortunately sometimes this tolerance is seen with foreign material if it is injected or entering in very large quantity, (which is capable to destroy all antibodies as well as lympho and plasmablast before their proliferation) or by injecting small quantities of antigen for fairly long time (since amount is too less to trigger immune system).

MONOCLONAL ANTIBODIES

Are artificially produced antibodies, designed to neutralise a specific protein (foreign) called antigen. Cloned cells (genetically identical) are stimulated to produce antibodies to target antigen. They are of multiple uses like to destroy cancer cells directly, they carry other drugs to combat cancer cells.

TRANSPLANTATION: TISSUE REJECTION

1. Any foreign cell transplanted into a recepient can cause immune responses and immune reactions. Though different antigens of RBC cause transfusion reactions but many more other cells are also found in the body which may lead to such type of reactions.
2. - *Isograft:* is a transplant of a tissue or whole organ from one identical twin to another.

- *Allograft:* Is a transplant from one human being to another; or from one animal to another animal of the same species.
- *Xenograft:* is a transplant from a lower animal to a human being; or from an animal of one species to one of another species.

Tissue Typing: HLA Antigen

It is the most common antigen for causing graft rejection.

- These are of three types:
  - —Class I: Present on surface of all body cells so mainly responsible for graft rejection. This is a group of about 150 different antigens located on cell membrane surface of all body cells. They are coded only for six separate genes, three on each chromosome of a pair. Genes are allelomorphic and can code for only six different HLA antigens in one man.
  - —Class II: Present specifically on surface of lymphocytic cells which is linked with immunity.
  - —Class III: Is concerned with formation of complement etc. required for immunity.
- They occur in WBC as well as in other cells.
- Some of HLA antigens are not severely antigenic.

Prevention of Graft Rejection

- Glucocorticoid hormones: They suppress the growth of all lymphoid tissue, thus decreasing the formation of antibodies and T cells.
- Lymphotoxic drugs: They block the formation of antibodies and T cells—(e.g. Azathioprine).
- Cyclosporin inhibitory effect on helper T cells, so T cell rejection reaction is blocked. Other immune processes are not blocked, so is most valuable drug.
- The incidence of cancer is common in a immunosuppressed person since this immune system is capable of destroying cancer cells before they start proliferation.

SUMMARY AND HIGHLIGHTS

- The ability of human body to resist almost all types of micro-organisms (infection) which can be harmful to body, is immunity. Phagocytosis, gastric HCl, resistant skin, lysozyme, complement, natural killer lymphocytes are gifts to human body by nature which constitute so called 'innate immunity.'
- Antigens are substances invading the body. They are protein in nature with a molecular weight 8,000 or more than this. They may be polysaccharides also—Antibodies are immunoglobulin (gamma globulin) of various types like IgG, IgM, IgA, etc. which are formed on invasion by antigen.
- Agglutination, lysis, neutralisation, precipitation are different ways by which antibodies inactivate antigen, or invading organism (including phagocytosis, opsonisation).
- The complement is a collective term to describe a system of 11 proteins (CI-C9; B; D) which acts like a cascade-means after activation, it binds CI proenzyme which activates other proteins. So a very small beginning causes a large amplified reactions.
- Acquired immunity is the product of body's lymphocytic system. Those lymphocytes that are eventually destined to form activated lymphocytes first migrate to and are pre-processed in thymus gland, are T lymphocytes are responsible for cell mediated immunity.
- The other population of lymphocyte—that are destined to form antibodies—are pre-processed in liver (mid foetal life), bone marrow (late foetal life). This population was first discovered in bursa of Fabricius—a structure not found in mammals, so called B-lymphocytes.
- T lymphocytes are categorised into helper, cytotoxic and suppressor T cells. Helper cells are numerous, they help in functions of immune system. This is achieved by forming a series of protein mediators called 'lymphokines and they are Interleukin-2 to 6, Interferon γ, granulocyte monocyte colony stimulating factors (G-CSF, M-CSF). Interleukin and helper T cells stimulate each other by positive feedback mechanism (vicious cycle). The HIV of AIDS destroy these T cells. These cells activate macrophages to cause more efficient phagocytosis. They also slow down migration of macrophages after they have been chemotactically attracted into the inflamed tissue area.
- Cytotoxic (killer) cells secrete hole forming protein that literally punch large round holes in the membrane of attacked cell. Then this cell releases cytotoxic substances directly into attacked cell. So the antigen gradually is swollen and dissolves shortly. Then it wanders for another cell. It is specially lethal to tissue cells that have been invaded by viruses.
- Suppressor T cells are capable of suppressing the functions of both above mentioned T cells and in this way they regulate the activities of other cells, so also called regulatory cells.
- Infusing antibodies, activated T cells called passive immunity which lasts only for 2 to 3 weeks.
- Injecting dead organisms (with antigenic power), attenuated, living organisms (not capable of causing disease) is called vaccination.

64 Inflammation

It is most common, most carefully studied and most important in changes that body undergoes during any disease and in essence it is a defence reaction.

INTRODUCTION

It may be defined as reaction of body tissues towards any injury. Early reaction followed by repair constitutes acute and if irritant may persist for a longer time then chronic inflammation is constituted which is characterised by the development of lymphocytes and new collagen fibres. The cardinal signs of inflammation are redness, swelling, heat and pain.

VASCULAR PHENOMENON

- Due to sudden irritating effect of the irritant, first effect to be seen is contraction of the vessel owing to stimulatory effect of it. It is the vascular dilatation which comes next and capable enough of drawing attention of the scientists; this dilatation is most marked in arteries, then in veins and last in capillaries. This paralytic vascular dilatation is associated with acceleration of blood stream and thus increasing the blood supply of part which explains the above mentioned cardinal signs as heat and redness. It is worth mentioning here also that due to this vascular effect the empty capillaries are also filled with blood thus increasing the active capillary bed and hence creating increased vascularity of the part concerned or involved.
- Normally blood flows inside the blood vessel in the way that red and white cells flow in its central part (axial stream) while plasma is flowing near wall of vessel but quietly separated from it (plasmatic zone). As the part gets inflamed, the leucocytes come out of their routine site axial stream and occupy the plasmatic zone dragging themselves with some difficulty. This arrangement is named as pavementing of leukocytes since vascular wall is paved by them with the strange that there exists no admixture of erythrocytes. This pavementing pattern is finally terminating into their emigration which is through diapedesis property. As leucocyte migrates into extravascular space, a new basement membrane is constituted between them and endothelium, with disappearance of outermost layer of basement membrane. One more interesting fact here is that due to vascular dilatation stasis or stoppage of circulation also results, so called sludging of erythrocytes since red cells stick to one another. This escape is not only confined to leucocytes but plasma also escapes into the tissues thus it contributes to the swelling designated as 'inflammatory oedema', of course the amount depends upon nature and severity of the irritating substance.
- As mechanism of above mentioned vascular phenomenon is concerned many theories have been put forwarded. Few of them are presented here—(i) Liberation of histamine like H substance in tissue destruction or inflamed part, is responsible for setting the cycle of vascular phenomenon. (ii) The leucocytes are coming out of the vessel because they are drawn out by chemotaxis. Out of all, polymorphonuclear leucocytes are most affected by chemotaxis; if irritant is a parasitic one; these are the eosinophils affected much. Lymphocytes are less affected because of less cytoplasmic content within them.
- The electric potential theory explains the attraction and adherence to vessel lining of leucocytes. In health erythrocytes, platelets and lining endothelium carry negative charge so repelling each other exists (white cells are also negatively charged but of low potential). As inflammatory process is initiated due to some irritant the endothelium becomes positively charged so naturally white cells are first to be attracted.

TISSUE CHANGES AS A RESULT OF INFLAMMATION

(a) If irritant is intense the tissue changes are in form of degeneration and (b) if it is mild then it releases stimulatory effect resulting in proliferation. As far as degeneration is concerned it may further result into local death of part (necrosis); the commonest examples are fatty—degeneration, cloudy swelling and albuminous degeneration.

Suppuration: When neutrophils, macrophages destroy bacteria by engulfing them, many of them also dies. After few hours to few days a cavity is constituted in inflamed region consisting of dead neutrophils, macrophages and necrotic tissue and such a combination is designated as pus. So the pus is fluid product of suppuration, generally alkaline in reaction, yellow coloured and constituted by pus cells and pus serum, together with bacteria, tissue destruction debris. Pus serum is inflammatory lymph together with products of cellular disintegration. Since fibrinogen of plasma is destroyed by leucocytic enzyme so it cannot coagulate.

Inflammatory exudate: The various leucocytes which are migrated, the blood plasma (emigrated) and mobile cells, all of these three constituents are accumulated at site of injury, constitutes so-called inflammatory exudate.

Neutrophil leucocytes: These are active cells in this aspect. They are chief constituent of pus. They constitute first line of defence against pyogenic bacteria. A leucocyte promoting factor is said to be liberated from inflamed tissues which diffuse into blood and on reaching bone marrow it leads to discharge of white cells as well granulocytic hyperplasia and together with discharge this substance causes increased production of white cells from bone marrow and thus increasing their population so called 'neutrophilia.' This substance is said to be a pseudoglobulin. These cells really act like a loyal soldier in the way that even after death, a substance is liberated which because of its proteolytic activity dissolves the dead tissue and thus hastening the recovery process. Cellular outline is sharp with distinct nucleus is observed in fresh exudate but with the advancement of degeneration process. Outline turns indistinct with disappearance of the nucleus as well as granularity of cytoplasm.

Mast cells: Their active function is observed in acute inflammation, where they lose their granules and become unrecognisable. (Mast-meaning food; a German word, since they found in connective tissue which is the site where due to lymph stasis nutrition is increased). It is a well known fact that these cells produce heparin (acid mucopolysaccharides). Bulk of histamine is also said to be contained within them. Small quantity of serotonin (5-hydroxytriptamine) is also present here. In conditions like urticaria or mast cell tumours there is a great increase in their population.

Lymphocyte cell: Next to neutrophils, these are the lymphocytes which are mentioned as far as population is concerned. It is a predominant cell in late acute and chronic inflammatory states. This cell is chiefly concerned with antibody formation. Together with plasma cells it constitutes so called 'round cell infiltration.'

Macrophage: *"Macrophages reach out great arms in two or more directions and at their arm end, clear protoplasm exists without flung steamers that wave and search for whatever can be seized; or whole advancing margin of cell flows out and comes back like a wave sucking in any particle coming in the way."*

Actually these are mononucleated large cells active in chronic inflammatory condition. In conditions where individual macrophage appears to be unable to deal with attacking elements they unite together to form multinucleated giant cells.

Eosinophil leucocyte: These cells are appearing early in inflammatory exudate and may also disappear entirely from the blood and this astonishing disappearance is further replaced by their surprising reappearance in the inflammatory exudate. On breaking down histamine is released resulting into increased capillary permeability with outpouring of more antibodies for neutralisation of antigen.

Plasma cell: In chronic inflammation it is present in large number but is non-mobile one. These are again important source of globulin antibody. Hypersensitivity leads to increase in number of these cells as well as hypergammaglobulinaemia also results into increased population of these cells. This is the cell with eccentric nucleus with more plenty of cytoplasm. Size is larger than lymphocyte. Cytoplasm is intensely basophilic creating clear space on side of the nucleus facing centre of the cell. Around the nuclear periphery chromatin mass is collected.

Lymph of exudate: Lymph escaping from vessels is thinner and containing less proteins due to selective endothelial permeability. There is remarkable increase in lymphatic flow of inflamed part. It accumulates in tissue spaces leading to inflammatory oedema as described earlier.

Fibrinogen of the plasma passes out of capillaries along with the lymph, which is acted upon by thrombin (source is disintegrated polymorphonuclear leucocyte) resulting in fibrin production, which is in the form of fine threads interlacing with each other. Fibrin is important as far as healing process is concerned as well as it acts as barrier for spreading infection together with the fact that it helps in localisation of infection.

Complaints of Patient with Inflammation

- Heat and redness, the one of the cardinal signs of inflammation is due to increased blood supply of the part (hyperaemia). Swelling is due to accumulation of inflammatory exudate the chief constituent of which is the lymph.
- Polymorphonuclear leucocyte discharge endogenous pyrogenic substance. This substance as well as bacterial toxins (endo or exo) are collectively considered as culprit for symptom of fever. Pyrogenic substance reaches to blood through thoracic duct where it regulates thermoregulatory centres.
- A pain producing substance identical with bradykinin (a polypeptide) found in plasma and present in inflammatory exudate. This as well as tension with pressure on nerve endings contribute for the symptom pain.
- Leucocytosis is chiefly due to release of a factor Leucocytosis promoting factor.

Types of Acute Inflammation

Serous inflammation	Serous exudate, e.g. pleurisy with effusion.
Fibrinous inflammation	Fibrin is chief element, e.g. dry pleurisy, diphtheria, pneumonia
Purulent inflammation	Suppuration
Catarrhal inflammation	Mild inflammation of mucous membrane
Membranous inflammation	Mucous membranous cells destroyed with the addition that false membrane is constituted by binding the entire necrotic layer with fibrin.
Allergic inflammation	If one is sensitised to bacteria by some previous inoculation, a repeated or subsequent injection of same organism will lead to local reaction with inflammatory changes which are extreme than previous one. Due to antigen antibody union within cells, tendency to necrosis and destruction together with large amount of exudate is characteristic one. Leucocyte as well as macrophage show high phagocytic activity.
Chronic Inflammation	Here the irritant is of low grade intensity and disease process does not run acute course. Lymphocyte, plasma cells and macrophages are characteristic cells of this type. At the periphery of lesion fibroblastic reactions are going on while in the centre polymorphonuclear cells are evident. Proliferating cells are fibroblasts. It is usually a sequel of acute stage. In fact acute and chronic are the two arbitrary terms. Fibrosis is more marked here so newly formed fibrous tissue will contract as it grows older and this is the cause of hardening as well shrinking of affected organ.

SUMMARY AND HIGHLIGHTS

a. Certainly inflammatory process is nothing but changes in tissues towards any injury. These changes appear in two forms, one cellular and other is chemical, and out of it cellular action is the leader commanding the action. The event stressing the minds of scientists is selectivity of antibacterial power of white cells; e.g. when staphylococci infect the body they liberate highly lethal toxins and as a result inflammatory process rapidly develops and with more intensity than these bacteria themselves multiply. On the contrary 'streptococci' don't liberate such high lethal toxin so inflammatory walling off process also comes slowly in action and so these bacteria develop or multiply continuously and hence they are more harmful than staphylococci since they do more destruction.

b. Phagocytosis is generally accompanied by increase in both intra- and extracellular acidity which itself can cause bacterial destruction. Energy for phagocytosis is coming from glycogen which through glycolytic fermentation yields lactic acid.
c. As far as metabolic reactions towards injury are concerned first of all immediate elevation of blood glucose occurs which naturally decreases level of glycogen in skeletal muscle and increases lactal and pyruvate level together with release of epinephrine and norepinephrine from adrenal medulla. This results further into increased blood amino nitrogen level through either decreased deamination in liver or due to loss of amino acids from muscle, all these lead to general blockage of carbohydrate breakdown and hence reduced output of energy. This also causes vasoconstriction to all these organs essential to life and all above mentioned changes lead to state of shock. After this, phase of recovery ensues characterised by excretion of urea nitrogen, sulphur and phosphorus.

BIBLIOGRAPHY

1. Galli SJ. New concepts about mast cell. New Eng J Med 1993;328:257.
2. Malech HL, Gallin JH. Neutrophils in human diseases. New Eng J Med 1987;317:687-94.
3. Metcalf D. Control of granulocyte and macrophages: molecular and clinical aspects. Science 1991;254:529.

65 Blood Groups

It is a fact that erythrocytes of an individual may be clumped when they are mixed with blood of others and lethal or dangerous situation may arise if transfusion is made. He was Karl Landsteiner in 1900 who told that all persons can be divided into four groups as regards the reaction of serum of one on red cells of another, and it comprises four groups namely A, B, AB and O (classical ABO system).

ABO SYSTEM

a. The red cells of all human beings can be grouped according to the presence or absence of two blood group substances called A and B. They are also called antigens or agglutinogens because they can stimulate antibody formation and there are naturally occurring antibodies to them (agglutinins).

b. It is evident that if an agglutinogen is present in erythrocytes of a person, corresponding agglutinin must be absent from plasma. If it does not hold true, agglutination of red cells can make circulation impossible (Landsteiner's Law).

c. *Agglutinogens:* Primarily there are two agglutinogens A and B. Group A is further subdivided into A_1 and A_2 and so also AB like A_1B and A_2B. They start appearing in sixth week of foetal life and their adult level is reached at the time of puberty. Besides erythrocytes; the other sites where they may be found are salivary glands, pancreas, lungs, liver and testes etc. They are protein mucopolysaccharides in nature chemically.

ABO Groups

Agglutinogens	*Agglutinins*	*Group*
A	β	A
B	α	B
Both A and B	None	AB
O	Both α and β	O

d. *Agglutinins:* There are two corresponding agglutinins alpha (α) and beta (β) present in plasma or serum, also called anti A and anti B respectively. Specific agglutinin starts appearing from round about tenth day after birth and their climax is seen in tenth year of life. Besides plasma, they can be detected in milk, lymph, exudates and transudates (body fluids rich in proteins) but not found in urine and CSF.

e. *Determination of blood group:* Take a clean glass slide and with glass marking pencil divide into two halves A and B. Put a drop of blood to be tested on each side.

Determination

Clumping	*Group*	*Comments*
A compartment	A	Agglutinin β and A agglutinogen
B compartment	B	α agglutinin and B agglutinogen
Both compartments	AB	None agglutinin and both agglutinogen
No clumping	O	Both agglutinins without agglutinogen.

Then add a drop of antisera A in A compartment and antisera B in B compartment. Mix the contents with separate glass rods. Observe for clumping by nacked eye or microscope.

f. *Universal donor and recipients:* When subjects belonging to either A, B or AB group are transfused with blood of group O, very little or no reaction occurs to the recipient in spite of the fact that it contains both agglutinins because they are diluted to such an extent as to exert no effect. So persons with group 'O' are called 'universal donors' since group 'O' person can give blood to anybody but can take from his own 'O' group.

Similarly persons with group AB are universal recipients because any blood may be transfused into them without ill effects as no reacting agglutinins are present.

Rh SYSTEM

i. After forty years of blood group discovery, Landsteiner observed that injection of red cells of Rhesus monkey into rabbits evoked the production of an agglutinin to these cells which would also agglutinate human erythrocytes almost in 85 per cent of white persons. This gave an idea of new factor called Rh system. These persons are called Rh positive because their red cells contain Rh agglutinogen and their serum naturally contains no corresponding agglutinin. The remaining 15 per cent are Rh negative, their serum also contains no agglutinin until they are transfused with Rh positive blood.

ii. There are three pairs (or six) agglutinogens Cc, Dd, Ee, C, D and E are Mendelian dominants while c d e are recessives. Common is D since C and E are rarely found.

Groups containing dominant agglutinogen D is Rh positive and recessive agglutinogen is Rh negative. Rh agglutinogen (mainly D) are strongly antigenic, i.e. they are capable of producing antibody and corresponding antibody is anti-D.

BLOOD GROUPS AND GENETICS

i. The various agglutinogens present in the members of one species are called 'iso agglutinogens and its presence in an individual is a hereditary character and is also attributed to the presence of a corresponding gene in one or both of paired chromosomes.

ii. Position of a gene on chromosome is called locus. A number of similar genes form an alternative allelic group. A particular locus on the chromosome can be occupied by any one amongst the group or alleles. Each of the paired chromosomes possesses a corresponding locus for genes amongst alleles. One is said homozygous in respect of his genetic character, if two genes in the two equivalent loci are of the same type. Description of his genes (genotype) and description of his blood or body character (phenotype) are exactly the same. An individual is said to be heterozygous if the two equivalent loci on the paired chromosomes are occupied by two different genes among alleles.

Genotyping groups

Blood group	*Genotype*
A	AA or AO
B	BB or BO
AB	AB
O	OO

IMPORTANCE

i. For blood transfusion purpose.
ii. They are studied for anthropogeny which means the study of origin and development of man as in racial distinction.
iii. Paternity test
iv. Study of human genetics
v. Association of blood group with various diseases.

Patients with carcinoma of stomach are more likely to belong to group A, while those with peptic ulcer are more likely to belong to Group O. The blood group substances are mucopolysaccharides which is present in larger amounts in group O persons than others. The mucopolysaccharides are present in much larger amounts in salivary and gastric secretion than in erythrocytes where they are antigens. It may be that mucopolysaccharides influence resistance to an exogenous ulcerogenic or carcinogenic factor, with group A protecting against ulcerogenic factor and group O protecting against carcinogenic factor. With group A the incidence of pernicious anaemia and diabetes mellitus are more than others.

Disputed paternity—MN grouping

Child group	*Parent's contributory group*	*Mother's group*	*Group absent in father*
M	M + M		N
N	N + N		M
MN	M + N	N	N
MN	M + N	M	M

BLOOD TRANSFUSION

Just like other medical devices viz. Antibiotics, anaesthetics, tranquillisers, immunisation, plastic surgery etc. blood transfusion is also a boon to the society or mankind but as good things are always criticised, transfusion is also abused.

Taking blood from a person and injecting into vein of another person constitutes what is known as transfusion. The person who gives the blood is donor and man who receives called recipient.

Indications

Whole blood transfusion should be ordered by medical authority:

a. To restore blood volume after acute haemorrhage or shock, and
b. To maintain the blood haemoglobin level upto normal level when anaemia is not treated by any measure.

c. To make haemophilic patients, non-haemophilic (through plasma transfusion)
d. To check antigen—antibody reaction by supplying complement to recipient through fresh plasma infusion.

Transfusion Reactions

According to famous saying, *'blood transfusion should be ordered when it is really essential,'* since:

a. Recipient may develop fever (pyrexia) of course, without destruction of erythrocytes. This reaction may be due to presence of certain proteins in donor's plasma to which recipient is allergic, and those are here acting as pyrogens;
b. Allergic manifestations may also occur in recipient sometimes because, foodstuff which donor has taken may be allergic to recipient's body and these allergens are quite notorious for such manifestations;
c. Every pint of transfused blood is said to contain approximately 200–250 mg of iron into body and this amount in excess is certainly not able to escape, constituting what is called 'haemosiderosis' involving vital organs like liver, spleen, kidney, heart, adrenals, pancreas and bone marrow, etc. Certainly, this state ensues when repeated transfusions are given;
d. Recipient may develop low blood calcium tetany since blood for transfusion is stored with citrate salts (anticoagulant) and this blood will combine with calcium ions making them non-ionizable. This tetany can even cause respiratory muscle spasm terminating in fatal results.
e. Occasional transmission of hepatitis or other bacterial/viral infection and now-a-days AIDS may also ensue.

Hazards of Mismatched Transfusion

i. *Certainly the thing which is beneficial at one place is injurious too at another site and so is true with blood transfusion.* If mismatched transfusion is given clumps of agglutinated red cells occur which blocks the capillaries resulting in haemolysis liberating haemoglobin into circulatory system. When mismatched transfusion is given, agglutination occurs by following mechanism—with mismatched transfusion, agglutinins are attached to erythrocytes and since these agglutinins are bivalent they can attach with two erythrocytes in one time and in this way many cells adhere with each other causing cells to clump and plug blood vessels throughout the circulatory system and after some time reticulo-endothelial cells destroy these cells terminating into so called haemolysis. Together with this sometimes 'anti A or anti B hemolysins' also develop in plasma which are notorious to cause haemolysis instead of clumping.
ii. The haemoglobin so released combines with a protein named haptoglobin still circulating without creating any harm upto approximately 100 mg/100 c.c. of plasma. Beyond this limit this red pigment of the blood is digested by reticulo-endothelial cells and dissociated into bilirubin and when its concentration rises above normal level, it leads to Jaundice.
iii. The ultimate end result is acute kidney shut down which results due to the fact that this above mentioned excess haemoglobin precipitates in kidney glomeruli and tubules thus blocking them; together with reflex renal vasoconstriction resulting from some toxic substances coming from haemolysing blood owing to antigen-antibody reaction. All this story finally ends in oligurea-anurea and renal failure terminating into life-threatening events within approximately fortnight time.

Rh Factor and Transfusion

This story starts from the fact that if mother is Rh negative and father is Rh positive, child inherits Rh positive characters from father and mother develops anti-Rh agglutinins which diffuse to foetus causing red cell agglutination. Generally no or not significant harm is created in first pregnancy but second or consequent pregnancies may cause sensitisation by the first child. This sort of disease with which newborn infant is effected by agglutination and phagocytosis of red cells is termed as erythroblastosis-foetalis.

Since anti-Rh-antibodies circulate in baby's blood so erythrocytes are destroyed liberating more and more pigment haemoglobin which then is converted to bilirubin so newborn baby is anaemic as well as jaundiced (haemoglobin level falls to 5-8 gm%). To compensate, liver and spleen again become active in formation of red cells as they perform in middle foetal life and due to their activation many early forms (erythroblasts) are produced and hence seen in blood which justifies the name of disease (erythroblastosis-foetalis). Sometimes this severe anaemia affects the motor areas of the brain. Precipitation of bilirubin in neuronal cells (leading to permanent damage) leads to what is known as kernicterus.

One thing should be clear at this moment that if one child is erythroblastosis foetalis it is not certain that other children will also develop this state since anti-Rh-agglutinins develops only when foetus is Rh positive and many of Rh positive fathers may be heterozygous causing many children Rh negative. Second protection from the state comes, when there is long interval between two pregnancies in such states where mother is Rh negative and father is Rh positive.

Second disease here may be 'hydrops foetalis' where foetus is oedematous one which may either die in utero or born premature dying within few hours.

Remedy

i. Before switching over to blood transfusion ABO as well as Rh grouping should be tested to avoid sensitisation.
ii. No Rh negative woman should be transfused with Rh positive blood otherwise sensitisation may occur leading to formation of anti D terminating into fatal results.
iii. Treatment of transfusion reactions (before kidney shut down stage)
   - Rapid fluid administration (intravenous route—to cause water diuresis)
   - Diuretics may help to control renal vasoconstriction as well as for prevention of water re-absorption).
   - Since alkaline tubular fluid can dissolve more haemoglobin than acid so alkalinisation of body fluid is preferred.
iv. How to treat haemolytic diseases?

Exchange Transfusion

The Rh positive cells which were available for destruction are removed and the same quantity of blood is replaced by Rh negative blood. This process is completed by inserting a polythene catheter into inferior vena cavae (umbilical vein is the way).

Direct Cross-matching

This is matching of recipient's serum against the cells of donor. Donor's cells are diluted in normal saline to know presence of ABO agglutinin and anti D. A second suspension also made in 20 per cent albumin and is also tested against recipient's serum.

BLOOD BANK

- First blood bank opening in New York in 1940 under the supervision of Dr. Richard C. Drew (1904–50).
- Another concept was at Moscow in 1938 at Skilfosovsky institute, founded by Prof. Sergei Yudun.
- The term blood bank was coined by Bernard Fantus who set up a centralise storage depot for blood in 1937 at Cook Country hospital-Chicago-Illinois.

Blood Substitutes

Solutions which can be administered in place of blood to perform the same functions are classed as substitutes of blood. Some of them are:

1. *Plasma:* In liquid form it can be stored for months together and in solid form for years together. It is more useful in traumatic shock and burn states. By adding sterile water plasma is reconstituted for use. Plasma is certainly having agglutinins but at the time of transfusion no attention is paid on this point since their titre is reduced to harmless levels but on large infusion certainly it is better to remove agglutinins from it and such plasma is conditioned plasma from which agglutinins are removed, storage of pooled plasma at 30°C for six months destroys even virus causing hepatitis.
2. *Crystalloids:* Small molecules of salt or glucose pass freely through the capillary wall by exerting negligible osmotic effect, and so injected fluid is retained in circulation. Little harm may be created since the fluid as it leaks into tissues carries plasma protein with it. It is particular with saline.
3. *Dextran:* A polysaccharide of high molecular weight is used for expending the blood volume. They are not of animal origin and are of low antigenicity and toxicity.

Stored Blood and Transfusion

Blood banks are instituted where blood is stored at 4°C temperature. It is better preserved in the presence of glucose which in fact provide a substrate for metabolism and hence aids in survival of cell. For ideal storage of blood ACD mixture is introduced (acid-citrate glucose blood diluent containing 20 ml of 15 per cent glucose to which 420 ml of blood added). It should be remembered that stored blood is not suitable for platelet as well leucocyte transfusion since both of them disappear within few days of transfusion.

If there is no time for matching, O negative blood should be used for transfusion.

Qualities of Donor

A person who wants to donate blood must possess some qualities viz. (a) he should not be suffering from anaemia, (b) he should not be a patient of hypertension, (c) he should not have any infectious disease, (d) his body weight should be more than 45-50 kg.

Chemical Risks of Transfusion

Besides many risks of transfusion listed above, there are some chemical risks, always to be kept in mind by medical authority when he gives the order for it viz. (i) With impairment of renal function, alkalosis may result since citrates are oxidised to bicarbonates by tissue cells, (ii) A risk of hyperkalaemia is always there.

Changes in Stored Blood

(a) Cell sodium (Na^+) increases and potassium (K^+) decreases with net increase in cell total base and water, (b) So cell shape turns to spherocytic—one readily can undergo haemolysis, (c) Inorganic phosphate may rise while ATP decreases due to disturbed balance between phosphorylation and dephosphorylation.

Coombs' Test

In determination of sensitised cells in erythroblastosis foetalis lies the main significance of this test. Rabbit is immunised against human red cells, rabbit's serum taken in test tube and to it 2 drops of 2 per cent saline red cell suspension added; mixture then incubated at 37°C for half an hour. Then it is centrifuged for two minutes and tested for agglutination which if present is suggestive of agglutinogen in red cells.

So to conclude it is better to say, though it is a priceless gift to the society, but it may prove hazardous if mismatched so it is to be ordered when it is really required and given with full care and supervision by skilled hands.

AUTOTRANSFUSION (AUTOLOGOUS TRANSFUSION)

- Patient's own blood is taken when any elective surgery is planned. If needed, then, this blood is infused, during operation.
- In such technique there is no risk of mismatched transfusion, along with transmission of diseases like AIDS, hepatitis etc.
- Approximately 1000–1500 ml can be withdrawn over 3 week period.

SUMMARY AND HIGHLIGHTS

- Blood group is a game of antigen (agglutinogen)—antibody (agglutinin) reaction. Karl Landsteiner divided (year 1990) the persons into four groups A, B, AB, O. According to Landsteiner's law 'for a specific agglutinogen corresponding agglutinin must be absent from plasma, i.e. opposite agglutinin must be present. Persons with group O are universal donors, while with group AB are universal recipients.
- Rh (Rhesus) factor was discovered by the same scientist forty years later (1940) in Rhesus monkeys. It contains six agglutinogens (common D) but without agglutinins.
- Blood transfusion should be ordered when it is really essential. It should be done under strict supervision of the doctor. The usual dangers of transfusion are—allergy, fever, haemosiderosis, overloading of cardiovascular system, transmission of infectious disease, nausea, vomiting, restlessness, shock etc. The hazards of mismatched transfusion includes agglutination (clumping), jaundice, anaemia, acute renal—shut down—which is due to reflex vasoconstriction, toxic matters, cortical ischaemia etc.
- Before transfusion, blood grouping of donor and recipient should be tested and matched. No lady before menopause who is Rh negative should be given Rh positive blood. This can lead to erythroblastosis foetalis, hydrops foetalis. Direct cross-matching and exchange transfusion are the remedies.
- Solutions which can be administered in place of blood to perform the same functions are called blood substitutes. Plasma, crystalloids, dextran are used as blood substitutes. Plasma from which agglutinins are removed is called conditioned plasma.
- Alkalosis (due to oxidisation of citrates into bicarbonates), hyperkalaemia are major chemical risks of transfusion.
- Cellular sodium increases while potassium decreases in stored blood which may change the shape of cell to spherical—one which is liable to be haemolysed. In stored blood inorganic phosphate may rise with a decrease in ATP.
- Two genes one on each side of two paired chromosomes determine ABO blood groups. These two genes are allomorphic genes that can be any one of three different types O-A-B. The possible combinations are- OO, AA, BB, OA, OB, AB. These different combinations of genes are known as genotypes. Person with genotype OO produces no agglutinogen at all and so group is O, person with genotype AA or OA produces type A agglutinogen and has type A. Similarly genotype BB or OB give type B and genotype AB give type AB.

BIBLIOGRAPHY

1. Grignani F, et al. Genotypic-phenotypic and functional aspects of haematopoiesis New York, Raven Press. 1987.
2. Hubbell RC (Ed). Advances in blood transfusion. Am. Blood Comn. Arlington Va. 1979.
3. Mohn JF, et al (Ed). Human blood groups. Karger New York. 1977.
4. Race RR, Sanger R. Blood groups in man. 1968; 5th Ed. Blackwell Oxford.

The Platelets (Thrombocytes)

From an inert particle which was thought to be an artefact, platelet has emerged as the most remarkable structure which possesses abundant metabolic equipment, some synthetic capability, a capacity to expend considerable energy; like muscle, the ability to contract when appropriately activated—more than 80 enzymatic activities of great variety have been recognised in this astonishing cytoplasmic particle.

INTRODUCTION

Platelets in circulating blood are oval, or rounded, round or dot shaped non-nucleated structures. These are colourless cells of 2–4μ in diameter. They bear some characteristic properties like easily clumping, sticking to water wettable surface and easily disintegration.

FORMATION AND LIFESPAN

From fragments of cytoplasm which are detached from cytoplasm of large polypoid cells of bone marrow called *"Megakaryocytes."* After detachment they enter the general blood stream. On examination with electron microscope, it is found that much of cytoplasm of megakaryocyte is divided up by membranes into areas about same size of platelets. These are certainly infolding of cell membrane which first appear as strings of vesicles that become arranged along future cleavage planes when such membrane vesicles coalesce, two membranes are provided, one to cover the detached surface of platelet that is leaving and other to cover the surface of cytoplasm by the cell where detachment occurred.

As shown by radioactive tracers lifespan of platelet varies between 5-9 days or even 12 days, worn out cells are removed by spleen, liver, bone marrow and phagocytic cells.

Control of Platelet Production

The normal process of producing platelets involves the development of megakaryocyte through *four overlapping phases* namely formation of identifiable polyploid cells from morphologically unrecognisable mononuclear precursors, nuclear replication within each cell (endo-reduplication), cytoplasmic maturation and demarcation into platelet subunits and platelet release into circulation.

Thrombopoietic Effect: Relation to Erythropoietin

Although increased erythropoiesis may be associated with an elevated platelet count but no correlation has been found with (a) Thrombopoietic plasma activity, (b) Hypoxia, (c) Polycythaemia

Thrombopoietic Effect: Role of Spleen

Early workers suggested that spleen might control the platelet count either by splenic destruction of platelets or by suppression of thrombopoiesis through a humoral inhibitory effect, i.e. hypersplenism. It is said that spleen contains both stimulatory and inhibitory factors. It is now known that beneficial effect of splenectomy in idiopathic thrombocytopenic purpura is due to removal of a major site of platelet destruction and hypersplenic thrombocytopenia is caused by pooling of platelets in enlarged spleen.

Thrombopoietic Effects: Other Hormones

- Large doses of corticosteroids for prolonged periods have been associated with decreased platelet counts in some patients with idiopathic thrombocytopenia.
- Some aplastic patients with severe threatening thrombocytopenia may show a modest but critical rise in their platelet counts following pharmacological doses of androgens.
- Menstruating females show a cyclic reduction in platelet counts most pronounced at or just before onset of menses.
- Platelets is the most fundamental factor in haemostasis since it appears to participate in all the known mechanisms utilised by the body to control the loss of blood.

FINE STRUCTURE

In a stained blood film two parts may be recognised, chromatomere—coloured part and hyalomere clear part (hyalo = glass). Coloured is named because it is brightly coloured (red or violet or even blue violet) after staining with Romanovsky stain; coloured part may be broken up into small granules which tend to occupy more or less central position in cell. On the basis of chemical studies it is said that considerable quantity of metabolically active ATP is present in cell. They also take up and carry serotonin. Ribosomes in coloured area has also been reported. On the whole platelets are found to contain ATP, ADP, adrenaline, histamine, phospholipid (clot promoting), 5HT in their granules as well as cell membrane. These cells are also said to contain 'thrombosthenin an actinomyosine like contractile protein.

TOTAL NUMBER AND VARIATION

Their total population in normal healthy blood varies between 200,000 to 500,000 cells per cubic millimetre of the blood. Generally the rise and fall in number is as follows.

Increased Number (Thrombocytosis)

Acute haemorrhage, fractures, iron deficiency anaemia, polycythaemia vera, chronic granulocytic leukaemia, after splenectomy, malignancy, myeloproliferative syndromes, haemorrhagic, various carcinomas like lung ovary, GIT.

Decreased Number (Thrombocytopenia)

It may be primary and secondary.
Primary may be idiopathic.
Secondary is due to ... chemical or drugs (sulphonamides, quinidine, phenylbutazone, digitalis, meprobomate, phenobarbitone, salicylates, chlorthiazide, gold etc.)

- Chronic lymphocytic or granulocytic leukaemia
- Aplastic anaemia
- Hypersplenism
- Disseminated lupus erythematosus
- Bone marrow infiltration.

FUNCTIONS

i. Their well known role in blood coagulation cannot be forgotten. This task is achieved partly by their tendency to stick to rough surface and partly by liberating factor III (thromboplastin) a major factor essential for coagulation.
ii. They also constitute first line of defence against bleeding of larger vessels through their characteristic property of collecting in groups around bleeding site as well as their property to retract and consolidate the clot and thus plugging the bleeding site.
iii. Leaks in capillaries are being sealed by these cells again through their basic property of aggregation and thus they are capable to repair the damaged delicate endothelium.
iv. They are supposed to contain some substances identical with ABO antigens.
v. Clot Retraction:
   i. It was postulated that retraction is brought about by a platelet ferment or enzyme. Retractozyme was the name given to this enzyme and a disease thrombosthenia was postulated caused by hereditary deficient platelets.
   ii. Mechanical explanation (Frank, 1915): Little clumps of platelets anchored in knots of fibrin net underwent shrinkage and in that manner caused a retraction secondarily of whole clot.
   iii. Intact platelets become adherent to the fibrin strands and in turn become the locus from which new needles of fibrin radiate. In this process twisting, bending and shortening of the fibres occur and as a result the reticulum shrinks.
   iv. The high concentration of ATP in platelets and the presence of glycolytic cycle lead to the logic conclusion that retracting force derives its energy in a manner similar to muscle contraction and in this bivalent cation (calcium) is essential.
   v. The physiological importance of clot retraction remains subjudice. It may play an important role in the growth of an intravenous thrombus.
   vi. Clot retracting force is weak and can be masked by external factors, e.g.
      - Higher the concentration of fibrinogen - less the retraction
      - Cell volume hampers the retraction.
      - It is poor in polycythaemia.
      - In a collodion coated tube no retraction occurs because of strong adherence of fibrin to the collodion wall.

Sum up, haemostatic function of platelets depends on their three fundamental activities of adhesion, contraction and secretion. When vascular endothelium is damaged and sub-endothelial tissue—collagen is exposed, platelets adhere to the site initiating the formation of haemostatic plug. Contact of platelets with collagen is a stimulus in itself for it. On contraction there occurs platelet release reaction leading to secretion of active substances from platelet granules; one is serotonin (aid in constriction of small blood vessels) and another is adrenaline (furthers the process of aggregation) together with ADP (activating role). The initial plug is of a lose texture but it soon consolidates and haemostasis is complete some three minutes after the injury. A rather less dramatic function of platelets is in the repair of minor gaps in epithelial lining of blood vessels by contributing material to damaged endothelial cells which hastens their restoration.

DETERMINATION OF ABSOLUTE NUMBER

This type of counting is done with the use of a special diluting fluid called 'Rees-Ecker's fluid' containing various constituents as follows. Sodium citrate (3.8 gm%) acting as an anticoagulant as well as fixative, formalin (2 cc) acting as fungi-bactericidal agent as well as preservative, brilliant cresyl blue (0.05 mg) responsible for platelet staining, and distilled water to make 100 c.c. solution together with acting as vehicle. Blood to be tested is taken in RBC pipette upto 0.5 mark and filled with diluting fluid up to upper most mark 101. It is mixed by rubbing pipette in between palms for 2–5 minutes. Then after discarding one or two drops, chamber is charged with all routine precautions. The counting is done in all 25 small squares of chamber. Platelets are then identified as small dots. Since first two drops are discarded so 0.5 mark blood actually diluted 100 times (101 – 1 = 100) So total dilution comes to 200 times.

Total volume of RBC counting area
= Length × breadth × depth
= 1 × 1 × 1/10 = 1/10 cu mm.
Suppose number of platelets counted are = x
1/10 cu mm area contains = x no. of platelets
1 cu mm area will contain 10x no. of cells.

Since dilution factor is 200 times so total cells = 10x × 200 or 2000x cells per cubic mm.

"Since platelets are having characteristic property to stick to water wettable surface so rinsing of pipette with diluting fluid before sucking blood into it constitutes main precaution of this experiment."

NOTES

Platelet Metabolism

Like erythrocyte it is also not containing nucleus but mitochondria are present due to which these cells are indulged in protein synthesis, fat metabolism, gluconeogenesis. Anaerobic glycolysis and oxidative phosphorylation are metabolic pathways and their metabolic activity is very high.

Structure (Electron microscopy)

- These cells are 3 μm long and 1μm thick.
- There is a peripheral trilaminar membrane with a unique and functionally important outer coat which is involved in the process of aggregation.
- Under this membrane there are helical coiled bundles of microtubules which are involved in platelet contraction.
- In addition there is a system of channels by which it is probable that products of secretory granules reach the exterior.
- Granules embedded in the matrix contain hydrolytic enzymes are rich in phospholipids having substances like fibrinogen, thrombosthenin, serotonin, adrenaline and noradrenaline, ATP, ADP, mucopolysaccharides, all of which are active in both platelet aggregation and initiation of blood coagulation.
- In general, platelets contain three types of granules—a granules, dense and lysosomal granules which in inactivated platelet are distributed randomly but on activation they move towards the centre. ADP, ATP, Calcium and serotonin are found in dense granules; while alpha granules are divided into :
  — Plasma protein group and is further subdivided into two groups—firstly albumin and IgG which are taken up by platelets; and secondly—substances including VWF, factor V, fibrinogen etc.
  — Proteins absent from plasma until secreted by activated platelets—This group includes thrombospondin, platelet derived growth factor (DGF), platelet factor IV, transforming growth factor (TGFb).

SUMMARY AND HIGHLIGHTS

- These cells are small, granulated bodies - 2-4μ in diameter. The giant megakaryocytes of bone marrow form platelets by pinching of bits of cytoplasm and extruding them into the circulation. Their production is regulated by colony-stimulating factors that control the production of megakaryocyte. Splenectomy causes an increase in the platelet count (thrombocytosis). Half-life is 8-12 days.
- Injury to blood vessel → Platelets adhere to exposed collagen (platelet adhesion) → Initiation of platelet activation by ADP and thrombin → Activated platelets change their shape, put pseudopodia out, discharge their granules and stick to other platelets called platelet aggregation → This aggregation is stimulated by PAF (platelet—aggregation factor—a

cytokine produced by neutrophil-monocyte and platelet itself. Chemically it is either phospholipid whose receptor is coupled to G protein) → which activates phospholipase C → Which leads to release of granules from platelets → which increases cytoplasmic Ca^{2+} and due to this phospholipase A_2 is activated → which leads to release of arachidonic acid and → it is converted into thromboxane A_2 → which further causes Ca^{2+} influx which further causes more release of granules.

- They contain many important substances in their cytoplasm viz. (1) Actin-myosin molecule with another contractile protein - thrombosthenin, (2) Endoplasmic reticulum and Golgi apparatus synthesise and store calcium ions, (3) Mitochondria capable of synthesising ATP and ADP, (4) Enzyme system which synthesise prostaglandins, (5) Fibrin stabilising factor (Factor 13th of coagulation), (6) a growth factor promoting growth of fibroblasts, vascular smooth muscle cells; Their membrane is made up of lipid-protein-complex. They secrete thromboxane A_2 which promotes vasoconstriction.

BIBLIOGRAPHY

1. Brien JR. Platelet stickiness. Ann Rev Med 1966;17:275-90.
2. Cooper HA, et al. The platelet : membrane and surface reaction. Ann Rev Phy 1976;38:501.
3. Frojmovie MM, Milton JG. Human platelets—size shape and related functions in health and disease. Phy Rev 1982;62:185.
4. George JN, Shattil SJ. The clinical importance of acquired abnormalities of platelet function. New Eng J Med 1992;24:27.
5. Philips DR, et al. The platelet membrane glycoprotein IIb-IIIa complex. Blood 1988;71:831-43.
6. Ruoslahti E, MD Piersch Bacher. New perspectives in cell adhesion. RGD and Integrins. Science 1987;238:491-97.
7. Ruggen ZM; TS Zimmerman. VWF and von-Willebrand's disease. Blood 1987;70:895-904.
8. Siass W. Molecular mechanism of platelet activation. Phy Rev 1989;69:58.
9. Turritio VT, et al. Factor VIII/VWF in subendothelium mediates platelet adhesion. Blood 1985;65:823-31.
10. Wagner DD, Marder VJ. Biosynthesis of VW protein by human endothelial cells: Processing steps and their intracellular localisation. J Cell Bio 1984;99:2123-30.

Haemostasis and Blood Coagulation

> The spontaneous transformation of fluid blood to solid clot has something in the nature of conjuring trick. It is like a firesprinkler system, unnoticed as long as everything goes well but ready for any emergency at a moment's notice.

INTRODUCTION

The subject of coagulation is becoming more complicated every year. The essence of the problem which means the bare skeleton on which super structure is built remains more or less the same and can be squeezed into single paragraph as, "In the process of coagulation thromboplastin acts on prothrombin in the presence of calcium ions to form thrombin, which in turn causes fibrinogen to change into fibrin."

a. Prothrombin $\xrightarrow{\text{Ca Ions and Thromboplastin}}$ Thrombin

b. Thrombin + Fibrinogen → Fibrin (Clot)

Blood is a fluid inside an intact healthy circulatory system. If it is taken out and kept in a tube without adding anticoagulant it will lose its fluidity and will set into a semi-solid jelly which is called clotting. On further keeping it is found to be shrunk, squeezing out clear straw or ambour coloured fluid called serum which will no more clot.

No Clotting in Normal Vascular System: Why ?

This is a common question which can puzzle the scientific minds. Here are few explanations:-

- It is the smooth endothelium which prevents contact activation of intrinsic clotting system.
- Inner surface of endothelium has got negatively charged protein adsorbed to its surface, repels the platelets and coagulation factors.
- When due to any cause this endothelial wall is damaged then above factors are lost, bleeding exists and clotting mechanism ensues.
- Heparin, the famous anticoagulant produced regularly from its intrinsic sources prevents coagulation inside the body.
- Fibrin threads formed during coagulation process as well as antithrombin (an alpha globulin) are again important parameters in this aspect. More clearly, thrombin which is formed from prothrombin in the first step of clotting process, adsorb to fibrin threads as they develop; thus preventing spreading of thrombin into remaining blood and in this way excessive spread of clot is prevented. Furthermore, the thrombin's portion not combining with fibrin threads, unites with antithrombin and becomes inactivated for few minutes.
- Last but not least important is fact that blood is actively circulating inside the body and as a law of Nature the thing which is active does not stand still easily. Flowing blood does not allow platelets to clump and agglutinate.

Blood Clot

It consists of a mesh of very delicate fibrils among which red and white cells together with fragmented platelets are entangled like a network. Fibrils are constituted by fibrins formed by alteration and polymerization of fibrinogen molecules. The fibrin threads usually stick to damaged surface of blood vessels and in this way it prevents blood loss.

Serum

Within say 30–60 minutes roughly retraction of clot occurs leading to release of serum. Platelets are said to be necessary for clot retraction to occur. Firstly due to their sticking property they act like a chain to attach different fibrin threads together. Secondly platelets are rich in energy currency of body—ATP and this high energy bond causes increased folding of threads, leads to decreasing their length and finally expressing serum from it.

Clot : Vicious Cycle

Once a clot is formed it acts as its own stimulant meaning by a positive feedback mechanism exists. Thrombin has got proteolytic action so it acts on prothrombin itself to form more and more thrombin from it and more thrombin will create more clot as well as more prothrombin activator. So once a critical amount of thrombin is formed, vicious cycle develops causing still more thrombin to be formed so clot continues till its growth is arrested by any means.

Nomenclature and synonyms for clotting factors

Roman Numeral	*Descriptive name*	*Synonym*
I	Fibrinogen	
II	Prothrombin	
III	Tissue factor	Thromboplastin
IV	Calcium ions	
V	Proaccelerin	Labile factor, AcG.
VII	Proconvertin	Stable factor
VIII	AHF antihaemophilic factor	AHG
IX	PTC Plasma-thrombo-plastin-component	Christmas factor, antihaemophilic β
X	Stuart-Prower factor	
XI	PTA (Plasma-thrombo-plastin-antecedant)	Antihaemophilic C.
XII	Hageman factor	Glass factor
XIII	Fibrin stabilising factor	Laki-Lorand factor
HMW-K-	High molecule weight kininogen	Fitzgerald factor
Pre K	Pre Kallikrein	Fletcher factor
ka	Kallikrein	
PL	Platelet phospholipid	

Clotting Factors—A Review

Factor I: Fibrinogen: It exists in plasma at a level of 100–7000 mg per cent formed in liver so in many liver diseases its level may decrease. Owing to its large molecular size (molecular weight 3,40,000), it may leak into interstitial spaces and hence due to its presence interstitial fluid may coagulate though poorly. Similarly when capillary permeability is increased pathologically this may enter tissue space and can cause lymph clotting too. Two low molecular weight peptides are removed when it combines with thrombin forming 'fibrin manomer' (activated fibrin—synonym); then many such manomers polymerise into long fibrin threads forming reticulum of clot and this whole channel is enhanced by Ca ions, protein stabilising factor as well as stability and strength to these fibrin threads. It can be precipitated by addition of one third saturated ammonium sulphate or half saturated sodium chloride, mixing with one-ninth part of ether and one-twelfth part of ethanol at 0°C.

Factor II: Prothrombin: It is present in plasma with its concentration as 15 mg per 100 ml (range up to 35 mg%). It is continuously formed by liver and also continuously used by body in clotting process. Vitamin K is essential for its synthesis by liver so in lack of vitamin K or presence of any liver disease, its level in blood so decreased enough to cause bleeding. It is an alpha globulin with molecular weight as 68,000. It can resist heat (55°C) for several hours. It is soluble in water and saline at pH 4.9. Acidity below pH 3.5 and alkalinity above pH 11 can inactivate it. It has a very shorter life in plasma and dicumarol—an anti-coagulant depresses its level in plasma. It can be separated from plasma by twenty times diluting followed by acidification of solution to pH 5.2. Prothrombin first splits into prethrombin and autoprothrombin C : latter immediately acts on former to change into thrombin. Such type of intermediate compounds and many others prothrombin activators are needed for its conversion into thrombin together with calcium ions and their quantity depends upon degree of injury to blood vessels.

Factor III: Thromboplastin: This is badly needed for conversion of prothrombin to thrombin.

a. *Tissue thromboplastin or Extrinsic system:* This is present in tissues (like lung, brain, testes, blood vessels, placenta etc.) liberated at time of injury or damage. It is extremely potent substance leading to quick conversion. It is formed by action of factors VII, X, V and Ca ions on a phospholipid.
b. *Blood thromboplastin or Intrinsic system:* Here platelets are source and thus playing an integral role in this process. Only this lacks the initiation so it requires interaction with several other factors; two are same of above (Factor V and X) with four additional factors as VIII, IX, XI and XII factors. Time required for its activity is 4–8 minutes. Both of these are lipoprotein complexes. Platelet extract contain mostly lipoid factor while tissue extract contains whole lipoprotein complex. Phospholipid in both fractions is either cephalin or its alike substance.

Factor IV: Calcium Ions: It acts actually as a cofactor in process of coagulation at step of conversion of prothrombin to thrombin as well for thromboplastin generation. In normal human, blood calcium is present in sufficient amounts.

Factor V: Labile factor: Easily destroyed by slight heat. It is essential for generation of both types of thromboplastins. It is present in normal plasma but completely adsorbed in the clotting process so absent in serum. It is present in its inactive form, becoming active during clotting process, and activated product is called 'Accelerin' (Factor VI), hence separate existence of VI factor is not there.

Factor VII: Stable factor (Proconvertin, Noble factor, synonyms): It is a protein identical or linked with prothrombin produced by liver. Dicumarol depresses its activity and is also one of the essential factors for thromboplastin generation. It is present in its inactive form but converted to active state called convertin.

Factor VIII: Anti-haemophiliac globulin (AHF, AHG): Is a protein linked with fibrinogen and unstable in stored blood. Its deficiency leads to haemophilia. It is not found in serum since completely utilised during coagulation process. It is also said to be essential for production of thromboplastin.

Factor IX: Christmas factor: Its deficiency leads to Christmas disease. Its activity can be treated in serum since it is not completely used up during coagulation process. It is a protein.

Factor X: Stuart-Prower factor: It is protein in nature Dicumarol is said to depress its activity. It is present in both serum and plasma. It is needed for generation of thromboplastin.

Factor XI: PTA (Plasma-thromboplastin-Antecedant): It requires factor XII for its activation otherwise present inactive. It also stimulates platelet clumping. Activates Christmas factor.

Factor XII: Hageman's factor: Is having strong affinity for adherence with foreign surfaces, which further is responsible for platelet clumping. Its role is still doubtful in generation of thromboplastin. It activates factor XI.

Factor XIII: Fibrin stabilising factor: It assures a firm-stable clot. Thrombin and calcium ions are said to be its activator.

Anticoagulants: Study Survey

Substances of biological origin inhibiting coagulation are anticoagulants.

1. *Heparin*
   a. *Nature:* It is mucopolysaccharide (Mucoitin-polysulfuric acid)
   b. *Source:* Mast cells scattered throughout the body but are more abundant in liver (Hepar = liver) and lungs. These cells are found in abundance in tissues surrounding capillaries of liver and lungs for the simple reason that these sites receive many embolic clots formed in slow flowing venous blood and in these circumstances this can prevent further new growths. Brain, muscle, intestinal walls, spleen, heart, thymus may also contribute. Minute quantities of this anticoagulant is produced by basophilic leucocytes but in fact, the number or percentage of these leucocyte is so low (0-1% in DLC) that their contribution is said to be negligible one.
   c. *Mechanism of action:* It is said to exert its anti-coagulant action in following ways. By preventing formation of intrinsic prothrombin activator; Action of thrombin on fibrinogen is prevented; By increasing rapidity with which thrombin interacts with antithrombin thus helping in deactivation of thrombin; by increasing the amount of thrombin adsorbed by fibrin; it inhibits agglutination as well lysis of thrombocytes, it acts as an anticoagulant because of its strong electronegative (acidic) SO_4 group; Heparin cofactor which is present in plasma is needed for its full action; it is said to bind ACTH and depress aldosterone.
   d. *Antidote: Protamine sulphate:* (1-1.5 mg per 100 units of heparin) which is found in germinative cells of some fish is the antidote to check its overaction. This substance being electropositive easily binds heparin which is of opposite charge. Hexadimethidine bromide (Polybrene) is another anti-heparin substance in action.
   e. *Duration and Excretion:* Instant effect is noticed on intravenous administration since destroyed if given orally owing to its protein nature. Peak level is reached after 2 hours of administration and action diminishes after 4 hours 'One unit is the quantity of heparin which exerts anticoagulant action of one ml of cat's blood for 24 hours. Enzyme heparinase found in liver destroys it and is mainly excreted through kidney.

      Its sodium salt is used for clinical purposes and it is non-toxic. It is also of use in vascular surgery and blood transfusion.
2. *Dicumarol:* Like vitamin K it is also a naphthoquinone derivative and hence it acts through competitive antagonism to vitamin K. Further its anticoagulant action is due to its inhibitory action on liver to form prothrombin, Factor VII and IX, X. More clearly when it is given to any patient it combines with some of chemical compounds in liver which normally combine with vitamin K. So in its presence vitamin K cannot combine with

them and hence cannot promote prothrombin formation. When it is administered, level of plasma thrombin falls to almost 50 per cent at the end of 12 hours Administration of large quantities of vitamin K is used when dicumarol therapy is discontinued. Initially it is used in high doses as 1200 mg followed by maintenance dose of 150 mg.

3. *Hirudin:* A leech extract coming from its buccal glands. It possibly prevents union between thrombin and fibrinogen to exert its anticoagulant action.
4. *Phenindione:* Mechanism is same as of dicumarol, i.e. vitamin K antagonist by inhibiting synthesis of factor VII, IX, X by liver. It is vitamin K antagonist.
5. *Decalcifying agents:* Citrates and Oxalates (sodium, potassium) are famous anticoagulants used in laboratories. Citrate ion combines with calcium in blood to cause unionised calcium compound, the lack of which prevents coagulation.

   Citrates are having advantage over oxalates that they are non-toxic and few quantity can be even administered intravenously while oxalates are toxic for the body. Furthermore, within few minutes citrates are polymerised into glucose by and in liver which then metabolised in the same way. If liver of recipient is damaged or citrates (along with blood) are transfused too rapidly, more and more depression of ionic calcium ensues with resultant tetanic convulsion and death, this also due to the fact that citrates are not removed as glucose due to liver failure or diseased.

   Addition of concentrated solution of neutral salts viz. sodium sulphate (half saturated mixed in 1:1 proportion), magnesium sulphate (1 : 4 proportion, 27%), sodium chloride (1 : 1; 10%) can also prevent clotting. They inhibit platelet disintegration as well as by preventing reaction between thrombin and fibrinogen. Zinc sulphate (0.5%) is also compound of this series. Sodium thiosulphate and cellulose sulphate and dextran sulphate are also in this group and act as anticoagulant due to sulphate group.
6. *Snake Venoms* (Cobra, Malayan pit vipour) act as anticoagulant due to its antithromboplastin effect along with depletion of fibrinogen. 0.01 mg per kg body wt of cobra venom is sufficient to check coagulation completely.
7. *Others:*
   - Cysteine due to sulphur content.
   - Peptones through liberation of heparin from mast cells.
   - Dyes like chicago blue, tryptan blue prevent coagulation.
   - EDTA (ethylene-diamine-tetra-acetate) acts by binding ionic calcium.

Factors Stimulating Coagulation

- Temperature (warmth) approximately 5°C above normal is capable of stimulating coagulation.
- Contact with water wettable surface.
- Contact of blood with water wettable surface is potentiated by gentle agitation.
- All above mentioned haemostatic agents.

Factors Depressing Coagulation

- Cold—below 5–10°C.
- Preventing contact with water wettable surface is an important factor in this aspect. Use of siliconed vessels (or paraffin, wax) comes under this section.
- Addition of decalcifying agents is of again paramount importance due to removing ionising calcium.
- By diluting blood roughly 20 times to its volume.
- All anticoagulants discussed above.

Physiology of Clotting

Fairy tale: Haemostasis prevents blood loss. This target is achieved under following steps.

Whenever wall of blood vessel is ruptured or traumatised, the pain impulses from site of trauma as well as from surrounding nervous tissue originate and reach to spinal cord which passes order signals to traumatised vessel through sympathetic nerves to cause spasm of the vessel. Local muscle also contribute to this spasm meaning that this vascular spasm is both neuro- and myogenic one. As the vessel wall is damaged the action potential develops along the vessel wall resulting in vessel constriction. This vascular spasm lasts for almost half an hour and it is said to be directly proportional to intensity of trauma. This explains that sharply cut blood vessels usually bleeds much more than does the vessel ruptured by crushing. Its importance also lies in the fact that persons in whom legs are severed by crushing trauma, develop such an intensive spasm which stops any serious bleeding.

As a result of trauma, certainly vascular endothelium loses its smoothness and non-wettability which provides enough ground for platelets to accumulate at injury site to form platelet plug. The persons lacking enough platelets, develop many haemorrhagic areas under skin and internal tissues. Roughly after two to three minutes plug becomes an effective seal though little leakage may be there. Within a very short time platelets in the plug are so tightly drawn together that they appear to loose their individuality by becoming a cohesive mass better described as 'viscous metamorphosis.'

Clotting mechanisms	
Extrinsic pathway	*Intrinsic pathway*
1. It is explosive in nature with severe tissue trauma; clotting can occur in 15 seconds.	It is slower to proceed requiring usually 2–6 minutes to cause clotting.
2. Begins with trauma to the vascular wall or the tissue outside the blood vessel.	Begins in the blood itself.

Next to it within few seconds to 2–3 minutes the clotting mechanism starts; within 5–7 minutes clot fills the gap and within 30–60 minutes clot retraction occurs. Development of thromboplastin is taken as first step for the sake of convenience of description. This factor is essential for conversion of prothrombin into thrombin. Thromboplastin requires both lipid and protein constituents for full activity. Silicon started a new era in this aspect.

Using siliconed glasswares it is possible to show that blood contains all the factors for generation of thromboplastin; it requires only a change in surface contact to trigger the mechanism. In intrinsic clotting system factor V, VIII, IX, X, XI, XII are required; factor XII when activated by surface contact initiates the reaction and then in presence of calcium ions other proteins are activated. Substance called 'thromboplastin inhibitor is present in plasma which inhibits its activity. Many anticoagulants can also depress its activity.

Now comes 'prothrombin activation.' Calcium ions are needed for prothrombin conversion to thrombin and factor V increases the rate of conversion. Thromboplastin needs factor X for its full activity. Prothrombin activator is formed in response to rupture of vessel or damage to blood itself. This activator then catalyses conversion of prothrombin to thrombin. Due to this description clotting process falls into two categories:

a. *Extrinsic mechanism:* That causes clotting when blood vessel is damaged since broken vessel wall exudes a tissue extract responsible for coagulation, so it is that mechanism in which an extract from damaged tissue is mixed with blood. The clotting substance in a tissue extract initiating clotting mechanism is thromboplastin which is chiefly composed of lipoproteins containing one or more phospholipids mainly cephalin. It requires Factor V, VII, X and calcium ions for itself to be changed into prothrombin activator.

b. *Intrinsic mechanism:* Is that in which blood itself is traumatised, more clearly it is that mechanism which initiates clotting in that blood which is removed from the body and held in a container. If its walls are made non-wettable (as siliconized) clotting process may be delayed. Here platelets play a leading role by liberating factor III (thromboplastin) after their disintegration. Several other factors are also needed besides factor III specially V, VIII, IX, X, XI, XII. Factor XI, and XII after coming in contact with rough or wettable surface they interact to form contact activation product which then activate other factors.

Conversion of fibrinogen to fibrin is probably the last step and this target is achieved by thrombin which acts enzymatically since it is a proteolytic enzyme having same sequence of amino acid as enzyme trypsin and pepsin. Presence of some antithrombin has been claimed by many workers by which normal plasma can neutralise thrombin and it is said to be some alphaglobulin in nature. By its action thrombin is not destroyed but neutralised and it is said to be slow in action.

Once a clot is formed either it can be invaded by fibroblasts which subsequently forms connective tissue throughout clot or it can dissolute.

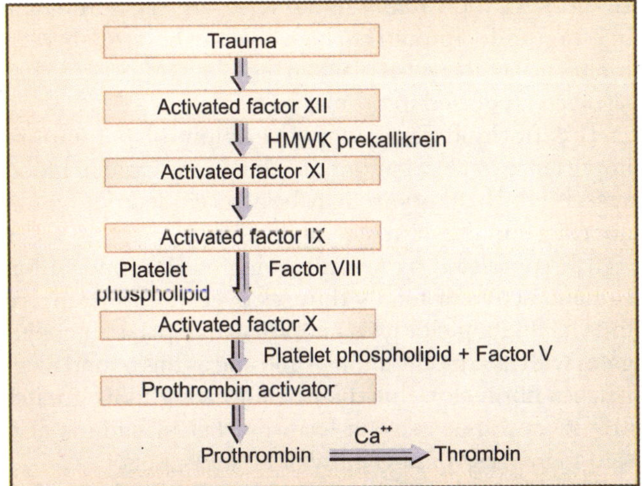

Schematic Diagram: Intrinsic pathway: Blood clotting

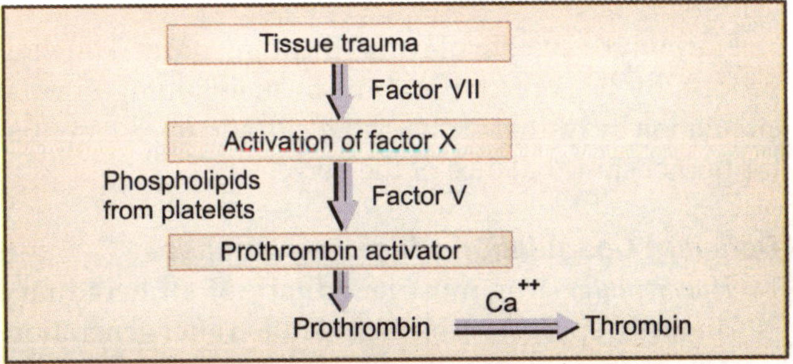

Schematic Diagram: Extrinsic pathway: Blood clotting

In effect, initiation of the extrinsic pathway for clotting secondarily activates the intrinsic pathway as well.

So it is to be told, 'clotting mechanism is a sequence of proenzyme enzyme transformation in which each enzyme activates the next until final substrate fibrinogen is involved.

Fibrinolysis : Fate of clot: As told earlier, once a clot is formed, it can be invaded by fibroblasts or it can dissolute: The plasma proteins are said to have a euglobin plasminogen or profibrinolysin which on activation changes itself to plasmin or fibrinolysin which is a proteolytic enzyme identical with trypsin of pancreatic juice and so it digests fibrin threads, fibrinogen, factor VIII, prothrombin, factor XII, V. So plasmin causes lysis of clot and other above mentioned clotting factors leading to hypocoagulability of blood. This as a whole is designated as fibrinolysis.

This main substance called plasminogen need activation because without proper activation it will not be changed into plasmin. An activator called urokinase found in urine is responsible for destruction of clot in urinary tract. Certain bacteria specially streptococci release an activator substance streptokinase so that in certain infection of streptococci, this activator dissolves clotted lymph and tissue fluids. Slight fibrinolytic activity is said to be increased with exercise, anoxia, adrenaline injection and serotonin but high levels of lipoproteins can inhibit it. Good level of plasmin inhibitor antiplasmin has also been reported in normal blood.

This fibrinolytic system is certainly of paramount importance in clearing minute clots from various blood vessels which otherwise may be all occluded if it would not exist and thus threatening the life.

It is completed by (a) Adsorbing of plasminogen on clot and activator totally diffuses over its entire surface thus facilitating clot lysis and, (b) active plasmin conjugates with its antidote antiplasmin and as this bound form reaches fibrin clot. It is dissociated owing to its greater affinity and thus causing lysis. Further plasmin is also said to increase permeability of blood vessels.

Blood from bodies after sudden death, blood after surgery, extensive burns show accelerated fibrinolytic activity.

Fibrinolytic system plays (a) In aiding normal healing process by lysis of clot and (b) In maintaining normal circulation by lysing intravascular clot and (c), Is essential for homeostatic balance of the body.

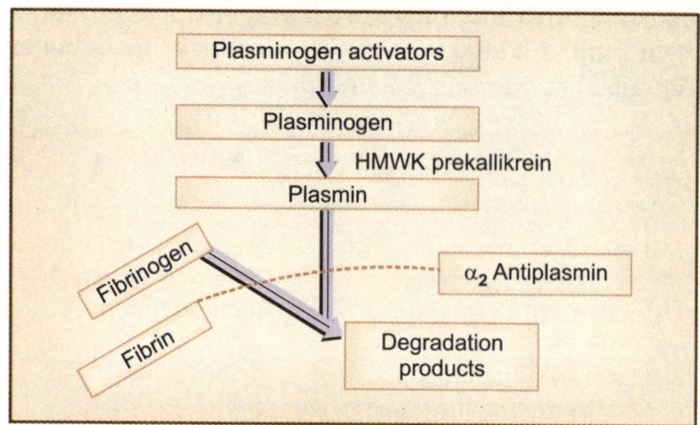

Fibrinolysis

Deficient Coagulation : Bleeding Diseases

1. *Haemophilia:* It is most hereditary of all hereditary diseases repeating itself in generation after generation. This disease originated like mutation in one of the parents of Queen Victoria. It is transmitted by females of the family and thus confined to males. A simple injury like tooth extraction or circumcision may lead to serious fatal haemorrhage or more better to say prolonged bleeding following a cut or trauma. Characteristic blood feature is prolonged clotting time but bleeding time is normal. The deficient factor VIII (AHF, AHG) is the primary cause of this disorder. Later on condition 'haemophilic joints' develop and main sufferer is elbow or knee joint and condition is identical with arthritis and in it haemorrhage into joints causes lack of absorption of blood which leads to proliferation of synovial membrane together with cartilage erosion. Females carrying the abnormal X chromosomes transmit disease to half their sons while remaining half daughters will be carrier. A haemophilic father is having normal sons but carrier daughters. The disease in not uncommon in domestic animals.
2. *Christmas disease:* Its more helpful name is haemophilia β. The lack of clotting factor PTC (plasma thromboplastin component) is said to be the causative factor. Thromboplastin generation test is single method of its detection.

GENETIC ASPECTS

Its gene is located on X-chromosome. Its gene is recessive, so it expresses itself only when it is paired. Is inherited as follows:-

Male ⓧy   *Female* xx

	ⓧ	y
x	xⓧ	x y
x	xⓧ	x y

Carrier daughter = two
Normal son = two

This carrier daughter is married to a normal man

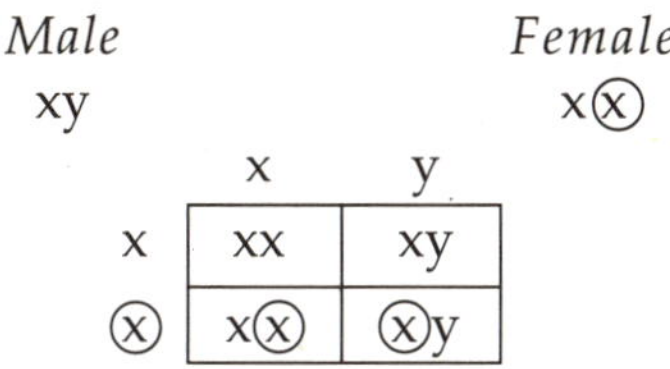

- one normal daughter
- one normal son
- one carrier daughter
- one diseased son
- Son gets disease from his mother and not from father.

3. *Afibrinogenemia:* Deficiency or absence of fibrinogen is the cause of this condition. In contrast to haemophilia there is no sex-incidences and the blood is incoagulable, not merely delayed as in haemophilia. Haemorrhagic diathesis from birth is the main characteristic feature. Of course existence of chronic arthritis may be a puzzling state. Fibrinogen may disappear in following prostate surgery, fibrinolysis process, abruptio-placenta, serious liver diseases etc.
4. *Hypoprothrombinemia:* Depression of blood prothrombin level is meant by it. Causative factor includes severe liver damage, malabsorption of vitamin K etc.
5. *Purpura:* It means haemorrhage into skin and mucous membrane specially nose, mouth, stomach, intestine, haemorrhage may be small or large. Bleeding time is prolonged while clotting time is normal. Thrombocytopenia is the striking change in blood but in severe cases platelets may even disappear. Splenectomy gives the best result. Leucocytosis and anaemia are other blood changes. Spleen moderately but liver is slightly enlarged together with redness or cyanosis of skin due to great vascular engorgement. Megakaryocytes are abundantly found in bone marrow but they fail to produce platelets due to arrest of maturation. This all includes thrombocytopenic purpura.

Thrombosis: Intravascular Clotting

Coagulation of blood within the blood vessel is thrombosis. Deposition of platelets occurs whenever there is any injury to blood vessel, constituting so called 'platelet plug.' On top of platelet nidus, fibrin threads are formed involving red and white cells which is called 'thrombus.' Portion of this thrombus which travels is called embolus, which may be lodged in lungs (pulmonary infarct), heart and cerebrum (cerebral and cardiac infarct).

Test employed

1. *Bleeding time:* This time is determined by getting a prick with all aseptic precaution either at finger tip or ear lobule. Drops of blood are wiped away every few (15 sec) seconds with filter paper. Cessation of bleeding is taken as end-point. Normally it ranges from 1–3 minutes. It is normal in haemophilia but prolonged in purpura.
2. *Clotting time (CT):* It is the time taken by shed blood to clot. Normally it is 3–8 minutes (average 5 minutes) and increased in haemophilia. After getting a prick with all aseptic precaution blood is filled in a capillary tube. After every few seconds, corner of capillary is broken till clot formation is there which is taken as end-point.
3. *Clot Retraction time:* With the help of a clean dry syringe almost 5 ml of blood is withdrawn in a clean dry sterile tube. It is then incubated at 37°C. Degree of retraction is recorded after 1, 18, 24 and 48 hours. Any discolouration or disappearance of clot is noted. Clot retraction appears almost within six hours and complete in 24 hours. It is normal in haemophilia but affected in thrombocytopenic purpura.
4. *Prothrombin time (Quickís one stage prothrombin time)*: When there is 20 per cent fall in normal prothrombin concentration bleeding ensues. This period is prolonged in deficiency of factor V, VII and X. Using a siliconed glass syringe approximately 4.5 ml of blood is drawn by using all aseptic precaution. It is then mixed with sodium citrate (0.5 ml of 3.8%) which is contained in another test tube. It is then centrifuged at 3000 r.p.m. for 15 minutes. 0.1 ml. of this citrated blood is put in a test tube in a water bath at 37°C and to it 0.1 ml of thromboplastic material (prepared from rabbit's brain) and 0.1 ml of 0.025 M solution of calcium chloride is added. The time from calcium chloride addition till onset of clotting is noted. Normal prothrombin time is 15–19 seconds.

Thromboplastin Generation Test

Fresh plasma containing factors V and VIII after removing other factors from it, serum containing factors VII, IX, and X after destructing other factors by incubating at 37°C and platelet extract for providing phospholipid component; all these three fractions are mixed and incubated at 37°C together with calcium ions. This will generate thromboplastin activity which will be tested at 1 minute interval. A thromboplastin generation curve can be obtained by plotting clotting times of substrates against amount of thromboplastin activity of samples.

This test is suggestive of haemophilia, Christmas disease diagnosis.

Partial thromboplastin generation test is simpler in comparison to above test. In it cephalin (phospholipid) is used instead of acetone treated brain for thromboplastin. It is also helpful in diagnosis of haemophilia. Kaolin is to be added to plasma for providing maximum activation of surface contact factors.

Even then it is said that, "No field of physiology is more complex or has been so confused by contradictory results, diversity of opinion, differences of interpretation as that of blood coagulation.

NOTES

a. Prothrombin:

i. Three distinct thrombin precursors have been obtained in laboratory. First one is Prothrombin which contains the precursor of thrombin and auto C; second one is DEAE—Prothrombin which does not contain the precursor of auto-C; a third one is 'prethrombin' which can be derived from above two.

ii. Prothrombin forms thrombin in physiological saline solutions with the addition of only auto C but the yield is small.

iii. *Autoprothrombin III:* With the knowledge that intact prothrombin would produce auto C and thrombin, next step was to dissociate prothrombin and isolate prethrombin as a precursor of thrombin and auto III as a precursor of auto C. Auto III is readily converted to auto-C in 25 per cent sodium citrate solution.

iv. *Prethrombin:* It is not converted to thrombin in 25 per cent sodium citrate solution but on addition of auto-C, thrombin is formed. Thus, it is clear that auto C is the enzyme which breaks one or more bonds in prothrombin to form thrombin. Ac globulin, lipids and calcium ion are needed for its accelerator activity in physiological integration.

PLATELET ACTIVATION

a. Diacylglycerol activates protein kinase—C-an enzyme which catalyzes transfer of phosphate from ATP to serine or threonine residues of proteins. The substrate is a 47-kD protein. Its phosphorylation is necessary for activation of platelets.

b. Inositol (1, 4, 5) tri phosphate (IP_3) leads to the entrance of calcium in cytosol from dense tubular system. This rising calcium concentration triggers.

- Activation of myosin light chain kinase which is needed for changing shape, secretion and contraction of platelets.
- Activation of calcium dependent protease (calpain) and through this other platelet enzymes are activated.
- Activation of phospholipase A_2.

BLOOD CLOTTING—AT A GLANCE

Initiation

- The exposure of blood (vitro) to a negatively charged surface (glass surface) starts the process with involvement of Factor XII, Factor XI, pre-kallikrein, and HMWK (high molecular weight kininogens). Factor XIIa activates prekallikrein to Kallikrein which further activates factor XII; which when generated in sufficient amount activate factor XI.
- The key event triggering blood coagulation during hemostasis is exposure of blood to tissue factor which is demonstrated on pericytes and fibroblasts in adventitia of blood vessels, on fibroblasts in loose connective tissue. Factor VII must bind to tissue factor for proper functioning. It is 30 KD transmembrane apoprotein, which becomes active on association with phospholipid of the cell surface membrane.
- It has been suggested that traces of factor VIIa exist in normal blood which can form a complex (VIIa—tissue factor) at a site of vessel wall damage and this complex will activate a minute amount of factor X. This represents convincing evidence for a basal, minimal continuing activation of factor X in normal individuals.

Thrombin Generation

- The two pathways of coagulation intrinsic and extrinsic come together at step of activation of factor IX; which is activated by factor XIa which is a significant reaction physiologically. To sum up, the activator of factor X are factor IXa, factor VIIIa, anionic phospholipid complex.
- Factor Xa is the known physiological activator of prothrombin, and other factor required in activation of factor Xa includes—factor Va, phospholipid, calcium ions. Further, factor Va must bind first to the platelet surface, where it constitutes 'platelet surface binding site' for factor Xa.
- A factor Xa/Factor Va/membrane phospholipid complex is also said to be formed on surface of cells other than platelets.

- Prothrombin binds to its activator on cell surfaces. First it binds to phospholipids in presence of calcium ions and to Factor Va.

Fibrin : Formation + stabilisation

- Thrombin activates Factor XIII which is an enzyme catalyzing the formation of covalent bonds between polymerizing fibrin molecules. Factor XIIIa stabilise fibrin and protect it from excessive fibrinolysis. Patients with deficiency of Factor XIII have a serious bleeding disorder.

FIBRINOLYSIS—AT A GLANCE

Plasminogen

i. It is a single chain 92 kD protein made in the liver and its plasma concentration is 100 µg/ml. with an intravascular half-life time of 2-2.5 days. It is converted into plasmin.

ii. Its activators are normally present in plasma in only trace amounts. These are released from vascular endothelium and is enhanced by exercise, catecholamines, vasopressin, venous occlusion etc.

iii. PAI-1 and PAI-2 (plasminogen activator inhibitors) are also present. PAI-1 is present within platelets (alpha granules) and its level rises after major surgery or trauma. PAI-2 is measurable only in third trimester of pregnancy. PAI-3 has also been reported in urine.

iv. The activators above mentioned are : tPA (tissue type plasminogen activator) and uPA (urokinase type plasminogen activator). Both are secreted by endothelial cells, and uPA is also secreted by epithelial cells, monocytes, fibroblasts and decidual cells since all of these possess a surface membrane receptor for uPA.

v. The formation and deposition of fibrin within vessels give rise to stimuli triggering release of plasminogen activity through activators from endothelial cells and initiation of secondary fibrinolysis.

vi. Plasmin inhibitors: Include α_2 antiplasmin (1µM concentration, made by liver, major) It also inactivates plasmin on fibrin but at a slower rate. This step is key for normal regulation of secondary fibrinolysis.

THROMBOSIS—CAUSES

1. *Injury to blood vessel:* Is first in this series and is caused by any trauma or application of irritant substance. It may be one of the mechanisms that damaged endothelial lining results into activation or release of some substances initiating the clotting process.
2. *Platelet deposition:* Is another factor. Just like sand is deposited at river's mouth or seashore when current is slowed down or like sticking of flies over fly paper platelets stick to damaged endothelium. The ADP present already causes rapid clumping of these cells. According to one hypothesis damaged endothelium releases ADP like substances which is capable of altering the platelet cell membrane making it enough to clump together.
3. *Slowed blood stream* is another causative factor. After surgical operation or childbirth or due to any other agent capable of slowing the circulation can promote thrombosis.
4. *Changes in blood* by any means promote thrombosis. Increased platelet number or increased fibrinogen level are considered as prethrombic state.
   - Regular active exercise to increase the venous return and proper anticoagulant therapy are amongst physiological basis of treatment of such type of states.

BIBLIOGRAPHY

1. Aoki N, et al. Congenital deficiency of α_2 plasmin inhibitor associated with severe haemorrhagic tendency. J Clin Invest 1979;63:877-84.
2. Baver KA, RD Rosenberg. The pathophysiology of prethrombotic state in humans : In sights gained from studies using markers of hemostatic system activation. Blood 1987;70:343-50.
3. Bevers EM, et al. Changes in membrane phospholipid distribution during platelet activation. Biophy Biochem Acta 1983;736: 57-66.
4. Biggs, Rossemary (Ed). Human Blood Coagulation, Haemostasis Thrombosis. Oxford Blackwell 1971.
5. Biggs and Macfarlane RG. Human blood coagulation and its disorders. Oxford Blackwell 1962.
6. Biggs R (Ed). Human Blood Coagulation: Hemostasis and Thrombosis. Lippincott, Philadelphia 1972.
7. Collen D, et al (Ed). The physiological inhibitors of blood coagulation and fibrinolysis. Elsevier, New York 1979.
8. Doolittle RF. Fibrinogen and fibrin. SC Americana 1981;245:126-35.
9. Furie B, Furie BC. Molecular and cellular biology of blood coagulation. New Eng J Med 1992;326:800.
10. Haber E, et al. Innovative approaches to plasminogen activator therapy. Science 1989;243:51.
11. Hoyer LW. Hoemophilia A. New Eng J Med 1994;330:38.
12. Kane WH, EW Davie. Blood coagulation factor V and VIII. Structural and functional similarities and their relationship to haemorrhagic and thrombotic disorders. Blood 1988;71:539-55.
13. Kaplan AP, M. Silverberg. The coagulation - Kinin-pathway of human plasma. Blood 1987;70:1-15.
14. Nemerson Y. Tissue factor and hemostasis. Blood 1988;71:1-8.

15. Nemerson Y, Nossell HL. The biology of thrombosis. Ann Rev Med 1982;33:479.
16. Nishizuka Y. Tumour of inositol phospholipids and signal transduction. Science 1984;225:1365-70.
17. Pannell RJ, et al. Complementary modes of action of tissue type plasminogen activator and pro-urokinase by which their synergistic effect on clot lysis may be explained. J Clin Invest 1988;81:853.
18. Quick AJ. The hoemorrhagic diseases: Pathology of Hemostasis. Thomas springfield III. 1974.
19. Repaport SI. Preoperative hemostatic evaluation: which tests if any. Blood 1983;61:229-231.
20. Rosenberg RD. Role of heparin and heparin like molecules in thrombosis and atherosclerosis. Fed Proc 1985;44:404.
21. Ruoslahti E, MD Piersch Bacher. New perspectives in cell adhesion: RGD and Integrins. Science 1987;238:491-97.
22. Ruggin ZM, TS Zimmerman. VWF and von-Willemond disease. Blood 1987;70:895-904.
23. Rittenhouse SE, CL Allen. Synergistic activation by colegin and PGH_2 of phosphatidylinositol metabolism and arachidonic acid release in human platelets. J Clin Invest 1982;70:1216-24.
24. Seegers WH. Blood clotting mechanism: Three basic reactions. Ann Rev Phy 1969;31:269.
25. Seligson UCK, et al. Activator factor VII: Presence in factor IX concentrates and persistence in the circulation after infusion. Blood 1978;53:828-37.
26. Sherry S, et al. Fibrinolysis and fibrinolytic activity in man. Phy Rev 1959;39:343-82.
27. Siess W. Molecular mechanism of platelet activation. Phy Rev 1989;69:58.
28. Stafford JL (Ed). Fibrinolysis. British Med Bull 1964;20:171-250.
29. Sprengers ED, C Kluft. Plasminogen activator inhibitors. Blood 1987;69:381-87.
30. Turrito VT, et al. Factor VIII/VWF in subendothelium mediates platelet adhesion. Blood 1985;65:823-31.
31. Wall RT, Harker LA. The endothelium and thrombosis. Ann Rev Med 1980;31:361.
32. Wagner DD, Marder VJ. Biosynthesis of VW protein by human endothelial cells: Processing steps and their intracellular localization. J Cell Bio 1984;99:2123-30.
33. Wion KL D, Kelly JA, et al. Distilution of factor VIII MRNA and antigen in human liver and other tissues. Nature 1985; 317:726-29.

Homeostasis—Blood Volume

The total amount of blood in circulation as well as in stores or reservoirs constitutes blood volume being expressed in relation to body surface and body weight. An average healthy person of 70 kg. body weight has 5 litres of blood in body.

VARIATIONS

Physiological

i. *Age:* During intrauterine life along with foetal growth the blood volume increases, but after birth a slow and steady increase is there till it reaches the adult level.

ii. *Sex:* Due to more surface area and body weight males are having more blood volume as compared with females (males 5 litres, females 4.5 or so litres).

iii. *Pregnancy:* Due to additional foetal mass as well as sodium retention the blood volume is increased but is said to fall slightly in last months.

iv. *Emotions:* It generally causes an increase in blood volume.

v. *Exercise:* Though regular physical exercise increases both blood volume as well as red cell count but a slight decrease is found after strenuous or vigorous exercise.

vi. *Surface area:* 2.8 litres per square meter of body surface is the average blood volume in this regard.

vii. *Body weight:* It is roughly 7 per cent of body weight.

viii. *Posture:* On assuming erect posture from recumbent position, hydrostatic pressure is increased leading to passage of some fluids from vessels to tissue spaces in lower limb, terminating into roughly 15 per cent or so reduction in blood volume.

ix. *Hypoxia:* This factor increases blood volume owing to increase in red cell volume under hypoxia.

x. *Temperature:* If one is having acute exposure towards cold, plasma water is lost to tissues leading to reduction in blood volume.

Pathological

1. *Hypovolaemia (Reduced blood volume):* In following conditions blood volume may be reduced -
   i. *Haemorrhage states* viz. injury or bleeding, haematemesis (blood in vomiting), haemoptysis, bleeding piles, antepartum and postpartum haemorrhages etc.,
   ii. *Haemolysis* Conditions leading to haemolysis terminate into hypovolaemia are famous mismatched transfusion, snake-bite, smallpox, measles etc.
   iii. *Myxoedema:* Blood volume is reduced due to reduction in red cells as well as plasma
   iv. *Shock:* It may be cardiac, neuro or psychogenic. One leads to hypovolaemia,
   v. *Anaemia:* Here red cell volume is certainly reduced but plasma volume is increased to compensate it and all this is sufficient to change blood volume,
   vi. *Anhydraemia (loss of fluid):* Like gastroenteritis, vomiting, pyloric obstruction, burns, excess sweating etc.,
   vii. Acute exposure to *cold.*
2. *Hypervolaemia* (Increased blood volume) This state is seen in (i) Hydration, (ii) Polycythaemia (iii) Leukaemia, (iv) Hyperthyroidism, (v) Congestive heart failure (due to sodium retention), (vi) Splenomegaly, (vii) Liver cirrhosis, (viii) Arterio-venous communication, (ix) Paget's disease, (x) Corticosteroid administration owing to salt retention.

DETERMINATION

Direct method (Welcker 1854; and Bischoff)

It is made upon animals. It is based on taking a small measured quantity of animal's blood and diluting it to 1 in 100 with normal saline. Animal is then bled and then vessels are washed out as blood ceased to flow, water was then added to the collecting fluid—blood and washings till its colour matches the tint of original diluted blood specimen. The total collected fluid divided by 100 gives the blood volume.

Indirect Methods

1. *Dye method*:
   i. *The principle (Keith, Rowntree and Geraghty)*: Consists of injection of a known amount of dye and then knowing degree of dilution in the plasma of it; colour of stained plasma is compared in a colorimeter with that of a standard dye solution of known concentration.
   ii. *Qualities of dye used*: It must not diffuse too rapidly from blood stream; it must colour only the plasma, it must not change its own colour on its entry in blood; it is not to be adsorbed by the cells of blood or blood vessel walls; it must not cause any haemolysis, it must be innocuous; it must be capable of mixing thoroughly with the plasma.
   iii. *Generally*: T-1824 (Evan's blue) is most commonly used, since with it error due to haemolysis is minimised and also it is eliminated very slowly from the circulation.
   iv. *A sample of plasma is obtained first*: Then a known amount of dye is injected (I.V.) and blood samples are collected at 10-20-30-40 and 50 minutes interval of time. Concentration of dye in plasma is measured. From the concentration of dye in sample and amount injected, dye dilution, plasma volume can be calculated.
   v. *Disadvantages*:
      - Repeated injections may cause some discolouration of skin and conjunctiva.
      - Repeated determinations may be inaccurate.
      - If haemolysis is present it is not satisfactory.
2. *Radioactive method*:
   i. I^{131} This has the advantage of requiring only two blood samples one of which is a control. It is not affected by haemolysis and it at the same time does not require specialised instrumentation. It is used at the bedside.
   ii. Fe^{55}, Cr^{51}, P^{32}, Fe^{59} are also used. Radioactive iron in the two samples is determined by Geiger counter.
   Total blood volume = Plasma volume × 100 ÷ (1 - hematocrit)
   Red cell volume can be calculated by subtracting the plasma volume from total blood volume.

NORMAL VALUES

i. The blood volume of a man of average weight (70 kg) is 5 litres.
ii. Blood makes up 7 per cent of body weight, plasma volume a little over 4 per cent and red cell volume about 3 per cent.
iii. Plasma volume of adult male is 40 ml, red cell volume is 29 ml and whole blood volume is 70 ml/kg.
iv. Rise in blood volume occurs in 'generalised oedema' (anasarca), polycythaemia vera, hypoalbunaemia, congestive cardiac failure, some kidney diseases etc.
v. Blood volume is a reflection of the volume of extracellular fluid (ECF). When it (ECF) decreased, e.g. vomiting, diarrhoea, water deprivation, severe burn etc. the blood volume is also shrinked.
vi. Out of total blood volume - 64 per cent is in veins, 13 per cent in arteries, 7 per cent in systemic arterioles and capillaries, 7 per cent in heart, pulmonary vessels 9 per cent.

LUNGS AS A BLOOD RESERVOIR

It approximately contains 450 ml of blood, i.e. 9 per cent of total blood volume of the circulatory system.

BLOOD VOLUME IN PREGNANCY

Increase in blood volume is characteristic of pregnancy.

Increase in plasma volume has been reported very early - (400 ml. increase in 8 and 900 ml. increase in 16 weeks of gestational age). It rises rapidly and so may cause 'physiological anaemia of pregnancy.'

Red cell mass also increases 20–30 per cent.

The mechanism for above changes are listed as: increased aldosterone secretion causes sodium retention which increases plasma volume. Increased 'erythropoietin' activity during pregnancy leads to increase in red cell mass.

Average gain in ECF	
Products of conception	1.5–2 litres
Uterus and breast	0.7 litres
Blood plasma	0.5 litres
Extragenital interstitial fluid	2.5 litres
Total	5.2 to 5.7

During greater part of pregnancy sodium is retained to the extent of 3 gm/week and this retention would lead to a rise in the osmotic pressure of extracellular fluid unless water were also retained. The retention of water and sodium may be related to the increased production of oestrogen in pregnancy since oestrogen therapy in woman has produced an increase of upto 20 per cent in blood volume with a lowered haematocrit.

EFFECT OF HAEMORRHAGE

- When more than 30 per cent of blood volume is lost rapidly body needs transfusion. On the contrary, on less than 30 per cent loss, compensatory mechanisms comes into action.

- 500 ml. of blood drawn out for transfusion purpose is replaced within an hour or so. Blood restoration in erythrocytes takes about 7 weeks on the average; of course administration of iron + protein may shorten this time.
- Early effects:
  1. If loss of blood is large, and of sudden occurrence as well as from an artery; there occurs prompt fall in blood pressure due to reduction in circulating fluid. On the contrary, a moderate loss (10 per cent of total amount) there is no significant fall in blood pressure. It is of significant occurrence when blood comes from a vein and the loss is gradual. In this case factors which maintain the compensation include - reduction in capacity of vascular bed, increased peripheral resistance and fluid entry from tissue.
  2. Haemorrhage → reduced blood flow → hypoxia → activation of chemoreceptors (aortic + carotid bodies) → increased rate and depth of respiration. Of course, on more blood loss complications in respiration may occur like Cheyne-Stokes breathing, air hunger, gasping respiration etc.
  3. Release of blood from blood reservoirs into circulation also help to restore the blood volume. As we know the reservoirs are spleen, liver, lungs, splanchnic venous vessels etc.
  4. Increase in heart rate is another accompaniment of severe haemorrhage. It is brought about through carotid sinus and aortic reflexes initiated by fall in blood pressure Anoxaemia of the cardiac centres is an additional factor. Liberation of adrenaline is the another cause. One hypothetical view is that increased heart rate may lower the central venous pressure which improves the pressure gradients in the veins; which would improve the venous return, which will correct the situation.
  5. Blood clotting occurs within a few minute which closes the opening in the blood vessel. A fall in blood pressure stimulates the clot formation. Platelets get deposited on injured surface and form a plug. They may liberate 5HT on disintegration which aids in haemostasis. Furthermore, on platelet disintegration, certain substances are released which are necessary for generation of thromboplastin and thus initiation of clotting. Clot retraction finally firms the clot; of course this process is also dependent on platelet population.
  6. If the wound is closed then flow of blood is slowed. If blood pressure has fallen, it rises again. This is the result of readjustment of capacity of vascular system. This is reduction in capacity of vascular bed which prevents initial fall of B.P. It is more or less initiated by reflex vasoconstriction in essential parts of the body, e.g. skin, mucous membrane, intestine etc. If haemorrhage is not severe, then this reduced vascular capacity will maintain the venous return/cardiac output/blood pressure etc. But if the haemorrhage is severe then there occurs fall of blood pressure.
- *Delayed effects:* Replacement of fluid which is lost occurs. Due to blood loss, there exists low hydrostatic pressure in the capillaries. So this facilitates the movement of the fluid from tissues to the capillaries. This dilutes the blood, and corpuscular concentration is also reduced. This fluid does not enter through lymphatics but it enters directly so protein concentration of plasma is markedly reduced. To compensate the protein deficiency here, protein is mobilised from stores.

  The extreme thirst felt by the patient of haemorrhage is actually the call of tissues for fluid. It indicates that their own fluid stores are being drawn into under filled vessels. The water administration will recover the water balance and will replenish the blood volume.

RECEPTOR RESPONSE AND REGULATION OF BLOOD VOLUME

It is necessary to match input and output of water and sodium each day in order to maintain the regulation of volume and osmolality of the body fluids.

STRETCH

Acute distension of whole left atrium

⇒ Diuresis

RECEPTORS

Factors included/participating in above reaction include:

a. Decrease in secretion of ADH due to increased activity of atrial stretch receptors.
b. Reduction in renal sympathetic nerve traffic.
c. Production and release of 'atrial-natriuretic factor (ANF) or polypeptide from atria which is stored as granules and they on release lead to hypotension, sodium diuresis and increase in haematocrit.

Atrial receptor stimulation → ANF release → Decreased reabsorption of Na^+Cl^- + H_2O → More water pass out from tubule into urine → Diuresis.

ADH AND BLOOD VOLUME

- This hormone released from supra-optic nuclei of hypothalamus, causes renal retention of water which increases blood volume. This leads to an increase in arterial blood pressure.
- This is compensated by excess sodium loss in the urine as well as by dilution of extracellular fluid done by excess water which is retained.
- So no significant alteration in blood volume is seen because of operation of compensatory mechanisms.

POLYCYTHAEMIA AND BLOOD VOLUME

In this condition the blood volume increases greatly.

i. Polycythaemia means increased number of red cells → Increase in peripheral resistance due to sluggish blood flow which is due to more viscosity → Reduced venous return.
ii. Compensatory changes are

Kidney retains the fluid → blood volume increase → high arterial pressure enough to provide necessary urinary output to prevent further fluid retention.

INCREASED CAPACITY OF CIRCULATION AND BLOOD VOLUME

- In a pregnant lady—the extravascular capacity of the uterus, placenta etc. increase blood volume.
- In very large varicose veins, the blood volume increases.
- Veins are 'large storehouse of blood' as compared with arterial system because of their large cross-sectional area.

EFFECT OF ANGIOTENSIN

Directly this hormone causes renal effects which leads to renal retention of salt and water. Indirectly it causes stimulation of aldosterone secretion. So only 5 per cent or so alteration in blood volume takes place on either its increased or decreased concentration.

ARTERIAL BARORECEPTOR REFLEX: VOLUME REFLEX

When blood volumes becomes too much great, it stretches the arterial baroreceptors which in turn causes reflex inhibition of sympathetic nervous system. This causes dilatation of renal arterioles which leads to increased urinary output. This is termed as volume reflex. In this connection it is to be remembered that total sympathetic denervation is not associated with a significant change in blood volume. This is because of the fact that on one side they exert renal retention of fluid but on another side they cause a simultaneous vasoconstrictor effect on blood vessels of decreasing the capacity of circulatory system.

ALDOSTERONE AND BLOOD VOLUME

- It causes strong reabsorption of sodium at distal segment of nephrone and this increased sodium also causes secondary reabsorption of water. This increases the blood volume and so the blood pressure.
- Now because of rise in blood pressure, the phenomenon of pressure diuresis and pressure natriuresis comes into action. So kidney begins to excrete same amount of sodium which was ingested, in spite of aldosterone. This is "aldosterone escape" by which increased blood pressure returns towards normal.

HEART DISEASE V/S BLOOD VOLUME

- A weak heart means myocardial infarction/valvular disease/congenital anomalies etc.
- The weak heart cannot attain a high enough arterial pressure to cause necessary urinary output of the fluid. So kidney retains the volume.
- This fluid retention is actually a compensation of myocardial weakness because this allows weak heart to pump a life sustaining level of cardiac output.

SUMMARY AND HIGHLIGHTS

- Blood is a part of extracellular fluid. A normal healthy adult male is having 5 litres of blood in his circulation. Body weight and surface area the two main factors on which it depends.
- Decrease in blood volume and red cell mass has been observed on prolonged stay in space.
- It can be measured by Dye method and direct method, as well as by using radioactive compounds.
- Hormones ADH, aldosterone, oestrogen, ANF are exerting a good influence on blood volume.
- So the basic theme is :- Increased blood volume → increase in cardiac output → increased arterial pressure → loss of fluid by kidneys and → blood volume returns towards normal.

BIBLIOGRAPHY

1. Albert SN. Blood Volume: springfield: Thomas.1963.
2. Bates ER, et al. The relationship between plasma levels of immuno reactive ANF hormone and hemodynamic function in man. Circulation 1986;73:1155-61.
3. Bishop VS, et al. Arterial and cardiopulmonary reflexes regulations of neurohumoral drive to the circulation. Fed Proc 1985;44:2377-81.

4. Clapp JF. Maternal physiological adaptation during early human pregnancy. Amer J Obst and Gynae 1988.
5. Gauer OH, et al. The regulation of extracellular fluid volume. Ann Rev Phy 1970;32:547-95.
6. Goetz KL, et al. Atrial receptors and renal function. Phy Rev 1975;55:157-205.
7. Gregerson MI, et al. Blood volume. Physiol Rev 1959;39:307-42.
8. Mayerson HS. Blood volume and its regulation. Ann Rev Phy 1965;27:307-22.
9. Milnor WR. In Medical Physiology edited by V. B. Mountcastle. St Louis CV Mosby. 1968;I:24-34. and 209-220.
10. Seitchik J. Total body water and total body density of pregnant woman. Obst Gynae 1967;29:155.
11. Shoukas AA, Sagawa K. Control of total systemic vascular capacity by the carotid sinus baroreceptor reflex. Cir Res 1973;33:22-23.
12. Zucker IH, Gilmore JP. Aspects of cardio-vascular reflexes in pathological states. Fed Proc 1985;44:2400-7.

69 Haemopoiesis

CONCEPT OF STEM AND PROGENITOR CELL

i. Haemopoietic *stem cells* possess two fundamental properties viz. self-renewal and an ability to differentiate into mature specialised blood cells. The frequency of stem cells in human bone marrow has been estimated as 1-2 per 1,000 nucleated cells; of course, small numbers also circulate in the blood.

ii. In some organs like spleen and marrow cavity, there are specific supporting tissues which permit growth and differentiation of stem cells and are referred as haemopoietic *microenvironment*.

iii. From a single cell, colony arises; this multitude of cells is called a *clone* and normal haemopoiesis is polyclonal.

iv. As stem cell differentiates, it becomes capable to produce specific cells. These properties suggest the existence of three functionally different stem cells namely pluripotent stem cells, myeloid stem cells giving rise to erythrocyte, granulocyte of all types, monocytes and platelets and a lymphocyte stem cell. This process is called *committation*.

v. As commitment progresses, the capability of a stem cell for self renewal diminishes. When it is markedly diminished or lost, the cell is no longer called a stem cell but is termed as progenitor cell, which are more numerous than stem cells and are present in both the bone marrow and the circulating blood.

vi. *CSF* (colony stimulating factor)
   - Is required for the growth of *CFU-GM* (colony forming unit—Granulocyte—monocyte).
   - CFU-GM is inhibited by prostaglandin E, which is produced by monocytes when they are subjected to the effect of CSF (feedback control).
   - Monocytes also produce 'acidic lactoferrin' which inhibits normal CFU-GM colonies in normal states but not in leukaemic states.

vii. A chemical *eosinopoietin* has been described specially in mouse which causes rise in eosinophil number in the peripheral blood.

HAEMOPOIETIC GROWTH FACTORS

i. These are *cytokines* which control growth, differentiation and function of blood cells. Chemically, they are distinct acid glycoproteins. (cytokines is a general term for proteins released by cells that act as intercellular mediators).

ii. *GM-CSF* (granulocyte-macrophage-colony stimulating factor)
   M-CSF macrophage - colony stimulating factor
   Interleukins (IL) (as IL-1, IL-2, IL-3, and so on) are materials affecting proliferation or function of lymphocytes or monocytes in immunology.

iii. IL-1 stimulates growth of T lymphocyte, which elaborate IL-3 and stimulate fibroblasts and endothelial cells to secrete GM-CSF and G-CSF-IL-1 also stimulates the release of neutrophils from bone marrow.

iv. *TNF* (tumor-necrosis factor)—is cytokine from macrophage.

v. *TGF* β (Transforming growth factor)—inhibit myeloid cell growth.

vi. Most of the growth factors are present in tissue fluids and blood in only minute concentration. They affect their target cells through binding to specific cell surface receptors.

ERYTHROPOIESIS

i. Two types of progenitor cells are recognised—viz. *'BFU-E'* (burst—forming—units—erythrocytes), *CFU-E* (colony forming units—erythrocytes).

ii. BFU-E forms large multilobulated colonies, where as CFU-E forms much smaller colonies.

iii. BFU-E requires the presence of *BPA* (burst promoting activator). Both IL-3 and GM-CSF stimulate the progenitor cellular growth. CFU-E is independent of BPA but requires erythropoietin for their full action.
iv. Haemoglobin synthesis requires three requisites—namely (a) adequate amount of mRNA for transcription and translation process of polypeptide chains; (b) iron for incorporation into protoporphyrin to form heme, (c) adequate amount of protoporphyrin.

GRANULOCYTE PRODUCTION

i. The growth factor IL-3 and GM-CSF can support the growth of colonies of eosinophils. IL-5 has been recently studied for directly stimulating the proliferation and maturation of eosinophils.
ii. A material called '*MBP*' (major basic protein) makes about 50 per cent of the mass of large granules. It is said to play a key role in the ability of eosinophil to damage the larva tissue stage of helminthic parasites and is extremely potent tissue toxin.
ECP (eosinophilic cationic protein)—a neurotoxic protein and an eosinophil peroxidase is also present in large granules. It also contains high concentration of aryl-sulfatase B, lyso phospholipase, which forms crystals called 'Charcot-Leyden crystals' in the pulmonary secretions of patients with asthma.
Eosinophils are increased in number when T cells are activated because of T-cell derived IL-5, IL-3 and GM-CSF.
iii. Basophils are produced from marrow stem cells. Hence, infusion of IL-3 is followed by increase in circulating basophils. Their surface membrane contains receptor for IgE molecules. In acute allergic reactions, a specific antigen reacts with IgE bound to basophils and they release their granular content. Basophils also contain chondroitin sulphate, proteoglycan etc.
iv. All granulocytes in post natal life are developed in red bone marrow. The most primitive (ancestor cell is CFU-GM (colony-forming unit granulocyte—monocyte).

THROMBOPOIESIS

Thrombocytes are derived from giant bone marrow cells called megakaryocytes which have large sized multilobulated nucleus and with abundant cytoplasm. Normal marrow contains 1 megakaryocyte per 500 nucleated red cells. They arise from a population of small to medium blast like cells called 'megakaryoblast.'

Mature megakaryocytes are amoeboid cells that extends cytoplasmic pseudopods through endothelial lining cells into the lumen of marrow sinusoids where pseudopods then fragment to form platelets.

Specific megakaryocyte progenitor cells may exist. It is under observation that GF-CSF may exist or not.

Thrombopoietin: stimulates megakaryocyte protein synthesis and the shedding of megakaryocyte cytoplasm as platelets but it does not support megakaryocyte colony growth.

TGF-β - a material that is released from alpha granules of platelets when they are activated inhibits the growth in vitro of megakaryocyte colonies and thus acts as a negative feedback regulator of platelet production.

In both acute and chronic thrombocytopenic states, the platelet production may be increased many times.

LYMPHOPOIESIS

However, the lymphoid cells have always been puzzling to haematologists; morphologically they are featureless consisting of featureless nucleus—a compact one. A nucleolus can be demonstrated along with varying amount of blue cytoplasm by electron microscopy.

Small round cells with the morphology of lymphoid cell may be the stem cell. From these stem cells some are destined to become T and others β lymphocytes.

The peculiarity in lymphocyte is that during their activities, they convert themselves back to lymphoblasts and divide, from β lymphoblasts plasma cells can develop which produce antibodies. Majority of lymphocytes circulating in our blood are T lymphocytes.

SUMMARY AND HIGHLIGHTS

- Haemopoietic stem cells possess two fundamental properties viz. self-renewal and ability to differentiate into mature specialised cells. From a single cell colony arises; this multitude of cells is called clone and normal haemopoiesis is polyclonal. As stem cell differentiates, it becomes capable to produce specific cells this is committation. When its size is shrunken or lost it is called progenitor cell.
- Cytokines are proteins released by cells that act as intercellular mediators and are haemopoietic growth factors. G-M-CSF, interleukins (1-5 so on) are materials affecting proliferation or function of lymphocyte or monocytes in immunology, TNF (cytokine from macrophage), TGF β (inhibit myeloid cell growth).
- For erythropoiesis two progenitor cells are required BFU-E and CFU-E. Haemoglobin synthesis requires adequate amount of mRNA, iron and protoporphyrin.

- IL-3 and G-M-CSF support growth for colonies of eosinophils. Basophils are produced from marrow stem cells so infusion of IL-3 is followed by increase in basophil number.
- Thrombocytes are derived from giant megakaryocyte whose progenitor cells exist. Thrombopoietin stimulates its protein synthesis.

BIBLIOGRAPHY

1. Beutter B, Cerami A. Tumour necrosis, cachexia, shock and inflammation: a common mediator. Ann Rev Biochem 1988;57: 505-18.
2. Donachue RE, et al. Human II-3 and GM-CSF-act synergistically in stimulating hematopoiesis in primates. Science 1988;241:1820-23.
3. Nathan CF. Secretory products of macrophages. J Clin Invest 1987;79:319.
4. Ogawa M. Differentiation and proliferation of haematopoietic stem cells. Blood 1993;81:2844.
5. Quesenberry P, L Levitt. New Eng J Med 1979;301:In 3 parts 755-60;819-823, 868-872.
6. Till JE, EA McCulloch. Haematopoietic stem cell differentiation. Biochem Biophys Acta 1980;605:431-59.
7. Weller PF. The immunobiology of eosinophils. New Eng J Med 1991;324:1110.

70

RE System

SPLEEN

For even many years it is classed as organ full of mystery. It is the real secret that how one of the largest of organs can be removed without producing any noticeable change in normal physiology of human body.

INTRODUCTION

Unlike the liver, kidney and pancreas it is a large abdominal organ without a duct. It is certainly considered as a vast reticulo-endothelial sponge with a supporting framework of trabeculae and reticulum, with certain amount of lymphoid tissue super added,—yes an apparatus appropriately designed to alter and detain the blood which is filtered through it. Its colour reddish purple, weight ranging between 150–200 gm, length being 12 cm, breadth 7 cm and thickness about 3 cm. Its consistency being soft and friable; located between stomach and diaphragm on left side of abdominal cavity.

GENERAL MICROSCOPIC STRUCTURE

It is roughly size and shape of a clenched fist lying in the shelter of 9th, 10th and 11th ribs with long axis parallel with them. If section cut at right angles of capsule and then examined microscopically lymphatic nodules are seen, which are chief sites of lymphocyte production. Red pulp which surrounds lymphatic nodules is having maximally erythrocytes in its mesh, an apparatus designed to act as a filter. Two major functions of this organ—lymphocyte production and filter tend to be segregated from one another—white pulp makes lymphocytes and red pulp filters. So over all is—

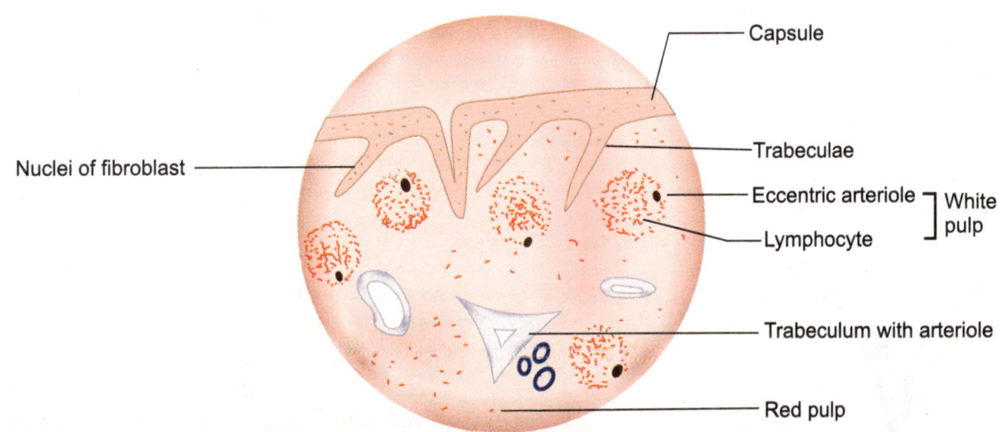

Fig. 70.1: Spleen

- Outer serous coat
- Structural framework made up of capsule, trabeculae and its network
- Red and white pulp

First two constituents (capsule and trabeculae) are made up of collagenous and elastic fibres together with smooth muscle fibres and reticular fibres. White pulp is made of central artery enveloped by lymphocytes and macrophages. Lymphatic sheath assume a capsular form called Malpighian corpuscles where lymphocytes are dealing with foreign antigen. Red pulp is made up of pulp cords and venous sinuses having all formed elements of blood, macrophages and mesenchymal tissues.

FUNCTIONS

a. *Spleen—a blood forming organ:* Before birth formed elements of blood are produced by spleen. Certainly after birth the function is exchanged by bone marrow. Here one thing still exists that if bone marrow is out of order due to any cause the function is again taken over by it. The lymphocyte variety of leucocytes is also manufactured here.

b. *Spleen—a blood destructive organ:* The aged, deteriorated or damaged elements of blood are destroyed by this organ, specially red cells which wander through infinite forest of its pulp and finally trapped by reticulo-endothelial cells. In pathological conditions spleen may become the predominant site of destruction. Platelets are also said to be destroyed here. On this functional property basis this may be questioned that whether it is a slaughter house or graveyard of erythrocytes? It is apparent that great reticulo-endothelial mass of pulp plays an active part in final destruction. Some abnormal cells as spherocytes of haemolytic anaemia have little chance of making their passage successfully.

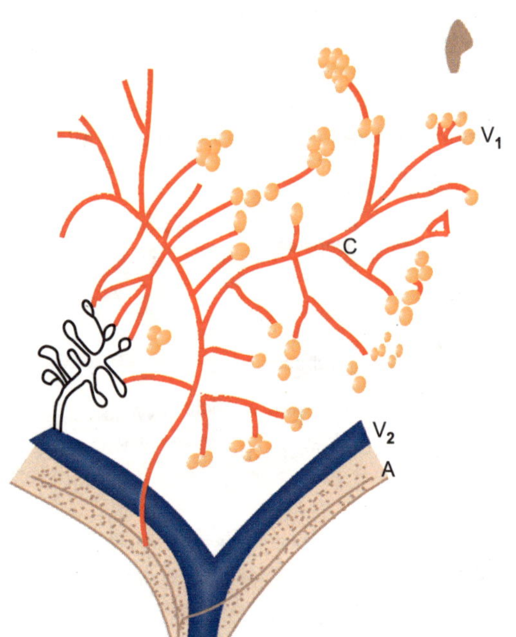

Fig. 70.2: Spleen (V_1 = Venous sinuses, C = Capillaries, V_2 = Vein, A = Artery)

c. *Spleen—as a great defence:* Splenic macrophages rapidly ingest bacteria or large parasites, also these macrophages are stimulated during immune response to produce precursors of lymphocytes and plasma cells which are truly antibody former cells of the body. The macrophages of germinal centre destroy lymphocytes releasing their gammaglobulin. As said Malpighian follicles manufacture lymphocytes.
Its phagocytic activity is also coming in class of defence functions, which is strongly stimulated by estrogenic materials and phagocytic activity is greatly depressed by cortisone. After splenectomy animal becomes more susceptible to certain parasitic and bacterial infections. Though spleen may hold only a small percentage of any particulate matter given intravenously, but it also can be stimulated to form more reticulo-endothelial cells and discharge them into circulation.

d. *Spleen as a storehouse:* It has been likened to a reservoir or blood bank (natural one) capable of emptying itself on a sudden demand like severe exercise, haemorrhage, asphyxia etc. This property is much more true for animals (cats and dogs) since they have got plenty of plain muscle as compared with man. The splenic blood was found to be richer in red cells and hence with splenic contraction, blood with amount one sixth of total blood volume and red cells equal to one fourth of body's total supply are expelled.

e. *Spleen influencive on number and structure of blood cells:* Spleen destroys abnormal cells certainly but normal erythrocytes are not destroyed until they have served their normal routine functions.

f. As regards sequestration of red cells is concerned there are two steps for convenience of description. One is culling which means ability of spleen to remove certain cells from circulation which don't meet minimum requirements like spherocytes, and another is pitting which means alteration of certain cells in their passage through spleen, like removal of granules from siderocytes.

g. In condition of thrombocytopenia, removal of spleen increases the platelet count possibly through megakaryocyte—the parent cell for these formed elements of blood. So it can be said that spleen has got some control over number of thrombocytes in circulation.
h. A factor is said to be released from spleen which stimulates bone marrow for releasing erythrocytes into general circulation.

SPLENOMEGALY—CHIEF CAUSES

a. Infections
   i. Bacterial (typhoid, tuberculosis, septicaemia, syphilis)
   ii. Viral (Infective hepatitis, infectious mononucleosis)
   iii. Protozoal (Malaria, kala-azar, trypanosomiasis)
   iv. Fungus (Histoplasmosis)
   v. Parasitic (Hydatid)
b. Haematological:
   i. Haemolytic diseases (hereditary spherocytosis, thalassemia paroxysmal nocturnal haemoglobinurea)
   ii. Malignancy (Acute leukaemia, chronic myeloid leukaemia, lymphomas, chronic lymphatic leukaemia)
   iii. Myeloproliferative diseases (Polycythemia vera)

SPLENECTOMY (SURGICAL REMOVAL OF ORGAN)

Inspite of a great debate this is an empirical form of treatment which may provide a great help in many conditions. Generally it is indicated in
a. Hereditary spherocytic anaemia (best results are obtained and gallstones are also prevented).
b. Thrombocytopenic purpura .... in which operation was followed by immediate cessation of bleeding, rise in platelet count and restoration of bleeding time.
c. Hypersplenism .... is completely relieved.
d. Rupture of spleen from trauma or disease, e.g. infectious mononucleosis.

Chief Effects

a. Diminished resistance towards infection,
b. Leucocyte population is increased,
c. Microcytic hypochromic anaemia results,
d. Loss of reservoir function so body's reaction to hypoxia - haemorrhage is slowed and
e. Erythrocytes become more resistant to hypotonic solution.

SUMMARY AND HIGHLIGHTS

- The spleen is an important blood filter that removes spherocytes and other abnormal red cells. It contains many platelets and plays a significant role in immune system. In the absence of spleen bacterial infections are more common and severe; Along with it malaria has higher mortality rate because deformed red cells containing malaria parasite are not removed.
- The unique circulation of spleen allows this organ to play an important role in extravascular haemolysis. As some of the small blood vessels enter red pulp of the spleen, they end in spaces called cords containing loosely meshed reticular and mononuclear phagocytes. The red cells are emptied into cords and must then percholate through the cords in intimate contact with mononuclear phagocytes and re-enter venous sinuses in the red pulp by squeezing between endothelial cells. These conditions favour the removal of red cells with decreased deformability of the cell membrane. Due to increased removal of red cells, the spleen usually enlarges in haemolytic disorders.

BIBLIOGRAPHY

1. Macphorsm. The Spleen. Thomas springfield III 1973.

LYMPHATIC SYSTEM

Lymphatic system forms one of the most all pervasive, important and indispensable parts of our anatomy, though it is very little in evidence in a state of health. Lymphatic first appears in round worm, they reach their highest development in amphibia and well developed in mammals in whom valves are present in vessels.

INTRODUCTION

Lymph capillaries are draining the tissue spaces and actually they are mesh work of delicate vessels in which lymph is moving towards great vessels. By the union of such small vessels large vessels are formed which swell in size and finally constitute right lymphatic and thoracic duct. These pour their lymph into blood stream by way of right and left subclavian veins. Lymph nodes are interposed in the course of large lymphatic vessels. These vessels upon reaching node or gland break into fine channels which piercing node enter its cortex part.

The permeability of lymph capillaries is increased by warmth, sunlight, mechanical or chemical stimulation, histamine etc. Lymphatic tissues are capable of regeneration. All of these are absent in central-nervous system where it is replaced by cerebro-spinal fluid and this is the cause that lesions like brain tumour don't spread throughout the body, i.e. outside the cranial cavity. *Lymph channels may be likened to an absorbent sponge, but nodes play the part of filter.*

LYMPH : COMPOSITION

- Lymph is a modified tissue fluid and both resembling blood plasma. Lymph of thoracic duct during fasting is faintly alkaline in reaction, yellow coloured, slow clotting tendency and transparent in appearance.
- As protein constituents are concerned. Albumin, globulin, fibrinogen and prothrombin are usual protein constituent but certainly lower than plasma and due to prothrombin it is slow clotting fluid. Generally speaking 2–4.5 per cent proteins are present but it also depends upon site and degree of activity.
- As fat constituents; they are low in fasting state but rises after a fat rich diet. Fats are present in form of chylomicrons. Cholesterol and phospholipids are bound with protein as called lipoproteins.
- Sugar level is up to 132 mg per cent.
- Amongst non-protein nitrogenous substances urea (23 mg%), creatinine (14 mg%) are present. Amongst anions, chlorides and bicarbonates are little higher than plasma and cations concentration is little lower than plasma.
- Overall composition comprises of 94 per cent water and rest 6 per cent is solid constituent in lymph is present.
- 1000–20,000 cells per cubic mm is total number of leucocytes present in thoracic duct lymph while in peripheral lymph only 550 cells/cu mm leucocytes are present. Out of it lymphocytes are in majority but occasionally plasma cells, monocytes are also found.
- 300–13,000 cells per cubic mm is the total number of erythrocytes present in thoracic peripheral lymph.
- The lymph coming from thoracic duct is mainly from intestine and liver so it will vary according to the respective digestive juices.

Differences

Blood	*Lymph*
1. Red coloured	Colour less
2. High protein content	Low protein content
3. More fibrinogen	Less fibrinogen
4. RBC present	No RBC
5. Less metabolic waste	More metabolic waste

LYMPH: FUNCTIONS

For enumeration purpose, its functions can be broadly taken as .

a. It returns nutrients specially proteins to the blood from tissues.

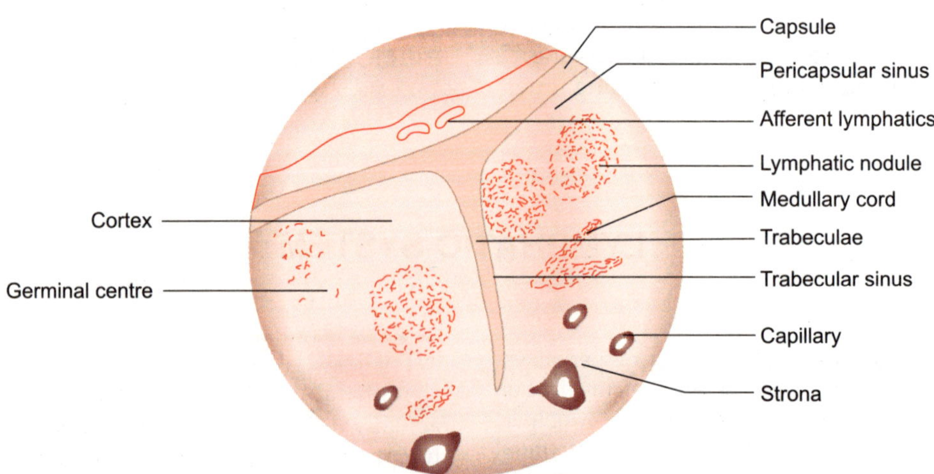

Fig. 70.3: Lymph node

b. It removes foreign particulate matter specially bacteria from tissues. This function is performed by monocytes and lymphocytes.
c. The task of redistribution of fluid in body (shifting fluid from one part to other in circulatory system) is also achieved by lymph.
d. Tissue integrity is maintained by lymph, e.g. if cardiac lymphatics are ligated it results into myocardial degeneration; hydronephrosis can be induced on tying ureter's lymphatics and degenerative hepatic changes are there on ligating bile duct.
e. It is one of the major channel for absorption specially of fats.

FORMATION, PRESSURE; FLOW

1. Any condition which increases the outpouring of fluid from capillaries into the tissues will tend to increase the flow of lymph.
2. The lymph capillaries are much more permeable than the blood capillaries.
3. The fluid which is transuded from blood at arterial end of capillary much of the water is reabsorbed at the venous end. Protein passes into the lymph. Lymph capillary is therefore a special channel by which protein is returned back to the blood. It is also serving the function of absorption of other colloids.
4. In mammals extravascular circulation of entire plasma albumin takes place in 20 hours. (In frog it is 50 times in 24 hours).
5. Rate of flow along human thoracic duct is 1–1.5 ml. per minute (0.46 c.c./mt. average flow in thoracic duct—and more than half of this, i.e. 0.26 c.c. is contributed by lymph vessels of liver). Pressure in thoracic duct is low.
6. Enlarging the capillary surface by vasodilatation, or increasing the number of patent capillaries, increase the leakage of protein from circulation. This occurs when saline infusion/dextran infusion is given. The protein of tissue spaces is returned to the blood by the lymph. This is important in regulation of fluid interchange modifying the balance of forces across the capillary wall.

RATE AND CONTROL OF LYMPH FLOW

In a resting man about 100 ml of lymph flows through thoracic duct and almost 20 ml flows through other channels. Total lymph flow is thus 120 ml/hr (1-1.5 ml/minute).

Lymphatic Pump and Control

Existence of valves in lymphatic vessels has been demonstrated. In large lymphatics valves exist every few millimetres and in smaller lymphatics valves are much closer located. The fluid always moves unidirectionally since valves open only in central direction whenever lymphatics are compressed by pressure due to any cause viz. contraction of muscle,' 'passive movement of parts of body,' 'arterial pulsation,' 'tissue compression from outside.' Lymphatic flow/pump becomes very active during exercise (4-15 times more than normal) but sluggish during resting conditions. During rest flow along lymphatic vessels is slight and lymph protein is hence high but during activity protein concentration falls since less transuded water undergoes reabsorption into blood and more is carried away by lymph channels. The contracting muscles exert pumping effect upon lymph driving it along the vessels.

Interstitial Fluid Pressure and Control

Whenever interstitial fluid pressure rises above its normal value of - 7 mmHg, there is increased flow of interstitial fluid into lymphatics thus increasing rate of lymph flow. This is the direct effect up to 0 mmHg pressure, above which increase is not there because interstitial fluid then start compression outside the lymphatic vessel so resistance in flow occurs. Factors which increase interstitial fluid pressure increases rate of lymph flow and in this series the most important factors are 'elevated capillary pressure,' 'increased capillary permeability,' 'decreased plasma colloid osmotic pressure, increased interstitial fluid protein.

Increased Functional Activity and Control

Little after commencement of activity of a gland or any part of body lymph flow increases through it which may be due to (a) formation of metabolites which increase osmotic effect of tissue fluid thus causing more fluid to leave the vessels, (b) vasodilatation, (c) anoxia, (d) more heat production or high temperature.

Interstitial Fluid Protein and Control

Generally, increase in tissue fluid protein increases rate of lymph flow and this washes the proteins out of tissue spaces, returning protein concentration to its normal low level. To explain this statement, small quantity of protein is present in fluid leaking from arterial ends of capillaries which is then absorbed at venous end so most of the protein is left behind. So protein continuously accumulates in interstitial fluid which in turn increases tissue colloid osmotic pressure, which increases interstitial fluid volume as well as increased tissue pressure which forces interstitial fluid into lymphatic channels and this fluid carries excess accumulated protein with it.

Isotonic and Hypertonic Solutions

By increasing the passage of protein and fluid from capillaries, lymph flow is increased by administration of isotonic fluids/saline. Protein is returned from tissue fluids by lymphatics. Returning lymph contains more protein.

The concentrated solution of sodium chloride, glucose etc. on intravenous administration causes increase in lymph flow.

During their way lymphatic channels are interrupted by lymph nodes. On approaching a lymph node, a lymph channel breaks up into several afferent channels which enter the lymph nodes. From here efferent channels emerge. So from here antibodies as well as lymphocytes are entering the blood in subclavian vein.

DYNAMICS OF OEDEMA

- It simply means presence of excess fluid in body tissues. It mainly accumulates in extracellular fluid but intracellular swelling is not uncommon.
- *Intracellular swelling:*
  - — The foremost important cause is lack of adequate nutrition to the tissues. When local blood flow of the tissue is depressed then automatically delivery of oxygen + nutrients is also diminished. It depresses the ionic pump of the cell specially the pump which removes the sodium ion. So due to retaining of sodium, water is also attracted through osmosis and thus increasing the intracellular volume.
  - — If cell is inflamed then because of inflammation, capillary permeability is increased which leads to diffusion of sodium ion etc. towards interior of the cell which leads to intracellular swelling.
- *Capillary pressure:*
  1. It is 25 mmHg if measured by direct canulation of the capillaries; while it is said to be 17 mmHg if it is in indirectly measured by isogravimetric method, and it is said to be the true functional capillary pressure.
  2. Oedema in heart failure: Reasons:
     - —Capillary and venous pressure both are increased because heart fails to pump blood normally from veins into the arteries. This leads to oedema.
     - —This decreases blood pressure, which decreases urinary output of water and salt by kidney—which terminates in oedema.
     - —Diminished blood supply to kidney leads them to secrete renin which cause formation of angiotensin II which causes secretion of aldosterone hormone by adrenal gland. All these factors lead to additional retention of salt and water by kidney.
     - —In left heart failure, blood is normally pumped into the lungs by the right heart; but it cannot easily escape from the pulmonary veins through the left heart. All this increases the pulmonary capillary pressure and so serious pulmonary oedema.

EXCESS CAPILLARY PRESSURE V/S OEDEMA

1. Excessive retention of salt + water by kidney
2. High venous pressure: heart failure, venous block.
3. Decreased arteriolar resistance: vasodilator drugs, excess body heat, paralysis of sympathetic nervous system.

Interstitial Fluid Pressure

1. It is -1 to +2 mmHg if measured by direct cannulation method by micropipette
   - — It is -6 mmHg when measured from implanted perforated capsules.
   - — It is -1 to -3 mmHg if measured by means of a cotton wick inserted into a tissue.
2. Role of proteoglycan filaments in interstitium:-
   - — Many nutrients don't diffuse readily through the cell membrane. So without the adequate spacing between the cells these nutrients or waste products cannot be exchanged between blood capillaries and cells. So they act as spacer in space between the cells.
   - — If they are not present then oedematous fluid will flow many times more easily than normal.
3. A sudden increase in total interstitial fluid pressure will increase the interstitial fluid volume. This extra fluid is a free fluid which form large fluid spaces which cannot be kept in tight proteoglycan filaments. This constitutes pitting oedema. One can press the tissue area by thumb to push the fluid out of that area into some other field. When thumb is removed a pit is left in skin for few seconds. This is in contrast with non-pitting oedema which occurs when the cells swell instead of swelling of interstitium or when fluid found in interstitium is clotted with fibrinogen so that it cannot move freely within the tissue spaces.

Plasma Colloid Osmotic Pressure

1. Proteins are only dissolved substances in the plasma which don't diffuse readily through capillary membrane. If any little quantity is diffused into the interstitial fluid it is immediately removed by lymphatic vessels. So concentration of protein is more in plasma (i.e. 7.3 gm/dl) as compared in the interstitial fluid (i.e. 2-3 gm/dl).
2. Now, these are the proteins which cannot pass through the capillary membrane will exert the osmotic pressure. It is called colloid osmotic pressure because protein solution resembles a colloid. On the contrary osmotic pressure which is exerted across the cell membrane is called total osmotic pressure.
3. Normal colloid osmotic pressure of plasma is 28 mmHg (19 mmHg contributed by proteins and 9 mmHg is the contribution given by cations.)
4. In renal nephrosis the glomeruli are damaged so they become leaky towards proteins which may pass into urine. This proteins loss decreases the colloid osmotic pressure which causes excessive filtration of fluid from tissue capillaries into interstitium. This is generally seen when their level reaches to 2-3 gm/dL.
5. These proteins are negatively charged. To balance electrically positive ions (sodium cations, Na^+) are attracted and bound to these proteins. These extra cations increase the number of osmotically active substances and so osmotic pressure is increased. This is the reason that colloid osmotic pressure of plasma is 50 per cent more than caused by proteins alone (Donnan equilibrium effect).
6. *Plasma contains following proteins:* albumin (molecular weight 69,000) globulin (molecular weight 1,40,000) and fibrinogen (molecular weight 4,00,000). Hence 1 gm of globulin contains only half as many molecules as 1 gm of albumin (and 1 gm of fibrinogen contains only 1/6th as many molecules as 1 gm of albumin). So
   Albumin - 4.5. gm/dl - exert 21.8 mmHg plasma colloid osmotic pressure
   Globulin 2.5 gm/dl exert 6.0 mmHg pressure
   Fibrinogen - 0.3 gm/dl exert 0.2 mmHg pressure
   So as regards capillary dynamics is concerned, it is only albumin which is important since 80 per cent of pressure is created by it. We must remember that osmotic pressure is determined by number of molecules dissolved in a fluid.
7. *Reflection co-efficient:* The plasma protein molecules that cannot cross the capillary wall; are said to be reflected—the opposite of filtered molecule. When all the molecules are reflected; they are said to create reflected co-efficient which is 1.0. It is said to be 0.0 when only one half are reflected. For brain it is 1.0, for liver sinusoids it is 0.0, and for muscles it approaches 1.0.

Interstitial Fluid Colloid Osmotic Pressure

1. The total quantity of protein in entire 12 litres of interstitial fluid is actually greater than total quantity of protein in plasma.
2. Because volume of this interstitial fluid is four times than plasma. So its average protein concentration is 40 per cent of that in plasma, i.e. 3 gm/dl.

SUMMARY AND HIGHLIGHTS

- Lymph is a tissue fluid that enters the lymphatic vessels. It drains into venous blood via the thoracic and right lymphatic ducts. Lymphocytes enter the circulation through the lymphatics and there are appreciable numbers of lymphocytes in thoracic duct's lymph. Its protein content is lower than plasma. Water insoluble fats are absorbed from intestine into lymphatics, and lymph in thoracic duct after a meal is milky because of its high fat content. It contains clotting factors and clots on standing in vitro.
- Lymph vessels have valves that prevent backflow. Skeletal muscle contraction push the lymph towards the heart. Such contractions plus contraction of walls of lymphatic duct are principal factors propelling the lymph. Agents increasing the lymph flow are called 'lymphogogues' which act by increasing capillary permeability and by increasing contraction of smooth muscles.
- The walls of the lymphatics are permeable to macro-molecules, and proteins are returned to blood stream through lymphatics (25–50% of total plasma proteins are returned daily). Transport of absorbed long chain fatty acids and cholesterol from intestine occurs through lymphatics.

BIBLIOGRAPHY

1. Leak LV. The structure of lymphatic capillaries in lymph formation. Fed Proc 1976;35:1863-71.
2. Leak LV, JF Burke. Ultra structural studies on lymphatic anchoring filaments. J Cell Bio 1968;36:129-49.
3. Zweifach BW. Microcirculation. Ann Rev Phy 1973;35:117-150.

QUESTION BANK

1. **Explain:**
   a. Nature has provided biconcave shape to erythrocytes. Why?
   b. Blood remains in fluid state within the body. How?
   c. Platelets seal the bleeding point. How?
   d. Red cell count is persistently higher at high altitude. Why?
   e. Clot is dissoluted after some time. How?
   f. Kidney shut down occurs with mismatched transfusion. Why?
   g. Stages of erythropoiesis. With labelled diagram/graph. (Raj. Univ. First M.B.B.S., 2001)
2. **Discuss the following:**
   a. Prevention and treatment of Rh incompatibility.
   b. Fate of erythrocytes.
   c. Plasma proteins. (Raj. Univ. First M.B.B.S., 1995)
   d. Physiological basis of diagnosis and treatment of anaemia. (Raj. Univ. 1992, M.D.)
   e. The mechanism of blood coagulation. Describe conditions in which defect in clotting mechanism produce excessive bleeding. (Raj. Univ. 1979, M.D.).
3. **Enumerate the differences between:**
   a. Large lymphocyte and monocyte.
   b. Haemophilia and purpura.
   c. Foetal haemoglobin and adult haemoglobin.
   d. Extrinsic and intrinsic pathway of coagulation.
   e. T and B lymphocyte.
4. **Write short notes on:**
   a. Immunity. (Raj. Univ. First M. B. B. S. 1995)
   b. Formation and function of Lymph.
   c. Functions of Spleen.
   d. Antigen-antibody reaction.
   e. Properties of leucocytes.
   f. Immunoglobulin. (Raj. Univ. 1996, M.D. 1995)
   g. Specific acquired immunity. (Raj. Univ. 1995, M.D.)
   h. Haemostasis. (Raj. Univ. 1994, M.D.)
   i. Iron channels (Raj. Univ. 1992, M.D.), Iron absorption. (Raj. Univ., First M.B.B.S., 1995)
   j. Rh factor. (Raj. Univ. 1992, M.D.)
   k. Haemophilia. (Raj. Univ. 1990, 1992, M.D.)
   l. Fibrinolysis. (Raj. Univ. 1980, 1990 M.D.)
   m. Tests for bleeding disorders. (Raj. Univ. 1992, M.D.)
   n. Autoimmune disease. (Raj. Univ. 1981, 1989, 1991, M.D.)
   o. Subgroups of ABO system. (Raj. Univ. 1990, M.D.)
   p. Thalassaemia. (Raj. Univ. 1990, M.D.)
   q. Agranulocytosis. (Raj. Univ. 1986, M.D.)
   r. Anticoagulants. (Raj. Univ. First M. B. B. S. 1995)
   s. Erythroblastosis foetalis. (Raj. Univ. First M.B.B.S., 2001)
   t. Erythropietin - BF/2003/08 M.D.
   u. Leucotriens - BF/2003/M.D.
5. **Describe blood groups. What are the hazards of mismatched blood transfusion? (Raj. Univ. First M.B.B.S., 1995)**
6. **Describe picture of normal bone marrow. What clinical information may be derived from its study. (Raj. Univ. 1982, M.D.)**
7. **Describe physiological basis and methods employed for storage of blood and its constituents for transfusion purpose. (Raj. Univ. 1982, M.D.)**
8. **What will happen and why: (Raj. Univ. First M.B.B.S., 2001)**
   i. To the clotting time in a patient with factor VIII deficiency.
   ii. To a patient with decreased platelet count.
   iii. To a patient with anaemic hypoxia.
   iv. To a patient with liver disease.
   v. To the urine colour in a patient of acute glomerular nephritis.

MULTIPLE CHOICE QUESTIONS : BLOOD

1. **Hypochromic microcytic anaemia occurs in all *except*: (AIIMS—1986, AI—1990)**
   a. Iron deficiency
   b. Thallasaemia
   c. Lead poisoning
   d. Chronic renal failure [ ]
2. **Microcytic anaemia is because of deficiency of: (UPSC—1983, PGI—1988, AMC—1987)**
   a. Iron
   b. Pyridoxine
   c. Vitamin B_{12}
   d. Folic acid [ ]
3. **Concentration of methaemoglobin in blood for cyanosis to manifest is: (UPSC—1986, PGI—1986, AIIMS—1987, AI—1988)**
   a. 5 gm per cent
   b. 2 gm per cent
   c. 1.5 gm per cent
   d. 0.5 gm per cent [ ]
4. **Best test for assessing the functions for platelet is: (AIIMS—1985)**
   a. Bleeding time
   b. Clotting time
   c. Clot retraction time
   d. Prothrombin time [ ]
5. **Human T and B cells originate from: (Delhi—1988)**
   a. Thymus and bursa
   b. Thymus and bone marrow
   c. Thyroid and bursa
   d. Thalamus and bone marrow [ ]
6. **In thrombocytopenia there is: (Delhi—1990)**
   a. Increased clotting time
   b. Increased bleeding time
   c. Both of the above
   d. None of the above [ ]
7. **Macrocytes in peripheral blood cells are seen in: (Delhi—1986)**
   a. Liver disease
   b. Aplastic anaemia

c. B_{12} and folate deficiency
d. CRF [ ]

8. In haemophilia B which factor is deficient: (Delhi—1983)
a. Factor V
b. Factor VII
c. Factor VIII
d. Factor IX [ ]

9. All are iron containing *except*: (PGI—1984)
a. Myoglobin
b. Catalase
c. Ceruloplasmin
d. Cytochrome oxidase [ ]

10. All are Vitamin K dependent factor *except*: (PGI—1982)
a. II b. V
c. VII d. IX [ ]

ANSWERS: MCQs

1 c **2** a **3** c **4** c **5** a **6** b **7** c **8** d **9** c **10** b

VIVA-VOCE : BLOOD

1. Enumerate the functions of Plasma Proteins
- i. Maintenance of colloid osmotic pressure
- ii. Maintenance of acid-base balance (Buffer)
- iii. Carriage of carbon dioxide (As carbamino-compounds)
- iv. Assisting in rouleaux formation through fibrinogen and globulin
- v. Immune body production
- vi. Maintenance of viscosity
- vii. Protein reserve
- viii. Assisting in repairing of damaged tissues
- ix. Fluid interchange between blood and tissue is regulated
- x. Carriage of some other substances (lipid, mucopolysaccharides cholesterol, steroids, phospholipids, bilirubin, hormones, metals, drugs etc.)
- xi. Blood clotting factors like fibrinogen, prothrombin are carried.

2. Why blood remains in a fluid state within the body?
- i. The blood remains in continuous circulation which does not allow platelets to agglutinate.
- ii. Smoothness of endothelium which prevents contact activation of intrinsic clotting system.
- iii. A monomolecular layer of negatively charged proteins adsorbed to inner surface of endothelium that repels clotting factors as well as platelets.
- iv. Fibrin threads which are formed during clotting process and an alpha globulin called antithrombin prevent clotting by removing thrombin from blood.
- v. Heparin formed by mast cells and basophils, prevent coagulation.

3. What are the peculiarities of foetal haemoglobin (HbF)?
Outstanding functional characteristic of it is that its oxygen dissociation curve shows a marked shift to left as compared with adult haemoglobin. As a result foetal blood can take up much large volumes of oxygen than adult blood at low oxygen pressure. Thus at 20 mm O_2 pressure foetal haemoglobin is 70 per cent saturated, at 40 mm. it is 90 per cent saturated.

4. Enumerate differences between Monocyte and large Lymphocyte :

	Monocyte	*Large Lymphocyte*
1.	Size-biggest (14–21 μ)	10–14 μ
2.	Nucleus cytoplasm ratio-2/3 part of cell is nucleus; remaining cytoplasm.	3/4 part of cell is nucleus and remaining cytoplasm
3.	Mostly eccentric nucleus	Mostly central nucleus
4.	Function highly phagocytic	Antibody formation
5.	Fine chromatin threads	Coarse chromatin threads
6.	In DLC-4-8 or 10 per cent	20-40 or 15-35 per cent (Including small lymphocyte)

5. What is Phagocytosis?
The neurotrophilic polymorphonuclear leucocyte along with monocyte and other RE cells constitute most important elements which body possesses for its defence against invading micro-organisms. Their power to attack bacteria and then to ingest it is phagocytosis (By Metchnikoff : Phago = I eat). Phagocytic vesicles thus formed fuse with granules of neutrophils. Granules contain various lytic enzymes and a system generating O_2 radical (Superoxide), H_2O_2 is formed and most bacteria are killed. It is also associated with marked transient increase O_2 consumption of cell and increased glucose metabolism via hexose monophosphate shunt.

6. What is erythrocyte sedimentation rate and tell about its variations?
In circulation red cells are uniformly suspended in plasma. But when a sample of citrated blood is taken and kept in a tube (standing); erythrocytes being heavier than plasma settle down, called sedimentation. It is of much prognostic value than diagnostic one. It is increased in various diseases like pulmonary tuberculosis,

malignancy, septicaemia, anaemia while decreased in allergy, protein shock. Specific gravity, rouleaux, viscosity, haemoglobin are factors determining it.

7. **What are the advantages of peculiar discoid shape of RBC ?**
   i. Gases can diffuse freely to every part.
   ii. RBC can mould their shape on passing through narrow capillaries
   iii. Haemoglobin remains distributed in a very thin layer
   iv. It allows considerable alteration of cell volume without increasing tension on cell membrane so it can resist haemolysis and can withstand considerable changes in osmotic pressure.

8 **What are hazards of mismatched transfusion?**
   i. Agglutination of red cells and haemolysis.
   ii. Jaundice due to breakdown of erythrocytes.
   iii. Haemoglobinurea (part of released haemoglobin is excreted in urine)
   iv. Renal failure (anurea; uraemia).

9. **What is Landsteiner's Law?**
   "If an agglutinogen is present in blood red blood cells, the corresponding agglutinin must be absent from plasma. if agglutinogen is absent, corresponding agglutinin must be present."

10. **Comment on haemolytic disease of newborn?**
   The changes in foetus may be termed as haemolytic diseases.
   a. Icterus-gravid-neonatorum-infant is haemolytic jaundiced. There may be no anaemia at birth since excess red blood cells destruction is compensated by intense normoblastic response of marrow with high reticulocyte count and presence of many nucleated cells (erythroblastosis foetalis). But anaemia may develop in first few days since rate of RBC destruction by anti D is maximal at birth. There may be severe neurological lesions involving basal ganglia which may stain bright yellow with bile pigment (kern-icterus). Liver may be severely damaged.
   b. Best treatment is exchange transfusion.
   c. If mother is Rh^{-ve} father is Rh^{+ve} foetus is Rh^{+ve} serious complications may occur. Cells containing D may pass across placenta from foetus to mother, latter responding by forming anti D which destroy foetal cells.

UNIT 10

Rhythm of Life

"Heart is a double cylinder pump. The Myocardium is unique among muscles that it can never rest for a period of time. If pump ceases to work, life ends."

Cardio-vascular System-I

71 Heart—Cardiac Muscle and General Concepts

INTRODUCTORY OUTLINE

a. Human heart is four chambered double pump; the right and left auricles and right-left ventricles.
b. It is located in middle mediastinum, placed obliquely behind body of sternum as well as adjoining portions of ribs and cartilage, in between two lungs.
c. 280–350 gm is the ideal weight of male heart while female heart weighs in between 250–280 gm (average 336 gm). It constitutes about 0.43 per cent of total body weight in males while 0.4 per cent in females.
d. It is enveloped in a double layered membrane called 'pericardium'. Thin slimy pericardial fluid is present between its two coats.
e. It is 12 cm from base to apex and 6 cm antero-posteriorly.
f. So called two auricles are separated from each other by 'interatrial septum' which is fibrous in nature. Two ventricles are partitioned by 'interventricular septum' whose upper one fourth is membranous while lower three fourth portion is muscular.
g. Functions of pericardium:
   i. Heart and adjacent structures are separated by it.
   ii. It is capable of resisting diastolic expansion which is more profound with right ventricle.
   iii. It is forming a receptacle.
   iv. Its inelastic resistant fibres are capable of protecting heart from sudden and excessive dilatation.

PATTERN OF CIRCULATION

a. The blood is pumped to entire body by left ventricle through aorta. This blood which is distributed to entire body gets impured (de-oxygenated). This blood from whole parts of body returns to right atrium from where it is pumped to right ventricle which pumps it to pulmonary arteries which takes it to lungs for oxygenation (since in lungs, gaseous exchange occurs). Re-oxygenated blood is returned to left atrium which pumps it to left ventricle which cyclically pumps it to distant cells of body once again. Left ventricle is the pumping station.
b. So, it can be better divided into
   i. 'Systemic or greater circulation' which begins at aorta extending to vena cava and emptying into right atrium; and
   ii. 'Pulmonary or lesser circulation' which consists of right ventricles, pulmonary venules, veins and left atrium.

HEART

It squeezes out about 2½ ounces of blood at every beat. It daily pumps at least 2,500 gallons of blood.

VALVES AND THEIR ACTION

i. It is desired that circulation should be unidirectional one, not allowing the arterial and venous blood to mix with each other and this is made possible by presence of valves.
ii. Mainly there are two sets of valve (total four); one is atrioventricular (AV valves) and second is semilunar valves. Amongst the first AV valves, one is that which guards opening between right atrium and right ventricle called 'tricuspid valve' and similarly left atrioventricular opening is guarded by 'bicuspid or mitral valve' (valve with two cusps). Amongst semilunar series—one is between left ventricle and aorta on left side and second is on right side between right ventricle and pulmonary artery.
iii. So in nutshell AV valves prevent backflow of blood from ventricles to atria during systole while semilunar valves prevent backflow from aorta and pulmonary artery into ventricles during diastole.
iv. *Atrioventricular valves* (tricuspid on right and bicuspid/mitral on left).

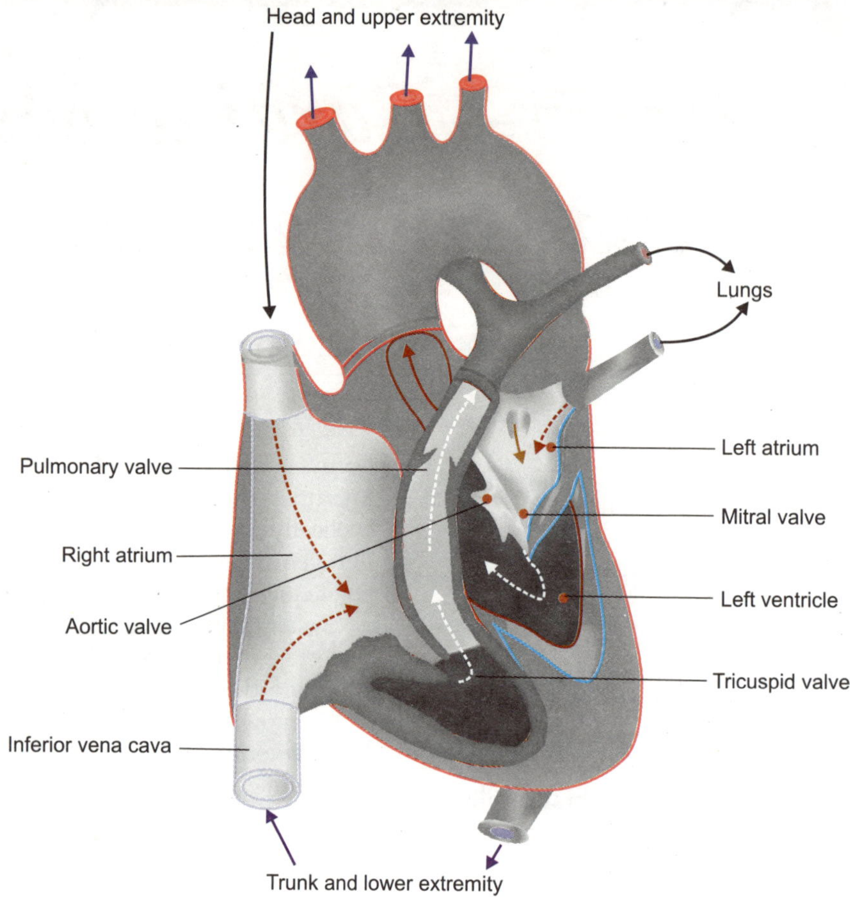

Fig. 71.1: Heart: An overview

- The valve between right atrium and right ventricle is made up of three cusps hence named, 'tricuspid valve' while 'mitral valve or bicuspid' is the name given to valve on left side located between left atrium and ventricle because of two cusps or leaflets.
- Means valve leaflets/cusps three on right and two on left side. These are attached by their bases to fibrous rings surrounding AV openings. Their free margins are connected through delicate tendons, i.e. chordae tendinae to the papillary muscles which prevent inversion of valves into the auricle during systole of ventricles.
- The leaflets are composed of double layer of endothelial lining of the heart. Few connective tissues have been also mentioned.
- The chordae tendinae are tightened at the commencement of systole by the contraction of papillary muscle.
- *Valve closure: A fairy tale:* During atrial systole, the leaflets of these valves occupy a mid position because of two currents of opposing nature. The inflowing blood pressing upon their atrial surfaces keep them open on the opposite side, eddies reflected in reverse direction from the ventricular walls strike their ventricular surfaces and tend to close them. In this way they float in a position of delicate balance.
- Now, at the end of atrial systole, a fall in intra-atrial pressure takes place; this incoming jet is diminished in force and it finally ceases. The eddies persist for a while and now being unopposed they cause approximation of the valves.

Semilunar valves

- The valves between right ventricle and pulmonary artery as well as between left ventricle and aorta are three cup like cusps attached to valve rings (semi = half; lunar = moon; so half moon shaped).
- The dynamics of their closure is also the same. The valves form three small pockets opening towards the arterial lumen. During ejection phase of systole, back eddies are set up which

prevent the contact of the valve with the arterial wall. As the ejection is complete the centripetal currents carry the valves into opposition. Higher pressure is also created upon their arterial surfaces and this facilitates their firm closure.

AURICLE

1. The two auricles (atria), are separated from each other by 'inter-auricular septum' which is made up of 'septum primum' (having an opening called foramen ovale) and 'septum secundum' (unperforated one).
2. Right auricle gets deoxygenated blood while left one gets oxygenated blood.
3. Auricular appendages is the name given to a flap like projection of atria when they are in a contracted state and it extends a short distance over the ventricle.
4. Since it receives blood from various parts of body it is called 'receiving chamber'.

VENTRICLES

i. Since it supplies blood to various parts of body it is called 'distributing chamber' so it functions as pump.
ii. It is comparatively more thick walled as compared to auricles.
iii. The two ventricles are partitioned by 'inter-ventricular septum' whose upper one-fourth is membranous while lower three-fourth is muscular.
iv. Its membrane is thrown into series of irregular muscular ridges named as 'trabeculae carneae', and are modified into 'chorda tendinae' between valve and wall of ventricle to regulate valve activities
v. On the whole it is a lower large thick walled well muscularised structure.
vi. 'Chordae tendinae' are modified into 'papillary muscles' to make them more powerful.

JUNCTIONAL TISSUES OF HEART

By this we mean some specialised tissues which are concerned with initiation and conduction of cardiac impulse through myocardium together with muscular contraction. These are two nodal tissues, bundle of His, Purkinje fibres.

Sinus-atrial Node (SA Node)

i. It is the place from where human heart starts its impulse so it is designated as 'pacemaker'.
ii. It is 1 cm long and 3 mm wide. Its fibres are of 3-5 microns in diameter. It is broad at one end while tapering below.
iii. It is shaped like English letter 'C'.
iv. Proof of pacemakership... Its inactivation or destruction results into slowing or cessation of auricular or ventricular contraction. If its temperature is raised heart rate is accelerated while cooling results into diminished heart rate.
It is the first part to become electrically active as compared to other parts of heart.
v. It generates so called cardiac impulse at the rate of 70-80/minute. This rate of impulse generation is certainly greatest as compared with other parts. Now this impulse is discharged or conducted to AV node and thence to Purkinje fibres. After this all these tissues start their recovery phase. The beauty is that SA node recovers rapidly or earliest and starts new impulse before other two tissues reach their threshold for further self-excitation. So more clearly an impulse from SA node will always depolarise these tissues before either of them could initiate a rhythm. Thus, it acts as a 'pacemaker'. A 'pacemaker' elsewhere than SA node is termed as 'ectopic pacemaker' and AV node as well as Pukrinje fibres generally become these sites.
vi. It is embedded in right atrial wall near entrance of superior vena cava. It is supplied by right vagus nerve.

Atrio (or Auriculo) Ventricular Node

i. It is located near the posterior margin of interatrial septum near the entrance of coronary sinus into the right atrium.
ii. Impulse is received by it from SA node, (through atrial muscle and internodal pathways) which further is transmitted to ventricles via atrioventricular bundle. When SA node fails, it is said to take over the function of it. So it is better to say that it can generate its own impulse but at a slower rate (40-60 per minute) which is called 'nodal rhythm'.

Bundle of His and Purkinje Fibres

i. It is the communication for propagation of cardiac impulse from atria to ventricles.
ii. From AV node, common bundle takes its origin which divides into right and left branch which courses on either side of inter-ventricular septum, of course through subendocardium, and lastly through heart muscles forming so called 'Purkinje fibres' the specialised conducting tissue of heart, which finally merges with ventricular musculature (of course penetrating into them for a short distance before merging).

iii. Left bundle branch is a long one while right branch is a small prolongation of common bundle. Base of anterior papillary muscle is the site where right bundle branch is first making its contact with ventricular muscle while on the contrary, left endocardial surface of inter-ventricular septum little away from aortic valve is the usual site where left bundle branch first makes its contact with ventricular muscle.
iv. Functions—On failure of both SA and AV nodes, bundle of His is capable of generating its own impulse, of course at a slower rate (30–40 per minute).
Impulse is conducted from atria to ventricles at a rate of 5 metres per second.

Internodal Tracts

- These are nothing but specialised tracts connecting SA node to left atrium and AV node. So these are preferential pathways for impulse conduction.
- The anterior tract is probably the main structure which further bifurcates into two towards left side. One branch extends over left atrium (Bachmann's bundle) along dorsal aspect of inter-atrial band while second merges with AV node by coursing through interatrial septum.
- The middle tract originates from posterolateral part of pacemaker SA node and reaches to AV node through inter-atrial septum.
- The posterior tract of course arises from SA node and reaches to upper border of AV node by passing along the crista terminalis.

NORMAL CARDIAC METABOLISM DETERMINANTS

- Cardiac muscle is having basic chemical patterns which is similar with skeletal muscle.
- Heart is choosing its fuel from foodstuffs like glucose, lactate, pyruvate, fatty acids-both esterified and non-esterified, acetate, amino acids etc.
- Under post prandial condition (after infusing glucose) myocardial metabolism is mainly glucose, lactate, pyruvate since its RQ is 0.9.
- During over night fasting heart derives energy from fat.
- Patients with heart failure/decreased cardiac work/ valvular disease, show an increased carbohydrate uptake by the heart.
- The heart of patients with diabeties mellitus derives energy from fats with a post absorptive RQ of 0.7, an increased uptake of fatty acids and a decreased carbohydrate uptake.
- The basal O_2 consumption of myocardium is 2 ml/ 100 gm/minute; while of beating heart is 9 ml/100 gm/minute. It increases during exercise. Increase in O_2 consumption requires increase in coronary flow.
- The O_2 consumption of the heart is determined by contractile state of myocardium, intramyocardial tension and the heart rate. Ventricular work per beat correlates with O_2 consumption. This work is the product of stroke volume and mean arterial pressure in the pulmonary artery for right ventricle and aorta for left ventricle.
- Since aortic pressure is seven times greater than pulmonary artery pressure, the stroke work of left ventricle is seven times more than right ventricle.
- In aortic stenosis intraventricular pressure must be increased to force blood through stenotic valve; whereas in aortic insufficiency, regurgitation of blood produces an increase in stroke volume with little change in aortic impedance. This is the reason that angina pectoris is more common in aortic stenosis than in aortic insufficiency.

ELECTROPHYSIOLOGY OF CARDIAC MUSCLE

i. It is well known fact that normally cardiac muscle possesses 80–85 mV's resting ***membrane potential*** and action potential is approximately 100–105 mV. It is worth remembering that cardiac muscle exhibits characteristic action potential. The membrane remains depolarised for roughly 0.15–0.3 seconds after the initial spike represented by so called 'plateau' and at the end of which repolarisation starts. All this causes increased period of contraction and action potential lasts for approximately 20–50 times as long as seen in skeletal muscle.
ii. *Cardiac muscle is refractory to restimulation during this spike of action potential.* This is better called 'functional refractory period (approximately 0.25 seconds long) meaning by 'the interval of time during which an action potential from another part of heart fails to re-excite an already excited area of cardiac muscle. Besides this there is also 'relative refractory period' (0.05 second duration) during which also the cardiac muscle cannot be re-excited. Due to this long refractory period heart muscle can neither be fatigued nor tatanized.
iii. *The cause of this above mentioned 'plateau' is two fold.* One view states that during plateau conductance of membrane for potassium is less than normal, (as compared with case of skeletal muscle), which impedes leakage of potassium out of fibre and hence recovery from depolarisation is checked. Second

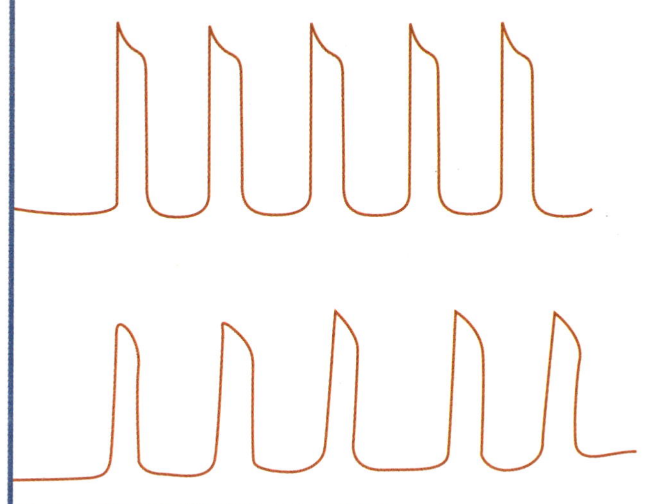

Fig. 71.2: Cardiac contraction: 'Plateau'

view holds that large quantities of calcium ions are diffusing inwards through membrane during depolarisation activity so depletion of calcium ions occurs outside the membrane. This is sufficient enough to further decrease membrane permeability to potassium.

Now as the 'plateau' ends and recovery starts, sufficient calcium ions diffuse to depleted area restoring normal permeability and thus leading to beginning of repolarisation process.

iv. *Excitation contraction coupling:* Besides above mentioned action potential, excitation and contraction are coupled and the bridging activity is performed by calcium ions. So along with depolarisation calcium ions are released which binds troponin, which then dislodges tropomyosine from myosin reactive sites, so leading to interaction between myosin and actin together with increased ATPase activity. It is worth recalling that calcium ions are stored normally in lateral sac of sarcoplasmic reticulum during resting state, together with the fact that extracellular fluid is additional source of these calcium ions in case of cardiac muscle. As depolarisation is gone these calcium ions return back to their original site, resulting in so called relaxation.

It is said that contraction in cardiac muscle begins, few millisecond after onset of action potential and it continues to contract for few millisecond after end of action potential.

It is also true that greater the strength of action potential with its longer duration, more will be the work output of cardiac muscle contraction.

viii. *Pacemaker potential (Pre-potential):* It seems astonishing at a glance that SA node the pacemaker bears membrane potential of 60 to 65 mV only (as compared with cardiac muscle–80-85 mV). The first explanation for this is 'high membrane conductance of these fibres for sodium' which results into rapid sodium leakage through membrane which is responsible for self-excitation of pacemaker, owing to re-establishment of resting potential each time. Then it declines and at this point suddenly action potential develops lasting for roughly 0.15 seconds. As action potential ends, membrane conductivity for potassium is increased resulting into discharge of positive charge outside (potassium) so terminating into increased negative charge inside fibres originating thus so called 'hyperpolarisation'. As conductivity for potassium is decreased, again rapid influx for sodium is occurring and in this way cycle continues keeping heart in rhythmic action.

CARDIAC PACEMAKER (ARTIFICIAL)

- It is used to correct an insufficient or irregular heart beat. It corrects the low cardiac rhythm through electrical stimulation which increases the contraction of heart muscle.
- It is weighing from 1–4.5 ounces (30–130 gm) and is a hermetically sealed titanium metal, and powdered by a lithium battery which can last for 2–15 years.
- A pacemaker has a gold or platinum electrodes, conducting wires and a pacing box (miniature generator). They are of two types—those implanted in chest or an external.
- In every case the electrode is attached to the heart's right ventricle, either directly through the chest, or threaded through a vein.

BASIC PROPERTIES OF CARDIAC MUSCLE

Cardiac muscle is possessing some inherent properties like:

a. *Rhythmicity:* Heart muscle contractions are rhythmic and it does not contract in half hazard way. SA node being pacemaker of heart generates impulse at highest rate of 70–90 beats per minute constituting 'sinus rhythm'. If it fails due to any reason, AV node generates impulse at comparatively slower rate 40–60 beats per minute constituting 'nodal rhythm'. If it too fails ventricular muscles are capable of generating impulse but at slowest rate 15–40 beats per minute. What actually to be told is that generation and transmission of cardiac impulse is existing in regular sequential contractile phenomenon.

b. *Conductivity:* Impulse generated normally from SA node, reaches AV node within 0.05 seconds (50 milliseconds) after spreading to atria. Here at AV node a delay of 0.08 second occurs and then this cardiac impulse reaches bundle. From here the cardiac impulse makes the ventricles its destination by exciting septum—papillary muscle in endocardial surface and then its epicardial surface. Then it travels to first outer walls of ventricles—first to left and then to right ventricle. From here impulse goes to lateral wall of left ventricle. It finally terminates to base of right ventricle somewhere in vicinity of left ventricle. It is worth recalling that conduction speed is maximum in Purkinje fibres as 4 metre per second, while atria conducts at 1 metre per second speed whereas speed of ventricle is only 0.04 metre per second.

c. *Excitability and Automaticity/Irritability:* As told previously it is the inherent quality of cardiac muscle to generate propagated action potentials spontaneously. The factors affecting excitability are as follows:

   i. *Nutrition:* This includes nutrients as well as oxygen. It is the diastolic pause which provides these nutrients since at this time, most of blood flow through coronary arteries occur. Heart needs approximately 450–550 ml of oxygen per minute. If oxygen supply is less than this, extrasystoles or premature beats occur. It is worth recalling that oxygen is required for proper utilisation of nutrients which will provide energy to myocardium of course if oxygen lack persists for a much longer time fatal results are met in the form of ventricular fibrillation and heart stoppage.

   ii. *Environmental temperature:* Temperature upto 40°C stimulates all the processes, i.e. de and repolarisation, while low temperature makes heart slow.

   iii. *Nerve fibres:* Cardiac muscle is not dependent on its nervous connections since no degenerative changes are observed in cardiac muscle on severing nervous connections. Excitability is said to be depressed on vagus stimulation or acetylcholine administration while it is accelerated on sympathetic stimulation.

   It is to be remembered that excitability is defined as ability of responding on any stimulus which may be electrical, thermal, chemical or mechanical one of course automaticity and rhythmicity are deeply inter-connected with each other. Excitability produces following changes in cardiac muscle viz. electrical, mechanical, thermal and chemical.

   Electrical ...... already dealt

   Chemical ..... ATP is converted into ADP and phosphoric acid. Myosin filaments slide past protein actin leading to breaking of bands which terminates into muscular contraction. As muscle relaxes, ATP is reformed.

   Thermal ...... Due to muscular contraction there occurs heat production.

   Mechanical ...... Shortening (increased tension) is the effect.

d. *Contractility and distensibility:* As already dealt the 'action potential' and 'excitation contraction coupling' are leading to contractility which means activity of cardiac muscle cell which either shorten or develop tension and perform work. Relaxation (coming back of muscles to their original length) is following the contraction which is distensibility. Following are some factors affecting contractility -

   i. *Stimulus intensity*: The stimulus of course must be of some threshold value.

   ii. *Initial tension:* It will better contract if initial tension is high as told by 'Starling law' that, 'energy for contraction is proportional to initial length of muscle fibre.'

   iii. *Stimulus timings:* This has been already dealt with importance of refractory periods.

   'Absolute refractory period' is lasting during entire depolarisation period and any stimulus will fail to excite cardiac muscle during this phase.

   Relative refractory period tends to discourage the occurrence of second contraction before sufficient time has elapsed to allow complete relaxation of muscle from a preceding contraction.

   Effective refractory period is the interval with the time of absolute refractory period during which cells produce graded response which is not conducted.

   iv. *Hypoxia:* Slight hypoxia accelerates contractility while it is depressed due to severe oxygen lack.

   v. *Drugs:* Adrenaline stimulates while acetylcholine depress it.

   vi. *Nerves:* Sympathetic accelerates while vagus inhibits.

   vii. *Temperature:* Temperature above 45°C leads to coagulation of contractile proteins so causes cessation of contractile process. Upto 40°C stimulatory effects are seen.

READ AND DIGEST: CARDIAC PECULIARITIES

Q. What are the peculiarities of excitation-contraction coupling mechanism in relation with T tubules?

Ans.

- Sarcoplasmic reticulum of cardiac muscle is less well developed than that of skeletal muscle and it does not store enough calcium to provide full contraction.
- Besides above weakness, Nature has provided following positive points for compensation-
  — Diameter of T tubules is five times greater,
  — Volume of T tubules is twenty five times greater
  — Inside T tubules, there is a large quantity of mucopolysaccharide which is negatively charged, so it binds positively charged calcium ions.

Q. The strength of contraction of cardiac muscle depends on Ca^{2+} ion concentration of extracellular fluid. How?

Ans. The ends of T tubules open directly to outside of cardiac muscle fibres. This facilitates the passage of extracellular fluid from cardiac muscle interstitium to T tubules. This causes availability of Ca^{2+}.

e. *Tonicity:* Tone is sustained minimal contraction of muscle in order to maintain posture as well as in regulating the volume of a substance contained in hollow organ. Cardiac muscle is not possessing true tone like that of skeletal muscle, since electrical impulses are generated just proceeding systole but not during diastole. But when ventricles are filled during systole, cardiac muscles are said to possess tone in order to regulate its volume.

READ AND DIGEST: CARDIAC IMPULSE

Q. How the cardiac impulse begins?

Ans. The action potential which develops in SA node, travel into surrounding atrial muscle fibres. It eventually spreads to AV node (velocity of conduction in atrial muscle is 0.3 m/sec.). There are three types of (anterior-middle and posterior) inter-nodal-fibres which conducts at a rapid velocity (1 m/sec.). This is because of the fact that there are present special conduction fibres mixed with atrial muscle. These fibres curve through the atrial wall and terminate in AV node.

Q. There is delay in AV node. How much and why?

Ans.

- The impulse reaches AV node 0.03 sec after its origin from SA node.
- Then within AV node, there is a further delay of 0.09 seconds.
- A final delay of 0.04 sec. occurs mainly in penetrating portion of AV-bundle. So total delay in AV nodal system is 0.09 + 0.04 = 0.13 sec.
- Causes of slow conduction are:
  — The resting membrane potential of these fibres is comparatively less negative than of normal cardiac muscle.
  — Very few gap junctions are existing. This provides great resistance for ionic movement from one fibre to the next.

Q. Then what happens to cardiac impulse?

Ans. Then there are Purkinje fibres which are coming into action. Their velocity of conduction is 1.5 to 4 m/sec. which means approximately five to six times that usually occurs in cardiac muscle or one fifty times of that occurring in transitional fibres.

Q. What can be the cause of this fast conduction?

Ans. The causes include:

- Increased permeability of gap junctions at intercalated discs between successive cardiac cells.
- Purkinje fibres have very few myofibrils.

Q. Can cardiac impulse be regurgitated?

Ans. No. Impulse is conducted one way. Impulse is prevented from entering in auricles from ventricles.

Q. How it is possible?

Ans. There is a fibrous barrier which separates atrial and ventricular muscles. This acts as an insulator.

Q. What is the next course?

Ans.

1. Purkinje fibres are distributed in the ventricles. The distal portion of AV-bundle passes downward in ventricular septum towards the apex of 'heart. Then bundle divides into left and right branches beneath endocardium. Each branch spreads downwards to apex of ventricle. There it divides into smaller branches which course around each ventricle and back towards base of heart.
2. It takes 0.03 seconds to travel from first entry at bundle to termination of Purkinje fibres.
3. The velocity of conduction in ventricle is 0.3 to 0.5 m/sec (1/6th of Purkinje system).
4. The cardiac muscle wraps around the heart in a double spiral fashion; of course fibrous septa are existing between two spiral layers. So, the cardiac impulse travels along direction of spirals. This transmission from endocardial to epicardial surface takes another 0.03 sec. So total 0.03 + 0.03 = 0.06 sec time is taken from initial bundle branch to last ventricular muscle fibre.

FACTORS AFFECTING CONTRACTILE RESPONSE

1. *Intensity of stimulation:* The existence of contractile response depends upon intensity of stimulus. If a normal silent ventricle is excited directly by electric shocks of increasing intensity, all stimuli above threshold result in contractions of the same amplitude, i.e. all or nothing response (Bowditch 1871).

2. *Spacing of stimuli:*
   - In the beating heart, stimuli are generally not effective during the period of contraction since the muscle remains depolarised throughout the period of contraction—(absolute refractory period).
   - During early relaxation, excitability increases progressively, but only stimuli still stronger than normal are effective—(relative refractory period).
   - These periods prevent the passage of a second impulse over the heart until the proceeding contraction is over. This relaxes the ventricles and allows them to fill with the blood before another contraction can occur. It also permits maximum development of tension by the myocardium.
   - The long refractory periods of cardiac muscle preserve the cardiac rhythm. The absolute period makes the summation of contraction and thus causes production of tetanus impossible. The relative refractory period leads to complete relaxation of muscle from the proceeding contraction.
   - The absolute refractory period—is shortened by a rise in temperature, by rapid heart action, and by vagal stimulation (only atrial).
   - It is also possible that an effective stimulus not coming from SA node affect the cardiac rhythm. A long pause follows the contraction caused by the artificial stimulus. This artificially induced contraction is called extrasystole/premature contraction. Compensatory pause is the name given to the long interval following the extra systole.
3. *Stretch and its effect:* When an isolated ventricular strip is stretched moderately then tension of it rises. If it is then stimulated electrically, the amplitude and duration of its contraction is increased. Or in other words "intraventricular pressure rises on increase of intraventricular volume"—which is increased by any one of the following means:
   - Vagal stimulation,
   - Exit of blood from the ventricle is blocked,
   - Blood return to the heart is increased.
4. Other factors:
   - Myocardial hypoxia, an increase in muscle temperature, an increase in blood calcium level—increase the force of contraction.
   - Factors decreasing the contractile force are—decrease in temperature, increased concentration of Mg^{++} and K^{+}, coronary occlusion etc.

STARLING LAW OF HEART

i. In a more formalised way Starling (1914) proposed that, energy for contraction is proportional to the initial length of muscle fibres.

ii. Whenever extra amounts of blood enter the heart chamber, certainly muscle contracts with a great force because of concerning interaction of actin and myosin filaments. All this is due to stretching of heart muscle which results into pumping extra quantity of blood into circulation. All this is classed as 'Heterometric autoregulation' of heart.'

iii. Besides this another mechanism in this respect is 'Homeometric autoregulation of heart' which states that it is the increased metabolism due to stretching which effects pumping capability.

iv. All this is known as 'Frank-Starling law'—two great. Physiologists (1895–1914) stating more clearly that, 'Quantity of blood pumped into aorta is directly proportional to filling of heart during diastole (venous return). Still in another way it can be explained as, 'within physiologic limits, heart pumps all the blood which is returned to it without excessive damming of blood in veins.

HEART TRANSPLANTATION

- Dec. 3, 1967 in Capetown South Africa—first heart transplant was performed by Dr. Christian Bernard with his 30 associates. The receiver was Louis Washansky—a 55-year-old wholesale grocer; and donor was Denise Ann Daval (25 years) who was an autoaccident victim. He lived for 18 days and died due to pneumonia.
- In USA, the first heart transplantation was on a 22 week old baby (male) by Dr. Adrian Kantrowitz on 6th December 1967. He lived for 6-7 hours. The place was Macmonides Hospital Brooklyn.
- The first adult in USA to receive heart transplant was Mike Kasperak (54 years) on January 6th, 1968 by Dr. Norman Shumway at Medical Centre in Palo Alto—California. He lived for 14 days.

TOBACCO AND HEART

- Means cigarettes, cigar, pipes, snuffs is more and more dangerous for health. This is associated with ten million cases of cardiovascular pulmonary diseases.
- The inhaled agent in cigarette smoke act directly on mucous membrane, may be swallowed in saliva or may be absorbed into blood stream from abundant capillary alveolar bed. They act on distant target organs, and thus cause disease.

- Maternal smoking damages foetus in various ways. Even ten cigarettes per day can lead to foetal hypoxia-higher foetal carboxy-hoemoglobin level. They all result in prematurity, low birth weight, increased incidences of abortion, premature rupture of membranes, placenta previa etc. etc.
- Lung cancer, bronchitis, emphysema, peptic ulcer, ischaemic heart diseases, hypertension, hypercholesterolaemia, stroke, pyloric reflux, accidents are all consequences of smoking.
- Inhaled cigarette smoke contains 43 known carcinogens—tar, nickel, arsenic, cadmium, chromium, acetaldehyde, phenol, irritants-like nitrogen dioxide and formaldehyde, cilia toxin like hydrogen cyanide and CO. Nicotine is its important constituent which is an alkaloid which readily crosses blood-brain barrier and stimulate nicotine receptor of brain. It is also responsible for addiction and its action is mediated through release of catecholamines.

CARDIAC CATHETERISATION

- It is done for detailed information, about heart, aorta and coronary vessels which cannot be obtained otherwise by other non-invasive method.
- It provides information about pressures in different cardiac chambers and also allows angiography to be carried out.
- It is an important method of determining the need for surgical valve replacement.
- Catheterisation of right heart permits accurate measurement of pulmonary artery pressure. The left atrial pressure is measured indirectly by wedging the right heart catheter in peripheral pulmonary arteriolar vessels.
- It plays an important role in congenital heart diseases. Anatomical site of intracardiac shunt can be defined by sampling the oxygen saturation.

CONCEPT OF LOAD (PRE AND AFTER)

Afterload

When left ventricle contracts blood is ejected in aorta. It is the hydrostatic pressure of the blood in aorta which opposes the ejection. So it acts as a load against ventricular shortening. This is "afterload" and is so named because it begins to operate after the onset of ventricular contraction. If it is on higher side, then force of cardiac contraction will be unable to overcome this afterload leading to isometric contraction of ventricles.

Preload

It simply means "end diastolic volume" Or load which operates before the beginning of contraction.

Preload	*Afterload*
1. It acts on muscle before it begins to contract.	It acts after it begins to contract.
2. Muscle contracts isometrically. Tension in it increases gradually.	Initially muscle contracts isometrically, but in later stages the contraction is isotonically.
3. Partial contraction of contractile component and then stretching of series elastic components.	Complete contraction of contractile component and no further stretching of series elastic components.
4. It is end-diastolic volume	It is the resistance against which ventricles pump the blood.

BIBLIOGRAPHY

1. Bozler E. The initiation of impulses in cardiac muscle. (Quoted by Best and Taylor in Physiological basis of Medical Practice, 1967, Williams and Wilkins). Amer J Phy 1943;133:273.
2. Burton AC. Importance of shape and size of heart. Amer Heart J 1957;34:801-10.
3. Dawes GS, JH Comroe Jr. Chemoreflexes from heart and lungs. Phy Rev 1954;34:167-201.
4. Degeest HMN Levy, et al. Depression of ventricular contractility by stimulation of vagus N. Cir Res 1965;17:222-35.
5. Dow P. Estimation of cardiac output and central blood volume by dye dilution. Phy Rev 1956; 36:77-102.
6. Downing SE, et al. Cardiovascular responses to hypoxia stimulation of carotid bodies. Cir Res 1962;10:676-85.
7. Downing SE, et al. Cardiovascular responses to ischaemia, hypoxia, and hypercapnia of CNS. Amer J Phy 1963;104:881-87.
8. Erashis. Excitation contraction coupling. Ann Rev Phy 1976;38:293-313.
9. Hoffman BF, et al. Electrophysiology of heart. McGraw Hill Book Co. New York 1960. (Quoted by Best and Taylor in Physiological basis of Medical Practice, 1967, Williams and Wilkins).
10. Katz AM. Physiology of heart, 2nd ed. Raven press. (Quoted by Ganong WF in Review of Medical Physiology—Lange Publications). 1992.
11. Lundin G. Mechanical properties of cardiac muscle. (Quoted by Best and Taylor in Physiological basis of Medical Practice, 1967, Williams and Wilkins). Acta Phys Scand 1944;7 supp: 20.
12. Mela Riker LM, et al. Regulation of mitochondrial activity in cardiac cells. Ann Rev Phy 1985;47:645.
13. Page E, et al. Permeable junction between cardiac cells. (Quoted by Guyton AC in Textbook of Medical Physiology—WB Saunders). Ann Rev Phy 1981;43:431.
14. Robb JS, et al. Normal heart: Anatomy and physiology of structural units. (Quoted by Best and Taylor in Physiological basis of Medical Practice, 1967, Williams and Wilkins). Amer Heart J 1942;23:455.

15. Rowell LB. Human cardiovascular control. Oxford University Press. (Quoted by Ganong WF in Review of Medical Physiology–Lange Publications). 1993.
16. Scher AM, et al. Spread of electrical activity through the wall of ventricle. (Quoted by Best and Taylor in Physiological basis of Medical Practice, 1967, Williams and Wilkins). Cir Res 1953;1:539.
17. Swynghedauw B. Development and functional adaptation of contractile proteins in cardiac and skeletal muscles. (Quoted by Guyton AC in Textbook of Medical Physiology - WB Saunders). Phy Rev 1986;66:710.
18. Vasalle M. Cardiac automaticity and its control. Amer J Phy 1977;233:H625.
19. Winegrad S. Calcium release from cardiac sarcoplasmic reticulum. (Quoted by Guyton AC in Textbook of Medical Physiology - WB Saunders). Ann Rev Phy 1982;44:451.
20. Winegrad S. Regulation of cardiac contractile proteins. Correlation between physiology and biochemistry. (Quoted by Guyton AC in Textbook of Medical Physiology - WB Saunders). Cir Res 1984;55:565.

72 Heart as a Pump: Cardiac Cycle

Heart works as a pump, with left ventricle working as pumping station. It is pumping the necessary volume of blood to impart to it a pressure sufficient to cause a continuous flow of blood through the vascular tree.

So cardiac cycle is defined as 'sequence of cyclic changes in each beat of heart with systole (contraction) and diastole (relaxation). Duration of one cardiac cycle is 0.8 second (60/75; heart beat per minute is 75). So it can be stated that all events in one cardiac cycle are repeated at an interval of 0.8 second.

PHASES OR SEQUENCE OF EVENTS

Atrial Events

Any way atrial systole and diastole are the two events:

a. *Atrial systole:* Its total duration is 0.1 second. Because of SA node (pacemaker), the first wave of contraction originates in right auricle and left atrium quickly follows it. This systolic phase is further subdivided into two; each lasting for 0.05 sec. - *dynamic phase*—here 70–80 per cent atrial fibres are contracting and approximately 70–80 per cent blood passes onwards to ventricles.- *adynamic phase*—during this time remaining fibres contract (20–30%) and remaining blood (20–30%) is passing towards ventricles.
b. *Atrial diastole:* 'It is an established fact that atrium collects the blood during first half of systole and emptying it during the second half.' AV valves remain closed to facilitate the auricular filling through vena cavae and pulmonary veins. So first half of atrial diastole is corresponding with ventricular systole. Its total duration is 0.7 second.

Ventricular Events

(Total duration 0.8 second). These are again subdivided into ventricular 'systole' (0.3 second) and 'diastole' (0.5 second).

a. *Ventricular systole:* (0.3 second; range 0.25–0.36 second). If the story of cardiac pumping is continued we find that by now atrial contraction is over and they are in a state of diastole or relaxation so pressure within them is falling, AV valves are open but semilunar valves (s l v) are closed and ventricles are being filled. Now story proceeds ahead, as ventricles are continuously filled with blood so pressure within them rises while pressure within atria is already falling, so to prevent regurgitation AV valves are suddenly closed producing well known 'first heart sound'. Semilunar valves together with AV valves closure are capable of changing these ventricles into more or less a closed cavity leading to increased tension within them which tends to increase hydrostatic pressure too, terminating into bulging of AV valves. This is termed as *'Isometric contraction phase'* lasting for 0.05 second (0.04–0.06 second).

   Now the pressure within both ventricles is increasing continuously. As it exceeds diastolic pressure of aorta (normally it is 80 mmHg) as well as pulmonary artery on right side (normally it is 10 mmHg), the semilunar valves on both the sides will be opened and blood passes onwards for circulation as well as purification purposes thus constituting *'Ejection phase'* so called, lasting in total for 0.25 second. For convenience this is further divided into following phases:

   i. *Minimum ejection phase*: Though it is not truly a significant event since it is merely beginning of this phase and it is said to last for 0.02 second.
   ii. *Maximum ejection phase*: This really extends from opening of semilunar valves to the point of maximum pressure and is lasting for 0.09 second (0.05–0.12 range). It constitutes the climax of blood ejection since maximum amount of blood is ejected.

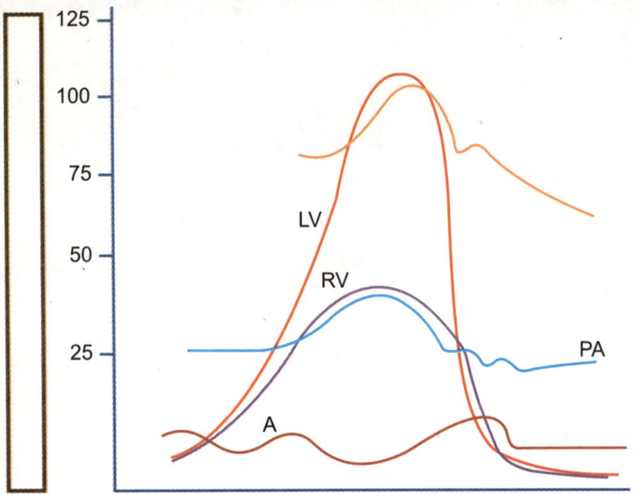

Fig. 72.1: Cardiac cycle (LV = left ventricle, RV = Right ventricle, A = Atria (left and right), PA = Pulmonary artery

iii. *Reduced ejection phase*: when outflow of blood is lessening owing to gradual decrease in pressure, the phase so constituted is of reduced ejection lasting for 0.14 second (range 0.06 to 0.14 second). It is due to the fact that most of the blood has already left the ventricles.

Ejection phase: A review .... So it begins with opening of semilunar valves and ending with beginning of ventricular diastole, since it ejects blood it is maintaining circulatory flow.

b. *Ventricular diastole*: Now ventricular muscles are relaxing. Due to their emptying, pressure within them is gradually decreasing and as it decreases more as compared with aortic and pulmonary trunk, blood may adopt backflow (regurgitation), i.e. from aorta or pulmonary trunk to ventricles back. To prevent this regurgitation the semilunar valves get closed suddenly, which is taken as appearance of so called *'second heart sound'* and this phase is designated as *'Protodiastolic phase'* which lasts for 0.04 second. *So to sum up protodiastolic phase is the interval elapsing between end of reduced ejection phase and closure of semilunar valves.*

By now atrias are being filled with blood so pressure within them is increasing gradually. On the other hand due to closure of both AV and semilunar valves the ventricles are turned into closed cavities and pressure within them is much reduced. This when falls below atrial pressure the AV valves open. This constitutes *'**Isometric relaxation phase**'* of cardiac cycle which lasts for 0.08 second. The word isometric here means that ventricles are closed—no blood is entering its cavity so length of fibres remain unchanged.

Now due to opening of AV valves a *'**third heart sound**'* is produced and blood rushes to ventricles for filling them once again from already filled auricles; thus constituting *'**Filling phase**'* which is further subdivided into following phases–

i. *First rapid filling phase (0.09 second):* Due to sudden opening of AV valves blood rushes from atria to ventricles almost 70–80 per cent of its total amount.
ii. *Slow filling or diastasis (0.19 second):* During this stage only small amount of blood is trickling from atria due to falling pressure within them.
iii. *Last rapid filling or auricular systole or presystole of ventricles (0.10 second):* Remaining approximately 10-20 per cent of blood finally rushes to ventricles due to atrial contraction and this event is capable of producing a sound called *'Fourth heart sound'*. So now ventricular systole once again begins.

Ventricular diastole .... A review .... Usually it begins with closure of semilunar valves and terminating in closure of AV valves; both third and fourth heart sounds are being produced here together with coronary circulation; it follows 'T wave' of ECG and 'v wave' of pressure curves.

END VOLUMES

- During diastole, filling takes place which increases the volume of each ventricle to about 110–120 ml. This is end-diastolic volume.
- On systole, volume decreases in ventricles to about 70 ml which is called stroke volume output.

PRESSURE, VOLUME EVENTS

The sequence of cardiac cycle can be considered in terms of pressures of auricles, ventricles as well as arterial side along with changes in volume due to emptying the cardiac cavities.

i. In one beat left ventricle pumps about 70 ml of blood but in fact 120–130 ml of blood is being filled in each ventricle during diastole, so the amount left in each ventricle even after pumping is 50–70 ml which is referred as *'End-systolic volume'*. During exercise or in any situation when heart contracts strongly this 'end-systolic volume' is reduced to 10–30 ml or so.

VENTRICULAR SHORTENING

1. Right ventricle resembles to a segment of sphere. Its small shortening will eject a large blood volume. If its volume is 130 ml and half is ejected, the diameter will decrease from 6.3 cm to 5.1 cm and circumference from 19.8 cm to 16.0 cm.
2. The reduction in diameter and circumference necessary to eject the stroke volume is different in two ventricles because of their shape and manner of contraction. But it is very small. Under normal circumstances; possibly half of their contained volume is not ejected with each contraction. If the left ventricle is regarded as a cylinder which ejects half of its volume of 130 ml, then diameter can decrease from 5.2 cm to 3.9 cm and circumference from 16.5 cm to 12.1 cm.
3. The wall of right ventricle is thin. So shortening of muscle fibres of lateral wall of right ventricle at different depths would be similar.

   But in left ventricle; the wall is thick. The deep constrictor fibres form a cuff of muscles and these fibres are circumferentially arranged. This thickness of the ventricular wall is so that inner layers near the endocardium have a much smaller radius and circumference than the outer layers near the epicardium. With the onset of contraction, the inner layers must shorten more than the outer layers in ejecting a particular volume. So it is presumed that no two layers of myocardial fibres shorten to the same extent during ejection.

READ AND DIGEST: CARDIAC PECULIARITIES

Q. Mention the characteristic of 'Isometric Contraction Phase' of cardiac cycle?

Ans. In ventricles sufficient pressure is built to open the semilunar valves. So contraction is occurring in ventricles, but there is no emptying, or tension is increasing in the muscles but not occurrence of shortening of muscle fibres.

Q. What is the characteristic of 'Ejection Phase' ?

Ans. When blood has been ejected by ventricle, it develops a momentum. As the systole progresses this momentum is decreased; which means → kinetic energy of momentum is changed into pressure in aorta → this makes arterial pressure a little more than pressure in ventricles.

Q. Mention the characteristic of 'Isometric Relaxation Phase'?

Ans. Ventricular muscles continue to relax though, there is no change in ventricular volume. Intraventricular pressure falls rapidly back to their low diastolic levels.

HEART SOUNDS

i. The sounds when they are produced during various events of cardiac cycle have been already mentioned. To pick up these waves of variable frequencies, 'clinical stethoscope' is used and put over chest. By this device only first and second heart sounds are audible while third and fourth sounds are inaudible.

First Heart Sound

i. It is heard like the syllable 'L-U-B-B (lub).
ii. It is having its duration as 0.9-0.16 second so having comparatively a longer duration.
iii. It is soft in quality with a low pitch.
iv. It marks the beginning as well as force of ventricular contraction so also referred as 'systolic sound'.
v. It is heard best and with its full intensity over 5th left intercostal space mid-clavicular line, i.e. area centred over apex beat.
vi. Cause of production—Sudden closure of auriculo-ventricular valves thus a tension is set up in leaflets of valves as well as in chordae tendinae due to increase in intraventricular pressure.
vii. Significance—Normal first sound is of great significance in the way that it is an indication of normal force of ventricular contraction, together with suggestive of ventricular systole, along with proper closure of AV valves and also signifies diastolic pressure in pulmonary and systolic circuits.
viii. Causes include:
   - Valvular element—i.e. closure of AV valves and tension set up in valve leaflets and chordae tendinae with the rise of intraventricular pressure.
   - Contraction of ventricular muscle.
   - Vascular element—i.e. rushing of blood from ventricles and shock transmitted to walls of aorta and pulmonary artery.
ix. Its intensity is conditioned by position of AV valves at the onset of ventricular systole.
x. Vibrations of first heart sound are increased in amplitude and number when tension developed by cardiac muscle is increased. Its intensity is directly related to rate of pressure rise within ventricle during isometric period. Its intensity is not dependent on volume of systolic discharge but upon diastolic pressure in pulmonary and systemic circuits.

Second Heart Sound

i. It is heard with a syllable of D-U-P-P (dup) by stethoscope. So sounds heard are lub and dup followed by a pause.

ii. Its duration is comparatively short (0.10 second).
iii. It is best heard in aortic and pulmonary area (aortic area is 2nd right intercostal space close to sternum while pulmonary area is at same level but on opposite side).
iv. Cause—It is mainly due to 'valvular element' which comprises with closure of semilunar valves owing to vibrations set up in blood column and arterial walls producing a tension for valves which finally leads to their closure.
v. Significance—Normal second sound is suggestive of end of ventricular systole, proper closure of semilunar valves.
vi. It is coarse pitched and harsh sound. It is also referred as 'diastolic sound'.
vii. In pulmonary area,. its two components are heard called 'split second sound.' In phonocardiogram, the first component represents the closure of aortic valve. Second component is caused by closure of pulmonary valve. The splitting of second heart sound widens during inspiration (0.05 second) and disappears during expiration (0.02 second).
viii. The conditions intensifying the second heart sound are mitral stenosis, left ventricular failure.

Third Heart Sound

i. It is heard 0.8 sec. after second sound and it lasts for 0.04 second.
ii. The causative factor of sound is rushing of blood into ventricles which sets the vibrations in ventricular wall. Another factor involved in its production is opening of AV valves leading to immediate ventricular filling.
iii. It is best heard at apex, i.e. mitral area.
iv. It is more clearly audible in athletes, children, i.e. with an excellent venous return, together with high cardiac output.

Fourth Heart Sounds

i. Causative factors involved in its production are two firstly, 'atrial contraction' and secondly, impact of blood coming from auricle against ventricular wall. It is a low pitched presystolic sound. It is absent in auricular fibrillation.
ii. *'Murmurs'* is name given to abnormal heart sound. Its character is serving as an important guide for valvular disorders. They are generally considered to be due to turbulent blood flow. The possible mechanisms for this production are—high flow through a normal valve (anaemia), normal flow through a constricted valve (mitral stenosis), abnormal flow through either an incompetent valve (aortic—regurgitation) or through an abnormal channel (patent ductus arteriosus).
iii. *Apex beat*: The movement appears as an impact or a thrust coming from interior of chest. The area over which this impact is visible is called 'cardiac impulse.' Lowest and lateral most area of cardiac impulse where it is seen or felt most forcibly is called 'apex beat'.

APEX BEAT: AN OVERVIEW

- It is the sensation of a thrust perceived by the palm of right hand placed on the left side of chest internal to mid clavicular line in left 5th intercostal space.
- It can also be seen as a pulsation in thin chest.
- It is important for studying:
  - — The size of the heart as well as its force of contraction.
  - — Change of position of heart, i.e. for any displacement.
  - — If there is fluid in left pleural space the apex is shifted to right and *vice versa*.
  - — If heart is bigger, its position is altered.
- It can be recorded by means of Marey's cardiograph, connected by a rubber tubing with a recording tambour.

DIFFERENT PHASES AND DURATION—A REVIEW: SUMMARY AND HIGHLIGHTS

A. *Auricular Events*
  I. Systole (0.1 second); dynamic and adynamic phase each lasting for 0.05 second.
  II. Diastole (0.7 second)
B. *Ventricular Events*
  I. Systole (0.3 second)
    - *Isometric contraction phase* ...... 0.08 second.
    - *Ejection phase* ..... Minimum (0.02 sec.), maximum (0.09 sec.) and reduced (0.14 second).
  II. Diastole (0.5 second):
    - *Protodiastolic phase* (0.04 second)
    - *Isometric relaxation phase* (0.08 second)
    - *Rapid filling phase* (0.09 second)
    - *Slow inflow or Diastasis* (0.19 second)
    - *Auricular systole* (0.10 second)

BIBLIOGRAPHY

1. Burns JW, JW Covell. Mechanics of isotonic left ventricular contraction. Amer J Phy 1972;223:1491-97.
2. Covel JW, et al. Comparison of force velocity relation and ventricular function curve as a measure of contractile state of intact heart. Cir Res 1966;19:364-72.
3. Craige E. Heart sounds, phonocardiography, carotid apex and jugular venous pulse tracings so systolic time intervals: In Heart diseases A textbooks of cardiovascular medicine edited by E. Brownwald Philadelphia, WB Saunders 1988;41-48.

4. Dock W. Mode of production of first heart sound. (Quoted by Best and Taylor in Physiological basis of Medical Practice, 1967—Williams and Wilkins. Arch Int Med 1933;51:737.
5. Dock W. The forces needed to evoke sounds from cardiac tissue, and the attenuation of heart sounds. (Quoted by Best and Taylor in Physiological basis of Medical Practice, 1967—Williams and Wilkins. Circulation 1959;19:376.
6. Irisawa H, et al. Left ventricle as mixing chamber. (Quoted by Best and Taylor in Physiological basis of Medical Practice, 1967—Williams and Wilkins. Cir Res 1960;8:183.
7. Leatham A. Splitting of first and second heart sound. (Quoted by Best and Taylor in Physiological basis of Medical Practice, 1967—Williams and Wilkins. Lancet 1954;2: 607.
8. Little RC, et al. The first heart sound in normal and ectopic ventricular contraction: mechanism of closure of AV valves. (Quoted by Best and Taylor in Physiological basis of Medical Practice, 1967—Williams and Wilkins. Cir Res 1954;2:48.
9. Rfushmer RF. Anatomy and physiology of ventricular functions. (Quoted by Best and Taylor in Physiological basis of Medical Practice, 1967—Williams and Wilkins. Phy Rev 1956;36:400.
10. Wiggers CJ, et al. The movements of mitral cusps in relation to cardiac cycle. (Quoted by Best and Taylor in Physiological basis of Medical Practice, 1967—Williams and Wilkins.Amer J Phy 1916;40: 206.

73 Heart as a Pump: Cardiac Output

As already told heart acts as a pump and so certain amount of blood is pumped by it to general circulation to meet the body demands which in turn is returned back to it. So following 'components' of 'cardiac output' must be made clear first (output = efficiency, workdone).

i. *Cardiac output*: It is the amount of blood ejected by each chamber of heart (ventricle).
ii. *Stroke volume*: (Systolic discharge)—It is output of heart per beat.
Normally in an average healthy individual 70–80 ml of blood is ejected by each ventricle per beat. So total is 140–160 ml of blood for both ventricles.
iii. *Minute volume*: It is the product of stroke volume and pulse rate' (so heart rate X stroke volume OR $75 \times 70 = 5$ litres). So it is the volume of blood ejected per minute by each ventricle.
iv. *Cardiac Index*: It is the volume of blood in litres ejected by heart per minute per square metre body surface area. (So it comes $5/1.8 = 2.8$ or 3 litres per minute; where '5' is normal cardiac output and 1.8 is whole surface area for adult of weight 70 kg). It is slightly lower for females but considerably higher for children.

Peripheral Circulation: Major Factor

Normally the cardiac output under resting condition is 5 litres per minute but heart may increase its output up to 13–15 litres per minute. The same quantity of blood is returned back to the right atrium of heart. So in more or other way it is the return of blood which is a dominant factor as compared with simple pumping action of heart. In trained athletes owing to sympathetic stimulation together with catecholamine liberation this cardiac output may increase upto 30–35 litres per minute and for this reason sometimes dilated heart is seen in athletes. The heart diseases of course are able to reduce the pumping capability of heart like myocardial infarction, valvular diseases, myocarditis, congenital diseases etc.

FACTORS INFLUENCING OUTPUT

Following are the factors greatly affecting cardiac output:

i. *Age:* It is said that cardiac output increases with the advancement of age. It is lowest in infants due to their low surface area.
ii. *Emotions:* anxiety, excitement or apprehension are said to increase the output while shock lowers output.
iii. *Temperature:* Since temperature is a cardiac stimulant so any rise of temperature above 30°C will increase output.
iv. *Digestion:* Cardiac output is said to be increased after meals attaining its peak level within three hours of meals and after it the level falls.
v. *Surface area*: It is a simple equation, i.e. 'larger the surface area, more is cardiac output and less surface area, less is the cardiac output.
vi. *Sex:* Since females are having less surface area so cardiac output is found less in females as compared to males.
vii. *Posture:* When one assumes erect posture blood is 'pooled out' thus diminishing the venous return and hence reducing cardiac output. Hence, it is comparatively more in sitting posture.
viii. *Pregnancy:* Little increase in cardiac output has been reported after 30th week.
ix. *Sleep:* In deep undisturbed sleep, it is said to be at basal level.
x. *Hyperthyroid states:* The more secretion of thyroxin hormone from thyroid gland is said to increase heart rate as well as output through increased metabolism.
xi. *Fever:* During fever, output is said to be increased due to increased metabolism.

xii. *Anaemia:* The anaemic persons in true sense are putting additional load over heart. This is because of the fact that heart has to increase its output in order to adjust with diminished number of erythrocytes which are unable to supply adequate oxygen to entire body tissues.

xiii. *Other factors increasing output:* Metabolic alkalosis produced as a result of sodium bicarbonate administration, low oxygen or high carbon dioxide in inspired air are capable of increasing cardiac output upto a significant extent.

xiv. *Drugs and Cardiac output*
Adrenaline increases the cardiac output.
Digitalis is said to increase cardiac output specially in conditions like congestive heart failure but not in normal individuals.
Very slight rise in cardiac output occurs with alcohol taken in moderate dose.

xv. *Conditions reducing output*: Atrial fibrillation, rapid heart rate, complete heart block due to myocardial degeneration and coronary sclerosis, congestive heart failure, etc. reduce output.

xvi. *Factors not influencing output:* Sleep, horizontal body position, menstruation, metabolic acidosis, mild or even moderate temperature variation, high altitude upto 15,000 ft high are some factors which don't change the cardiac output.

xvii. *Haemorrhage*: Loss of blood volume decreases the mean systemic pressure which can decrease the ability of blood to return to heart upto the extent that cardiac output is decreased.

FACTORS REGULATING CARDIAC OUTPUT

Now let us discuss the various factors regulating cardiac output:

Venous Return

i. It is the quantity of blood flowing from the veins into right atrium per minute and constitutes the major factor in maintaining pumping action of heart. Factors maintaining venous return are as follows -

ii. Whenever one individual is performing some exercise (running, cycling, walking etc.), muscles of legs are compressed against fascia which is compressed against skin and thus leg veins are compressed. This venous compression leads to flow of blood away from point of compression, i.e. towards the heart. Furthermore valves present within veins also facilitates the flow of blood towards heart. All this is collectively known as *'muscle or venous pump,'* on the contrary, those who

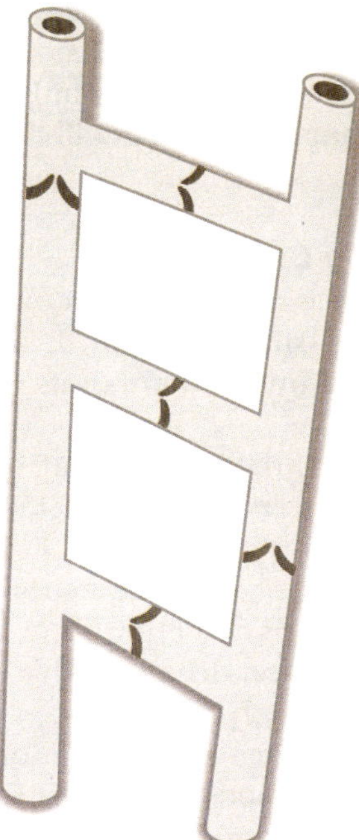

Fig. 73.1: Venous valve: Venous return

are not exercising (traffic police), the above mentioned 'muscle pump' is not operating which tends to increase the venous pressure in leg upto the extent that it crosses full hydrostatic values (90 mmHg) which increases capillary pressure causing leakage of fluid to tissue spaces terminating into 'leg swelling or oedema' together with fall in blood volume.

iii. *Respiratory pump* is another factor maintaining venous return. It assists in the way that during inspiration, increase in dimension of thoracic cage results which tends to increase the intrathoracic negative pressure (from normal negative 2 mmHg to negative 5 or 6 mmHg) terminating into sucking of blood into superior vena cavae and thoracic veins from all smaller veins owing to vacuum creation. So all this mechanism increases venous return during inspiration which increases cardiac output. So it is true that cardiac output increases during inspiration (but difficult to be demonstrated) but opposite is also true during expiration. The above explained mechanism is further assisted by rise of intraabdominal pressure during inspiration which presses abdominal veins and thus increasing venous return.

iv. As already told, blood moves from high pressure area to low pressure area so *'pressure gradient'* is another important factor controlling venous return.

It is an established fact that pressure in aorta is 100 mmHg; at arterial end of capillary it is 30-32 mmHg, at venous termination it is 18 mmHg and right heart side it is 0 mmHg so blood will flow from aorta to right atrium.

Heart's Pumping Capacity

i. This is once again another important factor controlling cardiac output. It means pumping efficiency of myocardium or its entire contractile apparatus.
ii. It is an established fact that on sympathetic stimulation heart acts as a better pump or appears with a greater efficiency due to liberation of catecholamines. Reverse action is noticed on stimulating parasympathetic nerves due to liberation of acetylcholine. This entire action is mediated through cyclic AMP.
iii. *Adequate nutrition* in the form of oxygen, food, blood glucose, non-esterified fatty acids (NEFA), sodium, potassium, calcium and other minerals are also necessary requisites for proper pumping of heart.
iv. If coronary circulation is inadequate the heart itself will receive less blood supply at the time of diastole. So any condition which reduces diastolic period, fatal results are expected since cardiac pumping suffers inversely due to lessened nutrition.
v. *Starling law:* already dealt
vi. *Pumping efficiency* or so called contractility is depressed by acidosis, hypoxia, hypercapnia and drugs like barbiturates.
vii. Through inhibiting breakdown of cyclic AMP, all xanthine derivatives (caffeine, theophylline etc.) increases cardiac output via improving pumping efficiency. Famous drug 'digitalis' (usually given to improve tone of failing myocardium) also serves the same purpose but through increasing the availability of calcium ions which on the other hand is achieved by inhibitory effect on sodium-potassium pump which tends to increase inter-cellular concentration of sodium ions.

Blood Pressure

It has also been studied that blood pressure if remains high, it is capable of damaging heart. It is 100 mmHg pressure in aorta which opens the semilunar valve to get the blood come out from left ventricle for circulation purpose. If one's blood pressure is higher than this 100 mmHg level, then left ventricle has to increase its pressure to get semilunar valve open and in this attempt, the length and mass of ventricular muscle increases leading to cardiac hypertrophy. So it is said that patients suffering from uncontrolled hypertension are having bright chance to suffer from myocardial infarction.

So to conclude, 'it is not the heart which is chiefly regulating cardiac output but tissues themselves as well as peripheral circulation are the primary controller.

CARDIAC RESERVE

i. Since heart is said to be 'rhythm of life' so according to body demands it is capable of increasing its output many times, to meet with situation.

   So cardiac reserve is defined as 'maximum percentage that cardiac output can increase above normal.'
ii. In an average healthy adult it is 300 per cent, while in trained athlete it is 500 per cent and in asthenic or sedentary person it is 200 per cent.
iii. Normal heart rate varies between 60–90/minute but reserve of it is 130–140 per minute extending to maximum as 210 beats per minute.
iv. The stroke volume reserve is 80–100 ml (Normally one ventricle ejects 70–80 ml while each ventricle contains 150–170 cc of blood).
v. Maximum cardiac output is 35 litres per minute in a man who is exercising upto the limit of exhaustion.
vi. The reserve work of the heart is 75 kg per minute. Maximum left ventricular work is about 80 kg per minute and resting left ventricular work is 5–6 kg per minute.

CARDIAC OUTPUT: EXERCISE-EMOTIONS

The parameters of importance are:

1. *Heart rate:* From rest to work, pulse frequency rises—from 160–180 per minute to even 240–270 per minute. This may be due to autonomic control. Vasodilatation takes place in active muscles which reduces blood pressure. This stimulates baro-receptors which causes elevation in blood pressure. Tachycardia is further due to regulation by higher centres.
2. *Ventricular volume and stroke volume:*
   - The left ventricular diastolic volume and stroke volume increases in recumbent position as compared to upright position.
   - In supine position the cardiac output increases with a decrease in heart rate. On assuming the upright position, the heart size decreases as well as the stroke volume.
   - Cardiac size decreases in exercise. Human heart at the end of systole contains 400 ml of blood equally divided into four chambers. This means

each ventricle contains 100 ml of residual blood in recumbent position and about 45 ml in upright position. This is used as ventricle becomes smaller with exertion. This causes a diminution in reserve volume of ventricles in severe exercise. This is compensated by blood volume of thoracic pool. The skeletal muscles of limbs and abdomen play an important role in translocating blood from periphery to central venous pool through their pumping action.

3. *Catecholamines:*
   - Human heart, possess strong adrenergic innervation. It contains stores of nor-adrenaline. The cardiac effects of stellate ganglionic stimulation can be mimicked by infusion of nor-epinephrine.
   - This is further evidenced by the fact that during stimulation of stellate ganglion, nor-epinephrine is recovered from coronary sinus.
4. *Haemodynamic variables:*
   - During heavy exercise (a large increase in cardiac output), there occurs many times increase in cardiac work index of left ventricle, increase in systolic blood pressure. There is a decrease in total peripheral resistance owing to vasodilatation in metabolically active beds.
   - In pulmonary circulation there occurs a moderate rise in arterial pressure while resistance is decreased or not significantly altered.
5. *Athletes* have lower heart rates, greater end systolic ventricular volumes and greater stroke volume at rest so they can achieve a given increase in cardiac output by further increase in stroke volume without increasing their heart rate.

METHODS OF DETERMINATION

In animals flow is measured by any flowmeter after cannulating aorta, pulmonary artery or great veins entering the heart.

1. *Starling heart lung preparation*: It was designed by Starling in the year 1910 to study the behaviour of isolated heart as well as to demonstrate functions of heart. Assembly is:

i. Thorax of an animal (usually dog) is opened, heart is exposed and artificial respiration is carried out.
ii. Vagi were severed to prevent variation of heart rate.
iii. Aorta is tied beyond innominate artery in which a cannula is inserted.
iv. All blood is diverted through innominate artery and cannula into an artificial resistance made of a rubber tube and is enclosed in a glass tube. The pressure on rubber tube can be voluntarily adjusted by a venous reservoir and a heater coil is wound around it for maintenance of temperature.
v. A screw clamp is provided on the main outflow tube from the heart so that arterial resistance can be increased or decreased.
vi. From the resistance blood is returned to right auricle and then to right ventricle which pumps the blood into lungs where blood gets oxygenated and is returned to left auricle and then to left ventricle and in this way circulation proceeds.
vii. Finally a special reservoir having air in its upper part and blood in its lower part is used which works as a elastic buffer to avoid fluctuations in blood pressure with each contraction of heart.

Comments

i. Firstly, relationship of end-diastolic volume to stroke volume output can be demonstrated by lowering and raising the venous reservoir; e.g. on raising the reservoir, rapid blood flow results in heart which is capable of distending its chambers; thus causing increased stroke volume output, which demonstrates Starling law.
ii. It further illustrates that within physiological limits aortic pressure has little effect on cardiac output. It can be concluded as increasing the arterial resistance does not greatly decrease stroke volume output if right atrial pressure remains constant.
iii. Heart rate is increased by various factors like increase in temperature, increasing load of inflowing blood, epinephrine administration while heart rate is decreased by injecting acetylcholine. So by such studies effect of different factors on heart rate is studied.
iv. Pressure, temperature, H^+ion concentration, inorganic ions etc. can be varied and their effect on cardiac output is also noted by such study.

Sarnoff's experiment: Broadly speaking there were two main drawbacks in Starling experiment; one is it is not fit to be applied in living body and second the volume of single ventricle could not be determined by cardiometer. So Sarnoff modified it and was directed to study the pressure volume relationship of single ventricle so it is a better guide to study ventricular pumping action.

2. Direct Fick Method:

$$\text{By this cardiac output} = \frac{\text{Oxygen consumption}}{\text{Arterio-venous oxygen difference}} \times 100 \text{ per minute}$$

The oxygen consumption is 250 ml per minute and was first measured by noting the oxygen concentration of the air going to lung by Douglas bag.

The arteriovenous difference of oxygen is 5 ml (19-14 ml at arterial and venous end respectively).

$$So = \frac{250}{5} \times 100 = 5 \text{ litres per minute}$$

- Mixed venous blood can be obtained from root of pulmonary artery. By puncturing brachial artery, arterial blood can be collected, by specialised arterial syringe after proper sterilisation. Routine procedure is of cardiac catheterisation (catheter No. 3, 8, 9) which is introduced through antecubital vein after proper sterilisation. Blood samples can be analysed for O_2 content (Van Slyke apparatus or photoelectric method).

Comments

i. The direct Fick method was first employed by Forssmann (1929-Germany) upon himself which was later on modified by Klein but it was popularised by Cournand.

ii. *Using oxygen:* Oxygen consumption per minute is determined by Douglas bag. Arterial oxygen content is also calculated from haemoglobin level. Oxygen percentage of right auricle blood (index of mixed venous blood) is determined by passing catheter through cubital vein. Then by using above formula output can be calculated.

iii. *Using carbon dioxide:* CO_2 output per minute is determined by Douglas bag. Alveolar air's CO_2 content is measured. For venous CO_2, alveolar air is again collected after breath holding for 5 seconds and its CO_2 tension is identical with venous blood.

iv. *Using foreign gases:*

- This is based on the principle that, if a person breathes an inert gas and if its absorption rate by blood, alveolar tension and stability are known the amount of blood flowing through lungs can be calculated by formula:

$$\frac{\text{gas absorption rate}}{\text{alveolar concentration of gas} \times \text{blood solubility}}$$

- Inert gases used are nitrous oxide, ethyl iodide and acetylene. It is selected on the basis that it must be dissolved in plasma but must not combine with haemoglobin, lipid or any other blood constituents.

v. This method is not applicable during exercise since in that situation arteriovenous oxygen difference changes because oxygen is used by tissues.

vi. Secondly the method is not of use during emotional crisis since this situation may increase heart rate or may lead to ventricular fibrillation.

3. Ballistocardiograph Method:

   i. The patient lies comfortably on a special table called ballistocardiographic table comfortably in supine position with his feet placed against a foot board. (ii) Now the method works on the principle, 'every action has an opposite and equal reaction'. It means when blood is pumped to aorta, i.e. systole there occurs 'headward thrust along with tailward recoil of body' while during diastole opposite reaction is seen. This gives rise to typical ballistocardiographic curve which can be taken as 'photo record' to magnify them to a great extent.

4. *Dye dilution method* (Stewart and Hamilton): By this technique the cardiac flow can be determined by following formula after injecting a known quantity of a dye (generally T-1824);

$$F = \frac{60\ A}{C \times t}$$

F = blood flow
A = amount of dye injected
C = mean concentration of dye in mg/litre of plasma
60 = Heart rate
t = time during which samples were collected; in seconds.

Every second the blood is collected. After 0.3 second dye appears in blood, then there is a fall since it is removed by aorta and then due to recirculation; again rise is reported.

Precautions to be kept in mind are:

1. The indicator substance or procedure must not cause any discomfort or injury.
2. Indicator substance must stay inside blood vessel till sampling is done.
3. Indicator substance should not diffuse into or out of erythrocytes during its passage.
4. Volumes of solution added or blood withdrawn for analysis should be minimum.

It is having merit over Fick Principle that

1. By it cardiac output can be determined from only few heart beats.
2. During exercise also, output can be measured.
3. Immobilisation due to intracardiac catheter is not required.

4. *Cardiometric method in animals:* Cardiometer is used in animals with open thorax. But its disadvantages are open chest and that inertia and friction of the moving parts deform the curve.
5. *Echocardiography:*
   i. This technique is still developing since requires expertisation. The theme consists of the fact that pulses of ultrasonic waves which are emitted from a transducer are applied to heart which are spreading in its various parts. These are reflected back and these echo waves are displayed on a screen over which entire activities of ventricular wall, septum and valves can be studied. So 'this technique' uses ultra-sound to image the heart and great vessels. Interconversion of electrical and mechanical sound energy is done by a transducer working in dual role, i.e. receiver as well as transmitter of sound.
   ii. Uses—this technique is useful in detecting valvular heart diseases, left ventricle examination (size, wall thickness, function), pericardial effusion, cardiomyopathies, congenital heart disease, cardiac masses etc.

REGIONAL DISTRIBUTION

i. In a normal body with 70 kg body weight 5–6 litres per minute is blood flow; with 250 cc per minute utilisation of oxygen (considered as 100%).
ii. 1,300 ml per minute blood flows through kidney with 20 ml per minute utilisation of oxygen. (Weight of kidney 0.33 kg).
iii. 800–1000 ml per minute blood flows through brain with 63 ml per minute utilisation of oxygen. (Weight of brain 1.54 kg).
iv. 1,500 ml per minute blood flows through liver (its weight 2.86 kg) with oxygen utilisation to 55 ml per minute.
v. 2–3 ml per 100 gm is blood flow through skeletal muscle with oxygen utilisation as 55 ml per minute (total weight considered as 34 kg). During exercise the blood flow is increased to 35 litres per minute with oxygen uses to 2700 ml per minute.

SUMMARY AND HIGHLIGHTS

Heart is not the passive servant of peripheral circulation. It does not pass on what it receives; but is capable of changing its performance at the same diastolic size. Thus, it is capable of circulatory modifications irrespective of primary changes in filling of the heart by venous return and in arterial resistance to flow. Its example is the nervous influences on heart, i.e. sympathetic and parasympathetic effects.

BIBLIOGRAPHY

1. Banet M, Guyton AC. Effect of body metabolism on cardiac output : Role of CNS. Amer J Phy 1971;220:662.
2. Bishop VS, et al. Cardiac function curves in conscious dogs. Amer J Phy 1964;207:677.
3. Bishop VS, et al. Quantitative description of ventricular output curves in conscious dogs. Cir Res 1967;20:581.
4. Cowley AW (Jr.), Guyton AC. Heart rate as a determinant of cardiac output in dogs with arterio venous fistula. Amer J Cardiol 1971;28:321.
5. Fermoso JD, et al. Mechanism of decrease in cardiac output caused by opening the chest. Amer J Phy 1964;207:1112.
6. Guyton AC. Regulation of cardiac output. New Eng J Med 1967;277:805.
7. Guyton AC, et al. Circulatory physiology: cardiac output and its regulations, 2nd ed. Saunders, Philadelphia 1973.
8. Guyton AC. Determination of cardiac output by equating venous return curves with cardiac response curves. Phy Rev 1955;35:123.
9. Prather JW, et al. Effect of blood volume, mean circulatory pressure and stress relaxation on cardiac output. Amer J Phy 216:467.
10. Sugimoto T, et al. Effect of tachycardia on cardiac output during normal and increased venous return. Amer J Phy 1966; 211:288.
11. Temini BA, Lee YC. Essentials of echocardiography. Medical economics co. 1976.
12. Weisel RD, et al. Current concepts measurement of cardiac output by thermodilution. New Eng J Med 1975;292:682.

74 Coronary Circulation Ischaemia—Angina

Coronary occlusion is a more challenging and perplexing problem for both doctors and the sufferers. It is important because many of us are certain to suffer from the condition, and it is challenging because of the various complications.

INTRODUCTION

- The resting coronary blood flow is 225 ml per minute which is 4–5 per cent of total cardiac output, or, 0.7 to 0.8 ml per gm of heart muscle. During strenuous exercise, this flow increases because of increasing cardiac output and all this increase is to supply extra nutrients needed by the heart.
- The left coronary artery supplies mainly left ventricle (anterior and lateral portion); while right coronary artery supplies right ventricle as well as posterior part of left ventricle. So in majority of cases, more blood flows through right coronary artery.

CONTROL

This coronary blood flow is controlled by many factors—Few highlights are :-

- *Oxygen demand:* When blood is supplied to heart musculature by coronaries naturally it loses oxygen to almost 70 per cent extent. So for supply of adequate blood and nutrients, much additional oxygen is to be supplied. This target is achieved by coronary dilatation.
- It has been postulated in this connection that at this time some vasodilator substances are released from muscle cells to fulfil the demand of oxygen which dilates the arterioles. These substances include adenosine (produced by degradation from ATP → ADP → AMP → adenosine), potassium ions, hydrogen ions, carbon dioxide, bradykinin, prostaglandins etc.
- This attractive theory is not fully agreed. When substances which prevent the vasodilator effect of adenosine are injected; then the vasodilatation is not stopped and secondly it has been established that vasodilatory effect of adenosine lasts only for one or three hours.
- The another concept in this aspect is that not only does the myocardial musculature but the arteriolar muscular wall itself suffers from oxygen deficiency and this causes local vasodilatation.
- *Nervous control*: Sympathetic nerves on getting stimulation releases catecholamines which are augmentor and accelerator nerves for the heart and at the same time these nerves dilate the coronary vessels and blood flow increases in proportion to the metabolic needs of the heart muscle.
- On the contrary, vagal stimulation releases acetylcholine which slows the heart and having a depressive effect on cardiac contractility.

RECEPTORS AND THE CORONARIES

- Both alpha and beta receptors exist in coronaries. Alpha receptors are constrictor while beta receptors are dilators. Generally, it is concluded that epicardial coronary vessels have a preponderance of alpha receptors, while muscular arteries are having preponderance of beta receptors.
- So sympathetic stimulation can cause either slight vasoconstriction or dilatation but usually more constriction.

ASSESSMENT OF ISCHAEMIA: MYOCARDIAL PERFUSION SCIENTIGRAPHY

1. Thallium-201, technetium-99m Sestamibi, tetrafosmin are frequently used.
2. Its indications are: (a) to distinguish ischaemic from infarcted myocardium, (b) when resting ECG makes an exercising ECG difficult to interpret (LBBB, baseline ST-T changes, low voltage etc.), (c) to

localize the region of ischaemia, (d) as a prognostic indicator in patients with known coronary disease (e) to assess the completeness of vascularisation following bypass surgery/coronary angioplasty.

3. This test provides images in which radionuclide uptake is proportionate to blood flow at the time of injection.
4. False positive test may occur as a result of diaphragmatic attenuation, or in woman, attenuation through breast tissue.
5. Defects observed when radio tracer is injected at rest, or still present 3-4 hours after an injection during exercise, or pharmacological vasodilation (IV adenosine) usually indicate myocardial infarction, but present with severe ischaemia.

Source: Current Medical Diagnosis & Treatment-2003 (Ed) by L.M. Tierney, Stephen J McPhee, Maxine A. Papadakis—Lange Medical Books/McGraw Hill.

ISCHAEMIA: INFARCTION: PATHOPHYSIOLOGY

- Ischaemia means insufficient blood flow. On coronary occlusion blood flow comes to an end in the coronary vessels. The area of muscle that has no blood flow or very less blood flow so that it cannot perform the cardiac function, it is said to be infarcted, and the over all phenomenon or process is called myocardial infarction.
- Onset of infarction → collateral blood supply into the infarcted area. This is coupled with dilatation of the local blood vessels. So the infarcted area is overfilled with stagnant blood.
- At the same time, haemoglobin is totally reduced and it turns into dark blue in colour so infarcted area takes this coloration.
- Later on, vessel becomes highly permeable and so leak the fluid, so tissue becomes oedematous and cardiac muscle cell begin to swell due to diminished cellular metabolism. Within few hours of no blood supply, the cells die.
- It is to be remembered that cardiac muscle requires 1.3 ml of oxygen per 100 gm of muscle tissue per minute to remain alive.
- The question often asked to physiologists is, why atherosclerosis is so much more common in coronary arteries than in other vessels of similar size? With every systole and diastole there is a change in length of coronaries. To meet this stress we find intimal supports of longitudinal muscles lying in matrix of the connective tissue. These supports are more developed in males than in females and they are the site of lipid accumulation.

CAUSE OF DEATH: CORONARY ISCHAEMIA

1. Overall pumping capability of affected ventricle is decreased; if some cardiac muscle fibres are not at all working/too weakly working. The force with which normal cardiac muscle fibres are contracting, actually forces the dead muscle fibres, which are pushed forwards, like a bag; this is called 'systolic stretch'.
2. The dead muscle fibres continue to degenerate and thin, till the heart ruptures.
3. On rupturing, the blood collects in pericardial space-so called 'cardiac temponad'—which means compression of heart by blood from outside. Ultimately the cause of death is decreased cardiac output since blood cannot flow in right atrium easily.
4. Fibrillations which are precipitated because of coronary occlusion is another contributing factor leading to death. The explanations are:
   - Loss of blood supply to cardiac muscle → rapid depletion of potassium from ischaemic muscles → increased potassium in ECF surrounding cardiac muscle → increased irritability of cardiac muscles.
   - Ischaemic muscles causes injury of current. This cannot repolarise its membranes. So it remains negative with respect to normal polarised cardiac muscle membrane. So abnormal impulses are generated leading to fibrillation.
   - Coronary occlusion → powerful sympathetic reflexes → irritability of cardiac muscle increases → fibrillation.

ANGINA PECTORIS

As I was walking about the room I cast my eyes on a looking glass and observed my countenance pale, my lips white and I had the appearance of a dead man looking at himself —John Hunter.

- It is characterised by transient episodes of pain that are usually precipitated by effort and that are relieved by rest and nitro-glycerine.
- Exercise, heavy meal, exposure to cold weather may precipitate the pain, which is generally described as crushing, dull, aching, squeezing, or oppressive.
- Variant angina is due to spasm of large coronary vessel occurring at rest or during normal activity. This spasm occurs in the absence of pre-existing atherosclerotic lesions of the coronary vasculature as well as in the presence of such lesions. This spasm is secondary to hypersensitivity of coronary artery to a localised atheromatous plaque.

- Alteration in sympathetic coronary innervation.
- Humoral agents (histamine, bradykinin).
- Anginal attacks are considered as forerunners of more progressive impairment/and,/or more severe changes within the myocardial wall. Therefore, therapeutic approach is correction of imbalance between oxygen supply, substrate delivery and demand placed upon the heart. β-adrenergic blockers and vasodilators are generally employed for purpose of providing greater coronary blood flow.
- As regards drugs are concerned, nitroglycerine or nitrates are drug of choice, which when administered sublingually leads to dramatic vasodilatation.
- Beta blockers (Propranolol) is used to treat anginal attacks. These drugs block sympathetic beta receptors which prevents sympathetic stimulation of heart rate and cardiac metabolism during exercise or emotions.

Surgical Treatment

Aortic coronary bypass: This surgical process has developed, for anastomosing small vein grafts to the aorta and to the sides of more peripheral coronary vessels. Long superficial saphenous vein removed from the leg is usually selected. Internal mammary artery is also a good selection for bypass.

Coronary angioplasty: The principle behind this technique is to open partially blocked coronary vessels before they become totally occluded. A balloon tipped catheter (1 mm diameter) is passed under radiographic guidance into the coronary system and pushed through the partially occluded artery until balloon portion of the catheter stretches the occluded part. Then balloon is inflated several atmospheric pressure which stretches the diseased artery almost to the point of bursting. With this technique the blood flow increases.

REST : THE PRIMARY TREATMENT

When metabolism of heart muscle is increased by any reasons like exercise, emotions or as a result of fatigue, the heart needs additional nutrients and oxygen for surviving. In extra active states, heart vessels are dilated so more blood flows through normal areas, so little blood is left for the infarcted area where the anastomosing channels are developing. This further spoils the condition of infarcted area. So rest avoids all these complications and hence it is the primary treatment.

The Recovery phase: Shortly after myocardial infarction (coronary occlusion), the muscle fibre die in the very centre of ischaemic area. Then in forthcoming days, the area of dead fibres grow. At the same time, collateral vessels grow into outer rim of infarcted area and so non-functional mass may become smaller and smaller.

EFFORT AND STRESS

It is true that sudden and unwanted exertion (specially in cold weather) may be followed by sudden death. This is because of intimal haemorrhage owing to sudden rise in blood pressure. The new capillaries are expected to come from minute vessels in adventitia. The excess demand of blood because of exertion and stress is not fulfilled because of narrow coronaries. Of course exercise is considered as protection against coronary (ischaemic) diseases but it should not be beyond the individual's cardiac efficiency.

THE GALLBLADDER

There are evidences that a patient of gallbladder diseases represent the symptoms of coronary occlusion or heart failure. Coronary sclerosis and gallstones were both present in the autopsy of John Hunter who suffered from recurring attacks of angina.

SUMMARY AND HIGHLIGHTS

Stress and strain of modern civilisation is blamed for coronary attacks. Government clerks often suffer from such attacks rather than a postman. Coronary bypass and angioplasty are the latest life saving measures. Exertion and emotions are basic causes of coronary heart diseases. Rest is the primary treatment which means complete physical and mental rest.

BIBLIOGRAPHY

1. Beller GA, et al. Contribution of nuclear cardiology to diagnosis and prognosis with coronary artery disease. Circulation 2000; 101:1465.
2. Epstein SE, et al. Dynamic coronary obstruction as a cause of angina pectoris implication regarding therapy. Amer J Cardiol 1985;55: 61B.
3. Furster V, et al. The pathogenesis of CAD and acute coronary syndrome. New Eng J Med 1992;326:242.
4. Gregge DE. Coronary circulation in health and disease. Lea and Febigir, Philadelphia. 1950.
5. Gregge DE. The natural history of coronary collateral development. Cir Res 1974;35:335.
6. Hutchinson. Prevention of coronary heart disease, Chicago Year Book Medical Publishers, 1985.
7. Klagsburn MD, et al. Regulation of angiogenesis. Ann Rev Phy 1991;53:217.
8. Klocke FJ, Ellis AK. Control of coronary blood flow. Ann Rev Med 1980;31:489.

9. Lee TH, et al. Clinical practice: Non-invasive test in patients with stable coronary artery disease. New Eng J Med 2001; 1840;344.
10. Marchelte G, Taccardi B (Ed). Coronary circulation and energetics of myocardium, Karger, Basel, 1967.
11. Ross R. A perspective for 1990's—Pathogenesis of atherosclerosis. Nature 1993;362:801.
12. Sharma B, et al. Intracoronary prostaglandin E_1 + streptokinase in acute MI. Am J Card 1986;58:1161.
13. Stone HL. Control of coronary circulation during exercise. Ann Rev Phy 1983;45:213.
14. Zaret BL, et al. Nuclear cardiology. New Eng J Med 1993;329: 855.

75 Informative of Heart—I Electrocardiograph (ECG)

Electrocardiograph may be defined as that branch of physiology which is concerned with the recording and analysis of electrical activity of the heart. It is an instrument which receives the electrical impulses as they vary during the heart cycle and transforms them into a graphic record called electrocardiogram. Records obtained directly from cardiac muscle are called electrograms.

Prior to or during each contraction an electrical impulse is generated in SA node which is then transmitted to AV node, His bundle, Purkinje fibres, ventricular muscle and surrounding tissues in which heart is bathed. Body is a volume conductor, and heart muscle being electrical generator with two opposite poles (dipole) is bathed in it. Under this condition electrical impulse which is initiated in cardiac muscle will be transmitted throughout the body. If suitable electrodes are placed (leads) on the body opposite to the heart and connected to a very sensitive galvanometer, with a recording device then electric potential can be recorded. The method of recording and analysis of electrical activities of the heart is known as 'Electrocardiography.'

HISTORY

Einthoven (1902-3) was pioneer and master mind of this field so he is known as father of electrocardiography.

FLOW OF CURRENT AROUND THE HEART

- Cardiac muscle is a syncitial mass. Prior to stimulation, the exterior of the muscle cells is positive while interior is negative. However, when this cardiac syncitium is depolarised, negative charges leak to the outside of the depolarised muscle fibre making the surface electronegative, with respect to remaining surface of the heart which is still polarised is electropositive. Therefore, a meter connected with its negative terminal on the area of depolarisation and its positive terminal on one of the still polarised area, records positive.
- Cardiac impulse first arrives in the ventricles in the septum and then to the endocardial surfaces of the remainder of the ventricles. This provides electronegativity on the inside of the ventricle and electropositivity on outer walls of the ventricles and current flows through the fluid surrounding the ventricles along elliptical paths. The average current flows from negative to positive side, i.e. from base of the heart to apex. At the very end of depolarisation the direction of current flow reverses for about 1/100 sec, i.e. from apex to base because it is outer wall of the ventricle which is last to be depolarised and it is near the base.
- So, if a meter is connected to the surface of the body, the electrode nearer the base will be negative, while electrode nearer the apex will be positive in ECG.
- As electrodes, (noncorrosive metal wrapped in cotton soaked in strong saline or by the use of special jelly) are put at different place, they constitute the term 'leads.'

By recording such ECG; we are having following *assumptions:*

i. The electric changes are considered as if they are occurring in a flat frontal plane.
ii. The electric charges occurring in the heart are caused as if by a single resultant dipole and from this dipole the electric field is conducted through the body tissues and blood, etc. to the surface of the body.
iii. These media conduct the electric field homogeneously in all directions.
iv. The body surfaces on which the electrodes are placed are so far away from the position of the manifest dipole of the heart that the electrodes are considered as at infinity and equidistant from it and therefore

also as forming an equilateral triangle with the dipole at its centre. This constitutes ***Einthoven's triangle*** which is drawn around the area of the heart. This is a diagrammatic means of illustrating that the two arms and left leg form apices of a triangle surrounding the heart. The two apices at the upper part of the triangle represent the points at which two arms connect electrically with the fluid around the heart, and the lower apex is the point at which the left leg connects with the fluid.

THE ECG LEADS

a. *Bipolar limb leads:*
   - *Lead I:* The negative terminal of electrocardiograph is connected to the right arm and positive terminal to the left arm. So when point on the chest where right arm connects to the chest is electronegative with respect to the point where the left arm connects, the ECG records positive which means above the zero base line.
   - *Lead II:* The negative terminal is connected to right arm and positive terminal to the left leg. So when right arm is negative with respect to the left leg, the ECG records positive.
   - *Lead III:* The negative terminal is connected to left arm and positive terminal to left leg. So ECG records positive when left arm is negative with respect to left leg.

b. *Unipolar limb leads (augmented = a):*
   - *aVR* — positive terminal is on right arm.
   - *aVL* — positive terminal is on left arm.
   - *aVF* — positive terminal on left leg.

   Recording of aVR is inverted normally; while aVL and aVF record similarly as that of bipolar leads.

c. *Precordial (chest) leads (V Leads):*
   - V_1 — 4th Intercostal space - right sternal border.
   - V_2 — 4th Intercostal space .... left sternal border.
   - V_3 — In between V_2 and V_4.
   - V_4 — Left 5th Intercostal space mid clavicular line.
   - V_5 — Left 5th Intercostal space anterior axillary line.
   - V_6 — Left 5th Intercostal space mid axillary line.

In leads V_1 and V_2 the QRS recording of normal heart are mainly negative, because chest electrodes in these leads is nearer the base of the heart than the apex, which is the direction of electro-negativity during most of the electric depolarisation process. On the contrary, QRS complexes in leads $V_{4,\,5,\,6}$ are mainly positive because chest electrode in these leads is nearer the apex, which is the direction of electro-positivity during most of depolarisation.

Leads — Importance
- V_1 activity of left and right atrium
- V_2 wall and cavity of left atrium
- V_3 Diaphragmatic surface of heart
- V_4 Anterior wall of heart
- V_5 Apex of heart
- V_6 Left ventricle
- aVL Left wall of heart

THE PEN RECORDER

- Special paper is used which does not require ink in the recording stylus. One such paper turns black when it is exposed to heat, the stylus itself is made very hot by electric current flowing through its tip.
- Another type turns black when electric current flows from the tip of the stylus through the paper to an electrode at its back. This leaves a black line everywhere on the paper that the stylus touches.

EINTHOVEN'S LAW

- If for example, it is assumed that lead I records a 'potential of + 0.5 mV' (–0.2 mV on right arm and +0.3 mV on left arm - So + .3 – 0.2 = +0.5). Lead III records a 'positive potential of 0.7 mV. So Lead II will record Lead I + Lead III, i.e. 0.5 + 0.7 = 1.2 mV.
- So Einthoven law states that, by summing up the electric potential of any two of the three bipolar leads; the electric potential of the third can be determined at a given instant.

ECG PAPER

- All recordings of ECG are made with appropriate calibration lines on the recording paper.
- Paper in the machine moves with a speed of 25 mm per second.
- Horizontal calibration lines are arranged so that ten small divisions upwards or downwards in the standard ECG represent 1 mV with positivity in upward and negativity in downward direction.
- The vertical lines are 'time calibration lines.' Each inch (in horizontal direction) is 'one second' and each inch in turn is broken into five segments by dark vertical lines; the intervals between these lines represent 0.20 second. These intervals are then broken into five smaller intervals by this lines, and each of them represent 0.04 second.
- The iso-electric line is a flat line used as a reference point for the measurement and configuration of all ECG complexes. It is considered to be in level with

that portion of base line between termination of T wave and beginning of P.

NORMAL ECG: OBSERVATION

Just like music is the game of seven notes *swara* by which we can compose western or Indian music, just similarly cardiogram is a game of six waves namely P, Q, R, S, T and U. So let us discuss them separately, after remembering the fact that P wave is an indication of auricular activities so it is called *'Auricular complex'* while QRST combinely called as *Ventricular complex* since it tells about ventricular activities.

a. *P wave:*
   i. It is the first upward deflection and is known to be due to auricular activities hence called auricular complex.
   ii. It is positive in lead I and II and is inverted in aVR. It lasts for 0.08 to 0.1 second attaining a maximum height of (2.5 mm) 0.5 cm (magnitude of 0.5 mV).
   iii. It is having a round summit. Voltage should not exceed 0.25 mV in lead II. It is due to atrial depolarisation.
   iv. Its beginning in ECG is indicative of fact that impulse has originated and travelled through auricles while its end is suggestive of the fact that auricles have come to a resting state.
   v. In fibrillation it is irregular while in flutter innumerable regular P waves are seen.
b. *Q wave:*
   i. The next negative wave is Q.
   ii. It is an indication of the fact that ventricles have been activated, preferably the septum.
c. *R wave:*
   i. It is the next sharp upward deflection.
   ii. When activating process travels through ventricles this wave is produced so its height denotes functional activity of ventricles.
d. *S wave:*
   i. The next downward deflection is S.
   ii. It is prominent in lead III and aVR.
   iii. It becomes deep and wide in abnormal conditions like ventricular hypertrophy and bundle branch block.
e. *T wave:*
   i. It is the last upward deflection associated with phenomenon of repolarisation. It is always positive in lead I and II, but negative in aVR.
   ii. Its duration is 0.24 sec, voltage is more as compared with P wave. At the end of wave S there is an isoelectric interval of 0.08 second and then wave T is produced. QRS complex represents ventricular depolarisation occupying 0.08 second and it must not exceed 0.12 second in health.

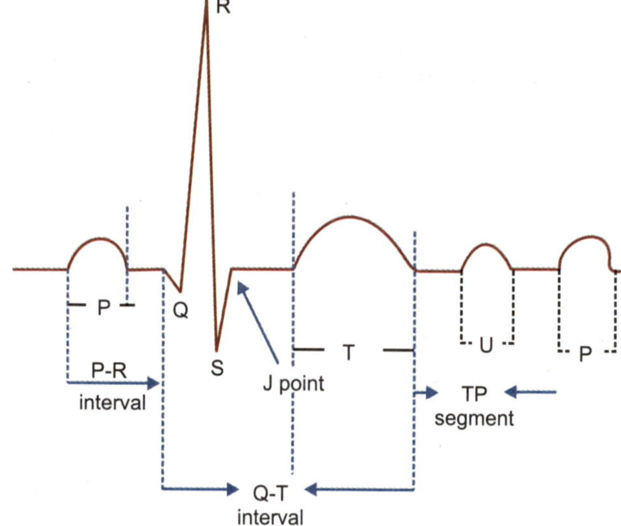

Fig. 75.1: Normal electrocardiogram (ECG)

f. *U wave:*
   i. Following T is the wave U appearing after another isoelectric interval of 0.08 sec.
   ii. Its duration is 0.08 second.
   iii. It is an indication of increased excitability of cardiac tissues.
   iv. Its voltage is approximately 0.02 mV.
g. *P-R Interval:*
   i. It is the time interval from beginning of wave P to beginning of wave R.
   ii. Normally it ranges from 0.13-0.16 second and must not exceed 0.2 second. It is prolonged in coronary artery disease, rheumatic heart etc.
   iii. Wolff-Parkinson-White syndrome (WPW).
      - ECG show shortening of PR interval + slurring of QRS complex.
      - There is an abnormal band of arterial tissue which connects atria and ventricles and can electrically by pass AV node.
      - Because of AV node and by pass tract have different conduction speeds and refractory period a re-entry circuit can develop leading to paroxysms of tachycardia.
h. *S-T segment:*
   i. While both ventricles are in contracted state this ST segment is written. It is that portion of tracing which immediately follows QRS complex. It is

isoelectric and may be elevated 2 mm or depressed 0.5 mm or less and still be considered normal.

ii. The J point is the point at which ST segment departs from the main body of QRS complex. Rather than forming a sharp angle with it, it normally curves gently into T wave.

i. *Q-T Interval:*
   i. It is measured from beginning of QRS to the end of T wave and varies with age, sex and heart rate.
   ii. Quinidine, procainamide, hypocalcaemia, CHF may prolong it, while, digitalis, hypercalcaemia and hyperpotassaemia may shorten it.

HOLTER-MONITORING (AMBULATORY ECG)

Is useful in detecting transient episodes of ischaemia/ arrhythmia. By this continuous recording of one or more ECG leads may be obtained by attaching them to small portable solid state or tape recorder. The recording is later played back at high speed and analysed.

HBE (HIS BUNDLE ELECTROGRAM)

A catheter containing ring electrodes at its tip is used and is passed through a vein to right side of heart. Three standard leads are recorded.

ELECTROCARDIOGRAPHY: VECTORIAL ANALYSIS (VECTOR CARDIOGRAM)

- Heart current flows in a particular direction at a given instant in the cardiac cycle. A vector is an arrow that points in the direction of electrical potential generated by the current flow with the arrow head in the positive direction. The length of the arrow is drawn proportional to the voltage of the potential (vector = direction of electric potential).
- Electric current flows between depolarised areas inside the heart (ventricular septum and parts of lateral endocardial walls) and nondepolarised areas on the outside of the heart. A considerable greater quantity of electric current flows downward on the outside of the ventricles towards the apex; which here is called 'Instantaneous mean vector; and is drawn through the centre of ventricles in a direction from base of the heart to apex. On the contrary small amount of current flows upwards inside the heart.
- When a vector is horizontal and directed towards subject's left side, the vector is said to extend in direction of 0 degree (zero reference point). From here the scale of vector rotates clockwise; which means above downward (+90°); left to right (+180°); upwards (–90° or +270°).
- Each lead is actually a pair of electrodes connected to the body on opposite sides of the heart. Direction from negative to positive electrode is called, axis of lead.
  — Lead I : Recorded between right arm (negative) and left arm (positive) in horizontal direction, the axis is 0 degree.
  — Lead II : 60°. Right arm connects to the torso in the upper right hand corner and left leg connects in the lower left hand corner.
  — Lead III : 120°.
  — aVF : 90° aVR 210°; and aVL –30°.

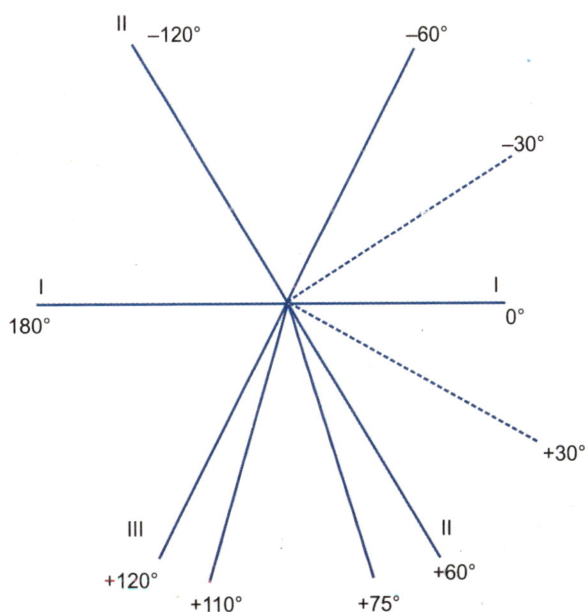

Fig. 75.2: Cardiac axis

AXIS DETERMINATION

- See lead I. If its net potential is positive it is plotted in a positive direction along the line depicting lead I. If it is negative it should be plotted on negative side.
- Do the same with lead III.
- Draw perpendicular lines from apices of two net potential of lead I and III respectively. Note the point of intersection. Draw a line, which denotes the axis.
- Normal axis is ranging from –30° to +110° and the mean is 59/60°.
- In left ventricular hypertrophy (hypertension) it is deviated to left; in right ventricular hypertrophy it is deviated to right. This is because-
  - More quantity of muscle is present on hypertrophied side as compared with normal on opposite side. It leads to excess generation of electrical potential on that side.
  - More time is required by the wave of depolarisation to travel through hypertrophied side.

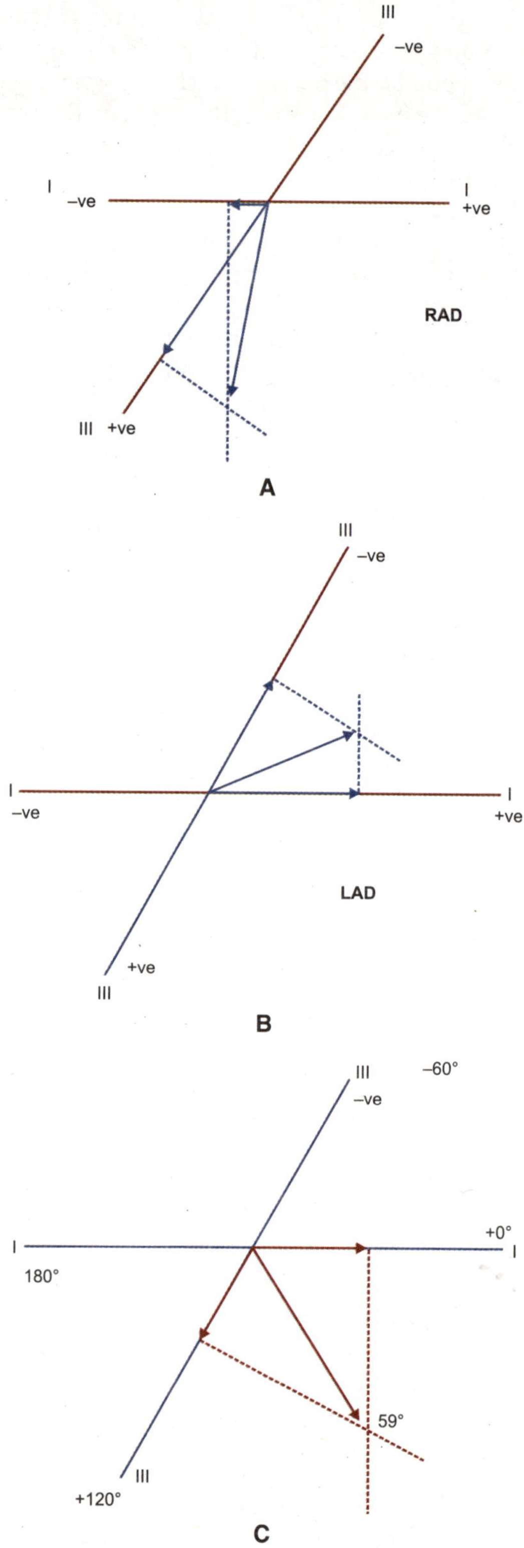

Figs 75.3A to C: Right axis deviation (A) Left axis deviation (B) Mean electrical axis (C)

ATRIAL DEPOLARISATION (P WAVE)

- Depolarisation of the atria begins in SA node and then spreads in all the directions over the atria. The vector remains generally in the same direction throughout the process of depolarisation.
- Vector of current flow during depolarisation in atria points in almost the same direction as in the direction of that in the ventricles. Because this direction is in direction of the axis of three bipolar leads I, II and III which means positive deflection. So record of atrial depolarisation is positive P wave.

REPOLARISATION (T WAVE)

- After depolarisation of entire ventricles, 0.15 second elapses before sufficient repolarisation begins. This process of repolarisation completes in 0.35 second after the onset of QRS complex.
- It seems a strange that septum and endocardial areas which are depolarised first of all, don't repolarise first of all; because of their longer period of contraction so it repolarises in the last.
- So the part to be repolarised first of all is entire outer surface of ventricle and specially near the apex of heart.
- Thus, the predominant direction of the vector through the heart during repolarisation of the ventricles is from base to apex. So T wave in three bipolar leads is positive.

CURRENT OF INJURY

- Because of some pathologic focus any part of heart muscle can be damaged. This damaged part due to new pathological focus causes the heart to depolarise all the time. In this circumstance, current flows between pathologically depolarised and normally polarised area. This is called 'current of injury.'
- The various causes include—mechanical trauma—(It makes membrane so permeable that process of repolarisation is checked), Infection (this damages the muscle membrane), Ischaemia of local areas of muscle because of coronary occlusion (due to non-availability of nutrient).

J (ZERO-REFERENCE POTENTIAL) POINT

- It is the exact point at which wave of depolarisation just completes its passage, through the heart. So it occurs at the end of QRS complex. Exactly at this point all parts of ventricles are depolarised so that no current is flowing through the heart. Therefore, potential at this point is zero voltage. This is J point. For analysis of electrical axis of the injury potential caused by a current on injury a horizontal line is drawn through ECG, at the level of J point.
- In old recovered myocardial infarction the Q wave of QRS complex develops in Lead I in anterior infarction, and in Lead III in the case of posterior infarction and this is because of loss of muscle in these respective areas.

QRS COMPLEX: DURATION AND DISORDERS

- Normal duration of QRS complex is varying between 0.06 - 0.09 seconds.
- Literary QRS complex means 'total duration of process of depolarisation which spreads through ventricles.'
- This period is prolonged when one or both ventricles are hypertrophied or dilated, bundle branch block etc.
- It takes 'Bizarre shape' when there occurs destruction of cardiac muscle in various areas throughout the ventricular system with replacement of it by scar tissue. It also seems to be evident when local blocks occur at multiple points in the ventricles.

ALTERATION IN ECG VOLTAGE

- Normally the voltage in the three standard bipolar limb leads is varying between 0.5 to 2.0 mV; as measured from the peak of R wave to the bottom of S wave. Lead II is recording highest voltage while lead III usually records the lowest voltage.
- In general, when the sum of voltages of all the QRS complexes of the three standard leads is greater than 4 mV it constitutes high voltage cardiogram; and on the contrary less than 4 mV is low voltage cardiogram.
- *Increased voltage cardiogram:* In cardiac hypertrophy there is increased muscular mass which occurs when there is an increased load on the heart. It is obvious that left ventricle hypertrophies because of hypertension as well as stenosis of aortic valve; while right ventricle is hypertrophied on account of stenosed pulmonary valve. The increased quantity of the muscle allows generation of increased quantity of electricity around the heart. Because of it electrical potential recorded in ECG leads are considerably greater than normal.
- *Decreased voltage cardiogram:* In cardiac myopathies (myocardial infarction, diminished muscle mass etc.) there is decreased voltage. Due to this, the wave of depolarisation moves slowly through the ventricles and thus major part of the heart is prevented from depolarisation. This prolongs QRS complex.
- *In lung emphysema:* There exists excessive quantities of air in lungs as well as enlargement of chest cavity. Because of these two alterations the lungs envelop the heart to a greater extent. In other words, they act as an insulator to prevent spread of electrical voltage from the heart to the surface of the body and this results in decreased voltage/potential in ECG leads.
- Normally the extracellular fluid conducts electric current with an ease. When there is pericardial effusion; this electric current is short circuited which reduces the voltage. Same thing occurs in pleural effusion.

ABNORMALITIES OF T WAVE

- T wave is normally positive in all the standard bipolar leads. The reason is explained earlier in this section. The T wave becomes abnormal when the normal sequence of repolarisation does not occur.
- Digitalis is the drug given to increase the strength of myocardial contraction during relative coronary insufficiency. However, digitalis also increases the period of depolarisation of cardiac muscle. In its overdosage, the depolarisation of one part of the heart may be increased out of proportion to that of other parts and this is responsible for non-specific changes in T wave like 'inversion' OR 'biphasic,' which is classed as 'digitalis toxicity.'
- In myocardial ischaemia, the depolarisation time of affected area is increased out of proportion as compared with other part. This is responsible for T wave changes.

ELECTROCARDIOGRAM: DISTURBANCES (CARDIAC ARRHYTHMIAS)

Common cardiac arrhythmias and their effects on heart pumping is very well diagnosed by Electrocardiography.

1. *Tachycardia:* Sinus tachycardia may be defined as a sinus rhythm with a rate in excess of 100 beats per minute in the average adult.
   Any condition that permits the pacemaker cells of SA node to reach threshold potential more rapidly can initiate sinus tachycardia.

Causes

a. Physiological mechanism in response to an increase in metabolic activity of the body in greater demand for oxygenation, e.g. maximal exercise, pain, emotions, heat application, ingestion of food, excess use of alcohol-coffee-tea, decreased vagal tone, increased sympathetic tone, psychic trauma, respiration etc.
b. As a compensatory mechanism in an effort to increase cardiac output, e.g. haemorrhage, shock, anaemia, CHF.
c. In drug induced, e.g. atropine, amphetamine, ephedrine, isoproterenol.
d. As a consequence of some pathology, e.g. infection, sepsis, fluid depletion, fever, embolic phenomenon, hyperthyroidism, myocardial infarction, neurosis.

2. *Bradycardia:* Means less than 60 beats per minute in an average adult, less than 100 beats in infant and less than 80 beats in children.

Causes

Includes:

a. In response to physiological changes, e.g. increase in carotid sinus and aortic pressure, vagal maneuvers, decreased metabolic needs (sleep, ageing process), conditioned training etc.
b. Increase in vagal tone, e.g. emotional trauma, eyeball compression, carotid massage, valsalva maneuver, mushroom poisoning, endotracheal suctioning etc.
c. Drug induced, e.g. narcotics, beta blockage agents, morphine, cardiotonic digitalis etc.
d. Pathologic changes, e.g. myxoedema, myocardial infarction, increased intracranial pressure, hypothermia, obstructive jaundice, hypopituitarism etc.
e. Bradycardia commonly found in athletes who train for a long period of time is attributed to the mechanism of slowing of intrinsic rate of SA node, and depression of tonic influence upon the sympathetic nerves. In non-athlete greater body activity is met by an increase in heart rate, whereas in long distance runner, there is a greater utilisation of stroke volume.
f. Excess quantity of blood is pumped by heart of an athlete. This gives birth to feedback circulatory reflexes which causes bradycardia at rest.

HEART RATE: DETERMINATION

- Find out R-R interval
- Suppose it is 0.8 sec (Four squares)
- Paper moves with a speed of 25 mm/sec
- So 60/0.8 = 75 beats/minute
  (Converting seconds into minutes).

SINUS-ATRIAL BLOCK

Sinus node has the fastest inherent rate and thus sets the tempo of cardiac rate. SA node may fail to discharge an impulse, OR; it may take longer for the impulse to activate the atrial myocardium; OR, an exist block may prevent the discharged impulses from reaching the atrial muscle. Dysfunction of this type are called sinus-atrial block.

ATRIO-VENTRICULAR BLOCK

- The AV bundle or bundle of His is the only means through which impulses can pass from atria into the ventricle.
- Types:
  — First degree block (incomplete block). Normally P-R interval ranges between 0.13 to 0.16 seconds. If it is prolonged; the patient is said to suffer from first degree block. It otherwise means - delay of conduction from atria to the ventricle (it is 0.30 sec).
  — Second degree (incomplete) block
    1. If P-R interval is ranging from 0.25 to 0.45 seconds and is characterised by dropped beats.
    2. Dropped beats means - normally one beat from atrium passes to ventricles. It may be comparatively weak sometimes that one beat from atrium may not pass to ventricle. This is causing alternate conduction and non-conduction. Atria beats faster than ventricles (dropped beats) giving rise to ratio like 2:1, 3:1 (atria beats twice or thrice for each ventricular beat).

— Complete block (Third degree block) - complete block of impulses from atria into ventricles. P wave is completely dissociated from QRST complex.

— Stokes-Adam syndrome—Sometimes, impulses are conducted from atria to ventricles; then, no impulses are transmitted. This total block period may be of indefinite duration. After sometime, "pacemaker of ventricle" is activated, which discharges impulses at rate of 15-40 per minute. This is vagal escape.

In its first part of story (means a period of block), the brain also gets no blood supply. Since brain cannot remain active for more than 3–5 seconds without blood, so person faints. This is followed by "vagal escape" which supplies enough blood to brain required for recovery. So recovery from fainting occurs. These periodic fainting spells are called "Stokes-Adam syndrome."

CONDITIONS LEADING TO AV BLOCK

- Ischaemia .... of AV node/bundle
- Inflammation ...... of AV node/bundle, diphtheria, rheumatic fever may lead to it.
- Calcification ...... of AV bundle may compress it.
- Vagal stimulation .... e.g. strong stimulation of baro-receptors with carotid sinus syndrome.

PAROXYSMAL TACHYCARDIA

- Paroxysmal means that the heart rate usually becomes very rapid in paroxysms, with its beginning suddenly and lasting for a few seconds, few minutes, or few hours or even much longer. They end as suddenly as they began.
- Ventricular paroxysmal tachycardia is more dangerous because it can initiate fibrillation which is a dangerous state. This tachycardia is seen in ischaemic states. It may result from digitalis toxicity.
- In such atrial tachycardia inverted P wave occurs before each QRST complex. This P wave is partially superimposed on the normal T wave of the preceding beat.
- It can also be treated by eliciting vagal reflex (application of painful pressure on eyeball).

VENTRICULAR FIBRILLATION

- *Introducing:* Sometimes due to any other reasons, one portion of ventricular muscle is contracting while another is relaxing. Therefore, co-ordination in contraction is lost in heart muscle which is required for a pumping cycle of the heart. Therefore, despite massive flow of stimulatory signals throughout the ventricles, the ventricles neither enlarges nor contracts but remain in an undeterminate stage of partial contraction pumping either no blood at all or negligible amounts. This is fibrillation.
- Treatment:
  - — Defibrillation - It is done by electric shock. Fibrillation can be stopped by 110 volts of 60 cycle AC (alternating current) which is applied for 0.1 second.
  - — Direct current (DC) of 1000 volts applied for a thousandth of a second can also stop fibrillation.
- *ECG in fibrillation:* Low voltage, irregular waves, or extreme bizarre showing no tendency towards a regular rhythm or must like an innocent child has written something on the paper which is not understood.
- Initially the voltage in fibrillation is 0.5 mV and they rapidly decay. Within 20-30 seconds they are of 0.2 to 0.3 mV. This voltage may further be reduced to 0.1 mV or even less in next few seconds.

CIRCUS MOVEMENT THEORY: VENTRICULAR FIBRILLATION

When a normal cardiac impulse has travelled to entire extent of ventricle then, it dies and heart is waiting for a new impulse. This is the normal happening. But:-

- If the distance is long (dilated heart) then the impulse will not die but it will continue again and again giving rise to fibrillation.
- If velocity of conduction is decreased (high potassium content, ischaemia, block in Purkinje system), then also fibrillation results.
- If refractory period is shortened (by epinephrine administration) then also fibrillation results.

ATRIAL FIBRILLATION

- Atria and ventricle are separated from each other, (rather insulated) by fibrous tissue. So fibrillation can occur in any one of them, independent from each other.
- Enlargement of atrium is the primary cause. It may be due to any valvular lesion which resist in emptying of atria, so leads to damming of blood. This constitutes long conductive pathway which manifests in fibrillation. The pumping capability of atria is reduced which supplies less blood (comparatively) to ventricles. So this is not so lethal as the ventricular fibrillation is:
- Treatment is the same, i.e. electroshock therapy.
- ECG picture includes:-
  - — Completely normal QRST complex, Either no P wave; or
  - — low voltage wave record.

VERTICAL HEART

aVF resembles V6
small r wave, large S and inverted T in aVR
Left cavity complex in aVL with QS, inverted T

LEFT AXIS DEVIATION

QRS axis>15
negative comples in LIII, aVF
upring in L1 & aVL

MYXEDEMA

Possible ECG effects include: bradycardia, prolonged P-R interval, low-voltage QRS complexes, low T waves
Note low QRS complexes and T wave

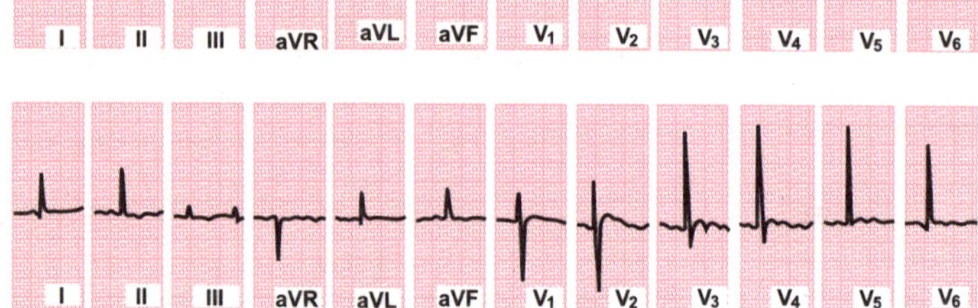

HYPERTHYROIDISM

Lead III shows rate of 125/min
Tachycardia is most characteristic finding; may produce non-specific T wave changes and ST elevation in left ventricular epicardial leads
Note interted T waves in I, II, III, aVF, V6 diphasic T waves in V2-5
Note: ECG also show LVH

Fig. 75.4

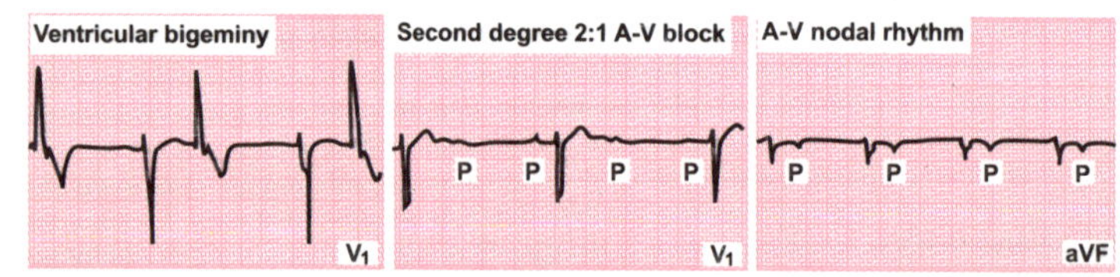

DIGITALIS TOXICITY

Unifocal or multifocal VPC's usually in bigeminy, varying degree of AV block
Junctional or nodal rhythms are the most usual arrhythmias due to digitalis toxicity

LEFT VENTRICULAR HYPERTROPHY

Deep S wave in V1, V2 and tall R in V5, V6
Left axis deviation
Tall R in aVL
Abnormalities of St-T segment in Left leads
Small equiphasic rS complex in aVF

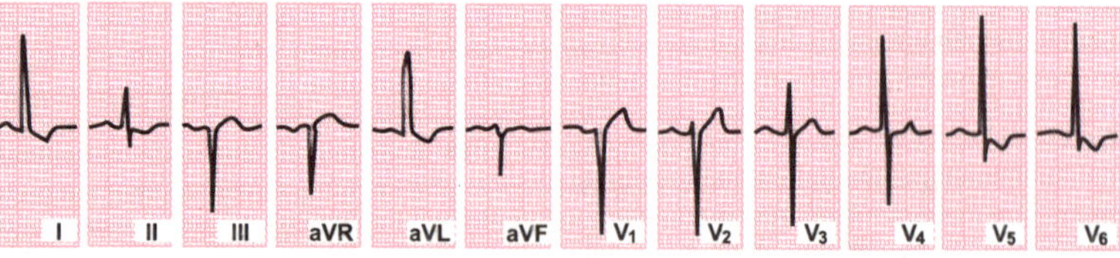

Fig. 75.5

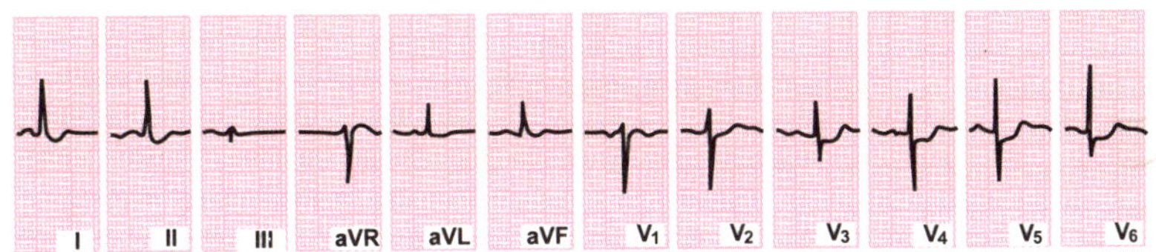

DIGITALIS EFFECT

ST segment depression commonly occurs with digitalization.
Not to be equated with digitalis intoxication
ST segment depression present I, II, aVF, and V2-6

RIGHT VENTRICULAR STRAIN

Vertical heart
Right axis deviation, tall 'R' and inverted T in V1-4 with or without depressed ST segment

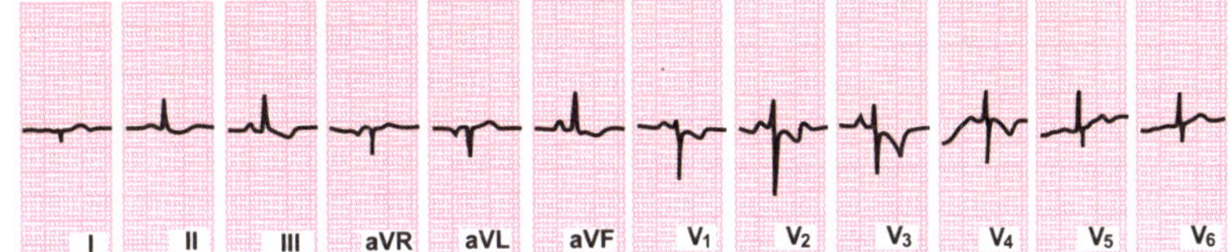

SINUS TACHYCARDIA

Sinus rhythm with rates above 100 beats per minute and below 160 (adult)

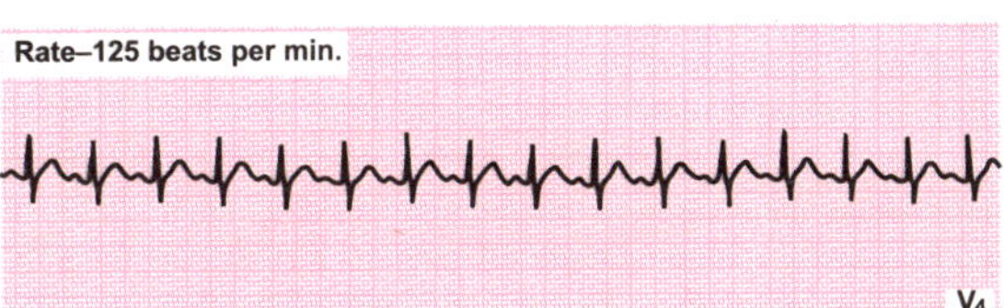

Fig. 75.6

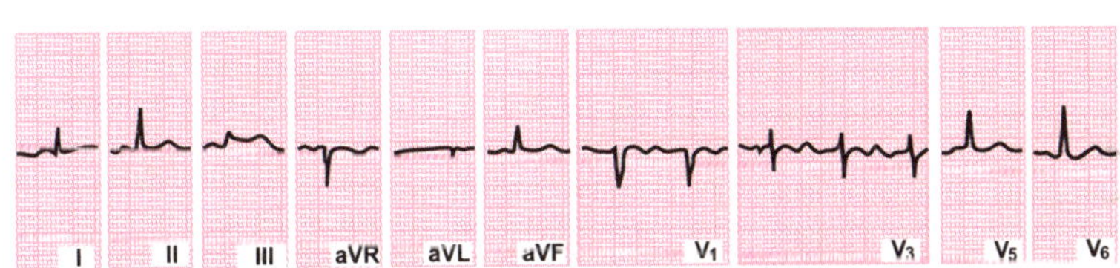

HYPOKALEMIA

T waves may become depressed, and prominent U waves are noted
Depression of ST segments in precordial leads is usual
QT appears prolonged in some leads where separation from U wave is not distinct

SINUS BRADYCARDIA

Sinus rhythm with rate below 60 beats per minute

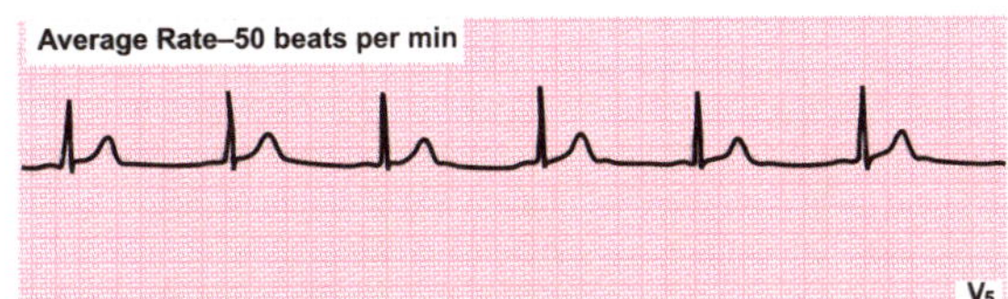

Fig. 75.7

VENTRICULAR FIBRILLATION

Rapid rate, irregular thythm
No discreate complexes chaotic and deformed deflections.
If untreated, is usually fatal.

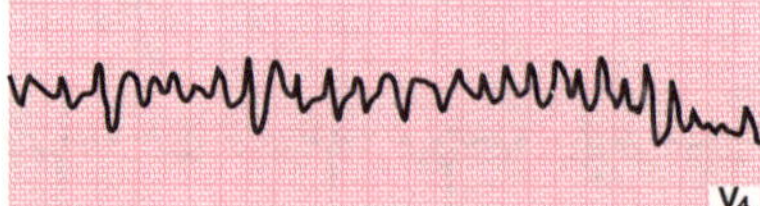

WOLFF-PARKINSON-WHITE SYNDROME (ACCELERATED CONDUCTION)

Short P-R interval
Wide QRS
Upstroke of R wave slurred in I, aVL, and V2-6
ST segment depression in I, aVL V2-6

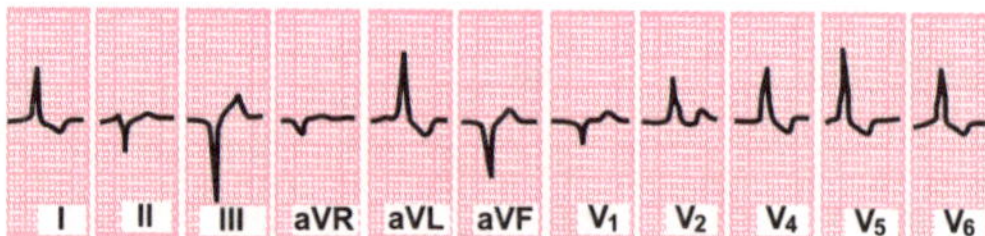

INCOMPLETE A-V BLOCK
(FIRST DEGREE BLOCK)

P-R interval 0.20 second
prolonged A-V conduction time only
ventricular rhythm regular
without dropped beats

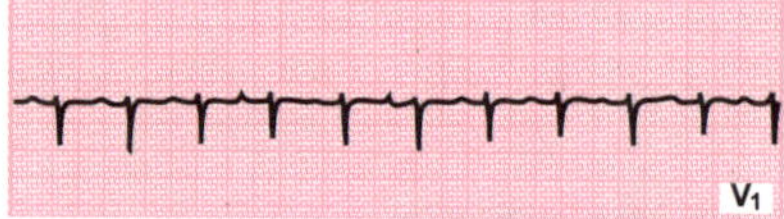

INCOMPLETE A-V BLOCK
(SECOND DEGREE BLOCK)

The example shows 2:1 block with alternate response of ventricle to atrial beats
Regular P-R intervals
when any but not all ventricular beats are dropped, 2nd degree A-V block exists

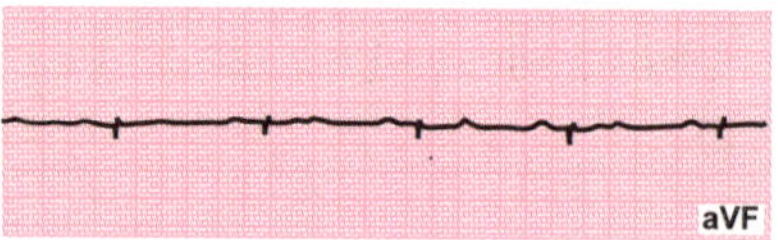

INCOMPLETE A-V BLOCK
(WENCKEBACH PHENOMENON)

Cyclic progressive lengthening of P-R interval in successive beats until a beat is dropped
Arrows - P wave

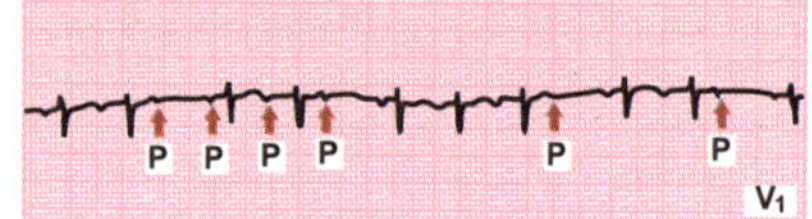

Fig. 75.8

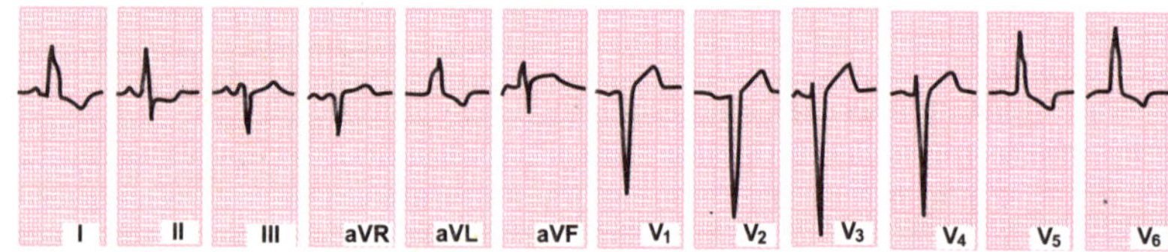

COMPLETE LEFT BUNDLE BRANCH BLOCK

QRS interval 0.12 Sec
wide slurred R wave in I, aVL, V5-V6
Absence of Q in I, V5-6
Lead similar to aVL and V5-6 with depressed ST segment and inverted T waves

COMPLETE A-V BLOCK
(THIRD DEGREE BLOCK)

Independent regular strial and ventricular rhythms
Atrial rate 72/min. ventricular rate 54/min
SA impulses do not depolarize the ventricles

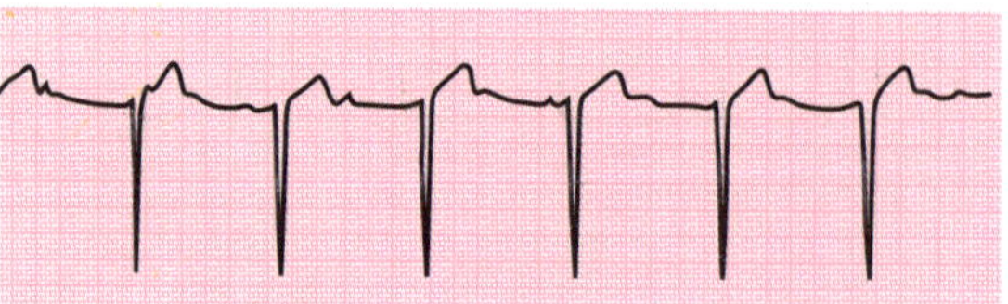

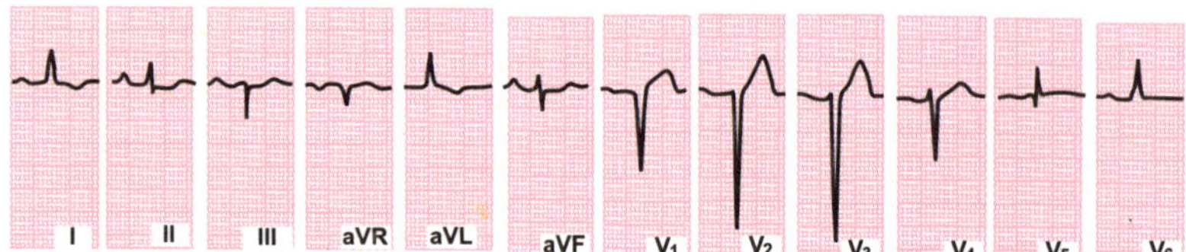

INCOMPLETE LEFT BUNDLE BRANCH BLOCK

Left axis deviation
QRS 0.09 sec. (less than 0.12 sec.)
VAT or intrinsicoid deflection shorter than 0.09 sec.
Inverted T in I and aVL
rsR' complex in V5
Slurred R in V6
Flat T in V5-6
Q waves not present in I, aVL, V5-6

Fig. 75.9

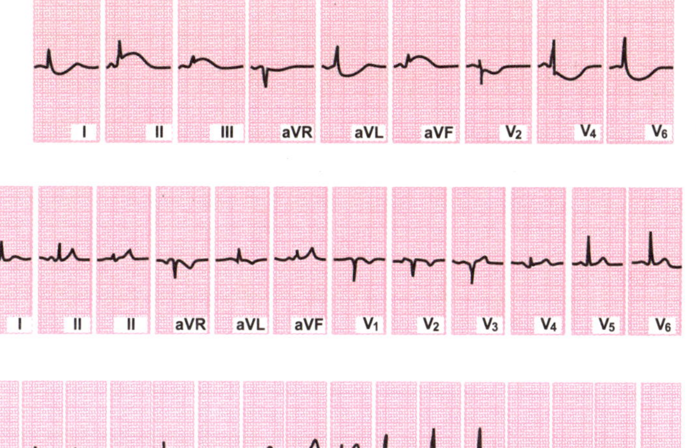

INFERIOR WALL INFARCTION
(Serial changes #1)

HYPER ACUTE STAGE
(Hours)

Elevated ST segment in II, III, aVF depressed ST segment I, aVL and V leads

OLD ANTEROSEPTAL INFARCTION

QS complexes in V1-3 with or without inverted T waves in V1, 2, aVL

OLD HIGH ANTEROLATERAL WALL INFARCTION

small, wide Q wave in I and aVL inverted T wave in I, aVL, V6
3rd interspace leads show QS complexes in 3V2, 3,4
(Poor 'R' wave progression)

VENTRICULAR TACHYCARDIA

Rate variable from 140 to 250 beats per minute
slightly irregular rhythm
Wide, slurred QRS complexes of ventricular premature beats
ST segment and T waves indistinguishable
There is an independent slower P rate, but the P waves are often obscured.

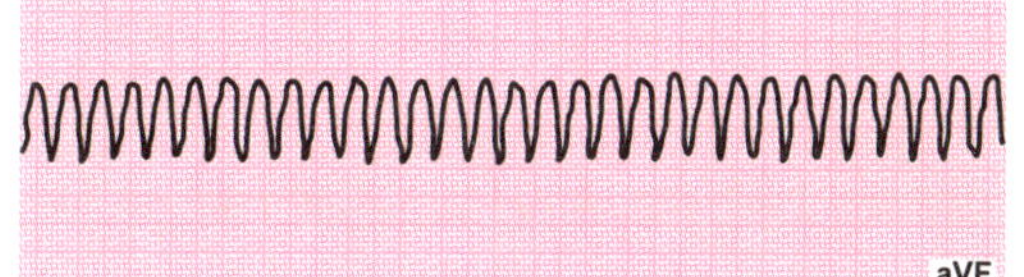

Fig. 75.10

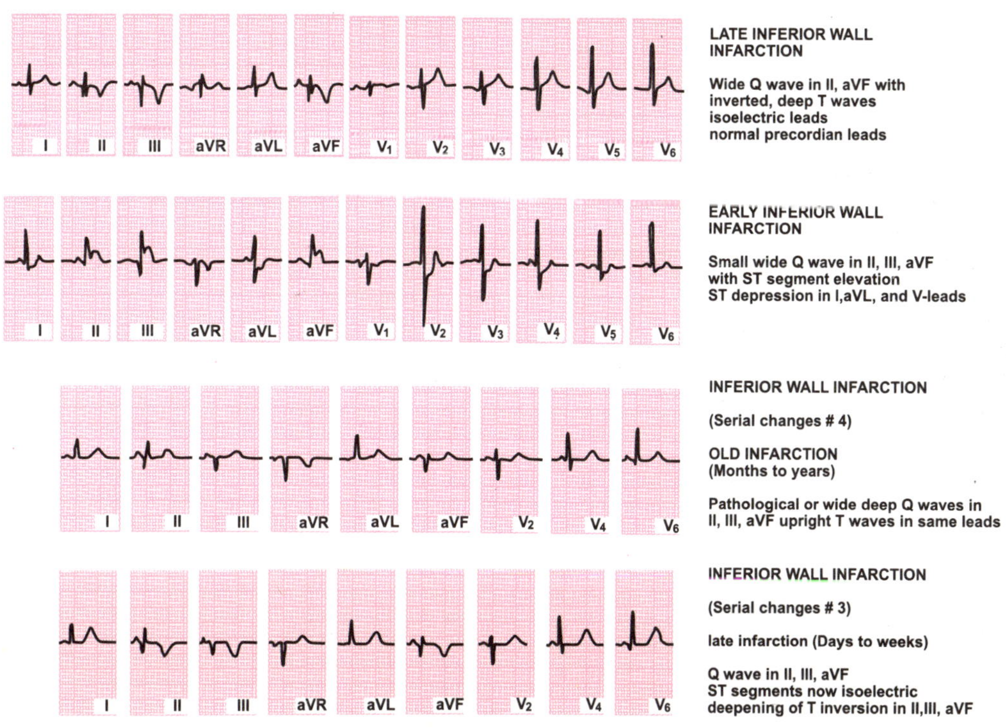

LATE INFERIOR WALL INFARCTION

Wide Q wave in II, aVF with inverted, deep T waves
isoelectric leads
normal precordian leads

EARLY INFERIOR WALL INFARCTION

Small wide Q wave in II, III, aVF with ST segment elevation
ST depression in I,aVL, and V-leads

INFERIOR WALL INFARCTION

(Serial changes # 4)

OLD INFARCTION
(Months to years)

Pathological or wide deep Q waves in II, III, aVF upright T waves in same leads

INFERIOR WALL INFARCTION

(Serial changes # 3)

late infarction (Days to weeks)

Q wave in II, III, aVF
ST segments now isoelectric
deepening of T inversion in II,III, aVF

Fig. 75.11

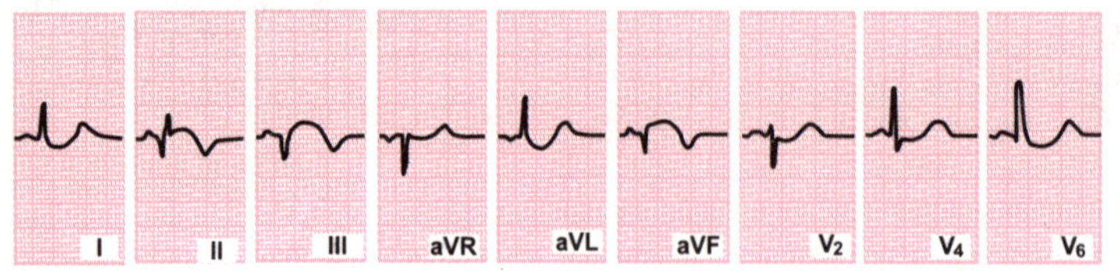

INFERIOR WAL INFARCTION
(Serial changes # 2)

RECENT INFARCTION
(Several bouns to days)

Appearance of Q wave in II,III, and a VF
Decreased elevation and depression of involved ST segments
inversion of T waves in II,III, aVF.

ATRIAL FLUTTER

Saw-tooth flutter waves may occur at rates of 220-350 per minute
Saw-tooth flutter waves seen in II,III,aVf
Regular atrial rhythm, 4:1 ventricular response
2nd flutter wave (indicated by arrows) altered by superimposition on T wave.

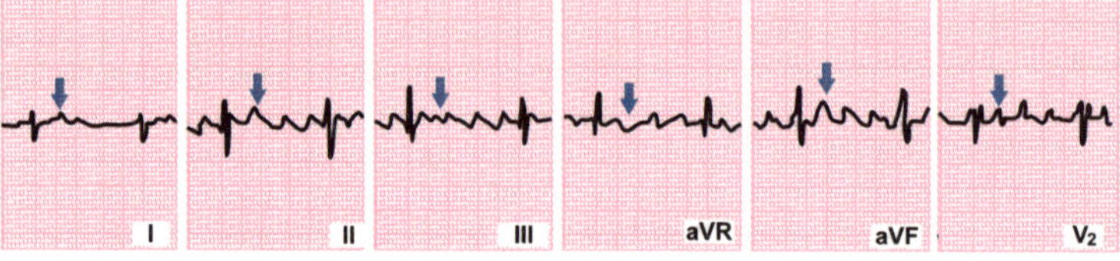

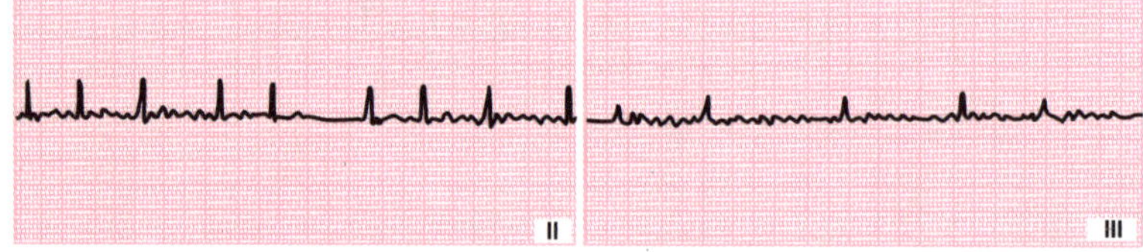

Fig. 75.12
(*Courtesy:* Nicholas Drug Company, Figs 75.4 to 75.12)

ECG: MYOCARDIAL INFARCTION

1. Elevation of ST segment because:
   - Membrane potential of infarcted area is greater than normal area. This makes normal region negative relative to infarct. So current flows out of infarct area into normal area.
   - Delayed depolarisation of infarcted cells causes infarcted area to be positive in relation to healthy tissue. This leads to ST segment elevation.
2. Appearance of Q wave in old infarction
   - After sometime ST segment abnormality disappear. Dead tissue is electrically silent. The infarcted area is hence negative in relation to normal myocardium.
3. T wave inversion.
4. Failure of progression of R wave. It fails to be successively larger in precordial leads.

BIBLIOGRAPHY

1. Burch GE, Winsor T. A primer of electrocardiography, 6th ed. Lea and Febiger, Philadelphia. 1972.
2. Chung EK. Electro cardiography, 2nd Ed. Harper and Row Hagerstown Md. 1980.
3. Goldman MJ. Principles of clinical electrocardiography, 12th edition, Lange publication. 1986.
4. Jelliffe RW. Fundamentals of electrocardiography, Springer-Verlag. 1990.
5. Johnson R, et al. A simplified approach to electrocardiography, Philadelphia, WB Sauders Co. 1986.
6. Lipman B. Clinical electrocardiography, Chicago year book medical publishers. 1984.

76 Informative of Heart—II Vascular System: Pulse

The pulse gives direct information regarding the condition of the vessel walls and amount and variations of pressure of the contained blood. By these observations valuable information regarding the state of the heart and circulation, as well as general state of the patient, can be obtained.

Don't examine the pulse as soon as the patient comes since exercise and emotions alter it. Give him little time to relax. Pulse is best felt when wrist is flexed and forearm is semipronated. It should be examined for one complete minute by putting three fingers on radial artery namely index, middle and ring.

OBSERVATION

Examine the pulse for following parameters

i. *Rate:* Simply means number of beats per minute. It is counted not when the fingers are first laid upon the pulse, but when any quickening due to nervousness of the patient has subsided and the pulse has resumed to normal state. The pulse rate is increased during exercise, fever, thyrotoxicosis, paroxysmal atrial tachycardia, atrial fibrillation flutter, etc.

   It is slowed somewhat in myxoedema, complete heart block.

   It should be remembered that normal pulse rate is ranging between 60-90 beats per minute; above 90 beats is referred as *'tachycardia'*, and below 60 beats is *'bradycardia'*.

ii. *Rhythm*

   Describe it in terms of *regular* or *irregular*. It simply means the time interval between two beats, which should be uniform throughout. Irregular rhythm with normal heart rate seen in multiple ectopics, slow atrial fibrillation, sinus arrhythmias.

iii. *Force and Tension*

   - Force corresponds to systolic pressure. Press the radial artery against the underlying bone with the more proximal of the two palpating fingers till the pulse wave is no longer felt with the distal finger. More the pressure required to obliterate the pulse, higher the systolic pressure.
   - Tension gives an idea of diastolic pressure. When tension is low, the artery is easily flattened and resumes its cylindrical shape without undue resistance. The pulse of low tension appears to collapse between the beats so that nothing is felt at this time. If the diastolic pressure is high, the artery is palpable both in systole and diastole.

iv. *Volume*

   Corresponds to amplitude and duration. Large volume in exercise, pregnancy, warm humid weather, pathologically in anaemia, fever, thyrotoxicosis, liver cirrhosis, hypertension, obesity, polycythaemia, nephritis, hyperkinetic states.

   Small volume - observed in

   - Decreased cardiac output (CCF, shock, pericarditis, myocarditis).
   - Peripheral vasoconstriction (hypovolemic shock).
   - Mechanical obstruction (MS, AS, coarctation).

v. *Condition of vessel wall:*

   For this purpose sufficient pressure should be exerted to empty the vessel of blood and then it should be rolled beneath the fingers against the underlying bone. In young persons the arteries cannot be felt or are soft. In older persons they are easily palpable. In arteriosclerosis they may feel hard or may be tortuous. It is a good practice to feel both radials and brachials.

DESCRIPTION OF A NORMAL PULSE

It is 75 beats per minute, regular in rhythm and equal in character. It is of moderate volume and is not collapsing in character. The arterial wall is just palpable, but is neither thick nor tortuous.

ABNORMALITIES OF PULSE

i. *Water Hammer pulse:* The pulse strikes with the palpating finger with a rapid forceful jerk and quickly disappears. It is classed as 'water hammer' because of its sudden impact and a collapsing quality because it falls away rapidly. The effect is accentuated if the pulse is examined with the patient's arm elevated because the radial artery is then in more direct line with the outflow stream from the aorta. It is seen in hyperkinetic circulatory states like anaemia, thyrotoxicosis, beri-beri, aortic in competence, liver cirrhosis, extreme bradycardia, Paget's disease, AV block. Physiologically it is found in pregnancy, hot water bath, alcoholism etc.

ii. *Pulsus alterance:* A strong and a weak beat. It results probably from alternate rather than regular contraction of muscle fibres of left ventricle, those which responds to one stimulus failing to respond to the next. It is seen in left ventricular failure, toxic myocarditis etc. In normal persons it may occur during paroxysmal tachycardia or for several beats following a premature beat.

iii. *Anacrotic pulse:* Seen in aortic stenosis where aortic valve is very small. Blood ejected is less during systole of ventricle due to obstruction. So this pulse is prolonged clinically with low pulse pressure. The ascent of pulse tracing is sloping and vibrating.

iv. *Dicrotic pulse:* Dicrotic notch becomes prominent due to diminished peripheral resistance. Two pulse beats are felt with one smaller. Heart rate is very slow. Seen in fever, vasodilatation states.

PULSE WAVE: TRACING

Tracing Itself

a. *Aortic:*
- The pressure rises abruptly at first (anacrotic limb)
- It reaches the peak which is rounded.
- Then it gradually falls (coinciding with last half of systole) until the closure of aortic valves, which is marked by dicrotic notch (incisura).
- Finally it is descending down slowly; coinciding with diastole (dicrotic wave). The descending part of the wave is catacrotic limb.

b. *Femoral/brachial*
- Delayed onset
- Rise of ascending limb is slow.
- The peak is sharp, (instead of round in aortic tracing).
- Quicker drop of descending limb
- Obliterated dicrotic notch with large dicrotic wave.
- Total events lasts shorter as compared with aortic tracing.

Methods of Study

i. With the help of catheter or needle connected with electronic pressure meters; it can be recorded. (ii) A pressure sensitive cup tambour may be placed over a superficial artery or vein connected with recording device. (iii) Peripheral pulse tracing is done by the instrument ***Dudgeon's sphygmograph***.

ii.
- ***Sphygmograph*** is an instrument specially used for recording pulse wave at wrist on radial artery.
- The record is written by a stylet which is moved by a metal button placed over the radial artery. The smoked paper moves through clock-work arrangements.

iii. Mackenzie ink polygraph is another device for it.

VENOUS PULSE

- Venous pulse tracing is called *Phlebogram.*
- It is due to pressure changes in the heart, which is imparted to the great veins at the root of the heart. It is mostly obtained from jugular vein.
- *Three upstrokes (positive waves) ...*
  - — The first up stroke is due to atrial systole when an impact is sent to the vein or engorgement of the vein which has failed to drain because of high atrial pressure during its contraction.
  - — Second upstroke is due to isometric contraction of ventricles because of which AV valves are swaying back to atrial cavity. Because of this the veins swell up temporarily and shows inability to drain.
  - — Third upstroke is because of increased pressure and stasis in Jugular vein during ventricular systole. Because of this, blood flow is impeded from neck veins into atrium, where pressure is rising.
- *Three down strokes (negative waves):*
  - — The first down stroke is due to atrial diastole.
  - — The second down stroke is due to suction of blood into atria because of ventricular contraction.
  - — The third down stroke is because of onset of ventricular diastole - opening of AV valves so blood flows from atria to ventricles.
- *Significance:*
  - — Guide for cardiac cycle
  - — First upstroke wave absent—atrial fibrillation

n
d

Arterial tracing (sphygmograph)
n = Dicrotic notch
d = Dicrotic wave

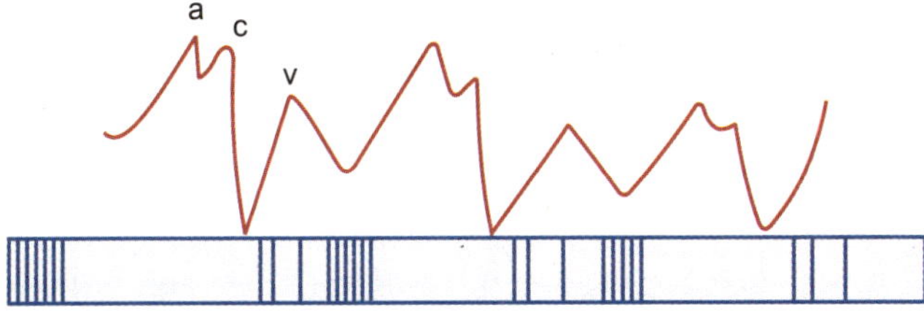

Fig. 76.1: Arterial tracing

— Numerous first upstroke waves—complete heart block
— Giant first upstroke wave—tricuspid stenosis.
— Giant third upstroke wave—tricuspid insufficiency.

- *Factors helping venous blood flow:*
  — Vis-a-tergo ... (Force from behind) - Is supplied by left ventricle contraction.
  — Vis-a-fronto- (Force from front) .. It draws in blood into right atrium.

SUMMARY AND HIGHLIGHTS

Don't examine the pulse as patients comes to you. Put three fingers on radial artery. The hand should be flexed and forearm should be semipronated. Examine for one complete minute. Put your observation under all the headings mentioned above.

77 Heart and Rheumatism
(Valvular Diseases)

> Rheumatism may lick joints, specially in children, but it certainly bites the whole heart. It is the valvular rather than myocardial damage which is the chief threat to the patient.

The causal agent is Group A haemolytic streptococci which sensitise the fibrous tissue in many parts of the body uniting with connective tissue protein to form an antigen. This, in turn, excites the formation of specific antibodies ensuring antigen-antibody reaction resulting in focal allergic neurosis with accompanying cellular response.

Rheumatic fever is therefore not a simple streptococcal disease like scarlet fever, because no bacteria can be demonstrated usually in blood or lesion, and an interval of 10-14 days elapses between initial throat infection and development of rheumatic fever. It is an allergic response to Streptococcus and its products. This response is accompanied by changes in plasma protein particularly hyperglobulinaemia, first of alpha and then gamma globulins. The C-reactive proteins which precipitates with carbohydrate of pneumococci is contained in alpha globulin.

When human body came into existence by nature, it was decided that it will be affected by various seasons. At least four times a year, the weather changes and the most common effect is a bad or sore-throat. It is due to infection caused by bacteria Streptococcus haemolyticus. It releases several proteins against which antibodies are formed. This antigen (M) - antibody reaction leads to various immunological damage, and the most sensitive part is the heart valves so called rheumatic heart disease.

In rheumatic fever large haemorrhagic, fibrinous bulbous lesion grow along inflamed edges of the heart valves. The mitral valve is often seriously damaged since it receives greatest trauma, and aortic valve is number two as regards the damage is concerned. Because of slight stress the pulmonary and tricuspid valves are less effected.

If because of this lesion the leaflets of the valve adhere to each other so extensively that blood cannot flow satisfactorily through them, this is called stenosis. On the other hand, when valve edges are so destroyed by scar tissue that they cannot close when ventricles contract; this leads to back flow or regurgitation of blood when valve should be closed.

DYNAMICS OF AORTIC VALVE DISORDERS

- In stenosis—left ventricle fails to empty its contents adequately.
- In regurgitation—blood returns back to the ventricle from aorta.
- So in both the cases, net stroke volume output of the heart is reduced; left ventricular pressure increases.
- To meet with the excess demand the left ventricle enlarges - so-called hypertrophy. Left ventricular mass increases and pressure may even rise up to 400 mmHg, and the pressure difference across the stenosed valve may be 100 mmHg. In severe aortic regurgitation, the hypertrophied muscle allows the left ventricle to pump a stroke volume output as high as 250 ml and this is the virtual fact that 3/4th part of this amount of blood returns back to left ventricle because of regurgitation.
- In such instances, the situation is compensated by increase in blood volume which tends to increase cardiac output and venous return; which in turn increases the ventricular end-diastolic volume and end-diastolic pressure, causing left ventricle to pump with extra power required to overcome the abnormal pumping dynamics.
- In aortic stenosis the pressure in left ventricle is raised and on pumping the blood towards aorta, because of its narrow size, a nozzle effect is created during systole with blood jetting at tremendous velocity

through the small opening of the valve. This turbulent blood impinging against the aortic walls causes intense vibrations and a loud murmur is heard throughout upper aorta and even into large arteries of the neck. It can be even felt as thrill by putting hand on upper chest and lower neck. It is so loud sound that is heard from a distance from the patient.

- In aortic regurgitation left ventricle has emptied its contents into aorta which means systole has taken place; so no sound is heard during systole. But the blood regurgitates into left ventricle which produces turbulent flow leading to production of blowing murmur (high pitch swishing quality).
- Stenosis of aortic valve may be classified as non-calcific or calcific. Former is predominantly due to rheumatic fever. The normal area of aortic valve is 3 cm to 0.5 cm. Those patients with aortic stenosis who are asymptomatic usually have a normal cardiac output and stroke volume. The systolic gradient of pressure between left ventricle and aorta is the diagnostic feature present in all the cases, (It may reach as high as 150 mmHg). The left ventricular end-diastolic pressure is usually normal.
- Haemodynamic picture: Aortic stenosis
  Because of obstruction between left ventricle and aorta; the left ventricular systolic pressure must rise to force blood through stenosed valve. The period of ejection is prolonged and blood is expelled at a high velocity. The percentage of left ventricular work in giving velocity to the blood rises sharply. An increased diastolic volume causes a more forceful systolic contraction with restoration of normal cardiac output. Left ventricular hypertrophy develops to compensate for the increased work load and may be the reason the left ventricle is able to sustain such high systolic pressure without failure.
- The left ventricular systolic pressure may rise very high but finally the end-diastolic-ventricular pressure must increase in an attempt to maintain cardiac output. One of the reasons for failure of left ventricle may be a decreased coronary supply. Elevation of left ventricular diastolic pressure may eventually lead to a rise in pulmonary circulation pressure through increased left atrial pressure, which puts increased workload for right ventricle leading to right sided heart failure.

Aortic Regurgitation

Aortic incompetence often results from rheumatic fever, or syphilis, rarer causes are bacterial endocarditis, trauma, dissecting aneurysm of the aorta or congenital defects of the valve. The murmur heard is pan-diastolic beginning early after closure of aortic valve. It is continuous throughout diastole because of persistent pressure difference between aorta and ventricle. This murmur is high pitched and usually of low intensity. An apical pre-systolic murmur identical of mitral stenosis is sometimes heard in such patients (discovered by Austin Flint). It is due to vibrations set up in anterior leaflet of mitral valve as blood regurgitates through aortic orifice into the path of the stream entering from left atrium.

Haemodynamics—Aortic Regurgitation

It is due to regurgitation of blood from the aorta into the left ventricle. In animals, it was demonstrated that magnitude of back flow varied with the size of leak and could be 50 per cent or more of the left ventricular output when the cusps were totally deficient. The pressure gradient existing in diastole between left ventricle and aorta, and the duration of diastole filling period are also important factors determining the amount of regurgitation. The left ventricle is called upon to accommodate in diastole, not only the blood from atrium, but that regurgitated as well. This leads to a high initial tension at the end of diastole, and a greater stroke volume during systole; in time dilation and hypertrophy develop to give a very large left ventricle.

MITRAL STENOSIS

The normal average circumference of the mitral opening is 10 cm. Anything less than 7 cm must be regarded as stenosis. It is much common in women than in men. The valve looks like a deep funnel, the walls of which are formed by fused cusps. This valvular opening may be a mere button-hole that hardly admits the tip of little finger. The thickened and sclerosed cusps may become calcified, so that valve can neither open nor shut, a combined condition of stenosis and incompetence. The chordae tendinae is so thickened and shortened that papillary muscles seem to be implanted on the valve.

- The blood rushing through this rigid funnel causes vibrations of its walls which is responsible for diastolic murmur.
- Mitral stenosis is the most common cause of haemoptysis (coughing up of blood). In severe cases, there may be great thickening of the basement membrane supporting both alveolar epithelium and vascular endothelium and space between them may become widened by oedema, so that the alveolar tissue may be many times thicker than normal. As a result there is a grave interference with gaseous exchange, the blood being separated from alveolar

air by so thick a partition. This explains why intense cyanosis may persist inspite of myocardial improvement.

MITRAL REGURGITATION

Blood flows backwards during systole through mitral valve. This leads to 'murmur' (high frequency blowing/swishing similar of aortic regurgitation). It is transmitted strongly into left atrium. But it is deeply situated so this sound is transmitted to the chest through left ventricle and is usually heard at the apex of heart.

Contraction of muscular ring at the base of mitral valve decreases the size of mitral leak during ventricular systole. Since the pressure gradient from left ventricle to left atrium is much larger than from left ventricle to aorta, regurgitation is favoured.

TRICUSPID STENOSIS

It may be due to rheumatic involvement or may be congenital. Its 'murmur' is like mitral stenosis (low pitched, rumbling, in its diastolic timings located parasternally in left fourth or fifth intercostal space; it increases in intensity with inspiration).

TRICUSPID INSUFFICIENCY

May be rheumatic or long congenital or may be due to bacterial endocarditis. Its murmur is pansystolic. The enlarged right atrium is with its increased pressure and so hypertrophied/dilated. This leads to high peripheral venous pressure with hepatomegaly, ascites, oedema etc.

SUMMARY AND HIGHLIGHTS

Rheumatic heart disease is predominantly a disease of childhood and youth (probably before age of 20). The patient may die from heart failure (a) during the first acute phase, (b) during a relapse, or (c) as a result of infection of valves.

By far the commonest valvular defect resulting from rheumatic fever is mitral stenosis. Infection seems to begin in valve rings, although primary focus in the case of mitral is probably the wall of atrium, and in the case of aortic the root of aorta. The condition usually is valvulitis - not merely an endocarditis.

It would seem that rheumatic carditis is mainly subclinical and that acute attacks of rheumatic fever are rare episodes in the course of disease.

BIBLIOGRAPHY

1. Agarwal AK. Aortic stenosis: Diagnosis and therapy of elderly patients. Geriatrics 1985;40:105.
2. Barry A. Aortic and tricuspid valvular disease. New York, Appleton-Century-Crofts. 1980.
3. Deplace NL, et al. Acute severe mitral regurgitation: pathophysiology, clinical recognition and management. Amer J Med 1985;78:293.

UNIT 11

Rhythm of Life

"Man is as old as his arteries."

Cardio-Vascular System—II

78 Haemodynamics Peripheral Resistance

PERIPHERAL RESISTANCE

It can be expressed as ratio between mean arterial pressure and the cardiac output or pressure flow ratio.

$$\text{Peripheral resistance} \propto \frac{\text{Mean arterial pressure}}{\text{Cardiac output}}$$

The mean arterial pressure depends upon amount of blood entering into arterial system and on the rate at which it leaves arterioles to run into capillaries and veins.

$$\text{Peripheral resistance} = \frac{90 \times 1332}{82} = 1{,}445 \text{ dynes sec cm}^{-5}$$

The term peripheral resistance unit is used so PRU

$$= \frac{mmHg}{ml / Sec} = \frac{100}{100} = 1.0$$

Normal range	0.25		4.0 PRU
(Systemic circulation =	(Intense vaso-dilatation)	–	(Intense vaso-constriction)

$$\text{PRU} = \frac{10}{100} = 0.1 \text{ in pulmonary circulation}$$

Normal range = 0.03 – 1.0

REYNOLD'S NUMBER

$$= \frac{rVd}{\eta}$$

r = radius of the tube/vessel
V = Velocity
d = density
η = viscosity

So, when it exceeds 1,000, the laminar flow changes to turbulent flow which produces sound.

Anaemia → less RBC → less viscosity → increased Reynold's number → turbulent flow → sound (murmur) produced.

POISEUILLE'S LAW (1842; French physician)

$$\text{Rate of flow} = \frac{P_1 - P_2}{8l} \times \frac{\pi r^4}{\eta}$$

P_1 and P_2 = Pressure at two ends of a tube
l = length of the tube
r = radius of the tube
η = viscosity of blood

If cross-sectional area decreases, there is increase in viscosity which cause increase in pressure due to increase in resistance.

The pressure at which blood flow stops is critical closing pressure.

MARQUIS-DE-LAPLACE LAW (France; famous "deterministic theory")

A. In a globular structure, e.g. lung alveolus

$$P = \frac{2T}{r}$$

P = Transmural force - or Sum total of all the forces trying to reduce diameter of the sphere.
T = Wall tension
r = radius

B. *Application in lungs:* When surface tension becomes high; or when radius of alveolus is narrowed then alveolus will collapse or, at the end of violent expiratory effort the respiratory bronchioles can collapse.

C. *Application in vascular system:*
- Small r means high P, which means collapse of arteriole
- When BP reduced then "r" falls, which leads to arrival of critical closing pressure; which causes closure of arterioles; which terminates into ischaemia or death of tissue.

D. *Application on heart:*
- Increase in "r" (excess blood at the end of diastole) will reduce the value of P. So efficiency of contraction, i.e. Cardiac output falls/reduced.
- Conversely reduction in "r" leads to an increase in cardiac output.
- On an increase in "r" leads to over distension of ventricles which may compress coronary vessels which may precipitate an attack of angina.

E. *Application in stomach:*
- Food in stomach increases its radius (r); so P (intra gastric pressure) does not rise. This explains "receptive relaxation."

CENTRAL VENOUS AND PERIPHERAL PRESSURE

- When a person is standing, the pressure in right atrium is 0 mmHg (lower limit is –3 to –5; and upper limit is 20-30 mmHg).
- In an adult who is standing absolutely; the pressure in the veins of feet is + 90 mmHg.
- In the arm veins, the pressure at the level of top ribs is about + 6 mmHg because of compression of subclavian vein as it passes over this rib.
- Right atrial pressure is also named as central venous pressure (Fig. 78.1). It is regulated by a balance between ability of heart to pump blood out of the right atrium; as well as tendency for blood to flow from peripheral vessels back into the right atrium.

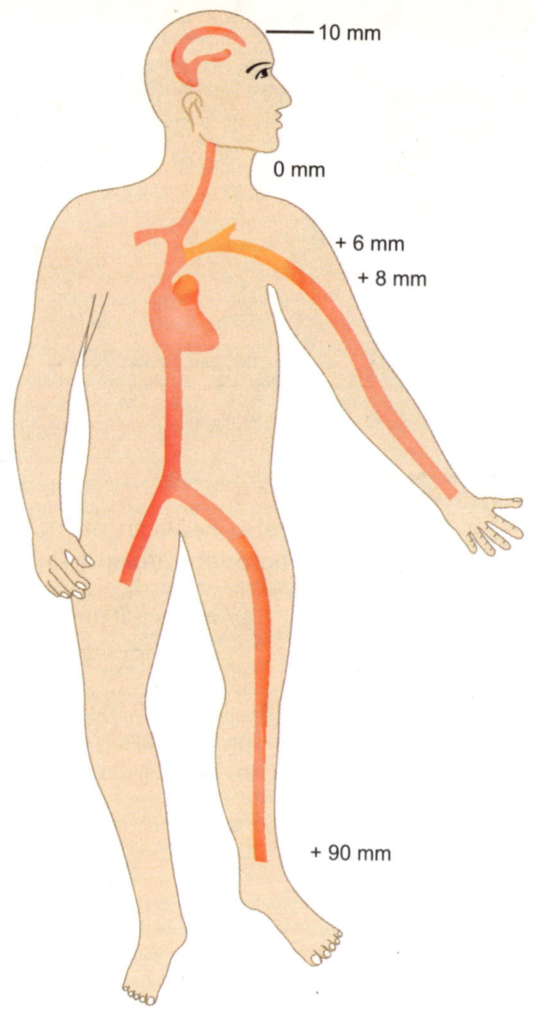

Fig. 78.1: Venous pressure

BLOOD FLOW

1. It means simply the quantity of blood that passes a given point in the circulation in a given period of time.
2. *Laminar flow (Stream line flow)* (Fig. 78.2)
   - Each layer of blood remaining the same distance from the wall.
   - The velocity of flow in centre of the vessel is far greater than that towards the edges.
   - Parabolic profile .... The fluid molecules touching the wall of the vessel adheres to it, so hardly moves. The next succeeding layers will slip over so fluid in middle of the vessel can move rapidly.
   - It is silent.
3. *Turbulent flow*
   - On some circumstances like blood passes through any obstruction, or when flow is very great, the blood flow takes a sharp turn, then it is called 'turbulent flow.'
   - It means whorls of blood/eddy currents.
   - Example—rapidly flowing river at a point of obstruction.
   - It is noisy.

Differences

Laminar flow	*Turbulent flow*
1. Characteristic of most of vascular system	Ventricles and aorta are main site. No small resistance vessels show.
2. Silent in nature	Noisy
3. Shows linear relationship with pressure	Given by Reynold's Number
4. Blood flow in large number of layers. Each layer remains at same distance from vessel wall	Blood flow in all direction and continuously mixing within vessel. Great energy loss is caused.

CIRCULATION TIME

Is the shortest time taken for any particle of the blood to travel from one point to another point in circulation.

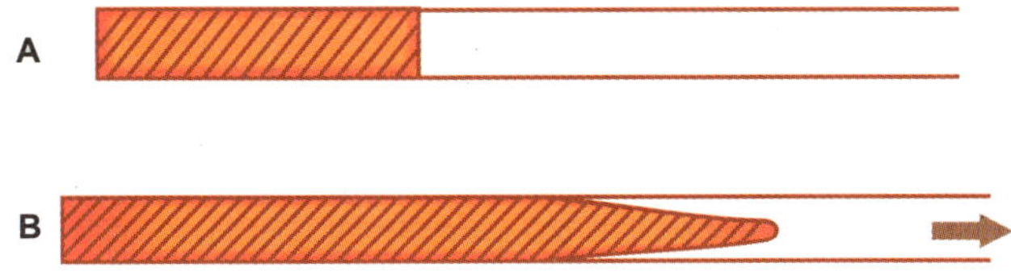

Fig. 78.2: Laminar blood flow

Methods

Name	Substance used	Endpoint	Normal
1. Arm to tongue	Decholine (5 ml of 2% soln.)	Bitter taste (13 sec.)	8-17 sec
2. Arm to lung	5 drops of ether + 5 ml 9% NaCl	Smell in expired air	4-8 sec/ 6 sec
3. Arm to face	Histamine 0.01 mg/kg	Flushing of face	24 sec
4. Arm to carotid body	Sodium cyanide 0.001 mg/kg	Gasping reflex	14 sec

Significance

a. Rough guide to the changes in circulation (volume flow, vasomotor changes);
b. Valuable diagnostic guide in congenital septal heart defects.

Increased Time

Low output failure, myxoedema, haemorrhage and shock, cardiac asthma, exposure to high barometric pressure.

Decreased Time

High output failure, hyperkinetic circulatory states like hyperthyroidism, fever, raised BMR, exposure to low barometric pressure.

ARTERIAL PRESSURE PULSE

i. Impact of blood ejected at one end of the vascular system (aorta) by the contraction of ventricle causes an expansion of vascular wall. It is transmitted to the periphery in the form of a wave with certain velocity.
ii. Pressure pulse reflects imbalance between the amount of blood discharged into the distended aorta and that leaving through the peripheral arterioles, leading to distension by which elastic recoil comes into play, resulting in its transmission as a wave peripherally. So pulse wave is better manifested in the arterial system, where the flow is intermittent, less so in the veins as the flow is continuous and practically nil in capillaries.
iii. Determinants of pulse wave are:
   - Intermittent discharge of blood from contracting left ventricles into aorta.
   - Resistance encountered by blood in its passage from arterioles into capillaries.
   - Elasticity of arterial walls.
iv. The velocity of pulse wave depends on : Elasticity of vessel wall and inertia of blood.

FUNCTIONAL ARRANGEMENTS : VASCULAR SYSTEM

a. *Windkessel vessels*: which convert pulsatile flow into continuous smooth flow.
b. *Resistance vessels*: vessels offering resistance to blood flow, viz small arteries, arterioles, to some extent capillaries.
   i. *Precapillary resistance*: offer bulk of resistance, e.g. small arteries and arterioles.
   ii. *Postcapillary resistance*: depending on veins and venules.
c. *Sphincter vessels*: terminal segment of small arterioles draining into capillaries. These can constrict or dilate and as such they control the area for capillary exchange.
d. *Exchange vessels are capillaries*: Incapable of active contraction but passively yield to alteration of resistance and calibre of sphincter vessels.
e. *Capacitance vessels*: are veins. Offer little resistance by changes in their calibre but can pool large amount of blood affecting venous return and cardiac output.
f. *Shunt vessels:* are arterio-venous-anastomosis, e.g. in palm, finger, ear lobule, nailbeds etc.

CONTROL OF LARGE ELASTIC ARTERIES (AORTA ETC.)

- Convert the fluctuation pressure (due to intermittent contraction of heart) with constant steady pressure.
- They have sensory innervation which monitor the stretching so that pressure is stabilised.
- The smooth muscle components are fairly innervated for this purpose. But the elastic component predominating the arterial wall of large sized vessel dilating easily without offering any resistance of flow.
- The smooth muscle also regulates sensibility of stretch receptor of large arteries and regulate their distensibility.

Differences

Arteries	*Veins*
1. Carry blood from heart to tissues	Carry blood from tissues to heart
2. Blood flows in jerks	Even flow of blood
3. Carry oxygenated blood	Carry deoxygenated blood
4. Deep seated	Superficially located
5. No valves	Provided with valves
6. Walls are thick, muscular and elastic	Thin and nonelastic walls
7. Small lumen	Large lumen
8. Blood flows fast due to high pressure	Flow not so fast

BIOPHYSICAL ASPECTS—I VOLUME FLOW

1. Diameter and cross-section area:
   - The diameter of left ventricle is 6 cm. The diameter and cross-sectional area of ascending aorta is 2.5 cm and 4.5 cm^2 respectively.
   - Vessels become narrow and short in periphery, their total cross-sectional area becomes very large because of large number of vessels involved.
   - The total cross-sectional area of arterioles (individual length 0.015 mm and diameter of .016 mm) is 400 cm^2.
2. *Blood contained:* Aorta contains about 100 ml (2% of total blood volume). The arteries contain 8 per cent of total blood volume; the arterioles about 1 per cent.

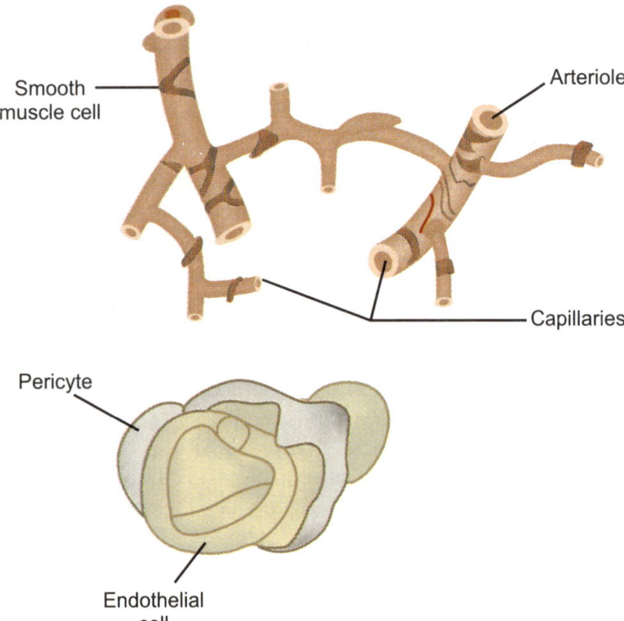

Fig. 78.3: Blood vessels

3. Aorta and its branches:
   - It is an elastic type of artery (i.e. abundant elastic tissue with rare muscle tissue). During systole and cardiac ejection, much of the pressure and flow are transferred to the periphery. Because of their greater distensibility owing to elastic tissue the walls of these large central arteries act as a compressive chambers which make the peripheral branches able to withstand this increase pressure and flow.
   - The left ventricle suddenly pumps blood into aorta by its powerful contraction. A considerable portion of the blood is stored locally by successive expansion of large vessels. It is estimated that up to one half of pressure and flow discharged during systole is stored here and this moves forward during diastole through elastic recoil of arterial walls. This allows a portion of blood to run off into capillaries during diastole.
   - The more peripheral arteries (carotid, brachial, femoral) are muscular type of arteries containing circularly arranged smooth muscle fibres which by shortening reduce the lumen of these vessels. Femoral artery dilates in response to contraction of the peripheral muscles.
4. *Arterioles:* Contain smallest blood volume but pressure and flow are more sensitive to minute changes in their blood content. They are final branches of distributing system, acting as stop cocks which control the run off of blood from arterial to capillary system. This strength is controlled by their developed smooth muscle fibres. They are supplied by vasomotor fibres which are controlled by centres located in medulla and spinal cord.

BIOPHYSICAL ASPECTS—II PRESSURE CHANGES

1. Different forms of energy:
   - On pumping of blood, the energy produced by left ventricle is potential energy (98%) and very less (1-2%) is kinetic energy. After pumping when blood enters aorta, its radius and length is increased. The branches of aorta stores this potential energy as tension in the arterial walls. Due to this velocity, some kinetic energy is also transferred to the blood.
   - Now imagine the event of muscular exercise or disease like aortic stenosis upto 50 per cent of the energy expanded by the heart is used for increasing blood velocity. So most of the potential energy is changed to kinetic energy to produce flow through vascular system, and is finally dissipated as heat through friction.

- Pressure in the aortic arch reaches a maximum during systole and minimum at the end of diastole. The numerical difference between these two is the pulse pressure.

2. Pulmonary circulation: Peculiarities
   - It is a low resistance circuit.
   - Arterioles are essentially absent.
   - These vessels supply only one type of tissue, i.e. alveoli, so vasomotor requirement is low.
   - Pulmonary blood volume is less.
   - The walls of pulmonary artery are one-third the thickness and their branches are much shorter and are of very small capacity.
   - There are numerous AV shunts.
   - The pulmonary veins are short containing less blood than the systemic veins.
   - The pulmonary bed is more distensible than the systemic circuit.
   - The blood volume here is only 800-1200 ml out of this 75-100 ml is in capillaries and rest is in arteries and veins.
   - Pulmonary vascular bed is an important reservoir of blood/a depot. With a change in posture 400 ml goes into or out of the lungs.
   - A marked pulsatile flow is retained in pulmonary capillary bed during rest and after exercise. During systole when blood is ejected in pulmonary artery by contraction of right ventricle and this imparts kinetic energy/energy of motion to the blood. As this blood enters/distends further in arterial tree, it acquires potential energy. This energy is also partially dissipated in small vessels by resistance to systolic flow. Now during diastole, this potential energy is partly lost in hysteresis and the remaining energy is dissipated in elastic recoil. By the end of diastole, the pressure in vascular bed is equal and leads to ceasing of capillary flow.
   - The resistance to blood flow in pulmonary circulation is slight as compared to systemic one (1/13th) because:
     - —There are high resistance arterioles.
     - —Pulmonary capillaries are large and numerous.
     - —Pulmonary vessels are easily distended passively.
3. Velocity is greater in systole than diastole, in distal part of aorta and its large arteries. However the vessels are elastic and there occurs forward continuous flow of blood due to recoil of vessel wall during diastole. This recoil effect is called *windkessel effect* (German elastic reservoir).
4. Basic structural view: The distensibility of the vessel is governed by their content of elastic and collagen tissue and smooth muscle. All blood vessels except the arterioles, capillaries and venules have prominent elastic tissue. In aorta, as much as 40 per cent by weight is elastic tissue. The elastic fibres due to great range of extensibility produce maintenance tension without expenditure of energy against the normal blood pressure. In wall of every blood vessel excepting-capillary, there are white collagenous fibres in a matrix. This collagen are stretched only at higher blood pressure so having a protective supporting role.

BIOPHYSICAL ASPECTS: CAPILLARIES

1. Its blood content is very small, i.e. 75-300 ml. Total filtering surface by capillary endothelium in adult is 6300 m^2 (68,000 ft^2).
2. The capillary wall is composed of a single layer of endothelial cell and is most tenuous structure. Not more than half a micron in thickness. The flat endothelial cells are joined at their fringes by intercellular cement which fills in between adjacent cells. The cement substance if washed is again renewed by endothelial cells. It is porous in nature and cementing substance is calcium-proteinate. Superimposed on this network is large adsorbed molecular component of protein which lines the inner surface. This capillary endothelial tube is supported by delicate membrane of fine fibrils derived from surrounding connective tissue. A freely moving fluid is contained between capillary and this membrane surrounding this in interstitial space is tissue fluid having gel like constituency.
3. The capillary wall is pierced with numerous ultra microscopic openings of diameter of 30 Å which are generally too small to allow the passage of plasma protein molecules, but are of sufficient size and number to allow water and NPN constituents of plasma. Lipid soluble molecules (O_2 and CO_2) can cross rapidly the plasma membrane. Passage of RBC and WBC occur through intercellular portion of the wall.
4. The capillaries of skeletal muscle are hundred times less permeable to water than glomerular capillaries.
5. At the ostia of each capillary is a small precapillary sphincter of smooth muscles controlled by sympathetic nerves. The meta-arterioles and their precapillary sphincters undergo periodic contractions at interval of 15 seconds to 2 minutes. When tissue is in resting state the constrictor phase of this rhythm is

dominant and thus leads to closure of precapillary sphincters. On the contrary, when tissue becomes active the opposite action exists, i.e. dilator phase of rhythm becomes dominant causing opening of precapillary sphincter. This cyclic opening and closing of precapillary sphincter is called *vasomotion*. Its constriction is stimulated by sympathetics and adrenaline.

BIBLIOGRAPHY

1. Alexander RS. The participation of venomotor system in pressor reflexes. (Quoted by Best and Taylor in Physiological basis of Medical Practice. Williams and Wilkins) Cir Res 1954;2:405.
2. Burton AC. On the physical equilibrium of small blood vessels. (Quoted by Best and Taylor in Physiological basis of Medical Practice. Williams and Wilkins). Amer J Phy 1951;164:319.
3. Burton AC. Physiology and Biophysics of circulation year book Chicago, 1965.
4. Coulter NA. Development of turbulence in flowing blood. (Quoted by Best and Taylor in Physiological basis of Medical Practice. Williams and Wilkins). Amer J Phy 1949;159: 401.
5. Glasser O (Ed). Medical Physics. Year Book, Chicago, vol. 2: 1944.
6. Kaley G, Altura BM (Eds). Micro-circulation, Univ. Park Press, Baltimore, vol. 2-3: 1977.
7. Lofving B. et al. Some aspects of basal tone of blood vessels. (Quoted by Best and Taylor in Physiological basis of Medical Practice. Williams and Wilkins). Acta Phy. Scand. 1956;37:134.
8. McDonald DA. lateral pulsatile expansion of arteries. (Quoted by Best and Taylor in Physiological basis of Medical Practice. Williams and Wilkins) 1953;119:28.
9. Peterson LH. Participation of veins in active regulation of circulation. (Quoted by Best and Taylor in Physiological basis of Medical Practice. Williams and Wilkins). Fed. Proc. 1951;10:104.
10. Rushmer RF. Cardiovascular dynamics. 3rd ed. Saunders, Philadelphia. 1970.

79

Homeostasis

CIRCULATORY CONTROL—I

The most important feature of circulation is that it is a continuous circuit. The blood vessels are a closed system of conduits that carry blood from heart to the tissues and back to the heart.

The circulation is divided into systemic and pulmonary. Since the systemic circulation supplies all the tissues of the body except the lungs, with blood flow, it is called 'greater or peripheral circulation.'

Arteries: Transport blood under high pressure to the tissues. This explains their strong vascular walls. The arterioles are the last small branches of the arterial system which act as a control valve through which blood is released into the capillaries and they are major site of resistance to blood flow and small change in their calibre cause large changes in the total peripheral resistance.

Capillaries: Function as exchange vessels which exchange fluid and nutrients between blood and interstitial spaces.

Venules: Collect blood from capillaries; they gradually coalesce into progressively large veins. Veins function as conduits for transport of blood from the tissues back to the heart.

Let us see in the following paragraphs how this circulation is beautifully maintained to ensure body'' homeostasis.

HISTORICAL NOTE OF BLOOD PRESSURE MEASUREMENT

It is well known that blood escapes from a cut artery under considerable pressure, and the first attempt to measure the pressure was made by Stephen Hales (1732). Now a days used sphygmomanometer is merely a developed method originally invented by Riva Rocci in 1896.

ARTERIES : TRANSPORT VESSELS

i. Arteries transport blood at high velocity and low energy cost from the heart to the periphery.
ii. Since most of the resistance offered by the circulation lies in the arterioles, changes in the calibre of these vessels cause much greater change in peripheral resistance than comparable changes in other vessels.
iii. The arteriolar walls are muscular. In transverse section of an arteriole, the ratio of the area occupied by muscle to the area occupied by lumen is about one to one and this ratio is called 'wall to lumen ratio. It is higher in arterioles than in other types of blood vessel.

CIRCULATION: LOCAL/AUTOREGULATION

i. *Metabolites theory:*
   - It has been shown that if blood flow is occluded/obstructed in a limb on resistance blood vessels; then on release of occlusion the blood flow is raised well above the resting level and then gradually returns towards the resting level. This increase in blood flow after occlusion is called, *Reactive hyperaemia.* The excess blood flow after release is sometimes referred to as 'blood flow repayment' for the 'blood flow debt' incurred during occlusion. Bigger the debt the bigger is the repayment. This phenomenon is restricted to occluded tissues only since it is not mediated by vasomotor nerves.
   - The same phenomenon occurs on exercise and is referred as *'Exercise hyperaemia.'* When exercise is stopped the blood flow is increased greatly above the resting level. Likewise it is

confined to only exercising muscle; and of course it is related to severity and duration of the exercise.

- This above mentioned phenomenon is of course related with increased concentration of metabolites in the tissues which causes vasodilatation. The accumulation of metabolites increases even after occlusion of vessel. When this occlusion is removed, the increased blood flow in already dilated vessel washes away these metabolites and blood flow returns to normal level.
- It is the local control of resistance vessels through metabolites which ensures that the blood supply to tissues is precisely regulated to meet their metabolic needs.
- Reactive hyperaemia in the skin can be decreased by cooling, tobacco smoking, epinephrine. Its amount and duration correlate with previous length of arterial occlusion. The blood flow or oxygen debt incurred during the period of occlusion can be calculated by multiplying the controlled blood flow or oxygen usage before circulatory arrest by the duration of occlusion.

ii. *Local temperature theory:*

- If parts like hand or feet is immersed in hot water at 45°C the blood flow of the part increases and this is independent of autonomic nerve supply and is due to local vasodilatation which also protects the part from damaging effect of heat. It is a direct local effect on the smooth muscle in the wall of the resistance vessel.
- Conversely if an extremity is immersed in cold water, it causes vasoconstriction which decreases blood flow in the part which may lead to local tissue death, so called necrosis.

iii. *Transmural pressure theory:*

- The pressure difference across the wall of blood vessel is measured by subtracting the external tissue pressure from the intravascular pressure. It is referred as 'transmural pressure' and it affects the changes in resistance vessels.
- As it rises the resistant vessels are dilated due to distension and increased blood flow. Of course, flow does not change very much when pressure is raised, which, suggests that the increase in transmural pressure elicits an increase in vascular resistance. The large increase in flow at a very high pressure is thought to be due to the distending forces overcoming the vasoconstrictor response.
- If the pressure is lowered below normal, the blood flow at first does not fall proportionately; this indicates that a fall in transmural pressure decrease the vascular resistance. However, at very low perfusion pressure the flow stops even while there is still a positive perfusion pressure head. "The closure of the vessels below a certain critical transmural pressure has been referred as critical closure." Over a very wide range of perfusion pressure the blood flow is relatively independent of the pressure head and this phenomenon is called 'autoregulation.'

Notes

- Whenever there is a decrease in oxygen supply of a tissue; there exists production of substances like adenosine phosphate, hydrogen ion, potassium ion, lactic acid etc. These are diffusing back to meta-arterioles, precapillary sphincters, etc. to cause vasodilatation. In this way blood flow increases which fulfils the tissue demand of O_2 and nutrients.
- At the origin of capillary; there is a precapillary sphincter. When a tissue needs oxygen then; this sphincter opens and blood rushes to that tissue. It remains open till its demand is fulfilled and then is closed; and remain closed till it uses that much oxygen (vasomotion).
- *Myogenic theory*: when arterial pressure is high → stretching of vessel wall→vascular constriction → reducing blood flow back to normal
- *On the contrary*: low arterial pressure → less stretching of vessel wall→relaxation of smooth muscle → increasing blood flow.
- *Long-term control*: By (a) Growth of new blood vessels (angiogenesis) by certain growth factors like fibroblast growth factor, ECGF (endothelial cell growth factor).

VASOMOTOR CONTROL: NERVOUS REGULATION

a. *Vasomotor centre*: In medulla there is a large number of cells and fibres concerned with transmission of impulses to blood vessels. So called 'Vasomotor centre.'

Afferents from all parts of the body e.g. mechanoreceptor cardiac and pulmonary centres in medulla itself.

Vasomotor centre is situated on the floor of fourth ventricle in the reticular formation at the level of calamus scriptorius. It forms a diffuse network of neurons; by extending from lower part of pons to the obex. It consists of two areas viz. *Pressor centre* leads to rise and other '*Depressor centre*' leads to fall in blood pressure; and is not the vasodilator centre, but it inhibits vasoconstrictor tone. Both of these are, in fact, constituting one functioning unit. The impulses are discharged from vasomotor centre, passdown the lateral white column of the spinal cord in cervical, thoracic and lumbar segment of spinal cord and form synaptic connections with lateral horn cells of the spinal cord.

b. *Vasoconstrictor nerves:*
   - These are nerves, which, when stimulated, cause blood vessels to constrict; and this action is mediated by release of nor-adrenaline which excites the smooth muscle in the walls of blood vessel. They were discovered by Claude Bernard (1852) who stimulated cervical sympathetic in rabbit and observed constriction of vessels of ear.
   - Their physiological rate of discharge is from 1-2 per second to 10 per second to maintain normal vessel tone. They mainly exert their effect on arterioles and adjacent smaller blood vessels where main drop of blood pressure from arterial to venous side occurs. So arteriole are controlled by constrictor fibres while capillaries are controlled by local factors. These fibres exert strong control over the size of the heart and veins. They thus alter the venous return and so influence the cardiac output. Veno-constriction has been reported in forearm, splanchnic area, on reflex sympathetic stimulation by cold/excitement etc. If these fibres are blocked by hexamethonium then these effects are abolished.
   - Hypothalamus role:
     - —In anterior hypothalamus a structure (centre) is located - only a few millimetres from relay station of sympathetic vasodilator fibres. Its topical stimulation leads to inhibition of sympathetic discharge which affect arterioles and veins. On its coagulation lowering of blood pressure results.
     - —There is a heat loss centre in anterior hypothalamus which plays a role in adjustment of blood pressure because it controls the discharge to vasoconstrictor fibres of cutaneous blood vessels. A rise has been reported through vasoconstriction when this centre is electrically stimulated or locally cooled; while a fall in blood pressure is seen through vasodilatation if this region is directly warmed. The vessels which are sensitively engaged are precapillary one, arterio-venous anastomoses and cutaneous arterioles.
   - *Cerebral cortex-role:* Stimulation of motor and premotor cortex leads to a rise in blood pressure through constriction of renal, splanchnic and cutaneous vessels; skeletal muscle vessels are of course dilated.

c. Vasodilator nerves:
   i. These are the nerves which lead to vasodilatation in blood vessels on stimulation; by releasing acetylcholine at their nerve endings.
   ii. Vasodilator fibres are not tonically active under normal circumstances. They appear to be brought into action whenever the need for them arises.
   iii. Parasympathetic vasodilators
      - Chlorda tympani to submandibular gland vasodilatation
      - Petrosal nerve to parotid gland vasodilatation
      - Lingual nerve to tongue vasodilatation
      - Pelvic splanchnic nerve to external genitalia vasodilatation
      - In skin and some exocrine glands the vasodilatation associated with these fibres is mediated by bradykinin.
   iv. Sympathetic vasodilators are:
      - Dilator fibres of coronary vessels.
      - Peripheral nerves
      - Stimulation of last anterior thoracic root leads to dilatation of kidney vessels.
      - Stimulation of right splanchnic nerve sometimes causes vasodilatation and fall of blood pressure.
   v. Antidromic vasodilator fibres:
      - It was demonstrated that stimulation of peripheral segments of cut posterior roots of the sacral nerves caused dilatation of vessel of experimental animal. Since such fibres don't convey the induced impulses to CNS, but rather the vasodilator impulses are conveyed along the fibres in a direction opposite to that in which ordinary sensory impulses travel; these are called antidromic.
      - The stimulus causing vasodilatation arise in dorsal root ganglia. It is to be conveyed antidromically to superficial blood vessels, (axon reflex). Its afferent and efferent limbs are formed by branching of a single nerve fibre. A stimulus applied to one branch sets an impulse which travels centrally to the point of division where it is reflected down the other branch to an effector organ. Various substances have been reported

to act as transmitter like acetylcholine, ATP, histamine like substances etc. The stimulants of local axon reflex include, trauma, cooling, frostbite, heating etc.

Veins: Capacity vessels

i. Veins are easily distensible and have little muscle in their walls. They possess resting tone and are capable of constriction and dilatation. Veins are constricted by adrenaline and nor-adrenaline.
ii. Veins transport the blood from periphery to heart with very little expenditure of energy. The veins offer very little resistance to blood flow.
iii. After passing slowly through the capillaries the blood speeds up as it passes through the venules and veins. This is because the total cross-sectional area of the venous bed is so much smaller than that of the capillaries.
iv. As the venules merge to form larger veins, they acquire a layer of connective tissue and then distinct muscle fibres. These vessels have a larger blood content than corresponding arteries. Their walls are much thinner containing less elastic tissue but having well developed muscular coat.
v. If 1,000 ml of blood is transfused; then about 990 ml of it will reside in extra-arterial places/low pressure system; of course 10 ml in arterial system. This means ability of venous system to take up blood is at least 100 times that of whole circulatory system.
vi. It has been indicated that venous system behaves like an elastic bag. When transfusion of 500 ml blood is made the pressure rises in central veins/ pulmonary artery/left atrium. Change of posture has no particular effect on their state of contraction.
vii. A minor trauma may completely close a medium sized vein. They are supplied with vasomotor nerves by which their distensibility can be changed.
viii. Changing from supine to erect posture results in veno-constriction; on resuming the supine position veno-dilatation occurs. Reduction of circulating blood volume (by means of phlebotomy) produce an increase in venous tone.

Venous Return

- Blood flows through the veins to the atria because the pressure in them is higher than it is in the atria, and it is usual that heart, unlike most pumps exerts no suction on the entering fluid. However, ventricular filling is very fast in early diastole, blood rushing into ventricles faster than it is ejected in systole. Further more, immediately after the end of systole the ventricles are not flaccid bags distended by the pressure within them, there is an elastic recoil of the contracted muscle which rapidly lowers the pressure in the chambers promoting an increased flow of blood from atria to ventricles.
- *Muscles pump:* Venous return is assisted by contraction of muscles all over the body, specially in legs. Due to this muscular contraction, blood is squeezed out of the capillaries and smaller veins within the muscles into the larger veins between the muscles. This blood flows towards the heart because of the presence of valves in the veins which acts as 'gate keeper' (they prevent back flow). The alternate contractions and relaxation of the leg muscles during exercise (walking, running, cycling etc.) serve to drive the blood back to the heart. A person standing rigidly in 'attention attitude' (traffic police, soldier) for a prolonged period of time may eventually faint because of impaired venous return to the heart by so called muscle pump results in diminished output of the ventricles. This is the reason that calf muscles are called "second heart" of our body.
- *Respiratory pump:* The Intrathoracic pressure (the pressure within chest, but outside the lung) is normally negative and this reduced pressure is exerted on the large veins and atria. Accordingly blood flows from the abdomen and other parts where the pressure is above atmospheric into the thoracic veins where the pressure is below atmospheric. The effective filling pressure of right side of heart is actually the difference between right atrial pressure and the intra-thoracic pressure i.e. $0 - (-5) = +5$ mmHg. The intra-thoracic pressure becomes more negative during inspiration and filling pressure therefore higher. During inspiration the descent of diaphragm causes an increase of intra-abdominal pressure which not only aids the return of blood to the thorax but also augments the flow of portal blood through the liver into the inferior vena cava. The importance of this respiratory pump is seen in performance of static effort (tug of war) or blowing a trumpet.
- Systemic veins act as a blood reservoir. When blood is lost from the body to the extent that blood pressure begins to fall, then pressure reflexes are elicited from the carotid sinuses and other pressure sensitive areas; which in turn cause sympathetic constriction of veins. Even after loss of 20-25 per cent of blood volume, the circulatory system functions normally because of reservoir function of the veins. The spleen, liver, large abdominal veins, heart and lungs itself, venous plexus beneath skin are considered as specific blood reservoirs.

SYNCOPE

- Means a transient loss of consciousness (fainting) due to reduction in cerebral blood flow. Along with it the tone of skeletal muscle is diminished and subject may fall on the ground; of course, fainting is a self-limiting one.
- Fainting occurs when fall of blood pressure is severe. This is due to the result of either a reflex vasomotor depression which produces marked vasodilatation; or the loss of baroreceptor reflex that normally maintain cerebral perfusion in the upright posture. Fainting therefore occurs most frequently when the person is upright, and consciousness usually returns quickly when he lies flat.
- Emotional fainting (vaso-vagal syncope) Due to strong emotions like road traffic accidents, surgical operation etc. These lead to vasodilatation of skeletal muscle which may be further due to increased circulating adrenaline and activation of cholinergic vasodilator fibres. Bradycardia, vasodilatation, hypotension constitute vaso-vagal syncope (Lewis). Other symptoms include pallor, cold sweating, nausea, yawning, hunger fatigue etc.
- Micturation syncope:- unconsciousness on passing urine.
- Cough syncope:- unconsciousness during coughing.
- Syncope may also be induced by depletion of circulating blood volume.
- When a subject stands up, blood is normally prevented from pooling in the legs under the influence of gravity by reflex adrenergic vasoconstriction. If for some reason, vasoconstriction fails to oppose the tendency of the blood to pool 'orthostatic hypotension' with syncope may result.
- Rarely, pressure on carotid sinus (tight collars) may lead to syncope via reflex vagal effects which leads to cardiac inhibition.

CAPILLARIES: EXCHANGE VESSELS

i. These are minute vessels (10 μ diameter) connecting arterioles with venules but differing from them in having no muscular coat. Each capillary consists of a tube of endothelium composed of a single layer of flat cells bound together into a continuous membrane by an intercellular cement probably elaborated by the cells themselves.

ii. *Permeability:* In defining capillary permeability it is necessary to know, the following factors which affect permeability viz. the volume/mass of substance passing through it, unit area, unit time, unit hydrostatic or osmotic pressure, per unit thickness of membrane. It is to be remembered that the rate of fluid transfer is affected by hydrostatic and osmotic pressure of the fluid outside the capillary.

   The impermeability of the capillary wall to protein (which is not absolute) depend upon integrity of inter-cellular cement; or; in other words, protein molecules leave the capillary by passing through the gap between endothelial cells. A fall in pH or absence of Ca^{2+} affects the cement substance in such a way as to promote the passage of protein molecules. If substances which damage the capillary endothelium (e.g. Narcotics, saponin) are added to blood perfusing capillaries, water and protein pass rapidly through their walls.

iii. *Fragility:* Refers to the production of minute haemorrhages (petechiae) in the skin when capillary pressure has been raised.

iv. *Blood flow:* The pulsatile flow characteristic of arterial system is absent in capillaries; the flow through these vessels is continuous. In the venules, the RBC pass along in a steady axial stream, leaving a clear peripheral stream of colourless plasma. The velocity of blood flow in the capillaries is about 0.5 mm/sec. (1000 times lower than that in aorta). This is because the total cross sectional area of the capillary bed is so enormous. The low rate of flow in capillaries provides a relatively long time for exchange to take place between the plasma and tissue fluid.

THE REAL FORCE/PRESSURE

The real force/pressure of the blood in the arteries depend on the proportion which the quantity of blood thrown out of left ventricle in a given time bears to the quantity which can pass through the arterioles into the veins at that time.

— Hales

BIBLIOGRAPHY

1. Alexander RS. The systemic circulation. Ann Rev Phy 1963;25: 213.
2. Bach LM. The reflex activation of vasodilatory fibres of dorsal roots and their role in vasodilator tone. (Quoted by Best and Taylor in Physiological basis of Medical Practice. Williams and Wilkins). Amer J Phy 1946;145:474.
3. Baler H. The anatomy and physiology of vascular wall : In Handbook of physiology section II, Vol. II page 865. Baltimore. The Williams and Wilkins Co. 1963.
4. Bohr DF. Peripheral circulation. Ann Rev Phy 1961;23:295.
5. Brody MJ, Schaffer RA. Distribution of vasodilator nerves in the canine hind limb. Amer J Phy 1970;218:470.
6. Carrier O, et al. Role of O_2 in autoregulation of blood in isolated vessels. Amer J Phy 1964;206.
7. Crowford DG, et al. O_2 lack as a possible cause of Reactive Hyperaemia. Amer J Phy 1959;191:613.

8. Duling BR, Kiltzman B. Local control of microvascular function. Role of tissue O_2 supply. Ann Rev Phy 1980;42:373-82.
9. Haddy FJ, Scolt JB. Active reactive hyperaemia and auto-regulation of Blood flow: In: G Kaley and BM (Eds): Micro-circulation Altura Baltimore University Park Press. Vol. 2. 1977.
10. Ranson SW, et al. Vasomotor reaction from stimulation of the floor of fourth ventricle. Studies in vasomotor reflex arc. (Quoted by Best and Taylor in Physiological basis of Medical Practice. Williams and Wilkins). Amer J Phy 1916;41:85.

CIRCULATORY CONTROL—II
INNERVATION OF HEART: HEART RATE AND REGULATION

A discussion of control of cardiac activity may be therefore subdivided into consideration of regulation of pacemaker activity and regulation of myocardial performance. However, the principal control of heart rate is related to autonomic nervous system. So let us now satisfy our scientific hunger in this present chapter.

PARASYMPATHETIC SUPPLY

a. *Effects or Actions*: Vagal effects on heart are enumerated as follows:
   - Slowing of heart rate (negative chronotropic)
   - Reduced force of contraction (negative ionotropic)
   - Less excitability of cardiac muscle (negative bathmotropic)
   - Slowing of conductivity (negative dromotropic)
   - It is universally recognised that vagus nerves exert profound depressant effects on cardiac pacemaker, atrial myocardium, atrioventricular conduction tissue and ventricles. It is due to liberation of a substance acetylcholine (vagustuffe).

b. Vagus nerves:
   - Are cardio-inhibitory and this action was discovered in 1845 by Weber brothers.
   - The cardiac fibres of the vagus separate from the trunk of the nerve in the neck. They enter into the formation of superficial and deep cardiac plexus and then they are continued to atrial muscle. Here they make connection with ganglion cells. Post-ganglionic fibres pass to the specialised tissue of SA and AV nodes. A rich plexus is formed here and exist in the form of boutons. These fibres don't enter the nodal tissue but terminate in atrial myocardium. None of the fibres enter ventricular myocardium. So the fibres are conveyed to special tissue of the heart and they form a centre in medulla (cardio-inhibitory centre).
   - Vagal tone. Is reflex in nature and is dependent upon afferent impulses flowing to the vagus centre specially along sinus and aortic nerves. It is a continuous restraint upon the action of heart or cardio-inhibitory action or action is similar to a dragging brake. So vagus possess an inhibitory tone and impulses passing from it in a continuous stream to the heart.
   - This tone can be explained by inhibiting vagus by atropine (1/20 to 1/15 grain). This leads to increase in heart rate upto 150-180/200 per minute. So 150-180/200 minus the normal rate of 70 per minute - this difference represents the vagal effect which is constantly exerted.

SYMPATHETIC SUPPLY

a. *Effects or actions*:
   Their effect over heart on stimulation is positive one in both chrono and ionotropic ways. Their action is mediated by the release of accelaranstuffe or catecho-lamine' together with increased force of ventricular contraction. So overall effects of sympathetics are listed as
   - Increase in heart rate (positive chronotropic action)
   - Increased force of contraction (positive ionotropic action)
   - Increased excitation of cardiac muscle (positive bathmotropic effect)
   - Increased conductivity of heart (positive dromo-tropic effect).

b. These accelerator fibres were first described by Von Bezold (1863). They are from thoraco-lumbar division of ANS. The cells constitute cardio-accleratory centre. The heart also receives accleratory fibres from the sympathetic chain as far as 4th, 5th, thoracic ganglion. The axons of cells of cervical ganglia (postganglionic fibres) form superior, inferior and middle cardiac nerves. The fibres of right side terminate into SA node while those of left side are distributed to AV node and His bundle.

- This superior cardiac nerve is distributed to large arteries at the base of heart; the inferior cardiac nerve is afferent.
- An accelerator tone also has been described like vagal tone. On excising stellate ganglion, slowing of heart followed.

READ AND DIGEST; CARDIAC INNERVATION

Q. These nerves are essential or not?

Ans. No. Pacemaker SA node originates cardiac impulse.

Q. If they are not essential, then why Nature has made them?

Ans. If vagus nerve is cut, then heart rate increases to 150-200/minute; If sympathetics are cut, then heart rate reduces to 40/minute. So they exert a 'tonic action and vagal tone is predominant in comparison with sympathetic tone.

Q. What is the mode of action?

Ans. They don't act directly but they act through chemicals (Otto-Loui-1921). "Vagus stuff or acetylcholine is the mediator from vagal endings - an inhibitory substance. "Adrenaline/catecholamine or acceleran stuff is the mediator substance from sympathetic nerve endings."

Q. What is vagal escape?

Ans.

- When vagal stimulation is continued, heart first slows down and then stops in diastole. After sometime again heart starts beating. This is vagal escape. It is due to 'idio-ventricular rhythm (30-45 beats/minute).
- On stoppage in diastole, blood gets stagnation in right side of the heart which is capable of stimulating cardiac muscle directly (mechanical effect).

Q. What is Bruler's law?

Ans.

- Law of specific nerve energy.
- Each nerve fibre is concerned with one sensation.

CONTROL BY HIGHER CENTRES

i. In the cerebral cortex the centres regulating cardiac functions are lying in anterior half of brain specially in frontal lobe (area 13), the orbital cortex, motor and premotor cortex, anterior part of temporal lobe, the insula and the cingulate gyrus. Stimulation of motor and premotor cortex leads to elevation in blood pressure with constriction of vessels like cutaneous, renal etc.

ii. In thalamus, tachycardia may be induced by stimulating ventral, midline and medial groups of nuclei. Variety of cardiovascular responses have been reported on stimulating H_2 fields of Forel in diencephalone.

iii. In medulla, distinct stimulatory and inhibitory centres are said to be present. Medially placed is 'cardio-inhibitory centre' which depresses heart on stimulation while little laterally placed is cardio-stimulatory centre leading to acceleration of heart on getting stimulation.

iv. It is said that heart rate can be varied by stimulating hypothalamus. Cardiac acceleration has been reported on stimulating 'posterior hypothalamus' while reverse is true if middle hypothalamus is stimulated. Hypothalamic centres are also involved in cardiac response to alterations in environmental temperature. Local temperature changes in preoptic anterior hypothalamus produce pronounced changes in heart rate.

v. Cardiac acceleration results if lateral horn cells of thoracic segments (1-5) are being stimulated.

FACTORS INFLUENCING HEART RATE

In healthy adults 60-90 beats per minute is considered as normal. Up to 100 per minute it is treated as high normal. An increase in heart rate (above 100 per minute) is called 'tachycardia' while decrease in heart rate is designated as 'bradycardia.' Under most conditions the SA node is under 'tonic influence' of both divisions of autonomic nervous system in the way that sympathetics exert a facilitatory influence on rhythmicity of pacemaker while parasympathetics are imposing an inhibitory effect. So changes in heart rate usually involve a reciprocal action of two divisions of the autonomic nervous system. In healthy resting individuals the parasympathetic tone is predominant. Abolition of the parasympathetic influences (by transecting vagus, atropine administration) leads to pronounced tachycardia while only slight slowing of heart has been reported on abolition of sympathetics. When both these autonomic divisions are blocked the heart rate in young adults averages to 105 beats per minute and intrinsic heart rate is the name given to the rate that prevails after complete autonomic blockade. So it can be concluded that, *'heart can go on functioning normally even after complete denervation so these nerves are not essential but they are said to exert a tonic action.'* Here are some factors influencing heart rate.

i. *Emotions; stress*

Any sort of emotions, excitement, anxiety are said to make the heart faster above 100 per minute. Fear, inferiority complex, frustrations varieties of stress can even decrease heart rate.

ii. *Higher centres*: Already dealt.
iii. *Sleep*: Normal sleep is capable of decreasing heart rate. It has been told that this effect is not met with disturbed sleep.
iv. *Muscular exercise*: On exercise decreased oxygen, excess carbon dioxide and H ion concentration, increased temperature results which together causes increase in heart rate. Due to autonomic stimulation heart rate increases even on thinking of exercise (not actual beginning). Athletes trained are having bradycardia.
v. *Meals:* Heart rate increases after meals. Heart rate is said to be a faithful follower of metabolic processes.
vi. *Age:* It is having somewhat inverse relation, i.e. as the age advances heart rate decreases, e.g. it is 140-160/minute in 5th week foetal life, after birth is 130-140/minute; adult level is attained at puberty time then it gradually declines.
vii. *Intracranial pressure:* This bears an inverse relation. Any condition which tends to increase the intracranial pressure will decrease heart rate through stimulating cardio-inhibitory centre.
viii. *Temperature*: Increased body temperature is capable enough to increase heart rate through directly stimulating SA node as well as cardio-acceleratory centre.
ix. *Body size:* This bears an inverse relation. In elephant it is only 25/minute while in canary (bird) it is 1000 per minute, in rabbits it is 250/minute.
x. *Barometric pressure*: It also bears an inverse relationship with heart rate as evidenced by slowing of heart rate in deep sea divers.
xi. *Role of hormones*: Adrenaline (through sympathetic stimulation), thyroxine (through raising general metabolism) and posterior pituitary extract are increasing the heart rate.
xii. *Respiration*: Heart rate is increased during inspiration; decreased during expiration. It is designated as *sinus arrhythmia*.
xiii. *Pathological states*: Congestive heart failure, myocardial infarction, anaemia, thyrotoxicosis, shock, adrenaline injection, haemorrhage, constrictive pericarditis, fever, auricular flutter and fibrillations are increasing rate while heart block, myxoedema, intracranial disorders, injection acetylcholine, decrease heart rate.

CARDIOVASCULAR REFLEXES AND REGULATION OF HEART RATE (FIG. 79.1)

a. Baroreceptor reflex:

i. Carotid sinus and aortic arch are the two best known such type of receptors. These two sets of receptors appear to be about equally potent in heart rate regulation.
ii. The afferent fibres running up from 'aortic arch' are called 'aortic nerve' and they are travelling along the vagus nerve to the vasomotor centre. These receptors are located in adventitial coat of arch of aorta. The efferent fibres descend from vasomotor centre to spinal centre reaching to the effector organs, i.e. heart and blood vessels.
iii. Since these receptors are sensitive towards any pressure changes (as the name suggests baro or pressure or mechano-receptors), an abrupt rise in pressure in aortic arch, results in bradycardia and hypotension due to stimulation of vagus centre (which terminates into lowering of heart rate and cardiac output) as well as inhibition of vasomotor centre (which leads to lowering of vasomotor tone which produces vasodilatation which finally causes fall of blood pressure). The reverse changes are also very much true when pressure within aortic arch is low which terminates into rise of blood pressure (due to vasoconstriction caused by stimulation of vasomotor centre), increased frequency of heart rate and increased cardiac output (due to vagal centre depression).
iv. The carotid sinus is a localised dilatation of internal carotid artery at its commencement opposite the level of superior border of thyroid cartilage extending down into distal part of common carotid artery. Its afferent fibres constitute sinus nerve which joins with glossopharyngeal nerve and finally through it reaches to vasomotor and cardio-respiratory centres. The dilatation of carotid sinus is due to its muscular deficiency. Its mechanism of action is also identical with aortic arch's one (above mentioned).
v. The above mentioned 'sino-aortic nerves' are also referred as 'buffer or stabiliser nerves' because they are said to maintain normal heart rate, respiration and blood pressure.
vi. In 1859, French physician *Etienne Marey* has developed the fact that heart rate and arterial blood pressure are inversely related with each other and it is often referred as '*Marey's law of heart*.' Of course this law is not applicable during exercise. It has been shown that alteration in heart rate evoked by changes in blood pressure were dependent on baroreceptors.
vii. *Bain bridge reflex:* In 1915, Bain bridge reported that any rise in pressure in right side of heart (by blood

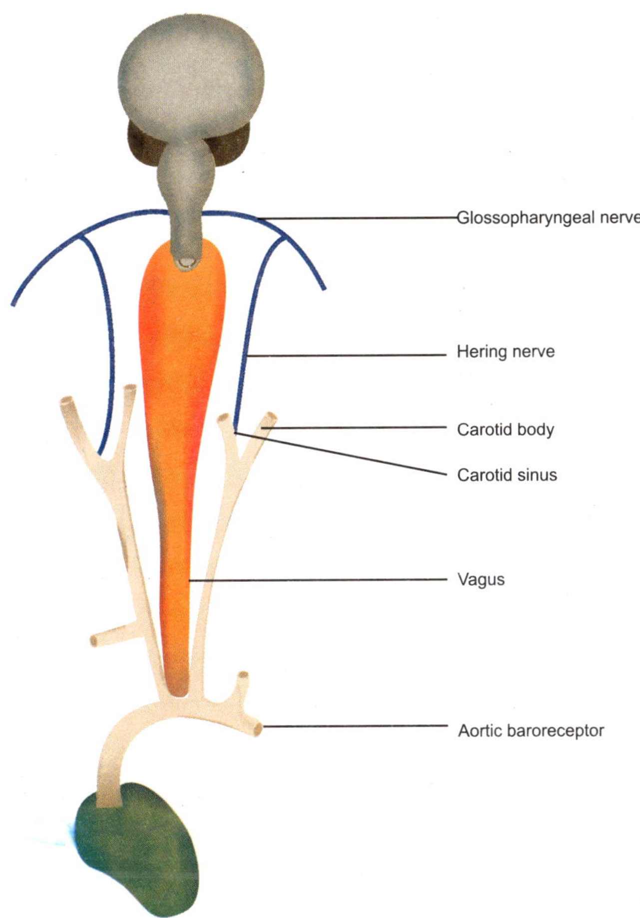

Fig. 79.1: Baroreceptor system: Arterial pressure control

or saline infusion) results in cardiac acceleration (tachycardia). He postulated that increased cardiac filling elicited tachycardia reflexly and afferent impulses were conducted by vagi so this reflex is abolished on cutting the vagi. If initially heart rate is high, the effect does not seem to occur.

In both atria the influencing receptors are said to be located and principally they are present at venoatrial junctions. When these receptors are distended, impulses are transmitted centrepetally in vagi. Efferent impulses are carried by sympathetic fibres to SA node which causes an increase in heart rate.

Two types of atrial receptors are known - type A are stimulated during atrial contraction while 'type B' are stimulated during diastole owing to passive dilatation of the atrium.

viii. Other arterial pressure receptors have been mentioned, in cranial cavity. It has been told that a sudden rise in intracranial pressure leads to systemic hypertension, and a sudden decrease in intracranial pressure causes hypotension. This is a proof of these receptors. Their importance is still a mystery.

ix. Baroreceptors also exist in other tissues like common carotid artery, thoracic and mesenteric arteries. These are not related to blood pressure homeostasis; but are engaged in local reflex adjustments of peripheral resistance and blood flow. Baroreceptor nerve endings are present in walls of caval veins, atria of the heart and in pulmonary circulation (cardio-pulmonary receptors).

x. Excitatory material which they secrete is glutamate while inhibitory one is GABA.

xi. It is important to remember that impulses generated in baroreceptor inhibit the tonic discharge of vasoconstrictor nerves and excite the vagal innervation of heart, producing vasodilatation, venodilatation, fall in BP bradycardia and a decrease in cardiac output.

xii. The receptors are located in adventitia. They are extensively branched, coiled, knobby and intertwined ends myelinated nerve fibres which are looking like Golgi tendon organs.

b. *Chemoreceptor reflex:*

i. Carotid body and aortic body are the sites where chemoreceptors are present. Innervation of chemoreceptor areas is equally rich but they are more richly vascularised.

ii. Carotid body is located in bifurcation of common carotid artery and is highly vascular structure (blood flow through it is said to be 2 litres/100 gm per minute) and is only 2 mg in weight. Afferent nerve fibres from carotid body join with sinus nerve of glossopharyngeal nerve.

iii. Aortic body are in fact two small nodular structures. On the right it lies between angle of left subclavian and left common carotid arteries while left body is located above aortic arch, medial to origin of left subclavian artery.

iv. When hypoxia has set in (blood oxygen is 80% or below) these chemoreceptors gets stimulated resulting into tachycardia owing to vasomotor centre stimulation.

Similarly when CO_2 concentration is in excess (above 35 mmHg) the chemoreceptors get stimulation and information is sent to cardiac, respiratory and blood pressure centres leading to increase in heart rate.

v. The fibres of aortic body run in the vagus while fibres of carotid body are branches of glossopharyngeal nerves.

vi. The aortic body is connected with a branch of fine artery arising from aorta beyond its arch.

vii. The carotid body is a small structure situated upon a branch of occipital artery. It is composed of rounded clumps of polyhedral cells, having a rich network of capillaries of sinusoidal character.

viii. Chemoreceptor activity is seen at CO_2 tension of 30-35 mmHg and oxygen tension of 80-90 mmHg. or less. With increasing pCO_2, decreasing pO_2; discharge of the chemoreceptor is diffuse.

It is doubtful that chemoreceptors exert any significant effect on circulation at rest. However, acute hypoxia causes systemic hypertension and vasoconstriction in the limbs and intestine. Responses are abolished if chemoreceptor areas are blocked—Heymans 1951-1960.

ix. The chemical changes exert their effects through central mechanism.

x. Chemoreceptors are also present in pulmonary and coronary circulation.

xi. In the presence of marked hypotension from haemorrhage chemoreceptors in aortic and carotid bodies are excited to induce vasoconstriction in capacity and resistance vessels.

xii. Hypocapnia can be produced by voluntary hyperventilation or by artificial respiration of anaesthetised animal.

In majority of human subjects, in standing position forced ventilation (hypocapnia) causes a fall in arterial blood pressure. This act interfers with venous return. Severe prolonged hyperventilation may lead to enough pooling of blood in dependent parts of the body which terminate into fainting and dizziness owing to decreased cerebral blood flow.

xiii. A moderate degree of hypoxia (at high altitude), leads to moderate increase in heart rate and increase in blood pressure. Breathing is stimulated so that a mild decrease in pCO_2 is noticed. Cardiac acceleration in response to hypoxia is mainly due to reflex stimulation of sympathetic centres by way of chemoreceptors.

xiv. When intracranial pressure is raised; it leads to persistent increase in blood pressure through compressing medullary vessels and so blood supply to vasomotor centres is interfered. The rise in pCO_2 in vasoconstrictor centre leads to an increase in its tone which leads to a rise in blood pressure. If rise in intracranial pressure is rapid then rise in blood pressure also occurs parallel along with decrease in heart rate which is elicited from pressure receptors.

xv. A combined effect of increased pCO_2 and decreased Po_2 is seen in asphyxia. Heart rate and blood pressure increased and so also cardiac output. On prolongation of asphyxia, the blood pressure is lowered because of decreased strength of cardiac contractions and conduction in AV portion of conducting system which is impaired.

xvi. Chemoreceptor discharge contributes to Mayer waves. These are regular slow oscillations in arterial pressure that occur at a rate of one per 20-40 seconds during hypotension. Here hypoxia stimulates the chemoreceptors which increases the blood pressure, by which blood supply in receptor organs is improved and it eliminates the stimulus to the chemoreceptors so that pressure falls and thus a new cycle starts. These Mayer waves should not be confused with Traube Hering Waves which are fluctuation in blood pressure synchronised with respiration.

c. *Other reflexes:*

i. A vast number of other cardiovascular reflexes have been described like 'Bezold and Jarisch reflex' elicited by certain drugs on receptors in ventricular wall. A drug 'veratrine when injected in left circumflex branch of coronary leads to hypotension and bradycardia. Vagus intactness is essential for this reflex which is commonly seen in cats and dogs.

ii. Pulmonary vessel reflexes

- Pulmonary reflex has also been mentioned. Inflation of lungs reflexly induces systemic vasodilatation and so decreased arterial blood pressure and reversely collapse of lungs causes systemic vasoconstriction and afferent fibres mediating this reflex lie in vagus nerve and their stimulation by stretching of lungs inhibits the vasomotor centre.
- Injection of certain drugs (veratridine, capsaicin, serotonin) into pulmonary artery leads to hypotension and bradycardia. This establishes the intactness of pulmonary depressor chemoreflex. Its concerning receptors are located in pulmonary veins. These drugs activates C-fibres ending close to capillaries in the lungs producing apnoea followed by rapid breathing.
- Respiratory arrhythmias: Mild inflation causes cardiac acceleration which is abolished by vagal section. It is thought that lungs are a constant source of impulses which exert an inhibitory influence on cardiac vagal centre, the influence being maximal during inflation and minimum

during deflation. Increase of CO_2 tension in the cerebral vessels increases the heart rate during each period of inspiratory discharge. It is yet to be decided that whether this central arrhythmia is due to decreased vagal activity during inspiration or stimulation/augmentation of sympathetic accelerator activity.

iii. Painful stimuli can elicit either pressor or depressor response. Decrease in pulse rate is found on pressing outer canthus of eyeball commonly known as oculocardiac reflex. Similarly distended bladder, rectum evoke blushing of face.

Abdominal Compression Reflex

Baroreceptor relfex→stimulation of sympathetic vasoconstriction→Vasomotor center and reticular area stimulation→Impulses to skeletal muscles specially of Abdomen→Their tone is increased so compression of venous reservoirs of abdomen→Translocation of blood out of abdominal vascular reservoirs towards the heart →Increased pumping of heart due to availability of more blood→Increased cardiac output and blood pressure.

So it becomes evident that persons having paralysed skeletal muscles are suffering from hypotension.

CNS Ischaemic Reflex

- Normally the baro and chemoreceptors are the reflexes producing organs which regulate blood pressure.
- When blood flow through VMC is decreased, i.e. cerebral ischaemia, the neurons itself are excited. This leads to an increase in systemic arterial pressure. All this is to compensate the decreased blood flow through this region which is not able to eliminate CO_2. This is CNS ischaemic response.
- It can elevate the mean arterial pressure many times. This reflex is one of the most powerful of activators of sympathetic system.
- It is operating when arterial pressure falls to a tremendously low level; in order to prevent further decrease and as well as to prevent brain damage.
- Suppose CSF pressure rises → blood supply to brain is cut off → initiation of CNS ischaemic response → rise in arterial pressure. (If blood pressure rises more than CSF pressure, blood flow restarts in brain vessels to get rid of ischaemia. This is "Cushing reaction" which protects vital centres of brain .
- It is to be remembered here that if cerebral ischaemia is continued for 3-10 minutes, the neuronal cells suffers badly. This thing further increases the value of CNS ischaemic reflex.

Effect of Respiration

Heart rate is increased during inspiration due to central factors plus Bainbridge response; whereas during late inspiration and expiration heart rate is slowed.

MECHANISM OF SYMPATHETIC INFLUENCES

i. Sympathetic nervous activity facilitates myocardial activities by increasing contractility of individual cardiac muscle cells.
ii. Norepinephrine released at nerve terminals involves exchange of calcium ions across myocardial cell membrane. It increases its permeability to these calcium ions which causes inward calcium ion current during plateau of action potential.
iii. This norepinephrine also raises cyclic AMPs intracellular levels, which promotes interaction of calcium ion with contractile protein and thus myocardial contractility is stimulated.
iv. Positive ionotropic effect on atria also facilitate ventricular filling.
v. Contractility is again stimulated by increased heart rate itself.

SUMMARY AND HIGHLIGHTS

So there exists no adequate substitute for reflex homeostasis of the circulation. Sympathetics are cardiac stimulatory while parasympathetics are cardio-inhibitory nerves. Both exert a tonic action 60-90 beats per minute is the normal heart rate.

BIBLIOGRAPHY

1. Abraham GJS. Carotid sinus reflex in cat : Effect of prior carotid artery clamping. Amer J Phy 1965;208:459.
2. Alexander N, et al. Sinoaortic baroreceptor reflex system and early pressure rise in renal hypertensive rabbits. Amer J Phy 1967;213:701.
3. Baccelli G, et al. Pressoceptive and chemoceptive aortic reflexes in decorticate and decerebrate cats. Amer J Phy 1965;208:708.
4. Brown GL, Eccles JC. The action of single vagal volley on the rhythm of heart beat. J Phy (London) 1934;82:242-57.
5. Burn JH, et al. J Phy (London) The relation of circulating nor adrenaline to the effect of sympathetic stimulation. 1960;150:295.
6. Calaresu FR, et al. Medullary basal sympathetic tone. Ann Rev Phy 1988;50:511.
7. Coleridge et al. In RJ Linden (Ed): Cardiac Receptors. London Cambridge University Press, 1978;117-137.
8. Davis DL. Sympathetic stimulation and small artery constriction. Amer J Phy 1964;206:262.
9. Dawes GS, JH. Comrol Jr. Chemo reflexes from heart and lungs. Phy Rev 1954;34:167-201.

CIRCULATORY CONTROL—III: BLOOD PRESSURE (BP)

'It is the lateral pressure exerted by blood on the vessel walls while flowing through it.'

TERMS

Systolic BP—Maximum pressure during systole.
*Diastolic BP*óMinimum pressure during diastole.
Pulse pressure—Difference between systolic and diastolic
Mean pressure—Arithmetic mean of systolic and diastolic blood pressure (diastolic pressure + $^{1}/3$rd of mean pressure).

PHYSIOLOGICAL VARIATION

a. *Age:* Blood pressure rises with age. viz. infancy (70-90 mmHg), childhood (90-110 mmHg), puberty (110-120 mmHg), old age (140-150 mmHg). It is associated with atherosclerotic changes.
b. *Sex*: In females, blood pressure is slightly lower than males.
c. Slight rise of systolic pressure seen *after meals*.
d. Blood pressure is elevated in *obese persons*.
e. *Emotions/excitement* raises systolic blood pressure.
f. There exists a precise relationship between respiration and blood pressure. At normal rates of breathing the blood pressure falls during most of inspiration but when breathing is slow, the inspiration is accompanied by a small rise in blood pressure.

   There is a slight acceleration of pulse during inspiration and a slight deceleration of pulse during expiration (*Sinus Arrythmia*). It can be explained on the basis that Inspiration→thoracic pressure falls and abdominal pressure rises→blood flow more readily into thoracic veins→rise of atrial and central venous pressure →acceleration of heart.
g. During *sleep* blood pressure may fall.
h. Slight variations in the readings on the two arms are not uncommon.
i. When the subject is supine the arterial pressures in brachial and femoral arteries are the same. With the subject's standing however, the femoral pressure is higher than that in the brachial artery, the difference being due to the pressure of the column of blood equal in height to the vertical distance between one artery and the other.
j. *Casual recording..* The blood pressure recording under ordinary conditions of life.
   Basal recording: Reading obtained 10-12 hours the last meal of the previous day, and after resting for half an hour in a warm room.
k. The pressure obtained by sphygmomanometer is affected by *thickness* of the arm - Thicker the arm, higher the value obtained.

NORMAL VALUES

Systolic pressure between 100-140 mmHg and diastolic between 60-90 mmHg (average 120/70 mmHg) is considered as normal. By nervousness, before the doctor or in hospital building, the blood pressure may be raised in few persons called *'white coat hypertension.'*

FUNCTION

Normal BP is required

i. To maintain a sufficient pressure head to keep the blood flowing
ii. To provide motive force at capillary bed so nutrition to tissue is assured and lymph and urine are formed.

FACTORS CONTROLLING

a. *Pumping action of heart*
   It is the effective contraction of heart which controls cardiac output, blood pressure and blood flow within the vessels. It is this pumping action of heart which is the main driving force of blood.
b. *Cardiac output*
   It directly affects blood pressure. It further depends on venous return, force and frequency of heart beat.
c. *Blood volume*
   - Increased quantity of blood will stretch the arterial walls and this will increase blood pressure.
   - Quantity of blood in arterial system: The arterial walls are distensible and elastic. Certain degree of stretching must occur within them before creation of considerable pressure. Greater the filling of arterial system more will be the blood pressure. So less of blood (due to haemorrhage etc.) if not compensated may cause fall of blood pressure and on the contrary, by increasing the total amount of circulating fluid (by blood transfusion/blood substitutes etc.) will increase the pressure.
d. *Viscosity of blood*
   - Alteration in blood viscosity will affect the diastolic pressure by its effect on peripheral resistance.
   - It means thickness of any liquid. So greater the viscosity, grater is the pressure required to force it along a length of a narrow tube in a given time.

If viscosity is high then internal friction resistance is also high. It depends upon the degree to which molecules or particles of a fluid cohere. Blood is five times more viscous than water. So greater the viscosity - greater will be the frictional resistance developed in this region and so less will be the quantity of fluid that will pass through in a unit of time.

e. *Peripheral resistance:*
'The blood has to overcome some resistance during its flow through the periphery and this is peripheral resistance. The chief site of peripheral resistance is arterioles.' It further depends on following factors viz.

a. *Velocity:* Pressure is always high in aorta in comparison of capillaries. A rapidly flowing stream will have more frictional effect than a slower one.

b. *Viscosity*
A more viscid blood will have higher friction than a lesser one. This explains the dominance of plasma transfusion over ordinary saline in order to maintain blood pressure.

c. *Lumen of vessel*
This bears inverse relation with peripheral resistance. Smaller the vessel higher will be the resistance.

$$\text{Peripheral resistance} \propto \frac{\text{Mean arterial pressure}}{\text{Cardiac output}}$$

d. *Elasticity*

- In old age, arterial walls become stiff since their normal elasticity is lost (atherosclerosis) and this explains rise in blood pressure as age advances. This also explains the fact that because of elasticity the arteries can accommodate considerable amount of blood with least alterations in blood pressure.
- Flow of blood is pulsatile in arteries. This flow is a continuous one beyond the arterioles (capillaries and veins). This conversion of pulsatile flow to a uniform one depends upon existence of diastolic pressure. At the usual diastolic pressure which exists, the walls are stretched and by virtue of their elasticity, they tend to recoil against the distending force. So elastic recoil of arterial wall acts as a subsidiary pump to push or drive the blood onwards in a continuous stream between the heart beats. So it is clear that any increase in elasticity of the arteries will lower the diastolic pressure.
- During systole the ventricular contents are thrown into vessel which causes its further distension since vessels are already having some amount of blood within them. As systole is over the elastic walls rebound, forcing the blood onwards through the peripheral vessels; so arterial lumen returns to its previous diameter and the energy which was stored during stretching of vessels is expanded during diastole.

SIGNIFICANCE: BLOOD PRESSURE

1. If blood volume is more, then systolic pressure will also be more. Systolic blood pressure is an indication of force of contraction.
2. If diastolic blood pressure is high, it suggests that there is much work load on the heart.
3. Pulse pressure is the index of cardiac output.
4. Mean pressure is related with flow of blood to different organs.
5. Diastolic is most important because (a) It is not influenced by routine factors by which systolic is affected; (b) If it is high then it means more work load on heart; by which heart can be diseased at any time.

REGULATION

a. Rapid control by baro, chemoreceptor + CNS ischaemic reflex

b. Long-term control - by *"renin-angiotensin system"* and *"fluid load system"* mediated by hormone aldosterone (described in detail at various places)

i. Decreased BP → renin secretion (JG apparatus-Kidney) → Angiotensin I $\xrightarrow{\text{Lungs}}$ Angiotensin II → Aldosterone secretion + vasoconstriction → Increased BP.

ii. Increased extracellular fluid → increased blood volume → increased venous return → increased cardiac output → increased blood pressure.

ARTERIAL HYPERTENSION

Hypertension is defined by Life Insurance Companies as any elevation of systolic pressure above 140 mmHg; and of diastolic pressure above 90 mmHg diastolic pressure is a true disease phenomenon while systolic pressure is not of a much significant importance.

Secondary Hypertension

i. *Renal hypertension*
He was Richard Bright who first recognised the relationship between chronic renal disease and elevated blood pressure. After a period of ninety years Harry Goldblatt provided experimental proof by producing hypertension by rendering both

kidneys of the dog ischaemic by means of clamps on the renal arteries which are slowly tightened over a considerable period. When the rat is used, unilateral renal ischaemia causes persistent hypertension together with arterial lesions of malignant hypertension in the opposite kidney.

Kidney has got two opposing functions in connection with blood pressure; one is 'hypertensive' and another is 'anti-hypertensive.' It is believed that ischaemic kidney produces a pressor substance, probably the enzyme 'renin,' which acts on a substrate 'hypertensinogen,' in the plasma to from 'angiotensin.' The Goldblatt kidney is a renin producer. Renin appears to be secreted by the granular cells of juxta-glomerular- apparatus. The renin acts as a trophic hormone on the zona glomerulosa of the adrenal cortex with the production of aldosterone. The 'renin-angiotensin system' may have a dual homeostatic role - regulating the blood pressure by the direct effect of angiotensin on the blood vessels; and regulating sodium and water through aldosterone.

Through the elaboration of renin, the kidney forms angiotensin II (AII) which alters blood pressure by increasing both peripheral resistance and blood volume. The former effect is achieved largely by its ability to cause vasoconstriction through direct action on vascular smooth muscle, the latter by stimulation of aldosterone secretion, which increases distal tubular reabsorption of sodium, and so also of water.

This Angiotensin II is rapidly inactivated by multiple blood and tissue enzyme called angiotensinase.

GOLDBLATT: ONE KIDNEY EXPERIMENT

- One kidney is removed and constrictor is placed on renal artery of remaining kidney.
- Response.
  - First phase–vasoconstrictor type of hypertension caused by angiotensin.
  - Second phase–hypertension; due to increase in fluid volume.

GOLDBLATT: TWO KIDNEY EXPERIMENT

- Artery to one kidney is constricted while artery to second kidney is normal.
- Hypertension results. Constrictor → decreased renal arterial pressure → retaining of salt + water due to renin secretion. This renin leads to formation of angiotensin which reaches opposite kidney through circulation to retain salt + water → hypertension.

Direct-renal effect: Angiotensin:- It constricts renal vessels→diminished blood flow through kidney→less fluid is filtered by glomeruli→slow fluid pressure in peritubular capillaries reduce their pressure→rapid osmotic reabsorption of fluid from tubules→less urine is excreted.

ii. *Endocrine hypertension*

The adrenals seem to play an important role in regulation of blood pressure. It is through adrenal medulla on one end, which secretes epinephrine which raises blood pressure; while on another end; the sustained or paroxysmal hypertension is associated with *'Pheochromocytoma'* (the chromaffin tissue tumour of adrenal medulla). In primary aldosteronism the salt retaining hormone, produced in excess by an adenoma of adrenal cortex, is associated with hypertension as well as with severe urinary potassium loss and renal damage. It is also a prominent symptom in pregnancy called *'toxaemia of pregnancy'* - a condition that may be caused by a pressure polypeptide secreted by placenta.

Vascular Hypertension

Elevation of blood pressure may be primarily due to narrowing of a main vessel (e.g. coarctation of aorta), or to a generalised constriction of small arteries and arterioles (e.g. polyarteritis nodosa). In coarctation of aorta, severe hypertension is produced in upper part of the body but in lower part of the body it usually remains in normal level.

ESSENTIAL HYPERTENSION

1. The mean arterial pressure is increased to 40-60 per cent.
2. Renal blood flow is decreased in later stages.
3. The resistance to renal blood flow is increased.
4. Cardiac output is normal.
5. Total peripheral resistance is increased in parallel with arterial pressure.
6. GFR is very near to normal.
7. The kidneys will not excrete adequate amounts of salt and water unless the arterial pressure is high.

Essential Hypertension

- *Increase in cardiac output*

  Basic and probably genetic defect is reduced renal sodium excretion in the presence of normal arterial pressure.

  Decreased sodium excretion → increase in fluid volume → rise in cardiac output → peripheral vasoconstriction → increased peripheral resistance → elevation of blood pressure (resetting of pressure natriuresis/autoregulation)

- *Vasoconstrictive influences*
  They include neurogenic factors, increased release of vasoconstrictive agents (like renin, catecholamine, endothelin), and a primary increased sensitivity of vascular smooth muscle, caused by a genetic defect in cell membrane transport of sodium and calcium, leading to increased intracellular calcium and contraction in the smooth muscle cells.

In early stages of essential hypertension, blood pressure elevations are intermittent and is triggered by over activity of autonomic reactions (e.g. cold, excitement) Later on, blood pressure elevation becomes sustained due to 'resetting' of barorceptor mechanism. Spasm of arterioles leads to hypertrophy of their musculature and there is some organic narrowing of the vessels.

Malignant hypertension is a syndrome in which necrotic arteriolar lesion develop with its usual complications like renal failure, papilloedema, cerebral symptoms etc. It is triggered by hypertension of any cause.

In essential hypertension, the underlying factor leading to increased peripheral resistance is vasoconstriction due to augmented intracellular calcium. This increase of intracellular calcium may be an inherited membrane defect, a primary or inherited change in the sodium-potassium -ATP-ase.

WHO IS HYPERTENSIVE?

- Above 140/90 mmHg BP at age of 20 years.
- Above 160/96 mmHg BP at age of 50 years.

FACTORS INFLUENCING ESSENTIAL HYPERTENSION

- Genetic and familial
- Socio-economic factors
- Dietary factors: obesity, intake of high salt, alcohol, and caffeine.
- Neurotransmitters: noradrenaline, acetylcholine, substance P, serotonin, dopamine, encephalin, neuropeptide Y.
- Hormonal: high renin, natriuretic peptide, effects of ADH.

Complications

- It influences other body parts and their functions. Generally the patient remains asymptomatic and the disease is diagnosed when some complications appear. This is the reason that it is classed as *'silent killer.'* Few highlights are :
- Stroke may result from cerebral haemorrhage. Carotid athermoa and transient cerebral ischaemic attacks are more common in hypertensive patients. Hypertensive encephalopathy is a rare condition characterised by a very high blood pressure and neurological symptoms including transient disturbances of speech or vision, disorientation, paraesthesia, fits and loss of consciousness.
- Retinal changes (Haemorrhage, may cause blindness
  Grade I
  Thickening, irregularity and tortuosity of arterioles. Increased reflection.
  Grade II
  Above changes with addition of constriction of retinal veins at arterial crossings.
  Grade III
  Above changes with addition of flame shaped haemorrhages and cotton wool exudates.
  Grade IV
  Above changes with papilloedema (bulging optic disc with blurred edges).
- Proteinurea and progressive renal failure are renal manifestations.
- Excess load on heart which leads to left ventricular failure.

BLOOD PRESSURE VARIATIONS V/S FACTORS DETERMINING

1. Altered heart rate: During cardiac acceleration, the diastolic period is shortened. This allows less time for the energy stored in elastic walls during systole to become converted into energy of flow during diastole. Since the elastic recoil tends to determine diastolic pressure, and in cardiac acceleration, next beat is arrived earlier than scheduled time; so a fall in pressure during diastole is halted at a higher level. The systolic blood pressure is not changed significantly, since quantity of blood entering the arteries per minute remains constant. A decrease in heart rate will exert opposite effect.
2. Blood amount discharged/minute by ventricle: Increase in output per beat will increase the systolic pressure. No significant change occurs in diastolic pressure, and consequently pulse pressure is increased. Due to high pressure at the end of ejection period, more energy is expanded in giving velocity to the blood so the pressure gradient during diastole is steeper.
3. Increased blood volume: Both systolic and diastolic pressures are increased due to greater stretching of

the arterial walls which are elastic + their overfilling.

4. Variation in elasticity of arterial walls: It is strange to say that when elasticity is lost, i.e. vessels behave like rigid tubes then diastolic pressure is lowered; provided same changes are not existing in peripheral vessels. If both large as well as peripheral small vessels loose elasticity then only diastolic pressure will be raised otherwise not. Diminished distensibility of the walls of aorta and larger artery leads to increase in systolic pressure.

Baroreceptor and Blood Pressure Regulation

As mentioned earlier, they have some characteristics as far as blood pressure regulation is concerned:

- They respond rapidly to changes in arterial pressure. If blood pressure is set at 150 mmHg of an individual and then it suddenly rises; then the rate of impulse transmission will be twice or even more in comparison of what it was at stationary level of 150 mmHg.
- Now say if one's blood pressure rises from 150 to 200 mmHg then as told above the rate of impulse transmission will be increased. But on next consecutive days this rate will go on decreasing till it re-comes at resting level. This explains that for long-term regulation of blood pressure, this structure is unimportant. This is called 'resetting' of baroreceptors (rapidly adapting).
- This mechanism prevents us from the effects of, 'postural hypotension.' From lying posture when one sits or stands, he tends to fall and to become unconscious due to decreased blood pressure. To compensate, due to falling pressure, these baroreceptors elicits an immediate reflex which causes strong sympathetic discharge which tends to raise the falling blood pressure.
- The primary purpose of it is to reduce the daily variation in arterial pressure.
- From raised arterial pressure, the arterial walls containing baroreceptors are deformed. If this deformation is prevented then baroreceptors will no longer respond to pressure changes.
- The buffer nerves (sino-aortic nerves) constitute an important mechanism for controlling blood pressure. The rise in diastolic pressure and an increase in heart rate which occur when body posture changes from recumbent to sitting or from sitting to standing position is brought about by these nerves.

EFFECT OF GRAVITY

- In standing position, the mean arterial blood pressure in feet is 180-200 mmHg and venous pressure is 84-90 mmHg. On the contrary the pressure in head is 60-76 mmHg while venous pressure is zero.
- If one is not moving at all 300-500 ml of blood is pooled in veins of lower extremities; fluid accumulates in interstitial spaces due to increased hydrostatic pressure in capillaries. Stroke volume is also decreased.
- This may reduce the cerebral blood flow and this cerebral ischaemia may lead to loss of consciousness.
- Compensatory changes:- Fall in blood pressure in baro-receptors starts these changes. Heart rate is increased which can maintain the cardiac output. There occurs immediate increase in levels of aldosterone and renin. The arterioles constrict which maintains the blood pressure. Fainting is also a compensatory/homeostatic mechanism since falling to horizontal position promptly restores the venous return, cardiac output and cerebral blood flow to adequate levels.

EFFECT OF EXERCISE

1. Even before exercise begins, the thought of exercise stimulates ANS which increases the heart rate and strength of contraction. Simultaneously it constricts the veins throughout the body; and this increases the mean circulatory pressure and thus pushing extra quantities of blood from peripheral circulation towards the heart. This increases cardiac output and so blood pressure.
2. At the very onset of exercise, the motor cortex transmit signals through sympathetic cholinergic nerve fibres to cause vasodilatation of muscle blood vessels. This leads to further instantaneous increase in cardiac output and blood pressure.
3. At onset of exercise, there occurs tightening of skeletal muscles and of abdominal wall around peripheral blood vessel. This additionally increases the mean systemic pressure, so cardiac output and blood pressure.
4. Also at the onset, motor cortex transmit signals directly into sympathetic nervous system to further intensify the sympathetic activity.
5. Finally, most important effect is direct effect of increased metabolism of muscle itself which causes increased usage of O_2 and other nutrients as well as formation of vasodilator substances. All causes marked vasodilatation which increases local blood flow. This local vasodilatation requires 5-28 seconds to reach full development after a person begins to exercise.
6. With the start of isometric muscle contraction, the heart rate rises. It just occurs with thought of perfor-

mance or even after infusion of neuromuscular blocking drugs. This is due to inhibition of vagal tone and increased sympathetic discharge. Within few seconds of the onset of an isometric contraction both systolic and diastolic blood pressure rises sharply, stroke volume changes relatively little and blood flow to steadily contracting muscle is reduced as a result of compression of their blood vessels.

7. In isotonic contraction, heart rate rises in the same way, but stroke volume is markedly increased. In addition there is a net fall in total peripheral resistance due to vasodilatation of exercising muscle. During exercise, systolic pressure rises but the diastolic pressure shows a less pronounced rise so that pulse pressure is increased (In trained individuals with severe exercise).
8. In light exercise systolic pressure rises to several millimeters but diastolic pressure may remain at normal level.
9. Immediately after the exercise the pressure drops momentarily to normal or even slightly below. It then mounts to its previous high level from which it gradually declines again, and in a healthy person reaches to normal within 1-4½ minutes. The evanescent drop in pressure is explained as being due to sudden relaxation of abdominal muscles. The blood is drained into venous reservoirs. These when deprived of their support (abdominal muscles) have their capacity increased and blood flow into right heart is temporarily curtailed

EFFECT OF POSTURE

- In standing position, as a result of effect of gravity on the blood, the mean arterial blood pressure in the feet of a normal adult is 180-200 mmHg, and venous pressure is 85-90 mmHg. The arterial pressure at head level is 60-75 mmHg and venous pressure is zero.
- If the individual does not move, 300-500 ml of blood pool in venous capacity vessels of lower extremities, fluid begin to accumulate in interstitial spaces because of increased hydrostatic pressure in capillaries and stroke volume is decreased upto 40 per cent. Symptoms of cerebral ischaemia develops when cerebral blood flow decreases to less than about 60 per cent of the flow in the recumbent position.
- The major compensation on assuming the upright position are triggered by the drop in blood pressure in carotid sinus and aortic arch. The heart rate increases, helping to maintain cardiac output. There is relatively little venoconstriction in the periphery, but there is a prompt increase in circulating levels of renin and aldosterone. The arterioles constrict helping to maintain blood pressure. Lastly CNS ischaemic reflex also initiates vasoconstrictor tone which is the last measure to raise the blood pressure.
- Prolonged standing represents additional problem because of increasing interstitial fluid volume in lower extremities. As long as the individual moves about, the operation of muscle pump keeps the venous pressure below 30 mmHg and venous return is adequate. However, with prolonged standing (military person in attention, traffic police) fainting may result.
- In some individuals, sudden standing causes a fall in blood pressure, dizziness, dimness of vision and even fainting called postural hypotension. Its causes include diabetes mellitus and syphilis, because of damage of sympathetic system, use of sympatholytic drugs.

HYPOTENSION

- It is said to be present when systolic pressure is below 90-110 mmHg.
- *Primary hypotension*: Absence of any underlying disease. Weakness and fatigue are the only symptoms. Patient is emotionally labile and asthenic. The patient is free from cardiovascular + renal disease, so it is a synonym of longevity.
- *Secondary hypotension*: Low BP may occur in conditions like myocardial infarction, pituitary insufficiency, tuberculosis, any debilitating state.
- *Postural (orthostatic) hypotension*:
  - Profound fall of blood pressure is seen on assuming standing position. Person suffers from syncope/dizziness.
  - CNS diseases:- diabetic neuropathy, tabes dorsalis, neuritis after infection, Wernicke's disease
  - After surgical sympathectomy
  - In late pregnancies, supine position may lead to hypotension and tachycardia.
  - Micturition hypotensions.
- *Dynamics of postural hypotension*:
  - It is not merely the pooling of blood in lower limbs but is an abnormal response to the usual shift in blood volume.
  - The abnormality consists in loss of reflex arteriolar and venous constriction which usually occurs on standing.

— It is not only the pooling of blood in lower extremity but abnormal fast rate of pooling, which, contribute in fall of BP.

— In such patients there is an absence of normal rise in venous blood levels of adrenaline and noradrenaline during upright tilting. Such patients also represent a hyper-reactivity to noradrenaline on its parentral administration. This suggests a failure of reflex release of noradrenaline from sympathetic nerve endings at effectors sites in vascular bed.

- *Treatment:*
  — Secondary diseases should be treated accordingly.
  — Helpful measures include abdominal binding, sympathomimetic presser agents, vasopressin, adrenal cortical sodium retaining hormones, high salt diet, elastic stockings etc.

SUMMARY AND HIGHLIGHTS

- Any pressure above 140-150 mmHg (systolic) and 90 mmHg (diastolic) is considered as elevated blood pressure.
- Blood pressure is determined by the product of cardiac output and the total peripheral vascular resistance. Cardiac output is controlled by factors like heart rate, ionotropic state which in turn are dependent on both neural and humoral effects of sympathetic-para-sympathetic nervous system and vasoactive agents. Cardiac output is also dependent on peripheral factors that influence venous return. Peripheral resistance is determined by both neurohumoral factors and it is also influenced by autoregulation in local vascular beds.
- The sympathetic nervous system influences blood pressure by producing changes in peripheral resistance and altering cardiac activity, as well as by changing the renal release of renin and influencing renal-pressure natriuresis. Drugs which inhibit adrenergic nervous system activity lower the blood pressure when administered to hypertensive patients. Major role of sympathetic nervous system lies in perpetuating high blood pressure by altering the normal relationship between blood pressure and sodium excretion by kidney; which plays a control role in hypertensive disorders.

BIBLIOGRAPHY

1. Bohr DF, et al. Vascular smooth muscle function and its changes in hypertension. Amer J Med 1984
2. Brown AM. Brief Reviews : Receptors under pressure an update on baroreceptors. Cir Res 1980;46:1-10.
3. Brown AM. Motor innervation of coronary arteries of the cat. J Phy (London) 1968;198:311-28.
4. Brown AM, et al. Plasticity of arterial baroreceptor in hypertension states. In DJ Reis (Ed): Disturbances in Neurogenic Control of Circulation. Bethesda: American Physiological Society, 1981.
5. Brubachor ES. Sodium deprivation and renin secretion in anaesthetised dogs. Amer J Phy 1968;214:15.
6. Careltero O, et al. Renin substrate in plasma under various experimental conditions in rats. Amer J Phy 1967;213:695.
7. Colins R, et al. Blood pressure : stroke and coronary heart disease. Lancet 1990;335:827.
8. Green HD, et al. Control of peripheral resistance in major systemic vascular beds. Phy Rev 1959;39:617.
9. Guo and Thames: Abnormal baroreflex control in renal hypertension is due to abnormal baroreceptors. Amer J Phy 1983;245(3):H 420-428.
10. Guyton AC, et al. Quantitative analysis of pathophysiology of hypertension. Cir Res 1969;24: I-1
11. Guyton AC, et al. Arterial pressure regulation: overriding dominance of kidney in long-term regulation and hypertension. Amer J Med 1972;52:584.
12. Guyton AC. Blood pressure control: special role of kidney and body fluids. Science 1991;252:1813.
13. Haas E, Goldblatt H. Kinetic constants of human renin and human angiotensinogen reaction. Cir Res 1967;20:45.
14. Horton EW. Hypothesis on physiological role of prostaglandins. Phy Rev 1969;49:112.
15. Johnson PC. Hoemodynamics. Ann Rev Phy 1969;31:331.
16. Johnston CE, et al. Plasma renin in chronic experimental heart failure 89 during renal sodium escape from mineralocorticoid. Cir Res 1968;22:113.
17. Kaplan NM : Systemic Hypertension : Mechanism and Diagnosis. In E Braun Wald (Ed): Heart Disease Philadelphia: WB Saunders Co., 1988;879.
18. Kezdi P. Baroreceptors and hypertension. New York, Pergamon press Inc. 1968.
19. Kruger EM. Time course of baroreceptor resetting in acute hypertension. Amer J Phy 1970;218:486.
20. Laragh JH, et al. Hypertension : Pathophysiology, diagnosis and management : New York: Ravin press 1990.
21. Levy MN. Influence of anomalous blood viscosity on resistance to flow in dogs hind limb. Cir Res 1956;4:533.
22. Ross R. Pathogenesis of atherosclerosis: A perspectives for 1990's. Nature 1993;362:801.
23. Rowell LB. Human cardiovascular control. Oxford university press. (Quoted by Ganong WF in Review of Medical Physiology. Lange Publication). 1993.

CIRCULATORY CONTROL—IV: HORMONAL- IONIC EFFECT

VASOCONSTRICTOR AGENTS

Catecholamines

- Adrenaline and noradrenaline are liberated from adrenal medulla which leads to increase in blood pressure. Noradrenaline is a general vasoconstrictor and, is present normally in the walls of arteries and veins, in the heart, aorta with an average amount of 0.5 µg/gm (rabbits). Here it lines along with vasoconstrictor nerve endings.
- Adrenaline causes constriction in cutaneous and other vessels but dilatation in vessels of skeletal muscle and the liver. The increased cardiac output causes rise in blood pressure (systolic) and the mean blood pressure may not be altered.

Vasopressin (ADH)

It is most potent constrictor substance in human body. It is formed in hypothalamus and is transported down the centre of nerve axons to the posterior pituitary gland where it is eventually secreted into the blood. It has two major roles; first is to maintain arterial pressure in the presence of reduced blood volume and, second is to regulate osmolality.

Angiotensin

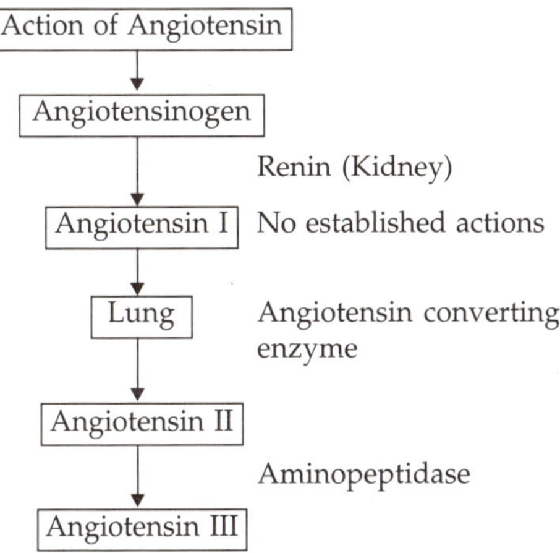

- The octapeptide Angiotensin II is having a generalised vasoconstrictor action. It directly acts on adrenal cortex to secrete aldosterone. It also increases water intake. It also acts on brain to increase blood pressure. It also facilitates the release of norepinephrine by a direct action on post ganglionic sympathetic neurons.
- Angiotensin II is the blood pressure regulating peptide while Angiotensin III is the natural aldosterone - stimulating peptide.

  Endothelin: Are active peptide. They constrict both arterial and venous smooth muscle in all vascular beds. Its arterial constriction augments arterial resistance. Cardiac output falls during infusion of endothelin. It exerts ionotropic effect on heart; and stimulates the secretion of ANP. The constriction caused by it follows a brief vasodilatation and is slow in onset and sustained. It opens a voltage sensitive Ca^{2+} channel.

VASODILATOR AGENTS

Histamine: It causes vasodilatation of resistance vessels, flushing of skin, and a fall in arterial pressure. It also increases capillary permeability which causes loss of protein and fluid from the circulation. It is released in every tissue of the body on damage, inflammation or due to some allergic manifestation.

Atrial natriuretic peptide (ANP): It antagonizes the action of various vasoconstrictor agents and thus lowers the blood pressure.

- It is secreted by heart. The muscle cells in atria contain some secretory granules which increase in number when extracellular fluid volume is increased or NaCl intake is increased. It is also found in adenohypophysis, brain (its site is extending from antero-medial part of hypothalamus to lower brainstem.
- Its actions include natriuresis, increasing effective surface area for filtration in glomeruli, promoting arterial and venous dilatation, reduction of blood pressure in dose dependent manner, Cardiac output decreased, blocking the effects of angiotensin II.
- Is a polypeptide with 17 amino acid ring formed by disulphide bond.
- Other analogues like BNP (brain-natriuretic-polypeptide) and CNP have been reported in brain.
- Three ANP receptors have been reported viz.
  - ANP R-A-for this ANP is having greatest affinity
  - ANPR-B -CNP is having greatest affinity
  - ANPR-C-binds all natriuretic peptide
- It acts through G proteins to activate phospholipase C and inhibit adenylcyclase.
- The atrial muscle release ANP when it is stretched. The rate of ANP secretion is proportional to the degree of stretch by increase in central venous pressure.

- Circulating ANP is having a short half-life. Is metabolised by neutral endopeptidase.
- A digitalis like steroid "ouabain" coming from adrenal glands, has been reported as ANP present in blood. It raises blood pressure by inhibiting Na^+K^+ ATPase.

Serotonin (5HT): It is present in high concentration in platelets, chromaffin tissues in large intestine and other abdominal structures.

Endothelium: Is important modulator of smooth muscle activity. EDRF (Endothelium - derived - relaxing factor) has been reported which diffuses into smooth muscle.

Kinins: Bradykinin: Kinins are small polypeptides which are split away by proteolytic enzymes from alpha 2 globulins in the plasma or tissue fluids.

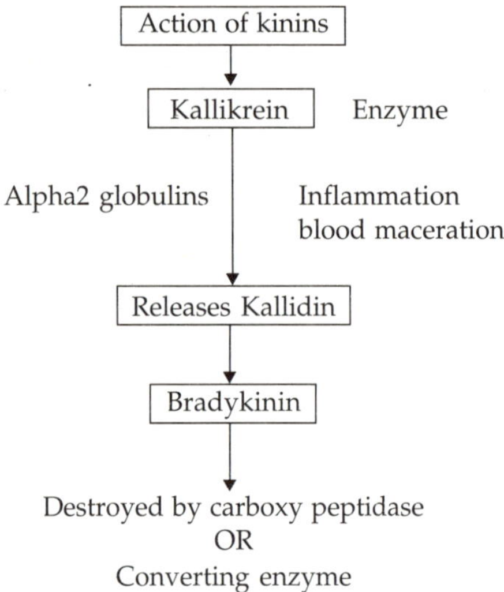

Bradykinin is famous because it causes powerful arteriolar dilatation and increases capillary permeability. It plays role in regulating blood flow in skin and GIT.

Prostacyclins: Is vasodilator derived from family of prostaglandins synthesised in endothelial cells. It exerts local effect and promote smooth muscle relaxation. Its synthesis is inhibited by nicotine. By acting synergistically with EDRF it inhibits platelet aggregation. Its synthesis is decreased in diabetes mellitus, atherosclerosis etc.

Endothelin: Are active peptide.

Alcohol: It causes a marked dilatation of blood vessels, as a depressant on vasomotor centre.

Acetylcholine: Coronary dilatation. Direct action.

PROSTACYCLINE + THROMBOXANE A_2

Th A_2 produced by platelets from their common precursor arachi donic acid through cyclo-oxygenase pathway. It promotes vasoconstriction and platelet aggregation. Just reverse, prostacycline leads to vasodilatation and inhibit platelet aggregation. This prostacy cline-Thromboxane A_2 balance is shifted towards the prostacycline on administration of aspirin. This explains the use of aspirin in myocardial infarction/ angina etc.

ENDOTHELINS (ET)

Most potent vasoconstrictor agents- a polypeptide. They are of three types ET_1, ET_2, ET_3.

ET_1: produced by endothelial cells and the enzyme involved is endothelin converting enzyme. On its intravenous administration it leads to fall in blood pressure, followed by a marked pressor response. It is released on stretching of blood vessels. It also activates phospholipase A_2 which increases production of prostacycline + Thromboxane A_2. It is present in circulating blood. It is a local paracrine regulator of vascular tone. There are endothelin receptors present in mesangial cells.

EDRF (Endothelium-derived relaxing factor)/NITRIC OXIDE (NO)

- NO is synthesised from arginine by the enzyme "NO synthase." NO activates the soluble "guanylyl cyclase" in cells producing cGMP which mediates relaxation of vascular smooth muscles.
- It is inactivated by haemoglobin. Acetylcholine will cause vasoconstriction if endothelium of membrane is striped off.
- Tonic release of NO is necessary to maintain normal blood pressure Its deficiency may cause hypotension and it is also involved in pathogenesis of arteriosclerosis/atherosclerosis.
- Ample work confirms that penile erection is produced by release of NO along with vasodilatation + engorgement of corpora cavernosa.
- EDRF is necessary for cytotoxic activity of macrophages, i.e. their ability to kill cancer cells. It is a major dilator of smooth muscle in GIT.

CIRCULATION: IONIC + CHEMICAL CONTROL

- Increase in Ca^{2+} concentration leads to vasoconstriction since calcium stimulate smooth muscle contraction.

- Increase in K^+ concentration leads to vasodilatation since it inhibits smooth muscle contraction.
- Increase in Mg^{++} concentration leads to powerful vasodilatation since they inhibit smooth muscle contraction.
- Increase in Na^+ concentration leads to mild arteriolar dilatation and this is due to increased osmolality of the blood.
- Mild degree of vasodilatation is caused by acetate and citrate.
- Increased CO_2 concentration leads to moderate vasodilatation in most of the tissues and marked vasodilatation in brain.
- An increase in hydrogen ion concentration (decreased pH) leads to arteriolar dilatation; slight decrease in hydrogen ion concentration leads to arteriolar constriction.

BIBLIOGRAPHY

1. Brown AJ, et al. Cardiovascular and renal response to chronic vasopressin infusion. Amer J Phy 1986;250:H 584.
2. Cantin M, Ganest J. The heart and ANF. Endo Rev 1985;6:107.
3. Collier HOJ. Kinins. Sc Amer 1962;207(2).
4. Emerson TE (Jr.) Vascular effects of angiotensin and norepinephrine in dog, cat and monkeys. Amer J Phy 1965;208:260.
5. Gerattini S, et al. Serotonin New York: American Elsevier Publishing Co. 1963.
6. Sliart L. Role of vasopressin in cardiovascular regulation. Phy Rev 1988;68:1246.
7. Vane JR, et al. Regulatory function of vascular endothelium. New Eng J Med 1990;327:27.

80 Disturbed Homeostasis: Shock

Shock is a clinical state resulting from an upset of normal physiological balance or homeostasis. Long ago it was defined as an expression of sympathy of the whole frame with a part suddenly subjected to serious injury.

Shock is liable to occur after severe injuries, extensive haemorrhage, extensive surgical operation and acute abdomen states viz. perforation of peptic ulcer, strangulated hernia, acute pancreatitis etc.

PRIMARY (NEUROGENIC) SHOCK

It is neurogenic or psychic in origin; nervous stimuli leading to widespread capillary paralysis, with vasodilatation of splanchnic vessels and pooling of blood, resulting in cerebral ischaemia and unconsciousness. It is a transient neurovascular collapse which may result from sight of blood, from pain (even from fear of pain e.g. person waiting for his turn for hypodermic needle prick).

SECONDARY SHOCK

It in essence the result of disparity between the volume of blood and volume capacity of vascular system.

Pathophysiology

The master word is ischaemia. When it becomes severe and persistent it may lead to anaerobic form of tissue metabolism which responds to ischaemia. The skin is resistant, most seriously effected is the liver because two thirds of oxygen normally used by liver comes in the venous blood of the portal vein.

- Two humoral vasotropic factors have been mentioned
  - — VEM (vaso-excitatory material). It is in the kidney.
  - — VDM (vaso-depressor material). It is in the liver and muscle. It is ferritin.
  - — Both are products of anaerobic metabolism resulting from ischaemia.
  - — During stress the production of VEM by renal cortex rises and power of normal kidney to destroy it is lost. When anoxia involves the liver and induces anaerobic metabolism in the liver, the production of VDM rises and power of healthy liver to destroy it is lost. VDM completely over shadows VEM since the vasoconstrictor power of epinephrine is neutralised by VDM.

CLINICAL PICTURE

Patient lies perfectly still and pays no attention in surroundings. The face is pale, large drops of sweat hang from eyebrow and skin is cold and clammy. The cardinal signs are subnormal temperature, shallow respiration, low blood pressure and feeble pulse.

BIOCHEMICAL CHANGES

- Reduction in blood volume and the dehydration are inherent in production of shock like state. Other changes like upset of electrolyte balance, acidosis and protein breakdown are dependent on the lesions in the kidney and liver.
- The fluid of the body is contained in three compartments namely in vessels, in interstitial tissue and in the cell. In rapid dehydration due to massive haemorrhage, or acute intestinal obstruction, it is the plasma and interstitial water that is lost.
- As the blood flow to the myocardium is reduced, so is the oxygen supply with a consequent change in metabolism of myocardium and a profound effect on work output of the heart. Glucose extraction falls, while pyruvate which is normally used by heart is given off in shock. The inability of heart to use pyruvate may be due to hypoxia and secondary inactivation of co-carboxylase essential for entrance of pyruvate into Krebs' cycle.

- It will be realised that collapse of shock with its accompanying hypothermia and hypotension may be regarded as protective devices calculated to slow down the metabolic fire, when carried to an extreme, they may become lethal however.
- Vascular tone is lost as a result of painful stimuli and a state of anxiety. As there are natural accompaniments of wounds, they are certain to increase the disparity between space and contents.

SHOCK: SOME EFFECTS

1. Muscular weakness:- due to diminished supply of oxygen and nutrients
2. Diminished tissue metabolism/cell deterioration
3. Reduced body temperature
4. Mental functions are depressed
5. Diminished renal efficiency/failure. Of course fluid retention by kidney may be useful.

SHOCK: CAUSES

Shock is an entity encompasses a complex array of reaction, no one of which can be said to represent the key factor leading to circulatory collapse.

1. *Reduction in Blood volume:* This may be due to blood loss which may be traced to (a) blood lost from injured part and (b) fluid lost into the injured part. The example is severe external or internal haemorrhage.

COMPENSATION OF HAEMORRHAGE

- Vasoconstriction (Venoconstriction)
- Tachycardia
- Increased thoracic pumping
- Increased muscle pumping
- Increased secretion of catecholamines
- Increased secretion of renin
- Activation of renin-angiotensin system
- Increased secretion of aldosterone
- Increased secretion of ADH
- Activation of baro-chemoreceptor and CNS ischaemic reflex
- Increased secretion of erythropoietin
- Increased plasma protein synthesis

2. So when blood volume is reduced because of any reasons, following body defensive mechanisms play their role to save the life namely -
   - Because of altered pressure baroreceptors get stimulated which elicit powerful sympathetic stimulation to raise the blood pressure.
   - The CNS ischaemic reflex further elicit more powerful sympathetic stimulation throughout the body. It is activated only when the blood pressure falls below 50 mmHg.
   - Because of decreased blood volume hypoxia may ensue which excite chemoreceptors which then elicit powerful sympathetic stimulation to raise the blood pressure.
   - Lowered blood volume and pressure stimulates release of renin from JG apparatus of kidney which leads to formation and triggering of renin-angiotensin system which by vasoconstriction of peripheral arteries and conservation of water and salt by the kidney, prevent the further progress of shock.
   - The ADH is also released (vasopressin) which also constricts the peripheral arteries and veins and also greatly increases water retention by the kidneys. Thus blood pressure rises.
   - Other defensive mechanism include - reverse stress relaxation of circulatory system, absorption of large quantities of fluid from GIT, increased thirst and appetite for salt etc.

In this way, the patient comes out from the critical situation and recovery takes place. This is called *compensated or non-progressive or reversible shock.*

The Opposite Side of the Picture

- Once shock has become severe enough, various factors are progressively decreasing cardiac output. Following may be the responsible factors-
- Because of decreased blood volume and pressure, the blood supply to the heart itself by coronaries is reduced. This causes reduction in oxygen and nutrition supply of the heart itself which results into further decrease in cardial output. In this way in the form of cardiac depression shock deteriorates itself by such vicious cycle.
- Inspite of above mentioned defensive factors, some times, blood supply of vasomotor centre itself is so reduced that first it becomes less active and then it turns to totally inactive. This is enough to deteriorate the situation.

SERIES EVENTS: PROGRESSIVE SHOCK

1. Cardiac depression: due to decrease in coronary blood flow → myocardium nutrition diminishes → repeated deterioration of myocardium.
2. Vasomotor failure: decreased blood flow to VMC→It becomes progressively less and less active.
3. Increased capillary permeability: leads to leakage of fluid.
4. Shocked tissue releases, toxins viz. histamine, serotonin etc. endotoxins are released from dead bacteria which leads to cellular depression.
5. Tragedy at cellular level:

- Decreased active transport of Na and K → swelling of cells:
- Depressed mitochondrial activity
- Lysosomes → release of hydrolases → intracellular damage

6. Acidosis: due to accumulation of lactic acid in the blood. This prevents normal removal of CO_2.
7. Tissue necrosis
8. Shock → sluggish blood flow in minute vessels → slugged blood.

SEPTIC SHOCK

- Causes: Generalised infection due to bacteria (Streptococcus/Staphylococcus etc.), spread of infection from intestine - urinary tract, peritoneum etc.
- It is characterised by high fever, high cardiac output, marked vasodilatation, sludging of blood.
- The end stage is just like a progressive shock which may threaten the life.

ANAPHYLACTIC SHOCK

- It is resulting from antigen antibody reaction.
- As a result histamine or histaminoid substances are released. This causes dilatation of arterioles, venous dilatation, increased capillary permeability.
- Due to remarkable decrease in venous return serious histamine shock results.

SHOCK MANAGEMENT: PHYSIOLOGICAL BASIS

1. Head down and feet up position to improve venous return
2. Oxygen therapy
3. Glucocorticoid therapy
4. Sympathomimetic drugs - specially in neurogenic and anaphylactic shock. They are of no importance in haemorrhagic shock.
5. In haemorrhagic shock - blood/plasma transfusion or administration of blood substitutes.

BIBLIOGRAPHY

1. Bernton EW, et al. Opioids and neuropeptides: Mechanism in circulatory shock. Fed Proc 1985;44:190.
2. Bond RF, Johnson G. Vascular adrenergic interaction during haemorrhagic shock. III Fed Proc 1985;44:281.
3. Califf RM, et al. Cardiogenic shock. New Eng J Med 1994;330: 1724.
4. Corewell JW, Guyton AC. Evidence favouring a cardiac mechanism in irreversible haemorrhagic shock. Amer J Phy 1961;201:893.
5. Guyton AC, Crowell JW. Dynamics of heart in shock. Fed Proc 1961;20:51.
6. Parillo JE. Pathogenetic mechanism of septic shock. New Eng J Med 1993;328:1471.

81 Regional Circulation

CEREBRAL

1. *Normal values*
   - Average blood flow 54 ml/100 mg of brain tissue per minute. Cerebral blood flow is 750 ml.
   - Blood pressure in cerebral arteries 100 mmHg. Systolic and 60 mmHg diastolic.
   - Total oxygen consumption is 50 ml/minute.
   - Respiratory quotient (RQ) is unity, i.e. carbohydrates are mainly used.
   - Cranial circulation time is 3 seconds.
2. *Factors affecting:*
   - Age higher in younger persons (first decade of life); falls rapidly with advent of puberty due to liberation of sex hormones.
   - It is directly varying with arterial blood pressure.
   - Any rise in intracranial pressure will reduce blood flow (brain tumour, meningitis).
   - Lack of oxygen will increase cerebral circulation through generalised vasoconstriction and local vasodilatation.
   - Decreased blood viscosity (anaemia) will increase the cerebral blood flow.
   - Sleep is induced because of cerebral ischaemia (less blood flow).
   - Increased CO_2 tension will increase cerebral flow.
   - Adrenaline increases the flow due to vasodilatation noradrenaline decreases the flow due to vasoconstriction.
3. Its measurement is done by nitrous oxide method on the basis of Fick Principle.

CAPILLARY CIRCULATION

1. *Peculiarities:*
   - No fixed direction of flow.
   - Because of its narrow size only a single file of cells can pass through. Red cells may be folded upon itself and squeeze through capillaries.
   - During rest the majorities of capillaries remain collapsed. When they become active they remain opened.
   - They adjust their diameter independent of arterioles and venules.
2. *Vascular response of skin*
   - If high stroke is applied on skin - it produces white line after a short latent period. After two or three minutes it fades away. It is due to this mechanical stimulus which causes capillary constriction.

Triple Response

- In hypersensitive persons response is little different
- At the point where skin is stroked a *red line* is first produced which is due to local vasodilatation. It is independent of nerves.
- Just after 15-20 seconds a *red flush or flare* appears which is due to arteriolar dilatation (antidromic axon reflex).
- Within five minutes *wheel* (*local oedema*) develops. This is because of increased capillary permeability which results into leakage of fluid which terminates into oedema.
- All above changes are because of liberation of histamine.

RENAL CIRCULATION

1. *Peculiarities*
   - Whole blood has to pass through glomerular tufts
   - It is a portal system of circulation
   - Rate of blood supply to kidney is comparatively high (1,300 ml/minute) 20 per cent of normal cardiac output.
   - Renal blood pressure is comparatively high, (75 mmHg) which is suitable for filtration.
   - There is no neurogenic vascular tone in kidney under basal state.

- Also neurogenic vasodilatation is not existing. Vasoconstriction can be produced by stimulating sympathetic nerve.
- Blood flow to the cortex is higher than medulla which is due to unusual length of vasa recta and increase in blood viscosity in medulla caused by transmembranous shunting of water from descending limb to ascending limb of vasa recta.
- It has got 'autoregulation.'

PERIPHERAL VASCULAR DISEASES

1. Raynaud's Disease (Described by Raynaud in 1862)
   - Young women are predominantly effected.
   - The attack is spasm of small arteries, i.e. fingers, less commonly toes.
   - The attack lasts for few minutes but may be prolonged up to one to two hours. The affected areas become cold, numb or cyanotic. The colouration starts from the tip and spread towards the bases of digits. Later on the numbness may be replaced by burning pain; and cyanosis by red hot. Thrombosis may terminate into ulcers or gangrene.
   - Generally, it is because of hyperactivity of vasomotor (constrictor) nerves. But according to some other workers the fault lies in vascular wall. According to other workers intense vasoconstriction + high concentration of catecholamines is secondary to incomplete destruction of amines liberated from peripheral nerve endings; in the vessel walls.
   - Ganglionectomy leads to a beneficial effect, of course, it does not remove the cause of disease. The attacks become less frequent and intense after the operation.
2. Buerger's Disease (Thromboangiitis-obliterans)
   - Buerger described high incidences of this disease in Jews. Excessive use of tobacco has been blamed as the main cause; some believe it of infectious in origin.
   - The disease is confined to the limbs. The vessels become stiff and hard. The adventitia is thickened and media shows muscular atrophy along with an increase in connective tissue. Thrombosis causes marked narrowing of vascular lumen.
   - The disease starts as fatigue of limbs on exertion, intermittent claudication, pallor, numbness, cyanosis or even dull pain in extremities. A reduction in blood flow occurs in limb.
   - With the advancement of the disease, the pulse disappears from wrist/popliteal/brachial artery and ultimately it terminates into ulcer/gangrene.
   - Amputation may be required.
   - Discontinuation of smoking causes a decrease in platelet adhesiveness. When vasospasm is existing then sympathectomy is of benefit.
   - ***"Either have cigarettes or have your limbs - choice is yours."***
3. Arteriosclerosis Obliterans
   Intermittent Claudication (Charcot, 1856)
   - It means organic narrowing of the arteries of a limb and thus restricting its blood supply. This causes pain/fatigue in muscles.
   - Pain disappears on rest but appear on exercise. Muscles are flaccid during the attack.
   - Muscular anoxia is the cause. Stimulation of sensory nerve by the metabolic product of muscular activity is another cause, because they accumulate in the presence of inadequate blood supply. These pain producing substances are "P substance."
4. *Frost bite*
   - Vasospasm and freezing occurs in small vessels of the part on prolonged exposure to cold. This arrests the circulation in the part.
   - All this increases capillary pressure which leads to an increase in capillary permeability which causes edema of the part.
   - If ischaemia is severe, gangrene may manifest.
   - Formation of ice crystals + dehydration of cell is the usual cause of damage.
   - This occurs specially in lobes of the ear and in digits of hands and feet.
   - As proverb states, "every cell wants to live, no cell wants to die." So on frost bite, sudden vasodilatation occurs, as manifested by a skin flush. This vasodilatation delivers warm blood to the skin. But this protective mechanism is less developed in human beings.
5. Immersion/Trench Foot (Story of 2nd World War)
   - It is a state of vessel/tissue of feet due to severe chilling from exposure to cold. Hands are rarely affected.
   - The feet are swollen, numb, pulseless, colour changes from bright red to deep blue/waxy white. After removal from exposure the feet becomes hyperaemic and painful which is of burning/stabbing in character.
   - Sailors working in wet boots, soldiers in wet trenches (trench foot) an example justifying the names.

82 Congenital Heart Anomalies

Malformation of heart and associated blood vessels during foetal life.

PATENT DUCTUS ARTERIOSUS
(Synonym - Left to right shunt)

a. Ductus arteriosus:
- Lungs are collapsed during foetal life.
- Because of collapsed alveoli, blood vessels are also collapsed; because of same elastic factors which close the alveoli, also close blood vessels.
- This increases pressure in the pulmonary artery during foetal life because of great resistance to blood flow through lungs.
- Pressure in aorta is less as compared with pulmonary artery because of low resistance to blood flow.
- This creates necessity of some other vessel in foetus called ductus arteriosus which connects pulmonary artery with aorta. In this way the lung is bypassed.
- The blood is oxygenated by placenta of mother in spite of the fact that lungs are collapsed.

b. After birth: no necessity of ductus:
- After birth, lung alveoli are no more collapsed, because lungs inflate. Resistance to blood flow is also decreased through pulmonary vascular tree. This causes a fall in pulmonary arterial pressure. Because of simultaneous delivery of placenta the aortic pressure rises, since blood flow through placenta is decreased. This leads to an increase in aortic pressure while a decrease in pulmonary vessel. This finally results into blood flow from aorta to pulmonary artery (backwards), while flow through ductus arteriosus comes to an end (forward). Within time to come which may be from few days to few weeks, the ductus gets occluded and finally closed.

c. Tragedy: persistence of ductus:
- If it so happens - means patent ductus arteriosus; generally no harm is seen in early months of infant life. But with the advancement of age; the situation may become more worse.
- In older children, with patent ductus the aortic blood flows through the ductus to pulmonary artery and then into left atrium through lungs and thence to left ventricle.
- Because left ventricle pumps more blood as compared with its normal action, its hypertrophy is common in such instances. So every thing may be normal in resting state but on moderate or severe exercise, the patient may be unconscious. Pulmonary congestion has also been reported in such cases because of high pressure in pulmonary area. On an average, lifespan is reduced.
- On auscultation doctor may listen a harsh blowing or machinery murmur. This is more prominent during systole when aortic pressure is high. On the contrary, its intensity is diminished during diastole because of diminished aortic pressure. So it waxes and wanes.
- Surgically ligating the patent ductus is the treatment.

d. Tragedy: tetralogy of Fallot:
- By birth few abnormalities have been noted, e.g. origin of aorta from right ventricle instead of left, blood may flow from left ventricle to right ventricle first and then to the aorta, highly developed musculature of right ventricle instead of left, stenosis of pulmonary artery. Because of these four abnormalities (tetralogy), the blood from right ventricle may pass into aorta (de-oxygenated). This gives blue coloration; originating the term blue or cyanosed baby. Another three characteristics of tetralogy are—high systolic pressure

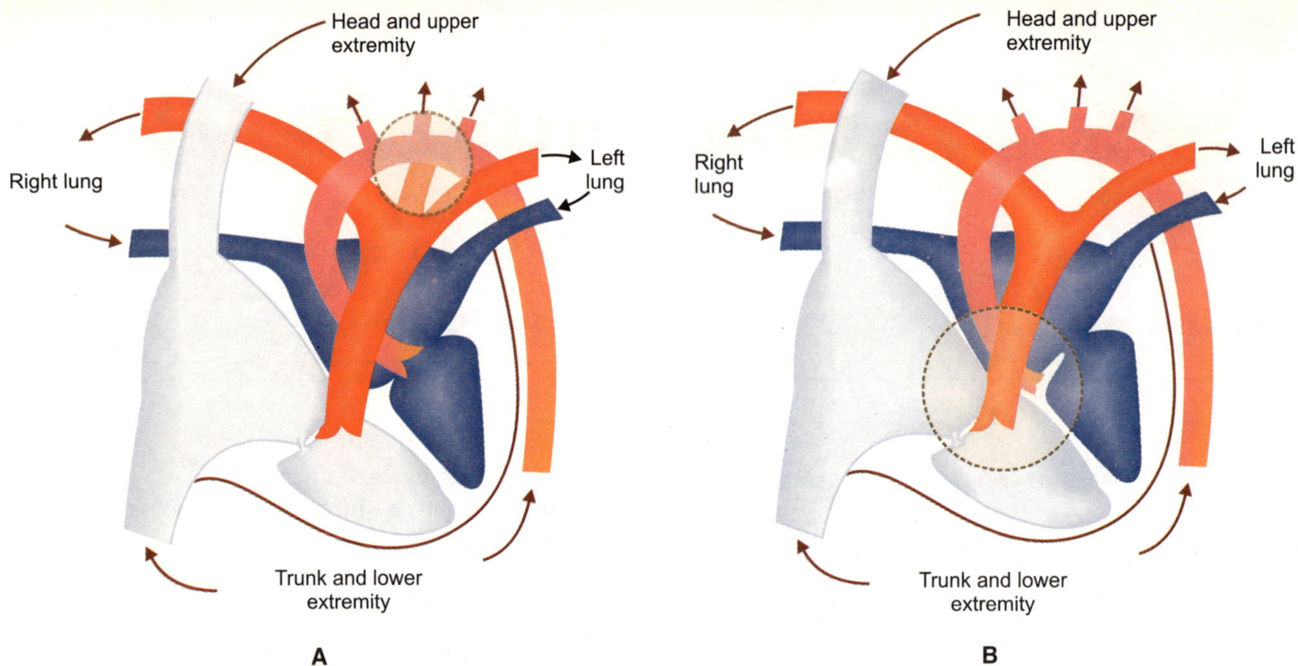

Figs 82.1A and B: Patent ductus arteriosus (A) Congenital heart disease (B)

in right ventricle, enlarged right ventricle radiologically, less blood flow through stenosed pulmonary artery.
- Treatment is surgical.

e. *Causes:*
- Viral infection of mother during early pregnancy, e.g. German measles.
- Congenital anomaly/hereditary.

TETRALOGY OF FALLOT: AT A GLANCE

A. Causes (Tetra = four) aorta originates from right ventricle, highly developed muscles of right ventricle, stenosis of pulmonary artery, blood flow from left to right ventricle.

B. Symptomatology (Tetra = four), blue baby, high systolic pressure in right ventricle, enlarged right ventricle, less blood flow through stenosed pulmonary artery.

C. Treatment Correction of pulmonary stenosis, allowing blood flow towards aorta, closing of septal defect.

BIBLIOGRAPHY

1. Grossman W (Ed). Cardiac Catheterization and Angiography. 3rd ed. Philadelphia: Lea and Febiger. 1986.
2. Heyman MA, Rudolf AM. Control of ductus arteriosus. Phy Rev 1975;55:52.
3. Olley PM, Coceani F. Prostaglandins and ductus arteriosus. Ann Rev Med 1981;32: 375.
4. Taussing H. Congenital malformation of heart Vol. I. General consideration. 2nd ed. Vol. 2: Specific malformation 2nd ed. Cambridge Mass: Harvard University Press. 1960.

Cardiac Failure

Failure of the heart results because of decreased pumping capability of the heart to satisfy the needs of the body. It may result in decreased cardiac output and damming of blood in the veins behind left or right heart.

DYNAMICS

Acute Effects

- Because of heart failure, the cardiac output is reduced which reduces arterial blood pressure. This decreased blood pressure activates baroreceptors which normalises the reduced blood pressure.
- Similarly chemoreceptors are also stimulated due to reduced oxygen concentration which also normalises the situation.
- The CNS ischaemic reflex is also activated to balance the situation.
- The strongest beneficial effect is sympathetic stimulation.
- All these actually make the heart a stronger pump. So patient feels only transient unconsciousness and a slight pain in cardiac region. So generally such persons ignore such attack and they cancel the visit to doctor. This is compensated cardiac failure.

CHRONIC STAGE

As the cardiac failure progresses following events ensues diminished cardiac output supplies less blood to the kidneys which suppresses the kidney functions which may lead to anurea, of course with retention of fluid; which in turn increases the blood volume; which leads to increase in mean systolic filling pressure which in turn, increases the pressure gradient for flow of blood towards the heart, i.e. increased venous return. This increases cardiac output. It certainly appears a beneficial effect.

But as the famous proverb is there, 'what is potent for good is also powerful for evil; so as the case exists here. If cardiac output is reduced to a very low extent then this extra fluid accumulation may lead to severe oedema throughout the body which may terminate into fatal results. This excess fluid may cause pulmonary oedema, over stretching of the heart etc. which may further deteriorate the situation. This is *decompensated stage* of cardiac failure.

As regards its management is concerned it should be directed towards (a) elimination of this extra fluid which is done by administration of diuretic drugs; and (b) improving the myocardial efficiency by drugs like digitalis (cardiotonic drug).

CHANGES IN DECOMPENSATED STAGE

- Progressive retention of fluid,
- Elevation of mean systemic filling pressure,
- Progressive elevation of right atrial pressure
- Heart becomes over stretched up to the extent that it is unable to pump even moderate quantity of blood.

The Kidneys and Heart Failure

- Reduced cardiac output → reduced arterial pressure → intense sympathetic constriction of kidney afferent arteriole → decreased GFR.
- Because of decreased cardiac output; renin-angiotensin-system is activated which further decreases blood flow through kidneys by acting directly on afferent arterioles of kidney.
- Increased reabsorption of water and electrolytes takes place and thus their quantity in body is increased.
- Angiotensin in turn, stimulates aldosterone secretion from adrenal cortex. Reduced renal function in cardiac failure elevates blood potassium level which also acts as a powerful stimulus for aldosterone secretion. This aldosterone in turn increases the reabsorption of water and electrolytes from renal tubules.

- Preventive role of ANF (atrial-natri-uretic factor) This ANF is a hormone released by atrial walls on stretch. During heart failure excessive stretching occurs which leads to release of ANF.

Chronic Heart Failure Leads to Pulmonary Oedema

Increased venous return → increased load on already weak left ventricle → blood damming up in lungs → increased pulmonary capillary pressure → small amount of blood transudate into lung tissues and alveoli → diminished degree of oxygenation of blood → weakening of the heart and peripheral vasodilatation → further increased in venous return → thus a vicious cycle goes on.

Basis of treatment: Bleeding the patient. A suitable diuretic is administered. A cardiotonic drug is to be administered. Oxygen therapy tourniquets may be put on all the four limbs.

Vicious cycle of deterioration: In chronic heart failure less blood is reaching to tissues and so less blood is returned back to the heart through coronaries and this is specially true for subendocardial surface of the heart. This part of the heart first dies and replaced by fibrous tissue. So heart becomes still weaker and weaker eliciting another such cycle which further weakens the heart. So after sometime it does not respond to any treatment.

CARDIAC RESERVE

- *The maximum percentage that the cardiac output can increase above normal is cardiac reserve.*
- Normally it is 300-400 per cent.
- Heart rate has upper limit of 210 beats per minute (130-140/minute).
- Oxygen reserve is 900 ml.
- Work of heart 75 kg/minute. Left ventricle at rest 5-6 kg per minute and during work, it may go to 80 kg/minute.
- Stroke volume 80-100 ml; capacity is 150-170 ml, normally 60-70 ml/beat.

HIGH CARDIAC OUTPUT FAILURE

In some cases, because of increased venous return, cardiac output increases which increases the load on heart which eventually terminates into cardiac failure. This is seen in

- *Thyrotoxicosis*: Due to increased production of thyroxine, basal metabolic rate is increased which leads to generalised vasodilatation which terminate into cardiac failure because of overloading of the heart.
- *Beri Beri:* This occurs because of deficiency of vitamin B_1 (thiamine). This causes poor metabolic utilisation of nutrients throughout the body. This causes dilatation of local blood vessels, which reduces total peripheral resistance so increasing venous return, and overloading the heart, terminating into cardiac failure.
- *Arterio-venous shunts*: In such instances blood is shunted directly from arteries to the veins which increases the venous return causing overloading of the heart which terminates into cardiac failure.

HEART FAILURE: CAUSES

- Valvular (obstructive + back flow lesion)
- Mechanical (pericardial disease)
- Myogenic (ischaemia + inflammation)
- Extrinsic
- a. Metabolic (beri-beri, hyperthyroidism, uraemia)
  b. Physical (systemic or pulmonary hypertension, Paget's bone disease).

QUESTION BANK—HEART

1. **Explain:**
   a. Cardiac muscle during contraction exhibits 'plateau'. Why?
   b. Sinus node controls the rhythmicity of heart. Why?
   c. Rest is valuable in treatment of myocardial infarction. How?
   d. The murmur sound in aortic stenosis is so loud that it can be heard several feet away from the patient. Why?
   e. Being a wave of re-polarisation T wave is a positive deflection in ECG. Why? How it becomes biphasic in digitalis poisoning.
   f. Heart rate increases during inspiration while it decreases during expiration. How?
   g. The athlete is having bradycardia. How? And sometimes a man wearing a shirt of tight collar becomes unconscious. How?
   h. A blowing murmur is heard in aortic regurgitation. Why?
   i. Left sided heart failure leads to pulmonary oedema. How?
2. **Discuss:**
   a. Causes of death following acute coronary occlusion.
   b. The mechanism of fibrillation and premature beats, and their treatment.
   c. Heart blocks.
   d. The working of baro and chemoreceptors.
   e. The mechanism of cardiac compensation during cardiac failure.
3. **Short Notes:**
   a. Venous return.
   b. Heart sounds.
   c. Bain bridge reflex and Bezold Jarisch reflex.
   d. Fick principle.
   e. Determination of axis in ECG and its clinical application.
   f. Heart rate and regulation.
   g. P - R interval in ECG.

QUESTION BANK—CIRCULATION

1. **Explain**
   a. In a patient of anaemia, murmur is heard. Why?
   b. Blood pressure is classed as silent killer. How?
   c. Long continued standing posture causes faintness. How?
   d. Exercise increases blood pressure. How?
   e. Sometimes the patient in shock recovers. How?
   f. What will happen to blood flow if radius of artery is halved.
   g. Blood flow in coronary arteries during diastole. (First MBBS, 2001, Raj Univ)
   h. ECG in bipolar limb lead II. (First MBBS, 2001, Raj Univ)
2. **Discuss:**
   a. Mechanism of circulatory shock and physiology of its treatment. (Raj. Univ. 1991, MD, First MBBS, 1995)
   b. Long-term regulation of blood pressure. Pathophysiology of essential hypertension. (Raj Univ 1982, 1995 MD)
   c. Local control of blood flow.
   d. Vasomotor centre and its control
   e. Immediate response of severe loss of blood from body and its management. (Raj Univ 1982, MD)
   f. Mechanism of reversible shock. What changes make it irreversible shock. (Raj Univ 1982, MD)
   g. Cardiac output during exercise. (First MBBS, 2001, Raj Univ)
   h. Sinoatrial node as pacemaker. (First MBBS, 2001, Raj Univ)
3. **Short notes:**
   a. Triple response
   b. Pulmonary circulation
   c. Determinants of diastolic BP.
   d. Humoral and ionic regulation of circulation.
   e. Neurogenic shock.
   f. Echo-cardiography. (Raj Univ 1994, MD)
   g. Starling law of heart. (Raj Univ 1997, MD)
   h. Autoregulation of blood flow in various organs. (Raj Univ 1996, MD)
   i. ECG. (Raj Univ 1994, MD)
   j. Baro-receptors. (Raj Univ 1994, MD)
   k. Arterial pulse. (Raj Univ 1980, MD)
   l. Heart sounds. (Raj Univ First MBBS, 1995)
   m. Venous return. (Raj Univ First MBBS, 1995)
   n. Pace maker potential. (Raj Univ First MBBS, 1995, 1989 M.D.)
   o. Electrocardiogram. (Raj Univ First MBBS, 1995)
   p. Cardiac catheterization. (Raj Univ 1982, MD)
   q. Vector cardiography. (Raj Univ 1979, MD)
   r. Circulation time. (Raj Univ 1979, MD)
   s. CNS ischemic response. (First MBBS, 2001, Raj Univ)
4. **Describe the mechanical events of the cardiac cycle and correlate them with the electrocardiogram. Illustrate with the help of diagram. (Raj Univ First MBBS, 1995)**
5. **What is heart rate? How is it regulated? (Raj Univ First MBBS, 1995, MD1995)**
6. **Discuss cardiovascular homeostasis in health and disease (Raj Univ 1995, 1996, MD)**
7. **Discuss dynamics of blood flow - or discuss the cardiovascular regulatory mechanisms. (Raj Univ 1996, MD)**
8. **How blood pressure changes with age and how it is regulated. Describe briefly Goldblatt experiments. (Raj Univ 1990, 1993, 1996, MD)**
9. **Discuss mechanism of abnormal underlying cardiac rhythms. (Raj Univ MD 1990)**
10. **Discuss the functional organisation of vascular bed. Discuss local and nervous control of vascular tone. (Raj Univ 1988, MD)**
11. **Describe ultrastructure of mammalian arterioles and pre-capillary sphincters. Correlate their structure with function. (Raj Univ 1988, MD).**
12. **Describe the basic design and evolution of CVS. (Raj Univ 1990, MD). Discuss comparative physiology of cardiac actions (Raj Univ 1982, MD)**

MULTIPLE CHOICE QUESTIONS: CARDIOVASCULAR SYSTEM

1. **Digitalis toxicity produce the following changes in ECG *except*: (AIIMS - 1988)**
   a. Inverted P wave
   b. Prolonged Q-T interval
   c. ST depression
   d. Prolonged P-R interval [ ]
2. **SA node is situated at: (PGI-1990)**
   a. Anterior medial aspect of junction of superior vena cava with right atrium
   b. Anterior lateral aspect of junction of superior vena cave with right atrium
   c. Anterior medial aspect of junction of inferior vena cava with right atrium
   d. Junction of anterior rough part and posterior smooth part [ ]
3. **Which of the following does not cause tachycardia: (PGI-1985 and 1986)**
   a. Thyrotoxicosis
   b. Shock
   c. Obstructive jaundice
   d. Digitalis poisoning [ ]
4. **Commonest cause of mitral stenosis is: (AMC - 1983, 1985, UPSC-1982, 1985)**
   a. Congenital
   b. Syphilis
   c. Rheumatic
   d. Hypertension [ ]
5. **Pulsus paradoxus is seen in: (PGI-1986)**
   a. Mitral stenosis
   b. Atrial fibrillation
   c. Aortic stenosis
   d. Asthma [ ]

6. **P waves are absent in: (Delhi - 1985, 1990)**
   a. Atrial flutter
   b. Atrial fibrillation
   c. Complete heart block
   d. Atrial ectopies [ ]
7. **Sinus bradycardia is seen in: (AIIMS-1986, Delhi-1990)**
   a. Hypothyroidism
   b. First degree heart block
   c. Graves' disease
   d. Adrenalectomy [ ]
8. **Which of the following is *not* a cause of collapsing pulse: (AIIMS 1985, 1988)**
   a. Patent ductus arteriosus
   b. Anaemia
   c. Malignant hypertension
   d. Thyrotoxicosis [ ]
9. **Opening of aortic valve is initiated by: (Delhi - 1986)**
   a. Contraction of atria
   b. Contraction of ventricle
   c. When ventricular pressure is more than aortic pressure
   d. None of above [ ]
10. **Vasovagal syncope is also called: (Delhi-1985, 1986)**
    a. Hypovolaemic shock
    b. Anaphylactic shock
    c. Emotional shock
    d. Septicaemic shock [ ]

ANSWERS

1 a **2** a **3** c **4** c **5** d **6** b **7** a **8** c **9** c **10** c

VIVA VOCE : CARDIOVASCULAR SYSTEM

1. **What is Frank Starling law of heart ?**
   - Greater the heart is filled during diastole, the greater will be the quantity of blood pumped into aorta.
     Or another way to express is
   - 'Within physiological limits heart pumps all the blood that comes to it without allowing excessive damming of blood in veins.'
   - It suggests that, 'energy for contraction is proportional to initial length of muscle fibres.'
2. **What is P-R Interval in ECG ?**
   It denotes time of passage of current from SA node to AV node. Normally it ranges between 0.13 - 0.16 second. If it exceeds 0.2 sec. it suggests heart block (delayed conduction of heart). It is between peak of P and R wave.
3. **Define stroke and minute volume?**
   Stroke volume is volume of blood ejected in each beat by each chamber. It is 70 ml so total stroke volume of both ventricles is 140 ml. Minute volume = Heart rate/min. × stroke volume (70 × 75 = 5250 ml or 5 litres approx.) It is the volume of blood ejected by each ventricle per minute.
4. **What is Bainbridge reflex ?**
   Bainbridge (1915), perfused right atrium with saline and found tachycardia which was abolished by section of vagi. It holds true only when initial heart rate is slow.
   Weak stimulus causes increase while strong stimulus leads to decreased heart rate.
5. **What is cardiac Reserve ?**
   The maximum percentage that the cardiac output can increase above normal is cardiac reserve. In normal individual it is slightly more than 300 per cent.
   Heart rate reserve is 130-140 beats/min., stroke volume reserve is 80-100 ml, potential reserve of oxygen is 900 ml, reserve work of heart is 75 kg/min., reserve blood flow is 30 litres/min.
6. **What is triple response and its cause ?**
   If the skin is stroked by a blunt instrument with hard pressure, after some latent period 'red line' along with line of stroke develops (due to liberation of histamine like substances) which is followed by formation of flare (due to local nerve reflex; axon reflex) which is crenated in appearance, resulting into 'wheel' which raises skin surface by 1-2 mm (due to liberation of histamine or histamine-like substances). It is a reaction of skin capillaries.
7. **What is sinus arrhythmia and what are its possible causes?**
   During inspiration heart rate is increased and opposite effect is seen on expiration. This is sinus arrhythmia.
   i. Inspiration → increased negative pressure in chest cage → increased pressure in abdomen due to descent of diaphragm → more blood flows from abdomen to thorax → increased venous return → stretching of heart → increased heart rate owing to Bainbridge reflex.

ii. Inspiration → Excess activity of respiratory centre → Impulse generation which overflows cardiac centre located near it → increased heart rate.

8. **What is cardiac index?**
Cardiac output per square meter of body surface is cardiac index. It average 3.2 liters.

9. **Mention the main determinants of coronary blood flow?**
   a. Mean aortic pressure.
   b. Tone of coronary arterial smooth muscle.
   c. Exerting tension of surrounding cardiac muscle mass.

10. **What is pulse and mean pressure?**
   a. Pulse pressure is the difference between systolic and diastolic pressure (120-80 = 40 mmHg; ratio 3 : 2: 1). It is index of cardiac output.
   b. Mean pressure = Diastolic pressure + 1/3 Pulse pressure.

BIBLIOGRAPHY

1. Barger AC. The kidney in congestive heart failure. Circulation 1960;21:124.
2. Braunwald E. Heart disease. Philadelphia: WB Saunders Co. 1988. (Quoted by Guyton AC in Textbook of Medical Physiology - WB Saunders).
3. Califf RM. Cardiogenic shock. New Eng J Med 1994;330:1724.
4. Francis GS. Neuro-humoral mechanism involved in congestive heart failure. Amer J Card 1985;55:15A.
5. Furster V, et al. The pathogenesis of coronary artery disease and acute coronary syndrome. New Eng J Med 1992;326:242.
6. Grossman WD. Diastolic dysfunction in congestive heart failure. New Eng J Med 1991;325:1557.
7. Hoffman JI, et al. Pressure flow relations in coronary circulation. Phy Rev 1990;70: 331.

UNIT 12

Emotions Greatly Affect Digestion

"Oh! You are young because your stomach is healthy. Good digestion waits on appetite and health on both."

84

Introduction

The entire alimentary canal is a long muscular tube extending from mouth to anus. Different organs are meant for specialised functions in connection with digestion and absorption.

SALIVARY GLANDS

The three pairs of glands are parotid, submaxillary or submandibular and sublingual and all of these are responsible for secreting saliva.

Parotids are located between mandibular ramus and mastoid process, and sternomastoid muscle, extending in front of internal auditory meatus. This lies in close contact with muscle masseter and mandibular ramus. Certainly it is largest salivary gland. The saliva produced by it is carried to vestibule of mouth through parotid ducts through piercing the buccinator muscle, opposite second molar.

Submandibular Located medially to mandible in submaxillary triangle. The salivary secretion is brought to caruncula sublingualis through submandibular ducts (Wharton's ducts).

Sublingual are lying little more medially underneath the mucous membrane in floor of mouth. Small ducts are carrying its secretion to sublingual folds as well as submandibular ducts.

The mouth particularly its mucous membrane reflects internal diseases of a general character; e.g. Koplik spots of measles, "blue lead line" of lead poisoning, haemorrhage in gums in scurvy. Mouth is also mirror of stomach and this explains the fact that tongue should also be examined with same care as pulse.

PHARYNX

It can be said as a conical chamber which conducts food from mouth to oesophagus with which its apex is continuous. It is serving as a passage way for both digestive and respiratory system "nasopharynx" lies above the level of soft palate and behind it is its "oropharynx" and from it laryngeal pharynx continues from below the level of hyoid bone into oesophagus.

OESOPHAGUS (GULLET)

As by one remark ***"Even if we don't live to eat but we should eat to live and hence oesophagus should be given a great importance since it is an organ through which food is conveyed to stomach. So it is a wonder that how little importance is given to this important organ."***

Any way it is a soft muscular tube about ten inches in length extending from lower border of cricoid cartilage to the hiatus in diaphragm (more simply from pharynx to stomach). Its only function is swallowing. The veins from its upper third drain into subclavian vein, from middle third of it to azygous vein and those from lower third by way of coronary, left gastric and splenic veins into portal vein, thus a communication is established between portal and systemic circulation which explains the development of oesophageal varies in cases of portal hypertension.

The "dysphagia" means discomfort on swallowing is commonest symptom of oesophageal disease, interferes with enjoyment of life more than is commonly realised (Benedict and Nardi, 1958).

STOMACH

It is composed of two units one is fundus and body while another is pylorus. Blood supply is derived from coeliac axis and is developing from foregut. The fundus is acid producing while antrum produces alkaline juice. It is considered as an expanded portion of GI. tract between oesophagus and small intestine. The fundus is described as that part lying above a horizontal line drawn through

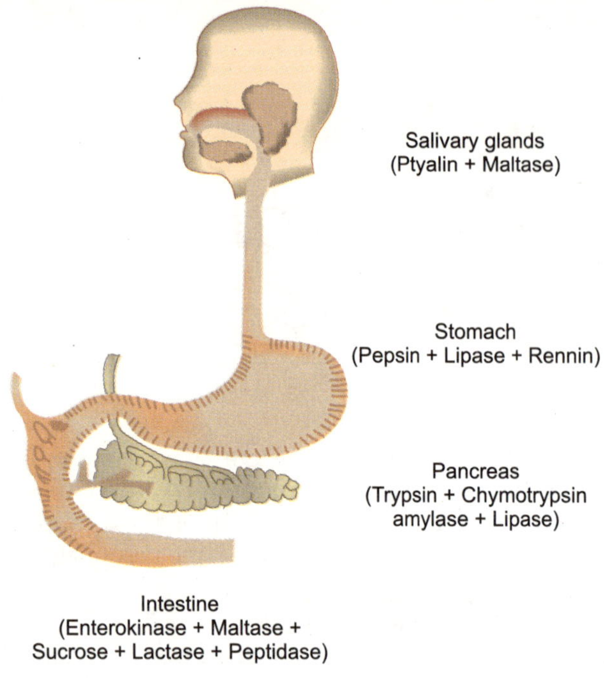

Fig. 84.1: GIT enzymes

the entrance of oesophagus and approximately remaining 2/3 portion is body while last one is pylorus (pylorus = exit or gate).

INTESTINE

- Small intestine is 20 feet long structure. Its first 10-12 inches constitute duodenum which is fixed in position not being suspended by mesentery. It is followed by horseshoe shaped course around pancreatic head to become continuous with Jejunum which constitutes next two-fifth part and the last three-fifth portion is ileum.
- The large intestine consists of caecum, vermiform appendix ascending, transverse, descending and pelvic colon and rectum opening to exterior through anus.

LIVER

It is the largest gland in the body consisting of lobes which further comprises lobule which are structural unit of it. It weighs 1400-1600 gm in males and 1200-1400 gm in females. Its colour is dark reddish brown or chocolate. Riedel's lobe is the name given to a tongue like process extending downwards from lower margin of liver external to gall bladder. As regards its consistency it is soft solid, friable, easily lacerated and when placed on a flat surface the dome like curve of upper surface appears flattened.

PANCREAS

It extends from inner duodenal curvature to spleen at 1st and 2nd lumbar vertebrae inside abdomen. It is compound recemose gland identical in pattern of salivary glands, having shape like a prism. The acini are ovoid or spherical in shape and a primary lobule is constructed by their union. It develops from outgrowth of primitive gut where ventral outgrowth grows into ventral and dorsal outgrowth grows into dorsal mesentery. Both the outgrowths unite at left duodenal border; ventral duct along with common bile duct (after uniting with it in ampulla of Vater) enters duodenal papillae at left side of second part of duodenum, the orifice, of course is surrounded by sphincter of oddi; dorsal duct enters duodenum 2 cm above duodenal opening of main pancreatic duct and thus forming duct of santorini (accessory pancreatic duct). It is supplied by both sets of nerves—parasympathetic (vagus) as well as sympathetic.

BIBLIOGRAPHY

1. Johnson LR (Ed), et al. Physiology of Gastrointestinal Tract 3rd ed. Raven Press, 1994.

85 Salivary Secretion: Digestion in Mouth

Saliva is not essential to life, but its absence results in number of inconveniences.

SALIVA: INTRODUCTION

It amounts to be 1000-1500 cc in 24 hours. Its secretory rate is high at meal time but reduced during sleep. Its specific gravity ranges between 1.002-1.012. Parotid gland's contribution is 25 per cent, submaxillary contributes 70 per cent and sublingual 5 per cent. Water is said to be 99.5 per cent and CO_2, O_2, N_2 gases are present.

Inorganic Constituents

- Bicarbonates increases with flow rate and its concentration is directly influenced by Pco_2 of arterial blood so any thing increasing Pco_2 will increase bicarbonates but bicarbonates have got reciprocal relation with chlorides. So with increased Pco_2 (arterial) bicarbonates enters saliva and exchange for chlorides.
- 'Phosphates' is about two-fold than plasma and majority of it is in inorganic state and is independent of flow rate. 'Chlorides' also vary directly with flow rates. Bromides are similar to chlorides but nothing significant is known about 'fluorides'.
- Sodium concentration is also dependent upon flow rate. Potassium concentration is high and exceeds that of plasma. Calcium concentration also increases with flow rate.
- Calcium and phosphorus are important inorganic constituents. Their concentration in saliva are even more than in blood.
- Sodium, potassium, magnesium, chloride, sulphate, thiocyanate (more in smoker's saliva) are also present in detectable amounts. Minute traces of fluoride, iodide, bromide, nitrite and copper have also been detected. Thiocyanate is having an antibacterial action, but it also acts as a cofactor for a protein in saliva which is exerting antibacterial action.

Organic Constituents

- 'Salivary proteins' are responsible for appearance of this secretion. Saliva from parotid gland has low viscosity and so watery while saliva obtained from submaxillary gland is viscous owing to its mucoprotein constituents. The main proteins are albumin, mucoprotein and mucin etc.
- Free amino acid, urea, uric acid, creatinine are also found here.
- Kallikrein an enzyme acting on plasma proteins to produce a vasodilator polypeptide called 'bradykinin or kallidin. Blood group substances have also been isolated in saliva.
- Glucose is not found in saliva even in a patient of diabetes.
- Lysozyme is bacteriolytic enzyme in saliva and chemically is mucoprotein in nature. So it performs an antiseptic action specially against strepto-staphylo-meningococci.
- The pH of human saliva varies between 6.35-6.85. (wide range being 5.5-7.5).

Enzymes and their action: Salivary amylase or ptyalin is the chief enzyme which acts on boiled starch converting them to maltose, entire reaction can be summed up as—

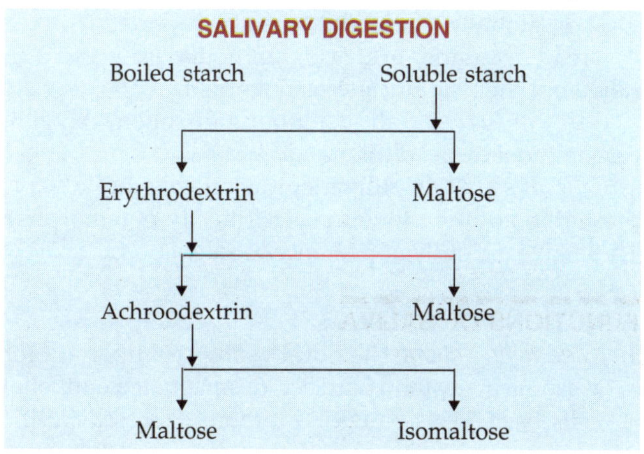

Erythrodextrin = red colour with iodine, Achrodextrin = no colour in response of iodine.

This ptyalin enzyme requires neutral or faint acid or faint alkaline medium for its full action. This enzyme has no action on cellulose and probably for this reasoning starch is cooked in order to break cellulose envelops.

Maltose as further acted upon by another enzyme *Maltase* to be changed into glucose. The starch is digested even in stomach by ptyalin before the atmosphere becomes strongly acidic.

PHYSICAL PROPERTIES OF SALIVA

Specific gravity	1.002 - 1.012
Surface tension	15.2 - 26.0 dyne/cm.
Osmotic pressure	0.151 - 0.301
Viscosity	1.06 - 2.4 (ostwald method) : It is due to mucin saliva is a viscous fluid.
pH	5.5 - 7.5 (average 6.7)
Secretion rate	0.01-2.0 ml./min. unstimulated 0.5 - 7.0 ml./min. stimulated

Other Constituents

i. The agglutinogens A, B and O which are soluble polysaccharides are found in saliva of about 80 per cent of persons (secretors).
ii. Most of the water soluble vitamins can be detected in saliva.
iii. Glucose is absent.

Salivary Proteins

Salivary mucins are synthesised by the mucus acinar cells of the paired submandibular and sublingual glands. So in nutshell, 'The oral environment, like other mucosal surfaces of the body, is coated by a slimy, viscoelastic coat termed mucus. This adherent layer, consisting predominantly of salivary glycoproteins, proteins and lipids, forms a jelly like blanket that represent the perimeter defence of the tissue/environmental interface.

The γ globulin (antibodies) are also reported.

Urea, creatinine, uric acid, ammonia are present in saliva but their significance is unknown.

Gases in Saliva: Saliva contains nitrogen, oxygen, carbon dioxide, in solution.

Cells in saliva: In saliva, epithelial cells are always present in addition to leucocytes (mostly polymorphs). These give a cloudy appearance to saliva.

FUNCTIONS OF SALIVA

a. *Cleansing action*: The flow of saliva is important for washing away food particles, desquamated epithelial cells, bacteria etc. Saliva in addition, possesses specific bacteriostatic or bacteriocidal properties. The bacterial flora of the saliva in the mouth exert production of some agents which inhibit some other bacteria (lysozyme is famous name in this series; its concentration is higher in combined submaxillary and sublingual glands than in parotid. 'Catalase' and peroxidase' are other names).

b. *Moistening and lubrication*: Soft tissues of oral cavity are moistened and lubricated by saliva and in this way they are prevented from drying. This is necessary not only for digestive and protective purpose but for articulate speech, as experienced in states of anxiety or fright when the salivary reflex is inhibited.

c. *Digestive function*: Digestion of carbohydrates begins in the mouth through the action of amylase. It hydrolyzes starches to various dextrins and sugar, mainly maltose; which in turn can be hydrolyzed either by maltase or bacteria.

d. *Preparation of food for swallowing*: The food is altered in its consistency. It is moistened and lubricated. In this way, it is converted into a plastic mass 'bolus' which facilitates the swallowing. Salivary mucin plays an important role by its lubricant action on the mucosa and the food.

e. *Regulation of water balance*: Drying of oral mucous membrane arouses the sensation of thirst which forces one individual to drink water which maintains the water balance. According to this view, thirst may be felt and water consumed even with normal stores of water whenever mucosa becomes dry, for instance, in fear, after injection of atropine etc. On the other hand, in a dehydrating individual, thirst may be alleviated by moistening the mucosa with water. So it was pointed out that salivary glands like other tissues must suffer when water is lacking in the body. Dehydration and loss of blood also evoke thirst.

f. *Excretory function*: Salivary glands are usually described as having an excretory function. Substances, e.g. iodine, thiocyanates, mercury, lead, alkaloids like morphine, antibiotics (like penicillin, chloramphenicol, streptomycin, aureomycin), are excreted from saliva. Ethyl alcohol is eliminated through the salivary glands and its estimation in saliva is done for medicolegal purposes.

g. Saliva, is having a special importance as a *'solvent'* since taste buds are stimulated only when the effective substance is in a liquid state (dissolved). Saliva dissolves many solid foods, thus aiding in appreciation of food and stimulation of taste buds with resultant reflex secretion. Some substances are said to give rise to a more persistent taste sensation (iodides, saccharine) which may be due to the fact that they are excreted in the saliva.

h. Saliva keeps the teeth moist and acids in their preservation by virtue of its chemical composition. So it aids in fixation of dentures.

i. The dog's lickling of its wound-promote healing. In cats, spitting is one of the bodily expression of rage....... elicited through sympathetic nerves.

j. *Arousing sensation of taste*: whenever any substance will be in solution form, it will be capable of producing its taste so saliva keeps edible substance in solution form to arouse its taste.

REGULATION OF SECRETION

It is regulated by nervous system, or it is a reflex process. Glands are innervated by both sympathetic and parasympathetic fibres.

Sympathetic Stimulation

When these nerves are stimulated it results into

a. Constriction of blood vessels supplying gland,
b. Serous cell stimulation, and
c. Contraction of myo-epithelial cells. (Salt and water secretion).

Parasympathetic Stimulation

On stimulating parasympathetic the results are:

a. Dilatation of blood vessels,
b. Due to stimulation of mucous cells, water and salt secretion results (hydrolytic effect) and
c. Enzyme secretion.

Paralytic secretion: Claude Bernard (1864) observed that when chorda tympani nerve is sectioned in dog or cat initially thick viscous secretion takes place which increases upto 7th day and finally diminishes by 6th week or so. It is due to the fact that secretory cells are sensitised by adrenaline.

Conditioned reflex: When only sight or smell of food causes salivation without actual food in mouth, the reflex is conditioned one. In one of his experiments I.V. Pavlov used to sound a gong before giving food to his experimental animal dog. This is called conditioned reflex where sound of gong acted as stimulus for it.

Unconditioned reflex: In this food is actually present acting as stimulus for salivation. It may be categorised as:

a. *Mouth salivary reflex:* Any stimulus (food, jaw movements etc.) can result into salivation. Stimulation of taste sensation is also dominant here.
b. *Oesophagosalivary reflex:* Passage of food through oesophagus, inflammation or malignancy of oesophagus can result into excessive salivation.
c. *Gastrosalivary reflex:* Irritation of stomach, infection, malignancy, gastritis all lead to excess salivation.
d. *Other organs:* Distension of uterus in pregnancy can also induce salivation.

EFFECT OF DRUGS AND CHEMICALS

i. Sympathomimetic drugs (adrenaline, ephedrine) causes salivation and so also parasympathomimetic agents (acetylcholine, pilocarpine, physostigmine, muscarine).
ii. Sympatholytic agents as well as parasympatholytic agents (atropine, scopolamine) depress salivary secretion.
iii. Quinine depresses secretion.
iv. Anaesthetics (chloroform, ether) reflexly stimulate salivary secretion. Now since excessive salivary flow may produce problems for anaesthetics so atropine and scopolamine have been long used as premedication to anaesthesia to inhibit or reduce salivary flow.

SALIVA: FORMATION

- It was formerly thought that formation of saliva is similar to formation of urine. Saliva is considered as ultra filtrate of blood.
- It is a procedure that requires energy for the work of secretion of organic substances; and active transport of inorganic substances across the cell membranes against concentration gradient by the duct epithelium.
- Source of energy for salivary gland metabolism is glucose.
- Saliva is hypotonic to blood serum.
- There exists a reciprocal relation between bicarbonate and chloride which is controlled by Pco_2.
- The bicarbonate-chloride exchange may occur in more distal part of salivary ducts.

CLINICAL PHYSIOLOGY

a. *Xerostomia or aptyalism* means complete stoppage or cessation of salivary secretion. The causes may be absence of salivary glands or congenital hypoplasia making speech troublesome and difficulty in chewing,

b. *Hyposalivation* means decreased salivation and may be due to X radiation or surgery.

c. *Hypersalivation or sialorrhoea*: Excess salivation may be due to inflammation or malignancy of stomach, oesophagus, buccal cavity, gastric or duodenal ulcer, parkinsonism, psychoneurosis.

SUMMARY AND HIGHLIGHTS: SALIVA NUTSHELL DESCRIPTION

- *Introduction:* Quantity per day 1000-1500 cc specific gravity 1.002-1.0125, pH 6.35-6.85, water 99.5 per cent, solids 0.5 per cent, gases (CO_2, O_2, N_2), Inorganic solids 0.2 per cent (sodium chloride and bicarbonate, potassium chloride and carbonate, calcium phosphate, acid and alkaline sodium phosphate), organic proteins (serum albumin, globulin, mucin, bradykinin), Enzymes (ptyalin or amylase, maltase, traces of Lysozyme), other organic substances (Urea, uric acid, amino acids, creatinine, ABO like blood group antigen substances).
- *Functions:* (a) Mechanical (moistening of mouth, protection by diluting the irritants, helping mastication leading to bolus formation, cleans mouth, helps speech), (b) Digestive (boiled starch converted finally to glucose and maltose), (c) Helping in sensation of taste (by dissolving edible substances), (d) Maintain water balance (by producing thirst), (e) Body temperature maintenance (animals particularly), (f) Blood reaction maintenance.
- *Mechanism:* Purely reflex phenomenon, no humoral regulation. Conditioned reflex (salivation on sight smell or thinking of food without presence of food) as well as unconditioned reflex (food actually present in mouth; oesophagosalivary reflex, gastrosalivary reflex and reflex from other distended or hollow organs like pregnant uterus.

BIBLIOGRAPHY

1. Fawcet DM, Kirkwood S. Role of salivary glands in extra thyroidial iodine metabolism. Quoted by Physiology of mouth by G Neil Jenkins (1966) - Third ed. page 288-357. Oxford: Blackwell scientific publication. Science 1954;120:547.
2. Gottschalk A Biochim, et al. Studies on mucoprotein. Biophys. Acta 1961;43:81, 91, 98.
3. Jenkins GN. The physiology of the mouth: 3rd ed. Oxford: Blackwell. 1966.
4. JW Puteny Jr. Identification of cellular activation mechanisms associated with salivary secretion. Ann Rev Phy 1986;48:75.
5. Lawrence A. Tabak: In defence of the oral cavity: structure, biosynthesis and function of salivary mucin. Ann Rev Phy 1995;57:547-64.
6. Melvidlle Schachter and Susanne Beilenson. Gastro enterology. Kallikrein and vasodilation in the sub maxillary gland. 52:401, No. 2, 1967.
7. Nour Ehdin F, JF Wilbinson. The blood clotting factors in human Saliva. Quoted by above book. J Phy 1957;136: 324-32.
8. Peterson OH, Gallacher DV. Electrophysiology of pancreatic and salivary acinar cells.Ann Rev Phy 1988;50:65.
9. Physiology of salivary glands by ASV Burgen and NG Emmelin. London. Edward Amol publishers ltd.
10. Putney. Identification of cellular activation mechanisms associated with salivary secretion. (Reference 8 and 10 quoted by Guyton AC in Textbook of Medical Physiology - WB Saunders). Ann Rev Phy 1986;48:75-88.
11. Schneyer LH, et al. Secretory mechanism of salivary glands. London : Academic Press, 1967.
12. Sreebny LM, Meyer J. Salivary glands and then secretion, vol. 3 of monograms on oral biology. Oxford: Pergamon, 1964.
13. Stromblad BCR. Observation on amine oxidase in human salivary glands. Quoted by above book. J Phy 1959;147:639-43.
14. Young JA, et al. The morphology of salivary glands. Academic Press 1978 - Quoted by Ganong WF in Review of Medical Physiology - Lange Publications.

86 Stomach: Gastric Juice and Digestion

Stomach is just like a sensitive receiving set, it cannot protect itself from weeping even when its neighbour is in trouble and when it itself is in trouble, its voice is more louder.

GASTRIC JUICE : INTRODUCTION

The total amount of stomach juice varies between 1200-1500 c.c. in 24 hours. Its nature is strongly acidic due to secretion of hydrochloric acid (HCl) by parietal cells located here. The enzymes present here are pepsin, rennin, lipase, cathepsin, carbonic anhydrase, gelatinase, lysozyme, urease etc. The other organic constituents of the secretion includes intrinsic factor of Castle, mucus and blood group substances. The inorganic constituents include chloride, bromides, iodides, sodium, potassium etc. Intrinsic factor is a glycoprotein chemically with a molecular weight 60,000 responsible for proper absorption of extrinsic factor (cyanocobalamine, vitamin B_{12}).

Details of Gastric Enzymes

Pepsin is the chief proteolytic enzyme present here responsible for protein digestion converting them into proteoses, peptones and few amino acids and polypeptides. This enzyme becomes active only in acid medium (optimum pH is 2.0 for full activity) and at pH round about 5, peptic activity is abolished. The chief powerful stimulus for its secretion is vagal stimulation and hence by vagus stimulation or insulin hypoglycaemia gastric juice of high peptic activity is obtained while reverse effect is seen with histamine. This enzyme is secreted from chief cells of fundic glands where in zymogen granules it remains in a dormant state called *pepsinogen* and when it is stimulated it starts producing the enzyme. When protease appears in urine it is known as *uropepsin*.

- Rennin or milk curdling enzyme is of doubtful existence in human beings where milk curdling function is said to be performed by pepsin itself. For milk curdling action calcium ions are necessary and optimum pH required is 6.0-6.5 and it is the gastric mucus which makes this resultant curd softer in consistency. The soluble casein of milk is first changed into paracasein (proteose like substance; soluble) by enzyme rennin at body temperature. Then with combination of calcium, calcium paracasein is formed which precipitates like curd. This resulting curd is becoming softer in consistency by mixing with mucus.
- Lipase a weak fat splitting enzyme, a tributerase is also reported in gastric juice. Its optimum pH is reported between 4-5.0 being inactive at 2.5 pH.
- Other proteolytic enzymes include
  - — Gelatinase acts on gelatine.
  - — Cathepsin (optimum pH 4.0), Parapepsin I and II
  - — Gastricin (optimum pH 4.0)
  - — Urease causes hydrolysis of urea producing ammonia (negligible role here).
  - — Carbonic anhydrase found in parietal cells playing a leading role in HCl formation, also reported in desquamated surface epithelial cells.
  - — Lysozyme a carbohydrate splitting enzyme found in small amounts and its amount is increased in ulcer or other inflammatory states. Its optimum pH is said to be 5-5.5.

GASTRIC MUCUS

i. It occurs as a visible sheet covering the entire stomach wall and is the mucinous part of residual gastric contents. Its sources are—epithelial cells of stomach wall, the chief neck cells, and the pyloric glands.

ii. *Chemistry:* Its major component is glycoprotein, i.e. conjugated protein to which small polysaccharides are linked as individual prosthetic group. The gastric mucus has the character of egg white and microscopically it appears as branching threads. The physical properties of mucus are dependent on pH (pH of pure mucus is around 7.2) and electrolyte concentration. The opacity of pure mucus is proportional to the content of gastric epithelial cells. Though serum proteins and serum mucoproteins have been detected in gastric juice, the muco-substances, native to gastric juice, are complex. Chondroitin sulphate and heparin (acid mucopolysaccharide); neutral glycoproteins, blood group substances, sialic acid and acid glycoproteins (glycoproteins) are present.

In man insulin or an acid gastric content may cause mucus to be secreted.

iii. *Mucus: a protective material*: It has long been assumed that visible mucus layer of the gastric epithelium protects it from gastric digestion. The ability of mucus to swell and secretion of fresh mucus to replace that which has been digested are also two possible explanations for its protective action. Impairment in this regenerative process can be a factor in ulcer formation. Small defects in mucosa (e.g. loss of few cells) are repaired by flow of surrounding cells into the gap with reformation of tight junctions and all this repair process occurs within 30 minutes, i.e. very shortly.

- It has been shown that surface epithelial cells of stomach secrete bicarbonate and its constant entry into unstirred layer of gel mucus increases its ability to maintain a high gradient of hydrogen ion concentration between bulk luminal fluid and the apical surfaces of the cells.
- The main characteristic of mucus is its hydrophobic character on biophysical standpoint. The surface property is region specific; so high values are seen in stomach and colon, where barrier properties against noxious agents in lumen are important. This hydrophobic property is due to its lipid constituents and presence of phospholipid-surfactants, that are synthesised, stored and secreted by gastro-intestinal mucus cells.

WHY STOMACH DOES NOT DIGEST ITSELF?

There are many questions coming in mind while studying gastric physiology. In many persons more acid is formed (hyperchlorhydria) even then ulcer is not occurring so what may be the cause of this immunity; furthermore, why this acid hydrochloric is not able enough to destroy stomach's own mucosa? The only reliable and convincing reply is gastric mucus which makes a considerable thick covering over stomach wall and is impermeable to pepsin too, because of its absorptive power. Furthermore due to its great cohesive power it sticks to the walls with a great tenacity. We must further look at the beauty that if a layer of mucus is broken down due to any cause a fresh layer is immediately formed due to regeneration power. This gastric mucin is having a high acid combining power and is glycoprotein in nature. *Visible mucus* is thick, viscous and jelly like produced by gastric mucosa's epithelial cells and is forming 2-3 mm thick coating over gastric mucosa. On the other hand *soluble mucus* is produced by pyloric, cardiac glands and mucus neck cells of fundus of stomach. Its antipepsin activity is said to be due to its mucoitin-sulphuric acid constituent. It lubricates and protects gastric mucosa from any sort of injury.

Besides mucus other less reliable explanations of this question are summarised below:

a. Enzyme urease combines with urea to form ammonia which is said to neutralise acid;
b. An antipepsin substance is also reported which prevents auto-digestion;
c. H^+ provide alkalinity to blood circulating through gastric regions;
d. A gastric secretory inhibitor substance has also been reported which aids in this protective mechanism.

STOMACH POUCHES

For study: Experimentally a pouch means to separate a portion of stomach with keeping mucous membrane intact.

Some of this type of study are as follows (after the name of discoverer) (Fig. 86.1).

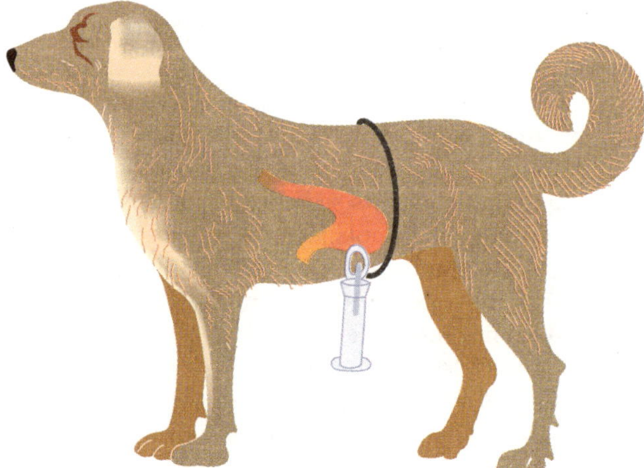

Fig. 86.1: Historical Pavlov's pouch in dog for studying gastric secretion

Heidenhain's pouch: In his study blood supply was kept intact, vagus supply cut while sympathetics escaped injury. It really gave response of hormonal type since original blood supply was severed after establishment of its own supply.

Bickel's pouch: It is a completely denervated pouch.

Pavlov's pouch: This preparation is having blood and nerve supply intact so both nervous and humoral mechanisms can be studied. In his experiment mucous membrane was exposed together with dissection of a portion of muscular wall (isthmus). It was kept in continuation with the main body by stitching the outer body, thus a cavity was formed with an outer opening whose edges were stitched to anterior abdominal wall so that secretions can come out for study purpose.

Fremont's pouch: End to end anastomosis was made by him by suturing oesophagus to duodenum and by cutting cardiac as well as pyloric stomach end. A fistulous opening was made into stomach by stitching cut end through abdominal wall.

Hollander and Jamerin pouch: This pouch was made by keeping blood and nerve supply intact.

- *Farrel and Ivy's pouch (stomach transplantation)*: Here dog's stomach was transplanted in subcutaneous tissue of abdominal wall, of course, it was denervated one. After sometime it became able enough to get blood supply from transplanted site. It is considered as the best for study purpose.

MECHANISM OF GASTRIC SECRETION

For the sake of convenience gastric secretion is divided into four phases:

a. *Cephalic phase*: This phase is activated by thought, sight, smell and taste of the food. Its efferent pathway is the vagus nerve, which contributes long preganglionic neurons, that originates in dorsal motor nuclei, travel to the stomach and terminating near short postganglionic neurons. These neurons are innervating parietal cells in body of the stomach and gastrin cells in antrum.

As the bolus of swallowed food enters the stomach it induces distension; which activate stretch receptors; which results into initiation of neural reflexes. This entire pathway involves short intramural fibres plus vago-vagal pathways.

So stimulation of vagus results into increased acid and pepsin secretion possibly by two mechanisms—one is direct stimulation of oxyntic glands and another is by stimulating the release of gastrin from antral gland area.

On the contrary vagotomy abolishes gastric acid and pepsin secretion.

Gastric acid secretion		
Phase	*Secretory stimulus*	*Secretagogue*
CEPHALIC	Psychic stimuli conditioned reflex	Cholinergic vagal impulses
GASTRIC	Gastric distension Food in antrum	Hormonal (gastrin)
INTESTINAL	Food in duodenum and jejunum	Hormonal

Since this phase is dependent on mental state, it has been termed as 'psychic or appetite juice'. Its amount is said to be roughly 50-150 ml/20 minutes; and it begins within five minutes and lasts upto 1-1½ hours. Delicious foodstuffs stimulate this phase while nauseating foodstuffs inhibits this phase; so it has forced to prompt that, *'Good digestion wait on appetite and health on both.'* This juice is rich in acid hydrochloric, and pepsin; and; is stimulated by sense of hunger as well as insulin administration when blood sugar reduces. So it has got both conditioned and unconditioned reflexes.

b. *Gastric phase:*

- As the bolus enters the stomach, hormone gastrin is liberated from pyloric antrum. Its secretion is stimulated by certain substances present in food, specially protein. It has been shown that although intact proteins are poor stimulants, peptic hydrolystate of the same protein and individual amino acids are potent secretagogues. It has been observed that amino acid decarboxylation may be a crucial step before gastrin stimulation. Antrum is said to be a major source of gastrin, upper small intestine is also said to contain this hormone which is released into circulation under the effect of some chemical stimuli.
- Antral acidification (upto a pH 2 or even less) causes gastrin inhibition and thus gastric phase of gastric secretion is inhibited. Antral distension on the other hand results into both stimulatory and inhibitory effects.
- This phase of secretion begins within ten to fifteen minutes as the food enters the stomach and it amounts to be 220-350 ml/5 hrs.
- For a much longer time this phase was considered to be due to histamine but since this phase is not destroyed/inhibited by histaminase enzyme neither and nor it lowers the blood pressure as histamine does-so this histamine hypothesis is not accepted.
- Its commercial preparation pentagastrin is used as clinical test material. Gastrin release directly varies with serum calcium level.

- For maximum secretion of gastric juice; both vagal stimulation as well as gastrin release are required. It was reported long back that extracts of pyloric mucosa stimulated gastric secretion when injected intravenously. It was suggested that active principle gastrin exercised a hormonal role in stimulation of gastric secretion following a meal. A new method was described for preparation of hormone gastrin in a potent and highly purified state from hog antral mucosa.
- Stretch receptors have been reported in stomach and their response is related to the degree of distension. They are located in smooth muscle fibre coat. The receptors are connected to medullated A fibres (1.8-3.6μ diameter). These afferent fibres are providing signals on distension of stomach. So at meal times or after water intake large number of receptors are excited and it reaches to maximum when stomach is fully distended. These are slowly adapting receptors. Therefore, number of impulses are continuously reaching the brain and these impulses gradually decrease until stomach is fully empty/emptied. Gastric stretch afferent fibres are making connections with hypothalamic nuclei which are exerting a regulatory function on food intake and satiety.

c. *Intestinal phase:*

- It refers to the fact that a secretion of gastric juice may be stimulated by the introduction of certain kinds of food into the upper portion of intestinal tract.
- This secretory phase lasts for 2-3 hours but sometimes extended to 8-10 hours and it amounts to be 200-300 ml/5 hours. Certain substances (like milk, alcohol, histamine, adrenaline, 10% glycerine, magnesium sulphate etc.) when present in intestine initiates and stimulates this phase; but the most potent stimulus is products of protein digestion. Fats when present in intestine are considered to be potent inhibitor of this phase; but this inhibitory action lasts till fats are present; as they are absorbed; this inhibitory effect is abolished and actually it terminates with profound increase in gastric secretion. This is called *'biphasic action of fats'*, or *'rebound phase of fat inhibition'*. This also explains the use of fat rich diet in treatment of peptic ulcer. This inhibitory action of fat is also due to liberation of a hormone *enterogastrone*; secreted from mucosa of upper small intestine; which also inhibits gastric motility. *Urogastrone* is the term applied to urinary excretion of this hormone.

d. *Interdigestive or Basal*: Here, acid is secreted in the absence of an external stimulus, although acid output may be affected by individual's emotions. Basal and stimulated acid output are higher in males than females because of greater parietal cell mass in males and diminished sensitivity of parietal cells to endogenous gastrin in females.

Gastric secretion—phases

Phases	*Amount (ml.)*
1. Cephalic	50-150 ml/20 minutes
2. Gastric	225-350 ml/5 hours
3. Intestinal	200-300 ml/5 hours
4. Interdigestive	30-60 ml/hours

Effecting drugs—Gastric secretion

Stimulants	*Depressants*
1. Histamine (most powerful)	1. Belladona
2. Pentagastrin	2. Atropine
3. Alcohol	3. Synthetic anticholinergic agents, e.g. tertiary and quarternary amines
4. Tea/coffee	
5. Insulin	
6. Parasympathomimetic agents (acetylcholine, pilo carpine, nicotine)	

SUBSTANCES IN DUODENUM BUT AFFECTING GASTRIC SECRETION

i. The introduction of fats in duodenum is the most potent inhibitor of gastric secretion and motility. Soaps have a greater inhibitory effect than fatty acids and both are potent than neutral fats. The mechanism is certainly hormonal (enterogastrone) but is also having neuronal reinforcement. Fats are having longer latent period and longer duration of effect, as well as a biphasic action.

ii. Introduction of acid in duodenum inhibits gastric secretion. Hydrochloric acid is comparatively weaker as compared with H_2SO_4 or acetic acid in this aspect. This acid inhibition is largely controlled by neural mechanism. On the contrary, stimulation of gastric acid secretion has been observed to result from introduction of weak alkalis into the duodenum.

iii. Duodenal distension inhibits motor activities in stomach. Incomplete digestion is associated with gastric hypersecretion.

iv. On introduction of hypotonic solutions in duodenum, inhibition of gastric function is observed, and the mechanism is operating through both the channels, i.e. neural and hormonal. Hypertonic solution of sugar, saline, peptones are also having inhibitory effects on gastric motor and secretory functions. The receptor for this pressure sensitive response are similar to those in RBC.

SECRETORY DEPRESSANTS

- Absorbable alkalis given in large doses exert depressant effect and favourite alkali from this point of view is sodium bicarbonate. After discontinuation of alkalis hypersecretion may result termed as acid rebound phenomenon and for this purpose non-absorbable substances viz. aluminium hydroxide and magnesium silicate are preferred. Actually these alkalis are collectively called *'ant acids'* which means their ability to buffer or neutralise gastric acidity. Furthermore absorbable alkalis can disturb acid-base balance resulting in alkalosis but it is not true with non-absorbable alkalis.
- Acids depress the gastric secretion. Administration of 1 per cent solution of acid hydrochloric causes inhibition of gastric secretion. It may be due to the fact that acidification causes depressed production of hormone gastrin.
- Belladona alkaloids (atropine, hyoscine, hyoscyamine) are classed under secretory depressants, although, but they are not used clinically for treatment of acidity due to their side effects viz. pupil dilatation, increased heart rate, accomodatory paralysis etc.
- Synthetic - anticholinergic agents (tertiary and quaternary amines) are used for inhibiting hyperacidity. They are safe of course minimal side effects have been observed like dryness of mouth, blurring of vision, slow urinary stream, etc.

SECRETORY STIMULANTS

1. *Histamine* is the most important gastric stimulant. It is destroyed by enzyme histaminase which is not present in gastric region. 0.5 mg histamine subcutaneously gives significant response. Histalogue which is an analogue of histamine is also used and is with minimum side effects. Stomach is so sensitive with histamine is that even immersion of hand in cold water (10°C) gives significant secretory response within 10-15 minutes (endogenous histamine liberation). If dose of histamine is increased step by step then parietal cells give maximum response from secretion point of view.
2. *Caffeine and alcohol* are secretory stimulants. This secretion is too rich in pepsin, acid and mucous too. They are possibly acting through histamine liberation. It is presumed that smoking two or three cigarettes stimulates while more number and that too for a much longer time depress the secretion. This may be due to stimulation of the autonomic ganglia with small nicotine doses while depression with high doses.

VITAMIN - HORMONES AND GASTRIC SECRETION

i. Achlorhydria has been reported in vitamin B_1 (thiamine) deficiency and it responds the administration of vitamin A.
ii. Excess administration of vitamin D can lead to decreased gastric secretion.
iii. Insulin hormone, through reducing blood sugar level of body then stimulates vagus nerve which finally leads to increased acid pepsin secretion. It is also suggested that hypoglycaemia activates both sympathetic as well as parasympathetic centres.
iv. Adrenal cortical hormones (steroids), ACTH are considered as powerful gastric stimulants. Gastric acidity and pepsin are said to be diminished by adrenalectomy.
v. Serotonin a substance or hormone produced by intestinal mucosa inhibits gastric secretion but it increases the intestinal motility.
vi. 10 mg. per cent is the optimum blood calcium level and it is said that if this level is significantly increased or decreased gastric secretion is decreased. So on these grounds effect of vitamin D and parathormone can be presumed.

EMOTIONS AND GASTRIC SECRETION

Stomach is a veritable sounding board of emotions and with emotional bombardments it suffers from all secretory, neurogenic abuses, so it is like a sensitive receiving set tuning to distant stations.

a. Famous American army surgeon Beaumont (1883) showed on his patient Alexis St. Martin that on taking food reddening of gastric mucosa results owing to increased HCl secretion. These observations were made through gastric fistula in that French Canadian patient.
b. Wolff and Wolff (1943) showed some observations on their patient Tom Little with chronic fistula. They observed that fear, depression caused reduced gastric secretion while worries, anxiety etc. causes increased parasympathetic activity while resentment leads to increased secretion as well as motility.

In the lights of above classical and historical experiments it is evident that stomach is greatly affected by emotions and its central mechanism lies in hypothalamus - the head ganglion of the body widespread connections are there between cerbral cortex and hypothalamus.

There are connections from cerebral cortex to hypothalamus and vice versa both through thalamus, in the form of so-called 'reverberating circuits' which means closed chains of neurons over which impulses can be maintained even long after the stimulus.

Through another mechanism emotions after disturbing hypothalamus affect pituitary adrenal axis and adrenal corticoids and ACTH are quite notorious to cause increased acid pepsin secretion terminating into fatal results of ulcers.

FUNCTIONS OF GASTRIC JUICE

i. Main is the digestive function in which pepsin, gastricin etc. all are proteolytic enzymes converting proteins into peptones, lipase is a weak-fat splitting enzyme, of course no carbohydrate splitting enzyme here but salivary amylase (ptyalin) continues to act on boiled starch till level of HCl rises sufficiently to block the reaction.
ii. The intrinsic factor helps to absorb extrinsic factor which is essential for maturation of erythrocytes otherwise in its imbalance pernicious anaemia results.
iii. Gastric mucus prevents its own wall from autodigestion from HCl.
iv. Heavy metals like bismuth, lead, toxins, drugs are excreted through gastric juice.
iv. Gastric HCl acts as an antiseptic by destroying many bacterias coming along with food but parasitic ova are not affected by it.
v. By its alkaline tide it helps to maintain acid-base equilibrium.
vi. Other functions of HCl are hydrolysis of cane sugar to glucose and fructose, activation of pepsinogen to pepsin, conversion of collagen protein to gelatine, providing suitable acidic environment for enzyme activation, providing proper environment for gastric emptying, dissolution of protoplasmic covering of fat globules etc.

HYDROCHLORIC ACID PRODUCTION: A MECHANISM

a. These are the parietal cells of gastric glands responsible for the secretion of this hydrochloric acid which first appear in secretory canaliculi which communicate with lumen.
b. The source of H^+ is though not clear but it is said to be ionisation of water as well as from substrate like glucose through flavoprotein - cytochrome - respiratory - enzyme chain. For each H^+ secreted, an OH^- remains in the cell, so OH^- is neutralised by H^+ formed by carbonic acid dissociation and it is the hydration of carbon dioxide which replenishes H_2CO_3 supply.
$NaCl + CO_2 + H_2O \rightleftharpoons NaHCO_3 + HCl$
Hydration of CO_2 is catalysed by an enzyme carbonic anhydrase present in abundance in gastric mucosa. If large quantities of diamox is administered the whole reaction can be inhibited since it is a powerful inhibitor of carbonic anhydrase enzyme.
c. The source of Cl^- is parietal cell and is secreted against chemical and electric gradient. H^+ and Cl^- are then coupled.
d. The energy for this activity is derived from oxidation most probably of glucose. According to one estimation, it is suggested that secretion of 1 gm molecular equivalent of HCl requires expenditure of 10,000 gm calories of energy.
e. For every hydrogen ion produced, a bicarbonate ion is released into the blood which requires continuous CO_2 supply which is coming from sources like circulating blood and metabolism of parietal cell itself. After meal when gastric acid secretion is high, sufficient H^+ are secreted capable of raising pH of systemic blood and thus making urine alkaline.

HYDROCHLORIC ACID SECRETION: A SUMMARY

- It is secreted by parietal or oxyntic cells of fundic glands.
- $H_2O \rightarrow H^+ + OH^-$ (within parietal cell)

$$CO_2 + H_2O \xrightarrow{\text{Carbonicanhydrase}} H_2CO_3 \rightarrow H^+ + HCO^-_3$$

$$NaCl \rightarrow Na^+ + Cl^-$$

$$HCO^-_3 + Na^+ \xrightarrow[\text{(from NaCl of plasma)}]{} NaHCO_3$$

- Cl^- thus released meet with H^+ inside canaliculi and together form HCl. This movement of Cl^- is against the concentration gradient and hence requires a great expenditure of energy, and it constitutes chloride pump.

H^+ are pumped out into canaliculi (called proton pump). This is an active transport since within the canaliculi the concentration of H^+ are much greater than that in parietal cell. So it requires energy which is supplied from ATP. The H^+K^+ ATPase enzyme is specially required for pumping out the H^+ ions (from interior of parietal cells to canaliculi).

When gastric secretion is increased after meals, sufficient H^+ may be secreted to raise the pH of systemic blood and to compensate this threatening situation; some of alkali are thrown out by body through urine. This makes urine alkaline after heavy meals which have been named as postprandial alkaline tide.

Stomach has a negative respiratory-quotient (RQ) which means that the amount of CO_2 in arterial blood is greater than the amount in gastric venous blood.

Acid secretion is stimulated by Histamine viz. H_2 receptors which increase intracellular cyclic AMP. Histamine is originating from cells in mucosa which resemble mast cells.

Acid production is also stimulated by acetylcholine (via M_1 muscarinic receptors; it is coming from endings of postganglionic cholinergic neurons innervating parietal cells) and gastrin (via gastrin receptors in membranes of parietal cells).

Anti-inflammatory drugs → inhibit prostaglandin synthesis → increase acid secretion and so ulcer (Fig. 86.2).

PHYSIOLOGY OF GASTRIC ACID SECRETION

- One of the hallmark of gastric function is its ability to secrete hydrochloric acid. As hydrogen ions are secreted the intragastric pH decreases to less than 3 which facilitates the conversion of zymogen pepsinogen to active proteolytic pepsin enzyme. In this connection it is to be remembered that acid and pepsin are required for hydrolysis of proteins.
- Approximately one billion parietal (oxyntic) cells are located in the walls of midsection of oxyntic glands—the secretory unit of gastric mucosa. Parietal cells are characterised by plenty of mitochondria (which are essential organ for generating energy for hydrogen ion secretion), tubulovesicular and canalicular structures. When the cell is dormant (nonsecretory phase) its cytoplasm is filled with tubulovesicular structures (hydrogen ion pump—a unique hydrogen-potassium-ATPase—that exchange hydrogen for potassium ions across apical membrane). On getting stimulation these tubulovesicles coalesce into expanded canaliculi which become filled with elongated microvilli. All this change increases membrane area of canaliculi which prepares the cell for acid secretion. When cell returns to resting state the canaliculi collapse, microvilli recede and tubulovesicular structure becomes evident.
- Muscarinic receptors have been shown in gastric mucosa which are localised to parietal, mucous and endocrinal cells. They increase hydrogen ion, pepsinogen and mucous through stimulating phosphoinositide second messenger system. Recently, subclasses of these receptors have been demonstrated viz. M_1, M_2 and M_3. M_1 receptors are present within postsynaptic neurons but they are not seen on parietal cells. Their over expression is responsible for increased output of acid and pepsinogen and therefore produce a pathophysiological base for peptic ulcer. M_3 subtype mediate acid secretion.
- Ingestion of meal → decrease in pH (intragastric) → inhibition of gastrin (between pH 1.5 - 3). As regards inhibition of gastrin, it is possibly through—(a) Intramural cholinergic and non-cholinergic neurons; (b) Somatostatin—a potent inhibitor of gastric acid secretion directly as well as the fact that it inhibits the antral release of gastrin. Muscarinic receptors regulate the function of somatostatin cells; (various regulatory peptides emanating from small intestine (gastric inhibitory peptide, enteroglucagon, peptide YY).

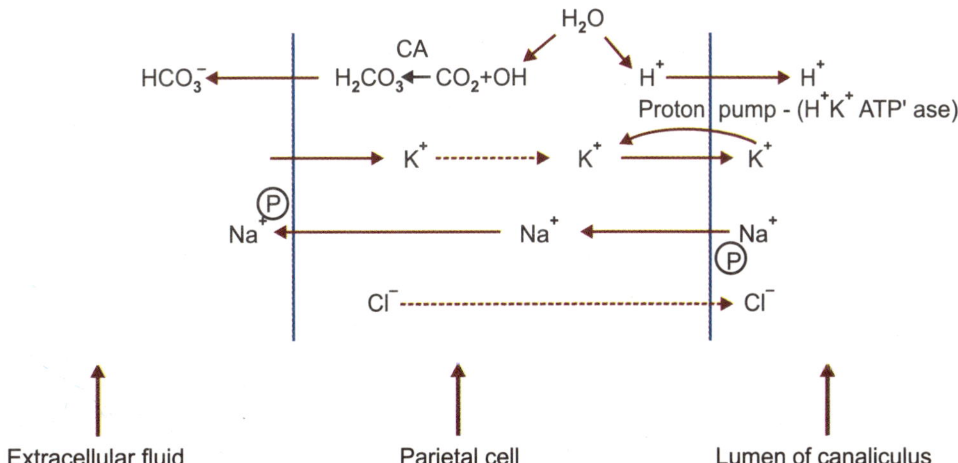

Fig. 86.2: Postulation of HCl secretion by stomach

- Reduction in acid secretion ....
  i. Histamine H_2 receptor antagonist - *cimetidine*. These agents selectively and competently inhibit the stimulation of parietal cell by histamine at H_2 receptor site on basolateral membrane of cell.
  ii. Antimuscarinic agents. Various side effects (dry mouth, visual disturbances, constipation, urinary retention, drowsiness, cardiac arrhythmias) are limiting their use. Selective muscarinic M_1 antagonist (pirenzepine) can be used.
  iii. Prostaglandins (E series) inhibit acid output through diminishing cyclic AMP production. It has lost popularity due to side effects like diarrhoea, smooth muscle contraction, induction of abortion etc. Endogenous prostaglandins may modulate basal gastric mucosal blood flow. Pentagastrin increases the output of vasodilatory and acid inhibiting prostaglandins.
  iv. Substituted benzimidazoles are potent inhibitors of acid secretion. They act through antagonizing the proton pump which exchanges hydrogen for potassium ions at tubulovesicular structures of the parietal cell.
  v. Somatostatin and its synthetic analogue—Octreotide sandostatin are potent inhibitors of gastric acid secretion as well as release.
  vi. Omeprazole—effective in healing duodenal ulcer. It inhibits H^+K^+ ATPase enzyme (proton pump) causing severe depression of gastric HCl secretion.

GASTRIC FUNCTION TESTS (GASTRIC JUICE ANALYSIS)

Indications

1. To determine whether patient can secrete any gastric acid (useful in patients of neurological sign and macrocytic anaemia or other signs and symptoms of pernicious anaemia.

   Patients suspected of suffering from pernicious anaemia.

   Exclusion of a simple peptic ulcer with suspicious ulcerating lesion of stomach.
2. To measure amount of acid produced by a patient with suspected duodenal ulcer who has no radiological demonstrable lesions.
3. To reveal the presecretory phase characteristic of Zollinger Ellison syndrome.
4. To determine the completeness of vagotomy by Insulin test
5. To determine proper type of surgical procedures for peptic ulcer.

Test Meals

- After stomach has been emptied the patient is given a small meal known as test meal.
- Types—300 ml of oat meal gruel
- A piece of dry toast and a cup of tea.
- A shredded wheat biscuit or a piece of toast with 350-450 ml of water.
- Two slices of bread without crust or 2 pieces of Zwieback with 350 ml water (Ewald test meal).
- Eight arrow root cookies with water 400 ml (modified Ewald meal).

Gastric Analysis

a. *FTM (Fractional Test Meal of Rehfuss)*: Patient is called in laboratory in early morning without any food taken since previous evening. A rubber tube (Ryle's tube) is swallowed by patient into fasting stomach and fasting contents are withdrawn by a syringe. Then he is given a pint of thin gruel (test meal) which stimulates the gastric secretion. After approximately half an hour of its ingestion, the samples are again taken every 15 minutes upto 2½ hours. The samples are tested for volume, acidity, peptic activity etc. The other test meal includes a dry toast and cup of tea, shredded wheat biscuits, piece of biscuit or toast with 300-400 ml water.

b. *Histamine stimulated gastric secretion*: For gastric juice stimulation purposes 0.5 mg of histamine is injected subcutaneously since it is a powerful secretogogue since it directly stimulates the parietal cells and more favourable thing is that enzyme histaminase responsible for its destruction is absent from gastric mucosa. Its slow intravenous administration is also effective but rapid administration is not. Its analogue—Histalog (3β amino-ethyl pyrazol) is more effective gastric stimulant since it produces no side effects as compared with histamine proper.

c. *Insulin stimulated gastric secretion* : 7-10 units of Insulin are sometimes given to stimulate gastric secretion since it too is regarded as a potent gastric stimulator (0.3 unit/kg body weight). The test is useful to see the result of vagotomy.

d. *Nocturnal secretion:* On the same day at noon the patient is given a liquid diet as well in evening about at 5 o'clock or so and round about 7 or 8 p.m. Patient is intubated and juice is collected in this 12 hours nocturnal (8 p.m. to 8 a.m.) period. During this time there should be no sight or smell of the food and the tube is connected to a low pressure vacuum pump at negative pressure of 30 inches of water along with the precaution that tube should not be plugged with mucus. For normals, the output of HCl (free) is 29 clinical units (660 mg) and volume is 580 c.c. while everything is increased in ulcer patients.

Analysis Proper

a. *Acidity:* Indicator dimethylamino azo benzene is used and then by titrating with N/10 NaOH solution the acidity can be found by change of colour from red to yellow. Similarly phenolpthalein as an indicator can also be used which changes to pink colour. Results are in clinical units which means number of N/10 NaOH base required to titrate 100 ml of gastric contents. Free acidity varies between 0-30 ml, while total acidity varies between 10-15 ml (30-70 units). Increased acidity is observed in duodenal ulcer and psychoneurosis.
b. *Volume:* Normally 20-100 ml but increased in pyloric stenosis decreased in pernicious anaemia, hour glass stomach, chronic alcoholism.
c. *Blood presence:* Normally blood is not present but if it is there, is suggestive of bleeding ulcer or malignancy, trauma, growth. Small number of RBC may be due to trauma caused by tube.
d. *Mucus excess:* It is suggestive of inflammation. It is seen as small flocculation of spherical/snail like bodies.
e. *Bile absence:* It shows absence of regurgitation of bile i.e. pyloric obstruction.
f. *Time factor:* Gastric stasis (pyloric obstruction) is indicated when food residues, starch sugar etc. are present in samples even after five to six hours or more since it is an established fact that ordinary food leaves stomach within four hours.
g. *Few terms:* Achlorhydria ... absence of free acid.
   True anacidity : No acid secretion even after histamine administration.
   Achylia gastrica ... Absence of acid and pepsin from gstric juice.
h. *Colour:* Normally opalescent, colourless. Abnormally it may be deep yellow green (intestinal obstruction), Red/coffee ground (oesophageal varices, peptic ulcer, carcinoma), greenish turbid (large quantities of old bile).
i. *Odour:* Odourless or slightly pungent normally. Abnormally odour of ammonia (uraemia), putrid foul (ch. gastritis, peptic ulcer).

Microscopic Findings

- *Pus*: Present in acute or chronic diffuse suppuration of the stomach, abscess in stomach, in few cases of gastric carcinoma.
- *Food residue*: Suggestive of atony or pyloric stenosis.
- *Epithelium*: Squamous cells from oesophagus, columnar from stomach and malignant cells in carcinoma.
- *Ova-Parasites*: Giardia Lambli, Ascaris Lumbricoides.
- *Yeast cells*: Large number suggestive of retention and fermentation.
- *Crystals*.
- *Bacteria*: Normally "Ubercel bacilli'; Boas oppler bacillus' are present.

Tubeless Method

1. *Dyes used:* Azure A; quinine (diagnex blue - azure A plus resin). Diagnex.

Advantages

- Safe and accurate. Discomfort of tube is avoided, so it is useful in debilitated patients.
- But the test is not quantitative one.

Tubes for Tube Method (FTM)

i. Ewald..... Hard rubber tube; 12 mm diameter.
ii. Rehfuss... Soft rubber tube; 3-4 mm diameter.
iii. Levin... Soft rubber tube, plain catheter end with several opening near the tip, used for alcohol test meal.
iv. Ryle's .... Rubber tube, 42 inches long, 2 mm inner bore. Marking at 14", 20", 25", 29" corresponding to cardiac, fundus, pyloric end and first part of duodenum.

Test Meals

i. Ewalds ... Two slices of bread (35 gm) without butter and 400 ml of water or tea without sugar modified.... eight arrowrot cookies and 400 ml of water.
ii. Reigel's test meal... Beef Broth add washed potatoes.
iii. Oatmeal gruel.... Oat meal boiled in water.

Barium meal: It remains the method of choice for investigation of a patient suspected of peptic ulcer, since radiological findings are conclusive.

Gastroduodenoscopy: It is a complementary to radiology and requires special training. Whole of oesophagus, stomach and duodenum can be thoroughly visualised and scrutinised by it. It is valuable in the diagnosis of shallow gastric ulcers not visible on radiography, in checking the result of medical treatment in cases of chronic-gastric ulcer, to differentiate between chronic ulcer and carcinoma, in detection of certain forms of gastritis, and in the diagnosis of duodenal ulcer.

The *fibrescope* is an instrument in which glass fibre provides the image transmission system. *Gastrocamera* has been developed now-a-days.

Serum gastrin: Can be estimated by radio-immuno-assay. It is increased in duodenal ulcer, achlorhydria, megaloblastic anaemia, after gastric surgery etc.

PEPTIC ULCER: PHYSIOLOGIC BASIS

- It is the disease of stress and strain increasing day by day with the advancement of civilisation. As the famous statement, 'It was once rare but now common, previously gastric ulcer was common but now duodenal, formerly females were most affected but now males or both sexes equally, previously only ulcer was common but now its complications are increasing.' The basic cause of the disease is too much secretion of gastric HCl in comparison of mucous secretion which is a protective factor. So ulcer is in fact an excoriated area of mucosa caused by digestive action of gastric juice. According to its location/place, ulcer falls into following groups:
- *Types:*
  - — *Gastric ulcer:* It involves pyloric antrum; most frequently on lesser curvature near incisura angularis. Ulcers are rarely seen in its fundus dome or upper part of greater curvature.
  - — *Duodenal ulcer:* It occurs exclusively within first few inches and on its anterior or posterior wall.
  - — *Oesophageal ulcer:* It occurs in lower part of oesophagus where most of acid gastric juice regurgitates, also cardia of stomach.
  - — *Diverticulum ulcer:* Occasionally found in Meckle's diverticulum.
  - — *Mann Williamson ulcer:* It is an experimental ulcer in dogs occurring in jejunum just beyond pylorus, named after discoverer.
  - — *Stomal ulcer:* It may occur in Jejunum mucosa after "gastro" Jejunostomy, i.e. in the region of anasto-mosis.

Pathophysiology

- Neurogenic factor is most important in this aspect. Constant worry, tension, anxiety, anger, frustration and all other types of stress precipitate an attack of the disease. During stress hypothalamus discharges impulses stimulating pituitary which aggravates adrenal's secretion finally terminating into ulceration by more HCl secretion, more vascular spasm, ischaemia, initial necrotic area.
- Chemical factor is another important cause, which means action of excess acid. Hyperacidity constantly occurs in ulcer patients though it does not occur in old cases. It does not occur in acid producing area.
- Blood groups are having relation with the disease. The persons with group O are being more liable to ulcer while persons with A group are liable to cancer stomach, owing to the fact that blood group substances are mucopolysaccharides in nature which is more in amount in O group found abundant in gastric and salivary secretions. Further it has been stated that mucopolysaccharides of O group offer resistance against carcinogenic factors while this substance of A group offers resistance against ulcerogenic factors.
- Hematogenic infection with organisms of low grade virulence is another factor concerned in this aspect. Due to such invasion digestion of gastric mucosa necrosis occurs due to inflammatory foci terminating into atrophic gastritis and finally ulceration.
- Hormones are said to be one of the causative factors of the disease. Hyperparathyrodism is directly linked with the disease; Adreno-cortical hypersecretion is the basis of ulceration as stated, long continued use of cortisone and other adrenocortical steroids is accompanied by ulcer development.
- Food deficiency is also classed amongst causative factors as said, Food is the normal stimulus for gastric juice manufacture on one end, while at another end it is the chief agent which protects gastric tissues from corrosive effects of acid. This explains the abundance of disease in south India where main foodstuffs are rice and curry, poor in all vitamins etc.
- Histamine—the most powerful gastric stimulant is again one of the culprits in this aspect. In severe burns, histaminoids are liberated which are accompanied by acute ulceration specially in first part of duodenum—a state termed as "curling ulcer".
- Caffeine and alcohol are strong secretory stimulants. Tobacco smoking also stimulates gastric secretion. The analgesics specially "aspirin" is also said to be quite notorious for ulceration as well as bleeding from gastric mucosa.
- Peptic ulcer is believed to result from a breakdown in mucosal resistance to the erosive action of acid activated proteolytic enzymes in gastric juice. The factors contributing for normal mucosal resistance are—protective mucus barrier, the maintenance of normal blood flow and vascular state, the activity of intra-cellular enzyme system and the remarkable regenerative capacity characteristic of mucosal epithelium. To sum up, 'An increase in acid-pepsin, a decrease in mucosal resistance, or a combination of these two factors can lead to the imbalance which

produces ulcer. Decreased mucosal resistance must be the dominant factor in majority of patients with both duodenal and gastric ulcer.

- Decreased blood flow through back diffusion of acid into mucosa can lead to a mucosal injury.
- Patients with duodenal ulcer have an average of about 1-9 billion parietal cells and can secrete about 42 mmoles of acid per hour compared with 1 billion and 22 mmoles for normal subjects.
- The tendency for acid hypersecretion in duodenal ulcer patients is associated with a parallel tendency for hypersecretion of pepsin and this is proved by increase in plasma pepsinogen I level.

Physiology of Symptoms

- Pain in epigastrium region is the leading complaint of disease which is of burning quality. In gastric ulcer it occurs soon after eating as acid juice is immediately in contact with ulcerated surface while pain originates 2-3 hours after food in duodenal ulcer which is the time when target amount of acid has been secreted in food response together with the fact that acid has acted for sufficient period to stimulate visceral pain nerves carrying muscle spasm.
- Contact of acid with ulcerated surface initiates a reflex, mechanism resulting in muscle spasm of smooth muscle in the vicinity of ulcer and due to inflammatory process greater excitability of sensory nerves is caused.

General Consideration

i. Peptic ulcers occur only in those parts of the digestive tract that are exposed to the acid and pepsin secreted by stomach. This includes lower end of oesophagus, the entire stomach, the first part of small intestine (first part of duodenum), those Meckel's diverticula which contain acid-pepsin secreting mucosa, and those parts of the tract which have become exposed to gastric acid and pepsin as a result of surgical procedure.

ii. The disease is widespread throughout the world. The disease is caused by a combination of stimuli provoking an ulcerous response, depending in part upon the genetic factors in the host. It is difficult to separate fully the environmental and constitutional facets. The results of occupational surveys are consistent with a psychosomatic basis for duodenal ulcer. It seems that those in position of considerable responsibility are at a greater risk. It is better to conclude in the way that, *'It is the disease increasing day by day as the civilisation is increasing.'*

iii. The famous dictum, *No acid no ulcer is correct.* Acid pepsin is an indispensable factor in ulcer formation. Ulcer occur only in mucosa bathed by gastric acid-pepsin. Duodenal ulcer has never been reported in a patient who does not secret readily detectable amounts of acid.

Physiology of Treatment

a. Reduction of acidity together with relief of pain, this target can be achieved by administration of alkalis called 'ant acids' with the preference of non-absorbable type of ant acids.

b. Avoidance of stress is advised since it is the main etiologic agent. Rest and placid way of life is safe.

c. Alcohol, smoking, aspirin, chillies are to be avoided, yet may be permitted by some in moderation.

d. Small meals at frequent intervals is best regime, together with avoidance of food which may cause gastric stimulation with mechanical irritation of ulcer (raw vegetables and fruits etc.).

e. As far as surgical treatment is concerned it is constituted by partial gastric resection with re-establishment of gastrointestinal continuity (gastroenterostomy). In this operative process, anastomosis is made between stomach and jejunum, thus bypassing duodenum. In gastrojejunostomy the continuity of intestinal tract is established, by leaving ulcer undisturbed through closing duodenal stump. Vagotomy (or vagectomy) is also appreciated where severing of vagus nerve below diaphragm as well as vagal trunks to avoid regeneration is done in order to eliminate cephalic phase of gastric secretion. By this gastric motility and tone are reduced. Generally after this surgery *'Dumping syndrome'* ensues characterised by weakness, sweating, flushing after meal mainly due to sudden passage of food into small intestine which may show distension along with plasma volume reduction, bradykinin release and hypoglycaemia.

TREATMENT OF PEPTIC ULCER

- A variety of ant acids, most of which contain aluminium hydroxide, magnesium hydroxide, calcium carbonate.
- H_2 receptor blocker drugs like—cimetedine, ranitidine, famotidine, nizatidine etc.
- Gastric H^+ - K^+ ATPase (proton pump) inhibitor like omeprazole.
- Antibiotics - For treating bacterial infection of H.pylori.
- Muscarinic receptor blocker (M_1)... atropine; pirenzepine
- Sucralfate - An aluminium salt of sucrose octasulfate - it increases the resistance of mucosa.
- PGE agonists (misoprostol) - long acting.
- Surgically - Vagotomy + gastrojejunostomy.

f. There are two kinds of histamin receptors viz. H_1 and H_2. The antihistaminic drugs block H_1 receptors to check allergic manifestations while H_2 receptor blocking drugs (cimetidine) have got marked gastric secretory inhibiting effect,
g. Milk is said to be the best ant acid so it should be given to ulcer patient many times a day.
h. Fat rich diet is also recommended to ulcer patients since it acts as a non-irritant to ulcerated surface along with the fact that it stays within stomach for a much longer time so neutralises the acid, together with the fact that it on reaching to intestine inhibits gastric secretion through liberation of hormone enterogastrone from upper small intestine mucosa.
i. Worst effects of ulcer pain are seen in night due to diminished protective factors which can awake patient and pain is relieved by taking milk and biscuit or so.

The disease in nutshell is precipitated by hurry, worry and curry.

SUMMARY AND HIGHLIGHTS—GASTRIC JUICE

Introduction: Amount 1200-1500 c.c. per day, pH 1.2 specific gravity 1.006-1.009, free HCl 0.4 - 0.5 per cent, water 99.4 per cent, Inorganic solids 0.16 per cent (NaCl, KCl, $CaCl_2$, $Mg_3(PO_4)_2$, organic solids 0.14 per cent (mucin, Castle's intrinsic factor regurgitated bile and saliva, and enzymes are pepsin, rennin, lipase, gastriscin, cathepsin etc.).

Functions

a. Digestion (pepsin is the main proteolytic enzyme converting them to peptones, rennin causes milk caseinogen to change into insoluble casein while lipase is weak fat splitting one).
b. Intrinsic factor helps in proper absorption of extrinsic factor.
c. Mucous protects gastric mucosa from corrosive action of HCl.
d. Alkaline tide of blood during HCl secretion helps to maintain acid-base balance.
e. HCl acts as an, antiseptic, hydrolyzes cane sugar to glucose and fructose, activates pepsinogen into active pepsin, provides acidic media for full activity of enzymes, convert collagen protein into gelatine.
f. Mucin also helps in lubricating any irritant.

Mechanism

a. Cephalic or nervous phase (before food actually reaches stomach secretion starts called psychic juice which is rich in pepsin and HCl produced by both conditioned and unconditioned and unconditioned reflex, accelerated by psychic influences like good pleasant flavour atmosphere as well as insulin while unpleasant flavour dirty atmosphere inhibit it)
b. Gastric phase (gastrin hormone is said to be chief controlling agent coming from pyloric mucosa).
c. Intestinal phase (some substances stimulate gastric secretions while present in intestine like proteins, water, alcohol, histamine, adrenaline glycerine etc. but fats when placed in intestine inhibits gastric secretion due to liberation of hormone enterogastrone coming from upper small intestine mucosa.

BIBLIOGRAPHY

1. Allen A, et al. Gastroduodenal mucosal protection. Phy Rev 1993;73:823.
2. Berglindh T. The mammalian gastric parietal cell in vitro. Ann Rev Phy 1984;46:377.
3. Cheli R, et al. Gastric protection. (3 and 4 references quoted by Guyton AC in "Textbook of Medical Physiology - WB Saunders), New York: Raven press. 1988.
4. Davenport H We. Physiology of the digestive tract, 3rd ed. Chicago: Year Book, 1971.
5. Dragestedt LR. Pathogenesis of gastroduodenal ulcer Arch Surg 1942;44: 438.
6. Feldman EJ, Grossman MI. Liver extract and free amino acid equally stimulate gastric acid secretion. Amer J Phy 1980;239:G-493-96.
7. Feldman M, et al. Inhibition of gastric acid secretion by selective and non-selective anticholinergics. Gastroenterology 1984;86: 361-66.
8. Feldman M, Richardson CT. Partial shamfeeding release gastrin in normal human subjects. Scand J Gastroenterology 1981;16:13-16.
9. Feldman M, Richardson CT. Role of thought, sight, smell and taste of food in cephalic phase of gastric acid secretion in humans. Gastroenterology 1986;90:428-33.
10. Forte JG, et al. Mechanism of gastric H^+ and Cl^- transport. Ann Rev Phy 1980;42:111.
11. Forte JG, Lee HC. Gastric ATP : A review of their possible role in HCl secretion. Gastroenterology 1977;73:921.
12. Garner A, Flemstrom G. Gastric HCO_3 secretion in the guinea pig. Amer J Phy 1978;234, E 535 - E 541.
13. Grossman MI. Regulation of acid secretion in Physiology of GIT, Vol. I by LR Johnson et al. New York: Raven Press, 1981;659-72.
14. Grotzinger U, et al. Effect of atropine and proximal gastric vagotomy on the acid response to fundic distension in man. Gut 1977;18:303-10.
15. Guth PH. Stomach blood flow and acid secretion. Ann Rev Phy 1982;44:3.
16. Guth PH, et al. Measurement of gastric mucosal blood flow in man. Gastroenterology 1978;74:831-34.
17. Hollander F. The mucus barrier in stomach. In David Sandweiss (Ed). Peptic Ulcer, WB Saunders Company, Philadelphia, page 65. (1 and 2 references quoted by Best and Taylor in Physiological basis of Medical Practice 1967- Williams and Wilkins).
18. Harper AA, et al. Gastric blood flow in anasthetized cats. J Physio London 1968;194:795-807.

19. Herawi M, et al. Different binding propertive of Muscarinic Mz receptors subtypes for against and antagonist in porcine gastric smooth muscle and mucosa. Gastroenterology 1988;94: 630-37.
20. Hogben DAM (Ed). Gastric Secretion of HCl, A symposium. Federation Proceeding 1965;24:1353.
21. Rabon EC, et al. The mechanism and structure of gastric HK - ATPase, quoted by Ganong WF in Review of Medical Physiology. Lange Publication. Ann. Rev. Phy. 1990;52:321.
22. Soll All. Pathogenesis of peptic ulcer and implications for therapy. New Eng J Med 1990;322:909.
23. S Paintal. A study of gastric stretch receptors. Their role in peripheral mechanism of satiation of Hunger and Thirst. J Phy 1954;126:255.
24. Woelfe MM, et al. Zollinger. Ellison Syndrome: Current concepts in diagnosis and management. (3 and 4 references quoted by Ganong WF in Review of Medical Physiology, Lange Publications). New Eng J Med 1987;317:1200.

87 Pancreatic Secretion and Digestion

Pancreas is a double organ; on one side it is a digestive gland secreting most powerful of all digestive juices while on another side it is one of the endocrine glands for islets of Langerhans form one of the chief regulators of carbohydrate metabolism.

INTRODUCTION (FUNCTIONAL ANATOMY)

It is an elongated gland which extends from duodenum obliquely upward behind the stomach, across the posterior abdominal wall to the spleen, at the level of first and second lumbar vertebra.

A matter of considerable clinical interest is the relation of pancreatic duct to the common bile duct at the point of their common entrance into the duodenum. They may enter separately or form a conjoined bile and pancreatic duct, which as it passes through the duodenum, dilates to form the ampulla of Vater which opens into duodenal papilla.

- Microscopically, the pancreas is seen to be made up chiefly of group of cells forming acini which tend to be spherical or ovoid in general contour but in closely packed tissue of the pancreas are actually polygonal. Groups of acini form primary lobules, also polygonal in contour, which are imperfectly separated from other primary lobules by incomplete connective tissue septa. Numerous adjacent primary lobules form a secondary lobule.
- The pancreatic tissue proper is composed of acinous cells, islet cells and duct cells. The acinous cell owing to the spheroid shape of acini, tend to be pyramidal with the truncated apex of the pyramid directed towards the lumen of acinous. They are large cells with a well developed nucleus, nucleolus and granular cytoplasm. The granules 'zymogen', vary in number and position in the cell depending on the state of activity of gland but tend to be more abundant in apical region of the cell. When very abundant they may occupy the major portion of cytoplasm, displacing the nucleus to the base of cell, but there is generally a zone free of zymogen granules near the base. Secretory canaliculi have been described in the acinous cell.
- So, exocrine pancreas consists of a system of anastomosing tubules or ducts. The ductal tree is terminated by groups of acinar cells, forming the acini and by irregularly shaped ductular cells or centro acinar cells wedged between acinar cells. Intercalated ducts arise from acini and subsequently fuse into intra- and interlobular ducts and finally into main duct. The cells of ductal tree are structurally similar to centro acinar cells. Ductular cells are small having few mitochondria, poorly developed endoplasmic reticulum, a small Golgi complex and moderate number of secretory granules and lysosomes. The cells are attached to each other by junctional complexes. Acinar cells contain numerous secretory granules, an elaborate network of RER (rough-endoplasmic reticulum) and a Golgi complex close to the nucleus. Junctional complexes with tight junctions are present at the apical pole of acinar cells. The acinar cells synthesize store and secrete digestive enzymes. The duct cells as well as centro acinar cells contain carbonic anhydrase which is important for their ability to secrete bicarbonate. The main pancreatic duct and interlobular ducts also contain mucus secreting cells.

PANCREATIC JUICE : INTRODUCTION

In the twenty-four hours time total quantity secreted is 500-1200 ml. It is a colourless, viscous fluid, alkaline in reaction owing to presence of sodium-bicarbonate. Its pH varies between 8-8.3 and specific gravity is ranging between 1.010-1.018.

Electrolytes: In contrast to gastric acid here is sodium bicarbonate. This is in order to maintain acid-base balance of rest of the body. It is well established fact that bicarbonates and chlorides have got a reciprocal relationship. In addition to bicarbonate and chloride, pancreatic juice also contains phosphate but less than blood plasma level.

The principal bases: Here are sodium, potassium mainly with small amounts of calcium, magnesium and zinc. Sodium and potassium level is equal with that of blood plasma and independent of secretory rate.

Enzymes: Pancreatic juice is in fact capable of digesting all types of foodstuffs since it contains all types of enzymes viz. proteolytic, amylolytic, lipolytic.

Proteolytic enzymes: Trypsinogen is the chief name here with molecular weight as 25,000. It hydrolyses those peptide bonds whose carboxyl group is contributed by an amino acid having positively charged side group as arginine or lysine. It also increases coagulation of blood where it acts like thrombokinase but it mildly acts with milk clotting. The trypsinogen is activated by enzyme enterokinase secreted from intestinal mucosa. Trypsinogen changes into trypsin in the presence of acid or due to certain enzymes called kinases.

Chymotrypsinogen is other enzyme with molecular weight 25,000 and it is converted into chymotrypsin by active trypsin as well as by enterokinase. It can coagulate milk but blood cannot be clotted. Its optimum pH is 8-9.

Peptidases and carboxypeptidases are other proteolytic enzymes present here digesting peptides further. Carboxypeptidase is basically exopeptidase and activated by trypsin.

Ribonuclease and desoxyribonuclease are also reported meant for hydrolysis of corresponding nucleic acid into mononucleotides and its optimum activity is said to be on pH 7.

Elastase and collagenase are also reported in this juice. **Lipase** is the enzyme for emulsification and hydrolysis of fats particularly triglycerides are changed to free fatty acids and glycerol. Its activity is optimum at alkaline side of pH. It acts best in presence of bile salts but this is also true that excess amount of bile salts inhibit its action.

After Lipase there is **amylase** which is like salivary amylase, with molecular weight as 45,000 and amylotic activity consists of hydrolysis of starch to maltose. Optimum pH for its full activity runs between 6.5-7.2. The activating ion is chloride.

REGULATION OF SECRETION

It is both under nervous as well as humoral control.

A. *Nervous-regulation*: Effect of parasympathetic stimulation is (vagus stimulation) increased enzyme secretion but no or very little effect on bicarbonate production and hence atropine or vagotomy are capable of blocking this action. Insulin induced hypoglycaemia is also capable of inducing such effect. Sight, smell, chewing of food all stimulate juice reflexly to some extent. Leaving aside the role of vagus, these are local-cholinergic-mechanism which also sufficiently influence this secretion. Within few minutes of taking food the secretion starts which continues for 10-20 minutes.
B. *Humoral regulation*: In 1902 Bayliss and Starling proved that pancreatic secretion was continue even after sectioning nerve supply of organ so any hormone was thought to be responsible for its secretion. Two hormones are said to be existing —

1. *Secretin* is with molecular weight 5000 responsible for secretion which is rich in alkalies but poor in enzymes. It is destroyed by another enzyme termed as secretinase found in blood and urine. It is also said to stimulate intestinal juice as well as bile from liver but may have depressant effect on gastric secretion. It is polypeptide chemically. Acids and it itself are two best stimulants for its secretion. Its source is mucosa of upper small intestine.
2. *Pancreozymin* is another hormone 'responsible for thick viscid secretion of small quantity but rich in enzymes, through its action on acinar cells. It is a polypeptide having 33 amino acids so it is effective

Regulation of pancreatic secretion

Phase	*Stimulus*	*Mediator*	*Response*
Cephalic	Sight and smell of food	Vagus gastrin release	Enzyme secretion Enzyme secretion
Gastric	Food in stomach, distension, acid discharged to duodenum	Gastrin vagus	Enzyme secretion Enzyme secretion
Intestinal	Acid in intestine, amino acids peptides, fatty acid	Secretin CCK vagus	HCO_3^-, H_2O secretion Enzyme secretion Enzyme secretion

on intravenous administration. Its action is like vagus but differing from the point that it is not blocked by atropine.

Distilled water, HCl, peptones, soaps, carbohydrates, fats present in intestine all are stimulant, acting in a little different way. HCl produces abundant secretion of dilute alkaline fluid without significant enzymes while fatty acids and soaps produces juice rich in enzymes and proteins are also acting like fats.

PHASES : A SUMMARY

a. *Cephalic phase*: All conditioned reflex is seen, i.e. secretion due to sight smell, tasting, chewing stimulate secretion through vagal stimulation by exciting vagal nucleus. According to another concept gastrin hormone is also released which result into HCl production which becomes cause of release of secretin and CCK-PZ which causes pancreatic juice liberation.
b. *Intestinal phase*: Food when enters the intestine causes release of CCK-PZ and secretin from upper small intestine which liberates the juice.

CONCEPT OF HYDROLYTIC AND ECBOLIC SECRETION

As the food enters the intestine, secretin hormone is released from upper intestinal mucosa which causes pancreas to secrete fluid (thin watery flow) rich in bicarbonates but low in chloride and this copious fluid flow is termed as hydrolytic secretion and is devoid of enzyme. Due to this following reaction occurs:

$$HCl + NaHCO_3 \rightarrow NaCl + H_2CO_3$$

$$H_2CO_3 \rightarrow Co_2 + H_2O$$

In this way it appears that acid delivered from stomach is neutralised and thus it acts as a natural protection against duodenal ulceration. Secondly this mechanism provides suitable alkaline medium (pH - 8.0) for better activity of pancreatic enzymes. In above mentioned reaction CO_2 is absorbed by body fluids.

On the other hand presence of products of protein digestion in intestine stimulates the release of another hormone 'pancreozymin' from upper small intestine mucosa, which leads to increased enzyme secretion in pancreatic juice, better termed as ecbolic secretion.

CONCEPT OF TRYPSIN INHIBITOR

It is an established fact that pancreatic enzymes remain inactive till they are poured into small intestine. So it may happen that trypsin along with other pancreatic enzymes may damage or digest pancreas itself while remaining inside pancreatic cells, just like HCl can digest stomach itself. But just like mucus protects the stomach, a substance 'trypsin inhibitor' is produced by same cells which produce trypsin which protects the organ by self or auto-destruction. This substance is stored in cytoplasm of glandular cells enveloping the enzyme granules and functioning as an agent which prevents trypsin activation both inside secretory cells as well as in acini and ducts. Due to any cause if the activity of this inhibitor substance is blocked then actually secretion accumulates and organ digests itself terminating into fatal results like life long pancreatic insufficiency or shock. This is the physiological basis of acute pancreatitis.

PANCREATIC ENZYMES

The pancreatic juice contains enzymes capable of digesting or degrading proteins, lipid, starch and nucleic acid. It is an interesting fact that three proteolytic enzymes are secreted in an inactive form.

a. *Trypsin*
   i. It is a protein. It hydrolyses native protein producing peptones and peptides, but do not cause the release of amino acid.
   ii. Its inactive precursor is trypsinogen. It exhibits no proteolytic activity.
   iii. It accelerates coagulation of blood in which it acts as a thrombokinase, but has only a feeble action in clotting milk. Its optimum pH for digestion of casein lies between pH 8.0-9.0.
   iv. The activation of trypsinogen to trypsin may be mediated enzymatically by the intestinal enzyme enterokinase.
   vi. Change of trypsinogen to trypsin is accelerated by acid or by exposure to concentrated $MgSO_4$, $CaCl_2$ active trypsin, or to one of a group of enzymes called kinases.
   vii. Inhibitors of trypsin have been also reported. These are found in colostrum, egg white, soyabeans, cell wall of 'Ascaris lumbricoides.
b. *Chymotrypsin; chymotrypsinogen:*
   i. Chymotrypsinogen is a protein substance present in pancreatic juice. It is converted to chymotrypsin by active trypsin but indirect activation can be accomplished by enterokinase if trypsinogen is also present to form trypsin.
   ii. Chymotrypsin is a proteolytic enzyme.
   iii. It coagulates milk but not blood (Chymo = clotting action on milk).
   iv. Its optimum activity occurs in the same pH range as that of trypsin.
   v. Chymotrypsin is also an endopeptidase.

c. *Pancreatic lipase:*
   i. Due to presence of lipase, the pancreatic juice is able to emulsify and hydrolyse fats to fatty acids and glycerol. The fatty acids are hydrolyzed one after another, and thus mono and, diglycerides are intermediates in the reaction sequence. This hydrolysis of fats by lipase is done in the presence of bile salts.

d. *Amylase:*
   i. It is secreted in active form.
   ii. The enzyme digests glycogen as well as starch; and end product in both instances is maltose. It acts on both boiled and unboiled starch.
   iii. Its small fraction is absorbed by blood and appears in urine; so urinary amylase is an indicator of pancreatic activity.

e. *Peptidases*: (erepsin is old term) (i) One is carboxy peptidase, an enzyme which hydrolyzes peptides containing a free carboxyl group but no free amino group.

f. *Others*: Collagenase, elastase (dissolves elastin in aorta wall leaving the collagen unchanged).

MECHANISM OF SECRETION

a. *Fluid and electrolytes*:
   i. This juice is isotonic with plasma. Bicarbonate concentration increases with flow rate and chlorides have got inverse relationship with bicarbonates. As regards sodium and potassium concentration, it is the same with plasma.
   ii. As far as bicarbonates are concerned CO_2 is coming from metabolism while HCO_3^- are poured from blood plasma. These bicarbonates are further originating from intralobular ductule cells and not in acinar cells. Furthermore, it has been proved that pancreas contains 'carbonic anhydrase enzyme' which yields bicarbonate and with the use of diamox (acetazolamide) - carbonic anhydrase inhibitor the bicarbonate secretion is said to be diminished.
   iii. If by any means Na and K concentration is increased in blood, their pancreatic contents also found to be increased.

b. *Enzymes:* The first step is *synthesis* in acinar cells. Amino acids required for synthesis are tryptophane, lysine, leucine, arginine, isoleucine, histidine, valine, phenylalanine, threonine, tyrosine, D-L valine is said to be a powerful stimulant for pancreozymine. So it can be concluded that for proper and adequate synthesis amino acid's availability is necessary. It was found that trypsin and lipase contents are more with a profound protein rich diet. *Storage* in the form of zymogen granules within the cell is another step which reaches within 45-60 minutes. Due to some stimulation these granules diminish in number and size and enzyme is poured into circulation. *Discharge* is accompanied by union of plasma cell membrane with zymogen granule's membrane.

Synthesis of enzymes: It results in elaboration and storage within the acinous cells, of the characteristic pancreatic enzymes or their precursors. Accumulation of zymogen granules within the cell is visible evidence of this process. It has been concluded that the synthesis of enzymes proceeds within the cell until a dynamic equilibrium is established between the zymogen material and the various substances that enter into reactions involved in its synthesis. It is an interesting fact that granules appear in the acinous cells of developing pancreas, as soon as acini are formed, on 17th or 18th day of development in embryo. Granules appear first in basal zone of the cell on or near mitochondria and then migrate to the apical zone where they become enmeshed in the Golgi apparatus and come to rest.

Secretion of enzymes: Following changes in appearance of cell during and after secretion as compared with resting cell are described :- (a) Entire cell was reduced in size, (b) The granular inner or apical zone was diminished in size more than the outer clear zone, (c) The zymogen granules of the inner zone were smaller in size and fewer in number than in the resting cell and those that remained were congregated near apical border of cell.

ASSESSING : PANCREATIC FUNCTIONS

A. Following tests can be employed:
   1. *Serum amylase*: Normal value—80-200 somogyi units/100 ml. It is increased in acute pancreatitis as well as in perforated peptic ulcer, renal insufficiency, ruptured ectopic pregnancy, intestinal obstructions, gallstones, mumps, morphine and morphine like drugs non-penetrating abdominal trauma.

      Low values seen in liver abscess, acute hepato-cellular damage, liver cirrhosis, cholecystitis, liver cancer etc.

      This is absent in newborn. It starts appearing at the age of two months and reaches its normal level at the end of first year.
   2. *Urinary amylase*: Normal 1-3 ml/minute. Has no renal threshold but is slightly altered by water induced diuresis. Its value is elevated in acute

pancreatitis, pancreatic duct obstruction, pancreatic carcinoma.

3. *Serum lipase*: Normal value 1.0 units (Tietz method). It rises parallel with serum amylase but it rises later and lasts longer. Conditions of rising value are the same as that of amylase but its increase is more pronounced.
4. *Urinary lipase*: Its level is elevated in hemorrhagic pancreatitis and in some cases of renal impairment.
5. *Fat Absorption Test*: Normal functioning of pancreas causes normal absorption of fats.
   - The test comprises of normal absorption of 1^{131} triolein and oleic acid on separate days and determination of percent I^{131} found in blood.
   - Absorption of only oleic acid is suggestive of impaired pancreatic function; while its failure of absorption is suggestive of malabsorption syndrome of non-pancreatic origin.

B. *Examination of pancreatic juice*
   - *Volume* In 60 minutes period 135-250 ml (2 ml/kg); children (0.8 ml/kg). Quantitative deficiency is seen in pancreatic duct obstruction. In pancreatitis qualitative deficiency occurs in which volume of course remains normal but enzyme secretion and bicarbonate are diminished.
   - *Bicarbonate concentration* Maximum is 90 m Eq/L.
   - *Amylase secretion* 6.0 units/kg.
   - *Trypsin secretion* Children 39 units; infants 59 units normally.
   - Presence of blood is suggestive of gastrointestinal bleeding.
   - Microscopically, presence of bile stained leucocytes is suggestive of chronic inflammatory process.

C. *Cytologic test*
   This is specially for malignant cells.

D. *Vitamin A tolerance test*: Normal serum vitamin A level is 15-60 µg/100 ml. Low level after oral administration of vitamin A is found in pancreatic insufficiency, cystic fibrosis of pancreas in children.

E. *Faecal fat excretion:* It is quantitative measurement of faecal fat excretion. Normally not more than 6-7 gm of fat per day is excreted by one individual. Patients with pancreatic insufficiency may excrete upto 50 gm per day.

F. *Secretin-pancreozymin test:*
   - First of all the sufferer should be tested for any hypersensitivity towards secretin-pancreozymin.
   - A double lumen tube is passed through mouth or nose. One lumen opening into stomach for draining gastric juice, while another opens into duodenum for collecting pancreatic/duodenal secretion. Gastric juice is aspirated continuously by a low pressure vacuum pump while the duodenal contents are aspirated manually. Samples are taken as an average interval of 10-20 minutes. After a control period of 30 minutes - Secretin in a dose of one clinical unit per kg body weight is given by I.V. route over 4-5 minutes period. After 10-20 minutes duodenal contents are collected for 10-20 minutes. Volume, pH, bicarbonate contents determination of enzyme is done.
   - In some places secretin and pancreozymin in 30 minutes are given. Sometimes pancreozymin is given first which is followed by secretin administration (after 10 minutes).
   - With normal functions, there is a rapid increase in flow rate following injection of secretin.
     [Ivy et al. 1926 to 1930; Ann. clini. Med. (1926) 4:798. Agren C, et al. 1936 - Acta Med. Scand. 90:224. (source:- Physiological basis of medical Practice by Best and Taylor, 1967, Williams and Wilkinson)].

COMPLETE PANCREATIC EXTIRPATION

a. Pancreatic lipase is certainly an important enzyme so in its absence fat digestion will be seriously effected. It leads to bulky greasy pale faeces due to disturbed fat absorption so they are excreted in stools.
b. The removal of pancreas (pancreatectomy) further leads to increased faecal nitrogen (roughly eight times above normal) due to incomplete proteolysis,
c. Certainly there is loss of calorific value of ingested food.
d. Such state of removing entire pancreas may exist in carcinoma, congenital pancreatic fibrocystic diseases.

> Pancreas is just like an automatic pistol with its handle nestled in the loop of duodenum and its barrel pointed at the hilum of the spleen. It is called 'an abdominal salivary gland. It cuddles the left kidney, tickles the spleen, hugs the duodenum, cradles the aorta, apposes the inferior vena cava, hids behind the posterior parietal peritoneum of the lesser sac and wraps itself around the superior mesenteric vessels.

SUMMARY AND HIGHLIGHTS

PANCREATIC JUICE—AN ABSTRACT

Introduction: Amount per day 500-1200 ml specific gravity 1.010-1.018, pH 8-8.3, water 97.5 per cent, total solids 1.5-2.5 per cent enzymes (trypsin-chemotrypsin-carboxypeptidases-nuclease-deoxyribonuclease-elastase, collagenase are as proteolytic, lipase as fat splitting which needs bile for activation and amylase splitting starch to maltose and glucose and is more active than salivary amylase, needing chloride for action).

Inorganic solids (Na^+, K^+, Ca^{++}, Mg^{++}, HCO_3^-, Cl^-, SO_4^-, HPO_4^-)

Functions:

a. Digestive (Proteins are finally changed into peptones proteoses - polypeptides by proteolytic enzymes, by the action of amylase amylolytic activity is completed turning even unboiled starch to maltose and glucose, lipolytic action is performed by lipase which causes emulsification and hydrolysis of neutral fats).
b. Neutralising gastric acid (due to its bicarbonate content).
c. Acid tide occurs in blood where anion rises and hence excreted in urine.

Mechanism:

a. Nervous control (vagus stimulation leads to enzyme rich juice, poor alkali content and small volume, this action blocked by atropine like vagal blocking drugs but vagus like action is noticed with parasympathomimetic drugs viz. acetylcholine, pilocarpine, physostigmine. Secretion also occurs with sight or smell of food, i.e. conditioned reflex.
b. Hormonal or chemical control (secretin hormone coming from upper small intestinal mucosa leads to copious watery secretion rich in alkalies but enzyme contents are poor. It also stimulates bile and succus entericus secretion but depresses gastric flow, can be destroyed by enzyme secretinase. Its best stimulant is gastric HCl; Pancreozymine another hormone acting like vagus, i.e. leads to enzyme rich secretion but not inhibited by atropine, of course secretion is thick and viscid. Chemically it is polypeptide identical with cholecystokinin so combined name CCK-PZ sometimes used.

BIBLIOGRAPHY

1. Case RM. Synthesis intracellular transport and discharge of exportable proteins in pancreatic acinar cells and other cells. Bio Rev 1978;53:211-354.
2. Folsch UR, Wormsley KG. Pancreatic enzyme response to secretin and CCK-PZ in the rat. J Physiol London 1973;234:79-94.
3. Fushiki T, Iwai K. Two hypothesis on feedback regulation of pancreatic enzyme secretion. FASEBJ 1989;3:121.
4. Gardner JD, Jackson MJ. Regulation of amylase release from dispersed pancreatic acinar cells. J Physiol (London) 1977;270: 439-454.
5. Go VLW, et al. Exocrine pancreas : biology : pathobiology and disease. New York: Raven Press. 1986.
6. Gregory RA, Tracy HJ. The constitution and properties of two gastrins extracted from hog antral mucosa. Gut 1964;5:103-117.
7. Harper AA. The control of pancreatic secretion. Gut 1972;13:308-317.
8. Hopfer U, et al. Proton and bicarbonate transport mechanisms in intestine. Ann Rev Phy 1987;49:51.
9. Irene Schulz, Hans H. Stolze. The exocrine pancreas : The role of secretagoues, cyclic nucleotides and calcium in enzyme secretion. Ann Rev Phy 1980;42:127-156.
10. Jerry D. Gardner. Regulation of pancreatic exocrine function in vitro: Initial steps in actions of secretagogues. Ann Rev Phy 1979;41:55-66.
11. Jerry D. Gardner, Rober T Jensen. Receptors and cell activation associated with pancreatic enzyme secretion. Ann Rev Phy 1979;48:103-117.
12. Kuypers GAJ, et al. The mechanism of fluid secretion in rabbit pancreas studied by means of various inhibitors. Biochim-Biophys. Acta 1984;778: 324-31.
13. May RJ, et al. Actions of peptides isolated from amphibian skin on pancreatic acinar cells. Amer J Physiol, 1978;235:E 112-118.
14. Schultz I, Stolze HH. The exocrine pancreas: The role of secretagogues, cyclic nucleotides and calcium in enzyme secretion. Ann Rev Phy 1980;42:127.
15. Steinburg W Tenner. Acute pancreatitis. (Quoted by Ganong WF in Review of Medical Physiology - Lange Publications). New Eng J Med 1994;330:1198.

88 Liver: Biliary System

Liver is a misleading organ, each cell is jack-of-all-trades. It is the master cook making the food digestible while on another end, it is also a storehouse, chemical factory and a receiving depot together with unique power of repair.

BILE: INTRODUCTION

- Since liver is a combined secretory as well excretory organ, hence bile is also a mixture of secretion as well excretory product from liver. This digestive juice (bile) first enters bile capillaries then it travels through cystic and hepatic ducts from where it finally reaches to gall bladder which is storehouse of bile. It should also be remembered that expulsion of bile from gall bladder into intestine is intermittent process having no dependency on bile formation by liver.
- It is yellowish green coloured juice with bitter taste. It appears that of viscous jelly like fluid. It amounts to be 600-1000 cc daily with the beauty that it is completely devoid of any digestive enzyme. Liver bile has a pH of 8.0-8.6 while gall bladder bile is either neutral or very slightly alkaline.

Bile salts: The acids of human bile are glycocholic and taurocholic acid. Bile salts pass to the intestine where they undergo reabsorption along with the fats which pass to lymph vessels while through portal circulation bile salts are taken back to liver for their re-excretion constituting what is called *'entero-hepatic-circulation'* and bile salts on reaching liver excite more cells to produce bile—a property called choleretic. This cycle is repeated nearly 10-14 times till more than 94 per cent bile is reabsorbed by liver.

Bile proteins: are also present. Gamma globulin, albumin and lipoproteins are the main protein constituents so far detected.

Bile electrolytes: The main cations are sodium and potassium while main anions are bicarbonates and chlorides. Their source is also two-fold one from liver itself and second from re-excretion of bile salts.

Bile pigments: 'Bilirubin' (chief pigment of human and carnivore bile) and biliverdin (oxidative derivative of bilirubin) are the main biliary pigments.

Lecithin and cholesterol: In liver bile lecithin (0.02-0.05%) and cholesterol (0.04-0.16%) is present. Ratio of cholesterol to bile salts is estimated as 1 : 20-1 : 30 but when this ratio falls to 1 : 13 or so cholesterol is precipitated which marks the basis of gall stone disease.

EVACUATION OF GALL BLADDER

For proper evacuation of gall bladder following are the requisites. One is relaxation of sphincter of Oddi and secondly, contraction of gall bladder musculature to produce sufficient pressure to move bile forwards in common bile duct. Following are the views put forwarded time to time to explain this phenomenon —

a. Mucous membrane of upper small intestine release a hormone 'cholecystokinin' immediately on entry of fat foodstuff in intestine and this hormone causes contraction of gall bladder musculature. It is free from histamine and other vasodilator substances.
b. As far as foodstuff is concerned it is the fat acting as a effective stimulus for discharge of bile specially cream, egg yolk or olive oil etc. Pure protein and carbohydrates are without such effects. Products of fat digestion, hydrochloric acid of strength comparable to that in chyme when enters intestine cause contraction of gall bladder musculature and relaxation of sphincter of Oddi.
c. Nervous control of gall bladder evacuation is comparatively less important than hormonal one. Vagus is the chief affecting nerve in this aspect which gets stimulated as food enters the stomach as well as smell, taste of food together with some psychic factors also cause vagal stimulation.

d. As regards drugs or chemicals adrenaline, histamine, stimulate gall bladder's smooth musculature whereas morphine, ergotamine and atropine are said to be inhibitory.
e. Duodenal ulcer, pregnancy, pernicious anaemia are the diseases which prolong the emptying time of gall bladder.
g. As the food enters the intestine, it undergoes peristalsis and when wave of intestinal peristalsis reaches nearby sphincter of Oddi it gets little relaxed in exchange and meanwhile certain amount of bile escapes from gall bladder and enters the intestine.
h. Gall bladder can store 40-70 ml of bile at a time. The bile duct can withstand 30 cm of water.

BILE: REGULATION

a. First of all it is the food which acts as best stimulus for biliary secretion. This explains more bile secretion in day time than in the night since food is taken in day time. Secondly moreover in food it is protein foodstuff which effects biliary secretion positively otherwise fats have got; no significant effect and carbohydrates moreover depress or inhibit the secretion.
b. As regards nervous regulation is concerned, on stimulating the vagus nerve biliary secretion is increased but on the whole effect of autonomic nerves on biliary secretion is said to be inhibitory.
c. As regards hormone role is concerned it is hepatocrinin which is secreted from upper small intestine mucosa stimulates biliary production.
d. *Cholagogue* means any agent which increases flow of bile into intestine, while *choleretic* word means agent which increases output of bile from the liver without changing its concentration, that means a choleretic will increase output of both bile solids and liquids (bile salts have got a powerful choleretic action), and word *hydrocholeretic* means agent increasing volume of bile without correspondingly increasing output of bile solids. Above mentioned terms should be clearly understood in relation with bile flow.

GALL BLADDER: FUNCTIONS

a. It stores and concentrates the bile approximately ten times so gall bladder bile may have ten times more total solids than bile collected from hepatic duct,
b. Excretion of cholesterol,
c. Reduction in bile alkalinity,
d. Equalisation of pressure within biliary system,
e. If bile ducts are obstructed by ligation and gall bladder tied off, it results in production of clear, colourless fluid named as '*white bile*' and the peculiarity is that it contains no salt, pigment or cholesterol and bears no relation with bile,
f. Secretion of viscous jelly like mucus
g. It protects the liver by acting as a reservoir since liver cells may be damaged if pressure in bile duct rises every time and sphincter remains closed.

BILE: FUNCTIONS

a. The main function of bile is digestion and specially of fats,
   i. This function is performed through their surface tension lowering property by which emulsification of fat is made easier rendering increased surface area for lipase enzyme to act.
   ii. Bile helps in digestion of fats by its hydrotropic action (by helping conjugated products formed with fatty acid and cholesterol which helps lipase action.
   iii. Bile also activates enzyme lipase which breaks fat molecules.
   iv. It is also a good solvent providing fluid medium for lipase to act.
b. Absorption of fats and fatty acids, fat soluble vitamins, calcium iron etc. function is also performed by bile. This function is performed by hydrotropic action and solvent property of bile.
c. It stimulates intestinal peristalsis so it acts as laxative.
d. Its mucin acts as a buffer as well as a lubricant.
e. It acts like autostimulant (choleretic effect) which means stimulation of its production by liver.
f. Of course, it maintains suitable pH by neutralising gastric acid through its alkaline nature.
g. It helps in solution formation of fatty acids, cholesterol and lecithin.
h. It also acts an antiputrefactive agent in intestine.
i. It also acts like an antiseptic by inhibiting growth of certain bacteria.

PHYSICO-CHEMICAL PROPERTIES OF BILE CONSTITUENTS

Normal human gall bladder contains 80-279 gm total solids per litre. Bile acids and lipids make up 53-71 and 23-29 per cent respectively of total solids. Electrolytes, proteins and bile pigment don't comprise more than 15 per cent of total solids. Bile lipids mainly consist of phospholipid and cholesterol. Lecithin accounts for over 80 per cent of the phospholipids in human bile. Cholesterol esters, glycerides and free fatty acids are present in traces only. Cholesterol concentration in liver bile is 150-220 mg per cent while in gall bladder bile is 400-800 mg per cent. Cholesterol, which is insoluble in water, is present in bile as water soluble complexes with other bile constituents. Cholesterol in bile is held in water solution by complex formation between cholesterol, lecithin and bile salts. Bile acids are weakly bound to the complex and can be easily dissociated.

Cholecystography is a specialised diagnostic technique for observing this organ.

PARTIAL EXTIRPATION OF LIVER

Liver cells are provided with masterpiece power of regeneration. It has been studied in dogs that if 80 per cent of liver is removed normal excretion of bile results since it is found to regenerate within 6-8 weeks time. As regards other biliary functions they are also said to be normal if nutritional states are made normal in that experimental animal.

COMPLETE EXTIRPATION OF LIVER

a. Blood sugar level may tremendously fall even to 40 mg per cent so-called hypoglycaemia,
b. Blood urea level also falls, but
c. Rise in blood amino acid level,
d. Jaundice ensues increasing bile pigments and bile salts level,
e. Certainly blood coagulation becomes defective due to fall in prothrombin, fibrinogen and albumin level, and more fatally,
f. Liver failure ensues characterised by vomiting, dyspnoea, anurea, coma and neurological signs.

FUNCTIONS OF LIVER : ENUMERATION

a. *Secretory functions*: Bile along with bile salts and pigments (also from blood) and bile is one of the important digestive juices,
b. *Synthetic functions*: Many substances of utmost importance are synthesised here like heparin, albumin, fibrinogen, prothrombin etc.,
c. *Excretory functions* : Certain heavy metals (bismuth, lead, arsenic etc.), cholesterol and bile pigments, bacterial toxins (typhoid), virus (yellow fever) are some of the main substances excreted through this channel,
d. *Hemopoietic functions*: Liver is the place where erythrocytes are formed in early foetal life as well as destruction of these cells occur here due to the presence of reticuloendothelial cells. It also acts as a storehouse or reservoir of blood. It is also said that some blood group substances are manufactured here,
e. *Metabolic activities* :
   i. *Carbohydrate:* Site of neoglucogenesis, helps in glycogenesis, helps in maintaining blood sugar level and helps in glycogenolysis.
   ii. *Proteins:* Helping deamination of amino acids, helps in urea formation, helping in transmethylation, concerned with specific dynamic action, help in purine and pyramidine metabolism, helps in new amino acid formation from carbohydrates and fats through process of transamination.
   iii. *Fats:* Helping fat oxidation, ketone formation, synthesis of phospholipids, fat storage.
f. *Detoxicating functions* :
   i. Because of reticuloendothelial cells foreign bodies are directly engulfed through phagocytosis.
   ii. Toxic products are further destroyed by it through conjugation with sulphates or by glucoronide formation.
   iii. Likewise benzoic acid is turned into hippuric acid by conjugation with glycine, it also protects the body by turning toxic elements into non-toxic one through formation of a harmless conjugate,
   iv. Antibodies are also formed here,
   v. Certain drugs (strychnine, barbiturates, adrenaline) are inactivated here through formation of inactive metabolic degraded products.
g. *Storage function*: Glycogen, vitamin A, D, folic acid, B_{12}, hematinic principal, iron are stored here.

Differences : Liver and gall bladder bile

Constituents	*Liver bile*	*Gall bladder bile*
1. Water	98%	89%
2. Specific gravity	1.010 - 1.011	1.026-1.032
3. pH	7 - 7.6	8 - 8.6
4. Bile salts	0.72%	6%
5. Fat and fatty acids	0.07%	0.82%
6. Cholesterol	0.06%	0.38%
7. Total solids	2%	11%

LIVER FUNCTION TESTS

a. Introduction:
   1. Detection of liver damage in absence of jaundice.
   2. Differential diagnosis of jaundice.
   3. Differential diagnosis of hepatic enlargement.
   4. Excessive haemolysis (investigation of anaemia).
b. Summary of tests:
   1. Bilirubin metabolism.
   2. Metabolic tests .... Carbohydrate, protein, lipid.
   3. Enzyme levels of blood
      —Alkaline phosphatase
      —Transaminase SGOT, SGPT
      —Cholinestarase.
   4. *Serum metals:* Serum iron and iron binding capacity, Serum copper, Serum Mg.
   5. Tests based on vitamin economy
      — Vitamin A, Vitamin B_{12}, Vitamin D
   6. *Detoxification and synthesis:* Hippuric acid excretion, prothrombin level and vitamin K response.
   7. *Foreign substance excretion:* Rose bengal, excretion, sulfobromophthalein excretion.
   8. Liver biopsy.

c. Tests based on excretory function:
 1. Van den Bergh Reaction.
 2. Bilirubin excretion tests: It indicates excretory power of liver. A standard amount of bilirubin is given I.V. and its concentration is determined in plasma from time to time. Normally not more than 5-6 per cent of pigment should be retained after 4 hours.
 3. Test for urobilinogen in urine: On the whole liver function is deficient. Positive test two things denote—Urobilinogen reabsorbed by intestine since it cannot be excreted by liver and bile is entering the intestine.
 4. Bromsulphalein excretion tests: A standard amount of dye is given I.V. and in blood its concentration is estimated time to time.
 5. Rose-Bengal excretion.

d. Tests based on metabolic function:
 1. Galactose (glucose) tolerance test (GTT)
 2. Estimation of plasma phosphatase in obstructive cases it increases.
 3. *Plasma protein concentration:* Since liver manufactures plasma protein so in deficient liver function protein mainly serum albumin globulin ratio is changed.
 4. *Prothrombin time:* It is a sensitive test. If this time increases even after vitamin K administration, it shows liver deficiency.
 5. *Taka and Ara reaction:* Mercuric chlorides, acid fuchsin and sodium carbonate when added to abnormal serum, mercuric chloride is precipitated. Positive reaction indicates parenchymatous liver damage.
 6. Serum colloidal gold test: Positive reaction indicate liver damage due to faulty globulin formation by liver.
 7. Thymol turbidity test: Normal 4-6 units. About 8 ml of thymol reagent added to 0.05 ml of abnormal serum. In liver disease precipitating of globin appears.
 8. Laevulose tolerance test: 40 gm of laevulose along with 250 ml of water is taken by fasting patient. Blood is taken after every half an hour for two hours and blood sugar level is determined. In case of liver damage blood sugar is found to be high in all the sample and does not come down in normal level within 2 hours.
 9. Flocculation test: Cephalin cholesterol-flocculation test. Aqueous emulsified mixture of cholesterol (300 mg) and Cephalin (100 mg) obtained from brain is added to dil. serum and allow to stay for 24-48 hours. In liver disease a clear supernatant with deposition occurs. Test is positive in liver disease.
 10. Cinnamic acid tolerance test: (lipid metabolism) The normal liver oxidises cinnamic to benzoic acid which is conjugated to glycine to form hippuric acid. The decrease hippuric acid excretion is seen in liver diseases.
 11. Transaminase estimation: (serum enzyme)
  a. Serum-glutamic-oxaloacetic transaminase (SGOT) normal 6-40 unit/ml of serum increased in liver diseases, posthepatic jaundice, CO_2 poisoning.
  b. Serum-glutamic-pyruvic-transaminase (SGPT) Normal 6-36 units/ml of serum increased in same conditions described as above.

e. Tests based on detoxification by liver:
 1. Oral hippuric acid excretion test: Not commonly done.
 2. I.V. hippuric acid test: A standard amount of sodium benzoate is given I.V. and after one hour hippuric acid is estimated in urine. Normally 0.7-0.95 gm is excreted as hippuric acid in first hour.

f. Estimation of serum metals:
 1. Serum copper: Normal 90-120 micro gm per cent. Increase in Wilson disease.
 2. Serum iron: Normal 80-140 microgm/100 ml. Elevation follows liver damage. It is not done routinely since haemolysis, bone marrow activity and abnormal absorption also effect blood level.
 3. Other metals: Potassium levels decrease in hepatic coma. Magnesium levels decreased in cirrhosis.

g. Other tests:
 1. Blood ammonia: Normally upto 1 microgm/ml. It is of value in study of a drowsy patient with known liver disease.
 2. Blood lipids and sterols: Normal cholesterol 150-250 mg per cent. Normal serum ester cholesterol is 60-140 ml per cent. Biliary obstruction caused a rise of free cholesterol. Parenchymatous liver damage will cause lowering of total serum cholesterol.
 3. Electrophoretic pattern of serum proteins: in obstructive jaundice there is increase in alpha and beta globulins whereas in liver cell jaundice there is a rise in gamaglobulins.

h. Selection of tests:
 1. To find out presence or absence of jaundice.
 2. For differential diagnosis of jaundice.
 3. In liver disease without jaundice: Any positive result may be significant.

With minimal liver change urine urobilinogen test useful.

In established cirrhosis - Serum albumin values below 2 gm per 100 ml indicate bad prognosis.

Common liver function test

Test	*Normal value*	*Remarks*
Total serum bilirubin	Less than 1 mg/100 ml	Increased in age, biliary obstruction
Serum cholesterol	150-250 mg/100 ml	Raised in intra- and extrahepatic obstruction
SGOT	Less than 40 units 5-17 international units	Increased markedly in acute liver cell damage
SGPT	Less than 35 units 4-12 international unit	Increased in early liver cell damage. Values may exceed 500 units in viral hepatitis (early stage)
Serum proteins albumin globulin	3.5-4.5 gm/100 ml	Diminished in chronic liver damage (reversed A/G rates)
	2.0-3.0 gm/100 ml (Normal A/G ratio–1.5:1.0)	Increased in chronic liver damage
Alkaline phosphatase	International unit 21-85. King Armstrong Unit–Less than 13 Bodansky units less than 4	Markedly increase in intra- and extrahepatic obstruction. Higher values suggest obstructive jaundice
Urinary urobilinogen	0.5-1.5 mg in 24 hours	Increased with liver cell damage. Diminished with intra- or extrahepatic obstruction

SUMMARY AND HIGHLIGHTS—THE HEADLINES

Introduction

Quantity per day 600-1000 cc, specific gravity 1.010-1.011 pH 8-8.6, water 97.5 per cent, inorganic solids 40 per cent (sodium, potassium, Ca, Mg, bicarbonates, chlorides), organic solids 60 per cent (bile salts, pigments, lecithin and cholesterol, fatty acids, others include glucose, urea, creatinine).

Functions

a. Digestion (specially of fats through reducing surface tension, activating lipase and by hydrotropic action),
b. Absorption (of fats, fatty acids and fat soluble vitamins through hydrotropic and solvent action),
c. Laxative (by accelerating intestinal peristalsis),
d. Choleretic action (stimulating its own secretion),
e. Mucin acts as buffer,
f. Antiseptic (natural detergent checks bacterial growth),
g. Gastric acid neutralisation thus pH maintenance,
h. Performs antiputrefactive action,
i. Secretin secretion gets stimulated.

Regulation

a. Food is primary stimulant so its secretion is much in day time as compared with night secretion, fats stimulate gall bladder contraction and thus bile's output too but proteins are considered as best stimulant.
b. Sometimes secretion is accelerated on vagus stimulation but overall autonomic stimulation is said to be inhibitory one.
c. Heptatocrinin hormone produced by upper small intestine mucosa is said to stimulate bile production by liver.

BIBLIOGRAPHY

1. Arne Norman. Physicochemical properties of bile constituents. In The Biliary System: Edited by W Taylor Blackwell scientific publishers, Oxford. 1965.
2. Bean JM. Micro structure of gall stones. Gastroenterology 1979;76:548.
3. Braver RW. Mechanisms of bile: secretion. Gastroenterology 1958;34:1021.
4. Caldwell FT. Dietary induction and dissolution of gall stones in mice. - JAMA 1964;188:437.
5. Caroli A, Lemonnier C, Charpentier B. Plessier. The inhibition of CCK: In The biliary system Ed. by W Taylor Blackwell Scientific publiation Oxford page 303.
6. Diamond Jared M. Mechanism of water transport by gall bladder. J Phy 1982;16:503.
7. F Magee. Physiology of gall bladder emptying. In: The biliary system, edited by W. Taylor. Blackwell Scientific publications Oxford : page 233. 1965.
8. Gerald Salen, Sarah Shefer. Bile acid Synthesis. Ann Rev Phy 1983;45:679.
9. Heintz K, et al. Gall bladder water and electrolyte transport and its regulation. Gut 1983;24:579-93.
10. Howard PJ, et al. Gall bladder : emptying patterns in response to a normal meal in healthy subjects and patients with gall stones: ultra sonographic study. Gut 1991;32:1405-11.
11. IVAR Sperber. Biliary secretion of anions and its influence on bile flow. In: The biliary system: Edited by W. Taylor. Blackwell scientific publications oxford. 1965.

12. Klaassen CD, et al. Mechanism of bile formation, hepatic uptake and biliary excretion. Quoted by WF Ganong in Review of Medical Physiology - Lange Publications Pharm Rev 1984;361:1.
13. La Morte WW. Biliary motility and abnormalities associated with cholesterol chole lithiasis. Current opinion in Gastroenterolology 1993;9:810-16.
14. Moorey EW, et al. Gastroenterology 1989;96:A 632.
15. Moorey EW, et al. Pathogenesis of Ca. PO_4 containing gall stones. Gastroenterology 1989;96:A623.
16. N Plevris, IAD Bouchier. Defective acid base regulation by gall bladder epithelium and its significance for gall stone formation. Gut 1995;37:127-31, 1.
17. O'Donnel LJD, Faviclough PD. Gall stone and gall bladder motility. Gut 1993;34:440-43.
18. Pelvris JN, et al. Mechanism of acid secretion in bovine gall bladder epithelium: Evidence of Na^+/H^+ exchange. Gut 1990;31:A 1215.
19. Plevris JN, et al. Evidence of H secretion from Human gall bladder in vitro. Gut 1992;33:554-59.
20. Reuss L, Stodard JS. Role of H^+ and HCO_3^- in salt transport in gall bladder epithelium. Ann Rev Phy 1987;49:35.
21. Shifman ML, Moorey EW. Acidification of gall bladder bile is defective in patients with all types of gall stones. Gastroenterology 1984;94:A 591.
22. Zakim D, Boyer TD (Ed). Hepatology. A textbook of liver disease, Saunders 1982. Quoted by WF Ganong in Review of Medical Physiology - Lange Publications.

89 Intestinal Secretion (Succus Entericus)

Functions of small intestine are digestion, absorption while of large intestine are storage and movements of contents.

INTESTINAL JUICE : INTRODUCTION

In general this juice is colourless or slight straw coloured, containing mucus. It appears cloudy due to mucus and cellular debris. Its pH varies between 6.3 to 9.0, so certainly an alkaline fluid. Its bicarbonate contents are higher than plasma or interstitial fluid of body.

Colonic secretion: It appears like a watery fluid with clumps of mucus so it appears viscid and opalescent. Reaction of juice is alkaline due to sodium bicarbonate. Enzymes present here are similar with that of succus entericus but with the exception of enterokinase which is not existing here. The large quantity of mucus as well as capacity of epithelial surface to produce mucus is a defensive factor against bacterial infection or use of irritant cathartics, though mucus secretion is an active process which utilises oxygen.

Enzymes

i. Protease is a proteolytic enzyme similar to pepsin but comparatively weaker in action.
ii. Peptidase performs final reduction of proteins to amino acids.
   — aminopeptidases act on peptide linkage of terminal amino acid having free amino group.
   — tri and di peptidase act on tri and di peptides respectively.
iii. Disaccharidases are maltase, sucrase and lactase.
iv. Enterokinase responsible for conversion of trypsinogen to trypsin of pancreatic juice.

Functions

a. Digestion of various foodstuffs by enzymes present.
b. It provides plenty of water for digestion which on the other hand acts as a solvent, medium of suspension, transport for solids dissolved in chyme.

Duodenal Secretion

a. It prevents duodenal ulceration. (Brunner's gland secretion).
b. It helps in emulsification and suspension of fat.
c. It, due to containing enterokinase helps in conversion of trypsinogen to tyrpsin.
d. Because of containing intrinsic factor it naturally helps in absorption of extrinsic factor (Vit B_{12}).

CONTROL OR REGULATION

A. *Nervous regulation*:
- It is stated that moderate amount of intestinal secretion is produced within a latent period of 1 to 1½ hours on stimulating vagus nerve. On the contrary significant amount of juice is found to be produced on cutting the sympathetic supply which is designated as 'paralytic secretion' which is inhibited by atropine and stimulated by drug like physostigmine. The phenomenon is explained by the fact that vasodilatation is produced on severing sympathetic supply, thus increasing blood flow, and furthermore motility is also increased which sometimes leads to messaging effect on intestinal mucous membrane.
- Local nervous reflexes are here said to be the most important stimuli since distension of intestine, irritation, amount of food or any tactile stimulation leads to copious secretion.

B. *Humoral regulation*: 'Enterocrinin' a hormone secreted from intestinal mucosa controls the secretion and enzymes too. Enzymes are said to be controlled by both—the enterocrinin hormone as well as parasympathetic nerves.

Control of Duodenal (Brunner's gland) Secretion

i. The chief controlling nerves are here again vagus. It is found that secretion from these gland is increased on stimulating parasympathetic nerves (vagus) or by administration of parasympathomimetic drugs (physostigmine, pilocarpine). It is not found to be stimulated by sympathetic nerves.

ii. A hormone 'duocrinin' has been isolated from its own mucous membrane which regulates the secretion.

Nervous Control of Colonic Secretion

i. Nervi erigentes' (supplying distal colon with parasympathetic fibres) on stimulation, causes a secretion from colon which is full of mucus, and rate of the secretion has been estimated to 5 ml/hour.
ii. Acetyl choline and pilocarpine drugs augment the secretion while atropine has got a blocking action.
iii. On histamine administration, slight increase in secretion has been noticed which is inhibited by anaesthetics.
iv. Paralytic secretion on cutting sympathetic supply is not noticed here.
v. Mucous colitis is an abnormal state in which excess mucus appears in stool, the condition is said to be emotionally originated, i.e. psychosomatic one. Mucous contain little or no faecal matter and comes up after every half an hour.

FUNCTIONS OF MUCUS IN LARGE INTESTINAL SECRETION

i. It protects the intestinal wall against any excoriation,
ii. It provides alkalinity to secretion,
iii. It helps in holding faecal matter,
iv. Acids formed in faeces becomes noncapable of attacking delicate intestinal walls,
v. It protects intestinal wall from bacteria.

FUNCTIONS OF LARGE INTESTINE

It consists of caecum-appendix, ascending colon, right colic flexure, transverse colon, left colic flexure, descending colon, pelvic or sigmoid colon and rectum opening into anal canal.

i. *Absorption:* It is a chief site for absorption.
   - 'Water' is absorbed 80 per cent (400-500 ml), 'sugar' is absorbed at 5 per cent solution; 'alcohol' is absorbed but amount is not significant, 'amino acid' though absorbed from small intestine but little or escaped amount is absorbed here, 'drugs' like sedatives, anaesthetics, paraldehyde, steroids are also said to be absorbed here but again quantity is not significant, 'amino acids' which escaped from small intestine are absorbed here.
ii. *Excretion:* Heavy metals like bismuth, lead, arsenic are excreted.
iii. *Synthesis:* Vitamin K, folic acid, B_{12} are synthesised here through bacterial flora.
iv. *Secretion:* Mucus and various electrolytes of various uses are secreted here.
v. *Movements:* Through their characteristic movements defecation act is facilitated.

BACTERIAL FLORA OF INTESTINE

Along with other bacteria colon bacilli are also present here. Vitamin K, thiamine, riboflavin, B_{12} are formed by their action together with flatus formation. They are also said to digest small quantity of cellulose too thus assisting in supplying little calories to body per day. Certain bacteria can lead to some fermentative changes which result into formation of lower fatty acids similarly acid producing bacteria creates a protective function. Since they need carbohydrates for their full action, so when these foodstuffs are lacking putrefaction may ensue. With the use of antibiotics this bacterial flora is either destroyed or made sterile so vitamins will be lacking so vitamins need to be supplemented along with antibiotics. The food which is escaped from routine digestion as well absorption is here acted upon by bacteria but products so formed are highly toxic. *E. coli,* aerobacteria aerogens, *Clostridium welchii* and many coccus are few bacterial names in this connection. At birth usually no bacteria is present here but afterwards bacteria grow by themselves taking entry through faecal contamination while passaging through vagina.

FUNCTIONS OF ILEOCAECAL VALVE

Backflow of faeces from colon to small intestine is prevented chiefly by this valve which acts as gatekeeper. Ileocaecal sphincter is the name given to thick muscular coat over ileal wall which precedes this valve.

Control

i. Degree of contraction of ileocaecal sphincter is augmented whenever caecum gets distension resulting into delaying the emptying of any more food chyme from ileum to caecum,
ii. This sphincter is also said to be constricted when caecum gets irritation viz. in appendicular inflammation, caecum undergoes severe spasm upto the extent that emptying of ileum is totally blocked. Similarly same results can also be obtained by irritation of other abdominal organs like kidney peritoneum etc.

ABSORPTION PROCESS: LARGE INTESTINE

- It can absorb as large as 5-7 litres of fluid-electrolytes everyday.
- Bicarbonate ions are secreted by its mucosa. In exchange it absorbs chloride ions - so-called exchange

transport process. This bicarbonate neutralises the acidic component in colon.

- The tight junctions between epithelial cells are comparatively much tighter here than small intestine. By this structural peculiarity, back diffusion of ions is prevented. It facilitates more complete absorption of sodium ions against a much higher concentration gradient.
- The absorbed sodium and chloride ions create an osmotic gradient across its mucosa, which causes water absorption.

GAS IN INTESTINE: FLATUS

a. These gases include carbon dioxide, methane and hydrogen. Explosive mixture is sometimes constituted by union of methane hydrogen and oxygen. Majority of gases are found in intestine but stomach also may contain and the source is swallowed air which is expelled through belching.

b. The source of intestinal gases is bacterial fermentation as well as diffusion from blood. Since nitrogen is not easily absorbed into blood owing to its high P_{N2}, so it is present in high concentration in gut while the gases which are passed in flatus comprises of CO_2, methane, hydrogen etc.

c. Approximately 8-10 litres of gases are formed each day in intestine and expelling amount is very little, i.e. 0.5-1 litre, the remainder amount is absorbed by mucosa.

d. Foodstuffs like onion, cauliflower, cabbage, venegar etc. are said to be quite notorious for gaseous formation, i.e. more flatus expulsion since they act as a good medium for bacterial growth.

e. As mentioned above it is the notorious nitrogen which escapes absorption and hence this can be treated by pure oxygen breathing which will reduce high P_{N2} creating a situation for proper absorption of it by blood, but such treatment is a long one because diffusion of nitrogen is a slow process.

f. Overall, composition of these gases is N_2 (80%), CO_2 (7.5%), O_2 (3%), hydrogen, methane and others 9.5 per cent.

g. There are three possible sources of CO_2—
   a. Diffusion from blood into lumen,
   b. Neutralisation of acid by bicarbonate and
   c. Production by intestinal bacteria.

h. In contrast to hydrogen which is produced within 48 hours of birth, methane production has not been detected in children under 2 years of age but it is at climax at 10 years of age.

MALABSORPTION SYNDROME

"*My bowel moves once a day but whenever they move, a bucket is filled driving every body out of the house and my stools are so bulky and greasy that they float on lavatory pan*" is the opening sentence of the patient to his doctor. Here the main defect lies in absorption of fats and due to their defective absorption they are passed in stools—'steatorrhoea'. It is being recalled that absorption mainly depends on good adequate intestinal mucosal surface required for absorption, healthy functioning mucosa itself, providing proper time for absorption and here in this disease these are the intestinal mucosal cells which are considered as main culprit since they are found to undergo atrophy and blunting of villi. This disease is of following types:

a. *Sprue*: It again falls into two categories 'tropical' (found in tropics, south united states) and non-tropical. The main symptoms of disease include abdominal distension, epigastric pain, flatulence, though steatorrhoea foul watery stools are common feature. Due to defective fat absorption, the fat soluble vitamins are also defectively absorbed (vitamin A, D, K). Again due to faulty absorption of vitamin B_{12} (anti-anaemic principle) patient also suffers from anaemia. The frothy nature stools are actually due to fermentation of unabsorbed carbohydrates.

b. *Celiac disease:* It is the disease of young children. Stools are bulky rich in fats, pale coloured due to bile absence, foul smelling due to excess fermentation, stench and stinking. The calcium is lost in great amount in stools which results into low blood calcium as well as tetany. In this condition abdominal wall gives a characteristic appearance because of its more thinness owing to loss of subcutaneous fats making gaseous distension more prominent. The main culprit (causative factor) are deficiency of succinic dehydrogenase enzyme deficiency in bowel cell as well as deficiency of Paneth cells in mucosa.

c. *Whipple's disease*: Characterised by steatorrhoea, abdominal (intestinal lipodystrophy) distension, asthenia, anaemia, arthritis. The lipids are deposited in intestinal mucosa as well in mesenteric lymph nodes. It is said to be due to lymphatic drainage obstruction together with faulty fat absorption.

ULCERATIVE COLITIS

This is one of the chronic and distressing disease having symptoms like diarrhoea and stools are containing mucus, blood as well as pus. The frequency is quite variable between 4/5 to 30 or even more. The patient also develops anaemia owing to blood loss, diminished erythropoiesis which is due to secondary infection. The main causative factors include stress and strain as well as food deficiency so both body and mind should be treated regularly since disease is characterised by exacerbations and remissions. Immunological factors are also said to cause the disease process. Sometimes the ulcer may rupture also terminating into peritonitis which may end fatally. Removing of entire colon surgically or to perform iliostomy may be the last measures.

SUMMARY AND HIGHLIGHTS—ROUND UP SUCCUS ENTERICUS

- Introduction: Quantity per day 1-2 litres specific gravity 1.010, pH 6.3-9.0, water 98.5 per cent, Inorganic solids 1-1.1 per cent (Na, K, Ca, Mg, chloride, bicarbonate, phosphates), organic solids (enzymes are protease-peptidases, - nuclease - nucleotidase - nucleosidase, lipase, amylase, maltase - lactase - invertase - alkaline phosphatases - nucleophosphatases, arginase. Activator is enterokinase. Others include albumin-globulin-mucin - shaded epithelial cells - urea etc. EREPSIN is name given in previous times to group of enzymes acting on peptones and polypeptides).
- *Functions:* (a) Digestion (Proteolytic enzymes complete protein digestion by yielding amino acids, while all amylolytic enzymes act on disaccharides to change them into monosaccharides while lipase is a fat splitting enzyme, (b) Absorption (due to more volume and more surface area), (c) Protection (mucus protects surface epithelium from injury etc.) (d) Hydrolytic function (due to plenty of water better transport of foodstuffs, ready water supply is possible required for hydrolysis purpose as well water is a famous vehicle for fat emulsification) (e) Intrinsic factor is also present in duodenal secretion) (f) Enterokinase activates inactive trypsinogen into trypsin.
- *Mechanism:* (a) nervous phase - Local nerve plexus are chief controller, after sectioning sympathetic nerves 'paralytic secretion ensues which inhibited by atropine but accelerated by parasympathomimetic drugs (b) enterocrinin hormone responsible for bringing out intestinal secretion and coming from its mucosa. Special hormone 'duocrinin' has been isolated for Brunner's gland secretion control. (c) Parasympathetic nerves help in toning up the local nervous reflex.

BIBLIOGRAPHY

1. Michael D, Levitt, et al. Volume composition and source of Intestinal gas. Gastroenterology 1970;53:921.
2. Sleisenger MH, Brandborg LL Malabsorption. Saunders 1977 quoted by Ganong WF in Review of Medical Physiology - Lange Publications.
3. Specian RD, et al. Functional biology of intestinal goblet cells quoted by Ganong WF in Review of Medical Physiology - Lange Publications. Amer J. Med. 1991;260:C1183.
4. Wormsley KG. Reaction to acid in intestine in health and disease. Gut 1971;12:67-84.
5. Wormsley KG. The source of duodenal asparate in man. Gut 1980;9:398-404.

90

Movements of Alimentary Canal (Mechanics of Digestion)

MOVEMENTS OF GIT: FOOD IN MOUTH

Two types of actions are listed here.

a. Mastication or chewing, and
b. Deglutition or swallowing

Mastication or Chewing

The food is broken into smaller masses thus decreasing its size. Biting or crushing of food (simple closing of mouth) is accomplished by masseter, temporal, internal and external pterygoid muscles while opening of mouth is accomplished by digastric and myloid muscles, while grinding movements of molar teeth are accomplished by rotational jaw movements, pterygoid muscles. Side to side movement of jaw completed by contraction of pterygoids of one side, forward jaw movement by contraction of both pterygoid while backward movement of jaw is completed by temporalis and geniohyoid muscles.

Effects

a. Harder food elements are broken into small pieces facilitating deglutition which are moistened by saliva so food is changed into 'bolus' (a plastic mass).
b. Saliva is thoroughly mixed so taste sensations are created since foodstuff is in a solution state.
c. A sense of pleasure and satisfaction is created ultimately leading to satiety.
d. It also starts cephalic phase of gastric secretion.
   - It is controlled by a centre in medulla.
   - Large food particles can be digested but they cause strong and painful contractions of muscles of oesophagus.

DEGLUTITION (Swallowing)

Both the process, i.e. 'mixing' (by chewing/mastication) and 'propulsion' (deglutition) are different and therefore takes optimum time to occur.

a. *First oral stage*: It consists of passage of material through the oral cavity into the pharynx. The food material is changed into a plastic mass called 'bolus' because food is rolled on upper surface of tongue by its movements, and saliva is also mixed with food. After this the front portion of tongue is retracted, mastication comes to an end, reflex inhibition of respiration occurs, slight elevation of hyoid is seen, back portion of tongue is elevated and retracted against the hard palate. This initiation of first stage is voluntary. Because of involvement of above structures, any inflammatory conditions or neoplasm of tongue and other oral structures like lips or palate may create difficulties in this first stage.
b. *Second pharyngeal stage*: Here, the main objective is to prevent 'respiratory tract' and to use the 'digestive tract' since both these are crossing each other in the region of pharynx.
   i. Regurgitation of food in mouth is prevented by high pressure in this region.
   ii. Soft palate is stiffened and is pressed against the posterior pharyngeal wall; so food is not allowed to enter the nasopharynx.
   iii. By union of vocal cords, laryngeal opening is closed and in this way larynx is protected from entry of food.
   iv. Reflex inhibition of respiration is again a preventive factor in this aspect. So larynx is elevated, upper oesophageal sphincter relaxes epiglottis diverts the bolus to one side or other of larynx and bolus enters the oesophagus. Pharyngitis, laryngitis, neoplasm or tuberculosis of both these parts are the main pathological states which can interfere in the process. Both first and second stage of swallowing are completed within less than one second time and once initiated it proceeds as a co-ordinated involuntary reflex.

c. *Third oesophageal stage*: Upper and lower oesophageal sphincters are acting like 'gatekeepers'. When bolus enters, the upper sphincter opens and it is closed when bolus has passed. Then peristaltic waves propel the food in aboral direction which is helped by action of gravity.

d. *Disturbances*

   i. *Achalasia:* Here, relaxation of lower oesophageal sphincter is not occurring, so food is not processed or propelled from oesophagus to stomach. It becomes massively dilated. Its causes include—increased resting lower oesophageal sphincter tension, incomplete relaxation of this sphincter during swallowing, weak peristalsis of oesophagus etc. This condition is due to lack of VIP containing neurons in lower oesophageal area.

   ii. Hiatus hernia: It is due to anatomical alterations of oesophageo-gastric junction.

   iii. Reflux oesophagitis: Here acid gastric juice is regurgitated into oesophagus. It leads to burning pain in middle of chest and neck (heart burn). It is due to lower oesophageal sphincter incompetence. It may lead to ulceration and stricture due to scarring. It can be treated as usual by the drugs like Omeprazole, H_2 receptor blockers etc. and surgically by fundoplication (making a fold of gastric tissue).

e. *Swallowing centre* (group of neuron in floor of IV ventricle): An area within the reticular formation of the brainstem has been identified as 'swallowing centre'.

DEGLUTITION

- It is a reflex response, triggered by afferent impulses in trigeminal, glossopharyngeal and vagus nerve.
- Efferents - pass to pharyngeal musculature and tongue through trigeminal, facial, and hypoglossal nerve.
- Impulses are centred/integrated in nucleus ambiguous and tractus solitarius.
- With open mouth swallowing is difficult.
- It begins as a wave of involuntary contraction in pharyngeal muscles which propels the food forwards into oesophagus.

MOVEMENTS OF GIT : FOOD IN STOMACH

a. *Tonus of stomach*: As with smooth muscles, it refers to relation between length of muscle and tension which it maintains. So it means either tension in the muscle maintained at constant length or length assumed by muscle at a constant tension. During emptiness of stomach the tone is minimum. Series of hunger contractions raise tone which when superaided with peristalsis due to food ingestion the vigorous contraction results. So during rest pressure is 1-2 cm of water but with peristalsis this rises up to even 15-30 cm of water. Stomach tonus increases during prolonged fast so this organ becomes tubular in shape but when it is filled with food, it recovers due to receptive relaxation. Furthermore; shape of stomach is related with volume of its contents, e.g. in upright position it is of 'J' shape owing to descending of mid portion. 'Systole' (contraction) and 'diastole' (relaxation) terms have also been discovered and it occurs after approximately every 20 seconds and during every systole peristaltic wave is increased.

b. *Gastric filling and emptying (Control of pyloric sphinctre):*

   - Normally pyloric sphincter remains relaxed. It closes when food enters.
   - As food enters the stomach, its acidity increases which opens this valve. As the acid chyme enters the duodenum, its acidity decreases while acidity increases in duodenum, which closes the valve. This process moves on alternately till stomach becomes empty. This attractive theory is not universally accepted because persons suffering from achylia gastrica shows normal activity of sphincter.
   - When the peristaltic wave is stronger the sphincter opens which leads to emptying of stomach, when anti-peristalsis in duodenum becomes stronger the sphincter also opens up causing duodenal regurgitation.
   - As digestion proceeds, concentration of peptones-proteoses increase which open the valve. The food is then pushed to duodenum. It decreases their concentration in stomach, which closes the valve. In this way the cycle proceeds.
   - When osmotic pressure of gastric content approaches that of saline constituents of plasma, the sphincter opens. On progressive digestion, the number of dissolved particles are increased which causes a rise in osmotic pressure which is capable of opening of sphincter.

c. *Hunger and appetite:*

   - Hunger is a natural desire for food while appetite is a psychological phenomenon. Appetite is the sensation of anticipated pleasure of eating hence it persists even after hunger.
   - Ingestion of food, chewing or swallowing, alcohol, smoking, emotions of high degree all are the factors inhibiting hunger sensation. Sleep does not inhibit hunger.
   - When stomach is empty, i.e. in active, then mild peristaltic contraction begin which gradually increase in intensity and even painful. This is

hunger contraction. They are associated with sense of hunger. They also regulate appetite. In hypothalamus, laterally located is feeding centre and medially is satiety centre (ventro medial nucleus). It appears that feeding centre is chronically active and its activity is inhibited by activity in satiety centre after ingestion of food.

- Appetite regulation: glucostatic hypothesis... It is the level of glucose within these centres, which regulate appetite. When their glucose utilisation is low (or a-v-glucose difference across them is low) then their activity is decreased and so the individual is hungry. On the contrary, when glucose utilisation is high, their activity is increased, which inhibits the feeding centre and satiety is felt.
- The transmitter involved here are neuropeptide "Y" and catecholamines.
- Activation of α_2-adrenergic receptors in medial hypothalamus increases appetite. While activation of β-adrenergic receptors (and dopaminergic too) in lateral hypothalamus decreases appetite. So drugs commonly used for weight loss purposes (i.e. amphetamine) thus acts on lateral hypothalamus.
- Cholecystokinin and calcitonin decrease the appetite. Two types of receptors have been identified.
  - —CCK-A- receptors in periphery.
  - —CCK-B- receptors in brain.
- Other factors affecting appetite:
  - —Distension of GIT inhibits appetite
  - —Contraction of empty stomach stimulate appetite.
  - —Cultural environment, past experience of eating, sight/smell/taste etc. all affect the appetite.
  - —A cold environment → thyroid stimulation → more thyroxine→more BMR→increased appetite. A hot environment decreases the appetite.
  - —According to one data, it is stated that an average woman gains weight of 11 kg between age of 25-65 years and this is due to excess food intake of 350 mg/day.

ANOREXIA

- Means loss of appetite.
- Anorexia nervosa means intense fear of being fat. It usually affects teenage or young adult females. This leads an individual to self imposed starvation and emaciation (extreme thinness) to the point that one-third body weight is lost. So later on in extreme stages, one dies due to starvation or suicide.

d. *Peristalsis*: It is a contractile event followed by relaxation moving away from mouth. It is weak in body and fundus owing to weak musculature. During first half an hour it is weak then increases with the rate of 1 cm per sec. and at antrum becomes 3-4 cm/sec.

Due to these movements food is macerated and digested at pyloric region while body and fundus are acting as reservoirs. This is followed by relaxation of first part of duodenum so stomach contents passes from pylorus to duodenum.

e. *Vomiting:*

- It is a reflex phenomenon through which gastric contents are expelled out through mouth. Its main associated symptoms are nausea, increased heart rate, rapid irregular breathing, sweating; pallor etc.
- Sequence of events:
  - —At the onset, nausea is felt. Then nasopharynx is shut off, glottis closed, but soft palate is raised.
  - —Then there occurs, relaxation of cardiac sphincter, oesophagus as well as body of stomach. The pyloric sphincter remains closed. The pylorus contracts and so flushes its contents into relaxed stomach.
  - —Then there occurs a sharp rise in intra-abdominal pressure, owing to contraction of muscles like expiratory, abdominal and diaphragmatic. All this compresses the relaxed stomach. This constitutes the chief motive force of vomiting. The vomitus passes to oesophagus from where it is expelled out, via. mouth. Antiperistalsis have been reported in oesophagus during ejection.
  - —This process remains continue till stomach is empty. In the end, the diaphragm relaxes along with contraction of expiratory muscles. Because of closure of glottis, the intrapulmonary pressure is raised which causes compression of oesophagus. It aids in expelling the last remnants of vomitus out.
  - —Vomiting is a reflex process. Centre lies in medulla in close association with vagal nucleus. The afferent impulses may arise in throat, stomach, intestine, uterus or some other viscera. The efferent impulses both excitatory and inhibitory are carried in vagus.

Causes of Vomiting

i. *GI tract* any irritation in duodenum, mucous membrane of stomach, irritating mucous membrane of mouth and pharynx, appendicitis.

ii. *Abdominal visceral causes* gall bladder (cholecystitis etc.), renal calculi, uterine distension.
iii. *Special sense organs* eyes (dirty scene viewing), smell (offensive odour), taste (unpleasant taste).
iv. *Ear* motion sickness, sea sickness, car sickness, psychic vomiting.
v. *Central vomiting* due to stimulation of vomiting centre in medulla due to increased pressure or injury.
iv. *Drug* apomorphine, picrotoxin etc. They act by stimulating chemo-receptor-triggor zone.
vii. *Metabolic* hyper-emesis-gravidarum or motion sickness.
viii. *Injury* increased intracranial pressure (brain tumour, cyst) lead to projectile vomiting, i.e. vomiting with a great force.

Mechanism of act: Contraction of duodenum followed by contraction of pyloric sphincter; all these lead to squeezing intestinal contents of duodenum into pylorus. The body and fundus, cardiac sphincter are relaxed, glottis is closed after deep inspiration, abdominal muscles then contract, diaphragm descend down and forcing out stomach contents by jerky abdominal movements. Throughout afferent nerves are vagus and sympathetic while efferent are phrenic, vagus, sympathetic fibres and few somatic nerves supplying anterior abdominal muscles and nerves forming pharyngeal plexus.

f. *Summary*

i. *Chyme* fluid mass is formed from the food ingested by powerful contraction of stomach muscles which breaks up the big food particles. Due to these movements a small amount of broken food, partly digested chyme and gastric juice can pass to duodenum. Slow and less vigorous movement of body and fundus suit them to act as a receptacle. Vomiting centre lies at floor of 4th ventricle in dorsolateral part of reticular formation in medulla.

FUNCTIONS OF STOMACH

a. *Secretion*: The well known gastric juice is secreted composed of acid, mucus and enzymes.
b. *Digestion*: Due to various enzymes present here protein, fats of food are digested. Carbohydrates are digested continuously here till atmosphere (pH) becomes fully acidic.
c. *Absorption:* Water, alcohol as well as hemopoietic factor are said to be absorbed by gastric mucosa.
d. *Storage or reservoir*: As food is taken, it begins to be arranged in concentric ring fashion. The body of stomach bulges outwards to accommodate large quantity of food termed as 'receptive relaxation' and its uppermost limit is said to be approximately one litre in this aspect and this property of body is owing to its little tone in muscular wall. One peculiarity is further found in this organ and that is in spite of its remarkable distension due to food or any other cause, the inside pressure increases very slightly—this is attributed due to property of plasticity which means the ability of this organ to increase its own length without remarkable change in tone. This explains maintenance of low pressure till maximum capacity of receptive relaxation (1 litre) is attained.
e. *Mixing or mechanical function*: As the food is mixed with digestive juice completely, the weak mixing waves (tonus waves) starts at the rate of approximately one in twenty seconds, of course, begin at cardia and terminates at pylorus. Certainly the purpose of such type of waves is to propel this food towards antral part where these waves become more stronger to get food and digestive juice to be mixed thoroughly.
   Yet another powerful mixing mechanism is again evident here which is due to peristaltic waves.
   The chyme is the name given to the fluid mass moving downward towards gut from stomach after mixing food with gastric juice and it is milky-semi fluid or paste like in appearance and its intensity of fluidity of course depends upon amount of gastric juice and food as well as rate of their mixing.
f. *Hemopoietic function*: Due to production of intrinsic factor from pyloric mucosa, extrinsic factor (vitamin B_{12}, cyanocobalamine) is absorbed, failing which pernicious anaemia may result which may terminate fatally.

Gastric slow wave: It is also known as pacemaker for antral peristalsis. These types of waves are, in fact wave of depolarisation of smooth muscle cells, beginning from middle of stomach to pylorus occurring after every 20 sec. and are co-ordinating antral peristalsis. These are said to play a major role in gastric emptying.

Nausea

It precedes the vomiting act and reported by patient as sinking sensation in epigastrium, together with sweating. It is said to occur when any irritant enters the alimentary canal.

Regulation of hunger: Feeding centre is found to be located in lateral area of hypothalamus while satiety centre is said to be located in medial area of hypothalamus. The above mentioned areas for food intake control are said to be rich in ATP, creatine phosphate, i.e. high energy phosphate compounds. Drugs (amphetamine etc.) which are given to inhibit feeding centre are actually increasing the activity of satiety centre, while opposite action can be seen when substances are given to improve appetite.

MOVEMENTS OF GIT: FOOD IN SMALL INTESTINE (Fig. 90.1)

Segmentation

i. These are actually mixing movements which causes proper admixture of food with digestive juices.
ii. These are local constrictions immediately followed by relaxation, and so intestine is divided into short segments. At the next movement, each of these segments is subdivided by a fresh batch of constriction, and the previous group disappears in the mean time. In this way the process proceeds.
iii. In man, the rate of segmenting contractions has been reported as 12 per minute in duodenum, and 8-9 per minute in ileum; and this depends on distance from pylorus.
iv. These contractions are said to be myogenic in origin independent of all nerves.
v. These movements also help in process of absorption by causing close contact between food and mucous membrane. They also increase the vascular and lymphatic supply of the part.

Peristalsis

i. It is a translatory movement travelling down the gut in an aboral (away from mouth) direction. It is a composite wave of relaxation followed by a wave of constriction. (peristalsis = variety of contractile phenomenon having one thing in common and that is direction of travel).
ii. It is a propagatory movement which propels the food onwards. Usually peristaltic waves are superimposed upon rhythmic segmenting contractions in such a way that two are present simultaneously.
iii. Stimulation of vagus increases peristalsis while of sympathetics inhibits it. Besides this nervous effect, local nerve plexus helps in co-ordination of peristaltic movements. In the same way acetylcholine helps to maintain the intestinal tone; while 5 H.T. (serotonin) stimulates intestinal movements. Thyroxine excites while adrenaline inhibits the movement. So it is evident that these movements are influenced by both nervous and chemical stimuli.
iv. Metabolic gradient theory:
   - Put forwarded by Alvarez.
   - Excitability, frequency of movement, strength of contraction and tone of intestine gradually diminish from above downwards along the intestinal canal.
   - The latent period of intestinal muscles gradually becomes longer in the lower parts of small intestine.
   - This peculiarity is due to the difference in the degree of metabolic activity between upper and lower parts of intestine. It is greater in upper part than in lower part. This gradient mainly affects this difference.
   - In abnormal states like infection/obstruction etc., the metabolic rate of diseased part becomes higher, so antiperistalsis starts which travels towards stomach.

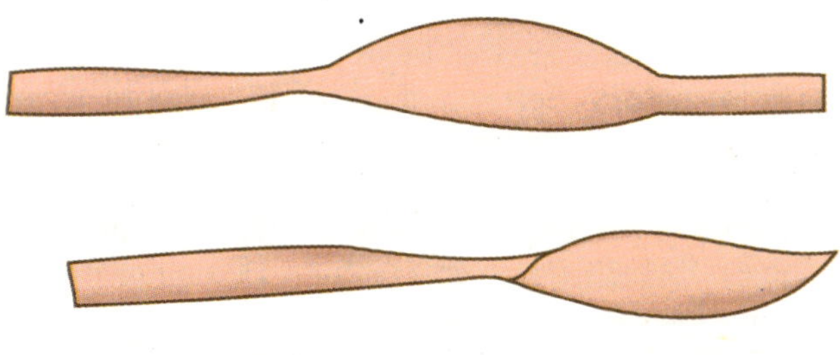

Fig. 90.1

Pendular movements: These have also been reported. It is a side to side movement (to and fro like a pendulum) and purpose of it is to rearrange the intestinal coils within the limited space of abdominal cavity.

Antiperistalsis type of movement has also been reported, which moves in oral direction. It may therefore lead to duodenal regurgitation into stomach. It is said to be present in second and third part of duodenum.

Law of Intestine

- Peristaltic waves characteristically travel in one direction, i.e. aborally.
- Bayliss and starling (1889, 1901): The response of small intestine to local stimuli consists of a contraction of smooth muscle proximal and relaxation distal to stimulated area. Canon (1912) added that myenteric reflex is responsible for law of intestine.
- Synonym - Polarity of intestine, law of gut, receptive relaxation theory.

NEURAL CONTROL: GIT MOTILITY

- The entire nervous system is existing from mouth to anus. The number of neurons is equal to the neurons existing in spinal cord.
- Two nerve plexuses are there:- (a) outer myenteric or Auerbach's and (b) inner Meissner's plexus or submucous one.
- The myenteric plexus controls GIT movements; the Meissner's plexus controls GIT secretion + local blood flow.

- The myenteric plexus controls motor activities, e.g. on stimulation the results are: increased tone of gut, increased intensity of rhythmic contraction, increased velocity of conduction of excitatory gut waves, increased rate of rhythm of contractions. It is not solely excitatory. VIP neurotransmitter—an inhibitory one is supposed to be secreted from its fibres.
- The Meissner's plexus is concerned with local effects like secretion, absorption and contraction of local muscles.
- Tonic contraction is exhibited by GIT smooth muscles. It is continuous lasting for a longer time. It is caused by repetitive series of spike potential. It may also be due to some hormones which is capable of doing depolarisation of muscle membrane. A continuous entry of Ca^{++} is not related with this.

MOVEMENTS OF GIT: FOOD IN LARGE INTESTINE

Haustrations - (mixing movements) (haustra = pockets):

i. It is identical with 'segmentation' of small intestine. Because of combined contraction of circular and longitudinal muscle (tineae coli); the unstimulated portion of large intestine protrudes outwards like 'bag' called 'haustrations'. These contractions are moving towards anus, reaching to their climax within thirty seconds; and, of course they disappear within next sixty seconds.
ii. New haustral contractions then appear after few minutes in near vicinity of previous haustrated area. This entire process leads to 'duging' and 'rolling' of faecal matter.

Peristalsis: It is a propulsive movement consist of those which propel the colonic contents analward and includes mass peristalsis with itself. Its forward progress depends on integrity of myenteric plexus. It is of great intensity in descending colon. Slow weak peristaltic movements have been reported in transverse colon along with alternating shortening and elongation.

Gastro-colic reflex: Increases in colonic motor activity following a meal. Even sight/smell/taste of food can induce this reflex.

Gastro-ileal-Reflex: Terminal ileum becomes hyperactive following meal. Its purpose is to drive gastric contents and ileal contents into caecum.

Notes

i. Colon agitates its contents by means of segmenting contractions like of small intestine; Haustral contractions in which colonic walls roll back and forth; Kneading movements in which large segments can contract while adjacent segments are relaxing to be followed by contraction and relaxation in reverse phase, and lastly by means of alternate peristalsis and anti-peristalsis.

DEFECATION

i. Usual stimulus is taking a glass of water (warm), or a cup of tea or coffee, or smoking cigarette. Defecation act is also induced by many persons by straining efforts which may raise the mercury pressure by 200 mmHg.
ii. It further consists of voluntary effort which is due to a particular posture which causes voluntary relaxation of external anal sphincter and compression of abdominal contents due to straining efforts.
iii. This reflex is under voluntary control. Centres are located in hypothalamus in lower lumbar and upper sacral segments of spinal cord and in ganglionic plexus of gut.
iv. *Defecation reflex:* Rectum is usually empty. When it receives faecal matter its walls are distended and initiates afferent impulses which travels through myenteric plexus to give birth to peristaltic waves in descending and sigmoid colon. In this way faecal matter is pushed or forced towards the anus. If external anal sphincter is relaxed, defecation occurs.
Initially this defecation reflex is weak. It is gaining more intensity through spinal cord (sacral segments) because afferents from distended rectum are reaching to this place of the cord. Spinal cord, in turn, send impulses back to sigmoid, descending colon and rectum through parasympathetic nerves, which finally leads to intensification of peristaltic waves.
v. Some persons are in a habit of straining effort. They take a deep breath, closes glottis and they force the abdominal muscles to contract. In this way faecal contents are pulled downwards.

LARGE INTESTINE : AT A GLANCE

i. It has been made 'seat of absorption' by Nature. It includes absorption of water, saline, glucose, amino acids and certain drugs like anaesthetics. 60-80 per cent water is absorbed here and therefore stools are formed.
ii. It is also a 'residence of bacteria of friendly attitude.' This 'bacterial flora' synthesises vitamin K, folic acid, B complex vitamins etc.
iii. It is also a place of secretion of mucus which is a famous lubricant. It has an alkaline reaction of pH 8.4.

ILEOCAECAL VALVE : AT A GLANCE

i. The wall of the ileum for several centimetres immediately preceding the ileocaecal valve has a thickened muscular coat called 'Ileocaecal sphincter.'
ii. It serves following important functions viz.
   a. To prevent the contents of ileum from passing into caecum before completion of digestive processes; and
   b. To prevent backflow of faecal contents from colon into small intestine. In this way small intestine is prevented from contamination.
iii. It is an oval or round opening from 2-3 cm in diameter situated in the centre of a small papillae. When it is tightly closed it does not allow passage of a finger even.
iv. It can resist reverse pressure of 50-60 cm of water. Emotions, excitement or swallowing of food increase the frequency of ejection.

CONSTIPATION

i. Accumulation of large quantities of dry and hard faeces in descending colon and this leads to slow movements of faeces through the large intestine. This is constipation.
ii. Neglecting the call to defecate' is the primary cause of constipation. If rectal contents are increased from 15-25 ml a natural desire for defecation is generated. If one is not visiting the toilet at this movement, the adaptation to this level is produced and then one requires some increase in pressure to provoke an urge. If this continues, then irritability of rectum is so reduced that an urge is no longer felt. This is the basis of constipation and at this stage one requires the use of a 'cathartic.'

DIARRHOEA

i. It is opposite of constipation which means rapid movement of faecal matter through the large intestine.
ii. During examination time, a student going for examination suffer from diarrhoea. Same thing happens with soldier going to battle ground or an unemployed man going for interview before a 'board.' All this is classed as 'nervous or emotional diarrhoea.' Emotional states lead to excessive stimulation of parasympathetic nervous system which leads to increased motility and secretion of mucus in colon, and it is also associated with loss of large quantities of water and electrolytes.

Infections diarrhoea is the main. Due to any sort of infection in large intestine; the mucous membrane is irritated which leads to increased secretion as well as motility. Due to increased propulsive movements this fluid is directed analwards.

GAS IN DIGESTIVE TRACT

i. Variable amount of gas is always reported in alimentary tract. Its main sources include swallowed air, gaseous formation due to bacterial action, and gases diffusing from blood to GI tract.
ii. The average composition is - CO_2-7.5 per cent, O_2-3 per cent, N_2-80 per cent, Methane-hydrogen etc. 9.5 per cent.
iii. Gases present in stomach include nitrogen and oxygen which are derived from swallowed air. In large intestine bacterial actions constitute the main source of gases and these are CO_2, methane and hydrogen. An explosive mixture is constituted by union of oxygen and methane + hydrogen.
iv. On an average daily 7 to 10 litres of gases are formed per day; but only 0.5-1 litre is expelled while remainder is absorbed by intestinal mucosa.
v. There are three possible sources of carbon dioxide
   a. Diffusion from blood into lumen;
   b. Neutralisation of acid by bicarbonate and
   c. Production by intestinal bacteria. This CO_2 is most predominant gas in flatus which results from ingestion of beans or other non-absorbable carbohydrates. Patients with small bowel disease may fail to absorb carbohydrates which normally are readily absorbed, and which leads to H_2 formation, Poorly absorbed proteins may also serve as substrate for bacterial fermentation and H_2 liberation. Methane (CH_4) formation has not been detected in children under 2 years of age and after this age, incidence of its production is increasing and climax is reached at ten years of age. Beans, cabbage, cauliflower, onion, corn, vinegar are amongst those foodstuffs which cause greater expulsion of flatus from large intestine.
vi. The highly emotional persons, when they hyperventilate they may swallow large amounts of air by process of eating/drinking. This is aerophagia. Some amount of it is regurgitated called belching.
vii. The gases are expelled out as flatus. Its characteristic smell is due to sulphides.
viii. This gas in intestine may cause cramps, rumbling noises (borborygmi) along with abdominal discomfort.

BACTERIAL ACTION IN LARGE BOWEL

- We don't live in a germ-free environment but in a world heavily populated by micro-organisms. It is true that we are being protected by these non-invasive micro-organisms normally populating skin and mucosal surface which are fighting against invasion by pathogenic organisms.

- They defend the body by two ways
  a. *Direct:* Which includes process like bacteriocidin production, depletion of essential nutrients, degradation of toxins, induction of low oxidation - reduction potential, and
  b. *Indirect:* Enhancement of antibody production, phagocyte stimulation, augmentation of interferon production etc. They also synthesise vitamins specially B_{12}, B_1, B_2, K.
- Some bacteria synthesise vitamin B complex and K as well as folic acid.
- It is the bile pigment from intestinal bacteria which provides brown colour to the stools. In their absence, the stools may be white.
- Some of the gases of the flatus are formed by bacteria. They also form organic acids from carbohydrates— so pH of stool is 5-7.0. They also play their role in cholesterol metabolism.
- They produce indole, skatol, sulphides which give aromatic odour to the stools.
- Ammonia is produced and absorbed in colon. In diseases of liver this is not damaged, which leads to hepatic-encephalopathy.
- They are E. coli, E. aerogenes, bacteroides fragilis, gas gangrene bacilli.

FAECES AT A GLANCE

- Total amount— 75-170 gm daily on average diet.
- pH— 7.0 to 7.5.
- Water— 70-75 per cent; solids 25-30 per cent.
- Organic constituents— cellulose, proteins and fats.
- Inorganic constituents— Calcium phosphate and oxalate, iron phosphate.
- Enzymes— Pancreatic amylase and trypsin, maltase, sucrase, lipase, lysozyme, nuclease.
- Brown colour is due to 'stercobilin and urobilin' the derivatives of bilirubin.
- Aromatic unpleasant odour is due to Indole, skatol, hydrogen sulphide and mercaptans.
- Average fats are: neutral fat 7.3 per cent of dry weight of faeces; free fatty acids 5.6 per cent; and soaps 4.6 per cent.
- Others— Desquamated epithelial cells, mucus, unabsorbed intestinal secretions.

BLIND LOOP SYNDROME

- It is a surgical operation in which blind loop of small intestine is constructed.
- Symptoms like macrocytic anaemia, vitamin B_{12} malabsorption, steatorrhoea appear.
- It is because of overgrowth of intestinal flora. Though they are symbiotic but also follows "excess of every thing is bad."
- The ingested vitamin B_{12} is taken up by these bacteria and so its deficiency leads to anaemia. These bacteria also cause excessive hydrolysis of conjugated bile salts. It constitutes the cause of steatorrhoea.

SUMMARY AND HIGHLIGHTS

MOVEMENTS OF SMALL INTESTINE

1. *Segmentation:* A portion of intestine is divided into segments. Contraction is at the site of maximum relaxation. Contraction is followed by relaxation. A segment is halved and halved unite to form a new segment. It is myogenic, independent of nerves. Duodenum 17/minute, ileum 12/minute. It is fundamental property of intestinal circular muscles. Its purpose includes proper mixing of food with digestive juices and facilitation of proper absorption and an improvement in intestinal circulation.
2. *Peristalsis:* Caused by both nervous and chemical factors (neurogenic) dependent on myenteric plexus. Its purpose is the propagation of food onwards. It consists of a composite wave made up of a wave of relaxation and contraction which follows law of intestine.

BIBLIOGRAPHY

1. Ardran GM, et al. The protection of laryngeal airway during swallowing. British Journal of Radiology 1952;25:406-16.
2. Bass P, Code CF, Lambert EH. Motor and electric activity of duodenum. Amer J Phy 1961,201:287.
3. Bosma JF. Deglutition: pharyngeal stage. Phy Rev 1957;37:275-300.
4. Bosma JF. Symposium on oral sensation and perception. Springfield III : Thomas. 1967.
5. Christenson J. The Control of gastrointestinal movements : some old and new views. New Eng J of Medicine 1971;285:85-98.
6. Christenson J, et al. The small intestinal basic electrical rhythm (slow wave) frequency gradient in normal men and in patients with a variety of disease. Gastroenterology 1966;50:309-15.
7. Fyke FE, et al. Resting and deglutition pressure in pharyngo oesophageal region. Gastroentrology 1955;24:29.
8. Giannella RA. Pathogenesis of acute bacterial diarrhoeal disorders. Ann Rev Med 1981;32:341.
9. Gonella J, et al. Extrinsic nervous control of motility of small and large intestine and related sphincters. Phy Rev 1987;67:902.
10. High Tower NC. Jr. Motility of alimentary canal of man. In disturbances in Gastrointestinal motility. Charles C Thomas springfield III. 1959.
11. Weisbrodt NW. Gastro intestinal motility quoted by Ganong WF in Review of Medical Physiology - Lange Publications. Ann Rev Phy 1981;43:7.

91 Digestion and Absorption

DIGESTION OF CARBOHYDRATES

i. *Digestion in mouth*: First of all when food is in mouth it is acted upon by saliva which contains 'amylase or ptyalin enzyme' which causes hydrolysis of starch to maltose. This can be personally felt by chewing bread piece for minutes together and then sweet taste is produced owing to liberation of maltose from starch. Since all natural starch are having a cellulose covering which cannot be digested so ptyalin will only act when this protective covering is destroyed by cooking. Two types of amylase has been found 'a-amylase' (acting at random inside polysaccharide molecule resulting in formation of maltose and glucose) and β-amylase (acts on polysaccharide molecule resulting in formation of quantitative amount of maltose only).

ii. *Digestion in stomach*: The digestion by salivary amylase continues even food has left mouth and entered stomach. It continues almost upto 30 to 50 minutes till the medium becomes acidic since it cannot act when pH falls below 4.

iii. *Digestion by pancreatic amylase*: As food leaves the stomach and reaches intestine pancreatic amylase is mixed with it which is actually more powerful than salivary amylase because it can even digest uncooked starch. So the starches which were not splitted by saliva are digested here with formation of maltose and isomaltose.

iv. *Intestinal digestion*: Maltase forms two molecules of glucose, 'sucrase' forms one molecule of glucose and fructose each by acting on sucrose, 'lactase' acts on lactose forming one molecule of glucose and galactose each.

The final products of digestion is monosaccharides which are then absorbed.

DIGESTION OF PROTEINS

Actually proteins are made of long chain of amino acids united together by so-called 'peptide linkages' and this site is attacked by digestive enzymes which are named 'peptidases.' Two types of such enzymes are known, one being 'endopeptidase' (splitting peptide linkage in interior of the molecule) and another being 'exopeptidase' (acting on peripheral peptide linkage).

i. Since no proteolytic enzyme is present in saliva, these foodstuffs are not acted upon by saliva.

ii. *Digestion in stomach*: Pepsin, Rennin, gastricin and other proteolytic enzymes are present in gastric juice out of which pepsin is the main. Pepsin is acting on all proteins (native as well denatured) in acidic media producing 'proteoses,' 'peptones' as well as acid metaproteins, through hydrolysis process existing at peptide linkages between amino acids. if food remains in stomach for a shorter time, more 'proteoses' are formed and conversely if it remain for longer duration of time more peptones are formed. The striking thing is that this enzyme can also act on 'collagen' which is a major constitutent of all intercellular connective tissue of meats and astonishing view further is that it is very little effected by other enzymes.

iii. *Digestion by Pancreatic juice*: When proteins in form of peptones, proteoses, polypeptides etc. leave the stomach and enter the intestine they are acted upon by 'pancreatic TRYPSIN' which exerts dual action—hydrolysis of all partially broken down products of protein as well as some of them are hydrolyzed to final amino acid stage. Another enzyme 'chymotrypsin' present here is catalysing the hydrolysis process of different peptide linkages almost acting similar with trypsin. 'Carboxy polypeptidases present here is capable of hydrolyzing polypeptides to amino acid. This enzyme is of A and B type and is converted into active state by trypsin whereas type A acting on peptides having aromatic side chain while type B is acting on peptides having terminal arginine or lysine residue.

iv. *Digestion by succus entericus*: The enzyme responsible for final hydrolysis are mentioned as 'amino polypeptidases', dipeptidases, (they break tri and di peptides respectively to monopeptides which are then attacked by carboxy peptidases, and these peptidases finally breaks peptide linkage to free amino acids). Enzyme 'erepsin' is, in fact name given to mixture of all peptidases and responsible for finishing digestion process by forming amino acids.

v. *Digestion of nucleoproteins*: Protein from nucleic acid is splitted by pepsin and then chain of react on is

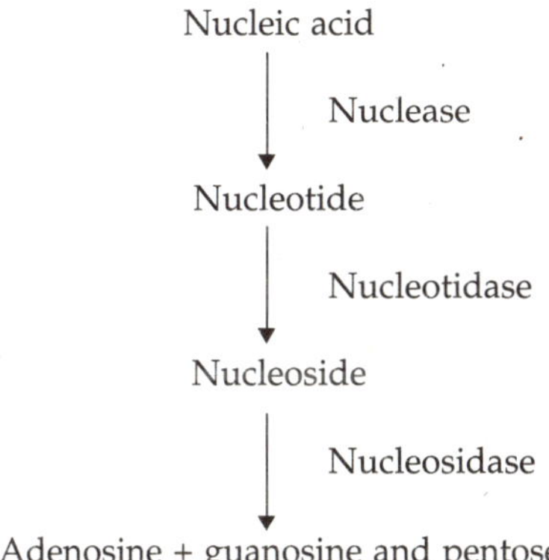

Almost all proteins are changed into amino acid while very few remains as peptone, proteoses, polypeptides while very few are not digested at all—is taken as conclusion.

DIGESTION OF FATS

All triglycerides of diet are finally broken into fatty acid and glycerol.

i. Since no fat splitting enzyme is found in saliva so fatty foodstuffs are not acted upon here. Of course, 'Lingual lipase' is first enzyme which hydrolyzes triglycerides. It can act within the stomach.

ii. *Digestion in stomach*: Though fat splitting enzyme lipase is present here but is comparatively very weak. Its action is also doubtful since its action is best reported in neutral medium (it is to be remembered that gastric juice is highly acidic) and it best acts on fine emulsified fat molecules.

iii. *Digestion by pancreatic lipase*: It is most potent, activated by intestinal juice. It is said to be of two type, one is esterases (acting on esters of monovalent alcohols) while other is acting on glyceryl ester of higher fatty acids and cholesterol esters. Another enzyme present here is phospholipase A which is capable of converting lecithin into lysolecithin which is known as detergent as well food fat emulsifier. Intestinal lipase acts similarly to cause fat's hydrolysis.

iv. *Role of bile*: Most important function in this series is performed by 'bile salts' and that is emulsification which means breaking fat globules into smaller sizes to enable digestive enzymes to act on fat globular surfaces. This important function is performed by bile salts through mechanism by reducing interfacial tension of fat which is achieved by their own structure, i.e. carboxyl part of bile salt is water soluble while sterol part is fat soluble and with this property upper action is achieved when bile salts aggregate at fat globular surface. Now when this interfacial tension is low even the nonsoluble fluid is broken down into small particles (which might have been more difficult if this tension is high), and every time diameter of fat globules is decreased almost fifty per cent.

INTESTINAL ABSORPTION: A REVIEW STUDY (Fig. 91.1)

There exists three structural peculiarities in tube-like small intestine, namely:

i. *Finger-like villi*: Projections of mucosal layer, 1 mm in length, more frequent in duodenum and jejunum than in ileum;

ii. *Valvulae conniventes (kerkering)* which are nothing but prominent mucosal folds in duodenum and jejunum more and less frequent in ileum.

iii. *Striated border of upper part of absorptive epithelium and consists of microvilli:* (1 μ long and 0.1 μ wide) and their number is 1,700 per cell. Human columnar cell is 25-30 μ in height and its width is less than one-third of its length. It becomes more taller as it migrates towards villus. Mucous secreting duodenal glands are classed as mucoid as compared with goblet cells which are purely mucous cells.

CARBOHYDRATE ABSORPTION

i. They are absorbed in the forms of monosaccharides.

ii. Absorption of monosaccharides is a complex process, viz.

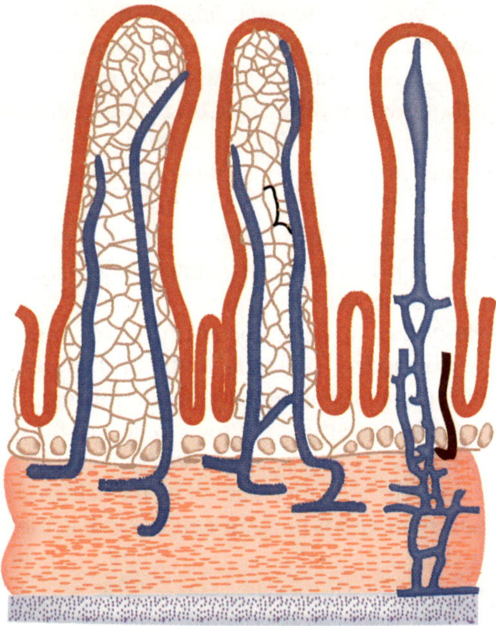

Fig. 91.1: Intestinal absorption

a. *Specificity*: The process of absorption represents a high degree of chemical specificity, since hexoses are absorbed at different rates, glucose and galactose are absorbed at similar rate but faster than mannose while fructose occupies intermediate position.

b. *Saturation:* The rate of absorption of some sugars does not increase proportionally with increase in concentration but approaches a maximum rate at high concentration.

c. *Competition*: The rate of absorption of one sugar can be reduced by presence of another sugar. This establishes a competition for a specific site in transport process.

d. *Inhibition*: The absorption of sugar can be inhibited by some of metabolic inhibitors interfering with the production and utilisation of energy. They include 'iodoacetate and fluoride' (which reduce glycolysis), fluoroacetate, malonate and arsenite' (exerting effect on citric acid cycle), 'dinitrophenol and chlorbutorl' (which uncouple oxidative phosphorylation; and an aerobiosis which blocks citric acid cycle), 'phlorrhizin' (exert an effect by acting on a mechanism responsible for glucose movement across the membrane on luminal side of the epithelial cell and also by inhibiting aerobic oxidation).

e. *Ionic dependence*: Absorption of sugar is mainly influenced by sodium ion. In support of this view—ouabain—an inhibitor of sodium movement in several tissues including intestine, also inhibits sugar absorption. Na^+ dependent mobile carrier system exists for sugar transport in brush border membrane. It was concluded by Robert Crane (1960) that two steps are occurring in active transport of sugars:
   - An energy independent but sodium ion dependent entrance into cell with considerable specificity, and
   - Energy and sodium ion dependent intracellular accumulation of sugar against a concentration difference. Potassium is not affecting more but transport is not dependent on K concentration but on Na:K concentration ratio.

f. *Active transport*: During absorptive process, active transport is said to occur. According to some physiologists 70-80 per cent of glucose disappearing from intestine is accounted for as glucose in mesenteric venous blood; 7-17 per cent as lactic acid and insignificant amount as CO_2, alanine and pyruvic acid. So it was concluded that glucose entered the mesenteric blood when blood glucose concentration was higher than luminal concentration.

g. *Electrical activity*: Some alterations in electrical activity of intestine has been observed during absorption of sugars.

iii. *Mechanism of monosaccharides*: It is mainly based on carrier hypothesis. A carrier is coupled with a energy source (usually sodium) which affects the supply of energy from ATP to transport process through influencing the activity of membrane ATPase. According to Crane, R.K. (1962) this sodium-sugar-carrier complex moves across luminal membrane in response to the difference in sodium concentration between lumen and the cell. It is further stated that concentration of sodium influences the affinity of the carrier for sugar.

iv. Absorption of sugar takes place only from small intestine. Gradient of glucose utilisation is exactly proportional to gradient of absorbing surface but gradient of glucose absorption rises sharply with distance from ileocaecal valve.

v. Effect of temperature has been studied. At low temperature absorption ceases or better to say cells at low temperature become relatively impermeable to sugars. Similarly optimal pH of the intestinal contents for absorption to occur lies near neutrality and buffers are rapidly neutralised by intestinal secretion.

vi. No role of hormones of adrenal cortex in active absorption of sugar.

Absorption: General view	
Substances absorbed	*Quantity per day*
Carbohydrate	250-450 gm (Sugar 120 g/h maximum rate of absorption)
Fat	100-160 gm
Amino acid	50-100 gm
Ions	50-100 gm
Water	7-8 litres

vii. *Absorption of disaccharides*: Sucrose absorption is dependent on concentration on mucosal side and is not actively absorbed. The activity of disaccharide splitting enzyme is reported to be greatesc in duodenum, and it decreases rapidly with distance from pylorus.

viii. *Fructose absorption*: It is not actively absorbed. It is however converted into glucose up to large extent and then absorbed. "Phlorizin" does not inhibit fructose absorption and, nitrogen and dinitrophenol inhibit the conversion of fructose to glucose but not its absorption. Fructose must be phosphorylated in order to pass through the epithelial layer. There are possibly two pathways for its conversion to glucose; first; in which initial reaction is formation of fructose-6-phosphate catalysed by hexokinase and second; in which fructose-1-phosphate is catalysed by fructokinase. It does not require metabolic energy for transport; but it requires a carrier system.

GLUCOSE/GALACTOSE ABSORPTION: SODIUM ROLE (SODIUM CO-TRANSPORT/SECONDARY ACTIVE TRANSPORT OF GLUCOSE)

A carrier protein for transport of glucose/galactose is present in brush border of epithelial cell. Glucose transport will not occur in the absence of sodium transport, i.e. carrier will also refuse to work in that situation. Both these are coupled together so they move with each other. Or in other words, glucose is dragged along with sodium. This increases intra-cellular glucose concentration more than normal level. It so then diffuses through basolateral membrane of epithelial cell into extracellular fluid by process of facilitated diffusion.

GLUCOSE TRANSPORTERS

1. SGLT 1 (Sodium dependent): It causes active uptake of dietary glucose from lumen of small intestine. Its usual sites are small intestine and kidney.
2. GLUT 1 (Facilitative glucose transporter): It causes basal uptake of glucose by cells as well as its transport across blood tissue barriers. Placenta, brain, kidney and colon are its usual sites.
3. GLUT 2 (Facilitative glucose transporter): It causes uptake and release of glucose across blood tissue barriers. Its usual sites include liver, pancreas, small intestine, kidney.
4. GLUT 3: It too is facilitative glucose transporter. It causes basal uptake of glucose by all cells along with brain. Brain, placenta and kidney are its usual site.
5. GLUT 4: It causes insulin stimulated glucose uptake. Skeletal and cardiac muscle are its usual site.
6. GLUT 5: Its site is jejunum. It causes sugar absorption from lumen of small intestine.

GLUCOSE TRANSPORTERS

- Glucose transport is an example of secondary, active transport. The transport of some sugar is directly affected by amount of sodium ion on intestinal lumen, i.e. a high concentration of Na^+ on mucosal surface of cell will facilitate; while a low concentration of Na^+ will inhibit sugar molecule's movement into the epithelial cell. This means, glucose and Na^+ share the same co-transporter. This molecule is SGLT-1, (sodium dependent - glucose transporter).
- Intracellular Na^+ is low in cells of intestine and kidney. Na^+ moves into the cells along its concentration gradient. Glucose moves with Na^+ and is released in the cell. Na^+ is transported into intercellular spaces and glucose is transported by GLUT-2 into interstitium and then in the blood.
- If this co-transporter of Na^+ and glucose is defective then diarrhoea results.

ABSORPTION OF FATS

a. Lipase hydrolyzes triglyceride by acting superficially on α ester bonds and form free fatty acid and monoglyceride. The extent of hydrolysis is dependent on amount of lipase, pH, presence of bile salts etc.

b. Entry into mucosal cell: Cell membrane engulfes small lipid droplets present at base of villi to get them entered into cell by a process of pinocytosis. Fat enter the cell mainly as fatty acid and monoglyceride with very little amount of diglyceride and unhydrolyzed triglyceride. This mechanism is energy dependent. Within the cell, the droplets are surrounded by endoplasmic reticulum.

c. Resynthesis of triglyceride takes place after entering the mucosa. For it fatty acids needs activation to form 'acyl Co A' which changes it into triglycerides in the presence of 'glycerophosphate'. To conclude, this resynthesis of triglyceride involves two steps (i) formation of a new glyceride-glycerol backbone by acylate of L-3 glycerophosphate, (ii) utilisation of dietary glyceride glycerol backbone by direct acylation of absorbed monoglycerides by fatty acids. Intra-cellular triglyceride synthesis from fatty acids and partial glycerides in intestinal mucosa may be facilitated by conjugated bile salts.

d. Chylomicron
   - Protein coating of chylomicron represents a specific synthetic step and is not a simple adsorption of protein on to a triglyceride emulsion. Moreover this protein covering helps in exit of chylomicron from epithelial cell.
   - Long chain fatty acids are transported by lymphatic route after being esterified by intestinal mucosa, while short chain fatty acids (which are poorly esterified and more water soluble) pass through the mucosal cell and are transported by the portal vein; while medium chain triglycerides can be transported by either route. The factors affecting this partition between blood and lymph are not known.
   - Muscle contraction of stomach—particularly peristalsis against a closed pylorus and squirting of fat through a partially opened pyloric canal—produce the shear forces sufficient for emulsification. The major source of gastric lipolytic activity originates in a group of serous glands beneath the circumvallate papillae of the tongue.
   - The products of large intestinal bacterial fermentation include volatile fatty acids namely acetate, propionate and butyrate. Most of them are absorbed across the colonic wall and could provide appreciable metabolizable energy for humans whose diet contain large amount of plant fibre. The upper gut of average healthy person absorbs over 98 per cent of the ≅ 150 g of lipid ingested as well as 15-40 gm of endogenous lipid (biliary, sloughed cell and secretion) entering the intestinal lumen. There is no evidence of absorption of fat (long chained lipids) in the colon. During transit many bacterial modification occur viz. hydrolysis of glycerides, phospholipids, cholesterol ester by bacterial lipases, hydroxylation of double bond of fatty acids and dehydrogenation, epimerization and deconjugation of bile salts.

e. This is greatest in upper parts of small intestine but ileum also absorbs a significant amount.

f. According to one data, 95 per cent of ingested fat is absorbed, only 5 per cent of fat is contained by stools. Faecal fat is derived from cellular debris and micro-organisms.

g. Infants are unable to absorb 10-15 per cent of fats which they ingested. So it is said that process of fat absorption is not completely mature at birth.

h. Cholesterol is readily absorbed by small intestine. But closely related sterols of plant origin are poorly absorbed. A pretty significant amount is incorporated in chylomicrons which enter the circulation.

Theories of Fat Absorption

1. *Lipolytic theory (Pfluger, Verzar and McDoughall 1936)*
   - All fat is hydrolysed in the intestine to fatty acids and glycerol by the action of lipase (gastric pancreatic, intestinal).
   - Prior to hydrolysis the fat is emulsified by the action of bile; and after sometimes by soaps produced by the interaction of liberated fatty acids with the alkali of intestinal fluids.
   - Fatty acids are made soluble chiefly through formation of complexes with the bile acids, glycocholic and taurocholic acid. These complexes enter the mucosal cells where bile acids are split off and mostly they are returned to the lumen.
   - The fatty acids are recombined with glycerol to form triglycerides which are transferred to lymphatics then after.
   - Process of phosphorylation is essential to the synthesis of triglycerides.
   - Some fatty acids may be absorbed through portal vein.

Lipolytic theory

Dietary triglycerides

↓ Lipolysis (Lumen)

Glycerol

| Re-synthesis (Cell)

2. *Partition hypothesis (Frazer, 1946)*
   - Bile and soap are not adequate emulsifying agents under the conditions found in the intestine because of acid reaction in duodenum.
   - According to him, the important step in the process is not lipolysis, but emulsification.
   - The chylomicrons are small fat particles, not exceeding 0.5 μ in diameter. They enter the

epithelial cells as triglycerides and are directly transferred to lymphatics. Each chylomicron is having a coating consisting of lipoprotein and phospholipid.

- According to him, resynthesis of fat in epithelial cell is not a necessary step in this process.

Partition hypothesis

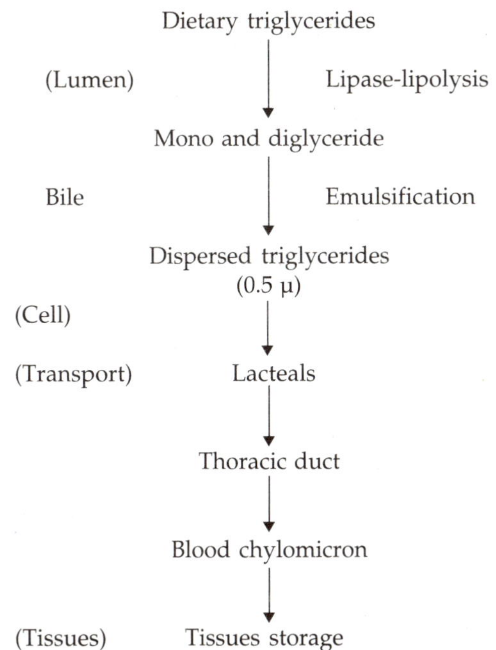

Source: Turner (1958) Amer J Dig Dis 8:594

Modified view

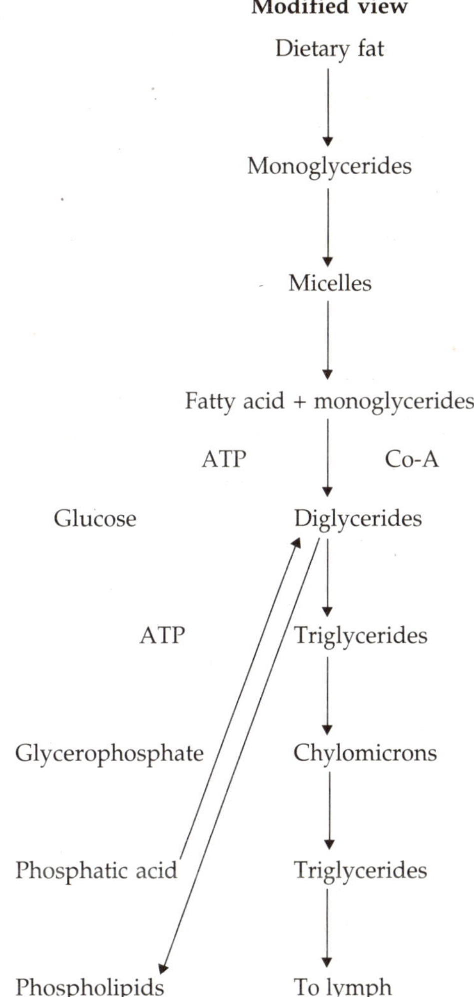

Source: Issel Bacher and Senior (1964) Gastroenterology 46:287.

3. *Modified view:*
   - Ingested fat is hydrolysed in upper small bowel by action of pancreatic lipase in presence of bile acids. Pancreatic lipase having affinity with triglycerides; produce free fatty acids and β-monoglycerides. Probably only 20-50 per cent of glycerides in the diet are completely hydrolysed to free fatty acids and glycerol.
   - These free fatty acids + monoglycerides combine with conjugated bile salts present, to form "micelles"—which are extremely small fat particles. They are not abundantly containing di-triglyceride+ cholesterol. Fat in this form is ready to be absorbed by epithelial surface. The conjugated bile acids are turned back to the lumen of the gut and are reused in the formation of new micelles.
   - Main function of small intestine is re-synthesis of triglycerides from fatty acids and monoglycerides and they are in the form of chylomicrons. The synthesis of triglyceride requires energy which is supplied in the form of ATP from glycolysis or oxidative phosphorylation. Mg^+ and CoA are also required.
   - The fatty acids are first activated by CoA. So they become more reactive and water soluble. Glycerophosphatate (is formed as a result of glucose breakdown) combines with activated fatty acids to form phosphatic acid which then changes into diglycerides which are then esterified to triglycerides/phospholipids. The process of forming triglycerides directly from monoglycerides is called mono-glyceride shunt. If activated fatty acids are not available for combining with monoglycerides, then they can be hydrolyzed into glycerol and fatty acid.

- The chylomicrons are covered by a fine coating of proteins. This protein covering amounts to less than one percent of the weight of chylomicron. They leave the epithelial cell at the level of nucleus passing into intercellular spaces. They pass across the basement membrane and into lymphatic vessels by passage between endothelial cells.
- Fats are mainly absorbed by upper small intestine. It is seriously affected on adrenalectomy because of deprivation of steroids + loss of salt.

Cholesterol Absorption

- Normally 2-3 gm of it is absorbed by small bowel per day (0.5 gm in diet per day + 2-3 gm endogenous cholesterol coming from bile, and desquamated epithelial cell).
- Bile and pancreatic lipase play a leading role in its absorption. In absence or deficiency of either of the two, the mechanism is seriously affected. Fat in the diet stimulate cholesterol absorption.
- Cholesterol in diet is in the form of esters. In small intestine they are hydrolysed by cholesterol esterase present in pancreatic juice. These are not as readily absorbed as free cholesterol.
- Once inside the cell (by simple process of diffusion) cholesterol is slowly esterified, then released for transport via lymphatic to thoracic duct.

ABSORPTION OF PROTEINS

i. Dietary proteins are normally hydrolyzed within the lumen of alimentary canal and are absorbed mostly as amino acid or small peptide units.

ii. Competition has been demonstrated between different amino acids in absorption. Four groups of amino acids have been distinguished namely—neutral (monoamino-monocarboxylic), basic, dicarboxylic (absorbed passively) and N-methylated acids.

iii. The absorption is specific and not a matter of simple diffusion. Two mechanisms of absorption have been extensively studied—first relates to mechanism of active transport and second relates to the bio-directional flux mechanism which establishes a steady state amino acid distribution ratio between intra- and extra-cellular compartments.

   a. Active transport of neutral amino acid: In one of the studies it was noted that effective inhibition among four of neutral amino acid occurs—glycine, L-proline, L-methionene and L-leucine and all were actively transported. All four were judged to share a common carrier mechanism for which methionene and leucine had much stronger affinity. Additional carrier for glycine and proline was suggested. Methionene has exerted a greater inhibitory effect on the transfer of glycine and proline than did glycine or proline on the transfer of methionene.

   b. Active transport of three diamino mono-carboxylic acids—L-lysine, L-ornithine and L-arginine has been studied. The dibasic amino acids are believed to share a common transport system since they represent competitive inhibition in intestine as well as in kidney cortex. It is also true that some of the neutral amino acids have an affinity for this carrier mechanism and will inhibit transport of dibasic forms in varying degrees.

iv. Protein passes more or less continuously into the alimentary tract in the form of digestive enzymes, mucoproteins and serum proteins. It appears that food protein is swamped by endogenous sources of protein and endogenous protein is more slowly digested than exogenous proteins.

v. It declines with age.

vi. Protein absorption also gives rise to food allergies after eating certain foods. Absorption of protein antigens (bacterial and viral proteins) take place in M cells (microfold cells); which are specialised intestinal epithelial cells and are overlying the "Peyer's patches' of intestine. They activate lymphoblasts which secret IgA in response to subsequent exposure to the same antigen.

vii. Absorption of amino acid is rapid in duodenum and jejunum but slow in ileum. Some of the ingested protein enters the colon and is digested by bacterial action. The protein in stool is not of dietary origin but is coming from bacteria and cellular debris.

viii. A congenital defect in transport of basic amino acid leads to cystinurea. "Hartnup disease" is the name given to a congenital defect in mechanism of transport of neutral amino acids in intestine and kidney tubules.

ix. A neutral amino acid carrier, a phenylalanine and a methionene carrier, and an amino acid carrier in brush border, are sodium dependent. The sodium in dependent carriers in brush border are carrier for basic amino acid and a carrier for neutral amino acid which prefers hydropic side chains.

x. The transported amino acid + those produced by intracellular hydrolysis of di and tripeptides accumulate first in mucosal cells and then by way of diffusion/facilitated diffusion, etc. they enter ECF. The small peptides entering the portal blood include proline, hydroxyproline, carnosine and anserine etc.

xi. Glutamic and aspartic acid may undergo transamination with pyruvic acid so that alanine is produced and released into portal blood. Transamination is complete if absorption rate is slow; while it is less during rapid absorption rate. Thus, the mucosa of intestine is capable to modify a particular amino acid mixture, i.e. amount can be reduced if it is already more in digestive mixtures and vice versa.

xii. During the process of absorption amino acid accumulate in mucosal cell. It may raise their intracellular concentration as compared with lumen. With accumulation within the cell, a favourable concentration gradient is established for diffusion out of the cell into portal blood.

xiii. Peptidases of intestinal secretion are intracellular enzymes which appear in the secretion as a result of breakdown of shaded epithelial cell (not actually secreted). Peptide can get through the epithelial cell in considerable quantity without being reduced to amino acid.

xiv. Native proteins are absorbed through a process of pinocytosis.

xv. "Phloridzin" which inhibit glucose absorption does not interfere with amino acid absorption. Amino acids are said to compete with sugars, i.e. sugars are absorbed more slowly from a sugar amino acid mixture than from a pure sugar solution.

ABSORPTION OF VITAMINS

a. Vitamin B_{12}: This vitamin is confined to animal food stuffs. Its requirement is about 1 µg per day. It is highly stored in liver (2000 µg lasting for several years). Intrinsic factor is produced in fundus and body of stomach by acid secreting parietal cells. It is mucopolypeptides or mucoproteins of high molecular weight. It promotes absorption of vitamin B_{12} as well as possessing a powerful binding ability for the vitamin B_{12}. According to many investigators ileum is the main site for intrinsic factor dependent vitamin B_{12} absorption but it is also evident that some absorption might occur in upper small intestine. The stages of absorption are:
   i. Separation of vitamin from material which are binding it and binding it with intrinsic factor.
   ii. Attachment of B_{12} intrinsic factor complex to special sites on luminal membrane of intestinal epithelial cells. This step requires calcium ions.
   iii. Transport into cell by mechanism still not known but possibly may be pinocytosis.

b. There occurs rapid absorption of ascorbic acid from proximal small intestine and absorptive capacity is high.

c. Thiamine is also rapidly absorbed from proximal small intestine but absorptive capacity is restricted. Riboflavin and pyridoxin are absorbed from upper small intestine.

d. Free folic acid is rapidly absorbed from proximal small intestine with a large absorptive capacity.

e. Absorption of water soluble vitamin is rapid. If absorption of fat is depressed, then absorption of fat soluble vitamin will also be depressed.

f. Most vitamins are absorbed in upper small intestine.

ABSORPTION: REMARKS

i. The primary function of intestine is absorption of nutrients, salts and water. These molecules move across the epithelium by several carrier mediated or passive transport mechanisms. The substances then enter the interstitial space and are carried away by the blood flow near the absorptive site. Epithelial transport can be divided into facilitated, carrier mediated transcellular transport through the membranes of the cell and passive paracellular transport through the tight junction and lateral space. In general, blood flow acts on carrier mediated transcellular transport through delivery of oxygen to support cell metabolism.

ii. The simple physico-chemical or biophysical forces governing the process of absorption includes diffusion.

iii. Regulation of blood flow and absorption:
   a. *Glucagon* - It can decrease intestinal absorption despite an increase in total blood flow and oxygen consumption and it is suggestive of a cholinergic mechanism of action. It increases total intestinal blood and lymph flow, capillary pressure and permeability. Increased capillary permeability to macromolecules, an increased capillary hydraulics, conductance and increased capillary hydrostatic pressure are primary mechanisms by which glucagon alters capillary fluid balance.
   b. *Somatostatin:* This increases net Na and Cl absorption across rat ileum. In human, it decreases jejunal glucose and amino acid absorption without affecting net Na and water absorption. It decreases total gut blood flow and glucose

absorption in diabetics.

c. *Vasoactive Intestinal Polypeptide (VIP)*: It increases active chloride and sodium secretion *in vitro* via stimulation of a cyclic AMP mediated process and thus effects transcellular transport. *In vivo*, it reduces net sodium and water absorption or increased secretion from small intestine and colon.
d. *Opiates*: They don't increase absorption but can reduce secretion. It causes an increase in absorptive side blood flow which increases the washout of absorbed salt and water.
e. *Role of nerves*: Cholinergic stimuli and reduction of adrenergic stimuli reduce intestinal absorption or increase secretion; while, adrenergic stimuli or reduction of cholinergic stimuli increase absorption. Vasoconstriction and pale villi are observed on vagotomy while engorged and vasodilated villi are observed on sympathectomy.
f. *Prostaglandins*: It may increase intestinal secretion due to stimulation of cyclic AMP, as well as through increased hydrostatic capillary pressure. They act as a stimulus for functional hyperaemia following ingestion of food.

ABSORPTION IN COLON

- Its absorption capacity is great.
- Many compounds when administered by rectal route are absorbed rapidly by colon like steroids, sedatives, tranquillisers, anaesthetics etc.
- When enema is given to a constipated person, much water may be absorbed sometimes to cause water intoxication.
- Na^+ is actively transported out of colon and water follows along osmotic gradient. There is a net secretion of K^+ and HCO_3^- in the colon.

DIETARY FIBRE

- Cellulose, hemicellulose, lignin, various gums, algal polysaccharides, etc. are important component of dietary fibre.
- They reach to large intestine in an unchanged state because there occurs no appreciable digestion of these substances in human GIT.
- They increase the so-called "bulk." So they act as bulk laxative since they provide a larger volume of indigestible material to the colon.
- Persons taking large amounts of vegetable fibre may not suffer from cancer colon or diverticulitis, coronary artery diseases, or diabetes mellitus etc. The cause still remains to be searched.
- Some persons are able to break down this cellulose (a component of dietary fibre); so this bulk is reduced in amount. This causes a complaint of chronic constipation in them.

ABSORPTION OF ELECTROLYTES

i. In man, gastrointestinal secretions present to the intestine a daily load of water and salt which considerably exceeds the dietary intake.
ii. When hypotonic solutions are introduced in lumen, NaCl moves from the blood until the intestinal contents become isotonic while in lower small intestine, net absorption of NaCl occurs from hypotonic solution.
iii. There is a net transport of Na inwards across the cell from the lumen; which is continue although a potential difference exists across the whole wall. Whole of this phenomenon constitutes a movement against an electrochemical gradient which suggests of active transport of ion.
iv. Na transport depends upon cellular aerobic metabolism.
v. Intracellular accumulation and transport of amino acid and some sugars by intestine are closely linked to Na transport. Thus, transport of sugar and amino acid is stimulated when Na absorption is in progress and vice versa. The energy for all this is derived from movements of Na and K ions down an electrochemical gradient which is maintained by a process involving hydrolysis of ATP. Replacement of lumen Na by K will abolish the ionic gradient across the mucosal border of the cell and therefore abolish the transport of sugars and amino acid. So it is evident that, Cl and K transport are also coupled with Na.
vi. Cl transport can also follow Na translocation through the cell in a passive fashion. The rates of Na and Cl absorption differ and the difference depends upon site of absorption, e.g. in rats, Na is fastly absorbed in jejunum while Cl is fastly absorbed in ileum and colon.
vii. Intestinal mucosal cells possess high intracellular concentration of K ions. Maintenance of high cellular K in rat jejunal mucosal cell is dependent upon a cellular metabolism requiring glucose as substrate. Furthermore, it is said that sugars unable to act as substrate causes loss of K ions by the mucosa.
viii. The Basolateral membrane of intestinal absorptive cell contains Na-K-ATPase (The Na pump) and has a parallel K permeability. A large electrochemical

gradient for Na entry across the apical membrane is thus formed which facilitates secondary active absorption of a variety of ions and non-electrolytes. In Jejunum Na entry occurs by (i) Na/H exchange; (ii) Na substrate cotransport, (iii) Na and PO_4; Na and SO_4 cotransport. In mammalian ileum Na and Cl transport are linked and Na substrate mechanism is less prominent. Since acetazolamide (Carbonic anhydrase inhibitor) inhibits linked NaCl transport in brush border vesicles as well as in ileum, it becomes evident that carbonic anhydrase present in brush border membrane is involved in the process. The crypt is the major site of Cl secretion (goblet cells and immature columnar cells). Intracellular Ca^{2+} is a major regulator of mammalian electrolyte transport. In colon of rat and ileum of rabbit increasing cellular Ca^{2+} decreases neutral NaCl absorption but don't alter Na-glucose or Na-amino acid absorption. Ca^{2+} activates basolateral K conductance. Furthermore, intracellular calcium stores appear to be involved in regulation of basal and at least some stimulated electrolyte transport. Furthermore, increase in intestinal cyclic AMP alter active Na, Cl and K transport; cholera toxin, VIP, secretin, bile salts, prostaglandin PGE_2, ATP, ADP, AMP and adenosine etc. are agents which increase intestinal cyclic AMP and hence electrolyte transport.

Increase in cyclic AMP → inhibits linked NaCl absorption; and increase Cl and K secretion.

ix. Major root of K movement is active and transcellular and variety of agents are regulating this transcellular K fluxes. Active transport by colon is regulated by endogenous mediators via modulation of intracellular cyclic AMP and calcium levels.

x. When one becomes dehydrated, then adrenal glands start secreting hormone aldosterone in large quantities. It in turn, enhances all the enzymes and transport mechanisms for all aspects of sodium absorption by intestinal epithelial cells. Secondary absorption of chloride and water, etc. is also increased. This effect of aldosterone is specially important in colon because it allows no loss of sodium chloride in faeces + very little water loss.

xi. Active absorption of bicarbonate ions: They are abundantly present in pancreatic secretion and bile. On absorption of sodium ions, moderate amount of hydrogen ions are secreted into the gut lumen (exchange for sodium). Then these hydrogen ions combine with bicarbonate ions to form carbonic acid i.e. $H^+ + HCO_3^- = H_2CO_3$. It then dissociates as— $H_2CO_3 = H_2O + CO_2$. The water remains as a part of the chyme and CO_2 is readily absorbed into the blood and expired through the lungs.

xii. Why diarrhoea in cholera?: (a) Some immature epithelial cells are present deeply in crypts of Lieberkuhn. Normally they secret NaCl and water into the intestinal lumen. This secretion is immediately absorbed by older cells. (b) But on getting cholera infection; the toxin so liberated is attached with chloride channel proteins of crypt cells in apical membranes. This leads to rapid flow of chloride ions from interior of the cells to crypts. This in turn, activates the sodium pump which activates sodium ions to be pumped along with chloride ions. This accumulation of NaCl causes extreme osmosis of water into the crypts. All this results into very rapid flow of fluid along with the salt. On one side it may be helpful in excreting more bacteria while on another side it may cause dehydration.

xiii. Absorption of calcium:
- Active transport of Ca^{2+} out of intestinal lumen occurs in upper small intestine. Passive diffusion is also a route of absorption.
- This process of active transport is facilitated by 1, 25-dihydroxy cholecalciferol—a metabolite of vitamin D formed in the kidney.
- Its absorption depends upon its level in the blood. If its level is increased then absorption is decreased; if its level is decreased then absorption is elevated.
- Its absorption is inhibited by phosphates and oxalates since they form insoluble salts with Ca^{2+}.
- Proteins facilitate the absorption of magnesium.

ABSORPTION: IN NUTSHELL

Enterocytes are mucosal cells in intestine. Here they have a brush border made up of numerous microvilli lining their apical surface. Enzymes are in abundance in the brush border. The glycocalyx is the name given to a layer which is rich in neutral as well as amino sugar and is lining along luminal side. Next to it, is unstirred layer. Solutes have to diffuse across this layer to reach to mucous cells. Substances pass from lumen of GIT to interstitial fluid and then to the lymph and blood by diffusion, facilitated diffusion, active and secondary active transport and endocytosis etc.

BIBLIOGRAPHY

1. Bengt Borgstrom. The dimensions of bile salts micelle: measurements by gel filtration. Biochem Biophys Acta 106:171.
2. Bensen JA, et al. GIT absorption. Ann Rev Phy 1966;28:207.
3. Bernard Throens. Facilitated glucose transporters in epithelial cells. Ann Rev Phy 1993;55:591.
4. Brown AL. J Cell Bio 1962;12:623.
5. Burnant CF, et al. Fructose transporter in human spermatozoa and small intestine in GLUT 5. J Biol Chem 1992;267:14523.
6. Clark B, Hubscher G. Biochem Biophys Acta 1961;46:479.
7. Csaky TZ, Hara Y. Amer J Phy 1965;209:467.
8. Cummings JH. Scand J Gastroenterology (Supp) 1984;93:89. Colonic absorption: The importance of short chain fatty acids in man.
9. Curran PF, Macintosh JR. Nature Lond, 1962;193:347.
10. Wright EM. The intestinal Na^+/glucose co transporter (quoted by Ganong WF in Review of Medical Physiology - Lange Publications). Ann Rev Phy 1993;55:575.

92 GIT Hormones

PRINCIPAL HORMONES

Gastrin

- It is produced by G cells located in antral portion of gastric mucosa (lateral wall of the glands). It is also found in islets of pancreas in foetal life. They are sometimes called APUD cells (amine-precursor-uptake decarboxylation); since they take up amine precursor and decarboxylate them.
- TG cells are another cells producing gastrin; they are present throughout stomach as well as small intestine (G 34 present; G 17 absent).
- G 14 and G 17 have half lives of 2-3 minutes, G-34 has half-life of 15 minutes.
- G cells are flask-shaped, a broad base having gastrin granules; a narrow apex reaching mucosal surface.
- Its secretion is stimulated by presence of products of protein digestion (particularly tryptophan and phenylalanine). Its secretion is affected by contents of stomach, rate of discharge of vagus nerve.
- Its various actions include—stimulation of gastric acid and pepsin, growth of stomach and intestine's mucosa, stimulation of gastric motility, contraction of musculature causing contraction of gastro-oesophageal junction, stimulation of insulin.
- It leads to increased secretion of HCl which inhibits further gastrin release by negative feedback mechanism.
- Factors inhibiting gastrin secretion are—acid in lumen, and secretin. GIP: VIP glucagon-calcitonin in blood.
- Factors stimulating gastrin secretion are—gastric distension, products of protein digestion, increased vagal discharge, increased level of epinephrine and calcium in the blood.

Secretin

- It is secreted by S cells lying very deep in the glands of mucosa of upper small intestine.
- Its half-life is 5 minutes.
- It leads to secretion of alkaline pancreatic juice. Its action is mediated via cAMP. It decreases gastric acid secretion and causes contraction of pyloric sphincter.
- Secretin release → stimulation of alkaline pancreatic juice → acid gastric juice is neutralised by it → further secretion of secretin is inhibited (feedback control).

CCK-PZ (CHOLECYSTOKININ-PANCREOZYMIN)

- It is a single hormone secreted by cells in mucosa of upper small intestine.
- The half-life of CCK is 5 minutes.
- It is also found in brain neurons (cerebral cortex), nerves in distal ileum and colon.
- Its actions include—secretion of pancreatic juice rich in enzymes, inhibition of gastric emptying, increasing secretion of enterokinase, enhancing motility of intestine and colon, stimulating contraction of pyloric sphincter, stimulation of glucagon secretion, trophic effect on pancreas etc.
- Its secretion is stimulated by products of protein, digestion presence of fatty acids in duodenum,

CANDIDATE HORMONES

1. *Motilin:* polypeptide. Having 22 amino acid residues. Secreted by EC cells (entero-chromaffin cells) and M cells (cells passing antigen to gut associated lymphoid tissue). It causes contraction of smooth muscles of intestine.
2. *VIP:* 28 amino acid residue. Also found in blood (half life 2 minutes). Found in GIT (nerves). Its actions include—stimulation of intestinal secretion mainly electrolytes + water, relaxation of intestinal smooth muscles, dilatation of peripheral vessels, inhibition of gastric acid secretion, etc. It aggravates the action of acetylcholine in salivary glands.

3. *Neurotensin:* 13 amino acid residue. Polypeptide. Produced by cells present in ileum. It increases ileal blood flow while GIT motility is inhibited.
4. *Substance P:* In endocrine cells of GIT. By it motility of small intestine is increased.
5. *Somatostatin* (growth hormone inhibiting hormone): Secreted by D cells in pancreatic islets and GIT mucosa. It is of two types—somatostatin 14 and 28. Its secretion is stimulated by acid in lumen. It inhibits exocrine secretion of pancreas, gastric acid-motility, and gall bladder contraction + absorption of glucose, amino acid and triglycerides.
6. *Guanylin:* Recently isolated. Polypeptide. Binds C type guanylyl cyclase. Secreted by Paneth cells. It regulates Cl^- secretion by intestinal epithelial cells.
7. *GIP:* 43 amino acid residues. Produced by mucosa in duodenum (K cells) and jejunum. It inhibits gastric secretion and motility in large doses. Also known as GDIP (glucose dependent insulinotropic-polypeptide).
8. *Caerulein:* Decapeptide. Isolated from skin of australia frog. (Hyla caerulea). Similar with gastrin and CCK. It leads to contraction of gall bladder during cholecystography.

Gastrointestinal hormone

Hormone	*Cellular location*	*Stimulus for Release*	*Action*
		(A) Established hormones	
1. Gastrin	G cells of antrum and duodenum	Gastric distension and protein in stomach	Stimulates gastric acid and peptic secretion. Stimulates growth of gastric mucosa and lower oesophageal sphincter
2. Cholecystokinin Pancreozymin (CCK-PZ)	Mucosa of entire small intestine	Fat, protein and their digestive products in intestine	Stimulates gall bladder contraction, stimulates pancreatic enzyme secretion. Inhibits gastric emptying; stimulates pancreatic growth
3. Secretin	Mucosa of duodenum and jejunum	Low pH in duodenum	Stimulate pancreatic and biliary HCO_3^- secretion. Augments actions of CCK (PZ) on pancreatic enzyme secretion
		(B) Candidate hormones	
4. Gastric inhibitory polypeptide (GIP)	Mucosa of duodenum and jejunum	Glucose or fat in duodenum	Stimulates release of insulin from pancreas. Inhibits gastric motility and its H^+ secretion.
5. Vasoactive intestinal polypeptide (VIP)	Mucosa of entire small intestine and colon	?	Inhibits gastric H^+ and pepsin. Stimulate pancreatic bicarbonate and secretion from intestinal mucosa. Inhibits gastric and gall bladder motility.
6. Motilin	Mucosa of duodenum and jejunum	Alkaline pH (8.2) in duodenum	Stimulates gastric motility, increases GI motility
7. Enterogastrone	Mucosa of small intestine	Fat in intestine	Inhibits gastric H^+ secretion
8. Chymodenin	Mucosa of small intestine	Fat in intestine	Specific stimulation of chymotrypsin by pancreas
9. Bulbogastrone	Duodenal bulb	Acid in duodenal bulb	Inhibits gastric H^+ secretion
10. Enteroglucagon	Mucosa of small intestine	Glucose or fat in intestine	Glycogenolysis
11. Villikinin	Mucosa of small intestine		Causes movements of intestinal villi (side to side, pumping)
12. Duocrinin -	Mucosa of small intestine		Causes stimulation of duodenal secretion
13. Hepatocrinin	Intestinal extracts		Increases biliary flow
14. Enterocrinin	Mucosa of upper intestine		Stimulus for intestinal juice

BIBLIOGRAPHY

1. Thompson JC, et al (Ed). Gastrointestinal endocrinology. McGraw Hill 1987.
2. Walsch JH (Ed). Gastrin, Raven Press, 1993.

(Bibliography 1 and 2 quoted by Ganong WF in Review of Medical Physiology - Lange Publications.)

93 Summary Chart: Mechanism of Secretion Digestive Juice

A. *Salivary secretion*

i. It is purely a reflex process which are of two types:

a. Conditioned reflex in which even sight or smell of food stimulates the secretion. Pavlov used to sound a gong at the meal time and experimental dogs showed salivary secretion.

b. Unconditioned reflex-stimulus arises chiefly in the mouth, but it may also arise when food passes down the oesophagus (oesophago-salivary reflex); in stomach (gastro-salivary reflex) and from other viscera (distended uterus during pregnancy).

ii. Increased flow of saliva has been observed after section of chorda tympani nerve by Claude Bernard which he named as *Paralytic secretion* which is said to be due to increased sensitivity of the gland towards adrenaline after sectioning chorda tympani nerve.

iii. Salivary centre consists of superior and inferior salivary nuclei in reticular formation of the brain stem. Salivary gland receives double nerve supply—both from sympathetic and parasympathetic, stimulation of parasympathetic nerve supply causes profuse secretion of watery saliva with relatively low content of organic material along with pronounced vasodilatation in gland while stimulation of sympathetic causes release of small amount of saliva rich in organic constituents.

B. *Gastric secretion*

i. Sham feeding and Pavlov's pouch are two classic experiments for study.

ii. Three phases

a. *Cephalic (nervous, appetite juice):* It is a reflex process involving both conditioned and unconditioned reflex, secretion begins within five minutes and continue for 1.5 hours with an amount of 50-150 cc/20 minute. It can be prevented by section of vagus nerves.

b. *Gastric:* It starts after half an hour of entrance of food in stomach, at a rate of 225-350 cc/5 hour. It is due to liberation of a chemical or hormone gastrin elaborated by pyloric mucous membrane of stomach. It is powerful stimulant of acid secretion. Effective stimulus for this phase is presence of food, in antrum.

c. *Intestinal:* It starts when food enters the duodenum. Presence of fats in the duodenum inhibits gastric secretion due to liberation of a hormone enterogastrone and when it or its derivative is excreted in urine, it is called urogastrone. All above three phases are inter-related, one initiates the next.

C. *Pancreatic secretion:* Two Phases

i. *Nervous:* Secretion begins one to two minutes after taking food. Reflex is purely unconditioned. Stimulation of vagus (parasympathetic innervation) results in secretion of enzymes but has little or no effect on the secretion of bicarbonate. The mediator is acetylcholine. Vagotomy and atropine markedly depress the enzyme secretion by pancreas.

ii. *Chemical:* Two hormones secretin and Pancreozymine are responsible and both of these can be extracted from the mucosa of duodenum and upper small bowel. Dilute HCl in the duodenum is a potent stimulus for the release of secretin while peptones or products of protein digestion serve equally well for release of pancreozymin. Secretin acts on ductile or centroacinar cells to stimulate them to secrete water and bicarbonate while pancreozymin stimulates the acinar cells to secrete enzymes. HCl produces an abundant secretion of dilute alkaline fluid having minimum amount of enzymes; Fatty acids and soaps increase enzyme concentration; whereas products of protein digestion produce only small amount of secretion which is highly concentrated in enzymes.

D. *Bile secretion*

i. It is secreted continuously. It is a product of both secretion as well as excretion. More bile is secreted during day light than night hours.

ii. Natural bile salts have a powerful choleretic action on liver.

iii. Fats have some tendency to increase bile output. Glucose given orally tended to decrease the bile output provided the bile secreted was not returned to the intestine.

iv. A specific hormone hepatocrinin increases bile flow, is coming from intestinal extracts.

v. Secretion of bile is increased by vagus stimulation but principal effect of autonomic innervation on bile secretion appears to be inhibitory.

E. *Succus entericus*

i. *Nervous:* Moderate secretion starts after a latent period of 1.5 hours. Stimulation of sympathetics causes no secretion but cutting the nerves result in marked increase in secretion called Paralytic secretion; inhibited by atropine. One of the most effective stimuli for intestinal secretion is mechanical stimulation of mucosa.

ii. *Chemical:* Enterocrinin- a hormone produced by intestinal mucosa is acting as an important stimulus for this juice.

Digestion is a process of enzymatic conversion of undiffusible form of food into diffusible or simpler form which are needed to carry on the metabolic activities for energy supplying in the form of heat as well as to supply the needs for repair and growth.

QUESTION BANK: DIGESTION

1. **Explain:**
   a. There is an increase in pH after meals (alkaline tide). Why?
   b. Stomach does not digest itself. Why?
   c. Stress is primary cause of stomach troubles. How?
   d. Food does not enter the respiratory tube on passing through pharyngeal cross roads. How?
   e. Auto-digestion of pancreas is normally prevented. How?
   f. A student going to examination hall often suffers from diarrhoea. Why?
2. **Enumerate:**
   a. Functions of colon
   b. Functions of liver
   c. Functions of saliva
3. **Describe secretory, regulatory and absorptive functions of duodenum?**
4. **Discuss :**
   a. HCl secretion in stomach
   b. Filling and evacuation of gall bladder
   c. Digestion and absorption of fats
   d. Factors stimulating parietal cells. (Raj Univ First MBBS, 2001)
5. **Describe various GIT hormones in detail?** (Raj Univ 1981, 1986, 1992, 1996, MD)
6. **Give differences between:**
   a. Hepatic, pre- and post-hepatic jaundice.
   b. Segmentation and peristalsis
   c. Serum bilirubin and bile bilirubin
   d. Cholagogue, choleretic and hydrocholeretic
   e. Gall bladder bile and liver bile
   f. Secretin and pancreozymin
   g. Hunger and appetite
7. **Short notes**
   a. Entero-hepatic circulation
   b. Gastric emptying and motility (Raj Univ First MBBS, 1995)
   c. Bile salts
   d. Liver function tests
   e. Peptic ulcer
   f. Jaundice
   g. Gastric analysis
   h. Deglutition
   i. Gastric emptying (Raj Univ 1980, 1988, 1994, MD)
   j. Van den Bergh Test (Raj Univ 1994, M.D.)
   k. Movements of Small intestine (Raj Univ 1993, MD)
   l. Peristalsis (Raj. Univ. 1992, M.D.)
   m. Secretin and cholecystokinin (Raj Univ 1990, MD, First MBBS, 1995, 2001)
   n. Iron absorption (First MBBS 1995)
   o. Enterohepatic circulation of bile salts (Raj Univ First MBBS, 1995)
   p. Segmentation movements (Raj Univ First MBBS, 1995)
   q. Gastroileal Reflex (Raj Univ First MBBS, 2001)
8 **You have taken a glass of milk with one egg and bread in your breakfast before coming to examination hall. Describe how it is going to be digested?**
9. **Describe formation and applied physiology of bile pigments.** (Raj Univ 1994, MD)
10. **Explain how gastric secretions are regulated? Discuss the cause and treatment of peptic ulcer.** (Raj Univ MD 1981, 1988, 1992, 1993)
11. **Enumerate important liver function. What is the basis of liver function tests ?** (Raj Univ 1980, 1991 MD)
12. **Describe the physiological basis of various investigations and therapy suggested in hyperacidity.** (Raj Univ 1983, MD)
13. **Describe hormonal regulation of gastric acid secretion. How stomach of cow differs from a man?** (Raj Univ 1979, 1983, MD)
14. **Describe the composition, functions and the regulation of secretion of pancreatic juice.** (Raj Univ First MBBS 1995)
15. **Discuss the mechanism of HCl secretion from stomach cells. Give a brief account of current concepts in diagnosis and management of Zollinger-Ellison syndrome.** (Raj Univ 1999, MD)

16. **Describe the role of bile in digestion. What are the factors involved in regulation of biliary physiology?** (Raj Univ 1999, MD)

MULTIPLE CHOICE QUESTIONS : DIGESTION

1. **Acute pancreatitis is best diagnosed by:** (AIIMS - 1982, Delhi - 1983, 1988, AMC - 1983, 1990)
   a. Serum amylase
   b. Serum lipase
   c. Serum LDH
   d. SGOT [ ]
2. **Peptic ulcer is associated with all *except*:** (AIIMS - 1990)
   a. Hyper-parathyroidism
   b. Pernicious anaemia
   c. Cirrhosis
   d. Zollinger-Ellison [ ]
3. **Milk is first acted upon by:** (Delhi - 1986)
   a. Rennin
   b. Pepsin
   c. Trypsin
   d. Enterokinase [ ]
4. **Gastric secretion is not influenced by:** (Delhi - 1986)
   a. Diet
   b. Gastrin
   c. Secretin
   d. Cholecystokinin [ ]
5. **Heart-burn is characteristic symptom of:** (PGI-1982)
   a. Myocardial infarction
   b. Pulmonary infarction
   c. Reflux oesophagitis
   d. Mediastinal tumour [ ]
6. **The normal faecal fat excretion is:** (AIIMS - 1987)
   a. Less than 5 g/day
   b. 8 g/day
   c. 10 g/day
   d. 15 g/day [ ]
7. **Clay coloured pale stools are seen in:** (AMC- 1985, AIIMS - 1984, 1986, UPSC - 1984, 1985)
   a. Haemolytic jaundice
   b. Hepatic jaundice
   c. Obstructive jaundice
   d. Amoebic hepatitis [ ]
8. **The main aim of vagotomy for peptic ulcer is to decrease:** (AIIMS - 1984, 1985, 1987; AMC - 1985, 1986; PGI - 1982, 1983, 1986)
   a. Emptying
   b. Pepsin secretion
   c. HCl secretion
   d. Mucous secretion [ ]
9. **Hour glass deformity of stomach is seen in:** (AIIMS - 1985)
   a. Carcinoma stomach
   b. Peptic ulcer
   c. Duodenal atresia
   d. Congenital pyloric stenosis [ ]
10. **Commonest site for carcinoma stomach is:** (PGI-1984, 1985, Delhi - 1984, 1990, UPSC-1983)
   a. Fundus
   b. Greater curvature
   c. Lesser curvature
   d. Antrum [ ]

ANSWERS

1 a 2 b 3 a 4 c 5 c 6 a 7 c 8 c 9 b 10 d

MULTIPLE CHOICE QUESTIONS : DIGESTION

1. **The pH of saliva varies directly with:**
   a. CO_2 content of blood
   b. O_2 content of blood
   c. Sodium content of blood
   d. Potassium content of blood [ ]
2. **The enzyme plays a significant role in HCl formation:**
   a. Gastric lipase
   b. Pepsin
   c. Carbonic anhydrase
   d. Gastric rennin [ ]
3. **Receptor for histamine in gastric glands are:**
   a. H_1 receptor
   b. Muscarinic receptor
   c. Nicotinic receptor
   d. H_2 receptor [ ]
4. **The best stimulus for greatest release of hormone secretin is:**
   a. Rice
   b. Vitamin A
   c. Proteins
   d. Hydrochloric acid [ ]
5. **The most effective stimulus for discharge of bile from gall bladder is:**
   a. Fatty food
   b. Rice
   c. Potato
   d. Bread [ ]
6. **The final product of protein digestion is:**
   a. Albumin
   b. Proteases
   c. Polypeptides
   d. Amino acid [ ]

7. **Fats are absorbed in the form of:**
   a. Neutral fats
   b. Cholesterol
   c. Fatty acid and glycerol
   d. Phospholipids [ ]
8. **The end product of carbohydrate digestion is:**
   a. Polysaccharides
   b. Sucrose
   c. Monosaccharides
   d. Tetrasaccharides [ ]
9. **Water absorption is mainly function of:**
   a. Small intestine
   b. Appendix
   c. Colon
   d. Stomach [ ]
10. **Swallowing centre is located in:**
   a. Cerebellum
   b. Pons
   c. Mid brain
   d. Medulla [ ]

ANSWERS

1 a 2 c 3 d 4 d 5 a 6 d 7 c 8 c 9 c 10 d

VIVA VOCE : DIGESTION

1. **How airway is protected while food is passing the pharyngeal cross-roads during deglutition?**
   When food is in the mouth following are the possibilities:
   a. It may return to mouth from oropharynx. This does not generally occur because of high pressure in this area as well as due to the position of tongue against the roof of mouth.
   b. Food bolus may pass up to nasopharynx. This set of event also does not occur normally because of two muscles namely 'tensor-veli- palatani and lavator veli-palatani' which help in separating the oral and nasopharynx by stiffening the soft palate and pressing it against the posterior pharyngeal wall.
   c. Food may proceed forward and may enter larynx. This possibility is prevented by approximation of true and false vocal cords. Inhibition of respiration during second stage of swallowing is another step preventing respiratory tract.
2. **Why does not the stomach digest itself?**
   i. The mucus barrier
   ii. Urea-urease mechanism
   iii. Alkalinity of blood flowing through vessels of gastric tubules due to loss of H ions
   iv. Presence of an antipepsin
3. **Describe the gastric mucus barrier?**
   i. 'Visible' mucus which is viscous and jelly like produced by surface epithelium of gastric mucosa. It forms almost 2-3 mm thick layer. Its secretion is stimulated by alcohol, rubbing mucosa, roughage in diet etc.
   ii. Cardiac glands and pyloric cells on the other hand produce 'soluble mucus' which is tenacious, viscous, mucoid and transparent.
   iii. Mucin protects the gastric mucosa from action of HCl by its high acid combining power. Its antiseptic activity is due to its 'mucoitin sulphuric acid' content. Due to its high viscosity it lubricates easily and thus protects gastric mucosa. It has got regeneration power if its one layer is destroyed by any cause.
4. **Comment on hunger and appetite?**
   i. Hunger is a physiological phenomenon while appetite is a psychological one.
   ii. Hunger is usually taken as sensation of emptiness of stomach resulting from abstinence of food while appetite is conditioned phenomenon.
   iii. Hunger is a unique sensation, symptoms of which are unpleasant starting within a few hours of birth so it is a physiological need for food, while appetite is acquired sense, emotional desire to eat associated with pleasurable past experience of eating.
5. **What is white bile?**
   It is clear, colourless fluid which does not contain any bile salt, pigment, cholesterol thus it has no resemblance with bile. It is produced after ligating the bile ducts as well as tying the gall bladder.
6. **What is gastrocolic reflex?**
   Rectal contractions are initiated due to distension of stomach by food, all of this terminates into defecation desire. This is gastro colic reflex due to which desire to defecate after meals is regular feature in children but in adults this much depends upon habits. It is conducted through myenteric plexus from stomach down along wall of small intestine. It increases excitability, motility and secretion of small intestine.
7. **How fats are being digested?**
   a. No digestion in mouth since saliva does not contain any fat digesting enzyme.
   b. Very slight or non-significant digestion by gastric lipase in stomach.
   c. Emulsification action by bile salts.
   d. Hydrolysis of fat is done by pancreatic lipase (most important enzyme for fat digestion) and intestinal lipase.
   e. Neutral fats (triglycerides, cholesterol etc.) are the common fats of diet. The final products of fat digestion are fatty acid and glycerol in which form they are absorbed.

8. How proteins of the diet are digested?

a. No digestion in mouth occurs since no proteolytic enzyme is present in saliva.

b. Pepsin of gastric juice is proteolytic one, splitting proteins into proteoses, peptones and large polypeptides, though process of hydrolysis at peptide linkage. This pepsin acts in acid media which is provided by HCl secretion by chief cells of stomach.

c. Then in duodenum, it is further digested by trypsin enzyme of pancreatic juice which converts them into peptides (di or poly). 'Carboxy polypeptidase' enzyme present here is capable of changing them up to final amino acid stage. 'Chymotrypsin' present here is capable of catalysing hydrolysis of different type of peptide linkages.

d. Intestinal proteolytic enzymes (Erepsin, amino polypeptidase, dipeptidase) are finally hydrolysing into amino acids, and in this form proteins are absorbed.

9. How carbohydrates are being digested?

a. Digestion in mouth by salivary enzymes.

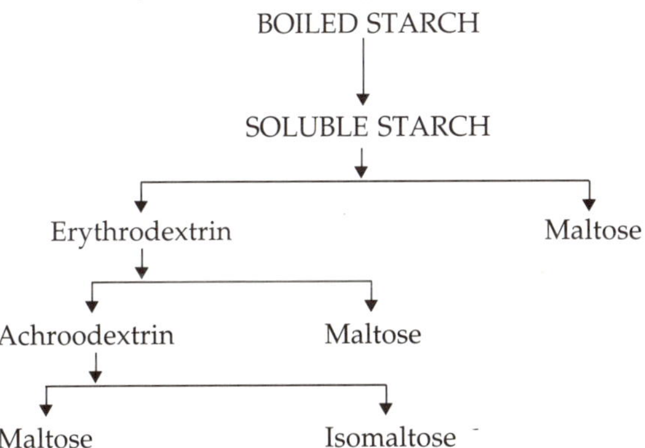

It has also been suggested that gastric HCl is capable of slight hydrolysis of starch and disaccharides. Digestion of carbohydrates continue in stomach till food is thoroughly mixed with gastric contents, i.e. 30-60 minutes after food has entered the stomach.

b. As food enter the small intestine, pancreatic amylase further acts on starch which has not been split by salivary enzyme. This is said to be more powerful since it is capable of digesting uncooked starch, like protective cellulose coverage etc.

c. The intestinal lactase, maltase, isomaltase, sucrase acts on respective carbohydrate and final product formed is glucose and constituent monosaccharide.

10. Why pH of urine is high after a meal?

Gastric mucosa contains abundance of carbonic anhydrase the enzyme catalysing hydration of CO_2. The amount of CO_2 in arterial blood is greater than amount in gastric venous blood. Blood coming from stomach is alkaline having a high bicarbonate content. When gastric secretion is increased after meals, sufficient H^+ may be secreted to raise pH of systemic blood and make the urine alkaline. It constitutes probable explanation of high pH of urine excreted after meals called post-prandial alkaline tide.

UNIT 13

Story after Digestion

“One must eat to live; but one must not live to eat. A rich dining table is the enemy of a man in this machinery age.”

Metabolism

94 Energy of Life: Metabolism

ATP (ADENOSINE-TRIPHOSPHATE) : ENERGY CURRENCY

i. It is present everywhere in the cytoplasm and nucleoplasm of all cells; essentially all the physiological mechanisms that require energy for operation, obtain this directly from stored ATP. In turn, food in cells is gradually oxidised and the released energy is used to reform ATP, thus always maintaining a supply of this substance; It is a combination of adenine, ribose and three phosphate radicals. Removal of each phosphate radical liberates 8,000 calories of energy; thus after losing one phosphate radical the compound becomes ADP and with the loss of second it becomes AMP.

ii. *Metabolism* means simply all chemical reactions in all the body cells; metabolic rate is normally expressed in terms of rate of heat liberation during chemical reactions.

iii. *Calorie* is the unit for expressing the quantity of energy released. One calorie (c) is the quantity of heat required to raise the temperature of 1 gm of water 1°C.

iv. *Creatine phosphate* which also contain high energy phosphate bonds is many times more abundant. High energy bond of it contains 8500 calories per mol. under standard conditions. It can be actually called as ATP sparer.

CARBOHYDRATE METABOLISM

i. These are for the most part, polymers of hexoses, of which most important are galactose, fructose and glucose. Once glucose enters the cells (since it is principal product of carbohydrate digestion as well as main circulating sugar), it is normally phosphorylated to form 'glucose-6-phosphate' and the enzyme catalysing this reaction is hexokinase (enzyme glucokinase has also been reported in liver having greater specificity for glucose and increased by insulin while starvation decreases it). Glucose-6-phosphate is either polymerised into 'glycogen or catabolised.' *Glycogenesis* means the process of glycogen formation while *Glycogenolysis* means of glycogen breakdown; and the breakdown of glucose to pyruvic acid or lactic acid or both is termed as *Glycolysis*. Glucose catabolism proceeds in two ways via cleavage to triosis, or via oxidation and decarboxylation to pentoses. Embden-Meyerhof pathway is the pathway to pyruvic acid through trioses and pathway through gluconic acid and pentoses is the *Hexos-monophospahte shunt* (direct oxidative pathway). Pyruvic acid is converted to acetyl Co-A.

ii. *Citric acid cycle* (Krebs', tricarboxylic acid cycle) : It is a sequence of reactions in which acetyl Co-A is metabolised to CO_2 and H atoms. This cycle is the common pathway for oxidation to CO_2 and H_2O of carbohydrate, fat, and some amino acids. The major entry into it is through acetyl Co-A but pyruvic acid also enters by taking up CO_2 to form oxaloacetic acid. This cycle requires O_2 and is not functioning under anaerobic conditions.
Acetyl Co-A is first condensed with a 4-carbon acid, oxaloacetic acid to form citric acid as HS-Co-A. In a series of seven subsequent reactions, $2CO_2$ molecules are split off, regenerating oxaloacetic acid. Four pairs of H atoms are transferred to flavoprotein-cytochrome chain producing 12 ATP and $4H_2O$, $2H_2O$ are used in the cycle.

iii. *Phosphorylase*: Glycogen is synthesised from glucose-1-phosphate via UDPG (Uridine diphosphoglucose) with the enzyme glycogen synthetase. Phosphorylase is catalysing cleavage of 1:4 a. Phosphorylase is activated in part by the action of epinephrine on β adrenergic receptors in liver. Protein kinase is activated by cyclic AMP and catalyses transfer of phosphate group to phosphorylase kinase converting it to its active form. Phosphorylase kinase in turn catalyses the phosphorylation and consequent activation of phosphorylase. Glycogen synthetase is active in its dephosphorylated form and inactive when phosphorylated. Glycogen is also broken down; break down is mediated by intracellular Ca^{2+} involving an activation of phosphorylase kinase independent of cyclic AMP.

PROTEIN METABOLISM

i. The principal constituents of proteins are amino acids. 21 of which are present in the body in significant quantities. Each amino acid has an acidic group (-COOH) and a nitrogen radical lying in close association with the acidic radical represented by amino ($-NH_2$) group. Amino acids are linked into chains by 'peptide bonds' joining the amino group of one amino acid to the carboxyl group of the next.

ii. Removal of the amino groups from the amino acids is called *'Deamination.'* It can occur either by *'Transamination'* (transfer of amino group to some acceptor substance or conversion of one amino acid to the corresponding keto-acid with simultaneous conversion of another keto-acid to an amino acid) and oxidative deamination (an amino acid is formed by dehydrogenation and this compound is hydrolysed to the corresponding keto-acid with the liberation of ammonia and occurs in liver).

iii. The ammonia released during deamination is removed from the blood by conversion into urea;

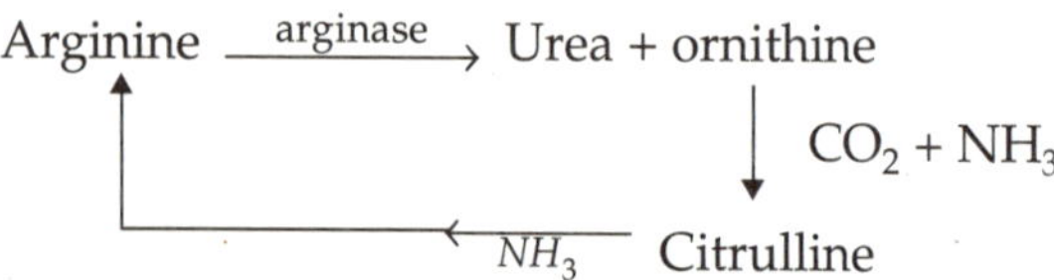

Essentially all urea formed in human body is synthesised in liver.

iv. Once amino acids have been deaminated the resulting keto-acid products can be oxidised to release energy for metabolic purposes.

v. The conversion of amino acids into glucose or glycogen is called *gluconeogenesis* while *ketogenesis* means conversion of amino acid to keto-acids or fatty acids.

vi. Carbohydrates and fats are called *'protein sparers.'*

LIPID METABOLISM

i. A number of different chemical compounds of the food and body are classified together as lipids which include neutral fat (triglycerides), phospholipids, cholesterol and few others. Chemically the basic lipid moiety of both the triglycerides and phospholipid is fatty acids which are simply long chain hydrocarbon organic acids. Triglycerides are used in the body mainly to provide energy for the different metabolic processes, which is shared equally with carbohydrates.

ii. *β oxidation* (Degradation of fatty acid to acetyl Co-A):
   a. Fatty acid molecule first combines with Co-A to form fatty acyl Co-A molecule.
   b. Fatty acyl Co-A loses two hydrogen atoms from alpha and beta carbons leaving a double bond at this point.
   c. A water molecule reacts at this site of double bond so that a hydrogen atom from the water attaches to alpha carbon and remaining hydroxyl radical attaches to a beta carbon.
   d. Two additional hydrogen atoms are removed, one from beta carbon and one from hydroxyl radical. Removed hydrogen atoms combine with DPN and are oxidised.
   e. Compound splits between alpha and beta carbon, the long portion of chain combining with a new molecule of Co-A while shorter acetyl portion remains combined with original Co-A in the form of acetyl Co-A.

iii. The acetyl Co-A molecule formed by beta oxidation of fatty acids enter into citric acid cycle, combining first with oxaloacetic acid to form succinic acid which then is degraded into CO_2 and H atoms. Hydrogen is subsequently oxidised by the oxidative enzymes of the cells. Thus, after initial degradation of fatty acids to acetyl Co-A their final breakdown is the same as that of acetyl Co-A formed from pyruvic acid during glucose metabolism.

iv. When fatty acid chains have been split into acetyl Co-A; two molecule of acetyl Co-A condense to form one molecule of aceto acetic acid, which then freely diffuses through the liver cell membranes and is transported by blood to the peripheral tissues.

NOTES

1. 1 gm of carbohydrates yields 4.1 calories, while 1 gm of fat yields 9.3 calories of heat, 1 gm of protein yields 4.1 calories of heat.
2. Normal G:N (glucose nitrogen) ratio is 3.65: 1.
3. Normally in males creatinine coefficient is 20-26.
4. Respiratory quotient of fat is 0.70, Carbohydrates is 1.0

RESPIRATORY QUOTIENT (RQ)

Introduction: It is the ratio between volume of CO_2 evolved and volume of O_2 absorbed during a given time (CO_2/O_2 ratio).

Normal value: It is 0.85 with a mixed diet.

Importance: It guides us about the type of food burning in the body/organ.

- It is helpful in determining metabolic rate.
- It helps in diagnosing various abnormalities like acidosis, alkalosis etc.
- It can determine the proportion of three basic food-stuffs.

Factors Affecting

a. *Diet:* with carbohydrate it is unity, since ... $C_6H_{12}O_6 + 6O_2 = 6CO_2 + 6H_2O$. R.Q. 6/6 = 1.0 with fats it is lowest about 0.7 since they are poor in oxygen - since oxygen taken in from outside is used for oxidising C + producing CO_2, and for oxidising H giving H_2O. So volume of CO_2 evolved will be less than volume of O_2 utilised. With protein it is 0.8.

b. The RQ rises in ***acidosis*** since breathing is increased by it and so washing more CO_2 without increasing O_2 consumption. Conversely ***alkalosis*** leads to a fall in RQ through depressing the respiration and thus retaining CO_2 inside.

c. It will fall in advanced stages of ***diabetes mellitus*** because of little burning of carbohydrates. So mainly energy is supplied from fats, of course on administration of insulin it will rise.

d. It may increase on rise of body temperature because of increased breathing in ***fever***.

e. The situation in ***starvation*** has already been discussed elsewhere.

f. ***Voluntary hyperpnoea*** → excess CO_2 washing → without/no corresponding increase of O_2 utilisation → RQ above unity

g. *Muscular exercise:*
   - It is un-altered on moderate exercise.
   - With violent exercise → lactic acid enters the blood → acidosis → raised ventilation → washing more CO_2 → RQ rises (up to 2).
   - During recovery, reverse changes take place so it goes back to the normal.

h. In ***thyrotoxicosis***, BMR is raised. Both O_2 intake and CO_2 evolution are increased in equal proportion. So RQ will not change.

i. Food interconversion: When carbohydrates are changed into fats (OR O_2 rich substances are changed into O_2 poor substances); RQ rises.

FUNCTIONS

A. *Carbohydrates*
   1. Main source of energy
   2. Act as constituent of cell membrane.

B. *Fats:*
   1. Richest source of energy.
   2. Can be stored in the body for subsequent use
   3. It forms important constituents of certain hormones (sex).
   4. Some fats supply essential fatty acids.
   5. Essential for absorption of fat soluble vitamins
   6. Help in forming structure material of cells and tissues, e.g. cell membranes.

C. *Proteins:*
   1. For building new tissues.
   2. Enzymes are nothing but proteins
   3. Antibodies are protein.

LACTOSE IN TOLERANCE

1. It is the principal sugar in cow's milk and found in dairy products.
2. It requires enzyme lactase for human digestion.
3. When this enzyme is not produced in adequate amounts by small intestine, then this condition is evident.
4. It causes abdominal cramps, diarrhoea, bloating and excessive gas when little amount of milk is ingested.
5. This problem can be managed by reducing the consumption of milk, and drinking milk during meals.

95 Vigour of Life: Nutrition-Vitamins

OBESITY — THE MOST COMMON NUTRITIVE DISORDER

It is associated with increased mortality, predisposes to development of important diseases, and diminishes the efficiency and happiness of life. It is a curse. On one side the flabby appearance of the body forces the viewers to pass a smile while on another side it invites many big diseases.

Complications

a. *Psychological:* Many obese people, specially young adult female are ashamed of their unattractive appearance and so develop many psychological problems.

b. *Mechanical disability*: Extreme obesity may terminate into flat foot, osteo-arthritis, abdominal and diaphragmatic hernias, external breathlessness, varicose veins, respiratory infections, accidents etc. The miserable sufferer always remains on mercy of others.

c. *Cardiovascular disorders*: Hypertension is common in obese. Extra wide sphygomanometer cuff must be used. Obesity increases work done by the heart, enlargement of heart, cardiac output, blood volume, stroke volume etc. Ischaemic heart diseases are also common with obesity.

d. *Metabolic disorders*: *obesity is open door for diabetes:* Other such disorders common in obese includes gall stones, hyperlipidaemia, hyperuricaemia, gout etc.

AETIOLOGY/CAUSES

a. *Age*: obesity is generally common in middle age. But no age can be classed as free from obesity. Menopause age in female is quite notorious for fat accumulation.

b. *Energy balance*:
   - Physical inactivity has an important role in development of obesity. Physical activity is less in obese than in lean, but it may not because, but is a result of it.
   - *Social factors,* business/advertising parties may contribute a lot in causing somebody obese. Some unhappy persons eat more.
   - If a person eats a slice (27 gm) of bread that is not needed each day or goes by car instead of walking for 15 minutes, the daily extra 60 kcal, will build up over four years to 10 kg of fats deposited (according to one statistic).

c. *Endocrines*: Diseases like hypothyroidism, hypopituitarism, Cushing syndrome, hypogonadism are notorious to cause obesity. Pregnancy is characterised by an increase in body fat.

d. *Drugs:* The use of oral contraceptive, insulin, steroids, phenothiazines may lead to obesity.

e. *Heredity*: obesity may run in families. It is difficult to separate environmental and genetic component.

f. *Socio-economic*: Obesity is common in lower socio-economic group. In developing countries it is more common in elite and prosperous group. Airline pilots and fashion designers must remain slim.

Investigation

1. *Body mass-index (BMI)*

$$= \frac{\text{Weight}}{\text{height}^2\,(\text{m})} \text{ (see the table)}$$

2. *Skin fold thickness (non-invasive method)*
   Several varieties of callipers (Harpenden skin callipers) are available for it. The sites where the measurements are taken include: mid triceps, biceps, subscapular and suprailiac regions. The sum of these measurements should be less than 40 mm in boys and 50 mm in girls.

3. *Other include:* Total body water, total body potassium, body density
4. *Waist-hip-ratio (W/H; WHR):* The hip circumference is measured at the maximum circumference around the hips; and, waist circumference is obtained at the level of umbilicus with subject supine. Normal - WHR-Males-Females.

Table 95.1: Activity v/s calories consumed

Activity	*Calories consumed (per hour)*
Sitting	100
Tennis (double)	300-350
(Single)	420-480
House work	180
Gardening	200
Digging	350-450
Football	500
Jogging (5-10 mph)	500-800
Bicycling (5 mph)	210
Standing	140

Table 95.2: Body weight in adults

Height (ft. - inches)	*Weight (kg.) Range*	*Obese*	*Acceptable lowest*
4 - 9	42 - 53	63	34
4 - 10	44 - 55	66	35
4 - 11	45 - 56	68	36
5 - 0	46 - 58	69	37
5 - 1	47 - 59	71 - 73	38 - 39
5 - 2	49 - 61	75	40
5 - 3	50 - 62	77	41
5 - 4	51 - 64	79	42
5 - 5	52 - 66 (55 - 69)	81 - 83	43 - 44
5 - 6	43 - 67 (56 - 71)	85	45
5 - 7	55 - 69	87	46
5 - 8	56 - 71	89	47
5 - 9	58 - 72	93	50
5 - 10	59 - 74	95	51
5 - 11	61 - 76	97	52
6 - 0	62 - 77.5	99	53 - 54
6 - 1	69 - 86	104	55
6 - 2	71 - 88	106	57
6 - 3	72 - 90	108	58
6 - 4	74 - 92	111	59

Table 95.3: The vitamins

Vitamin	*Deficiency effect*	*Daily requirement*	*Source*
		(A) Fat soluble	
Vitamin A	Keratinization of epithelial structure, night blindness. xerophthalmia	5000 IU	Cod liver oil, milk, butter, egg, fish, carrots, spinach, yellow fruits, green leaves
Vitamin D	Rickets, Osteomalacia, Tetany in infants, defective teeth formation	400 IU	Fish liver oils, butter, milk, egg
Vitamin E	Sterility, muscular dystrophy	15 - 20 mg	Egg, milk, fish, vegetable seed oil viz. wheat, soyabean, corn.
Vitamin K	Bleeding	5 mg. given in bleeding states	Cabbage, spinach, tomato, soyabean
		(B) Water soluble	
Thiamine (B_1)	Beri beri, polyneuritis	1.8 mg	Cereals, pulses, nuts, yeast, carrots, cauliflower, polished rice, wheat flour, egg yolk.
Riboflavin (B_2)	Loss of weight and appetite, corneal vascularization (cheilosis, dermatitis)	1.8 mg	Milk, liver egg white, muscle, whole grains, green leafy vegetables.
Nicotinic acid	Pallegra, dermatitis, dementia	1.8 mg	Peas, tomato, beans, wheat, green vegetables
Pantothenic acid	Chicks dermatitis alopecia, hypofunction of adrenal cortex, skin cornification		Meat, egg yolk, wheat, pea, potato
Biotin (Vitamin H)	Dermatitis GIT symptoms, lassitude, rise of blood cholesterol	300 mg	Egg yolk, kidney, liver, cauliflower, pea
p-Aminobenzoic acid	Graying of hair, ricketesial Graying of hair, ricketesial infection		Animal sources, wheat germ, rice, milk
Folic acid	Macrocytic anaemia	0.5 mg	Liver, kidney, green vegetables.
Vitamin B_{12}	Pernicious anaemia, hyperglycaemia, nervousness, irritability	1 µg daily	Liver, kidney, eggs, milk, absent in plants.
Vitamin C (Ascorbic acid)	Scurvy, bleeding gums, malformation of bone and teeth	75 mg daily	Citrus fruits, cabbage, cauliflower, pulses, germinating grams
Vitamin P	Haemorrhage of scurvy		Citrus fruits, cabbage, cauliflower, pulses, germinating grams

Table 95.4: Foodstuffs: Nutritive value

Name	*Calories*	*Protein (gm)*	*Fat (gm)*	*Vitamin C (mg)*	*B_1 (mg)*	*Iron (mg)*
			Cereals			
Wheat	336	8.2	1.6	0	0.74	4.9
Bajra	361	11.6	5.0	0	0.32	5
Rice (raw)	345	6.8	0.5	0	3.1	3.1
			Fats oils			
Ghee (cow)	900	0	81.0	-	-	-
Butter	729	0	81.0	-	-	-
Coconut oil	900	-	100	-	-	-
			Fruits			
Apple	59	0.2	0.5	-	-	-
Mango	7	0.6	0.4	16	0.08	1.3
Grapes	71	0.5	0.3	1	-	0.5
Guava	51	0.9	0.3	212	.03	1.4
Tomato (ripe)	20	0.9	0.2	27	0.12	0.4
Orange	48	0.7	0.2	30	-	0.3
Pineapple	46	0.4	0.1	39	0.20	1.2
			Milk Products			
Cow's milk	67	3.2	4.1	2	0.05	0.2
Curd	60	3.1	4.0	1	0.05	0.2
Cheese	348	40.3	24.1	-	-	2.1
Kheer	176	6.9	12.2	3	0.12	-
			Miscellaneous			
Biscuit (salty)	534	6.6	32.4	-	-	-
Biscuit (sweet)	450	6.4	15.2	-	-	-
Honey	319	0.3	0	4	-	0.9
Pappad	288	18.8	0.3	-	-	17.2
Jaggary	383	0.4	0.1	-	0.02	11.4
Bread (white)	245	7.8	0.7	-	0.07	1.1

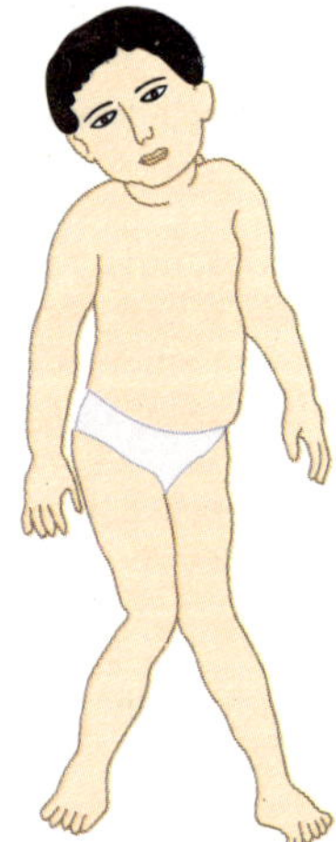

Fig. 95.1: Note deficiency of vitamin D (Rickets)

Prevention and Control

1. Dietary changes: The fats should be reduced. Fibre content of the diet should be increased.
2. Physical activity: should be increased.
3. Drugs: (a) Amphetamine - not widely accepted because of cerebral stimulation
4. Surgical (a) Surgical by pass - gastroplasty (b) Jaw wiring

Historical Notes

- Discovered by Lunin (1881)
- Term introduced by Dr. Casimir Funk (1912).
- Eijkman (1897) discovered Beri beri.
- Vitamin A discovered by Mc Collum and Davis.
- Term B_6 was given by Gyorgi to pyridoxin.
- Nobel prize was given to Dorothy Crowfoot Hodgkin in 1964 for chemistry of structure of B_{12}.
- Vitamin E discovered by Sure.

BIBLIOGRAPHY

1. Chamey E, et al. New Eng J Med 1976;295:6.
2. Garrow JS. In Recent Advances in Medicine. vol. 18 Churchill Livingstone. 1981.
3. Hager A. Br Med Bull. 1981;37(3):287.
4. Oliver MF. Br Med Bull 1981;37(1):49.

96 Metabolism: Normal-Special Circumstances

METABOLIC RATE (METABOLISM = CHANGE)

The metabolism means all chemical and energy transformation which occur in the body. The amount of energy liberated per unit of time is metabolic rate. 1 kcal means 1000 cal.

BMR (Basal metabolic rate)

a. The metabolic rate determined at rest in a room at a comfortable temperature in a thermoneutral zone, 12-14 hours after the last meal is called BMR. The term 'basal' denotes widely acceptable and known standard conditions.
b. In females it is slightly lower than males. It is high in children but declines with age. It is increased by anxiety/emotions because of increased release of adrenaline + over tension on muscles. Patients under depression have low BMR. During febrile conditions BMR rises. Due to prolonged starvation there occurs a fall in BMR. After feeding BMR as well as sympathetic functions are increased.
c. *Basal conditions:* The person must be empty stomach for the last twelve hours, he must have enjoyed a sound sleep last night, he must not have performed any strenuous exercise; there should be no excitement in his behaviour. These are the conditions which one should fulfil before going for measurement of BMR.
d. BMR is expressed as calories per hour per square meter, i.e. in proportion to body surface area.
e. As one remains healthy, it remains constant, in the same person.
f. When it is expressed as +25 which means - it is 25 per cent too high; OR -15 which means - 15 per cent too low.
g. Metabolator - measuring BMR: (Benedict Roth's apparatus for BMR measurement) (Fig. 96.1)

- The apparatus contains a floating drum having an oxygen chamber connected to a mouthpiece by two rubber tubes. A valve is present in one of these two tubes which allows the air to pass from oxygen chamber into the mouth. The air passing from mouth back to the chamber is directed through another valve through second tube.
- Expired air from the mouth flows through a lower chamber containing pallets of soda lime which combine with CO_2 in expired air.
- Now, oxygen is used by the person, and CO_2 is absorbed by soda lime then the floating O_2 chamber which is balanced by a weight, sinks in the water, due to O_2 loss. This is provided with a pen which writes on a moving drum.

Factors Affecting Metabolic Rate

a. *Exercise:* Strenuous exercise produces one hundred times more heat for a few seconds.
b. *Thyroxine*: This also increases metabolic rate 50-100 per cent above normal. Conversely its diminished secretion reduces the metabolic rate.
c. *Growth hormone*: It also increases metabolic rate by 10-20 per cent since it effects metabolism.
d. *Sleep*: It reduces metabolic rate due to decreased tone of skeletal muscle + diminished sympathetic activity.
e. *Fever:* Because of overall increase in metabolism the fever increases metabolic rate.
f. *Malnutrition*: Because of lack in necessary substances, metabolic rate is decreased.
g. *Age*: The metabolic rate of young child in relation to his size is twice that of an old person. This is because of his high rates of cellular reactions along with rapid growth.
h. *Season*: Metabolic rate is found to be lower in tropical regions than in arctic regions. This is because in cold thyroid gland is stimulated.
i. *Stimulation of sympathetics*:
    - Because of this, adrenaline is secreted which causes glycogenolysis + increased intracellular activities.

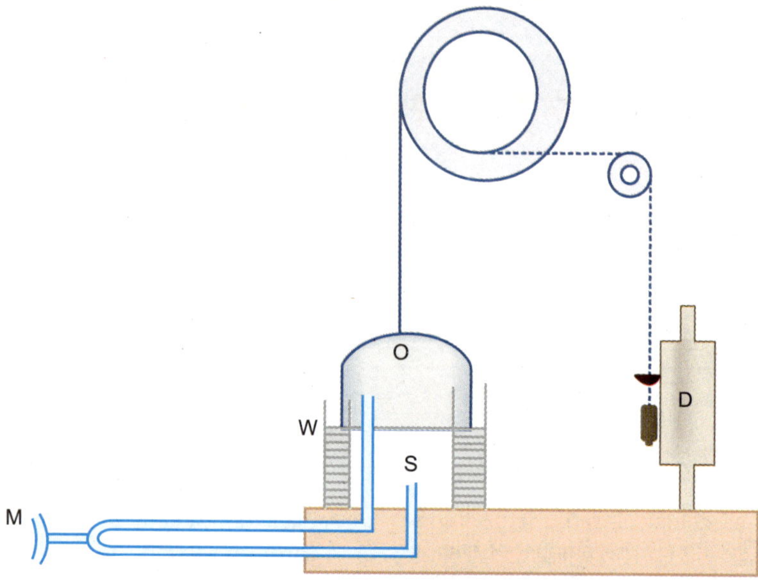

Fig. 96.1: Metabolator
(O = Oxygen, W = Water, S = Soda lime, D = Recording on drum, M = Mouthpiece)

- A special type of fat tissue is brown fat. It contains large number of mitochondria and many small globules of fat instead of one large fat globule. When these cells are stimulated by sympathetics; the mitochondria will produce more heat but no ATP. So almost all the released oxidative energy becomes heat. The neonate body is rich in such cells, so called 'non-shivering - thermogenesis. No brown fat in adult but it may come into existence after cold adaptation.

j. *Proteins: specific dynamic action:* On a heavy protein diet, the metabolic rate rises within one hour and it lasts for 3-12 hours. This is SDA of protein. On the contrary, the metabolic rate rises only slight on carbohydrate and fat diet.
k. *Pregnancy*: In later half of pregnancy there is a marked rise in BMR.
l. *Surface area*: It varies directly with surface area.
m. *Emotional excitement*: Raise metabolic rate.

Conditions Increasing BMR

Hyperthyroidism, fever, cardio-renal diseases, leukaemia, polycythaemia

Conditions decreasing BMR: starvation, under nutrition, hypothyroidism, Addison's disease, lipid nephrosis

Bedside measurement of BMR: (Read's formula)
BMR = 0.75 (Pulse rate + 0.74 x Pulse pressure)-72

It is correct within a range of ±10 per cent Above 10 per cent - Is higher, below 10 per cent is lower.

Importance of BMR: (a) For diagnosis of various diseases (b) To prescribe a diet of adequate calorific value (c) To study the effect of various drugs and food on BMR.

BMR

Metabolic rate of the body is expressed as kilo calories of heat dissipated per square meter body surface per hour. The metabolic rate of body while a person is at complete mental and physical rest is called "basal." It is 6-8 hours after the last meal. Food during assimilation leads to an increase in metabolic rate, called SDA.

- Adult male = 40 calories/square meter body surface/hour
- Female = 37 calories/square meter body surface/hour
- Children = 45-50 cal/square meter body surface/hour

METABOLISM IN STARVATION

Complete deprivation of water, salts and food means starvation. In one week, the animal dies if deprived from water only, while deprived from salt only death results in two weeks, while food starvation may take 3-4 weeks to die. The longest period of survival is 9-10 weeks.

Metabolic Stages

1. *First stage (stage of carbohydrate depletion)*: This is depleted in first two days. Blood sugar is maintained at a steady state which may be due to neoglucogenesis by the liver. R. Q. is highest.
2. *Second stage (stage of fat depletion)*: Fats of adipose tissue is utilised first. Because of non-availability of carbohydrates, fat oxidation is incomplete so producing ketosis (acidosis). Ketones from liver

passes into blood and thence ketone bodies appear in urine.

3. *Third stage (breakdown of proteins)*: Tissue protein is broken down and amino acid is formed after hydrolysis; constitute amino acid pool. The amino acid undergoes deamination in the liver and non-nitrogenous part helps in maintenance of blood sugar level. The amount of nitrogen excretion during first few days is directly proportional to amount of protein intake before starvation. This stage lasts for less than one week. RQ continuously diminishes.

General Condition

During first two days there is craving for food which later on subside. Gradually desire for food vanishes with increase in weakness. Later on subject becomes semiconscious. Pulse and body temperature remains normal; sleepiness increases with slower respiration. Before death temperature falls. Amount of urine decreases + urea content also.

Table 96.1: Body changes: Starvation

i. *Blood*: acidosis with diminished alkali reserve, low blood sugar, raised potassium, increased blood fat

ii. *Urine*: Less volume, fall in nitrogen volume, rise of potassium, increased excretion of ammonia, increased acidity.

iii. *Grave*: Loss of body weight, fall of body temperature, rise of nitrogen excretion.

METABOLISM IN DIABETES MELLITUS (Glycosuria accompanied with hyperglycaemia)

I. Carbohydrate

- Glycogen content of liver will be low but glycogen formation diminished. In muscle, glycogen content diminishes and its synthesis during recovery is depressed. In heart, glycogen content increased. Insulin corrects all these changes.
- Rate of neo-glucogenesis increases. Activity of enzyme "transaminases" is increased which is responsible for conversion of glucogenic amino acid to carbohydrates intermediates. So hyperglycaemia is enhanced.
- Lowered glucose tolerance
- Glucose combustion is depressed so-
  — RQ is about 0.7. Arterio-venous glucose difference is very low. This shows that fats are burning and very little glucose is used.

II. Protein

- Disturbed. Since insulin is absent or in adequate, then growth hormone acts unopposed. Glucose is formed from non-carbohydrate sources at a faster rate in liver. If enough proteins are not given in diet, then tissue proteins will be mobilised, deamination will take place in liver and may be converted into sugar. D/N (dextrose and nitrogen) ratio is 3.6. Anti-ketogenic amino acids are converted into sugar. Loss of weight and impaired protein synthesis seen in Juvenile diabetes.

III. Fat

- Mobilisation of depot fats.
- Liver is loaded with fat.
- Formation of ketone bodies
- Rise in blood cholesterol
- RQ falls to 0.7
- Glycerol is converted to sugar.

IV. Blood

- Rise in blood sugar
- Blood fat is increased.
- Increased cholesterol level
- Ketosis-acidosis
- Rise in blood phosphate.

V. Urine

- Presence of sugar and acetone
- Increased urine volume
- Raised ammonia coefficient
- Increased loss of nitrogen.

A person is said to be suffering from diabetes mellitus if fasting blood sugar level exceeds 126 mg/dl and at 2 hours to 200 mg/dl—WHO.

Notes:

- In children, oral glucose is given on the weight basis (1.5 to 1.75 g/kg.)
- In pregnant lady, 100 gm oral glucose is recommended.
- In mini GTT, fasting and 2 hours ample of blood and urine are collected instead of ½ hour interval.

Table 96.2: Differences

IDDM	NIDDM
1. Onset at childhood	Predominanly in adults
2. Normal or low body weight	Obese
3. Mild/moderate genetic based	Strong genetic basis
4. Insulin deficiency due to destruction of β cells	Impaired production of β cells
5. Frequently found auto-antibodies	Rarely found auto-antibodies
6. Ketosis very common	It is rare
7. Rare diabetic complication	They are 10-20 per cent
8. Oral hypoglycaemic are not useful	They are suitable
9. Insulin administration required always	It is usually not necessary
10. Symptoms exist from weeks	They exist from months to years

UNIT 14

The Remote Control

"…….Every structure appears childish when compared with brain and spinal cord. Certainly human brain is dominant over infinite numbers of computers………"

Central Nervous System

97 CNS: Remote Control of Body Organisation

Human beings are finest creation of God; this holds true because of single aggregated structure—'the brain.'

To be familiar with structural and functional beauty, we must consider following titles—

SENSORY DIVISION (Fig. 97.1)

When any sensation (like pain, hot, cold, or touch etc.) is there; the stimulus is first taken up by the 'receptors' (identical with a receptionist in a hotel or a big administrative block) which are nothing but information agents or specialised bodies which are sensitive towards special messages. These receptors code the information called 'impulse' which travel through afferent nerves to higher centres which lead to some response called 'sensation' and this entire division is called 'sensory system'.

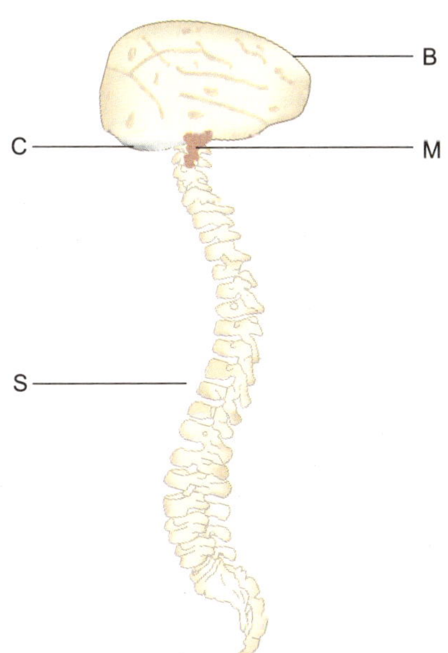

Fig. 97.1: Showing brain and spinal cord—The basic organisation of nervous system.
B = Brain, C = Cerebellum, M = Medulla, S = Spinal cord

MOTOR DIVISION

After receiving information, all higher centres then regulate muscular and glandular actions through special nerves called 'motor or efferent.' It results in muscular contraction and secretions from exo or endocrine glands, which are called 'effectors'.

'Neurophysiology deals with functional aspect of nervous system with transmission of nerve impulses, motor control, reflexes and; even with perception, emotions and mentation.'

So nervous system is a self-organising, self-regulating, signal processing system, continuously working throughout the life. It functions with approximately ten million afferents, fifty billion control and a half million efferent neurons. A ratio of 20:1 exists between sensory and motor channels. On many of these neurons there may be thousands of synaptic endings.

FUNCTIONAL ORGANISATION IN RELATION TO ANATOMICAL LEVELS

a. *Spinal cord level*
   It is the lowest integrative part acting as 'gateway' for voluntary activities. It receives all sensory informations and transmit it either into motor response called 'reflex action' or towards higher centres upwards.
b. *Brainstem or subcortical level*
   Here all subconscious activities are controlled like blood pressure, respiration, heart rate etc. Here centres of emotions, sleep, feeding, pleasure, secretion of digestive juices are also located.

c. *Brain or cerebral cortex level (highest centre)*
It is vast information storehouse and highest centre. It is seat for higher functions, skilful movements, complex voluntary activities. It is also a centre for conscious sensation of general as well as special sensibilities.

SOME ELEMENTARY FEATURES

- Structural and functional unit of nervous system is neurons.
- Nervous system is broadly classified into peripheral and central.' CNS means that part of nervous system which occupies the central axis of the body. Peripheral nervous system means part of nervous system lying in periphery or outside CNS and it includes various nerve fibres in limbs, trunk, head and neck, sympathetic and parasympathetic.
- Sensory nerve (afferent) means the nerve which is bringing information to CNS; while motor nerve (efferent) means a nerve bringing the order from various centres to effectors (muscles; exo-endocrine gland).

BRAIN: GENERAL APPEARANCE

It is a large oval mass divided into two hemispheres by great longitudinal fissure. The curved elevations or convolutions are 'gyri' which are separated by fissures called 'sulci.' It consists of two massive lobes 'cerebral hemispheres' which are separated by 'corpus callosum'. The cerebral cortex is divided into various lobes.

FRONTAL LOBE

Occupies front part of hemisphere. It extends back as far as 'central sulcus'. Cerebral cortex covering this lobe is concerned with individual's personality and voluntary movement. 'Precentral gyrus' is called its 'motor area', with foot, leg and thigh having representation at the highest level on gyrus. It is divided into agranular and granular cortex and later is 'prefrontal area' concerned with body movements.

PARIETAL LOBE

It is located between frontal and occipital lobe extending from central sulcus in front to an arbitrary line posteriorly which is continuous with parieto-occipital-fissure, 'sensory or somesthetic area' is located in its 'post-central gyrus'.

OCCIPITAL LOBE

Highly developed in man. It is located at posterior pole of hemisphere. It is in this area where visual sensations

SUMMARY AND HIGHLIGHTS—THE BRAIN

Part	*Subdivision*	*Functions*
Telencephalon or cerebrum	Cerebral-hemisphere	Sensory impressions are synthesised into perceptions. Area for control of all motor activities. Many impulses are stored as memories.
Diencephalon (Fore-brain or Prosencephalon)	- Thalamus	- Important relay station, sorting the impulses and relaying them to cerebral cortex.
	- Lateral geniculate body	- Here fibres of optic nerve are terminating and then sent to occipital lobe (visual area).
	- Medial geniculate body	- Important relay station for auditory pathway and sending fibres to temporal lobe.
	- Basal nuclei	- Important relay station between cortex.
	- Mammillary bodies	- Concerned with olfactory reflexes.
Mesencephalone (Mid-brain)	- Cerebral peduncles	- Connecting the spinal cord with cerebrum.
	- Superior colliculus	- Giving rise to tectospinal pathway.
	- Inferior colliculus	- Concerned with auditory reflexes.
	- Red nucleus	- Concerned with righting and postural reflexes.
Rhomboncephalon (Hind brain)	- Pons	- Relay station from medulla to higher centres. Connect two halves of cerebellum. Having nuclei of V, VI, VII, VIII cranial nerves.
	- Cerebellum	- Concerned with equilibrium and orientation. Skilled muscular movements are controlled. Integration of proprioceptive impulses.
	- Medulla	- Many vital centres and nuclei of cranial nerves are present. - 'Brainstem' includes all portions of brain except cortex and underlying white matter of cerebral hemisphere and cerebellum.

are analysed and integrated into perceptions which forms visual memory.

TEMPORAL LOBE

Primary cortical centres for hearing and smell are located here. These areas are unilateral, i.e. in left handed persons it is on the right, while in right handed persons it is on left side. It is seen to project forwards forming a 'flap' or cover called 'operculum'.

So brain is divided into two 'hemispheres' and each is subdivided into 'lobes' and cerebral cortex of each lobe is further delineated into 'areas' which are designated by 'numbers'.

BIBLIOGRAPHY

1. Bekhtereva NP. Neurophysiological aspects of human mental. Oxford University Press, New York, 1978.
2. John Carew Eccles. Neurophysiological basis of mind. Oxford Clarendon Press.
3. Joseph G Chusid, Joseph McDonald. Correlative neuro anatomy and neurology, Lange Medical Publication, 13 ed. 1967.
4. Russell B. Human knowledge : Its scope and limits. London 538, p.162, 1948, quoted by Neuro-physiological basis of mind. Oxford University Press by John Carew Eccles.
5. Sherrington CS. Integrative actions of nervous system. Yale University Press, New Haven 411 (pp. 109, 151, 181), quoted by John Eccles, Neurophysiological basis of mind. Oxford University 1906.
6. Sidney Ochs. Elements of Neuro-physiology, 1965. John Wiley and Sons, Inc. New York - London - Sydney.

98 Propagation of Message

MESSAGE - I

The major function of nervous system is to process incoming information in such a way that appropriate motor response occur. First of all we collect 'information' from the surrounding world which is then converted into 'nerve impulse' which is then travelling in big ocean of neurons called 'neuronal pool'. Suppose we are viewing an exhibition; we are looking at many stalls but only one or two are remembered by us for a pretty longer time. This confirms that 99 per cent of informations are unimportant and irrelevant. To understand this important function of our nervous system we divide our study into following components.

a. CNS : as a head post office
b. Synapses
c. Receptors

CNS : AS A HEAD POST OFFICE OR A TELEPHONE EXCHANGE : THE HIGHLIGHTS

- A particular part of the body is innervated by a large number of nerve fibres, each of which arborizes into hundreds of minute 'free nerve endings' which are receptor for pain sensation. It is certain that number of endings is larger in the centre of the field as compared with its peripheral part. When any painful stimuli (pin prick) is applied in centre of field; then it will stimulate more number of fibres causing greater sense of pain. This is phenomenon of ***'spatial summation'***. Another possibility for transmitting signals of increasing strength is by increasing the frequency or amplitude or strength of stimulation. Such a phenomenon is named as ***'temporal summation'***.
- It should be kept in mind that on stimulation, neurotransmitter is released by discharge of single excitatory presynaptic terminal; which stimulates post-synaptic neuron. It should be remembered here in this connection that discharge of a single excitatory pre-synaptic terminal is not capable of stimulating post-synaptic neuron. For proper stimulation either large number of terminals must discharge on same neuron or they must discharge on rapid succession. Such neurons which are excited but not discharging are called 'facilitated neurons' and the phenomenon is known as ***'Facilitation'***. On these grounds stimulus may be of a threshold or subthreshold value.
- Many informations from different parts of the body reaching to one same place, just like the letters from all sub-post offices are reaching finally to head post office. Interneurons of spinal cord receives signal from peripheral nerve fibres entering the cord, corticospinal fibres, propriospinal fibres, from one segment of the cord. From interneurons all these informations are sent to single common site 'anterior motoneurons' to control muscular activity. This is ***'convergence'***.
- When letters are converged to head post office, then they are dispatched and delivered in different direction. Identical to this here is the phenomenon of ***'Divergence'***. One way is information from spinal cord passes to cerebral cortex, thalamus, cerebellum etc. called ***'Multi direction divergence'***. Second way is that they are controlling the contraction of at least 10,000 muscle fibres, called ***'amplifying divergence'***.
- Sometimes the output neuron sends a collateral branch back to its own dendrite or some to re-stimulate itself again and again. This will keep the neuron discharging for a longer time thereafter. Later on this so-called ***'Reverberation circuit'*** becomes complex and constituted by facilitatory and inhibitory

fibres. Due to this property input stimulus is lasting for only one millisecond while output can last for several milliseconds or even minutes.

Here is elaboration of this phenomenon which are quite identical with posting letters for distant stations in letter box from where they are taken out, sorted out, dispatched and delivered to respective places.

PROPERTIES OF REFLEX ACTION (SORTING OUT PROCEDURE) SUMMATION

i. *Temporal*: Repetition of a subliminal stimulus may produce a reflex response due to gradual building up of a 'central excitatory state' in the central neurons, which reaching a threshold value, fire off. Each EPSP lasts for fifteen milliseconds, and if a second discharge appears before it ends, new EPSP will be added or summed up with old.

ii. *Spatial*: Simultaneous excitation of successively greater number of excitatory terminals leads to progressive increase in post-synaptic potential and it is named as 'spatial summation.' It occurs over entire membrane of the soma, dendrites and of initial segment of axon all at the same time.

iii. *Localisation*: The particular 'locus' where a stimulus is applied is constituting 'localisation' and which is then capable of evoking the desired response (e.g. Knee jerk).

iv. *Delay*: When any stimulus is applied, it takes some time to elicit the desired response. This time gap is 'delay;' called 'reflex time' which normally averages between 18-25 m. sec. (for a flexor reflex).

iv. *Fractionation*: It is established fact that maximal response by a muscle is obtained on stimulating motor nerve; but when corresponding sensory nerve is stimulated, the response will be a fraction of total response given by motor nerve. This is so-called 'fractionation.'

v. *Irradiation*: If incoming stimulus is spreading, it constitutes so-called 'irradiation.' It involves additional motor neurons responsible for reflex contraction; e.g. on stimulating sole of foot, flexion of toes results but it also leads to contraction of flexor muscles of foot, ankle and leg too.

vi. *Reciprocal innervation*: When 'protagonist' muscles are contracting on stimulating afferent nerve, the 'antagonists' will always relax. All this is because of 'reciprocal innervation.'

vii. *Facilitation*: Sometimes, when first stimulus is not of a threshold value, it will be exciting neurons but those neurons will not discharge. If second stimulus is applied immediately after the first, then reflex response will occur quicker—such neurons which are excited but not discharging are called facilitated neurons and the phenomenon is called 'facilitation'.

viii. *Rebound*: When a stimulus is applied, a reflex response is obtained. When response ceases, sometimes the same response is returned with full strength and magnitude. This is called 'rebound' and is possibly due to over excitation.

xi. *After discharge*: Due to persistence of response, repetitive discharges are noticed along the motor neuron called 'after discharge.'

x. *Recruitment*: When a motor nerve is constantly or repeatedly stimulated, it leads to 'tetanic contractions' but this tetanus is produced quickly as well as the fact lies that it will disappear on discontinuing the stimulation. On the other hand, on stimulating corresponding sensory nerve such tetanus persists for some time on withdrawing stimulation as well as the fact that its development is also slow. This is due to recruitment.

xi. *Fatigue*: On first stimulation the response is at its climax which gradually becomes weaker till it finally ceases. This phenomenon is fatigue and anoxia, ischaemia or anaesthesia are blamed as causes for it. It occurs most readily at synapses.

xii. *Inhibition*: When protagonist muscle contracts on stimulating sensory neuron, antagonists get inhibition. It also shows synaptic delay, after discharge, recruitment, fatigue and summation. It appears to act on motor neurons. Similarly, the knee jerk in a spinal preparation can be inhibited by single break shocks to an ipsilateral afferent nerve.

xiii *Subliminal fringe*: Afferent neuron acting individually, gives rise to a response. When they are stimulated simultaneously then a response is generated which is more than the sum of the two individual responses.

xiv. *Occlusion:* When two afferent sensory neurons are stimulated, simultaneously, the sum total response is sometimes much less than the sum of the two individual responses when stimulated separately. It is 'occlusion' and is said to be due to central overlapping of afferent neurons.

xv. *Drug susceptibility*: Reflex excitability is diminished by chloroform, ether, alcohol, nitrous oxide, morphine and synthetic hypnotic, through an increase in synaptic resistance, while strychnine produces convulsions.

SUMMARY AND HIGHLIGHTS

CNS : AS A HEAD POST OFFICE

This process is quite identical with posting letters for distant stations in letter box from where they are taken out, sorted out, sent and delivered to respective places. Same is the case here with our brain. Thousands or indefinite informations are feeded which are being responded in their respective way.

MESSAGES - II

Our brain is working quite identical with head post office and truly speaking it is more busy than a big telephone exchange of this world.

We collect information from the surrounding world and every information is first taken up or received by sense organs called 'receptors/detectors.' They code this message and convert it into 'nerve impulse' which travels into big ocean of neurons called 'neuronal pool' and is finally sent to CNS which is the 'sole interpreter and integrator' of this coded message. It decides some thing by its own wisdom/intellect and then the appropriate order is transmitted to particular muscle or gland, for appropriate response, suitable for necessary adjustment. To understand this thing we divide this study into three, components of this mechanism namely:

1. Receptors
2. Synapse and
3. Transmission properties.

THE RECEPTORS (Fig. 98.1)

i. *Introduction*: These are specialised end organs located at peripheral end of a sensory/afferent nerve. It is responding most effectively to one or other type of stimuli.

ii. *Classification*: Broadly they are divided into two groups namely 'exteroceptors' (those receptors which respond to stimuli arising outside the body like eye, ear, skin etc.) and 'interoceptors' (receptors lying in mucus lining of the body).

Exteroceptors are again subdivided into 'taleoceptors' (receptors carrying information from a distance, e.g. situated in visual, auditory or olfaction sensation and therefore also called distant receptors), and 'cutaneous receptors.'

Interoceptors are further subdivided into 'proprioceptors' (receptors carrying information from muscles, joints and tendons, etc. to collect informations regarding the position of the body in movement or rest; also called Kinaesthetic receptors) and visceroceptors.

iii. *Generator/Receptor potential*

- The electrical response of a receptor may be studied by isolating a single fibre from a sensory nerve trunk and applying the appropriate stimulus to the end organ. Nerve ending can be stimulated by either deforming it or by chemical means. This leads ions to diffuse through the nerve membrane, which causes a local flow of current. This is 'generator potential' because nerve fibre itself generates current and the voltage. The maximum amplitude that can be achieved by generator potential is around 100 mV.
- Another parallel term is 'receptor potential' which is caused by specialised, non-neuronal receptor cells which are lying either in near vicinity of these nerve fibres or it may be entwining these end organs.
- Their main purpose is to convert various forms of energy (which stimulate them) into electrical energy in sensory nerve endings. Depletion of sodium from the receptor greatly reduces the generator potential and so stops it. So potential is linked with permeability of unmyelinated nerve endings for sodium.

RECEPTOR POTENTIAL: AT A GLANCE

- It is non-propagative.
- It is confined within receptor.
- It does not obey all or none law
- It is monophasic
- It is not action potential; it is similar to EPSP in synapse/end-plate potential in myoneural junction/electronic potential in nerve fibre.

iv. *Properties*

a. *Excitability*

It can be stimulated by any form of energy. On stimulation ionic changes take place leading to depolarisation and generating receptor potential, or generator potential. It is better to class a receptor as an 'excitable unit.'

b. *Specificity*
As told above receptor is an excitable unit, but, it is excitable only in respect to a specific stimulus. For example, the principal sensations which we feel in our daily life are pain, temperature (including both hot and cold), touch, vision, audition etc. are called *'Modality of sensation.'* In this respect, it is said that when a pain fibre is stimulated it will cause feeling of pain sensation; and if touch fibre is stimulated, person perceives the sensation of touch and like this the statement is true for other sensations also. The specificity of nerve fibres for transmitting only one modality of sensation is called *"law of specific nerve energies."*

c. *Adaptation*
- When a continuous sensory stimulus is applied, the receptor responds at a very high impulse rate at first, then progressively less rapidly, until finally it does not respond at all. This is adaptation and is characteristic of all receptors.
- On the basis of adaptation; receptors are again divided into two groups, namely:
  a. *Rapidly adapting* - because they react 'when a change is actually taking place.' Again, the number of impulses transmitted is directly

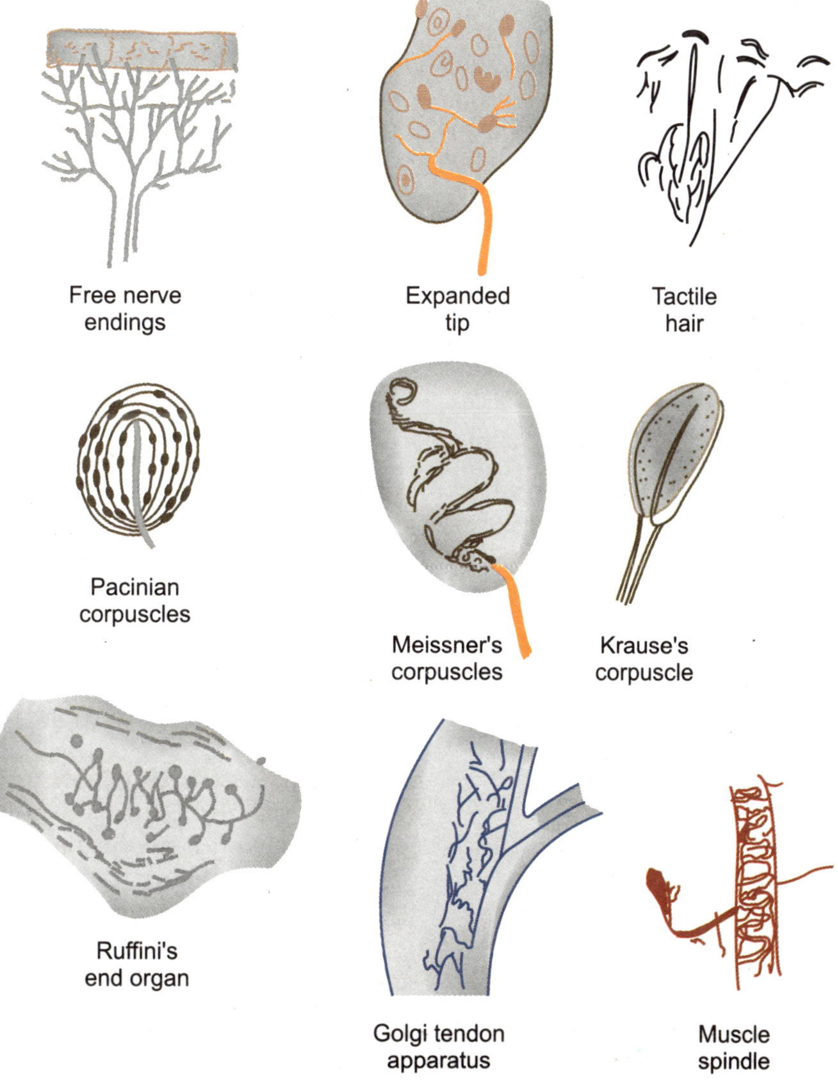

Fig. 98.1: Sensory nerve endings

related to 'rate at which change takes place,' so they are also designated as 'rate/movement/ phasic receptors.' Pacinian corpuscle—a mechanoreceptor is the example of such class of receptor.

b. *Poorly adapting or tonic* - are those which adapt very slowly and continue to transmit impulses to the brain as long as stimulus is present. The examples are muscle spindles, Golgi tendon organs, macula in vestibular apparatus, sound receptors of ear, carotid and aortic bodies (chemo-receptor) etc. In this way, brain is having up-to-date information about status of body and its relation to surroundings. They are also known as tonic receptors because they continue to transmit impulses for many hours.

c. Though it is doubtful to say that receptors can be 'fatigued;' e.g. if eyes are exposed on sun's eclips, retinal damage may occur which means that receptors present there are destroyed by too much stimuli; and, extremes of hot or cold stimuli evoke pain sensation.

CLASSIFICATION OF RECEPTORS

i. Exteroceptors	Present on surface fields of body. They make the individual aware of environment. It includes distance and contact receptor.
ii. Interoceptors	(Visceral receptors) - Responsible for sensation related with visceral activities governed by ANS.
iii. Proprioceptors	Lying on muscle, tendon, joints. Give rise to movement and position sense.

DIFFERENT RECEPTORS

a. For touch-pressure (tactile/mechano-receptive)	Merkel's disc, Meissner's corpuscles, Pacinian corpuscles, free nerve ending
b. Pain	Free nerve ending
c. Warmth	Free nerve ending, Ruffini's organ
d. Cold	Krause's end bulb
e. Proprioceptive	Muscle spindle Macula of vestibular apparatus of internal ear.
f. Interoceptors	Chemoreceptors (carotid and aortic body) Baroceptors - (carotid sinus, receptors for Hering-Bruer reflex, left ventricular mechanoreceptor)

v. *Description*

a. *Pacinian corpuscles* are distributed in subcutaneous tissues, tendon of muscles, capsular ligaments of joints, in the walls of mesenteries and blood-vessels. Their dimension is 1-4 mm long and 2 mm wide. Their shape is oval and are made up of concentric layers of lamellated connective tissue in which meduallated nerve fibre enter and also end within it in expanded extremity.

PACINIAN CORPUSCLES—A STUDY

- These can be easily dissected from mesentery of experimental animals.
- Tip of nerve fibre is unmyelinated which extends through the core of corpuscles. This tip is enveloped by concentric layers of the corpuscles.
- Pressure stimulus → compression of Pacinian corpuscle → change in its shape → deformity of central core fibre → opening of sodium channel→receptor potential → spread along unmyelinated part of nerve fibre → development of action potential in nerve fibre when it passes through node of Ranvier.

b. *Meissner's corpuscles:* An encapsulated nerve ending. It is concerned with perception of light touch sensation with discriminative judgement. They are abundant in fingertips, lips, dermis of hand/foot, nipple.

c. *Merkel's disc:* It is expanded tip tactile receptor looking like a cup like disc. It is concerned with light touch. They are existing in abundance in sensitive areas like lip, fingers, genitalia etc.

d. *Ruffini's bodies:* The end organ for heat sensation. They are distributed in dermis of skin.

e. *Pain receptors:* These are free nerve endings—axons splitting up into numerous branches in the form of a brush. Some of these filaments may enter epithelial cells. They are distributed in muscles, tendons, vessels etc.

SYNAPSES AND JUNCTIONAL TISSUES

i. *Introduction:* Synapse is a bridge between two neurons. It is conducting information from one neuron to another. It is identical with shaking hands between two friends.

ii. *Synaptic transmission:* An action potential is developed on stimulation of axon which travels down and reaches the area overlying the synaptic vesicles in the knob of presynaptic membrane. The synaptic vesicles thus on stimulation release

NERVE ENDINGS

A. SENSORY

Name - Introduction	*Distribution*	*Function*
1. Meissner's corpuscles (Elliptical-lamellated connective tissue body with soft central core)	Papilla of skin under epidermis specially hands and feet	Subserves touch sensation
2. Pacinian corpuscles (Large, oval, lamellated like onion shape. Gets deformed on getting adequate stimulus)	In dermis, specially of hands and feet. Also in deeper, structure like joints, tendons viscera/peritoneum	Carry pressure, stretch, kinaesthetic sensation
3. Krause's end bulb (spheroid connective tissue body, axis cylinder ends in basket like network)	Papillae of skin, conjunctiva, lips, tongue, genital organs, structures near joint	Carry cold sensations
4. Ruffini's end organ	Skin and subcutaneous tissue of finger	Carry heat sensation
5. Free nerve terminals (first forming deep and then superficial nerve plexus. Then terminal filaments pass to the surface)	Widely distributed (dermis, cornea etc.) between muscle fibres, tendons	Carry pain sensation and touch
6. Mechano-receptors	Carotid sinus and aortic arch	Blood pressure regulation
7. Chemo-receptors	Carotid or aortic bodies	Partial pressure of O_2 and CO_2 in blood is regulated
8. Osmo-receptors	Medulla oblongata, hypothalamus	Osmotic pressure of plasma is regulated
9. Thermo-receptors	Hypothalamus	Temperature regulation of blood
B. Musculo-tendinous receptors		
1. Muscle spindle	Between muscle fibre	Carry kinaesthetic impulses
2. Organ of Golgi	Found in tendons near the junction with muscle	Carry kinaesthetic impulses
Motor		
1. End-plate	In all voluntary muscles	Transmits motor impulses by liberation of acetylcholine
2. Free nerve terminal (only autonomic)	Involuntary and cardiac muscles, glands etc.	Transmits motor impulses

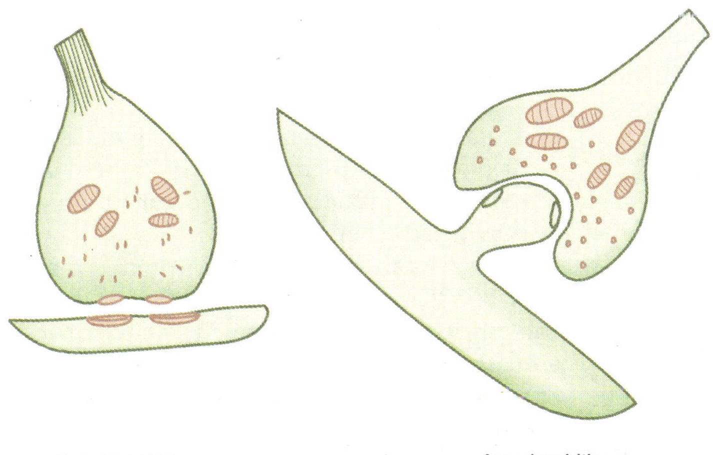

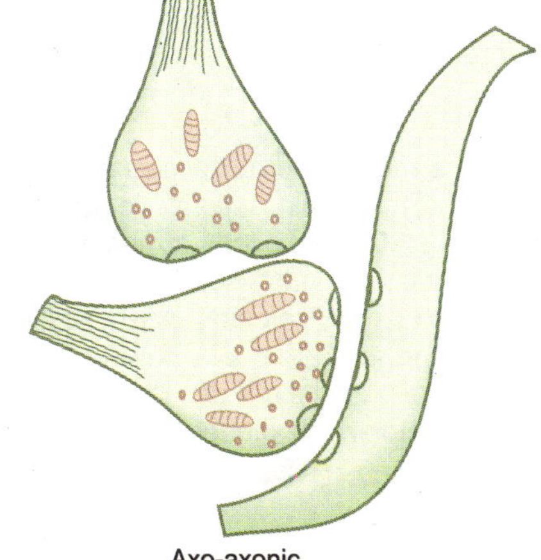

Fig. 98.2: Synapses

chemical transmitter from themselves. This transmitter substance leaves the membrane and by crossing the synaptic cleft combines with the receptors which creates so-called. synaptic potential in the post-synaptic membrane, which is of two types 'EPSP and IPSP' (excitatory and inhibitory post-synaptic potential).

a. *EPSP:* It is strictly localised, does not follow "all or none law," and is developing due to entry of all cations inside the cell; along with the fact that it is fore-runner of an action potential. When it exceeds threshold value, then nerve action potential in post-synaptic neuron is initiated.

EPSP—AT A GLANCE

- It is monophasic and non-propagating.
- It represents a depolarisation which is localised to the soma of motoneuron.
- It does not follow all or none law since it can be augmented simply by intensity of input volley.
- EPSPs of different inputs can sum on a post-synaptic cell to produce a greater depolarisation.
- Motoneuron membrane contains channels through which ions can flow to cause EPSP development. These channels are supposed to be additional to those serving as producers of the action potential.

b. *IPSP:* It is produced by movement of chloride ions from extra to intracellular fluid. When a motor neuron receives inhibitory impulses, there occurs hyperpolarisation of cell membrane, called IPSP, which exerts inhibitory influences on EPSP, leading to inhibition in setting up the nerve impulses.

During development of EPSP, simultaneous IPSP is developed by incoming nerve action potential. The propagation of nerve impulse by EPSP is dependent upon its intensity.

IPSP—AT A GLANCE

- When a motor neuron receives an inhibitory volley of impulses, hyperpolarisation of cell membrane takes place. This is IPSP. This exerts an inhibitory effect on EPSP; leading to inhibition of setting up the nerve impulse.
- It is because of increased permeability of post-synaptic membrane to K^+ and Cl^-, but not Na^+. The decreased excitability of nerve cell during IPSP is because of hyperpolarisation which hinders the membrane potential to reach to firing levels.

BEAUTY OF POTENTIAL

1. Soma of spinal motor neuron has got resting membrane potential of -65mV.
2. Resting membrane potential of larger peripheral nerve and skeletal muscle is -90 mV.
3. Decreasing the voltage to a less negative value (from -65 to -45 mV) makes the membrane more excitable, i.e. EPSP generation. Beyond this value, there is simultaneous discharge of many terminals leading to 'Summation'.
4. If potential becomes more negative, i.e. -75 mV (little more than normal) then inhibitory transmitter will lead to influx of chloride ions from extracellular fluids towards interior, as well as potassium ions towards exterior. This is hyperpolarisation.

NEUROTRANSMITTERS

One neuron is capable of secreting only one neurotransmitter but some specialised neurons are said to be capable of secreting more than one such neurotransmitter; this extra is called 'co-transmitter'.

a. *Acetylcholine:* As told earlier, it is secreted at autonomic ganglia, neuromuscular junction, postganglionic parasympathetic nerve endings, synapses and neuroterminals of brain, post-ganglionic sympathetic fibres supplying sweat glands and sympathetic vasodilators. Caudate nucleus and retina contains largest amount, while moderate amount is contained in brainstem, thalamic nuclei and cerebral cortex but least amount is contained in dorsal root, optic nerves and cerebellum.

b. *Dopamine:* There exists some 'dopaminergic neurons' in neuronal tract (nigro-striatal path). It is closely associated with disease Parkinsonism. Possesses inhibitory action. The PIH (prolactin inhibitory hormone) is dopamine by hypothalamus.

c. *Catecholamines:* Noradrenergic neurons are found to exist in post-ganglionic sympathetic fibres, in brain, causing mood elevation. They cannot cross the blood-brain barrier. Their concentration in brain is ranging between 0.1 to 0.5 μ gm/gm Large amount is found to exist in hypothalamus, olfactory bulb, limbic system, median eminence etc.

d. *Histamine:* As already known, it is produced by 'mast cells' and 'basophils' and hypothalamus is found to contain its notable amount. It is concerned with arousal, sexual behaviour, blood pressure, regulation of anterior pituitary hormones etc.

e. *Serotonin (5HT):* Its producer neurons are found in brainstem (hypothalamus, basal ganglia, spinal cord).
f. *GABA (Gamma-amino-butyric acid):* In brain and spinal cord (cerebral cortex, post-synaptic junction) it is widely distributed.
g. *Substance P:* Chemically it is a polypeptide with a molecular weight of 1600. Usual sites are dorsal root of spinal nerves, hypothalamus and substantia nigra.
h. *Others:* Glycine, Glutamate, asparate, prostaglandin, CGRP (calcitonin gene related protein), opioid peptides (non-inhibitory).
i. *Opioid peptides:*
   a. There exists two closely related pentapeptides called 'enkephalins' which binds to these opiate receptors. These enkephalins are working as 'synaptic transmitters.' They decrease intestinal motility, exert analgesic action when injected into brainstem.
   b. Other polypeptides include—vasopressin, oxytocin, bradykinin, angiotensin II, endothelin, insulin like molecules, gastrin—neurotensin and gastrin releasing peptides etc.

Other Transmitters

a. *Nitric oxide*—It also produced in brain.
b. *Carbon-monoxide*—A probable transmitter.
c. *Co-transmitters*—Many times neurons secrete two or three transmitters.

NITRIC OXIDE: A VIEW

- Is a neurotransmitter in CNS.
- It acts as a mediator for dilator effect of acetylcholine on small arteries.
- It is neither produced by neuronal cells nor stored in vesicles.
- It is produced by non-neuronal cells (e.g. endothelial cells of blood vessels). Then it diffuses into other cells.
- Nitric oxide → activation of guanylyl cyclase enzyme → formation of cGMP from GMP → smooth muscle relaxation + dilatation of arterioles.

NEUROPEPTIDES: A CONCEPT (SLOWLY ACTING TRANSMITTERS/GROWTH FACTOS)

1. These are different group of transmitters than small molecule transmitters.
2. Their action is usually slow.
3. They are not synthesized in cytosol of presynaptic terminal; but by ribosomes in neuronal cell body.
4. Protein molecule entering space inside ER

↓

Protein split into smaller fragment | Packaging of neuropeptide into small vesicles which release into cytoplasm (by Golgi body)

↓

Transportation of transmitter vesicle to the tip of nerve fibre by axonal streaming of axe cytoplasm

↓

Release of transmitter at neuronal terminals in response to action potential

↓

Autolysis of vesicle

5. They are many more times potent than small molecule transmitters.
6. They cause more prolonged action, viz. prolonged closure of calcium pores, prolonged changes in cellular metabolic machinery, activation/deactivation of specific gene in cellular nucleus, prolonged alteration in number of excitatory or inhibitory receptors.
7. They include releasing hypothalamic hormones (TRH, LRH), pituitary peptides (Beta endorphin, prolactin, oxytocin, vasopressin, MSH, ACTH), gut and brain affecting (CCK, gastric, VIP, insulin, neurotensin, nerve growth factor, glucagons and substance P) form other sources (angiotensin II, bradykinin, and calcitonin).

PROPERTIES OF SYNAPSES

a. *Synaptic response:* Synapse is acting as a relay station as well as an integrator and its mechanism is lying in cerebral cortex.
b. *Synaptic delay:* It is sum of synaptic latency and time taken for depolarisation which leads to a spike height in the neuron. This delay is due to release in chemical transmitter substance which then cross the synaptic cleft and then combines with receptor.
c. *Fatigue site:* It is considered as seat of fatigue which is due to exhaustion of neurotransmitter because of repeated presynaptic stimulation.
d. *Synaptic inhibition:* It is an active process which either prevents the onset of activity in a structure or totally stops the already existing activity.
   i. *Presynaptic inhibition:* Presynaptic depolarisation decreases the action potential which is propagating towards axon terminal and thus causing a decrease in amount of neuro-transmitter and this inhibition is nothing but presynaptic inhibition. It is responsible for the depression of EPSP since it reduces

the size of presynaptic impulse and thus decreases the liberation of excitatory material. It is seen only in sensory neuron.

ii. *Post-synaptic inhibition:* It is the inhibitory transmitter which causes such an inhibition since it is capable of changing permeability of post-synaptic membrane to either potassium or chloride or both of them. Any way this change in permeability leads to hyperpolarisation of post-synaptic membrane and therefore, action potential produced by excitatory stimulus will fail to occur. Acetylcholine is said to be a inhibitory transmitter of vagal effector organs.

iii. *Renshaw cell inhibition (Renshaw, 1941):* It is a normal sequence that A alpha motor neuron are arising from anterior horn cells which are supplying the muscles. Corticospinal or pyramidal tract fibres are also said to impinge on these motoneurons, and this is a fact that collaterals are emerging from alpha motoneurons which impinge upon 'Renshaw cells.' So on getting alpha fibres stimulated the Renshaw cell also is excited which then inhibit nerve cell soma of alpha neurons giving birth to phenomenon 'Renshaw cell inhibition'. Its importance lies in the fact that muscle is protected against too high frequency stimuli.

iv. *Direct inhibition:* Suppose the flexor group of muscle is contracting, the opposing (extensors) must relax to cause flexion (Reciprocal Innervation).

PRE-SYNAPTIC INHIBITION: OVERVIEW

1. Here in most of the time the inhibitory transmitter released in GABA.
2. It lies outside of pre-synaptic terminal nerve fibril, before their termination on post synaptic membrane.
3. This GABA leads to influx of chloride ions into terminal fibril.
4. These negative charged ions nullifies the effect of positive sodium ions.
5. This occurs in many sensory pathways.
6. Adjacent terminal nerves fibrils mutually inhibit one another.

RENSHAW CELL INHIBITION: OVERVIEW

1. Renshaw cells are large number of small interneurons.
2. These are located in ventral horns of spinal cord in close association with motor neurons.
3. As axons leaves the body of anterior motor neuron, collaterals from axons pass to adjacent Renshaw cell, which are inhibitory cells, transmitting inhibitory signals back to surrounding motor neurons.

SOME OTHER WAYS OF SYNAPTIC TRANSMISSION

a. *Diverging circuits:* It is the means by which nervous system can amplify weak signals into stronger one, e.g. motor pathway from motor cortex to the effector muscles. It further means that a single input neuron stimulates more and more neurons at successive stages.

b. *Converging circuits:* Impulses from many different sources are converging on a single output neuron. All sensory fibres can provoke reflexes, therefore several of them must converge to the same motor centre. Impulse conducted by different sensory neurons converge to a final common path.

c. *Reverberating circuits:* Impulses return to one of the early neurons and in this way, new impulses are being initiated which are reverberating around and around through the circuit, and therefore the output neuron will go on discharging impulses till reverberation persists. If by any means the neuronal pool is facilitated, the reverberating circuit will be proceeding continuously.

SYNAPTIC BLOCK

Inhibitory transmitter can be blocked at synaptic junction, e.g. strychnine and tetanus toxoid.

Ephapse (false synapse)

It is the process of transmission of an electrical impulse from one axon to another without having synaptic connection of any type.

DOPAMINE

a. It is a prolactin—inhibiting hormone secreted in the hypothalamus.
b. There is a genetic defect in schizophrenia, as a result of an abnormality in chromosome 5, which involves dopaminergic system.
c. Amphetamine, which stimulates secretion of dopamine and norepinephrine, produces psychosis. Major tranquillizers are capable of blocking D_2 receptors.

SEROTONIN

a. It may play an excitatory role in regulation of prolactin secretion.
b. It is involved in regulation of circadian rhythms since there exists a prominent serotonergic innervation of supra chiasmatic nuclei of hypothalamus.
c. Discharge in serotonergic neurons in dorsal raphe nucleus leads to migraine and antimigraine drugs inhibit this discharge.
d. Descending serotonergic fibre system inhibit transmission in pathway of pain in dorsal horn.

GABA

a. It is formed by decarboxylation of glutamate and the enzyme which catalyze this reaction is GAD (Glutamate decarboxylase). It is metabolised by the process of transamination and it is GABA-T (GABA transaminase) an enzyme which catalyzes the transamination.
b. There exist GABA receptors of two types—namely 'metabotropic' ($GABA_B$ receptors, act via G protein to increase conductance in K^+ channels), and ionotropic ($GABA_A$ receptors; made up of subunits like α, β, γ, δ, p classes).
c. The effects of GABA on Cl^- conductance are facilitated by benzodiazepins group of drugs. Metabolites of steroid hormones progesterone and de-oxy-corticosterone bind to $GABA_A$ receptors and increase Cl^- conductance.

MECHANISM OF RELEASE OF NEUROTRANSMITTER

Depolarisation opens specific 'calcium gates' in terminal axon membrane which leads to influx of calcium ions. These ions initiate 'quantal release reaction' after reaching to internal surface of axon membrane. The transmitter molecules are enclosed within synaptic vesicles which undergo frequent collisions with axon membrane, that calcium brings about attachment and local fusion between vesicular and axon membrane and this is followed by all or none discharge of vesicular content into synaptic cleft. The contents of the vesicle, i.e. neurotransmitter substance is released by the process of exocytosis.

POST-SYNAPTIC INHIBITION: ROLE OF IONS

Some of the synaptic vesicles are in close contact with membrane and one or more are caused by impulse to eject their contained transmitter substance into synaptic cleft. Diffusion occurs along cleft. Some of the transmitter becomes attached to specific receptors sites on post-synaptic membrane with the fact that some fine channels across the membrane open or in other words, subsynaptic membrane assumes a sieve like structure. Chloride and potassium ions move readily across membrane and this intense ionic influx produces IPSP which counter acts the depolarising action of excitatory synapses, and hence effecting inhibition.

ELECTRICAL—CHEMICAL TRANSMISSION

- Action potential → transmitter → diffusion across synapse → activation of post-synaptic membrane → EPSP → action potential
- The action potential travels along the presynaptic terminal causing a release of transmitter material. As far as acetylcholine is concerned, it is stored in packets (synaptic vesicles) at the terminals of presynaptic fibres. Action potential causes the release of acetyl choline. The released transmitter diffuses across the cleft in a very short time (0.6 msec.) to attach to receptor site on the post-synaptic membrane. Now, the depolarisation of membrane is produced and the flow of current through depolarised region give birth to EPSP. This current flow outward through the initial segment of axon hillock and set up an impulse in the post-synaptic axon. Then release, diffusion, attachment are the usual steps. After this inhibitory substance attaches to post-synaptic membrane producing hyper-polarisation which produces inhibition.
- Indication of chemical transmission are:
  - — Presence of choline acetylase in many nuclei of nervous system.
  - — Abundance of cholin-esterase.
  - — Anti-cholinesterase prolongs the activity of certain neurons like Renshaw cell.
  - — Other chemicals also have been identified like glutamic acid.
  - — There is synaptic delay of 0.5 msec. in vertebrates.
  - — These synapses are susceptible to anoxia and metabolic inhibitors.

TRANSMITTER SUBSTANCE: AT POST SYNAPTIC NEURON

1. Just like any guest comes at our residence, we receive him/her in two ways. Firstly, we put few steps ahead of our main gate and receive him. Identical to this is 'Ion channel'. 'Cation Channel' allows sodium ions to pass when opened since they are negatively charged so they attract positive sodium charge; but sometimes potassium or calcium ions too. 'Anion channel' allow mainly chloride ions to pass. The entry of positive sodium charge excites the post synaptic membrane so the transmitter released is 'excitatory', and entry of chloride leads to release of 'inhibitory transmitters' which inhibit the neuron. These channels close very shortly so they are not meant for causing prolonged post synaptic neuronal changes.
2. Second way of welcoming the guest is, we take him towards/inwards to our house after shaking hands. This is identical as 'second messenger' system. This is present in post synaptic membrane itself and most prevailing is 'G protein' which is attached to the portion of receptor protein which protrudes to the interior of the cell. The 'G protein' itself consists of three parts—'alpha' (the activator part); 'beta' and 'gamma' components (that attach G protein to inside cell membrane). The alpha component serves many functions like activation of cyclic AMP, activation of some intra cellular enzymes, activation of gene transcription, and opening of specific ion channel. This cause prolonged changes in neurons (from seconds to months/years), so used in memory process.

SUMMARY AND HIGHLIGHTS

So when an impulse reaches a synapse, conduction is slower, fatigability is greater, the threshold value of a stimulus has greater variability, there is much greater dependence on blood supply for oxygen, there is a greater refractory period; it is the place where summation of impulses may occur, it has got greater susceptibility to various drugs and anaesthetics and there is greater reinforcement and inhibition of one reflex by another. So by all above means and mechanisms, the sorting out process of different message/impulses/informations is taking place. So it is better to say that indefinite numbers of computers together cannot even dare to compete human brain.

BIBLIOGRAPHY

1. Adrian ED, et al. The impulse produced by sensory nerve endings. J Phy 1926-28;61:151.
2. Alverez Buylla R, et al. Local responses in pacinian corpuscles. Amer J Phy 1953;172:237.
3. Bruton J, et al. Hereditary hyperammonaemia. Brain 1970;93: 423-34.
4. Eccles C. Ionic mechanism of post-synaptic inhibition. Science 1964;145:1140.
5. Gray JAB, et al. Properties of receptor potential in pacinian corpuscles. J Phy 1953;122:610.
6. Ile F, Jack JJB. Ammonia: Assessment of its action on post synaptic inhibition as a cause of convulsion. Brain 1980;103: 555-578.
7. Katz. Quantal mechansim of neural transmitter release Science 1971;173:123.
8. Leslie L, Iverson. Dopamine receptors in brain. Science 1975;188:1084.
9. Lloyd DPC. Facilitation and inhibition of spinal motoneurons. J Neurophy 1946;9:421.
10. Lloyd DPC. Temporal summation in rhythmically active monosynaptic reflex pathways. J Gen Phy 1957;40:427.
11. Matchison, Zingg HH. Chloride dependent effect of GABA on Hypothalamo-neurohypophyseal axons in vitro in Rat. J Phy 1979;292:51.
12. Pixner B. Evidence for depression of post-synaptic inhibition by morphine in frogs. J Phy 1979;292:50.
13. Richards D, Snell CR. Evidence of a non-opioid inhibitory peptide in brain. J Phy 1979;292:43.
14. Solomen H Snyder, James P Benne. Neuro-transmitter receptors in brain: Biochemical identification. Ann Rev Phy 1975-76;38: 153-175.
15. Solomen H, Synder, et al. Drugs, neurotransmitters and schizophrenia. Science 1974;184:1243.

(1, 2, 5, 9 and 10 bibliography quoted by Physiological basis of medical practice by Best and Taylor, 1967- Williams and Wilkins)

99 Feelings: Sensation and Sensory System

DEFINITION

It is a conscious feeling generated by any stimulus which is a disturbance of environment.

BASIC PROPERTIES

These can be summed up as:

i. *Localisation:* Capacity of an individual in locating the exact spot from where a particular sensation is arising.
ii. *Quality:* Signifying the modality, e.g. pain, touch, temperature, etc.
iii. *Extent:* It is the area involved and so it depends on number of receptors involved.
iv. *Discrimination:* It means to differentiate between two responses in quality, intensity etc.
v. *Affect:* Subjective responses evolving out of sensation.
vi. *Intensity:* It depends on frequency of sensory impulses travelling up the sensory pathway.
vii. *Latent period:* There exists always a time interval between application of stimulus and onset of its response. This is called latent period.
viii. *Adaptation*: On application of a stimulus the response is at its climax at the onset but it is gradually decreased and finally it fades away.

MODALITIES OF SENSATION

Law of specific nerve energies:

- Each of different types of sensation which we are experiencing like pain, touch, temperature and sight etc. is called modality of sensation.
- Each sensory fibre is transmitting only one modality of sensation and this is called law of specific nerve energies.
- Each modality of sensation is subserved by a specific type of sensory receptor that has specific sensitivity for the type of stimulus that excites that particular modality of sensation.

SENSATION OF TOUCH

Touch sensation results from stimulation of tactile receptors; while pressure sensation is resulting from deformation of deeper tissues; and, vibration sensations are resulting from rapidly repetitive sensory signals. It is basically a cutaneous sensation.

Pathway

a. *Fine or epicritic or light localizable*
   - Merkel's disc, Meissner's corpuscles, hair bulb endings are the receptors.
   - Impulses from periphery pass along posterior root ganglia cells and enter the spinal cord, and ascend up in tract of Goll and Burdach in posterior funiculus; and this information is also carried by 'C' type of fibres (5-12 μ; 30-70 meter/sec. rate of conduction (first neuron).
   - The fibres of second neuron are arising from above two nerve tracts, cross the mid line as internal arcuate fibres. They are joined by nerve fibres carrying crude touch sensation at dorsally to pyramid of medualla oblongata. Both these fibres are ending by relay in posterolateral ventral nuclei of thalamus (second neuron).
   - Third neuron fibres are arising from thalamus and are finally terminating in post-central gyrus (area 3, 1, 2) where the particular sensation is felt.

b. *Pressure or Protopathic or crude touch*
   - Receptors are same of above with addition of Pacinian corpuscles.
   - Fibres enter the spinal cord in above mentioned way through posterior root and end by relaying into posterior grey column (first neuron).

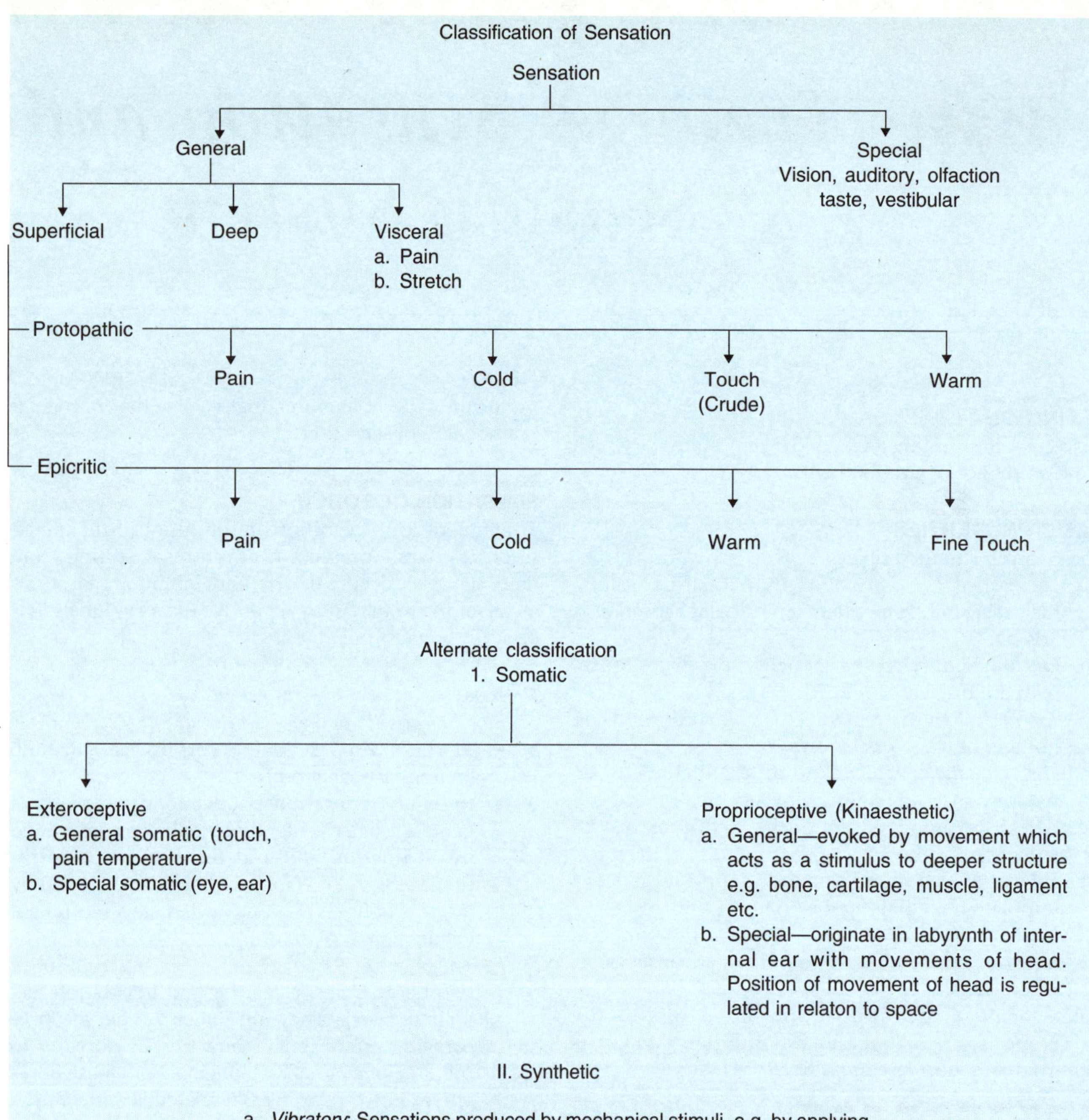

II. Synthetic

a. *Vibratory*: Sensations produced by mechanical stimuli, e.g. by applying vibrating tuning fork over tibia. These travel up to spinal cord through dorsal column. These are lost if dorsal column is damaged as in diabetes mellitus, anaemia pernicious, vitamin deficiency.
b. *Stereognostic*: is a discriminative sensation by which one is able to recognise size, shape and texture of familiar objects when placed in hand and he can also appreciate their weight without seeing them.
c. *Two point discrimination*: is the minimum distance at which two points of a compass can be identified as two separate points.
d. *Itching*: Damage to spinothalamic tract abolishes this sensation. Injection histamine produces itching which is the cause of itching.

- From posterior grey column fibres are originating, cross the opposite side forming ventral spino-thalamic tract. Then they ascend up and join fine touch fibres in medial leminscus and then end in posterolateral ventral nuclei of thalamus (second neuron).
- From here, fibres arise and then terminate in medial nuclei of thalamus where the sensation is felt (third neuron).

Transmission of Tactile Sensation

- Almost all specialised sensory receptors transmit their signals in type Aβ nerve fibres having velocity of 70 m/sec. Free nerve endings tactile receptors transmit the signals through Aδ myelinated fibres with a velocity of 5.30 m/sec.; while some transmit via C unmyelinated fibres at a velocity of 2 m/sec.
- *Tickling:* Sensitive, rapidly adapting mechano-receptive free nerve endings are eliciting tick and itch sensation. These receptors are found in superficial layers of skin. It is transmitted by small C type unmyelinated fibres. Itch sensation makes a man aware of mild surface stimuli, e.g. fly about to bite, or a flea crawling over the skin etc., which excite the scratch reflex, which relieves the sensation. The pain signals are believed to suppress the itch signals in the cord through lateral inhibition.

Notes:

a. Heating the skin raises and cooling diminishes the excitability of these receptors. On the other hand, excitability of tactile receptors is reduced by mechanical stimulation.
b. Main features of touch sensation include—accurate localisation, quick adaptation, two point threshold, two categories (fine and crude) and large action potential.
c. The most sensitive areas (as regards distribution of touch receptor) are—tip of tongue, tip of nose, midline of palm, volar surface of finger. Least sensitive areas in this respect are midline of neck and back.
d. Receptors for fine epicritic touch are characterised by rapid adaptation, low threshold, receptive field of 1.5-5 sq cm.
e. Along with feeling of touch sensation through spinothalamic system, arousal response is also felt owing to its connection with reticular formation. Together with this, psychic attitude accuracy is coupled with touch sensation because of projection of fibres to somatic area I.
f. Touch receptors can be stimulated by various ways; oldest is Von Frey's which is consisting in touching the skin with hair mounted on a wooden handle. Henson has used glass wool or nylon threads. Bishop has used high voltage low current sparks to stimulate single sensory units without skin deformation.
g. Fatigue and old age diminish sensitiveness to touch, specially the capacity to discriminate. Touch receptors are showing high degree of adaptation and having no after discharge.

SOMATIC SENSORY CORTEX/SENSORY AREA

It occupies the portion of cerebrum behind the central sulcus and can be divided into regions like those of motor areas in front of sulcus. By sensory aphasia is meant the condition of those who are unable to understand written, printed or spoken symbols of words although the sense of vision and that of hearing are unaffected.

Area I

On its excision following are the result:

- He is unable to judge critical degrees of pressure against his body.
- He is not able to localise discretely the different sensation in different parts of the body.
- He cannot judge the weight, shape or forms of the objects (astereognosis).
- In the absence of this area pain and temperature sensations are altered either in quality or intensity. They are poorly localised.
  — It lies in post-central gyrus (Brodman area 3, 1, 2). Each side of the cortex receives sensory information exclusively from opposite side of the body.

Area II

- This area is much smaller lying posterior and inferior to lateral end of somatic sensory area I. The face is represented anteriorly, arms centrally and legs posteriorly.
- Signals enter here from area I, both sides of the body, other sensory areas of brain.

Association areas:

Are Brodman area 5, 7 located in parietal cortex behind area I and above area II. It receives signals from somatic sensory area I, ventrobasal nuclei of thalamus, other thalamic areas, visual and auditory cortex.

Amorphosynthesis

- Means removing somatic association area
- He forgets about the existence of opposite side of the body
- If he is called to examine any object, he forgets to examine the opposite half of it.

MAJOR SENSORY PATHWAY

a. *Posterior column:*

i. Afferent neurons enter the spinal cord and turn up upwards to ascend on same side to medulla oblongata. These neurons make up a group of tracts called posterior column because of their position in back part of the cord.

ii. Neurons which constitute the posterior column end in medulla oblongata. In the medulla the impulse is transmitted across a synapse to activate a secondary fibre in the chain of this sensory pathway. The axons of these neurons cross medulla to the opposite side, turn up and ascend in a tract called medial lemniscus. This secondary neuron ends in thalamus which in turn, relays the impulse to cerebral cortex.

iii. It conveys sensation of touch, pressure and proprioception. If posterior funiculus is destroyed these sensory modalities will be lost on affected side. Touch and pressure are also transmitted in part by other pathways, therefore destruction of posterior column does not completely impair the ability to appreciate touch and pressure. Serious loss of proprioception is certainly there. Ataxia (lack of arrangement or co-ordination) results which means loss of usual high integration and smoothness of muscular activity.

iv. The beauty in this system is that each time a point in periphery is stimulated, a signal ordinarily is transmitted to somesthetic cortex. On an increase in intensity of this stimulation, the intensity at cerebral cortex is also increased simultaneously. Moreover when a discrete area of body is stimulated, the signal from this area is transmitted to highly discrete area of cerebral cortex. In its neuronal circuit, signals of different intensities are transmitted to cortex by means of spatial and temporal summation.

b. *Lateral spinothalamic tract:*

i. The afferent neurons which are activated by receptors specific for pain and temperature transmit the impulse into spinal cord through dorsal roots. These fibres end in dorsal horn of grey matter. The axon of secondary neuron arises from a cell body situated in nucleus of dorsal horn of grey matter. This axon crosses spinal cord at the same level and then turns upwards on opposite side to ascend through spinal cord and medulla to thalamus. From here fibres are projected to cerebral cortex.

ii. It differs from above medial lemniscus system in the way that velocity of transmission is comparatively less, less acute spatial localisation of signals transmitted, less acute gradation of intensities and unability to transmit rapidly repetitive sensations.

c. *The two pathways—functions:*

- *Dorsal column:*
  1. Touch sensations requiring a high degree of stimulus localisation.
  2. Touch sensation requiring transmission of fine gradation of intensity.
  3. Position sensation.
  4. Pressure sensation with fine degrees of judgement of pressure intensity.
  5. Vibratory sensation.
- *Anterolateral system:*
  1. Pain
  2. Thermal sensation,
  3. Crude touch and pressure sensation,
  4. Tickle and itch
  5. Sexual sensation.

"Mechanoceptive sensations are transmitted by both systems. Spinothalamic tract system represents a cruder type of transmission system. Pain thermal and sexual sensations are only transmitted by spinothalamic tract."

MUSCLE SENSE

i. Psychologically attention has been directed towards sense of muscle. This information is carried in, either, by usual tactile signals in deep tissue or by signals in motor cortex. Any way, this sense is originating in deeper structures as, muscle, ligaments, joints and bones.

ii. *Path:* End organs are muscle spindle and tendon organs. Posterior root ganglion contain cell bodies. A fibres are entering spinal cord or brainstem. Some of these fibres are travelling through posterior column and terminate into nucleus gracilis and cuneatus; while some fibres are terminating into internuncial cells of spinal cord and they are concerned with muscle tone, body posture as well as with maintenance of tendon jerks; while some other fibres are terminating into Clarke's column of cells forming spino-cerebellar tract which terminate round cerebellar cortex (First neuron).

— The second order neuron fibres are emerging from nucleus gracilis and nucleus cuneatus → forms internal arcuate fibres → cross mid line → ascend up brainstem and joined by ventral and lateral spinothalamic tract as well trigeminothalamic tract → finally terminating into posterior ventral nucleus of thalamus (second neuron).

— Third neuron fibres are emerging from thalamus and finally terminate in two ways—for crude sense in medial nucleus of thalamus while for conscious/vibratory/discriminatory sense in post-central gyrus and Betz cells.

iii. Betz cells are guided by information of position and movement during volitional activities like appreciation of weight, form and texture without vision.

TESTING

Position sense: Ask the patient to look away or shield their eyes. Doctor moves his finger up or down and then he is told to say the direction of movement.

Vibration's appreciation: Put vibrating tuning fork on the body surface and ask the patient about their feeling. This type of sensation may be lost in tabes dorsalis, in peripheral neuropathy.

Pain

- Pin prick or pressure on deeper structures (cutaneous stimulation) will elicit pain.
- Squeeze a distal muscle (Achilles tendon). Patient feels it. This sensation is abolished in "tabes dorsalis."
  — analgesia... absence of pain sensation.
  — hyperalgesia..... even a mild stimulus causes unnatural degree of painful sensation.

Temperature: Use test tubes containing warm and cold water. Touch with part to be tested turn by turn and ask about the feeling.

Tactile Sensibility

- Use a cotton wool/tip of index finger. Ask whether he is feeling touch or not.
- With the help of blunt divider, the discrimination between two points can be felt. The patient is asked whether he is feeling both the points or not. Normally two millimetre of separation of points can be recognised as two separate stimuli on the fingertips and slightly wider separation on the pulps of the toe. It is useful in posterior column lesion etc.

Size/shape Recognition

- Place objects of same shape on palm of the patient, but their sizes should be different (e.g. small rods/matches of different length). His eyes should be closed.
- For recognition shapes of familial objects are placed on palm. (coin, knife, scissors etc.) and patient is said to identify and describe them.

THERMAL SENSATION

- Cold, warmth and pain receptors are there. Pain receptors are stimulated at extremes of hot and extremes of cold.
- Cold and warm receptors are located immediately under the skin.
- Cold receptor is a small, Aδ myelinated nerve ending; and a branched structure. Some of the cold sensations are also transmitted in type C fibres.
- Cold receptor "adapts" rapidly but not completely.
- On stimulation of receptor by alteration in temperature; the signals enter the spinal cord. It travels in "tract of Lissauer" and terminate in dorsal horn. Then after travelling a long distance fibres cross to opposite antero-lateral sensory tract. It terminates into reticular area of brainstem, and thalamus (ventro-basal). Few fibres are relayed to sensory cortex I. So removal of post-central gyrus makes a man unable to distinguish gradation of temperature.
- Cold receptors respond between 10-38°C; and warm between 30-45°C.
- Sense organs are located subepithelially; so the temperature of subcutaneous tissue determines the response.

PAIN SENSATION (DARD)

Pain is usually regarded as a symptom of an underlying disease. Pain is a specific modality like vision or audition with its own central and peripheral apparatus -

- Pain is pain to an animal presumably, and all pain serious and significant —Beecher H.K.
- Pain is a passion of the soul, a feeling state, and not a specific sensation
  —Aristotle
- Sensation of pain is the psychical adjunct of an imperative protective reflex
  —Sherrington

TYPES

- Pricking pain is felt when a sharp object strikes the body surface, e.g. cutting of skin by knife or stucking of a needle into skin.
- Burning pain gives the impression of pain with burning.
- Aching pain is a deep pain with varying degrees of annoyance. It is characteristic of tissues like bones, joints and muscles.
- Besides these, cutting, tearing, crushing, stabbing typed pain may also be encountered.

RECEPTORS

These are *free nerve endings* which are widely distributed in superficial skin layers along with certain tissues like arterial walls, periosteum, joint surfaces, tentorium of cranial vault. Their distribution is punctiform.

PURPOSE AND REACTION

- In actual sense pain is a protective mechanism of and for the body, since it forces the suffering individual to remove pain stimulus.
- The effected individual reacts both ways—psychic as well as reflex motor reactions. Psychic includes crying, anxiety, depression, muscular excitation etc.; while reflex activities are quite identical with withdrawal reflex.

REFERRED PAIN

- It happens that, pain fibres from many viscera are synapsing with pain fibres from the skin, within the spinal cord. Due to this sort of synapsing, whenever pain fibres of viscera get stimulation, this pain sensation is spreading to that area of skin supplied by these neurons. Due to all this the patient feels pain sensation in skin itself. *This is referred pain which means that person feels pain in some area which is quite away from that tissue which actually is causing pain.* Reflex spasm of lumbar muscles due to ureteric pain is another example. On the other hand convergence of pain fibres (visceral and skin) at thalamic level is another explanation of it.

POSSIBLE CAUSES

- Due to damage of tissues, pain nerve endings get excitation which becomes the cause for release of some chemical substances which are called pain producers. Histamine and bradykinin are two notorious chemical in this series.
- Muscle spasm is said to be another cause for pain. Because of it, the blood supply is cut owing to compression of underlying vessel and resulting ischaemia (less blood supply) is terminating into pain. Moreover due to spasm, rate of muscle metabolism is also increased which adds to pain sensation.
- Tissue ischaemia is also a causative factor.
- Accumulation of some metabolites specially lactic acid is also responsible for stimulation of pain nerve endings.
- Of course, temperature at which tissue is damaged is also a causative factor and it is 45°C or above. It is said that tissues are completely destroyed if temperature remains at this level for an indefinite time.

PAIN PATHWAY

i. The receptors are free nerve endings.

ii. These pain signals are carried by both fast pain fibres (delta A type; 3-10 meters per second; carrying pricking pain sensation) as well as slow pain fibres (type C fibres; 0.5-2 meters per second; carrying burning and annoying/aching pain). This is the reason that sudden painful stimulus gives a double sensation—one is pricking and then burning sensation.

iii. These fibres enter the spinal cord. On entry, these fibres ascend for four or five segments in the tract of Lissauer and finally terminate into gelatinous substance forming the apex of dorsal grey column typing immediately deep to posterior lateral column (first neuron).

iv. From above gelatinous substance second neuron arises, crosses the opposite side (opposite lateral funiculus) and ascend upwards as lateral spino thalamic tract to be terminating into posterolateral ventral nuclei of thalamus, through medulla, pons and mid-brain (second neuron).

v. From thalamus, third neuron arises, which ascends up through internal capsule to be finally terminated into sensory cortex (area 3, 2, 1 in post-central gyrus). It is to be remembered that somatic sensory area II is more sensitive for pain than area I.

vi. If pain is in the lower part of body cordotomy in upper thoracic region relieves pain while bulbar tractectomy is suggested in patients where above surgery is not successful. In it, lateral spinothalamic tract is sectioned in brainstem.

vii. Visceral pain pathway
   - Many follow the above pathway.
   - From some organs like distal colon, rectum and bladder, fibres make their entry into spinal cord through sacral parasympathetic nerves and to central nervous system through cranial nerves, (glossopharyngeal and vagus).
   - When pain is referred, it is usually to a structure that developed from the same embryonic segment or dermatome as structure in which the pain originates. Say heart originates from neck and upper thorax (C_3 to T_5), stomach (T_7 to T_9), gall bladder (T_9). This is called 'dermatomal role.'

Few New Concepts—Pathway

- Type Aδ pain fibres terminate into lamina I of the dorsal horn and there excite second order neurone of neo-spinothalamic tract which gives rise to long fibres which cross the opposite side of the spinal cord and then pass upwards in anterolateral column. These fibres in majority terminate into thalamus (posterior nucleus) but few are also terminating in reticular formation.
- Type C fibres (slow, chronic pain) terminate in substantia gelatinosa (with few fast fibres too). Here long axons arise which joins the fibres of fast pain passing to opposite side and then pass upward in the same anterolateral pathway. The fibres are finally terminating into thalamus, (as well as, either to, reticular nuclei of medulla/pons/mesencephalon, tectal area of mesencephalon, or periaqueductal grey region surrounding aqueduct of Sylvius.
- Substance P-a neuropeptide is said to be released by type C fibres (where they synapse in the dorsal horn). This substance persists for many more seconds even after disappearance of pain because:
  — It explains persistence of pain even after removal of this stimulus.
  — It explains the increasing intensity of slow chronic pain with time.
- Pain perception is made possible by lower centres and cerebral cortex. Plays an important role in interpreting quality of pain.

Hyperalgesia

Sensitivity of pain receptors is altered on any injury or inflammation or due to any other stimulation. This is hyperalgesia. When pain fibres are facilitated due to low threshold stimuli, it constitutes primary hyperalgesia; while on the contrary, in so-called secondary hyperalgesia the pain threshold in affected area is raised but the pain perceived is severe, unpleasant, prolonged and extending well beyond site of injury.

Visceral Pain

- Ischaemia to viscera, chemical irritation (HCl from perforated ulcer can lead to peritonitis terminating into severe pain), spasm of hollow viscus, over distension of hollow viscus are said to be causative factors.
- Parenchyma of liver and lung alveoli are visceral areas which are entirely insensitive to pain while on the contrary, liver capsule, bile ducts, parietal pleura and bronchi are the structures which are very much sensitive to pain.

Measurement

- Clinically, skin is pricked with a pin or needle and subject's expressions are noted and compared on healthy side.
- Radiant heat of increasing intensity is applied to exposed part to know pain threshold.
- Mechanical device is pressure algometer.
- Pain sensation slowly adapts. It is intensified by asphyxia; and it is abolished with retention of other sensation in syringomyelia (dissociated sensory loss).
- The manifestation of pain in dog consists of (i) Somatic withdrawal reflex, (ii) autonomic responses like transient tachycardia, hypertension, hyperpnoea etc. and (iii) psychic reaction involving repeated vocalisation, struggling and biting behaviour (identical with flight or fright or fight).

NATURE OF PAIN RECEPTORS

It is clear that Sherrington would not regard the pain nerve endings as specialised receptor. Three types of receptors have been described as specific receptors for pain:

i. *Thermo-sensitive nociceptor.* It evokes pain when exposed to temperature of 45°C or higher. It may also cause sufficient tissue damage to reduce or prevent responses to subsequent stimulation.
ii. *Mechano-sensitive nociceptor:* Noxious deformation of skin receptor believing to evoke pain, constitutes 20-25 per cent of cutaneous receptors in primate and cat and is supplied by fine myelinated afferent fibres conducting at 5-28 m/sec. (primate). Adequate stimulus is noxious deformation of skin.
iii. *Chemo-sensitive receptors:* These are not nociceptors since chemical stimulus is not intense and evokes pain without causing injury. Intra-arterial injections of chemical agents like hypertonic salts, acids and alkaline solution, specific cations and anions will evoke pain.
iv. The free nerve endings have the most widespread distribution in the body, which are usually derived from medium size or fine myelinated axons, but some free endings originate from thick myelinated or non-myelinated fibres.

Notes

- There are two kinds of pain, viz. one is bright and sharp; and another is dull-intense-diffuse. These are also called first and second pain, OR fast and slow pain. The fast pain is due to activity of A (delta), while slow one is due to activity of C fibres.

- If blood supply of a muscle is occluded then its contraction causes pain, which persists after contraction until blood flow is re-established. It is said to be due to release of a substance P factor-(Lewis). Pain of angina pectoris is a classical example of this. When the blood supply is restored this material is washed out or metabolised with relief from pain.

Deep Pain

This type of pain is poorly localised, nauseating and associated with sweating and alteration in blood pressure. This pain initiates reflex contraction of skeletal muscles of near vicinity; which becomes ischaemic—which stimulates the pain receptors.

HEADACHE

The problem of headache is increasing with the advancement of civilisation. It must not be neglected but it should be always remembered that 'headache is felt when any part of our body is in trouble; means that its cause should be traced and it should not be treated with so-called routine pain killers.

Extracranial Causes

i. All sorts of emotions so-called 'stress.' In such tension headache the muscular spasm occurs in muscles attached to scalp, neck muscles attached to occiput.
ii. Retro-orbital headache is sometimes felt with poor vision. The ciliary muscles are under excessive contraction when such persons focus their eyes on to some objects.
iii. Some absorbed toxic products which have been accumulated in body as a result of constipation is also responsible for headache.
iv. Hang over headache after celebrating evening with alcohol is common. Its direct toxicity towards cerebral meninges is the real cause. It is said to exert the diuretic effect which results in loss of fluid.
v. Infection or irritation in nasal structures (sinuses) is also cause of headache which is referred behind the eye.

Intracranial Causes

i. Meningitis—a fatal disease due to inflammation of all the meninges can cause headache and pain is referred over entire head.
ii. Trauma (due to brain surgery, brain tumour) is also one of the causes. General location of an intracranial tumour can be assessed from the area of headache. Most of it results from meningeal irritation.
iii. Migraine—the real problem of modern civilisation is caused by emotional tension → vasospasm of brain arteries → ischaemia of affected portion → symptoms viz. nausea, visual disturbances, sensory hallucination etc. → blood vessels dilating and pulsating → excess stretching of walls of arteries → migraine pain.
iv. Low CSF pressure - stretches various dural surfaces and so produces pain.

CENTRAL INHIBITION

- A soldier in wounded state in battle ground is not feeling any pain; acupuncture technique has been long used in treating pain, it is also well known that touching the injured area relieves the pain. By these and many more examples we can know that pain mechanism may be inhibited at some or other places.
- Few terminology:
  - *Hyperalgesia :* Stimuli which normally causes mild pain will cause severe prolonged pain.
  - *Hyperpathia:* Threshold for stimulation is some what increased, but when reached sets off intense burning pain.
  - Causalgia: There is spontaneous burning pain long after trivial injuries. It is often associated with hyperalgesia and allodynia.
  - Allodynia: Gentle stimuli (e.g. touching the clothes etc.) causes an intense pain.
- Relief:
  - by analgesic drugs
  - For relieving chronic intractable pain, stimulation of dorsal column with implanted electrodes has been used. This pain relief is usually antidromic rather than orthodromic conduction.
  - Prefrontal lobotomy, i.e. cutting the deep connections between frontal lobes and rest of the brain.
  - Anterolateral cordotomy, i.e. knife is inserted into lateral aspect of spinal cord and swept anteriorly and laterally. By this technique lateral spinothalamic tract and anterolateral system pain fibres are cut while ventral spinothalamic touch fibres are kept intact.
  - Cingulate gyrectomy
- Dorsal horn is the important site of inhibition of pain transmission. It is really the gate through which pain impulses reach the lateral spinothalamic system. Stimulation of those large fibre area from which the pain is initiated, reduces the pain. Collateral fibres from dorsal column touch fibres enter the substantia gelatinosa, and impulses in these collaterals/interneurons on which they end, inhibit transmission from dorsal root pain fibres to the spinothalamic neurons. It acts via presynaptic inhibition (Gate control).

- Morphine relieves the pain and produces euphoria. On, intrathecal administration it is partially effective. There are opioid receptors in substantia gelatinosa that may be on substance P containing terminals of nociceptive afferents and inhibit release of substance P.
- Enkephalin containing neurons terminate presynaptically at the site of receptors on these afferents but no presynaptic terminal has been identified. Naloxone is morphine antagonist.

Pain Control System (ANALGESIA)

1. Three components are: Periaqueductal grey area of mesencephalon and upper pons surrounding aqueduct of Sylvius
2. Raphe magnus nucleus: Thin midline nucleus located in lower pons and upper medulla
3. From here signals are transmitted down to dorsal horn of spinal cord. This is the point where pain can be blocked. Electrical stimulation in either of these regions completely suppress many pain signals entering by way of dorsal spinal roots.
   - Encephalin and serotonin are important transmitter substances involved in analgesia system. Encephalin is causing presynaptic inhibition of both incoming fibres, i.e. Aδ and C where they synapse in dorsal horn, through blocking calcium channels in membrane of nerve terminal. This analgesia persists for a much longer time. This can also block many of other cord reflexes that result from pain signals (withdrawal reflex). Similarly pain transmission to further areas is also blocked like to reticular formation and in thalamus etc.
   - β endorphin is present both in hypothalamus and pituitary. Dynorphin—having 200 times pain killing effect as morphine on direct injection into analgesia system.
   - On electrically stimulating large sensory fibres, intra-laminar nuclei of thalamus, periaqueductal area of diencephalon, pain can be inhibited.
   - Stimulation of large sensory fibres from peripheral tactile receptors depress the transmission of pain signals either from same area of body or located many segments away.

BIBLIOGRAPHY

1. Basbaum AI, et al. Endogenous pain control system: Brainstem spinal pathways and endorphin circuitary. Ann Rev Neurosc 1984;7:309.
2. Basson JM, et al. Peripheral and spinal mechanism of nociception. Phy Rev 1987;67:67.
3. Bond MR. Pain its nature, analysis and treatment. New York: Churchill Livingstone. 1984.
4. Bonica JJ, et al (Ed). The management of pain. 2nd ed. 2 vol. Lea and Tebiger. 1990.
5. Brown, REW Fyffe, JE Heavner, R Noble Morphology of collaterals from axons innervating pacinian corpuscles. J Phy 1979;24.
6. Cervero F. Sensory innervation of viscera. Peripheral basis of visceral pain. Phy Rev 1990;74:95.
7. Darian Smith I. The sense of touch: performance and peripheral neural process: In: Handbook of physiology sec. I. Vol. III. Bethesia Md American physiological society 739, 1984. (Quoted by Text of book of medical physiology by AC Guyton, WB Saunders).
8. Damasio H, et al. The return of Phineas Gage : clues about the brain from skull of a fomous patient. Science 1994;264:1102.
9. Edward R Perl. Somato sensory mechanism. Ann Rev Phy 1963;25:459.
10. Head H. Studies in Neurology Vol. II. London. Oxford University Press. 1920.
11. Kruger L (Ed). Neural mechanism of pain. New York: Raven Press. 1984.
12. Lewis RV, et al. Biosynthesis of enkephaline and enkephalin containing polypeptides. Ann Rev Pharm Toxico 1983;23:353.
13. Mc Clskey DI. Kinaesthetic sensibility. Phy Rev 1978;58:763.
14. Melazack R. The tragedy of needless pain. Sc Am (Feb.) 199__;262:27.
15. New Concepts in pain and its clinical management Edited by E. Leong Way. FA Davis (Company, Philadelphia).
16. O Bishop. Central nervous system : Afferent mechanism and perception. Ann Rev Physiol 1967;29:427.
17. Robert KS. Pain. Lim Ann Rev Physiology 1970;32;269.
18. Ryan RE. Headache—diagnosis and treatment. 2nd ed. St. Louis. CV Mosby Co. 1957.
19. Sherrington C. Integrative action of nervous system. New Haven Yale, University Press. 1947.
20. Shin Ho Chung and Anthony Dickenson. Pain—enkaphalin and acupuncture. Nature 1980;283:243.
21. Weiner SL. Differential diagnosis of acute pain by body region. McGraw Hill quoted by Review of Medical Physiology by WF Ganong. Lange Publication.1993.
22. White JC, Sweet WH. Pain : Its mechanism and neurosurgical control springfield: Illinois Charles Co. Thomas. 1955.
23. Whitear, M. Quoted by Touch heat and pain. A Ciba found action symposiums - Edited by AVS DE REUCK and Julie Knight, J and A Churchill Ltd. London 1966. J Anat. 1960;94:387-409.
24. Wolff HG. Headache and other head pains. 2nd ed. New York: Oxford University Press. 1963.

(Bibliography 2, 3, 4, 5, 7 and 9 quoted by Guyton AC in Textbook of Medical Physiology, WB Saunders)

100 The Obedience: Motor System (Muscular Activity)

INTRODUCTION

If we revise the evolution; the neural mechanism governing skeletal muscular activity is not dependent upon cerebral cortex and moreover, it is not present in birds and reptiles. In such animals spinal cord is playing a dominant role since there are two ways of execution—namely by reflex mechanism and by voluntary means (will). In human beings useful voluntary movements are dependent upon 'precentral motor - cortex' of course; we cannot deny the importance of sub-cortical centres (basal ganglia, red nucleus, substantia nigra, reticular formation, cerebellum, globus pallidus, corpus striatum), which are the chief controller in lower animals. To sum up, two mechanisms are existing as controller—one is already existing which is named as *'Extra pyramidal system'* and another is newly superimposed on it because of cerebral cortex is named as *'Pyramidal system'* responsible for controlling skilful voluntary movements affecting distal part of limb. From all grounds both these systems are functioning by establishing a good balance with each other, operating simultaneously; of course they are anatomically independent units.

CONCEPT OF MOTOR NEURONS

If a peripheral nerve which supplies a skeletal muscle is cut or destructed by any means; it may lead to muscle paralysis, no reflex activity and muscle wasting, all this is named as 'lower motor neuron paralysis'. The only drawback with this term is that it is having a counter part 'upper motor neuron' or its paralysis.

i. Nuclei located in cortex, on brainstem or even sub-cortical regions which are supplying impulses to lower motor neurons are termed as *upper motor neurons*. These are mother substances of both pyramidal and extra pyramidal tracts.
ii. Lower motor neurons are nothing but anterior horn cells of cord and their cranial homologues. They are said to supply the muscles at peripheral end.
iii. All muscle fibres supplied by single anterior horn cell, constitute motor unit. Range of movement along with magnitude of tension is determined by it. Motor neuron pool is constituted by union of several anterior horn cells for performing a particular action.

CONCEPT OF PYRAMIDAL SYSTEM

Motor control system is hence divided into two classes—Pyramidal (operating through cerebral cortex) and extra-pyramidal (employing a series of complex circuits involving basal ganglia and brainstem nuclei).

Pathway

- Fibres are arising from pyramidal cells including Betz cells of area 4, and also area 6, 8, 3, 1, 2, 5, 7. Neurons governing body movements are lying in pre-central gyrus (superolateral surface) and adjoining para-central lobule in such a way that body is represented upside down.
- Fibres are descending vertically downwards to corona radiata → Internal capsule (genu and anterior two-third of posterior limb) → mid-brain → pons (basilar part) → medulla oblongata. Most of the cortico-spinal fibres approaching medulla decussate in median plan with fellow fibres of opposite side and it descends to spinal cord as crossed pyramidal tract while few fibres are reaching the cord as direct pyramidal tract) → spinal cord (crossed fibres are running through lateral funiculus and named as lateral cortico-spinal tract while direct tract's fibres are descending through ventral funiculus as ventral cortico-spinal tract.
- As regards their termination fibres terminating in anterior horn cells by making synapses with inter-

nuncial cells are constituting cortico-spinal fibres; while those making synapses with cells of motor cranial nerve nuclei of opposite side by crossing median plane are constituting what is known as cortico-bulbar fibres.

A review study: As told earlier it is a newly superimposed controlling system, so it is developing later on along with fact that myelination starts at birth and hence it starts functioning after second or third year of life. The fibres composing this system are fine myelinated having their diameter less than 3 µ, along with slow conduction rate. It controls upper limb more, as well as dorsal half of spinal cord. Flexor muscles of body are more regulated by this system. It is said to be responsible for non-postural fine movements of small muscles at distal joints of limbs. On their lesion flaccid paralysis is evident with more disability. It discharges directly into lower motor neuron in anterior grey column of spinal cord. It is concerned with finalisation of work. All voluntary muscular activity is not completely achieved by these corticospinal fibres since it is not a multi- or poly-synaptic pathway. They terminate in cervical (55%), thoracic (20%) and lumbosacral region (25%).

Functional aspect: It is the initiator of skilled and fine voluntary activities. It provides the grace to the motion. It controls distal muscles by presiding over fine movements of distal joints. It is also supposed to impress some of the special type of reflexes.

Note: Betz cell of precentral gyrus is giving origin to only few percentage of corticospinal fibres. The majority or remainder are arising from cells in precentral gyrus, parietal cortex.

CONCEPT OF EXTRAPYRAMIDAL SYSTEM

i. *Components* : The parts constituting are cortical units (area 6, 4, 5, 22 as non-specific one; while area 8, 13, 19 as specific one) and sub-cortical units (corpus striatum, red nucleus, substantia nigra, reticular nucleus, pons, medulla, cerebellum).

ii. *Pathway from cortex*:
   - Cortico-strio-nigral tract which controls tone and posture since it carries impulses to lower centres; while cortico-ponto-cerebellar tract is meant to control activities of protagonists and antagonists and on their damage, it leads to intention tremor.
   - All descending tracts (reticulo-spinal, vestibulo-spinal, rubrospinal, olivospinal, tectospinal) are connecting lower motor neurons.

iii. *Review study:* Since it is already existing controller, so it is classed as old motor system and all this is because of the fact that before birth myelination starts and therefore, it starts functioning before birth. Just on the contrary, it controls lower limb and ventral half of spinal cord, and it is said that extensor group of muscles are mainly regulated by it. It is, of course, a multi-channel polysynaptic cortical pathway. It is influencing large muscle groups of proximal joints of limb and trunk. On their lesion less disability has been reported; of course paralysis with spasticity is resulting. It is having a faster conducting rate. Of course, it is mainly responsible for postural adjustment of body, automatic associated movements of body, regulation of reflex activity, synergistic voluntary movement of big muscle groups, making ground for skilled movements.

DIFFERENCES

Decerebrate animal	*Thalamic animal*
1. Spinal cord with medulla oblongata retained.	Spinal cord, hindbrain, midbrain and part of diencephalon retained.
2. Animal is unable to move without assistance.	Animal can rise without assistance.
3. Decerebrate rigidity present.	Decerebrate rigidity absent.
4. Animal cannot maintain equilibrium.	Animal can maintain equilibrium
5. Respiration is abnormal.	Respiration is normal.
6. Postural reflexes are found but righting reflex is absent.	Righting reflex is present due to reflex regulation of skeletal musculature.
7. Normal body temperature cannot be maintained.	Animal is capable of maintaining body temperature.

DESCENDING TRACTS (Motor or Efferent tracts)

A. Pyramidal tracts:

i. Is the longest tract starting from motor cortex and reaching up to the last segment of the cord. It is only present in higher animals and man where cerebrum has developed. It is composed of one million nerve fibres of which 50 per cent are myelinated, 40 per cent are non-myelinated.

ii. Why so named?

   a. The fibres arise from pyramidal cells of different sizes including Betz cells located in fifth layer of area 4, 6, 8, 3, 1, 2, 5, 7.

   b. The fibre bundle meant for spinal motor neurons are arranged in the form of two pyramidal swellings on the ventral aspect of medulla oblongata, one on either side of median plane.

iii. Course: The fibres from their origin descend downwards through:
   a. *Corona radiata:* Fibres are wide and broadly distributed.
   b. *Internal capsule:* In this structure fibres form a compact band. Here at this point, these pyramidal fibres are accompanied by extrapyramidal fibres. The fibres lie in genu and anterior two-third of posterior limb.
   c. *Mid-brain:* Middle 3/5th of crura cerebri contain corticospinal fibres, while medial fifth have cortico-nuclear fibres.
   d. *Pons:* Here fibres are arranged into discrete bundles in its basilar parts.
   e. *Medulla oblongata:*
      - Here fibres converge. Then they are arranged into two pyramid bundles; one on each side of median plan. Majority of fibres decussate in median plan with fellow of opposite side—so-called decussation of pyramid. Then it descends into spinal cord—so-called crossed pyramidal tract. Remaining least number of fibres remain uncrossed and descend into spinal cord—called - direct pyramidal tract.
   f. *Spinal cord:*
      - Fibres of crossed pyramidal tract descend through lateral funiculus—lateral corticospinal tract.
      - Fibres of direct pyramidal tract descend through ventral funiculus—ventral corticospinal tract. Most of the fibres cross.
   g. *Termination:*
      - Corticospinal fibres terminate in anterior horn cell and synapse with internuncial cells.
      - Corticobulbar fibres terminate by synapsing around motor cranial nerve nuclei by crossing median plane.

iv. Functions:
   a. It is initiating skilful voluntary activity,
   b. It controls distal muscles
   c. It provides precision, accuracy, fineness to the motion to make the movement graceful.
   d. Some reflexes are influenced by it.

DESCENDING TRACTS

1. *Rubro-spinal tract:*
   - It arises from nucleus magnocellularis (red nucleus). They cross the opposite side so-called Forel's decussation) ventral to sylvian aqueduct. During their descend—some fibres end in cerebellum + reticular nuclei of medulla. Spinal cord receives maximum number of fibres (Cervical part).
   - It lies dorsally in pons, ventrally in medulla.
   - It enters lateral white column of spinal cord and ending upon internuncial neurons at the base of anterior horn cells.
   - It exerts facilitatory influence over flexor muscle tone.
2. *Tectospinal/Tectobulbar tract:*
   - These take origin from deeper layers of superior colliculus (decussation of Meynert).
   - At medulla its fibres descend as low as cervical level.
   - They terminate upon anterior horn cells.
   - They convey impulses subserving reflex postural movements in response to visual + auditory stimulation.
3. *Reticulospinal tract:*
   - As the name suggests the fibres arise from reticular substance of pons and medulla and descend in anterior/anterolateral part of spinal cord.
   - Fibres of pontine origin are crossed and descend mainly in anterior funiculus of spinal cord so-called medial reticulo-spinal fibres.
   - On the other hand, medullary reticular fibres are uncrossed which primarily descend in lateral funiculus (anterior part). Most of the neurons end in anterior horn cells of spinal cord—so-called lateral reticulo-spinal fibres.
   - *Functionally:*
     — Pontine reticulo-spinal tract are concerned with facilitation. So voluntary movements are facilitated:- vasomotor effects and expiration also increased.
     — Medullary reticulo-spinal tract influences gamma motor neuron whose axons terminate in motor end plate of intrafusal fibres. Normally the area 4S (suppressor) inhibits motor activities of nucleus of medullary reticulo-spinal tract. Other effects seen on their stimulation include—deep inspiration and fall of blood pressure.
     — On stimulating brainstem reticular formation can either facilitate or inhibit voluntary movement, alter muscle tone, modification of respiration, altered blood pressure and alteration in central transmission of sensory impulses results.
4. *Vestibulo-spinal tract:*
   - *Lateral tract:* Takes its origin from Dieter's nucleus of medulla. It receives fibres from cerebellum as well as eight cranial, nerve (vestibular division). It ends in anterior horn cells (medial part) after descending in entire length of spinal cord.

- *Medial tract:* Fibres arise from inferior/medial vestibular nucleus. It reaches to anterior funiculus after descending up to upper thoracic spinal segment. Some fibres are also relayed to brainstem reticular formation.
- Lateral part is supposed to exert facilitatory influences on reflex spinal activities and also controls the muscle tone (spinal mechanism). Cerebellum also interferes with its activities because of its above mentioned connections. Medial part of this tract is concerned with nausea, vomiting, palpitation, perspiration, pallor of face, conjugate horizontal eye movements, integration of eye and neck movements, etc.

5. *Olivo-spinal tract (Bulbo spinal/Tract Helweg):*
   - Fibres arise from inferior olivary nucleus and terminate into anterior horn cells by travelling through anterior part of lateral white column. It is located only in cervical region. It is acting as an important pathway through which cerebrum and thalamus are inter-connected.
6. *Descending medial longitudinal fasciculus:*
   - It originates from medial vestibular nucleus, reticular formation, superior colliculus and Cajal's interstitial nucleus. It is present only in upper cervical segment of spinal cord. It descends in anterior funiculus of cord (posterior part). Its functions include—Co-ordination of reflex ocular movements + integration of eye and neck muscles.

Inter-segmental Fibres

a. *Anterior fasciculus*: This ground bundle connects anterior horn cells of one side with those of opposite side, or of the same side.
b. *Lateral funiculus:* Fibres originate from lateral horn cells. They then ascend upwards into medial longitudinal fasciculus.
c. *Posterior funiculus*
   1. *Posterior ground bundle:* Fibres originate from posterior horn cells.
   2. *Septo-marginal fasciculus:* Fibres originate from posterior horn cells and connect them with same types of fibres at lower level.

CONCEPT OF MOTOR NEURON PARALYSIS

a. Upper motor neuron lesion is caused by damage to crossed pyramidal tract. It is characterised by spastic paralysis, exaggerated deep reflexes with increased knee jerk, presence of ankle clonus, extensor plantar reflex, no reaction of degeneration and no wasting of muscles, rigid paralysed muscles due to increased tone, loss of superficial reflexes.
b. Lower motor neuron paralysis is mainly caused by damage to anterior horn cells. The condition is characterised by flaccid paralysis, absence of all reflexes, wasting of muscles, presence of reaction of degeneration.

MOTOR AREA

- The surface of the brain involved in the motor function is pre-central gyrus of frontal lobe (grey matter in front of central sulcus). Large pyramidal cells whose fibres form the corticospinal pathway are located in pre-central gyrus and arranged so that motor cells for toe movement are located in upper part and motor cells for face movements are located near lateral cerebral fissure.
- If area 4 is stimulated it is found that discrete muscles are caused to contract, (isolated contraction). When top of area 4 is stimulated, muscles in feet contract; when lower sections of area 4 are excited the facial muscles move. Thus, there must be an orderly arrangement of fibres from cortex to the brainstem and spinal cord (point to point relationship) on the whole along with it subcortical nuclei, basal ganglion, cerebellum, all are playing a co-ordinative and integrative role.
- There, however, exists a *'supplementary motor area'* on and above the superior bank of cingulate sulcus on the medial side of the hemisphere that reaches to premotor cortex on the lateral surface of the brain.
- The supplementary motor area projects to the motor cortex. It is involved in programming motor sequences. Its lesions produce awkwardness in performing complex activities and difficulty with bimanual co-ordination. It has been said that there occurs increased blood flow on increased neuronal activity.
- Premotor cortex on the other hand is concerned with setting posture at the start of a planned movement and with getting the individual ready to perform. So it projects to brainstem areas concerned with postural control and to the motor cortex and also towards cortico-spinal and cortico-bulbar outputs.
- Besides it, the somatic sensory area and related portions of posterior parietal lobe project to premotor area.

ABNORMALITIES OF VOLUNTARY MOVEMENTS

a. *Paralysis:* It means loss of voluntary movements. Generally two types:

i. *Flaccid*: There is not only loss of voluntary control but reflex movement is either absent or very weak, resulting in that, limb does not respond to stretch and it cannot be moved and is completely inert. It is seen in poleomyelitis. Limb appears to be little more than bones covered with skin.

ii. *Spastic:* It is seen in strokes (cerebrovascular accident). There is also loss of voluntary movement but reflex action not only persists but is unusually sensitive, so limb is thus rigid. The muscles retain their size so that structure appears normal.

b. *Tremors (trembling)*: It is an involuntary shaking. There is characteristic rhythmic muscular contraction and relaxation which is beyond individual's control (to inhibit) called *non-intentional tremor* or steady persisting trembling. Tremor appears only when fine muscular movements are executed called *'intention tremor.'* In some of the psychological states they are seen without the involvement of central nervous system. Essential tremor is most common movement disorder. There may be a disorder of motor control in addition to dysfunction due to tremor; it may lead to functional disability. It progresses slowly but serious physical, social and psychological disability may be caused by essential tremor.

BIBLIOGRAPHY

1. Asanuma H. The pyramidal tract. In Brooks VB (Ed). Handbook of Physiology. Sec. I, Vol II. Bethesda Med. American Physiological Society 1981;703.
2. Grillner S. Locomotion in vertebrates: Central mechanism and reflex interaction. Phy Rev 1975;55:247.
3. Kalaska JF, Crammont PJ. Cerebral cortical mechanism of reaching movements. Science 1992;255:1517.
4. Lisherger SG. The neural basis for learning simple motor skills. Science 1988;242:728.
5. Stein PSB. Motor system with reference to control of locomotion. Ann Rev Neurosci 1978;1:61.
6. Williain Koller, Nahil Biary, Sandra Cone. Disability in essential tremor. Neurology 1986;36(7):1001.
7. Weisendanger M, et al. Ascending pathway of low threshold muscle afferents to cerebral cortex and its possible role in motor control. Phy Rev 1982;62:1234.

(Bibliography 1, 2, 5 and 7 quoted, by Guyton AC in Textbook of Medical Physiology, WB Saunders)

101 Grace—Glamour: Posture—Equilibrium

It is the distribution of muscle tone responsible for setting a particular posture which further depends on various reflexes called postural reflexes which are controlled by centres located in brainstem. The homeostasis of posture is equilibrium.

(One must revise his knowledge on reflex arc, stretch reflex, muscle spindle, pyramidal and extra-pyramidal system and principal tracts of extra-pyramidal system etc. before going through present discussion). The purpose of posture is to make the movement smooth and accurate, as well as to maintain a constant line of gravity.

MUSCLE TONE: A VIEW

1. *Definition*: It is a state of tension present normally in tissues. It is due to this that parts are kept in normal shape during resting condition and are ready to act on application of stimulus.
2. *Tone in muscle*: May be taken as state of tension present in muscle during resting condition, consequent on continuous asynchronous discharge from neuro-muscular-apparatus.

Clinically it is assessed as active resistance offered by muscle to passive stretch given by examiner.

3. *Posture:* Signifies an unconscious adjustment of tone in different muscles during active movements so as to maintain line of gravity constant (equilibrium).

   OR

   It does not mean a movement OR it refers to adjustment in distribution of tone to the different groups of muscles, involved in a particular movement.
4. *Variation:*
   a. Increased in decerebrate animal, upper motor neuron lesion
   b. Unchanged in thalamic animal.
   c. Abolished by interrupting any part of reflex arc as follows: By destroying posterior root, anterior root, centre in spinal cord, by transection of spinal cord, by division of peripheral nerve entering a muscle.
5. *Importance:* (a) It makes the ground for skilled movements. (b) It is responsible for maintenance of posture, (c) It also helps in maintenance of look of a object.
6. *Mechanism of genesis:* Granit's theory
   a. There is gamma efferent activity which discharge impulses tonically to intrafusal fibres of muscle spindle. This leads to contraction of intrafusal fibres leading to stretching of nuclear leaf, causing distortion of annulospiral endings, causing set up of receptor potential.
   b. Now then, receptor potential is changed into action potential. Afferent discharge pass through primary and secondary afferents. This is transmitted to posterior nerve root of spinal cord.
   c. Afferent discharge from IA afferents pass to α motor neurons through monosynaptic path. This results into muscular contraction (a phasic reflex response). The tension of intrafusal fibres is released, which abolishes IA discharge.
   d. Group IA afferent discharge is followed by afferent discharge through IB fibres.

The contraction of extrafusal fibres is proportional to gamma efferent activity; which lasts as long as activity persists. Even passive stretching of muscle causes distortion of annulospiral ring leading to contraction as long as stretch is operative.

7. *Factors affecting*
   a. *Drugs:* Chlorpromazine, hypnotics, tranquillisers decreases tone while muscle relaxants (curare) will lead to loss of muscle tone.
   b. *Sleep:* Causes lack of inputs of sensory impulses to RAS which is responsible for alert and arousal. It causes damping effect on excitatory extrapyramidal tract causing inhibition of gamma-

efferent activity. Unconsciousness leads to loss of muscle tone.

DECEREBRATE RIGIDITY

- In this operation (firstly done by C.S. Sherrington), a transection is made in between superior and inferior colliculi. This leads to complete lack of communication between cerebral hemisphere and brainstem; so brain stem is not getting any message from these higher centres.
- Secondly, medullary inhibiting area is becoming more a non-functional entity.
- Thirdly, in decerebrate preparation, facilitatory impulses sent by vestibular nucleus are exaggerated. All such facilitatory impulses stimulate gamma efferent which increases tone.
- On the whole such animals stand hyper-extended with pillar like rigidity in all four limbs, tail and neck are hyper-extended along with hypertonia in both extensors and flexors of limbs, along with the fact that influencive control from cerebral cortex is lost on brain stem centres (e.g. release phenomenon).
- A spino- bulbo-spinal (SBS) reflex system has been investigated in decerebrate cats, dogs and man. Afferent sources are from cutaneous nerve while efferents are inflexor muscles. It depends upon relay through bulbar reticular formation and recurrent projection to spinal motoneurons.
- The main feature here is hypertonia of antigravity muscles meaning an exaggerated posture of reflex standing.
- Receptors—in muscles and tendons of affected muscles and in otolith organ of labyrynth.
- Efferent-pathway originates in Dieter's nucleus → vestibulo-spinal tract and large cells of reticular formation of pons and medulla → lateral reticulospinal tract → ventral horn cells.
- In human beings - it exhibits marked spastic rigidity of all four limbs, arched back, retracted neck (opisthotonus)

POSTURAL REFLEXES (Figs 101.1 to 101.3)

a. *Stretch reflex*: Receptors are muscle spindle, stimulation is stretch; centre lies in spinal cord and is giving response by causing contraction of muscles.

b. *Positive supporting or magnet reaction*: Pressure on sole (during standing) or palm is acting as a usual stimulation of proprioceptive receptors of lower limb muscles, which responds by causing extension of limbs in order to support the body. However, centre lies in spinal cord.

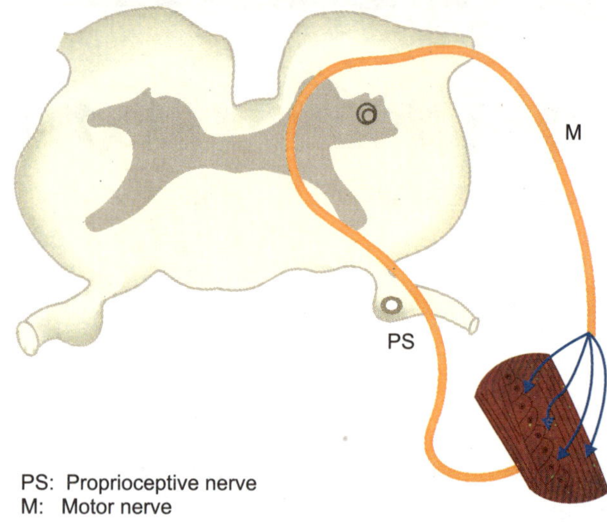

Fig. 101.1: Stretch reflex

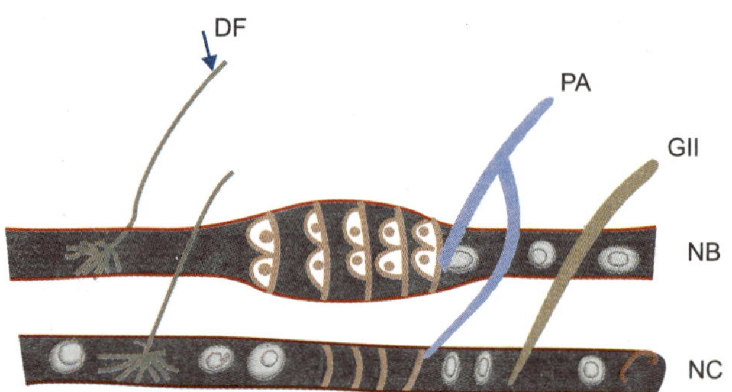

Fig. 101.2: Muscle spindle fibres

c. *Tonic neck reflex*: The usual stimulation is obtained by turning head to one side or any upward or downward movement of head. This stretches proprioceptors in upper part of neck which are receptors. This is responding in the way that extension of head leads to flexion of hind limbs and extension of forelimbs, as well as, flexion of head leads to extension of hindlimbs and flexion of forelimbs. However, centre lies in medulla.

d. *Righting reflex*: As the term is self-explanatory, it means correction, i.e. when posture becomes wrong/ abnormal, the animal tries to correct it.

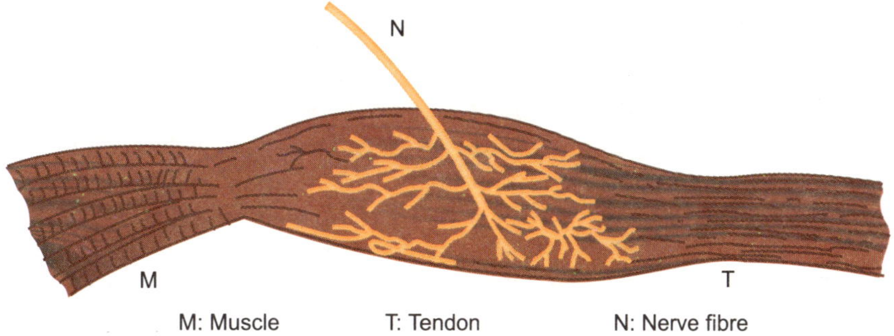

Fig. 101.3: Golgi tendon organ

i. *Labyrinthine (vestibular) reflex*: Tilting of head which is a usual stimulus; is detected by receptors in vestibular apparatus (otolith organs) and therefore the posture is corrected by compensatory contraction of neck muscles. Centre is located in mid-brain.

ii. *Optical reflex:* Eye receives the images of the surrounding objects that means usual stimulus is opening of eyes; responded by righting of head centre present in cerebral cortex.

Two more such righting reflexes have been demarcated viz. Body on head, and body on body. Stimulus for both is pressure on side of body; and receptors are exteroceptors while centre lies in mid-brain.

e. *Hopping reaction*: If animal is pushed laterally while standing, this act is a stimulus for it; and is responded by movements which keep limbs in position to support the body. Centre lies in cerebral cortex.

f. *Negative supporting reaction*: When any previously applied pressure from sole or palm is removed, this stimulates proprioceptors in extensors which is responded by release of above mentioned magnet reaction. Centre lies in spinal cord.

g. *Placing reaction*
   - Pressure events like touch or push is acting as a stimulus which is detected by proprioceptive, exteroceptive, and visual receptors. The response is given by limb which is replaced on supporting surface in position to support the body. The centre lies in cerebral cortex.
   - If a blind-folded animal is lowered rapidly, its forelegs extend and toes spread. This response to linear acceleration is vestibular placing reaction that prepares animal to land on floor.

h. *Grasp reflex*: Touching the palmar surface of hand is a stimulus which responds by flexion of hand which results in grasping the particular object. The beauty or characteristic feature is that if attempt of withdrawal is made, the grasping movement becomes more forcible. As known, it is present normally in newborn and pathologically in cerebral damage but is absent in normal adults. It is a cutaneous spinal reflex analogous to human flexor plantar response.

i. *Clasp knife (Lengthening reaction) reflex:* It protects the muscles from damaging contraction against strong stretching forces. If extended limb of a decerebrate animal is flexed forcibly then it resists initially, but if more force is applied then extended limb is suddenly collapsed. Since extensor muscles are lengthened so it is named as lengthening reaction.

AFFERENT FOR MUSCLE TONE AND POSTURE

- Kinaesthetic impulses are main
- Kinaesthetics from deeper parts of sole.
- Vestibular impulses.
- As per Romberg's sign, if a subject stands on tip toe with eye closed, balance becomes difficult; it is evident that retinal impulses are also playing a role.

CONTROL OF POSTURE, TONE AND EQUILIBRIUM

- The extra-pyramidal system is exerting its full influence on spinal motoneurons via descending extra-pyramidal pathways and with their help it controls the stretch reflexes. Postural reflexes are particular examples of total activity of extra-pyramidal system. So brainstem, reticular formation and spinal cord are playing essential role in maintaining muscle tone, posture and equilibrium.
- Any disease or injury to cerebellum (paleo and neo) disturbs the controlling system of posture and equilibrium; suggests that cerebellum also plays a significant role in it.
- In disorders related with basal ganglia; this beautifully controlled system is disturbed. This also

proves the role of basal ganglia in this system. (e.g. Parkinson's disease, chorea, athetosis).

- Vestibular nuclei is also having a significant role, since its unilateral destruction results into abolition of rigidity of some side. It is also said to exaggerate muscle tone in ischaemic decerebration.
- Cerebral cortex, being the highest centre is exerting a great influence on maintenance of posture and equilibrium since its injury or lesion leads to a defection in this equilibrium. The additional background activity necessary to bring potential postural patterns to successful expression are coming from somatic sensory inflow, from other spinal and brainstem level, from vestibular and reticular organs and from cortex and basal ganglia.
- Response by Golgi tendon organ: Signals from tendon organs play a role in reflex regulation of muscles. A tendon organ will respond to a contraction of single motor unit provided that some of the fibres of unit lie directly in series with receptor. Contraction of fibres which are not in series with the receptor can cause a tendon organ which is discharging to a passive force to pause during contraction.

ROLE OF VESTIBULAR SYSTEM IN POSTURE CONTROL

i. The vestibular apparatus comprises three semi-circular canals, utricle and saccule (otolith organ). Canals are arranged in three planes of space viz. horizontal or external, anterior or superior, vertical and posterior vertical. Utricle is united with saccule by ductus endolymphaticus.

ii. The principal central connections from labyrinth follow:

Fibres arising in labyrinth have their cell bodies in the vestibular ganglion and then pass as vestibular division of eight nerve to the upper part of medulla. The nerve enters the medulla ventral to inferior peduncle and terminates in superior and medial vestibular nuclei and in a group of cells in outer part of floor of fourth ventricle, the lateral vestibular or Dieters' nucleus.

- From lateral and superior nucleus fibres (axons) pass to cerebellum.
- From lateral vestibular nucleus fibres descend into anterolateral region of spinal cord as vestibulo-spinal tract.
- Connections are established with red nucleus.
- Ascending fibres from vestibular nuclei make connection with oculomotor nuclei and end in superior colliculi of corpora quadrigemina.
- Fibres from vestibular nucleus enter medial lemniscus and pass to the thalamus from which they are relayed to the temporal cortex.

iii. *Semi-circular canals:* Lateral, anterior and posterior are three such canals lying in three planes at right angles to one another. Each is beginning in a dilatation—ampulla which contains a broad projecting ridge—crista acustica. It is a specialised neuro-epithelial structure projecting into endolymph.

- It gives information about kinetic equilibrium, i.e. information about direction, degree and plane of movement of head. Thus, it aids in equilibrium. It also helps to maintain reflexly the tone of muscles. Head movements stimulate these canals. Lateral turning of head stimulates horizontal canals while backward and forward movements stimulate vertical canals. These canals are arranged so that movements of head causes increase in pressure of endolymph in one ampulla with a corresponding lessening of pressure in parallel canal of opposite side. The stimulation of sensory hair are transmitted by fibres to vestibular nerve. The changes in pressure in these canals stimulate fibres of vestibular nerve. As these fibres convey impulses to vestibular nucleus in medulla, from which impulses are relayed to motor nuclei of extrinsic muscles of eye, motion of eye takes place.
- On stimulation, a normal subject exhibits nystagmus in opposite direction, past pointing, vertigo.
- Head rotation: Role of semi-circular canals:
  1. When head begins to rotate in any direction (angular acceleration) the endolymph remains stationary due to its inertia while semi-circular canals turn themselves. This leads to fluid flow in canals in opposite direction of head rotation. Within a second or so of rotation back pressure from bent cupula causes endolymph to move with same speed as that of semi-circular canals. When rotation suddenly stops then oppositely—endolymph continues to rotate while semi-circular canal stops. The hair cell does not discharge because cupula is bent in opposite direction. After another few seconds endolymph stops moving and cupula returns to its original position.

     Thus, these semi-circular canals transmit signals when head begins to rotate as well as when it stops rotating.

2. Suppose a man is running forward very fast and then he suddenly begins to turn to one side then he feels to be falling off, until and unless appropriate balance is made quite ahead of time. This falling off tendency is predicted by the semi-circular canal and the information is conveyed to brain and in this way this malequilibrium is corrected.

iv. *Otolith organ (saccule + utricle)*
- Are neuro-epithelial elements, one in lateral wall of utricle, other on medial wall of saccule, and their surfaces are perpendicular to each other. Maculae acts as stretch receptor and gravity acts as a stimulus. Alteration in position of head in space causes otolithic membrane to pull on hair cells, saccule respond to a lateral tilt and, utricles to a ventral and dorsal flexion. So the otolithic organs are giving information about static position of head and are concerned with linear acceleration.
- *Linear acceleration: Role of maculae:*
  — When body accelerates, the statoconia having greater inertia than the surrounding fluids fall backwards on hair cell cilia. This is sending the information of malequilibrium to the brain. So one feels that he will fall down backwards. So he leans his body forwards until the tendency of statoconia is equalised. At this point of equilibrium; the brain detects the balance and then no more forward leaning is ordered by it. This work is done by maculae in this way.
  — It is to be remembered that maculae don't operate for detection of linear velocity. This explains the fact that when racer begins to run they lean forward to prevent backward falling; but once they attain a speed, they don't require further leaning.

v. *The principal functions of labyrinth are:*
- To influence postural activity in eyes, trunk and limbs
- To guide the cerebellum in its regulation of muscular activity
- To provide conscious sensation of position of movement of head.

LABYRINTH MAY BE CONSIDERED AS A SPECIALISED ORGAN OF PROPRIOCEPTION AND IN GENERAL, IT SUPPLEMENTS THE CONSCIOUS AND UNCONSCIOUS PROPRIOCEPTIVE PATHWAYS IN THEIR FUNCTIONS.

EXPERIMENTS: VESTIBULAR APPARATUS

1. *Barany's test (Past pointing test)*: A normal person who is able to put his fingers on a particular spot with eyes open, can also perform the act even after closing this eye. Then he is subjected to a rotational movement and then he is said to perform above act. He fails with eyes closed. His fingers deviate/past point the object.
   - *Barany's chair* is used which moves around a vertical axis. Subject sits on chair which rotates at the rate of one rotation per two seconds. Eyes are kept closed. At the end of rotation, the subject shows post-rotatory nystagmus which consists of quick rhythmic, jerky movements of the eyes in direction opposite to rotation.
2. *Labyrinthectomy in man:*
   - In animals this operation causes violent disturbances of equilibrium. It is not observed in man after division of vestibular nerve, of course, vertigo is noticed.
   - Streptomycin—an antitubercular drug—is causing degeneration of neuro-epithelium of maculae which results in transient vertigo.
3. *Ménière's syndrome:* is characterised by tinitus (noises/ringing in ear) along with progressive loss of hearing and vertigo. It is due to degeneration of neuro-epithelium of cochlea and semi-circular canals; so it affects the internal ear.
4. *Other methods of stimulating vestibular apparatus:*
   - Syringing the external ear with warm and cold water (43°C, and 12-30°C respectively) produces nystagmus, called caloric nystagmus.
   - On passing galvanic current through ear. So-called galvanic nystagmus is produced.
5. *Motion sickness:* Peculiar sensation while moving in train/vehicle/rolling on sea/aircraft during flight. It is characterised by pallor, vertigo, salivation, nausea, vomiting, drowsiness. Out of these many symptoms are due to vagal stimulation since it is inter-connected with vestibular nucleus and inhibitory control from vestibular system is withdrawn. Psychogenic factors aggravate the situation because inhibitory control of reticular formation from vestibular system is withdrawn earlier. An intact vestibular system is needed to produce motion sickness.
6. *Adaptation:*
   - Is a phenomenon in which repeated exposure to a new environment will not produce ill-effects.
   - Otolith organs show little adaptation when tilted to a new position in the earth's gravitational field.

These organs are stimulated by pattern of depression of macular substrate by otoconia. The nerve impulses are generated without any change with each new position of the head.

7. *Habituation:* It is seen that with repeated vestibular stimulation; many subjects develop relative sensitivity to subsequent vestibular stimulation.
8. *Coriolis effect:* It can be tested by asking a subject to rotate about his vertical axis in a clockwise direction and head is to be nodded forwards so as to make the chin to touch his chest. He feels that he is rolling clockwise to his right about antero-posterior horizontal axis.

NEURAL CONNECTIONS: VESTIBULAR APPARATUS

- Vestibular impulses are carried by vestibular division of eight cranial nerve (vestibulocochlear nerve).
- First neuron — The peripheral processes of bipolar cells of vestibular ganglion.
- Receptors situated in internal auditory meatus, begin at synaptic link with the bodies of hair cells of crista of semi-circular canals and ampulla of utricle and saccule. The axons of bipolar cells enter the brainstem and terminate in:-

Vestibulo-cerebellar Tract

a. Few fibres pass directly to flocculo-nodular lobe and fastigial nuclei of cerebellum via inferior cerebellar peduncle.
b. Majority of fibres terminate into superior, lateral, medial inferior nuclei of vestibular nerve located in vestibular area of floor of IVth ventricle at medulla oblongata. From here, the relay fibres follow:
   1. *Vestibulo-ocular tract:*
      - Fibres from superior vestibular nucleus join with median longitudinal bundle of same side.
      - Fibres from medial vestibular nucleus pass to the medial longitudinal bundle of opposite side.
      - Fibres from inferior vestibular nucleus ascend to medial longitudinal bundle of both the sides.
      - All these fibres terminate into nuclei of 3rd, 4th and 6th cranial nerve through medial longitudinal bundle. Through these connections reflex ocular movements along with movement of the head are performed.
   2. *Vestibulo-spinal tract*
      - Fibres from lateral (Deiters') and inferior vestibular nuclei descend to spinal cord.
      - Fibres from inferior vestibular nucleus join the lower part of median longitudinal bundle, extend downwards to upper cervical region where they end around anterior horn cells of spinal cord.
      - By this vestibular nucleus is connected with muscles of neck, trunk and limb through anterior horn cells.
   3. *Vestibulo-reticular fibres:* These connections are important for smooth voluntary movements. Impulses from both labyrinths are reorganised into excitatory and inhibitory impulses so as to influence the flexors and extensors of limb in accordance with principle of reciprocal innervation.
   4. *Vestibulo-cortical fibres:* Fibres terminate into cortex of temporal lobe (dog, cat, monkey) and is, concerned with conscious vestibular sensation.
   5. *Vestibulo-labyrinthine fibres:* Efferent fibres arise from lateral vestibular nucleus and terminate into hair cells of neuro-epithelium.

NYSTAGMUS—AT A GLANCE

- Normally, the right vestibule tends to move the right eyeball towards the left, and left vestibule tending to move the left eyeball towards the right; the eyes remain in normal straight head position by neutralising action of both vestibules.
- If one of the vestibular functions is lost because of any reason; the other tends to move the eye to the opposite side, but this tends to be corrected by jerky and swift movement of the eyes towards the same side producing nystagmus. So it is defined as jerky swift movements of eyeballs either on a horizontal or on a vertical axis due to dysfunction of one vestibular apparatus. This happens when eyes are allowed to move in a plane from central position to one side or other.
- *Pathway:* From intact vestibule the impulse pass through vestibular nerve to vestibular nucleus in medulla.
  - Slow component is due to impulses passing through the fibres from median longitudinal bundle and in reticular formation reaching nuclei for nerves supplying eye muscles.
  - The slow component of nerve fibres communicate with reticular formation and on reaching threshold they discharge to produce quick movements.

- The inhibitory part of reticular formation is stimulated simultaneously which cuts off the slow component discharge.
- The high threshold reticular neuron then stops discharging from vestibular nerve through medial longitudinal bundle.
- If due to any reason, inhibitory neurons in reticular formation are damaged then there occurs no jerky movement but occurs only conjugate deviation of eyeballs.

LABYRINTHINE DISORDERS

- This is manifested by symptoms like vertigo, dizziness, in co-ordination and ataxia.
- Such disorders are due to labyrinthitis, vestibular neuritis, abnormal fluid balance within system, local infection etc.
- Severe derangements may lead to progressive loss of hearing, tinitus.
- Drugs like streptomycin (2 gm daily for long period) may give rise to vestibular symptoms. It is due to its action on ventral cochlear nucleus.

ROLE OF CEREBELLUM

1. Extreme disturbances of posture and equilibrium are observed on damaging flocculo-nodular lobe as well as vermis. One of the causes is that it developed phylogenetically at the same time when vestibular apparatus came into existence.
2. The vestibular apparatus dictates the body position and rapid changes; while cerebellum maintains the balance between agonists and antagonist — muscles.
3. In performing the rapid movements, the signals from periphery of the body (foot) dictates the brain about position of different parts of the body during movement as well as about direction of the motion. This role of progression for next sequential movement is performed by cerebellum.
4. It computes the actual position of respective parts of the body at given time.
5. It assists cerebral cortex to co-ordinate the pattern of movement involving distal parts of the limb viz. hands fingers, feet etc.
6. It also helps cerebral cortex to plan the timing and sequencing of the next successive movement which will take place after completion of present movement.
7. After learning its duty, cerebellum provides turn on to agonists and turn off to antagonists group of muscles. This continues till one movement comes to an end. Where turn off signals are transmitted to agonists and turn on signals are transmitted to antagonists.

ASSESSMENT: VESTIBULAR FUNCTION

a. *Nystagmus:* Spontaneous vestibular nystagmus is enhanced by movement of the eyes in the direction of fast phase and diminished by movement in the opposite direction. In destructive vestibular lesion the activity of contralateral vestibular system predominates, driving the eyes in the direction of damaged side. This is slow phase interrupted by a fast saccadic compensatory movement in the opposite direction. This will be maximum while looking at opposite direction of lesion.

b. *ENG (Electro-nystagmography):* Measurement of eye movements. Changes in electrical potential recorded from two electrodes close to the eyes is monitored. It is recorded on a moving paper strip. Eye act as a dipole (cornea is positive with respect to retina).

c. *Romberg's test:*
   - Patient stands with feet close together, arms outstretched, eyes first open and then closed.
   - Disorder of posterior column—person sways or even may fall when eyes closed.
   - Central dysfunction—person sways to both sides.
   - Uncompensated unilateral labyrinthine dysfunction—instability to side of lesion.
   - This is a test for proprioception.
   - Patient may even fall and are severely disabled when walking in the dark.

d. *Gait:*
   - Patient is said to walk with eyes open.
   - Uncompensated peripheral vestibular disorders veer towards affected side.
   - Central pathology — First staggering and then veering to other side.

e. *Caloric testing:*
   - Patient lying in bed with head at 30° so as to bring lateral semi-circular canal into vertical plane.
   - External canal is irrigated with water at 30°C and then at 44°C for 30-40 seconds, respectively.
   - This thermal gradient produces convection currents within endolymph.
   - Cold water produces nystagmus away from ear, warm water produces nystagmus towards the ear.
   - Evoked nystagmus may be recorded by ENG.

f. *Electro-cochleography:* A needle is inserted through tympanic membrane under local anaesthesia. Cochlear nerve action potential, summating potential are recorded.

BIBLIOGRAPHY

1. Bazett HC, et al. A study of sherringtonian decerebrate animal in the chronic as well as in acute condition. Brain 1922;45:185.
2. Crosby EC. Nystagmus as a sign of CNS involvement. Ann Oto Rhinol and Laryngol 1953;62:1117.
3. Chakraborty - Ghosh and Sahana in Human Physiology.
4. Fitzgerald G, et al. Studies in human vestibular function I. observation on directional preponderance of caloric nystagmus resulting from cerebral lesion. Brain 1942;65:115.
5. Grillner S. Locomotion in vertebrates: central mechanism and reflex interaction. Phy Rev 1975;55:247.
6. Pearson K. The control of walking. Sci Amer 1976;235(6):72.
7. Peterson BW. Reticulo-spinal projection of spinal motor nuclei. Ann Rev Phy 1979;41:127.
8. Peterson BW, et al (Ed). Control of Head Movement. New York: Oxford University Press 1988.
9. Precht W. Vestibular mechanism. Ann Rev Neurosci 1979;2:265.
10. Preene W. Vestibular mechanism. Ann Rev Neurosci 1979;2:265.
11. Shick ML, et al. Neurophysiology of locomotor automatism. Phy Rev 1976;56:465.
12. Stein RB. Peripheral control of movement. Phy Rev 1974;54:215.
13. Wilson VJ, et al. Peripheral and central substrates of vestibulo-spinal reflex. Phy Rev 1978;58:80.

(Bibliography 1, 2, 4 quoted by Best and Taylor, in Physiological basis of Medical Practice, Williams and Wilkins).

(Bibliography 6, 7, 9, 11 and 12 quoted by Guyton AC in Textbook of Medical Physiology, WB Saunders).

102 First Button of Remote: Spinal Cord

INTRODUCTION

i. It is the lowest integrative channel.

ii. It is downward continuation of medulla, descending through the vertebral canal ending at level of lower border of L_1 vertebra.

iii. In cross-section appearance, it shows outer white matter (having tracts; descending-ascending) and inner grey matter (look like H). Three horns are seen—

- Anterior horn—contains nerve cell bodies giving rise to somatic motor nerves supplying skeletal muscles.
- Posterior horn—receives sensory nerve through dorsal root ganglia.
- Lateral horn—conspicuous in thoracic and upper lumbar segments of spinal cord. From here sympathetic fibres arise.

Central canal exists in central part of grey matter (H) and is direct continuation of 4th ventricle.

iv. It is ultimate authority to translate any voluntary action planned and initiated by higher centres.

v. *Grey matter:* Centrally placed. H shaped or like two wings of butter fly. Clark's column, is a well defined collection of cells occupying the inner part of base of posterior horn. It is also called dorsal nucleus since it is confined to thoracic region.

Reticular formation (formatio reticularis) is an area where strands of white matter and prolongations from main mass of grey matter intermingle. It is prominent in cervical region and is continuous with medulla and pons.

Substantia gelatinosa of Rolando is actually a cap of gelatinous material located at the apex of dorsal horn. It is said to contain group of small nerve cells with many dendrites. It receives fibres from posterior root.

vi. *White matter:* It is completely surrounding grey matter.

It is divided into two halves by anterior median fissure and posterior median septum.

- Anterior funiculus lies between anterior median fissure on one end, and, anterior horn and fibres of ventral roots on other.
- Dorsal funiculus situated between posterior horn and dorsal root fibres.

SPINAL NERVES AND ROOTS

i. It is divided into 31 segments each of which is giving rise to a pair of spinal nerves one from each side of the segment. So there are 31 pairs of spinal nerves namely C_8, T_{12}, L_5, S_5, coccygeal 1. Lower spinal nerves are arranged like tail of a horse called *'cauda equina'*.

ii. Each spinal nerve is constituted by the union of anterior (ventral or efferent) and posterior (dorsal or afferent) nerve root.

iii. Bell Magendie Law states that, 'posterior nerve root are carrying afferent impulses while anterior root are carrying efferent impulses.

iv. Each spinal nerve functionally is a mixed nerve meaning that possessing both motor and sensory function while morphologically they are containing somatic and visceral fibres.

v. *Anterior nerve root:*

- Composed of efferent myelinated fibre. Majority of fibres composing are alpha A. fibres, of course they are rapidly conducting fibres with an average thickness varying between 9-13 μ.
- C fibres are also seen to constitute these nerve fibres (thickness varying between 3-6 μ) and they constitute gamma efferents.
- Slowly conducting B fibres have also been reported (conduction rate 3-15 metres per

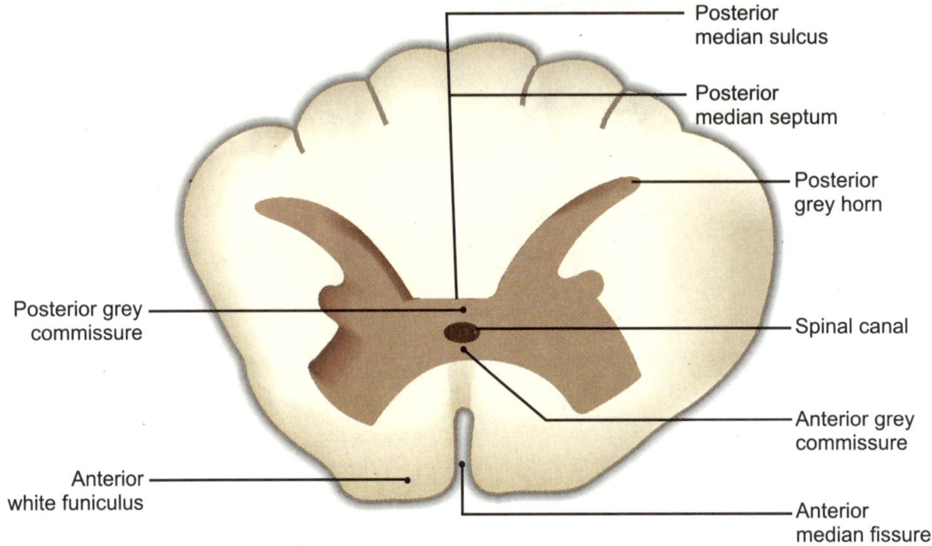

Fig. 102.1: Section of spinal cord

second; thickness 3-10 μ), which are confined to ventral root of all thoracic and upper two lumbar spinal nerves.

- On sectioning, the fatal results are in the form of complete loss of tone of muscles, complete paralysis of muscles, loss of reflex activity, presence of reaction of degeneration, trophic disturbances, alteration in excitability of affected muscles, but of course no sensory change.

vi. *Posterior nerve root:*

- Its fibres are varying between 0.5-20 μ and are having both myelinated as well as unmyelinated afferent nerve fibres.
- It is arising from posterior root ganglia.
- Constituting - A fibres (conduction rate 50-120 metres per second, 10-20 μ thick, carrying cutaneous touch and proprioceptive sensation).
- C fibres—(Unmyelinated, slow conduction rate, carrying diffuse pain sensation).
- B fibres—(Medium sized, thickness 0.5-10 μ, carrying less specifically pain and thermal sensation).
- On sectioning, loss of all forms of sensation, complete loss of tone of muscles in affected area, loss of reflex activity, vasodilatation, weakness and muscular in co-ordination and loss of protective sensory impulses results.

Functional significance: In nutshell, it can be remembered that, spinal cord is the main or central place through which all incoming and outgoing impulses are passing. Besides this, it is considered as main centre for reflex activities. On the whole 'trophic control over muscular system is also exerted by it.'

SPINAL MOTONEURONS

i. As told above it is the central place for all sorts of impulses, i.e. sensory signals enters it through sensory roots and they go on spreading through cord; while motor signals leave through motor roots. Between these two roots, motoneurons and internuncial cells are widely spread in good population to control nicely the reflex functions.

ii. Anterior motoneuron gives rise to A alpha nerve fibres (9-16 μ diameter) which controls contractile function of the skeletal muscle fibres. Gamma motoneuron (5 μ diameter) supply intrafusal fibres.

iii. The high level of phosphorylase activity in certain neurons (type F alpha motor neurons and large sensory neurons of lamina IV) suggests that they are more dependent on glycogen metabolism than rest of spinal cord neurons. Alpha motor neuron of fast motor units are defined by high phosphorylase and low succinate-dehydrogenase activities; while gamma motoneurons are having reverse histochemical typing, i.e. high SDH and no phosphorylase activities.

In nutshell, these are present widely distributed in dorsal and anterior horn as well as the space in between. They are firing at 1500/second. They are rich in properties like convergence, divergence, after discharge etc. These cells are also as numerous as motoneurons are.

PROPRIOSPINAL FIBRES (Intrinsic Spinal Fibres)

These are fibres arising and terminating wholly within the spinal cord and they are vast in number. These fibres exist everywhere throughout the white matter though they lack even distribution. In dorsal column they are small (1 μ) while in ventrolateral column fibres of all sizes are marked, many are large too, which are conducting impulses at rates up to 120 m. per second.

Thus, white matter of spinal cord consists chiefly of fibres extending longitudinally and, all sizes of myelinated as well as unmyelinated fibres are present.

SUMMARY OF ORGANISATION OF NEURONS IN SPINAL CORD

a. *Somatic motoneurons:* Group of motoneurons occupying large ventral horns. Axons existing through ventral roots to innervate skeletal muscles.
b. *Visceral motoneurons:* They activate sympathetic neurons innervating visceral effectors, smooth muscles and glands. They are sending axons through corresponding ventral roots to sympathetic ganglia. Another component is parasympathetic craniosacral autonomic ganglia.
c. *Propriospinal interneurons:* They stitch the spinal cord together horizontally as well as longitudinally. They are occupying broad base of dorsal horn and their axons are communicating with grey matter. They derive information from several neighbouring spinal segments and thus contributing integrated signals to all spinal segments and caudal brainstem.
d. *First order sensory relay and sensory control neuron:* It occupies tapering dorsal part of dorsal horn (sensory analysis) and thus it constitutes sensory relaying nuclei arranged in layers. Another is motor synthesis, on ventral motor side and organised like reticular formation.
e. *Second order sensory neurons:* Notable part of dorsal horn is substantia gelatinosa and its cells provide a spinal relay and controlling station relating to sensory input.

TRACTS OF SPINAL CORD

1. a. Long tracts—connecting the spinal cord with other supraspinal region of CNS. Ascending and descending type
   b. Short tracts—begin and end within spinal cord. (Intersegmental; ground bundles). They are communicating in between segments of spinal cord.
2. The dorsal spinocerebellar tract is characterised by a significant number of large fibres, the velocity of few of them is 120 m. per second.
3. Fibres comprising spinothalamic tract in anterolateral white matter are small. Some of the larger fibres (5 μ or more) in anterolateral white matter of lumbar segments are said to constitute ventral spinocerebellar tract having conduction rate 30-80 m./second.
4. The vestibulo- and reticulo-spinal tracts (descending) are of fairly uniform size conducting at rates comparable to those of large A fibres. The pyramidal tract contains fibres ranging through a wide band of fibre sizes, the largest conducting at rates of about 65 m/sec.

ASCENDING TRACTS OF SPINAL CORD (Sensory/Afferent tracts)

A. In dorsal (posterior) funiculus:

1. *Tract of Goll: Synonym: Fasciculus gracilis.*
   - It is made up of bipolar cells of posterior root ganglia.
   - It receives afferents from lower half of the body.
   - After entering the spinal cord the fibres run in the posterior column throughout the cord. Above the mid-thoracic level the fibres are pushed medially. They don't cross.
   - They end as:
     - Some fibres end round the posterior horn cells, then cross and join the ventral spinothalamic tract of opposite side.
     - Some fibres give descending branches to form comma tract of Schultze
     - Some fibres make reflex connections at different segments.
     - Majority of fibres end in medulla at nucleus gracilis. Here second order neuron arise.
     - Neuron axis is divided into external and internal arcuate fibres; external one are again subdivided into dorsal and ventral. Dorsal group end in cerebellum.
     - *Internal arcuate fibres* cross the opposite side, enter the medial lemniscus and end in thalamus (posterolateral nucleus. Here the third order neuron arise which end in sensory cortex (postcentral gyrus) by passing through internal capsule.
   - Functionally it carries following impulses from lower half of the body; fine touch, tactile locali-

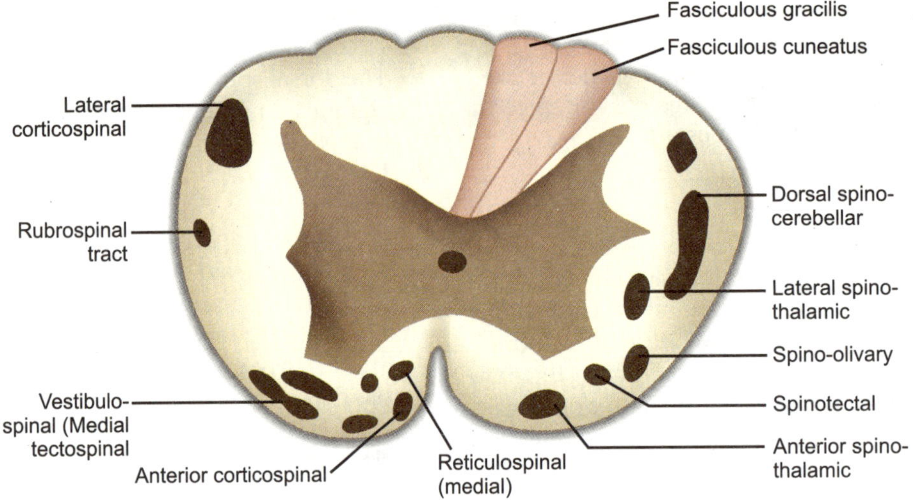

Fig. 102.2: Spinal cord tracts

sation and discrimination, kinaesthetic sensation, sense of vibration.
- Some unconscious kinaesthetic impulses passing to cerebellum through external arcuate fibres.
- Sensory pathway to superficial reflexes.

2. *Tract of Burdach*—Synonym: Fasciculus cuneatus.
   - It is quite identical with tract of Goll but the differences are:
     - Carry sensory impulses from upper half of the body,
     - Fibres end in medulla at nucleus cuneatus—lateral to nucleus gracilis
     - It is made up of posterior root fibres from upper half of the body
     - It is situated laterally in posterior column of upper thoracic and cervical regions.
3. *Comma tract of schultze:* Synonym: Tractus inter-fascicularis.
   - Short descending fibres from tract of Goll and Burdach constitute it.
   - It is situated in posterior column between tract of Goll and Burdach.
   - It appears like comma in transverse section.
   - Functionally
     - It is important to establish intersegmental communication.
     - They also constitute the reflex arc (short).
     - It also contains motor fibres.
     - Though it is sensory in function, but fibres descend.

B. Anterior funiculus:

1. *Anterior (ventral) spino-thalamic tract*
   - It extends from spinal cord to thalamus. Carry fibres from opposite side.
   - First order neuron: Fibres arise as central processes from the cells of posterior root ganglia and enter the spinal cord through dorsal/posterior nerve root. It ascends a short course in posterior funiculus of spinal cord. They end by synapsing with cells of chief sensory nucleus of posterior grey column of same side.
   - It is formed by axons of chief sensory nucleus of posterior grey column, crosses in anterior white commissure to reach anterior funiculus of opposite side of spinal cord and then it ascends upwards as the name explains itself to reach medulla oblongata (2nd order neuron).
   - In medulla oblongata it lies in close contact with lateral spinothalamic tract. It is to be remembered that they together constitute medial lemniscus. Its fibres end in postero-lateral nucleus of thalamus and finally the sensations are relayed to post-central gyrus (area 3, 1, 2).
   - It conducts crude touch, pressure sensibilities + tactile localisation from periphery of opposite side to sensory cortex, and cerebellum by passing through inferior cerebellar peduncle. Ventral group cross the opposite side to end in cerebellum on opposite side.

C. Lateral funiculus

1. *Anterior/ventral spinocerebellar tract*: Synonym: Tract of Gower.
   - It begins in upper lumbar region of spinal cord. Then it extends vertically to the upper part of pons. From here it passes to cerebellum through superior cerebellar peduncle.
   - The fibres arise from large cells of posterior grey column (Clarke's column) of mostly opposite side, but few fibres of same side too. The fibres ascend through lateral funiculus of spinal cord to pons (upper part) through medulla. From here the fibres enter the cerebellum through superior cerebellar peduncle to end in superior vermis of the same.
2. *Dorsal/posterior spinocerebellar tract*: Synonym: Tract of Flechsig.
   - First neuron arise from cells of posterior root ganglia; enter the spinal cord through posterior root; terminates in Clarke's column of same side; of course some fibres coming from same side. Fibres don't cross the opposite side but ascend on the same side.
   - It lies dorsal to anterior spinocerebellar tract and then ascends in lateral funiculus of spinal cord.
   - It enters the cerebellum through inferior cerebellar peduncle to end in vermis of cerebellum.
   - Both of them carry proprioceptive/unconscious kinaesthetic sensation from lower limbs and trunk to the cerebellum which adjusts muscle tone.
3. *Lateral spino-thalamic tract:*
   - It is formed by axons of cells of substantia gelatinosa of Rolando, which after ascending a short distance, cross to opposite side. The cells have their cell station in posterior root ganglia. After entering the spinal cord through dorsal root they ascend for a short distance in dorsilateral part (tract of Lissauer) and enter substantia gelatinosa.
   - Second order neuron arise from above cells + cells of substantia gelatinosa, run forward and medially across anterior white commissure to reach lateral funiculus of opposite side. Then they ascend in lateral spino-thalamic tract, lying in close relation with spinocerebellar and spinotectal tract.
   - It continues upwards through medulla oblongata, pons and mid-brain (spinal lemniscus) and ends in thalamus (ventral postero-lateral nucleus). It sends collaterals to reticular formation. From thalamus, third order neuron relay fibres, pass upwards through posterior limb of internal capsule to end in cerebral cortex (post central gyrus area 3, 1, 3).
   - Functions: It carries pain sensations from muscles, viscera. It conducts painful and thermal sensibilities from opposite side of body to anterior part of lateral thalamic nuclei and to sensory areas of brain. It subserves tickling, itch and sensation of muscle fatigue. It also subserves rectal and bladder sensation + sexual impulse.
4. *Spino-vestibular tract:*
   - Fibres run from spinal cord and end in lateral vestibular nucleus.
   - It extends in spinal cord (ipsilateral column) from the level as far as lumbar segments.
   - It is concerned with postural reflexes.
5. *Spino-cortical tract:*
   - Fibres largely arise from cervical spinal cord. They run parallel with corticospinal tract. Not clear in function.
6. *Spino-pontine-tract:*
   - Fibres are collaterals of spino-cortical fibres.
   - Terminate into pontine nucleus.
   - It is concerned with certain exteroceptive impulses to the cerebellum.
7. *Spino-olivary tract:* Fibres arise from dorsal grey column. Fibres ascend up in spinal cord. They terminate in inferior olivary nucleus of opposite side. They transmit proprioceptive impulses to cerebellum.
8. *Spino-reticular tract:* Fibres arise from cells of dorsal grey column, ascend in spinal cord. Most of the fibres terminate in 'nucleus-reticularis-giganto cellularis'; while few in 'nucleus reticularis' (pons), 'formatio reticularis' (mid-brain), thalamus and hypothalamus. These are concerned with alert and arousal.
9. *Dorsilateral tract:* (Tract of Lissauer)
   - The first neuron fibres originate from cells of posterior root ganglia and enter the spinal cord. Here, they divide into 'ascending and descending branches'. Former pass upto one or two segments in the cord and terminate around cells of posterior grey column of the same side.
   - The second order neuron arise from cells of posterior grey column of same side → pass to lateral funiculus of opposite side to constitute lateral spinothalamic tract.

- The fibres terminate in cells of posterior grey column of same side.
- Pain and thermal sensations are conducted and relayed in 'substantia gelatinosa of Rolando'.

EFFECTS: HEMISECTION OF SPINAL CORD

a. *In cervical region:*
   - Constriction of pupil on the same side. This is because of involvement of first second and third thoracic anterior roots; since pupil dilating fibres which come from medulla and pass out through this routes.
   - On involvement of 4th, 5th, 6th, cervical, there occurs loss of biceps, triceps, supinator-pronator jerk.
   - On involvement of 4th, 5th, 6th, cervical (phrenic nerve) diaphragmatic paralysis takes place of same side.

b. *Lumbar region involvement:*
   - On involvement of 3rd and 4th lumbar—the additional features include—loss of knee jerk along with few disturbances in micturition.

c. *Lumbo-sacral involvement:*
   - On its involvement the loss of sphincter control is the additional symptom.
   - On its lesion, ptosis may result because of involvement of third nerve nucleus, paralysis of ocular muscles, dilatation of pupil because of paralysis of sphincter-pupillae which is innervated by oculomotor nerve, loss of pupillary light reflex of same side, contralateral spastic hemiplegia results.

d. *Details of injury:*

   I. *Below the section:*

   a. *Same side*
   - Loss of fine touch, tactile localisation, tactile discrimination as well as kinaesthetic sensation (due to damage of tract of Goll and Burdach).
   - No effect on sensations like pain, temperature, crude touch (due to crossing of spino-thalamic tract/fibres).
   - Upper motor neuron type of paralysis, i.e. affected muscles are rigid due to increased tone, exaggerated deep reflexes, loss of superficial reflexes, positive Babiniski sign, absence of reaction of degeneration, no significant muscular wasting (due to damage of crossed pyramidal tract).
   - Temporary loss of vasomotor tone.

   b. *Opposite side*
   - Complete loss of pain, temperature and touch (crude) (due to damage of spino-thalamic fibres).
   - Persistence of kinaesthetic sensation, fine touch (due to not involvement of posterior column tracts of opposite side).
   - No significant paralysis.
   - "Evident is below the level of section there exists extensive sensory loss but non-significant motor loss, on opposite side. On the contrary on the same side there is significant motor loss but little sensory loss. All thus constitutes Brown Sequard syndrome."

   II. *At the level of lesion*

   a. *Same side:*
   - Complete anaesthesia (due to loss of posterior horn cells/spino-thalamic fibres cross the opposite side).
   - Paralysis of lower motor neuron (flaccid muscles due to loss of tone, loss of deep and superficial reflexes, presence of reaction of degeneration, muscular wasting).
   - Complete vasomotor paralysis.

   b. *Opposite side*
   - Some pain sensation lost
   - Very slight motor changes

   III. *Above the level*
   - Hyperaesthesia referred on opposite side.
   - A band of hyperaesthesia on same side.

SYRINGOMYELIA (syrinx = a tube; syringe)

i. The major lesion is a gliosis in the grey commissure and the base of posterior horns in the lower cervical and upper dorsal region. This lesion process may extend through the entire length of the cord and even up into the brainstem. The newly formed glial tissue becomes soft and liquefied to form a tubular cavity. This cavity is lined by a layer of ependyma.

ii. Symptoms complex includes
   - Loss of pain and temperature sensibility while sense of touch is retained and all this is named as dissociated anaesthesia, which is commonly seen in arms as lesion is commonly seen in cervical cord. The fibres for pain and temperature cross in grey commissure, so caught in destructive process while most of the touch fibres pass up in posterior column and so they escape.

- Spasticity of the legs with some loss of power is possibly due to pressure on pyramidal tract in cervical region.
- In the arms there is muscular atrophy of lower motor neurons type. The reason for this is obscure but trophic lesion are still more obscure. Root of trouble is anaesthesia which permits the tissue to be traumatised. Thus, burns on hands are of common occurrence, as patient is insensitive to heat.

iii. So it is a condition of excessive overgrowth of neuroglial tissue, accompanied by cavity formation involving grey matter round the central canal of spinal cord. It is rare disease of earlier part of life.

TABES DORSALIS

(Tabes = wasting) (locomotor ataxia)

It is a syphilitic disease of cord, a late manifestation coming on from two to ten years after primary infection.

The lesion is degeneration and disappearance of posterior columns of the cord and their replacement by neuroglial tissue. Posterior nerve roots are atrophied and shrivelled as compared with plump anterior roots. It is wasting of dorsal columns which gives the name to this disease.

Symptom complex includes

i. Sensory disturbances include pain, paraesthesia, loss of muscle and vibration sense. The patient feels as if he was walking on something soft like cotton wood. Lightning pains of extreme severity shoot down the legs.

ii. As both muscle sense and vibration sense impulse pass up in the posterior column, so naturally they are lost. When a vibrating tuning fork is placed on some bony prominence, the patient states that 'he merely feels a cold object in contact with his skin.'

iii. Loss of sense of position. When the eyes are shut, the position of foot is unknown and patient sways when standing (Rombergism, Romberg's sign).

iv. Incoordination which is due to interference with muscle sense. Stamping gait, i.e. patient is not sure of his position he walks unsteadily and with a wide base lifting his feet high and throwing them down forcibly.

v. Loss of deep reflexes. Knee jerk depends on integrity of 3 and 4 lumbar segments. It is due to interference with the short fibres which anastomose directly around cells of anterior horn. Light reflex in pupil is commonly lost though, contraction on accommodation is retained (Argyl—Robertson pupil). The lesion is in the subependymal region of aqueduct of sylvius.

vi. Visceral crisis are severe paroxysms of pain referred to various viscera.

vii. Trophic disturbances—Charcot's joints.

COMPLETE TRANSVERSE DIVISION

Any injury, inflammation or any other factor may cause either complete or incomplete tran section of the cord. Whatever the nature of damage, subject may have following three stages: (Spinal preparation)

a. *Stage of spinal shock:* Immediately following the injury there occurs complete loss of visceral and somatic sensations. The state is further characterised by loss of all reflexes (tendon jerks, abdominal reflex, plantar response), paralysis and flaccidity of muscles. Sphincters are at first paralysed but they regain their tone quickly. Cold and blue skin is having bright chance to have bedsores. This stage lasts for one to three weeks in human beings.

b. *Stage of reflex activity:* Depending upon general health and resistance of the body the stage of recovery starts. Spontaneous flexion movements are early and frequent. Flexor reflex returns first. Tone of flexor muscles on return leads to paraplegia in flexion (hip and knee flexed, ankle and toes are dorsiflexed). Knee jerk comes back first.

   Many times elicitation of flexor reflexes is associated with evacuation of bowel and bladder and this is named as mass reflex by many scientists; and this is not of much occurrence in incomplete transaction of cord.

   On the contrary if the cord is incompletely transacted the extension movements are early but flexor reflex return later but they are accompanied by crossed extensor reflex, i.e. gentle flexion of one limb causes extension of opposite limb (Philipson's reflex).

   Extension reflex return much earlier (extension thrust reflex) and knee jerk shows prolonged period of relaxation. Paraplegia in extension results, tendon jerks are exaggerated, patellar as well as ankle clonus can be easily elicited while abdominal reflexes are lost.

c. *Stage of reflex failure*: A poor state of nutrition or any infection or any other cause may overcome the above second stage. Therefore, poor sufferer may enter this stage characterised by more difficulty in elicitation of reflex, flaccid and wasting of muscles, bedsores, hypercalcaemia, urinary stones due to hypercalcinurea, abolition of mass reflex, cystitis, and disease finally terminates into fatal results via septicaemia, uraemia etc.

BIBLIOGRAPHY

1. Brinkman BM, Bush R, Porter. Deficient influences of peripheral stimuli on pre-central neurons and monkeys with dorsal column Lesions. J Phy 1978;276:27-48.
2. Carrea RME, Grundfest HJ. Neurophysiol 1954;17:203-38.
3. Campa F, King W. Engel Histochemistry of motoneurons and interneurons in the cat lumbar spinal cord. Neurology 1970;20(1): 559.
4. Hennemann E, et al. Functional organisation of motoneuron pool and its inputs: In Brooks VB (Ed). Handbook of Physiology section I, Vol. II. American Physiological Society 1981;423.
5. Hussan A, et al. Animal solutions to problem of movement control. The role of proprioceptors. Ann Rev Neurosc 1988; 11:199.
6. Mandell LM. Modifiability of spinal synapses. Phy Rev 1984; 64:260.
7. Rexed B. Cytoarchitective organisation of spinal cord in the cat. J Comp Neurol 1952;96:415-95.
8. Shimamura L. Longitudinal conduction systems serving spinal brainstem co-ordinations, Livingstone. J Neurophysiol 1963;26: 258-72.
9. Weisendanger M, et al. Ascending pathway of low threshold muscle afferent to cerebral cortex and its possible role in motor control. Phy Rev 1982;62:1234.

(Bibliography 4-6 and 9 quoted by Guyton AC in Textbook of Medical Physiology, WB Saunders)

103 Reflexes—Reflex Action

The motor behaviour in living beings is a complex action at one moment, while it is changed at another movement, for example, a cat running, suddenly turn to avoid an unfriendly dog, or, leap at a bird anticipating the position of the prey in flight. This aspects of behaviour is known as reflexes which were first clearly described by descartes in 17th century. Reflex action is an involuntary (automatic) motor response due to a sensory stimulus.

REFLEX ARC

Each reflex action (Fig. 103.1) is produced by a group of neurons. A combination of neurons involved in each reflex action is called reflex arc. It consists of:

- *Afferent limb* constituted by receptors and afferent or sensory neuron which transmit the impulse to the efferent limb through synapse.
- *Centre:* It consists of synapse between afferent and efferent neurons either directly or indirectly through internuncial neurons situated within CNS. Synapse is a neuronal junction responsible for unidirectional conduction of nerve impulse transmitted from afferent (sensory) to efferent (motor) neuron.
- *Efferent limb* is constituted by efferent (motor) neuron which receives the impulse from sensory neuron and then is transmitting to the effectors which may be muscles or glands.

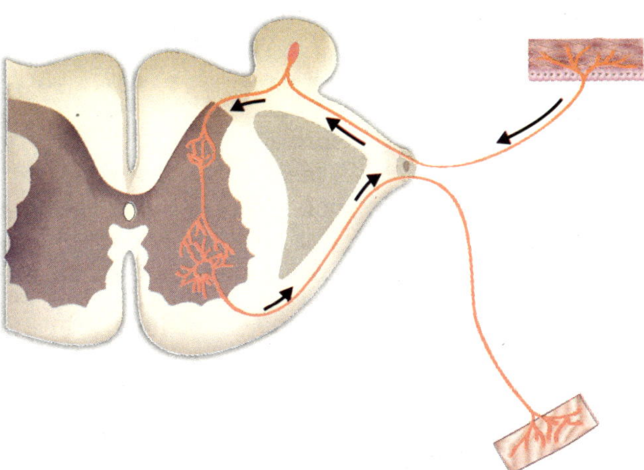

Fig. 103.1: Reflex action–various components

MODERN WAY OR CONCEPT OF CLASSIFICATION

a. *Monosynaptic:* (Two neuron reflex arc) Single synapse. Example is reflex controlling muscle tone. Synaptic delay is 0.5 m. sec. Usual time lag is 1 m. sec.

b. *Polysynaptic (Multineuron reflex arc):* More than one synapses are involved. Time lag is 3.5 m. sec. e.g. flexor reflex.

   i. *Crossed reflex arc:* Afferent limb is connecting itself with efferent neuron of opposite half of spinal cord and connecting neuron is also located in opposite side.

   ii. *Complex reflex arc:* Afferent neurons are connected with efferent through various collaterals which are sent by afferent neurons, e.g. referred pain.

   iii. *Intercalated reflex arc*: The interneurons are placed between afferent and efferent limbs.

c. *Clinically*

   i. *Superficial,* e.g. Plantar reflex

   ii. *Deep:* Elicited by taping over tendons : stretch reflex

   iii. *Visceral:* Obtained from deep lying structures, e.g. pupillary, carotid sinus reflex.

   iv. *Pathological:* Seen in diseased states, e.g. Babiniski's sign.

d. *Anatomically*

   i. *Segmental:* Where end of afferent and beginning of efferent neuron are in the same segment.

ii. *Intersegmental:* The above location is in different segments of spinal cord.
iii. *Suprasegmental:* Integrated part of centre extending from spinal cord to brain.

e. *Physiologically:* (i) Flexor and (ii) Extensor (iii) Conditioned and unconditioned.

STRETCH OR MYOTATIC REFLEX: KNEE JERK IS AN EXAMPLE

i. The patient sits comfortably on chair with one leg on another. Knee jerk is then taken. This indicates that when tendon of a muscle is stretched a contractile response is obtained, hence the name stretch reflex.
ii. On stretching the tendon, the muscle spindles are under tension and so discharges. This afferent impulse reach the spinal cord. This information is delivered to motor neurons of extrafusal fibres of muscle which responds by contraction.
iii. It helps in maintenance of posture. It is of monosynaptic variety.
iv. It shows all the properties of synapses viz. localisation, inhibition, recruitment, summation, facilitation, reciprocal innervation but it does not show after discharge and fatigue.
v. *Dynamic stretch reflex* is that which caused by sudden increase in stretch resulting into strong reflex. On the contrary, static stretch reflex is that which is caused by slow increase in stretch which results into weak reflex. With this we can understand that dynamic stretch reflex is wonderfully damping the muscular contraction. Hence with dynamic reflex, the movements are obtained without jerkiness.
vi. There also exists a negative feedback (negative stretch reflex). On shortening the muscle — rate of impulses reduced which inhibits muscle tone and excitation of antagonist muscles occurs.
vii. It should be remembered that, stretch reflex is there to control the length of muscle while tendon reflex is there to control muscle tension. Excessive load on muscle → increased stretching of muscle → muscle spindle stimulation—increased contraction of muscle to oppose the load → returning muscular length back to desired value.

Tension on muscle increased → inhibitory effects from tendon organ → sudden relaxation of entire muscle (lengthening reaction; prevent tearing of muscle).

On stretching a skeletal muscle with intact nerve supply, contraction results; this is stretch reflex.

Stimulus	—	stretching
Response	—	contraction of muscle
Sense organ	—	muscle spindle

Conduction of impulse by fast sensory fibres which pass directly to motor neurons which supply the same muscle. Neurotransmitter is glutamate.

A NOTE ON REFLEX

The time between application of stimulus and the response is reaction time; which for knee jerk is 19-24 ms in humans. Central delay is the time taken for reflex activity to traverse the spinal cord which in human for knee jerk is 0.6-0.9 ms.

MUSCLE RECEPTORS : THEIR ROLE

The muscles and their tendons are supplied abundantly with two special types of sensory receptors — (i) Muscle spindle—which are distributed throughout the belly of muscle. They detect length of muscle as well as rate of change of length of a muscle; (ii) Golgi tendon organ — which are located in the muscle tendons. They detect tension or rate of change of tension applied to the muscle.

Structure

i. Each spindle is constituted by small intrafusal fibres which are pointed at their ends (polar region) and are attached to surrounding extra fusal fibres. The midway area called "equatorial zone" is having

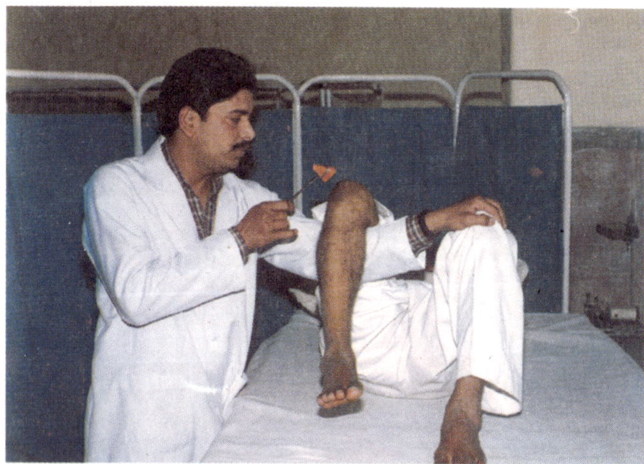

Fig. 103.2: Elicitation of reflex
(*Courtesy*: Department of physiology, SP Medical College and Associated Groups of PBM Hospital, Bikaner)

Table 103.1: Deep reflexes

Name of Reflex	*Elicitation*	*Response*	*Centre*	*Comments*
1. Biceps jerk	Sharp tap on biceps tendon in front of elbow joint	Flexion of elbow, contraction of biceps	5th and 6th cervical segment	
2. Triceps jerk	Tap/blow on triceps muscle just above ulnar olecranon process	Extension of elbow forearm. Contraction of muscle	6th and 7th cervical segments or upto 8th	
3. Supinator jerk	Tap/blow on styloid process of radius	Flexion of elbow. Contraction of supinator muscle	6th and 5th cervical segments	
4. Jaw jerk	Tapping chin with mouth partly open	Contraction and jerking jaw	Pons	
5. Knee jerk	In semiflexed knee joint, sharp tap upon patellar tendon by neurologist's hammer	• Forward movement of leg contraction of quadriceps • Enhanced when subject clenches his first or make other voluntary effort (reinforcement)	L3, 4, 2	Jerk is increased in decerebration or injury to descending motor pathways. It is abolished by injury or disease involving reflex arc or centre. It is effected less by anaesthetics, spinal transection, circulatory failures.
6. Ankle jerk	Sharp tap/blow upon tendo-Achillis	Quick contraction of calf muscles	First sacral segment	Under certain conditions a muscle or a group instead of contracting smoothly, may do so rhythmically in a series of rapidly repeated movements (clonus).

"primary and secondary receptors." The primary ending (also called annulospiral ending) is a type Ia fibre averaging 17 micrometers in diameter and its velocity of transmitting signals is 70-120 m/sec. to spinal cord. The Secondary endings (also called flower spray receptors) are type II fibres with an average diameter of 8 micrometers. This central equatorial zone with both these receptors does not contract along with contraction of both ends; because it contains very few or almost no actin and myosin filaments.

ii. Various types of intrafusal fibres have also been mentioned—(a) Nuclear bag fibres—extend from end to end of the spindle. Large number of nuclear fibres are present into an expanded bag in central portion of receptor area. (b) Nuclear chain fibres—Here, nuclei are arranged in a chain like fashion, averaging from three to nine in number.

Response

- The primary receptors (annulospiral) are very large in number and are sensitive too, so it starts discharging within fraction of millisecond of application of stimulus, and attains steady state also within a very short time; so it detects rate of change of length of muscle OR it discharges only when length is actually increasing. Secondary receptors are not much sensitive as compared with primary so it detects only length of muscle. So in nutshell, muscle spindles are length detecting device.
- A passive stretch to the muscle causes intrafusal fibres to contract → which stretches or stimulates primary and secondary receptors due to stress → this causes processing of information to spinal cord → which leads to stimulation of alpha motoneurons → which finally terminates into the contraction of main muscle belly.
- This mechanism is called *servo control* since it makes length of contraction less load sensitive, brain need not to expand much of the extra nervous energy, and it can compensate for fatigue.
- Gamma motor nerves (gamma efferents; Y) are also of two types viz. Y_1 (dynamic; gamma d) and Y_2 (static; gamma S).

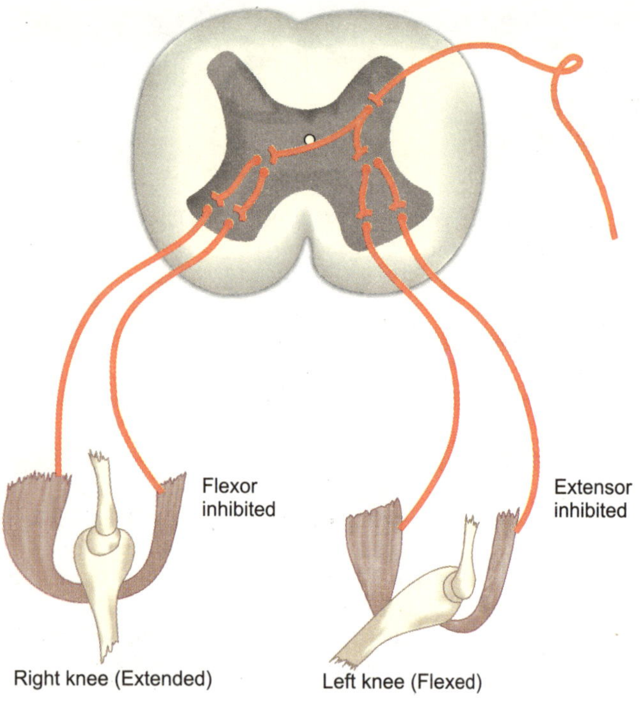

Fig. 103.3: Crossed extensor reflex

- Now, on above mentioned sequence of events, after stimulation of alpha motor neurons, the muscle belly contracts which may cause relieving of stretch of nuclear bag region, which leads to stoppage of discharge from alpha afferents which may finally lead to nullification of discharge from alpha motoneurons. In this way, these gamma efferents keep the muscle fibres sensitive for stretch reflex.
- Two local factors try to limit the self-energising effect of stretch reflex—slackening of muscle spindle when the muscle contracts and high threshold inhibitory effect (autogenic inhibition) of tension on the tendon organs. Therefore, each natural stretch reflex response is an equilibrium, in which there is a balance of proprioceptive excitation and autogenic inhibition. This equilibrium gives plasticity to the response so that an increase in length of muscle is followed first by an increase in its contraction; then some less contraction and immediately after this new length is achieved (lengthening reaction). Conversely any sudden shortening of muscle is associated with a cessation of discharge in many contractile units followed by recovery of some contractile units—(shortening reaction). The Golgi tendon organ being in series with extra fusal fibres will record tension equally to stretch and contraction.
- According to servo-assistance view of stretch reflex mechanism a major functional role for muscle spindle endings in a voluntary contraction is to provide supportive excitation to the contracting muscle. Thus, a change in load on a muscle is thought to induce corresponding changes in spindle feedback and appropriate changes in motoneuron discharge. On suddenly increasing the load, the compensatory response has been found to contain a mixture of voluntary and reflex activity, the latter composed of short and long reflex components. It is concluded that potentiation of reflex mechanism during contraction is not due primarily to a fusimotor action. Sudden decrease in load produced a pause in spindle discharge.

FLEXOR REFLEX (WITHDRAWAL; NOCICEPTIVE REFLEX)

i. When any nociceptive stimulus is applied, it leads to a contractile response which involves flexor muscles.
ii. It shows all the properties of synapses like synaptic delay, occlusion, after discharge, fractionation, fatigue, facilitation but recruitment is not seen. It is said to be propotent.
iii. This reflex is meant to withdraw the affected body part away from stimulus, so it is protective function.
iv. The receptors are located in the skin. The pain afferents enter the spinal cord and appropriate stimulus/impulse is sent through motor neuron supplying the concerning muscle for withdrawal. The main features are—diverging circuits to spread the reflex to necessary muscles for withdrawal, circuits to inhibit antagonist muscles and circuits to cause a prolonged after discharge.

EXTENSOR REFLEX

i. When due to a stimulus flexor reflex is elicited then, opposite limb shows extension. To elicit it, left lateral popliteal nerve is stimulated electrically, extension of right knee joint is observed.
ii. It shows all properties like localisation, facilitation, recruitment, after discharge, inhibition, reciprocal innervation but does not show fatigue.
iii. Signals from the sensory nerve cross the opposite side of cord to cause opposite reaction of flexor reflex. Many internuncial cells are in circuits between incoming sensory neuron and outgoing motoneurons of opposite side. It is the mechanism for crossed extension. Prolonged after discharge is again of benefit here to go away from painful stimulation.

Table 103.2: Superficial reflexes

Name of Reflex	*Elicitation*	*Response*	*Centre*	*Comments*
1. Normal plantar flexion	Light scratch applied to skin of sole	Plantar flexion of all the toes	First sacral segments	• If normal response is replaced by dorsiflexion of great toe and spreading or fanning of outer toes, it is named as Babiniski sign (extensor response), found in upper motor neuron lesion. • Oppenheim's reflex is modification of Babiniski's sign in which firm downward sliding pressure on skin of anterior border of tibia, shows dorsiflexion of hallux.
2. Abdominal reflexes	Light scratching the skin of abdomen	Contraction of abdominal muscles.	Thoracic segments 6, 7 upper-10, 12, lower abdominal	Abolished by any lesion interrupting afferent conduction from skin of abdomen, destroying anterior horn cells or motor pathways for abdominal muscles, lesion interrupting corticospinal pathway above 7th thoracic.
3. Cremasteric reflex	Light stroke applied to skin on inner aspect of upper part of thigh	Cremaster muscle contraction and elevation of testicle.	First or second lumbar segment	Abolished by corticospinal lesion or lesion of centre.
4. Anal reflex	Scratching neighbouring skin	Contraction of external anal sphincter	4th and 5th sacral segment; coccygeal segment	Lost after interruption of reflex arc
5. Gluteal reflex	Scratching skin of buttock	Contraction of gluteal muscles	4th and 5th lumbar and upper sacral segments	
6. Bulbo-cavernosus reflex	Stimulation of glans penis	Contraction of bulbo-cavernosus muscle	3rd and 4th sacral segments	Absent in lesions involving reflex arc centre

CLONUS

- A man in standing posture, suddenly drops downwards in order to stretch gastrocnemius muscle. So impulses are transmitted from muscle spindles into spinal cord. This causes reflex excitation of stretched muscle and in this way body is lifted back and falling is prevented.
- After some time this reflex dies out. Then second such oscillation occurs. Then third-fourth and so on.
- This continuous oscillation of stretch reflex for long period of time is clonus.
- It develops readily in decerebrate animals, because stretch reflex is highly facilitated.

BABINSKI'S SIGN

- When a firm tactile stimulus is applied to the lateral sole of foot; then the great toe extends upwards while other toes fan outwards. The Babinski's sign is used clinically to detect damage superficially in corticospinal portion of motor control system. So this sign does not occur when damage occurs in non-cortico spinal portion of motor control system.
- *Cause:*
  - Corticospinal tract is main controller of muscular activity for purposeful movements.
  - On the opposite side, non-cortical part is mainly protective from any damage.
  - So when non-corticospinal portion is functioning then such stimulus will cause withdrawal protective reflex.
  - But when corticospinal portion attains maturity, then above mentioned protective reflex is inhibited and higher order of motor function is excited.
- It is elicited best from outer border of sole.
- The dorsiflexion of great toe is due to contraction of extensor hallucis longus.

It is also called extensor response.

SUMMARY AND HIGHLIGHTS

- Suppose you are smoking a cigarette in front of a cigarette shop. Suddenly your father comes. You, all of a sudden run away to escape and throw the cigarette out of your mouth. This is a reflex action in our day to day life.
- Suppose you have put your hand on a hot stove. As you feel heat you suddenly remove your hand from the hot stove. This is flexor reflex.
- When you record reflexes with hammer, the patient should be kept busy in talking. He must not know about your technique.

BIBLIOGRAPHY

1. David Burke, et al. Muscle spindle responses in man to changes load during accurate position maintenance. J Physiol 1978;276: 159-64.
2. Derek Denny Brown General principles of motor integration. In Handbook of Physiology Section I : Neurophysiology Vol. II.
3. Eyzaguirre. The electrical activity of mammalian intrafusal fibres. J Phy 1960;150:169-85.
4. Granit R. The basis of motor control. London Academic Press. 1970.
5. Hunt CC, et al. Spinal reflex mechanisms concerned with skeletal muscle. (quoted by Guyton AC, Textbook of Medical Physiology, WB Saunders) Phy Rev 1960;40:538.
6. Hunt CC. Mammalian muscle spindle: peripheral mechanisms. Phy Rev 1990;70:643.
7. Jami C. Golgi tendon organs in mammalian skeletal muscle: functional properties and central actions. Phy Rev 1992;72:623.
8. Lee RG, Tatton WG. Motor responses to sudden limb displacement in primates with specific CNS lesion and in human patients with motor system disorders. Can J Neurol Sc 1975;2:285-293.
9. Marsden, et al. Servo action and stretch reflex in human muscle and its apparent dependence on peripheral sensation. J Physiol 1971;216:21-22.
10. Marsden, et al. Servo action in human thumb. J Physiol 1976;257: 1-44.
11. Matthews PBC. Mammalian muscle receptors and their central actions. London Arnold. 1972.
12. Muscle receptor and their reflexes in receptors and sensory perception by Ragnar Grainit. Yale University Press 1962;191-235.
13. SID Gilman, W Ian McDonald. Relation of afferent fibre conduction velocity to activities of muscle spindle receptors after cerebellectomy. J Neurology 1967;30:1513.

104 Path to Big Guns: The Brainstem

It comprises medulla oblongata, pons and mid-brain; along with ascending and descending fibres, collection of nerve cells, nuclei to reach to higher faculties.

MEDULLA OBLONGATA (SPINAL BULB)

i. It is continuation of cervical spinal cord extending from foramen magnum to the caudal border of the pons.

ii. In its lower third—ventrally—is the decussation of pyramidal tract.

Dorsally—is cuneate and nucleus gracilis on which the fibres of posterior column synapse.

Anterolaterally is descending rubro- and vestibulo-spinal tracts and ascending ventral spinocerebellar tract.

In mid medulla—central canal approaches the dorsal surface to open into fourth ventricle at calamus scriptorius. The inferior olivary nucleus lies dorsal to pyramids and from its hilum the fibres pass to cerebellum through superior and middle cerebellar peduncles mostly to opposite side, transmitting impulses from spinal cord, brainstem and cerebral cortex.

iii. *Functions*

- *Respiration:* Inspiratory centre is located in ventral reticular formation dorsal to inferior olive; while expiratory centre lies slightly cephalic and dorsal to former.
- *Cardiovascular:* Cardiac inhibitor and accelerator centre is located in floor of fourth ventricle near dorsal nucleus of vagus. Vasomotor centre is at apex of calamus scriptorius in floor of fourth ventricle. It is said that integrity of medullary centres is essential for maintenance of normal cardiovascular tone.

So medulla is said to be a vitally important part of CNS because of the fact that its disturbances may lead to respiratory and cardiac arrest.

- Deglutition and vomiting centres are also present here.
- It is also responsible for some other reflexes viz. sneezing, coughing, suckling, salivary etc.

PONS VAROLII

i. It lies between medulla and cerebral peduncles ventral to cerebellum.

ii. Nuclei pontis is an irregular collection of nerve cells and longitudinal and transverse fibres at its basilar part and, is occupying the space between bundle of nerve fibres.

iii. There lies transversely crossing bundles of middle cerebellar peduncle which are running from pons to opposite cerebellar hemisphere and vice versa.

iv. It is concerned with control of respiration. Pneumotaxic centre is lying in upper pons which produces a normal respiratory rhythm by controlling exaggerated activities of apneustic centre which is situated in caudal margin of trapezoid body—the border between pons and medulla.

v. Its posterior surface forms upper part of anterior wall of fourth ventricle. At the cephalic end the lateral walls converge to form the aqueduct of sylvius and gives rise to two bundles of nerve fibres—the superior cerebellar peduncles which are lying undercover of cerebellum and running from cerebellar nuclei to red nucleus.

MID-BRAIN (MESENCEPHALON)

i. It is situated between pons and diencephalon or better to say it connects forebrain with hindbrain.

ii. It is formed by cerebral peduncles and corpora quadrigemina. The cerebral peduncles contains cerebro-spinal fibres and fibres which connect pons and cerebellum with forebrain. It is related topographically to the aqueduct of Sylvius, which is the fluid channel connecting third and fourth ventricles.

iii. *Corpora quadrigemina* are composed of four rounded bodies forming dorsal part of mid-brain. Two bodies above are called superior colliculi which receive fibres from retina via optic tract, from visual area of occipital cortex and from spinal cord and it is concerned with visual reflexes which co-ordinate eye movements with those of head, body and limbs. Two bodies below are inferior colliculi, are connected with superior colliculi and acting as relay stations in hearing pathway, thus serving as reflex acoustic centres.

iv. *Substantia nigra*—The aqueduct of Sylvius is covered dorsally with superior and inferior corpora quadrigemina, the tectum, and ventrally by cerebral peduncles each of which is divided into two part by a layer of pigmented grey matter—the substantia nigra, which is considered as an important extra-pyramidal or non-pyramidal nucleus which is affected in Parkinson's disease since symptomatology of this disorder is caused by lesions involving it. It is extending in whole length of mid-brain and projecting into caudal diencephalon.

v. *Tegmentum*—Broad layer of central grey matter which is having less myelinated fibres but rich in diffusely grouped cells. It contains three important decussation viz. superior peduncles, rubrospinal tracts and tectospinal tracts.

vi. *Red Nucleus:*
   - It is a large oval mass of cells in the medial part of tegmentum, extending from cephalic border of superior colliculus into the hypothalamus. It is hence a mass of grey matter high in mid-brain, below thalamus, close to third nerve nucleus. Its colour is due to reddish brown lipochrome.
   - It sends efferents to - globus pallidus (rubro-striatal), thalamus (rubro-thalamic), inferior olivary nucleus (rubro-olivary), motor nuclei of cranial nerves, spinal cord (rubro-spinal) and reticular formation, pons and cerebellum.
   - It receives afferents from motor cortex (cortico-rubral), cerebellum of opposite side, vestibular nucleus of same side, globus pallidus of same side.
   - It believes to act as a centre for reception and reorganisation of impulses before they are sent on to the motor centres of spinal and cranial nerves. Through rubro-spinal pathway reflex postural adjustments are made.
   - *On the whole, mid-brain is concerned with integration of optic, auditory and postural reflexes. Stimulation of tegmentum causes alteration in posture and inhibits rigidity in decerebrate preparation.*

CRANIAL NERVES

Twelve pairs of cranial nerves emerge from under surface of the brain and pass through foramina in the base of cranium. They are classified as motor, sensory and mixed nerves.

i. *First or olfactory nerve* : It arises from central or deep processes of olfactory cells of nasal mucous membrane, where its fibres form a network and are then collected into twenty branches which pierce the cribriform plate of ethmoid bone and form synapses with cells of olfactory bulb. It carries the impulses for sensation of smell.

ii. *Second or optic nerve*: Axons of ganglionic cells of retina bending at right angles, converge towards a point on inner surface of retina known as optic disc and form optic nerve. Fibres partially decussate in optic chiasma and end in lateral geniculate body and superior colliculus. It is the special nerve for sense of sight.

iii. *Third or oculomotor:* It arises from a nucleus in the floor of cerebral aqueduct. It is the motor nerve for four of six extrinsic eye muscles and for the raiser of upper eyelid.

iv. *Fourth or trochlear:* Originates in mid-brain and innervates the superior oblique muscle of eyeball. Its chief function includes movements of eyeball and muscle sense.

v. *Fifth or trigeminal:* Largest cranial nerve. Fibres of motor root arise from two nuclei, a superior located in cerebral aqueduct while inferior located in upper part of pons. Fibres of sensory root arise from cells in trigeminal ganglion which lies in a cavity of dura mater near the apex of petrous portion of temporal bone. Motor fibres innervate muscles of mastication. Sensory fibres are distributed to skin of face, eyeball, mucosa of mouth and nose, teeth. Its proprioceptive component is chiefly concerned with muscle sense and fibres are distributed with muscle branches of V.

vi. *Sixth or abducent:* It arises in a small nucleus lying beneath the floor of fourth ventricle. Fibres are distributed to external rectus of eyeball.

vii. *Seventh or facial*: Mixed nerve. Motor fibres are supplied to muscles of face, part of scalp, pinna, muscles of the neck; while sensory fibres are supplied to anterior two-third of tongue, and few to the region of middle ear. Motor fibres are arising from a nucleus in lower part of pons while sensory fibres from geniculate ganglion on facial nerve.

viii. *Eight or acoustic (auditory):* Sensory nerve containing two distinct fibres—cochlear nerve is the nerve of hearing whose fibres originate in spiral ganglion of cochlea; and vestibular nerve which is a nerve for maintaining equilibrium and its fibres are emerging from vestibular ganglion of internal auditory meatus.

ix. *Ninth or glossopharyngeal*: Its motor branches supply the muscles of pharynx and the base of tongue. It supplies secretory fibres for parotid gland while its sensory fibres are supplied to tongue and pharynx and together with facial, it constitutes nerve of taste. Motor fibres arise from nucleus ambiguus situated in medulla while sensory fibres arise from superior and petrous ganglion.

x. *Tenth or vagus:* Mixed nerve having more extensive distribution. Motor fibres arise from nucleus ambiguus and are supplied to muscles of larynx and alimentary canal. Sensory fibres are arising from cells of Jugular ganglion and from ganglion nodosum located on trunk of nerve and are distributed to mucous membrane of larynx, lungs, trachea, oesophagus, stomach, gallbladder and intestine. Its inhibitory fibres control the heart.

xi. *Eleventh or accessory:* Motor nerve. Two parts—internal (cranial) and external (spinal). Internal arising from nucleus ambiguus and fibres are distributed to pharyngeal and superior laryngeal branches of vagus. External arising from spinal cord as low as 5th cervical and fibres to sternocleido-mastoid and trapezius.

xii. *Twelfth or hypoglossal:* It is motor nerve for muscles of tongue and larynx, and arising from hypoglossal nucleus.

CRANIAL NERVE TESTING

Olfactory Nerve

- Three bottles of pungent odours (peppermint oil etc.) and three bottles of common bed side substances like scent/fruit/soap etc. Irritating substances (ammonia) should not be used.
- *Anosmia* means absence of sense of smell. *Parosmia* means pleasant odours seem to be offensive; i.e. alteration in character of smell.
- *Hallucination* may also exist leading to epilepsy etc.
- Hyposmia means reduction of sense of smell.

Facial Nerve

In its lesion:

- Tell the patient to whistle. Impossible for patient with its lesion.
- Tell him to smile or to show the upper teeth. Mouth is drawn to the healthy side.
- Tell him to inflate mouth with air and then tap on cheeks which are inflated. Air escapes from mouth easily on weak or paralysed side.
- Tell him to shut eyes tightly. It is to be noted by the doctor that affected eye is either not closed at all, or if closed, then eyelashes are not so deeply buried in the face as compared on healthy side.
- Now doctor attempts to open them while patient wants to keep closed (means against the wish). It will be impossible to go against the wishes of the patient if oribcularis oculi are acting normally. This may draw the corners of the mouth upwards. In paralysis of lower part of the face, the corner on affected side is either not drawn up at all, or it is drawn on healthy side.

Glossopharyngeal Nerve

- Loss of taste in the posterior part of tongue occurs on lesion of its trunk.
- *Palatal reflex:* Tickle the back of pharynx and note its reflex contraction. This is absent on the side of damage of the nerve.

Vagus (Xth)

a. *Palate:*
    - Tell him to report any regurgitation of fluids through nose during swallowing. This happens in total paralysis of soft palate.
    - Difficulty in pronouncing words which require complete closure of nasopharynx (egg = spoken as eng, rub = as rum etc. etc.).
    - Watch the movements of palate during phonation.

b. *Larynx:* Paralysis leads to characteristic laryngeal stridor (bilateral). This is done by 'Laryngoscopy' i.e. visualisation of larynx with laryngoscope.

Accessory Nerve

1. Paralysis of upper part of trapezius—Ask the patient to shrug (shrug = to raise shoulders to express helplessness, a sign of *laachari* or *bebasi*) his shoulders while doctor presses downwards on them. The patient is unable to shrug his shoulders on affected side.
2. Paralysis of sternomastoid leads to weakness of rotation of chin towards the opposite side.

Hypoglossal Nerve (XIIth)

Tell the patient to put out the tongue as much as possible. On the paralysis of this nerve, the tongue is deviated over to paralysed side instead of its straight protrusion. Also tell him to move tongue side by side and to lick the cheeks and doctor must watch that it is done freely. Also note for wasting of tongue.

105 Basal Ganglia

These are paired sub-cortical masses (situated below cortex) of grey matter. In lower animals it acts as highest centre controlling muscular activity.

INTRODUCTION

For all practical purposes the term 'basal ganglia' includes 'caudate nucleus,' 'putamen', 'globus pallidus,' 'red nucleus,' 'substantia nigra,' 'subthalamic body of Luys.' The clasutrum may also be listed but till now nothing significant is known about it. In lower animals the basal ganglia constitute important part of nervous system which chiefly regulates the muscular activity. The caudate nucleus and putamen are collectively referred as striatum while putamen and globus pallidus are referred as lenticular nucleus, while globus pallidus referred as "pallidum."

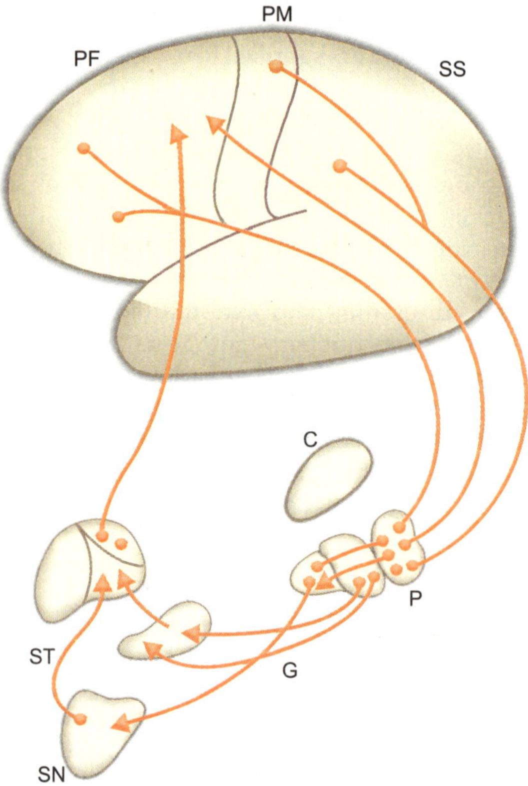

PF = Prefrontal cortex
SN = Substantia nigra
PM = Premotor cortex
SS = Somatic sensory
ST = Subthalamus
P = Putamen
G = Globus pallidus
C = Caudate nucleus

Fig. 105.1: Basal ganglia

VARIOUS PATHWAYS (Fig. 105.1)

1. Feedback system of servo control type is being operated here. It is said that various nerve pathways pass from motor parts of cerebral cortex to caudate nucleus and putamen which send fibres to globus pallidus and thence from here to ventrolateral thalamic nuclei which send fibres back to same motor regions.
2. Short neuronal connections among themselves are present within various basal ganglia. Again, globus pallidus (a lower basal ganglia) is said to project fibres into lower brainstem like reticular nucleus of mesencephalon and thence to red nucleus. It is presumed that through these circuits extra-pyramidal signals for motor cortex are conducted.
3. This is the established pathway that from motor cortex signals pass to pons and thence to cerebellum; this cerebellum sends signals back to same motor cortex through ventro-lateral nucleus of thalamus which is the same nucleus through which basal ganglia signals are relayed.
4. The basal ganglia are bypassed by large nerve fibres coming from motor cortex to reticular nucleus and pontine areas.

5. As told earlier, within the basal ganglia all parts are inter-connected with one another, viz. fibres are sent from globus pallidus to red nucleus, substantia nigra and subthalamic nucleus, also fibres are sent from substantia nigra to red nucleus, globus pallidus; together with the fact that subthalamic nucleus sends fibres to globus pallidus, red nucleus and substantia nigra. In this series it is stated that caudate nucleus and putamen are acting like primary receiving station of basal ganglia system whereas red nucleus and globus pallidus are acting like a relay station since caudate nucleus and putamen are receiving afferents from cerebral cortex, substantia nigra and ventral anterior thalamic nucleus while they discharge efferents to globus pallidus and substantia nigra; whereas red nucleus receives afferents from all basal ganglia's nuclei while sending efferents to reticular formation, ventro-lateral thalamus nuclei, spinal cord, oculomotor and inferior olivary nuclei as well as structures outside basal ganglia.

FUNCTIONS

For many years together it is a matter of debate that 'what is the function of basal ganglia'. Many persons abuse these structures by saying them as 'vestigial.' Fortunately after repeated studies few of its functions have been studied as mentioned here:

1. *Voluntary muscular activity:* There occurs loss of control of (role of substantia nigra) gamma activating system of muscle spindles if this structure is destructed so this part of basal ganglia is needed for proper excitation of gamma efferent nerve fibres. All this activity is needed for positioning of the part concerned in order to perform discrete motor function of either hands or limbs. All this is designated generally as 'mental make up or providing background muscular tone.
2. *Automatic Associated movements:* Basal ganglia are said to be exerter of a wide influence over these movements. The common example of such movement is swinging of arms in walking and it is said to be abolished if destruction of basal ganglia results. General poverty of movements is also seen leading to mask like face on destruction.
3. *Abnormal involuntary movements:* Such movements in the form of so-called tremor is seen on destructive lesion of these structures. It is believed that due to their destruction the natural inhibitory control is removed resulting into increased and abnormal behaviour of the part concerned. Tremors at rest are seen in destruction of substantia nigra and globus pallidus (Parkinsonism). Intention tremors are associated with destruction of dentato-rubro-thalamic-system which sends efferent to precentral motor cortex via ventro-lateral nucleus of thalamus.
4. *Functions of striate body (caudate nucleus and Putamen):* This part of basal ganglia are supposed to control (initiate and regulation) the intentional movements performed unconsciously by all of us. This function is performed nicely because of its connection with motor cortex.
5. *Motor tone inhibition:* Basal ganglia are said to inhibit muscle tone throughout the body. This act is completed by passing inhibitory sensations to facilitatory areas and stimulatory sensations to inhibitory area. So as destructive lesions to these structures occurs, muscular rigidity occurs due to over activity of facilitatory area along with under activity of inhibitory area.
6. *Role of globus pallidus:* When one individual wants to perform a work with one hand then first of all he in routine language prepares himself mentally for the same by taking respective position and then arm musculature will be tensed by so-called tonic contractions which involves globus pallidus part of basal ganglia.
7. *Basal ganglion:* Evolutionary aspect
   i. In birds basal ganglia totally replaces the cerebral cortex since it is very poorly developed.
   ii. In cats and dogs if cerebral cortex is removed the walk, sleep and wakefulness, fighting, eating, rage, sex activities are not at all effected but on the contrary if basal ganglia structures are removed all activities are more or less abolished with presence of only stereotyped movements.
   iii. In human beings if basal ganglia are destructed the opposite side of the body is almost totally paralysed while on decorticating no effect is observed on equilibrium, walking or any subconscious activity.
8. *Role of subthalamic areas:* Stimulation of these areas lead to rhythmic motions, and crude forward walking reflex. It is said to control forward progression. Experiment on cat illustrates the entire story when its brain was transacted below thalamus and above subthalamus. The animal was walking properly but if it comes in contact with any obstruction, it strikes its head and tries to remember the purpose of its own walking action means purpose of motion was disturbed.

BASAL GANGLIA: FEW MORE ASPECTS

1. These structures are essential for cognitive functions which means thinking processes of the brain. For example, if a violent mad person is suddenly visible on road then one may either run away of his sight, or he may try to take a shelter or to hide himself anywhere.
2. Above mentioned cognitive functions are existing because of their connections. Caudate nucleus is connected with entire cerebral cortex, i.e. anteriorly with frontal cortex, posteriorly through occipital and parietal lobes, and curving forwards again into temporal lobe. It also receives inputs from association areas of cerebral cortex. From here signals pass to globus pallidus and thence to thalamus (ventro-lateral and ventro-anterior) and finally back to cerebral cortex (pre-motor, pre-frontal and supplementary motor areas of cerebral cortex).
3. Basal ganglia are also concerned with intensity of movement, i.e. how rapidly it is to be performed, and scale of the movement, i.e. how large the movement will be?
4. The various neuro-transmitters functioning here are:
   - *Dopamine pathway:* From substantia nigra to caudate nucleus and putamen. Inhibitory transmitter.
   - *GABA* : From caudate nucleus—putamen to globus pallidus and substantia nigra. Inhibitory transmitter so functioning as stabiliser.
   - *Acetylcholine pathway:* From cortex to caudate nucleus and putamen. It is an excitatory transmitter, so it provides positive features of motor actions.
5. Its other functions include:
   - Helping cerebral cortex to execute subconscious + learned patterns of movements.
   - Helping in planning multiple parallel and sequential patterns of movements which is to be kept in view by cerebral cortex to complete a purposeful task.

CLINICAL MANIFESTATIONS

Now, on the light of detailed structure and function of basal ganglia, it is the right time to study some of the states owing to destruction of these structures:

1. **Parkinson's disease** *(The shaking palsy):* The disease is characterised by
   i. *Rigidity:* It involves all the voluntary muscles and in more practical grounds, 'the unfortunate sufferer turns as rigid as a block of marble. Finally articulation and swallowing too, becomes so difficult that they turn into anarthria and dysphagia respectively. Similarly due to rigidity patient becomes unable to even close the mouth leading to dribbling of saliva down the chin. Certainly this rigidity differs from decerebrate type, of rigidity in the following way.

      It is due to excessive impulses transmitted in corticospinal system leading to activation of alpha motor fibres to the muscles.

      It is said to be due to more activation of gamma efferents to muscle spindles.

   ii. *Tremor:* In more appropriate ways 'the hand fails to answer which mind wants to dictate.' It affects hand and fingers, originates at rest but disappears with the movement.

      Physiologic explanation—Firstly, in a normal schedule, substantia nigra has got inhibitory control on antagonist muscles, the nuclei of which resides in reticular substance of brainstem. Now due to destructive lesion of this part of basal ganglia this control exists no more and hence the part oscillates better called 'tremor' clinically; secondly, loss of inhibition of spinal cord, thirdly, if there is loss of basal ganglia impulses, the feedback in globus pallidus—thalamus—cortex route is increased leading to its oscillations which we name as tremor.

      Alternating movements of flexion and extension at wrist, or supination pronation at elbow and this tremor is much more pronounced in emotional states while not existing during rest or sleep or on hemiplegic side. The rhythm of these tremors has been mentioned as 4-8 per second. It may involve the entire body in severe cases. These are between agonist and antagonist muscles of the body.

   iii. *Attitude:* As regards this character, the patient adopts 'flexion attitude', i.e. head flexes on chest together with arms and wrist but knees are bent. The upper limbs are adducted at shoulders together with flexion at metacarpophalangeal and interphalangeal joints.

   iv. *Gait:* Patient is forced to take quicker and shorter steps thus assuming running pace : on the whole the gait is slow shuffling appearing that he is trying to catch up to his centre of gravity and doing her or his best effort to prevent himself from falling. If the sufferer is pushed either forwards or backwards, he cannot stop himself quickly but takes small but repeated steps in direction of pushing.

v. *Mask like face:* Patient loses automatic associated movements like swinging of arms during walking. Facial expressions are lost during emotions so face appears mask like. On the whole due to this loss the patient stands emotionless and rigidly like a statue.

vi. Post-encephalitic Parkinsonism is also said to present same symptoms but the disease runs a progressive course. The cause of this is lying in substantia nigra and red nucleus. It is better a extra-pyramidal disease since pigmented cells of substantia nigra disappears. Such patients are having same symptoms with the addition of ocular crisis (oculogyric crisis) as well as oily skin and sialorrhoea.

Exaggerated tendon reflexes with impairment of Babinski's sign is noted in the disease in arterio-sclerotic group of patients.

vii. *Basis of treatment*: It is an established fact that nerve endings of neurons in basal ganglia specially substantia nigra are secreting L-dopa derivative (dopamine). When these neurons are destructed this chemical transmitter substance is not secreted which results into these diseases. So administration of L-dopa is correct step to treat such patients.

viii. *Parkinson Disease: Few More Aspects*

- The tremor is called involuntary tremor—for it occurs during all waking hours. In cerebellar disease the tremor is intention type when person performs intentionally the initiated movements.
- Akinesia is often more distressing, i.e. to perform even simplest movement, one has to exert highest degree of concentration, or to say highest will power is to be executed. Then the movement so results is stiff and staccato in character (opposite of Smooth).
- Other drugs used for treatment besides L-dopa-
  - Dopaminergic agonists—Bromocriptine, piribedil, lisuride. With these dyskinesia is least prominent
  - Facilitator of dopaminergic transmission—Amantidine, selegiline.
  - Peripheral decarboxylase inhibitors—Carbidopa
  - Antihistaminics—Promethazine
  - Central anticholinergic—Benzhexol
- Surgical treatment of this disease is also available. It is destruction of ventro-lateral and ventro-anterior nuclei of thalamus by electro-coagulation.
- As far as treatment with dopamine is concerned:
  - Dopamine itself cannot be administered since it cannot cross blood-brain-barrier.
  - L-dopa is converted into dopamine within the brain which corrects the situation.

2. *Chorea:* It is of two types.

a. *Sydenham's chorea:* It is the commonest of such type of nervous disorders occurring in particularly girls before age of twenty years or so and is said to be a manifestation of rheumatic fever. Involuntary—jerky movements of face and limb's musculature is the chief characteristic feature. These movements are sustained and hence objects are dropped from hands and sufferer does not remain quiet; all this is labelled as "St. vitus-dance." Nerve cells in this disorders suffer from slight degeneration with significant hyperaemia but death rarely occurs. The lesion chiefly involves basal ganglia and cerebral cortex.

b. *Huntington's chorea*: This is a disease terminating fatally with marked hereditary tendency. It leads to jerky movements of upper limb, dysarthric speech, uncertain gait. Mental deterioration and irritability is of the extent that suicidal or homicidal tendencies spoils the life of unfortunate sufferer (cerebral dementia). The disease generally is found in fourth decade of life. The chief lesions comprise of atrophy of cortical cells, cells of putamen and caudate nucleus are destructed but mild damage to globus pallidus occurs.

To conclude this chorea consists of uncontrolled continuous contractions of different muscle groups. More clearly, unfortunate sufferer starts one sequence of movements for a while, then it is succeeded by another series of movements and then still another and in this way there occurs progression of movements.

3. *Athetosis:* To start with worm like movement, then followed by over extension of fingers and hands followed by flexion and terminating in rotatory twisting to side; all movements are slow but rhythmic and aggravated by emotions. Many times affected muscle exhibit a great spasm. The disease often begins in childhood due to asphyxia or injury at birth or encephalitis and is said to be due to destruction of basal ganglia specially caudate nucleus and putamen.

Sometimes *choreo-athetosis* may also occur leading to involuntary jerky quicker movements and said to be absent during sleep and abolished by alcoholic ingestion but are troublesome in waking hours specially during tension states. It may be a unilateral entity (causing hemiparesis) or bilateral one (athetosis double).

4. *Hemiballismus (hemichorea):* This is comprised of violent but uncontrollable movements of large body areas. To explain in a better way one leg undergoes sudden jerky movements or arm is pulled suddenly upwards. As one can easily predict that patient is liable to fall down if he is walking. Patient may even die due to exhaustion but these movements disappear during sleep. It usually occurs in old age since it is due to cerebral arterio-sclerosis and is resulting due to vascular lesion of subthalamic nucleus of Luys.
5. *Torsion spasm:* It also deserves description. It causes involuntary twisting movements involving neck, extremities and trunk turning body into bizarre postures.
6. *Progressive hepato-lenticular degeneration (Wilson's disease, 1912):* Normally on copper administration, it first attaches itself to serum albumin but within a very short time (approximately 24 hours) it shifts to globulin fraction called 'ceruloplasmin' owing to its blue colour. In this disease this copper fails to attach itself to globulin or it remains attached with albumin so ceruloplasmin level is decreased and this copper is deposited in liver, brain, kidney and cornea, raising serum copper level at these sites.

BIBLIOGRAPHY

1. Delong MR. Activity of pallidal neurons during movements. J Neuro-physiol 1971;34:414-27.
2. Duvoisin RC. Parkinson disease. New York: Raven Press, 1978.
3. Ferrante RJ, et al. Selective sparing of a class of striatal neurons in Huntington's disease. Science 1985;230:561.
4. Hoehn MM, et al. Parkinsonism: Onset progression and mortality: Neurology 1967;17:427.
5. Martin JB, et al. Huntington's disease: pathogenesis and management. New Eng J Med 1986;315:1267.
6. Nutt JG, et al. The ON:OFF phenomenon in Parkinson disease: Relation to levodopa—absorption and transport. New Eng J Med 1984;310:438.
7. Olsen RW. Drug interaction at GABA-receptor-ionophore complex. Ann Rev Pharma and Toxico 1982;22:245.

106 Silent Hunter: Cerebellum

(Small brain; diminutive brain: Little brain, Silent area)

INTRODUCTION

i. It consists of two "cerebellar hemispheres" joined by a "vermis."

ii. It is the large subdivision of hindbrain lying within the posterior cranial fossa. It bears a ratio of 1:8 with cerebrum in weight and in infant this ratio is 1:20. It is the "tentorium cerebelli" which separates it from posterior part of cerebral hemisphere.

iii. Peduncles
- *Superior:* Connects cerebellum with midbrain.
- *Middle:* Connects cerebellum with pons.
- *Inferior:* Connects cerebellum with medulla.

iv. Lobes

a. One view
- Anterior lobe (Paleo-cerebellum)
- Middle lobe (Neo-cerebellum)
- Flocculo nodular lobe (Archi cerebellum, oldest lobe)

b. Alternate view—Corpus cerebelli—which is further subdivided into anterior and posterior lobes with fissura prima running in between these two.

v. *Nuclei:* They are four deeply placed nuclear masses within its white matter, namely dentate nucleus (largest embedded in middle of each hemisphere), nucleus emboliformis (lying close to medial aspect of hilum of dentate nucleus), nucleus globosus (lying medial to N. emboliformis), and nucleus fastigii.

CONNECTIONS

a. *Afferent*
- *Spino-cerebellar tract:* From spinal cord. Through them, it gets information about degree and distribution of contraction of muscles, position of limbs in space as well as posture.
- *From vestibular nucleus:* It itself receives fibres from vestibular apparatus of internal ear. Through it, 'righting reflex' gets initiated.
- *From olive of medulla:* Olive itself receives collaterals from the pyramidal tract. Through it, pyramidal system activity is controlled.
- *From cerebral cortex:* Like temporal and occipital lobe.
- *From pontine nucleus:* It itself gets collaterals from pyramidal tract.

b. *Efferent*
- From 'dentate nucleus' efferent fibres are coming out to their destination viz. area 4, vestibular nucleus, reticular formation. The two paths are—dentato-rubro-thalamo-cortical path' and, cerebello-thalamico-cerebral-path.

- In this way, cerebellum receives impulses from cerebral cortex and in turn controls the pyramidal system. All this constitutes what is known as closed loop circuit (cerebro-cerebellar circuit).
- Efferent fibres from cerebellum cross to the opposite side before reaching the destination.

ARCHI CEREBELLUM (VESTIBULO-CEREBELLUM) (Figs 106.1 and 106.2)

- Phylogenetically oldest part.
- Components are: Flocculo-nodular lobe, nodulus and flocculi.
- *Afferents:* Vestibulo-cerebellar tract: Fibres are originating from vestibular nuclei lying in pons and medulla. It reaches to cerebellar nuclei after crossing the inferior cerebellar peduncle of the same side. From these nuclei fibres reach to flocculo-nodular lobe. It is worth recalling that vestibular nuclei receive fibres from vestibular apparatus in inner ear through eight nerve (vestibular division).

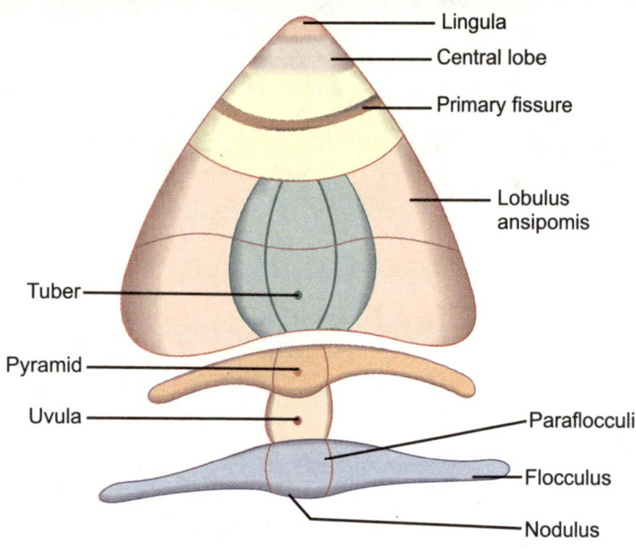

Fig. 106.1: Division of cerebellum

- *Efferents:*
  a. *Cerebello-vestibular fibres*: Fibres arise from flocculo-nodular lobe, cross the inferior cerebellar peduncle and terminate in vestibular nuclei of brainstem. This pathway forms extra-pyramidal system.
  b. *Fastigio-bulbar fibres*: Fibres from nodulus reach the fastigial nucleus, then they cross inferior cerebellar peduncle of same side and finally terminate on vestibular nuclei and reticular formation. They form extra-pyramidal system.
- *Functions:*
  - Maintenance of tone, posture and equilibrium
  - Controls linear and angular acceleration.

PALEO/SPINO-CEREBELLUM (Fig. 106.3)

- Connected with spinal cord
- *Components:* Cerebellar hemisphere, para flocculi, parts of vermis (lingula, central lobe, culmen, lobulus simplex, pyramid, uvula).

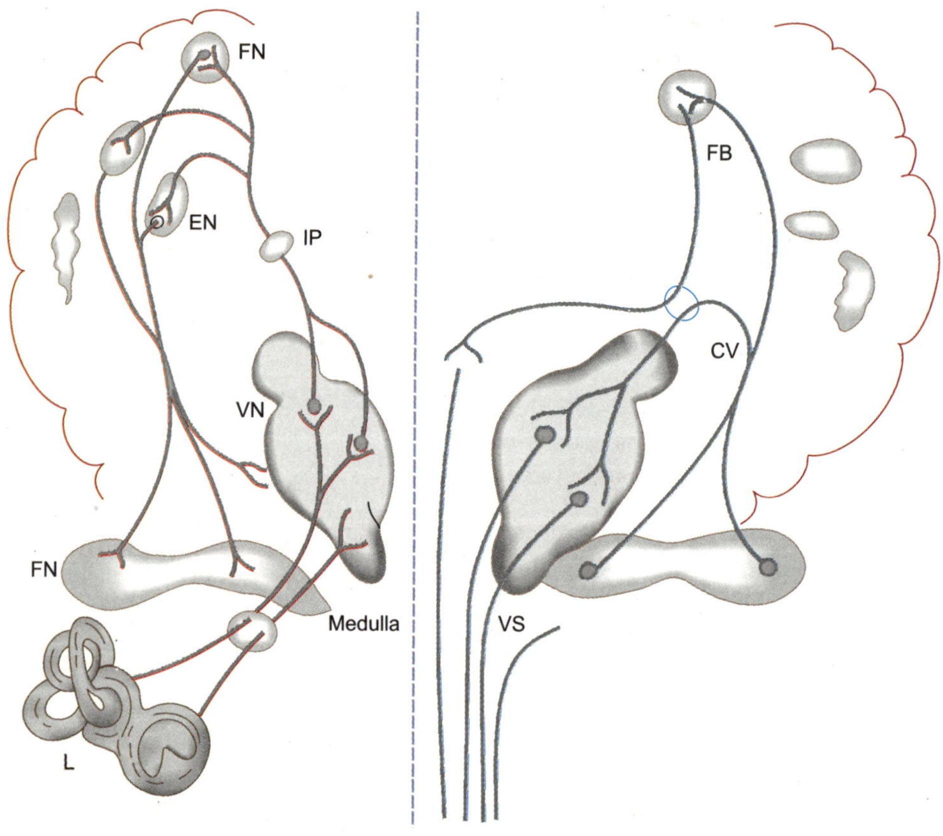

Fig. 106.2: Division of cerebellum

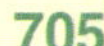

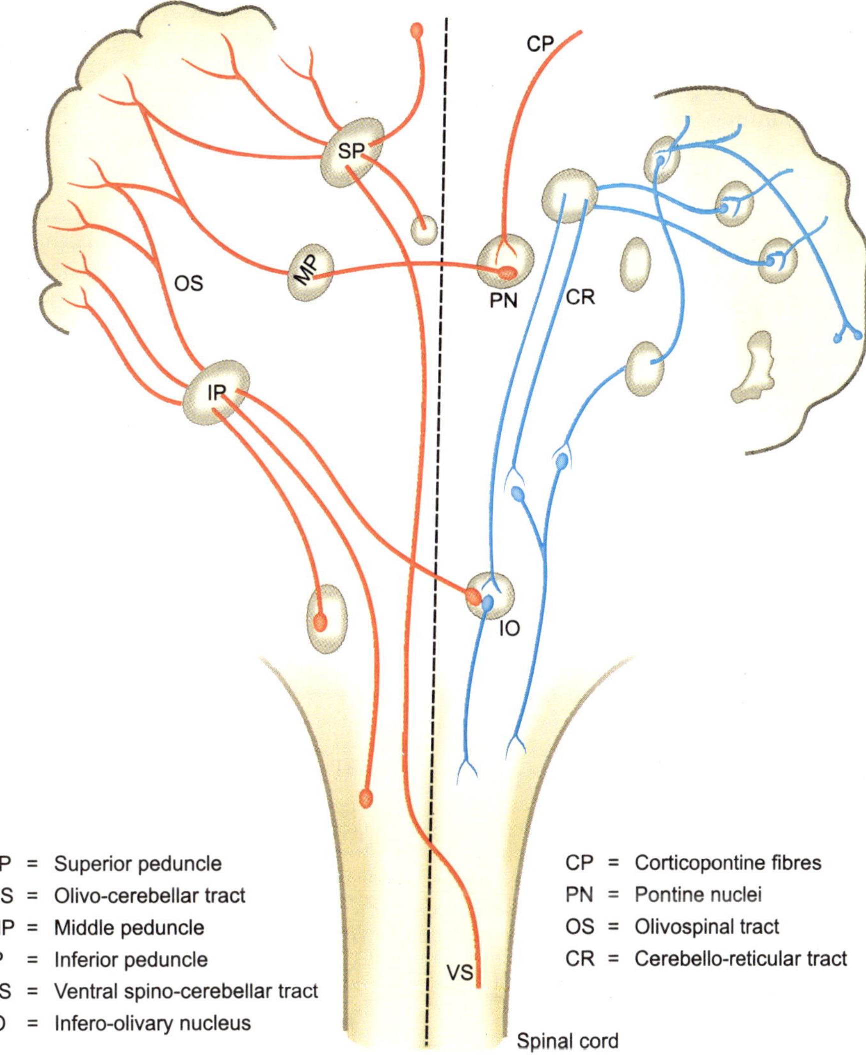

Fig. 106.3: Cortico-cerebellum

- *Afferents:*
  (a) Dorsal spino-cerebellar tract (b) Ventral spino-cerebellar tract (c) Cuneo-cerebellar tract (d) Olivo-cerebellar tract (e) Ponto-cerebellar tract (f) Tecto-cerebellar tract (g) Trigemino-cerebellar tract.
- *Efferents:*
  a. *Fastigio-bulbar tract*: Fibres arise from fastigial nuclei, end in reticular formation by crossing superior cerebellar peduncle
  b. *Cerebello-reticular tract*: Fibres arise from emboliform and globose nuclei and terminating in reticular formation. From here fibres go to spinal cord (reticulo-spinal tract) terminating into gamma motor neurons.
  c. *Cerebello-olivary tract*: Fibres arise from emboliform and globose nuclei and reaches to inferior olivary nucleus by passing through superior cerebellar peduncle. From olivary nucleus fibres descend to alpha motor neurons of spinal cord (olivo-spinal tract).
- *Functions:* It receives impulses of tactile, auditory, visual and proprioceptive types. Cortical impulses are also received here. Different body parts are represented here directly (in cerebral cortex inverse presentation occurs). Postural reflexes are regulated by modifying muscle tone. It facilitates gamma motor neuron which reflexly modify the activity of alpha neuron and thus muscle is regulated.

NEO-CEREBELLUM (Cortico-cerebellum) (Fig. 106.4)

- Largest part of cerebellum. Phylogenetically new.
- It is concerned with planning, programming and co-ordination of skilled movements, i.e. integration and regulation of well co-ordinated muscular activities. Apart from cerebral cortex, fibres are also received from proprioceptors in muscles.
- *Afferents:*
  a. Ponto-cerebellar tract
  b. Olivo-cerebellar tract
- *Efferents:*
  a. *Dentato-thalamic fibres*: Fibres originate from dentate nucleus—cross the midline (after passing through superior cerebellar peduncle) → form decussation with fibres of opposite side → terminate in lateral ventral nucleus of thalamus after passing through red nucleus → from thalamus fibres are projecting to cerebral cortex.
  b. *Dentato-rubral fibres:* From red nucleus fibres arise:
     - *Rubro-thalamic* - From red nucleus to lateral ventral nucleus of thalamus.
     - *Rubro-reticular* - Fibres end in reticular formation which projects into spinal cord (reticulo-spinal tract).
     - *Rubro-spinal tract* - Red nucleus is directly projecting to spinal cord.

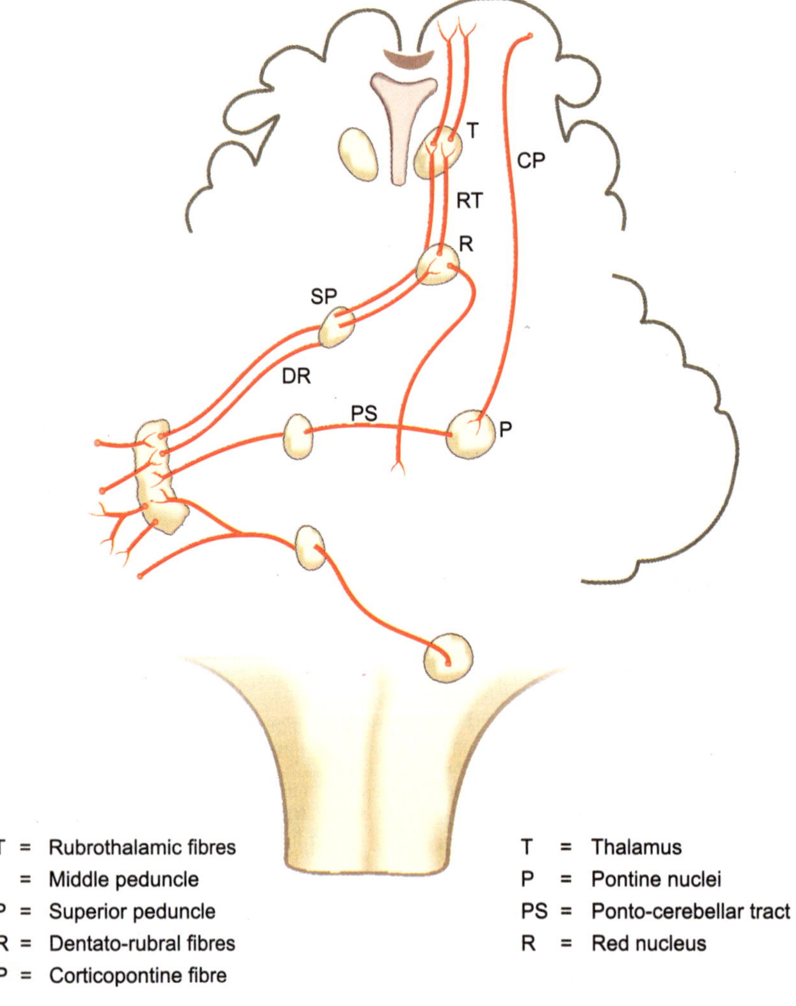

Fig. 106.4: Spinocerebellum connections

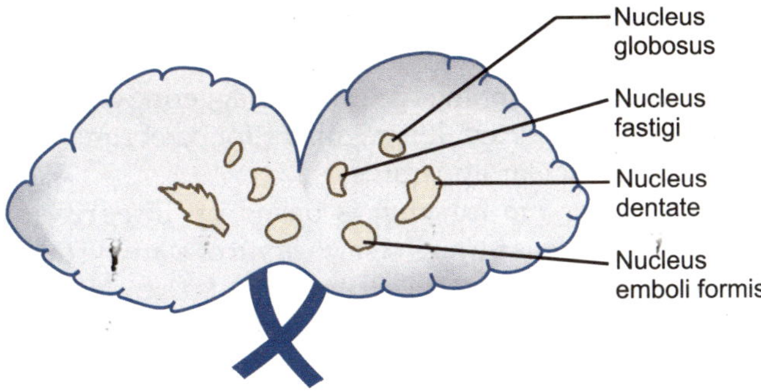

Fig. 106.5: Nuclei of cerebellum

MECHANISM OF CEREBELLAR ACTION (Fig. 106.5)

- The cerebellum sends impulses to cerebral cortex to discharge appropriate signals to respective muscles so that extra-muscular activity is prevented. So cerebellum acts like a *"brake"* on cerebral cortex. This is *Damping*.
- In some skilled work (e.g. dancing, typing, cycling some alternate movements take place called ballistic movements. Cerebellum plays a leading role in pre-planning these movements during learning.
- While performing any skilled activity (typing, dancing etc.) one performs chain of movements sequentially. So after learning process, it plans, programmes the activity like fixing the time for each event as well as their intervals. All these are transmitted to cerebral cortex where they are stored as memory.
- So after all this learning, the movements are executed in sequential manner without any interruption. This is *servo mechanism*.
- It receives informations from muscles (effectors) via proprioceptives as well as from cerebral cortex. Then it decides the intensity/severity of a particular movement. It also modifies the cerebral discharge. This is *comparator function*.

FUNCTIONAL SIGNIFICANCE AND DISORDERS (Fig. 106.6)

1. It is concerned with maintenance of normal tone of muscles. 'Decrease in tone' of peripheral muscles after loss of cerebellar hemisphere is observed which may result from loss of facilitation of motor cortex by 'cerebello-cortical pathways. It is said to regulate the tone in co-ordination with spinal cord and cerebral cortex.

   Asthenia (slowness of movement and early fatigue) is another condition due to involvement of corpus cerebelli.

   Due to disturbed tone body equilibrium is also deranged which is due to disruption of vestibular connection to the cerebellum. *It is worth to mention here that flocculonodular lobe is exerting leading effect in erect posture maintenance.*
2. It maintains body equilibrium in various positions like running, jumping, standing etc. One of the major function of cerebellum is automatic excitation of antagonist muscle at the end of movement while at the same time inhibiting agonist muscles that have started the movement.

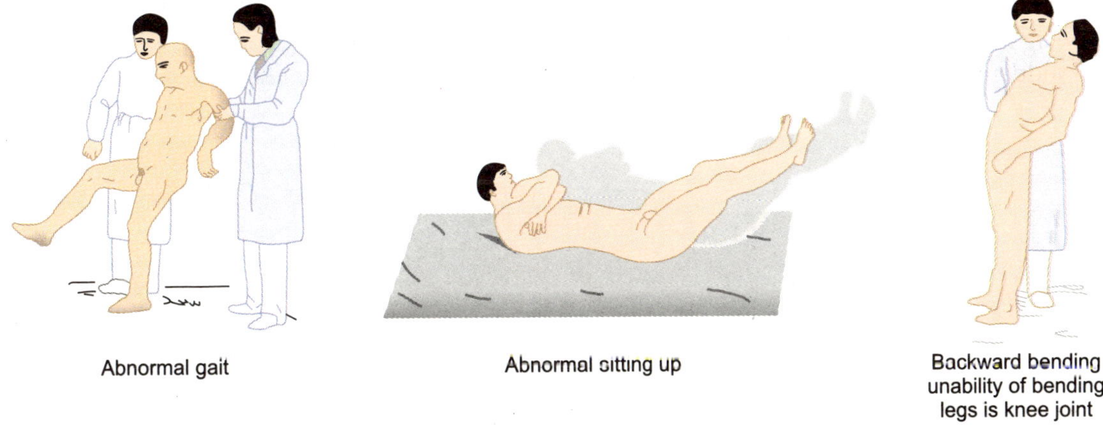

Fig. 106.6: Cerebellar disease—Motor disorders

Clinical application: Dysmetria is a condition in which there is loss of adjustment of the range of contraction which is necessary for the accomplishment of a particular act.

Ataxia is a condition of in co-ordinated movement.

3. It gives ability for *progression* from one movement to next in an orderly succession.

   Clinical application: When this function fails due to any lesion here, the person suffering loses the part during rapid motor movements. It leads to occurrence of a series of jumbled movements instead of normal upward and downward movements and state is named as, *'Dysdiadochokinesia'* which is said to be due to asynergia between protagonist, antagonist and synergists.

   This may also occur in form of *Dysarthria.* Some words are spoken very loud or some weak, some are spoken for short interval of time; on the whole jumbled vocalisation exists.

4. If it is intact, appropriate subconscious signals stop the movement at the intended point and thus overshooting of a particular movement is prevented, and intention tremor is checked (Tremor when appears in later part of act on an attempt to perform a particular movement).
5. *Cerebellar nystagmus* is a condition in which the patient is asked to follow an object with his eyes but when the direction of object is reversed the eyeball oscillates. It may be either due to damage of flocculonodular lobe or dysfunctioning of pathways through cerebellum from semi-circular canals.
6. Normal cerebellum powerfully sensitizes stretch reflex whenever any body portion begins to move in an unwilled direction. Clinical significance...... *Rebound* occurs due to loss of cerebellar component of stretch reflex when patient is asked to do—say flex the elbow against a resistance and if this resistance is released suddenly, the patient still makes effort to flex elbow, the whole limb shoots up towards the direction of movement.
7. On its lesion scanning speech and staggering gait have also been reported. It is regulator for cerebrum or of neuro-muscular apparatus.
8. *Cerebellum and learning* is based on integrity of olivary nucleus through which input of learning takes place. Each Purkinje cell receives inputs from 2,50,000-1 million mossy fibres, but each is having only one climbing fibre.

CEREBELLAR DISTURBANCES: DEMONSTRATION

1. The patient tries to put the tip of finger of outstretched hand on the tip of nose.
2. The patient is not able to perform rapid pronation and supination movements.
3. The patient moves on a zigzag path, i.e. he tends to deviate to the affected side and comes back in original line.
4. He is imperfect in execution of movements of laryngeal muscle and tongue. So speech is slow and lalling.

BIBLIOGRAPHY

1. Brooks VB, et al. Cerebellar control of posture and movements: In Bethesda, MD (Ed): Handbook of Physiology, sec I, Vol. II, American Physiological Society 1981;877.
2. Dow RS, Moruzzi G. The physiology and pathology of cerebellum - Minneapolis. 1958.
3. Gelman S, et al. Disorders of cerebellum. Philadelphia: Davis 1981.
4. ITO M. The cerebellum and neural control. New York: Raven Press. 1984.
5. Jenson J. Acta Physio Scand 41 Suppl. 1957;143.
6. Oscarsson O. Acta Physio. Scand. 42 Suppl. 145, 146.
7. Samson Wright's applied physiology: Revised by CA Keele and Eric Neil, Toronto: Oxford University Press.
8. Thach WT, et al. Cerebellum and adaptive co-ordination of movement. Ann rev neurosci 1992;15:403.

107 Loyal Association Thalamus (Diencephalon)

It is better to say that, 'it is a nuclear mass where all afferent fibres to the cortex with the sole exception of olfactory fibres, are relayed.' more or less it acts like PA of supreme command—the cerebral cortex.

It is a large oval structure located above mid-brain. The medial and lateral geniculate bodies, known as meta thalamus, are its parts relaying auditory and visual reflexes. Each thalamus is lying along the wall of third ventricle and the central aqueduct and bounded laterally by internal capsule. The thalami are joined in midline by massa intermedia. Thalami are two large oval convex cell masses, situated below cerebral hemisphere and above cerebral peduncles.

On hemi decortication initially all sensations are lost on opposite side of the body but after several days response to nociceptive stimuli is regained. Light touch, position sense and stereognosis are lost permanently. This can explain that thalamus deals with all crude sensations as well as there exists extensive ipsilateral sensory representation in it.

CONNECTIONS (Fig. 107.1)

a. *Afferent or input:*

i. Specific sensory fibres are received from spinal cord via medial lemniscus (convey proprioceptive and discriminative tactile sensation to posterolateral nuclei of ventral group); and spinal lemniscus (carry pain, heat, cold and touch sensation to posterior nuclei of ventral group).

ii. From opposite cerebellum (cerebellar efferents) fibres are terminating into intermediate nuclei of ventral group.

iii. Rubro-thalamic and cortico-thalamic fibres are also received.

iv. Olfactory sensations are carried through mammillo-thalamic tract to its anterior part.

v. Head sensory impulses via trigeminal nerve bringing touch, pain, temperature and gustation senses from nucleus tractus solitarius.

vi. Fibres are also received by hypothalamus, corpus striatum, substantia nigra.

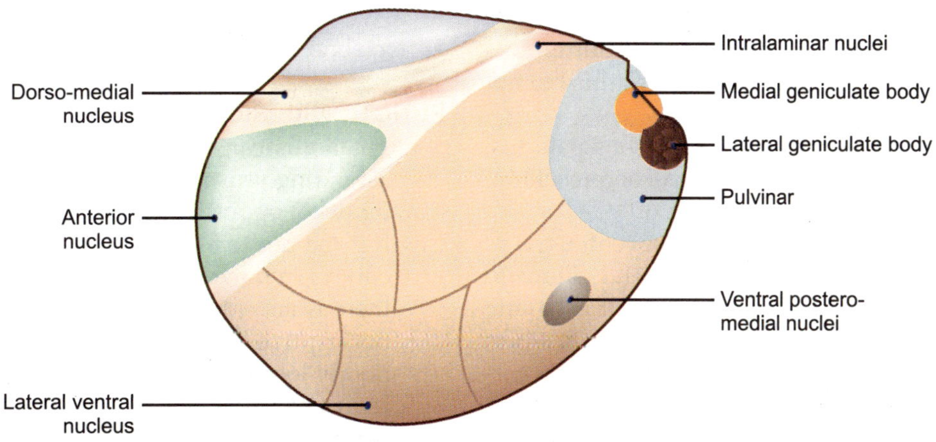

Fig. 107.1: Thalamic nuclei

vii. Impulses from viscera are also carried; which are terminating in mainly lateral group of nucleus; of course, few terminate in medial group too.

b. *Efferent or output*
   i. Fibres terminate into specific areas of sensory cortex (post-central gyrus; Brodmann's area 1, 2 and 3); called thalamo-cortical fibres.
   ii. Similarly, nonspecific thalamocortical fibres are terminating into cerebral cortex.
   iii. Efferents are also going to caudate nucleus, globus pallidus, hypothalamus, corpus striatum, intra-thalamic connections.

THALAMIC NUCLEI

Nuclei of Medial Mass

1. *Anterior nuclei*: It bulges into lateral ventricle. It receives fibres from mamillary bodies which convey olfactory impulses, i.e. mamillo-thalamic tract. It sends fibres to paracentral lobule and cingular gyrus (posterior part) on medial aspect of hemisphere.
2. *Dorso-medial nuclei*: is a dorso-lateral group of small cells and a medial group of large cells. The former dorso-lateral group project to prefrontal areas of cerebral cortex; and is serving as an association centre where visceral and crude somatic sensation are synthesised. It is also considered as a conscious centre for cruder (protopathic sensation) where sensation are integrated into feelings. The large cellular mass is connected with hypothalamus; and also projecting to corpus striatum.

Nuclei of Lateral Mass

a. *Dorsal group:* Synonym - lateral nucleus of thalamus divided into dorso-lateral and postero-lateral nuclei.

b. *Ventral group:*
   - *Anterior ventral:* Receiving fibres from globus pallidus and projecting to corpus striatum but not to cerebral cortex.
   - *Lateral ventral:* Fibres arising in globus pallidus, dentate nucleus of contralateral half of cerebellum. Efferents pass to area 4, and area 6.
   - *Posterior ventral:* It projects to post-central gyrus areas 3, 2, 1, 5 and 7 and it also sends fibres to hypothalamus and corpus striatum. It is having two parts viz. postero-medial which receives trigeminal fibres and postero-lateral which is thalamic station for medial and spinal lemnisci. It is the main subcortical centre for sensory impulses ascending in trigeminal, medial and spinal lemnisci.

Nuclei of Midline

Situated in massa intermedia and in adjacent part of medial mass forming upper part of wall of third ventricle. Phylogenetically oldest part. It is centre for primitive sensations, e.g. from viscera and other structures occupying axial regions of body. These nuclei are connected with other subcortical centres like hypothalamus, mid-brain etc. Few fibres are passing to cerebral cortex, body of Luys, red nucleus. It is also having intra-thalamic connections. It also receives fibres from corpus striatum.

Intralaminar Nuclei

Scattered group of cells. Located within internal medullary lamina. Well marked in primates. They receive trigeminal and fibres from medial lemniscus. They project to globus pallidus and also make many intrathalamic connections. Most prominent nucleus of this group is centro-median nucleus—an intrathalamic integrating centre.

Pulvinar Nuclei

Continuation of lateral nuclear mass. It projects to cortex, its inferior part comprises to an area of temporal lobe; rest part projects to parietal and temporal lobes.

MID-BRAIN/THALAMIC PREPARATION

- All connections of thalamus with cerebral cortex are removed by sectioning at level of mid-brain.
- All fine sensations are lost viz. touch, tactile discrimination and localisation along with conscious kinaesthetic sensation.
- Crude sensations are intact.
- Righting reflexes are retained. Muscle tone not affected.
- Co-ordination of reflex movement is not lost.
- Exaggeration of movements occur during emotional drive.
- No abnormal involuntary movements.

FUNCTIONAL SIGNIFICANCE

i. Thalamus can be regarded as a relay station on ascending sensory pathway. It represents sensory inputs of opposite half of body.

ii. It is the centre for cruder sensation. When cerebral cortex is removed on one side, (hemi-decortication), there is anaesthesia on the opposite side and then nociceptive stimuli are appreciated but they are poorly localised. Tactile sensation may return. The return of crude sensation is partly due to ability of thalamus on decorticate side to subserve crude sensation and partly to bilateral representation of touch and pain.

iii. It (the midline and intra-laminar group of nuclei, being connected with reticular formation) is concerned with alert and arousal reaction.

iv. Due to its projecting fibres to frontal lobe, it is concerned with emotions as well as personality and social behaviour of one individual.

v. Because of these widespread connections, cortex is helped by it in appraisal of various sensory inputs, and hence it causes conditioning of sensory impulses which are relayed to cortex.

vi. Since stimulation of cerebral cortex does not produce pain and removal of cortex does not produce permanent anaesthesia, it is usually said that pain is appreciated at thalamic level and not at cortical level. It may not be right to say that pain is entirely thalamic. So it is said that pain, heat and cold are distinguished in thalamus while touch and pressure are distinguished in cortex. So it can be concluded that it differentiates the modality of sensation.

vii. Since it is forming a connection or link between cerebellum, basal ganglia and cerebral cortex, therefore it is concerned with some complex motor activities.

viii. Through hypothalamus, it is concerned in perception of visceral sensation as well as with autonomic control of viscera.

ix. *Thalamic syndrome* (Dejerine and Roussay-1906): On destruction of posterior parts of the ventral and lateral nuclei this symptom complex is observed.

- Hemi-anaesthesia severe for cutaneous sensibilities (touch, pain, temperature) but marked for deep sensibilities with an exaggerated response to stimulation with painful or thermal stimuli. Pain is felt frequently intense on the side where there is anaesthesia, it is persistent having the characteristic of deep pain.
- Motor disturbances in contralateral limbs in the form of ataxia, choreoathetosis, hemiparesis, intention tremors and thalamic hands (flexion at wrist with hyper-extension of fingers with extension of whole hand).
- Sensory disturbances include astereognosis occurring on contralateral side of lesion, loss of tactile and thermal sensation over the face and some part of body, sensory ataxia (unability to localise a touching point), thalamic over reactions (spontaneous paroxysms of attack of pain with pain threshold either lowered or increased), thalamic phantom limb (unability to localise the position of limbs with an attempt to find them in air due to loss of sense of position).
- The pain threshold is very much reduced or increased. So intense pain is felt by patient. Sometimes light touch may be unpleasant. It is so severe that it resists the action of powerful sedatives like morphine. It is due to over activity of medial mass of nuclei which escape the lesion.
- *Amelognosia* is the illusion felt by the patient that his limb is absent—is felt by patient.
- It occurs due to blockage (thrombosis) of thalmogeniculate branch of posterior cerebral artery. Mostly postero-ventral nuclei are affected since this artery supplies this part.

BIBLIOGRAPHY

1. Jones EG. Thalamic connections. TPS Powell Brain. 1970;93:37-56.
2. Lemin RN. Thalamic pathway for rapid afferent input from hand motor cortex in monkey. J Phy 1979;55.

108 Supreme Command: The Cerebral Cortex

- It is the site of mind and the intellect—popular belief.
- It is the area which carries out a final integration of neural mechanisms—scientific thought.
- Cortex means bark, i.e. outer covering of a tree and so of brain.

The great wealth of fibre connections run vertically up and down rather than from side to side. It is an estimated fact that 12×10^9 cells in human brain, no less than 9.2×10^9 lie in cerebrum itself. All of them allow a great number of alternatives to be considered by the cerebrum; the decision taken are also represented. The sources of study of cerebral functions are from the study localised destructive lesions and surgical removal, from the sensations and physical responses of conscious patients when electrical stimulation is deliberately applied to different points on the surface of cortex and from the pattern of response in epileptic seizures arising from an irritative lesion in one part of the cortex. Its cells are arranged in six layers namely (1) molecular, (2) external granular, (3) external pyramidal, (4) internal granular, (5) internal pyramidal, (6) fusiform (from the surface inward).

- The bulkiest portion of CNS is cerebral hemisphere which occupy most of the cranial cavity. The two hemispheres are completely separated from each other by longitudinal cerebral fissure both in front and behind. Each cerebral hemisphere is subdivided into four lobes namely frontal, parietal, occipital and temporal as well as two sulci lateral and central.

FRONTAL LOBE AND FUNCTIONAL AREAS

It consists of pre-central gyrus lying in front of the *central sulcus* and behind the *pre-central sulcus* and superior middle and inferior gyri separated from one another by means of two anterio-posterior sulci superior and inferior frontal sulci. Olfactory sulcus containing olfactory bulb and tract is an anterio-posterior sulcus on orbital surface of frontal lobe, close to the medial border.

Pre-central Area

- *Area 4* is a tapering strip of agranular cortex lying in front of central fissure and occupying the posterior part of the precentral convolution. It is a centre for movement; giving origin to an important part of corticospinal tracts and also projecting to the pons, corpus striatum, red nucleus, thalamus and the subthalamus. Major part of it is buried for it is covering the anterior wall of central fissure.
- Damage to *area 4* produces loss of strength, flaccidity and diminished tendon reflexes with incapability to movements (and most sufferers are skilled movements). Irritative lesions involving *area 4* are originating localised clonic convulsive seizures. There may be localised facial twitching, or of finger/foot or it may become generalised (Jacksonian epilepsy).
- *Area 4S* (cortical inhibitory area) Inhibition of reflexly induced movements in anaesthetised animal is caused on stimulation of a narrow band of area 4.
- *Area 6* (premotor area) is confined to adjoining posterior portion of superior, middle and inferior frontal gyri—extending into medial frontal gyrus on medial surface of each hemisphere. It has got all the structural similarities with area 4 with the exception of absence of giant pyramidal cells in ganglion. Both area 4 and 6 are connected by intra-cortical fibres can lead to awkwardness of movements with negligible spasticity, increased tendon reflexes, forced grasping along with autonomic disturbances. Destruction of pre-central motor cortex (area 4 and 6) terminating into spastic hemiplegia.
- Functions of *pre-motor area* includes - (i) Co-ordination of activities of motor cortex for smooth and regular movement (ii) Area 6 is highest cortical centre

for extra-pyramidal system, (iii) on stimulation it causes motor responses, (iv) Removal of pre-motor cortex leads to increased muscular tone resulting into forced grasping—groping and exaggerated jerks and (v) temporary loss of acquired skill is seen in lesions affecting the pre-motor area, resulting into awkward movements.

- Functions of *excitomotor cortex* includes— (i) Control of opposite half of the body (initiation and organisation of purposeful voluntary movement). (ii) It has some control over muscular activities of the ipsilateral side specially in proximal joints of lower limbs. (iii) It also exerts some control over many visceral and vascular activities like heart rate, GIT motility, respiration, vasomotor activities etc.
- Functions of frontal lobe (*Pre-frontal area*) can be summarised as (i) it is a site for emotional stability, planned action, accurate judgement (*organ of mind*). (ii) It exerts full influence on autonomic reactions which are associated with emotions owing to its connections with brainstem and hypothalamus. (iii) It exerts inhibitory control over supramedial gyrus of parietal lobe of dominant side (ideomotor area).
- *Pre-frontal area* (orbito-frontal region): It embraces the part of frontal lobe in front of area 8 and 44. It is divided into different areas namely 9, 10, 11, 12, 13 which are also known as silent areas (association area) concerned with visceral rather than somatic sensation.
- *Area 44 and 45* (Broca's area; motor speech centre): It is as a distinguished region of pre-motor cortex playing essential role in speech production.
- *Area 8*: It is lying adjoining area 6. It forms one of the centres for extra-pyramidal system including frontal eye filed.
- Frontal lobes synthesise the information about the outside world received through the exteroceptives and the information about the internal states of body and that they are the means whereby the behaviour of organism is regulated in conforming with the effect produced by its action.
- Pre-frontal area is concerned with high associative or synthetic abilities and emotional feelings. After sectioning of fibres from these cells, individual may be restless and lack initiative and they are unable to work with abstract ideas.
- *Frontal Lobe Syndrome (Organ of Mind):*
  - *Frontal lobe:* Seat of intelligence.
  - Intelligence depends upon a knowledge of external world received through channels like visual, auditory, somesthetic perception etc. They all are stored in cerebral cortex. Tracts of association fibres link together these areas. These sensation are synthesised into complex memories. Thus with the progress of time these experiences become more integrated.
  - The main features of its destruction/lesion include:-
    1. Lack of restraint—Causes aggressiveness, boasting, hostility.
    2. Restlessness—Difficulty in fixing attention.
    3. Lack of initiative—Difficulty in planning any course of action.
    4. Impairment of memory—Only recent type.
    5. Impairment of moral/social sense—Loss of love for family.
    6. No realisation—False sense of well-being (euphoria).
    7. Hypermotility

    Flight of ideas—Emotional instability.

THE PARIETAL LOBE (The somesthetic area)

- The somesthetic area is sensory in function and is *post-central gyrus* (band of cortex lying behind including area 3, 1 and 2). A part of the temporal lobe which lies adjoining the occipital and parietal lobes is also included in it which constitute basal area.
- *Area 3* (somesthetic, somatic, primary sensory area) is anterior part of post-central area. This band of sensory cortex is turning over the upper border of cerebral hemisphere and extending down the mesial surface as far as the ungulate gyrus. The primary somatic area (somatic area I) receives sensory fibres carrying exteroceptive and proprioceptive sensibilities from opposite side of body through thalamus. Somatic area II lies in upper wall of sylvian fissure, i.e. below face area of somatic area I. The order of representation in sensory area II is the inverse to that of area I.
- The somesthetic cortical area is responsible for (i) stereognosis (recognition of similarities and differences like relative size—texture of objects, weights of objects, (ii) spatial recognition (recognition of position and passive movement of limb, (iii) recognition of relative intensity of different stimuli.
- Area 1 and 2 is posterior part of post-central area. On stimulation it produces numbness, tingling, prickling sensation etc. but not the pain.
- Parietal area (association area) is situated between visual area behind and post-central area in front and below is auditory area. Functionally, it is concerned with senses of stereognosis from the opposite half of body, spatial recognition from the opposite half of

body, general sensation from opposite half of body, appreciation of taste sensation.

- Motor speech centre is confined to inferior parietal lobule of both the hemispheres and is related with motor activities of parts like face, lip, tongue.
- *Sensory speech centre* is confined to inferior parietal lobule in angular gyrus, and is related with printing, writing and spoken words.
- *Pre- and post-central areas* are considered as one functional unit (sensiromotor cortex) e.g. stimulation of post-central area produces both sensory and various motor activities.
- *Area of taste* is the cortex at the lower end of somesthetic area which is lying near to motor cortex controlling masticating muscles. It receives fibres from taste nucleus of thalamus.
- On lesion of sensory cortex Jacksonian epilepsy is seen along with prickling sensation, pins and needle sensation and sensation of cold etc.
- Ablation of area 1, 2, 3 (post-central gyrus) resulted in loss of position sense, two point discrimination and position in space of opposite limb, specially in its distal part.

THE TEMPORAL LOBE

- It is obvious that within temporal cortex there are mechanisms which play an important role in act of remembering and of making comparisons between present sensory perceptions and past experience. Here alone electrical stimulation and epileptic discharge activate synaptic patterns. It is only in this region that such stimulation produces complex psychical illusions and hallucinations argues for some degree of localisation of intellectual function. Its unilateral ablation has no discernible effect on auditory, memory or equilibrium process.
- *Area 41 and 42* (audito-sensory area) is situated in anterior transverse temporal gyri which are confined in the floor of posterior ramus of the lateral sulcus which partly is extending to a narrow strip of lateral surface of superior temporal gyrus. It is centre for hearing so in its unilateral lesion, one gets difficulty to locate the sound source. So here fundamental auditory sensation (intensity and pitch) are appreciated. It is further sub-divided into area I and area II.
- *Centre for smell* is located in uncus and anterior part of hippocampal gyrus, amygdaloid nucleus and hallucinations regarding olfaction are seen on its stimulation.
- *Centre for equilibrium* is present in posterior part of superior temporal convolution.
- Its *bilateral extirpation* gives rise to a symptom complex constituted by visual agnosia, oral tendencies, hypermetamorphosis, tameness, hypersexuality, changes in dietary habits—all constitute *Temporal lobe syndrome in monkeys*.
- *Monkeys: Kluver-Bucy syndrome (1939) (Bilateral extirpation of temporal lobe including neocortex and rhinencephalon)*
- The characteristics are:
  1. Loss of recognition ability
  2. Very strong tendency to examine all objects with the mouth (oral tendency).
  3. Loss of sensation of fear (tameness).
  4. Increase in various sexual activities (hypersexuality).
  5. Tendency to take notice and to attend every visual stimulus (Hypermetamorphosis).
  6. Monkeys don't eat meat normally: but now they eat is along with an increase in their diet (altered dietary habits).
- While same in human being is represented by speech disturbances, auditory disturbances, dreamy state, vision, taste and smell disturbances, and memory loss, as described below:

Lesion: Temporal Lobe Syndrome in Man

It leads to

1. Speech disturbances: Disturbed understanding/expression/recall of name of objects. Lesion exists most likely in postero-superior part near the posterior part of Sylvian fissure (aphasia).
2. Paroxysmal attacks of tinitus (ringing sound in ear), auditory hallucinations, epileptic attacks are seen (auditory disorders).
3. Paroxysmal hallucinations of tastes and smell of unpleasant type (uncinate seizures).
4. Feeling of unreality: Attacks are similar to a dream. His activities are destructive, e.g. tearing the clothes of others, removing of his own clothes, wandering aimlessly (psychomotor seizures).
5. Visual hallucinations are in the form of objects.

OCCIPITAL LOBE

- Area 17 (Visuosensory or striate area) receives as well as recognises visual impressions like colour, illumination, transparency etc.
- Area 18 and 19 (Visuopsychic area) is storehouse of past experiences of visual impressions as well as it

helps in assessing distance as well orientation of an object in space. Area 19 contains an additional occipital eye field.

- Area 17 is concerned with perception of visual impulses so primary visual area; area 18 is concerned with its interpretation, so-called visual association area, area 19 (occipital eye filed) is concerned with movements of eyes.
- It receives afferent from lateral geniculate body; it sends efferents to superior colliculus as well as lateral geniculate body.

If two stimuli are given to an animal (The stimuli are very much alike and identical that they cannot be distinguished), the animal becomes upset and fails to co-operate and tries to escape. According to Pavlov it is experimental neurosis.

HEMISPHERE : AN OUTLOOK

i. The corpus callosum is having more than 200 million axons which are interconnecting neo-cortical system and is sending information from one hemisphere to be integrated with information in other. It deals with information from ongoing unilateral experiences crossing the midline to the contralateral hemisphere.

ii. Anterior commissure (connecting temporal lobe structures) is capable of instructing and stabilising memory experiences between two hemispheres.

iii. There is no symptomatology in persons with congenital agenesis of corpus callosum.

iv. Inferior parietal cortex (area 7) is a major region for sensorimotor activities. Following neurons for vision have been reported:
   - cells sensitive to visual stimuli
   - cells concerned with visual fixation
   - cells are neither sensory nor motor.

v. Left hemisphere, as it is, dominant for initiation, programming and monitoring of sequential tasks.

vi. If entire sensory cortex is removed from both cerebral hemispheres the individual is unable to appreciate any sensation. If sensory areas are removed from only one hemisphere, then sensation is lost only on opposite side of body.

DECEREBRATE PREPARATION

- Means—removing all the connection of cerebral hemisphere at the level of mid-brain, i.e. by sectioning in between superior and inferior colliculus.
- Characterised by decerebrate rigidity.
- Decerebrate rigidity:
   - Such an animal the caricature is extension of all four limbs, tail, arching of the back or hyper-extension of spine. This attitude is called ophisthotonus. Body posture cannot be maintained.

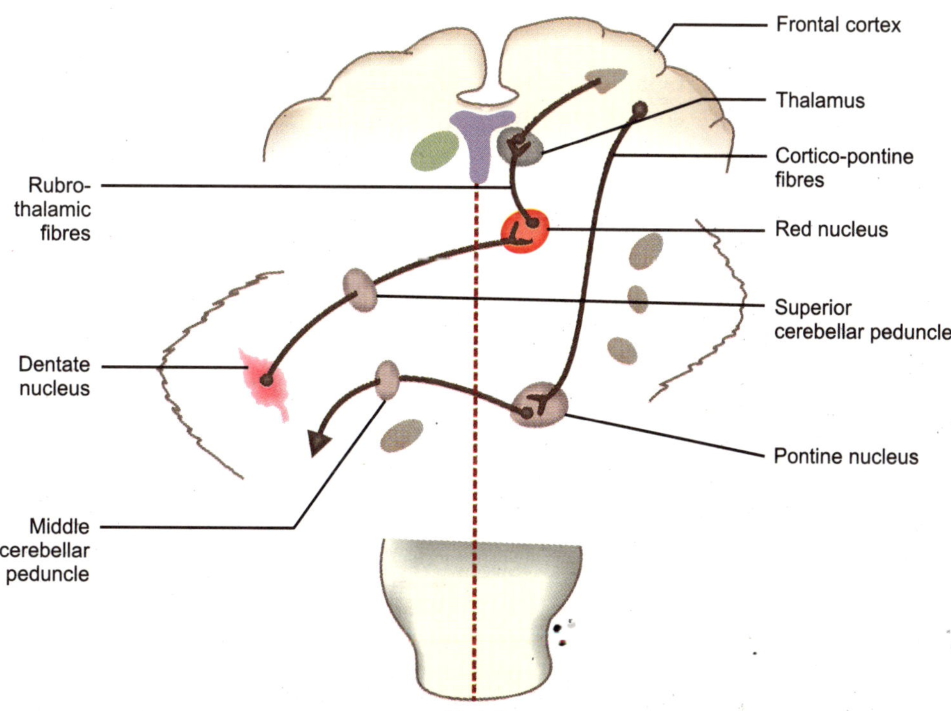

Fig.108.1: Cerebro-cerebellar circuit

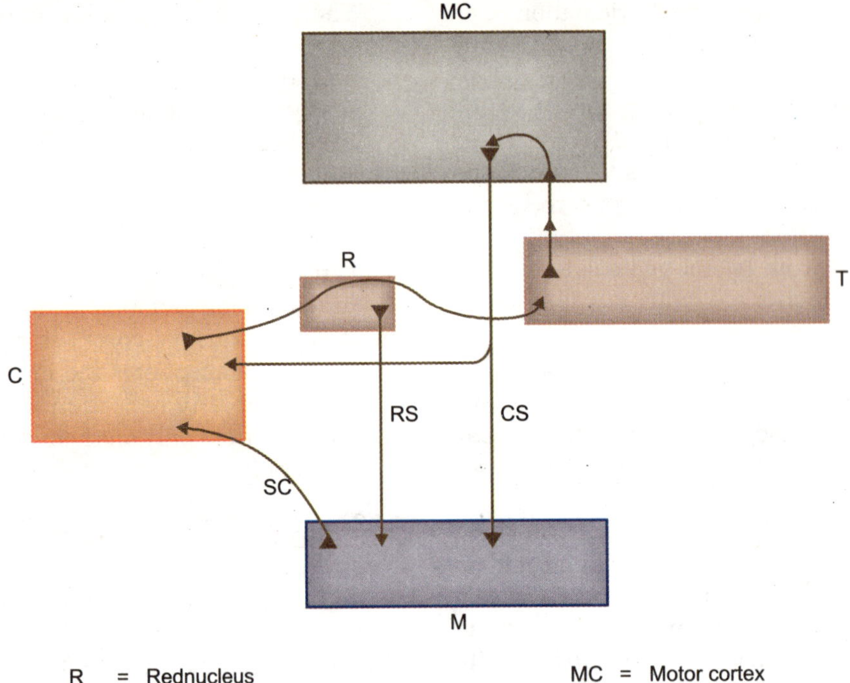

R = Rednucleus
M = Muscles
SC = Spino-cerebellar tract
C = Cerebellum
MC = Motor cortex
T = Thalamus
CS = Corticospinal tract
RS = Reticulospinal tract

Fig.108.2: Voluntary movements cerebro-cerebellar control

- Its cause is—release of centres, situated below the section from higher inhibitory control and this inhibitory area is 4S.
- This can also be produced by blocking blood supply to fore-brain, i.e. by occluding basilar/ common carotid artery.

DECORTICATE PREPARATION

- Produced by removing all the connections of cerebral cortex. Basal ganglia and brainstem are kept intact.
- If animal (dog/cat) is on its feet, posture is normal, muscle tone is distributed equally in both flexors and extensors. If animal is suspended in air, there is severe hyper-extension of all the limbs.
- In decorticate man, there is extension of lower limb and flexion of upper limb at elbow joint across the chest. The fingers and wrist flexed. Neck reflexes can be elicited when neck is turned to the right there occurs flexion of both limbs—upper and lower—on opposite side.
- This is due to lesion of corticospinal tract which exert inhibitory influence on extensor muscles.

CORRUS CALLOSUM: FEW MORE PECULIARITIES

- Fibres in corpus callosum connect most of the respective cortical areas with each other except for anterior portion of temporal lobes. So its most important function is to transfer the information stored in one hemisphere to another. On its cutting:
  - Informations from Wernicke's area of dominant hemisphere to motor cortex of opposite side is blocked. This leads to loss of control of intellectual functions (located in dominant hemisphere) over right motor cortex.
  - Corpus callosum is required for the two sides to operate co-operatively. Anterior commissure plays an important role in uniting the emotional responses of two sides of the brain.

DOMINANT HEMISPHERE: A CONCEPT

- In majority of persons left hemisphere is dominant. This means interpretative functions of Wernicke's area, and angular gyrus, functions of speech and motor, control areas are comparatively more developed in one hemisphere than in the other.

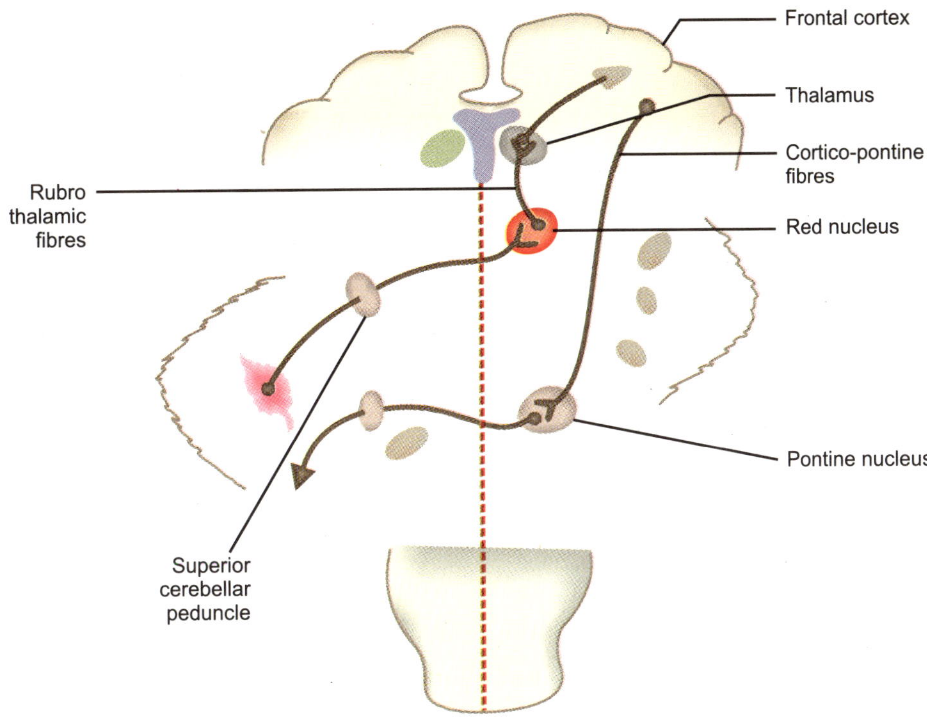

Fig.108.3: Connection between cerebellum and cerebrum

- Right from the birth left temporal lobe begins to be used to a greater extent than right. So this part is paid more attention. So this part grows rapidly while opposite side remains slight. So in majority of persons left temporal lobe and angular gyrus become dominant.
- Motor areas for controlling the bands are dominant on left side of the brain in majority of persons. This explains right handedness in majority of persons.

EXPERIMENTAL STUDIES: ANIMAL PREPARATION

1. Decorticate preparation
   - Cerebral cortex removed; basal ganglia corpus striatum intact
   - Dog and cat maintain normal posture without decerebrate rigidity; and performs reflex walking movements
   - Monkeys show full extension of hind limbs and semiflexion of forelimbs
   - If animal is looked after properly, it may assume erect posture with some awkward walk.
2. Decerebrate animal
   - Spinal cord with medulla oblongata retained
   - Decerebrate rigidity present
   - The animal cannot maintain equilibrium
   - Righting reflex absent
   - Normal body temperature cannot be maintained
   - Out of order respiration.
3. Thalamic animal
   - Spinal cord, hind-brain, mid-brain and a part of diencephalon retained
   - Decerebrate rigidity absent
   - Equilibrium, body temperature can be maintained
   - Righting reflex present
   - Normal respiration.

BIBLIOGRAPHY

1. Eccles JC. I to M, Szentagonthai J. (1967). The cerebellum as a neuronal machine. New York: Springer Verlag, 343.
2. Evarts EV, Thach WT. Motor mechanism of CNS: Cerebro-cerebellar Interrelations. Ann Rev Physiol 1969;31.
3. Galaburda, et al. Right left asymmetries in brain. Science 1978;199.
4. Herrick CJ (1915). An introduction to neurology. Saunders London 199. Quoted by Physiology of nervous system. London, New York - Toronto: Longmans, Green and Col, 1959.
5. Kalaska JF, et al. Cerebral cortical mechanisms of reaching movements. Quoted by Ganong WF in Review of Medical Physiology, Lange Publication. Science 1992;255:1517.
6. Luria. Higher cortical functions in man. II edition, New York: Basic Books Inc. Publishers. 1977.
7. Penfield W, Rasmussen T. The cerebral cortex of man. Macmillan. 1950-57.
8. Walsch EG and John Marshall Above book. 1959.

109 Higher Functions

Mental functions and disorders are really thrilling subjects. In organic diseases some structural disturbances are the main culprit while functional diseases are referred as mental by a common man since no organic lesion is there. On the whole the subject of higher functions and disorders is quite interesting and providing good scope for future investigation and real follow-up of patient.

MEMORY

i. *Definition*: It is defined as individual's ability to receive, retain as well as recalling any sensory impression once or many times.

ii. *Types:* For the sake of convenience it is divided into following categories:

a. *Instantaneous memory*: Any thing stored in mind for a short time is instantaneous or transient memory; e.g. if one moves in a car then he comes across many scenes/pictures or one goes across any exhibition or any industry or like that innumerable things, pictures are stored in his or her mind. Of course, exact mechanism cannot be manifested but few of the theories for its explanations are:

i. *Reverberating circuit aspect*: It is an established fact that cerebral cortex is connected with basal ganglia and subcortical nuclei (thalamus etc.) through reverberating circuits and when it will be stimulated it will go on discharging impulses as long as stimulation is continued and at the most up to one hour after withdrawal of stimulation.

ii. *Post-tetanic potentiation theory*: It is again a common belief that if tetanic stimulation to any neuron is given, it remains excited for even few hours. If the same neuron is again stimulated it gets hyper- excited. This is said to be responsible for such type of transient memory.

iii. *D.C. potential concept*: In the above mentioned concept on applying second stimulation the neuron's membrane potential is altered which further last for few hours. Cortex is said to originate such type of DC potential which is responsible for memory.

b. *Fixed memory*: It is once again composed of short-term and long-term memory. As the name suggests, fixed memory of whatever type can be recalled even after years.

Short term: As the name itself is suggestive it is remembered only for few days and is destroyed by electric shock and damage to temporal lobe.

Long term: As suggested by name it is remembered for years together but is not affected by either temporal lobe lesion or electric shock.

iii. *Explanation:* Many theories are there to explain it as follows:

i. *Synaptic change*: Fixation of any memory results from synaptic changes like alteration in number of pre-synaptic terminal, size, chemical configuration etc. Furthermore the active neurons of cortex are having synaptic connections which are increasing with age. Diminished activity can lead to thinning of cortex (specially visual area terminating into vision loss) while on the contrary, any over activity can lead to thickening of the concerned part. Further this sort of processing is adversely effected by cooling, diminished oxygen supply, drugs etc.

ii. *RNA-DNA hypothesis*: Since these are classed as code carriers so in this way they are capable of taking memories from generation to generation. Furthermore, it is also evident that if RNA synthesis mechanism are blocked fixing of memories is not interfered.

iii. *Glial and extra neuronal theory:*
It is an observation that many changes are occurring within glial cells during activity along with many

alteration in mucopolysaccharide or any other chemical changes around the synapses. This is another concept in field of memory, since all these changes are finally increasing the facilitation of synapses.

iv. *Memory: Molecular basis (synonym; memory engram/memory trace):*

1. *Facilitation:* Stimulation of facilitator + sensory neuron → release of serotonin from its terminal → binding with serotonin receptor → activation of enzyme adenyl cyclase in terminal membrane → formation of cAMP inside sensory presynaptic terminal → activation of a protein kinase $\xrightarrow{\text{phosphorylation of concerned protein}}$ Blocking potassium conductance → prolonged action potential since flow of these ions is necessary for recovery → more Ca^{2+} flow towards sensory terminal $\xrightarrow{\text{more release of transmitter}}$ facilitation of synaptic transmission.
2. *Habituation:* When sensory terminal is stimulated repeatedly and facilitator terminal is not activated then signal transmission is very great in the beginning, but later on it becomes less intense until it almost ceases. This is habituation and is a type of memory which leads the neuronal circuit to lose its response to repeated insignificant events.

v. *Memory-Abnormalities*

1. *Amnesia:*
   - Means loss of memory.
   - Due to lesion in hippocampus, there is no establishment of new long-term memories (antero grade amnesia).
   - When one fails to recall past remote long-term memory, it is retrograde amnesia; which is seen in temporal lobe syndrome.
2. *Dementia:* Means progressive loss of memory, as seen in Alzheimer's disease; (senile dementia) in which cerebral cortex is at fault with a decrease in acetylcholine synthesis as well as of adrenaline. Motor functions are also affected along with onset of psychiatric symptoms.

vi. *Notes:*

i. Now by considering all the aspects about memory process, three separate mechanisms are said to interact in its production, firstly; one which mediates immediate recall of moment events, secondly; one mediating events of minute or hours before and lastly mediation of remote events. Strangely events including in remote memories are found to be persisting even after severe brain diseases.

ii. The part played by temporal lobe in connection with memory process is further very interesting. On its stimulation memory is rewinded and particular or any special memory is coming up by stimulation of its special point. So it can be said that temporal lobe is the site where memories are present along with the fact that various points of temporal lobe are like keys which are unlocking memory traces found elsewhere in brain.

iii. Another interesting event in the temporal lobe role is that sometimes when stimulation is given to this part person's attitude is changed up to a remarkable state in the way that he may feel strange in homely or familial place or thinks that this thing has occurred with him previously in his life time. All this is called deja-vu-phenomenon (= already seen). In strange atmosphere one is alert while he may feel relaxed in familial atmosphere. Such events are noticed both in normal as well as in temporal lobe's epilepsy individuals.

iv. The entire discussion of memory will be considered incomplete if hippocampus's role is not viewed. If ventral hippocampus is destructed recent memory is inversely effected but remote memory remains intact. Of course change in recent memory is seen in some alcoholics with brain damage. Actually encoding or consolidation of memory needs hippocampus intact, along with its entire connections.

DIFFERENCES: MEMORY

Short term	*Long term*
1. Remembered for short time	Remembered throughout life
2. Loss of memory occurs on temporal lobe damage.	No interference of temporal lobe
3. Its loss occurs on giving electric shock.	No interference of electric shock
4. Different areas are concerned	Separate areas are concerned

SLEEP AND WAKEFULNESS

1. *Introduction*: It is temporary but reversible state of unconsciousness since one gets back to consciousness or wakefulness. Physiologically sleep and wakefulness are opposite to each other.
2. *Changes during sleep:*
   i. As common feeling, whole body is relaxed and of course muscles are in low tone and relaxed too.

ii. Pulse rate slows down. Cardiac output is reduced. Blood pressure occupies the basal level together with dilatation of skin blood vessels.

iii. Gastrointestinal motility is, of course, increased owing to augmented parasympathetic activity but otherwise entire digestive, metabolic and cardiac functions are slowed down. Basal metabolic rate also falls 10-20 per cent.

iv. As told above sympathetic activities decreases with occasional augmentation in parasympathetic activity.

v. All reflexes are also becoming sluggish. Extensor plantar response is sometimes seen in children during deep sleep.

vi. Deep but regular respiration is noticed. Alveolar pO_2 falls with rise in alveolar pCO_2.

vii. All body sphincters are said to maintain their normal tone but exception is in children resulting in wetting of bedsheets owing to relaxed sphincters.

viii. By sleep a good balance between different parts of nervous system is constituted together with the fact that behavioural activities are made smooth. Though there is less neuronal and cerebral cortex activity during sleep but blood supply to the cortex remains same.

3. ***Sleeplessness***: *Effects*—Certainly due to sleeplessness or prolonged wakefulness, nervous system is inversely effected in the form of behavioural and mind dysfunctions. Irritability, inability to solve mental problems, early fatigue, loss of attention, occasional fall in body temperature and pulse rate are few of its results.

4. ***Sleep and wakefulness:*** *Mechanism*—Various theories have been put forward to explain the exact mechanism of it as follows:

   i. Feedback theory and role of reticular activating system :

   - (RAS) Both reticular activating system and cerebral cortex are connected with each other. So if RAS is activated the degree of activity of cerebral cortex is also augmented and so also on activation of cerebral cortex in turn the activity of RAS is further intensified. In this way vicious cycle (positive feedback) exists and in this way a high degree of wakefulness is achieved. The pre- and post-central gyri (sensorimotor cortex), frontal cortex, hippocampus, cingulate gyrus, basal ganglia are important structures of cerebrum sending fibres to RAS.
   - Another mechanism playing a leading role in wakefulness is once again a positive feedback mechanism between RAS and sympathetic nervous system. When RAS gets excited, it stimulates sympathetic system which in exchange produces epinephrine which acting through brainstem—constituent of RAS—further stimulates it and this vicious cycle is capable of wakefulness.
   - In some other way another positive feedback is said to exist between RAS and peripheral/autonomic activities, to make one more alert or attentive.
   - Now, when wakefulness is achieved by any of the above mentioned mechanisms, the neuronal cells of this loop becomes less excitable or better to say fatigued and thus decreasing the excitation impulse throughout RAS and entire loop. Thus, a positive feedback of depression exists between RAS and cortex, RAS and sympathetic division, RAS and peripheral muscles etc. So when all components of feedback loop are set to decreased activity, sleep results.
   - After a particular time of diminished activity, the neuronal cells then regain their excitability. This regaining activity together with some arousal signals induce once again wakefulness which then persists owing to above mentioned vicious cycle.

   ii. *Role of Neuronal/sleep centres:*

   - Besides role of RAS, few centres are also there capable of altering sleep and wakefulness mechanism. Electrical stimulation of centre located in upper medullary and lower pontine area of reticular formation closely associated with superior fasciculus (upper part) induces sleep which can be studied in electro-encephalogram; together with the fact that if this area is destructed loss of sleep (insomnia) results.
   - Waking centre is also said to be located in posterior hypothalamus. It has been observed that if this part is stimulated it results into wakefulness while any lesion here terminates into sleep.
   - Cerebral anaemia is also said to be responsible for sleep. This is a discarded view since during sleep cerebral blood flow is not altered at all.
   - Some hormone is also said to be responsible for sleep induction.

5. *Varieties:* Sleep may also be classified as described below:
   i. *REM or paradoxical sleep (Rapid eye movement)*: It is characterised by rapid eye movements, skeletal muscle tone is decreased, inhibition of stretch and polysynaptic reflex, dreaming, increase in arousal threshold, teeth grinding, decreased heart rate and arterial blood pressure, uncontrolled muscular movements. This type of sleep occurs in each night for two to four times at interval of 1-2 hours and each sleep lasts from five minutes to one hour. Sleep cycle of infant is markedly constituted by this type. Truely speaking it gives plentiful or adequate rest to the individual since if the person is awakened each time during it, he feels, a sort of exhaustion together with some neurotic tendencies. The centre for it are oral and caudal reticular nuclei of pons, while rapid movements of eye controlled by vestibular nucleus. Its duration is decreased by barbiturates. Impulses coming from mediolateral pontine tegmentum are said to be the causative factor for hypotonus of skeletal muscles. It has been also noted that no adverse psychological effects are produced if drugs inhibiting REM sleep are given for a longer time. This type of sleep constitutes 25 per cent of total sleep time on an average, and is more towards morning. This type of sleep exists in all mammals and birds. If brain stem lesions are there REM sleep is suppressed since in that situation forebrain is depleted of norepinephrine due to interrupting adrenergic fibres.
   ii. *Non-REM sleep*: Just reverse of above is this non-REM type of sleep which is contributed by hypertonus of skeletal muscles; rapid eye movements are not said to exist. Low threshold for arousing is there and it is classed as deep sleep, without dreams. It is mainly due to lacking of desynchronising effects on motor cortex by RAS. Presence or production of serotonin is associated with induction of this type of sleep and is produced by neuronal loop (thalamus, pons, medulla, brainstem) projecting into limbic system and hindbrain.
   iii. *Narcotic sleep*: Sleep induced by alcohol, ether, chloroform, morphine opium, sleeping pills, e.g. barbiturates; electric shock is classed under this title.
   iv. *Abnormal or pathological sleep:* Cerebral anaemia, tumours or any other disease if induces sleep is classed here. Its prolonged duration is called coma.
   v. *Hypnotic sleep:* Induced by hypnotist through hypnosis.
6. *Electro-encephalographic attitude (EEG):* For the sake of convenience following stages have been described—

Non-REM Sleep

   i. *Stage A (Awaking stage)*: Alpha-waves of fast frequency and low voltage diminishing in amplitude and per cent of time.
   ii. *Stage B (Drowsy)*: Further diminishing and finally disappearing of alpha waves. Low voltage delta waves appear.
   iii. *Stage C (Light sleep)*: Appearance of waves in bursts at rate of 14/second. They are superimposed upon low voltage delta waves.
   iv. *Stage D (Medium sleep)*: Lowering of delta wave frequency with great amplitude with disappearance of spindle bursts.
   v. *Stage E (Deep sleep)*: More prominence of delta waves with long duration and high frequency.
7. *Disorders*:
   i. *Sleep walking (somnambulism):* The sufferer walks with open eyes and remove all obstacles coming before him but he remembers nothing on waking. It is usually associated with nocturnal enuresis (bed wetting). It does not occur in REM sleep but found in non REM type sleep.
   ii. *Narcolepsy*: It means an abnormal state in which the sufferer wants to sleep even in day time/waking hours. Person feels uncontrollable desire to sleep sometimes many times in a day. Episodes may last from few minutes to several hours.
8. *Notes*
   i. If human subjects are awakened every time during REM sleep, they become irritable and anxious. Prolonged REM deprivation does not have any physiological reaction.
   ii. EEG: REM sleep:
      a. Waves are irregular, frequency is high which replaces slow waves of non-REM sleep, i.e. alert/wakefulness pattern of EEG.
      b. PGO spikes (Ponto-geniculo-occipital spike)—Phasic potential of high amplitude appearing in groups (3-6) which originate from pons, geniculate body and occipital cortex.
   iii. Sleep is a cortical phenomenon but it is observed in decorticate animals.
   iv. Sleep depth: a view: Examples are: A mother wakes up immediately as her baby cries; a night duty telephone operator immediately wakes up at ring of telephone. It is measured by minimum noise which will awake a person.

9. *Snoring:* It is produced by vibration of soft palate. It is caused by any condition which hinders breathing through nose. More common when person is sleeping on back. It can reach up to 69 decibels.

Age-wise: sleep time (daily)	
1-15 months	16-22 hours
3-9 years	11 hours
10-13 years	10 hours
14-18 years	9 hours
31-45 years	7-8 hours
50+	5-6 hours

SPEECH PHYSIOLOGY

1. *In production of speech:* It is expiration act during which words are formed. Vocal cords also help by adopting the position of phonation, by being tense and thus glottis is closed also through laryngeal muscular contraction. It is also said that due to contracting thoraco-abdominal muscles, intra-tracheal pressure also rises.

   These are thyro-arytenoid muscle which are opening the glottis partially and at the same time it gives the desired shape to the glottis, for voice to be emitted.

   The vocal cords then separate causing air to escape under pressure through glottis.

   This sound (laryngeal sound) is modified in resonators which means that expiratory blast is checked as well as some overtones are checked. On the whole, we get characteristic sound.

   Audible sound is produced by imposition on air stream of modulating components, ranging from 80-16,000 cycles per second by vocal cords.
2. *Nervous mechanisms*: Auditory centre is located in temporal lobe, visual centre in occipital lobe. Association centres for the understanding of words, verbal expression are widely spread in the cortex of left hemisphere.

   Speech areas are situated in posterior part of third, or inferior frontal convolution through temporo-sphenoidal lobe and Reil island, and extends from here to posterior part of parietal lobe namely Brodmann's area 4, 44, 43, 41, 42, 22, 39.
3. Following are centres:
   - Area 44 (lower frontal area)
   - Upper frontal motor cortex over medial surface of hemisphere
   - Parietal cortex (posterior to post-central gyrus)
   - Temporal cortex (posterior)
4. *Aphasia:* It is a speech disturbance, mainly due to disturbed cerebral mechanism of understanding and expression, but fortunately mental disturbances are not reported. It literary means loss of power of speech. The term includes any marked interference with the ability either to use or to comprehend symbolic expressions of ideas by spoken or written words or by gestures, and any interference with the use of language in thinking.
   a. *Motor or expressive aphasia (Broca's aphasia)*: It means difficulty in speech and also in articulating words. Prefix - suffix - plurals are omitted leading to inadequate formation of sentences, but there is no paralysis. The lesion lies in posterior part of third or inferior frontal convolution, on left side (Broca's centre) in front of cortical motor centres of muscles participating in voice formation. Its attenuated form is pure motor aphasia where words cannot be articulated.
   b. *Sensory or receptive or Wernicke's aphasia*: The poor sufferer is unable to understand spoken language (word deafness) and lesion lies in superior and middle temporal convolutions contiguous to cortical centre for hearing. Loss of power to understand written or printed language (word blindness or alexia) is due to lesion in inferior portion of posterior parietal lobule, gyrus angularis and supramarginalis, contiguous to occipital visual area.
   c. *Verbal aphasia*: Formation, evoking and pronouncing of words is difficult.
   d. *Nominal aphasia*: Difficulty in finding correct words to name an object.
   e. *Syntactical aphasia*: Sentences are not properly formed while individual words are well constructed. They may be insane.
   f. *Semantic aphasia*: Because of loss of general significance conversation cannot be proper though words and short sentences are well constructed.

A child born deaf, is also dumb. Initial speech noises first appear in a child during second half of first year. By the end of first year, child puts his efforts to combine individual syllables into words.

   g. *Conduction aphasia*: It is associated with a highly distinctive structural pattern and that damage to the arcuate fasciculus is strongly associated with the syndrome. Pathway originates in the cortex of supra-temporal plane, arches around the back end of sylvian fissure and courses in superior longitudinal fissure over extreme capsule and insula to reach lower frontal region. Anatomically damage to three areas is important in connection with conduction aphasia namely Wernicke's area, supra-marginal gyrus and arcuate fasciculus area. On discussing possible mechanisms for its genesis two exclusively anatomical patterns are said to be capable for its production namely supra-marginal or arcuate fasciculus lesion and auditory region lesion.

h. Agnosia: Inability to understand the words OR he is unable to identify a known object.
i. Agraphia: Inability to write. No difficulty in hand-muscles.
j. Word blindness: Inability to read written words.

Dyslexia (Greek—Language difficulties)

- The patient cannot group the meaning of sequences of letters, words, or symbols, or the concept of direction. Normal intelligence may also be affected.
- Such children may reverse letter and word order, make bizarre spelling errors, or may not be able to name the colours, or write from dictation.
- It may be caused by minor visual defects, emotional disturbance, or failure to train the brain. 90 per cent are males.
- It was first discovered by Professor Rudolf of Stuttgart—Germany (1887). Its reference is found as back as 30 C.E. when Valerius Maximus and Pliny described a man who lost his ability to read after being struck on the head by a stone.

CONDITIONED REFLEX

i. Nobel prize winning investigations by Russian physiologist I.P. Pavlov and his successors have made significant contribution towards determining the neural mechanism involved in the learning process. The classic example is the conditioning of salivation. Saliva is reflexly secreted normally when food is chewed. Normally there is no salivary response to a sound like the ringing of a bell. But if bell is always rung when food is given, the animal will gradually develop a response to sound alone and eventually will salivate at sound even if no food is given. We can say that the animal has learnt to associate the bell and food or that the animal learns that ringing of bell means that food is forthcoming.

ii. *Characteristics*:
   - They are dependent on pre- existing unconditioned reflex.
   - For development conditioned stimulus must precede the unconditioned stimulus.
   - Intact cortical and subcortical centres are required for its development.
   - They are unstable, and are easily lost permanently.
   - Unlimited number of stimuli acting on any of the receptors can provoke them, but they always follow nerve paths used by inborn reflexes.
   - They appear after completion of a formative process.

iii. *Significance:*
   - This is an indication of various habits of an individual.
   - These are the basis of learning process.
   - They can be utilised clinically and psychologically.

iv. *Positive (excitatory) conditioned reflex:*
   a.
   - Stimulus that provoked the inborn reflex is called simultaneous conditioned reflex.
   - Sometimes response is obtained after a latent period called delayed conditioned reflex.

   b. *Properties:*
   - Long latent period.
   - Response is evoked by conditioned stimulus (specificity).
   - They are easily lost (instability).
   - Sense reinforce each other (summation)

   c. *Essential conditions for its establishment*
   - Stimulus must be of a threshold strength.
   - It must be applied repeatedly.
   - It must be periodically reinforced.

   d. They are used in the study of the capacity of sense organs of animals to respond.

   e. *Effect of drugs*:
   - Caffeine increases all conditioned reflexes. Similar action of strychnine has been reported.
   - Bromides have no effect but they increase the inhibitory process.
   - Hypercalcaemia causes quick extinction of excitatory conditioned reflex.
   - Alcohol in moderation leads to stimulation of excitatory process.

   f. *Negative or inhibitory conditioned reflex*: Conditioned reflex can be inhibited by two ways viz. external or internal inhibition.
   - *External Inhibition*:
     a. Sir I.P. Pavlov decided to demonstrate his discovery of conditioned reflex in general public but the thing turned to a tragedical end when animal—dog—has not responded by salivation and he could not demonstrate. But scientific world could get another discovery out of it and that is if another stimulus is

applied before the conditioned stimulus which is capable of diverting the attention of the animal, the response to conditioned stimulus is considerably diminished and this he named external inhibition. The public assembled there was making a noise and this noise (another stimulus) diverted the attention of dog and there was no salivation.

b. The delay between response and stimulus is called delayed conditioned reflex and it may be as long as 90 seconds.

- *Internal inhibition*: Here, it is necessary to apply the stimulus repeatedly before it becomes efficacious. Following are its varieties:
  a. *Extinction*: If an animal is conditioned to secrete saliva on listening to a tuning fork by applying this stimulus simultaneously with feeding or before it. The conditioned reflex is well established. Animal is made to listen the tuning fork repeatedly without being given the food, saliva is secreted progressively in decreasing amounts until the sound of tuning fork no longer provokes the salivary flow. This is extinction of reflex due to inhibition.

  So positive conditioned reflex that are not reinforced are soon lost. Extinction occurs most easily in recently established conditioned reflex than in long standing ones. Extinction is also having after effect.

  b. *Conditioned inhibition*: If a strong extra stimulus is applied simultaneously with a conditioned stimulus without reinforcing the latter, after this procedure has been repeated several times, a negative conditioned reflex will be established. It means that, application of extra-stimulus will inhibit salivary secretion though application of originally conditioned stimulus alone still provokes the salivary flow.

LEARNING

i. Learning is the ability to alter behaviour on the basis of experience; while memory is the ability to recall past events at the conscious or unconscious level.

ii. When first time a neural stimulus is applied then it evokes a response but on repeated application it evokes less response. The subject ignores the stimulus. It is habituation.

iii. But repeated stimuli may produce a greater or intensified response; if one stimulus is coupled with another stimulus which may be pleasant or unpleasant. This is sensitisation. It is composed of some arousal value. The example is the mother who can enjoy sound sleep in presence of many noises, but wakes promptly when her baby cries.

iv. Explanation:
  a. In certain invertebrate animals, habituation is due to a decrease in Ca^{2+} in the sensory endings that mediate the response to a particular stimulus. While, sensitisation is due to prolongation of action potential in these endings with a resultant increase in intra-cellular Ca^{2+} which facilitates the release of neurotransmitter by exocytosis.
  b. Post-tetanic potentiation (as already described) which is actually a prolonged facilitation of effectiveness of synaptic transmission is also triggered by Ca^{2+} accumulation in post-synaptic neurons.

v. • In learning and memory process, cerebral cortex is also involved. If we remember a thing which we have previously seen then increased activity in frontal, parietal, occipital lobe is observed (specially of right side) in response of spatial location of visual stimuli. Same increased activity has been observed when one learns some letters/ statement and then he rehearses these statement because he will be asked/questioned about it. This is encoding. For short-term memory hippocampus is not playing a leading role but for long term memory hippocampus, para-hippocample portions of medial temporal cortex are playing leading role. Striking defects in recent memory has been observed on bilateral destruction of ventral hippocampus.
  • Amygdala is not involved in encoding the memory process but is mainly concerned with emotions. Long-term memories are stored in various parts of neocortex. Stimulation of portion of neocortex in humans evoke detailed memories of remote past which are often beyond the power of voluntary recall.

vi. Temporal lobe is playing a very interesting role in memory process. On its stimulation, one may feel strange in a familial place (so one becomes alert or vigilant) or he may feel a familiar background (so he is less alert or vigilant). This is already seen (deja-vu-phenomenon = French words).

vii. The circuit: When one recalls the past events; it depends on activity distributed in relevant association areas of neocortex activated by incoming sensory stimuli. It projects to medial temporal lobe (particularly to para-hippocampal gyrus). From here it enters the hippocampus.

- Mammillary bodies are connected with hippocampus through fornix. It is the mamillothalamic tract which causes projection of mamillary bodies to thalamus. From thalamus, memory fibres project to prefrontal cortex and from here to basal forebrain and from here diffuse projection occurs to neocortex, the amygdala, hippocampus.

Alzheimer's Disease

- It is a primary degenerative cerebral disorder with a characterised neuropathology. It results in widespread cerebral atrophy specially involving cortex and hippocampus. Neurochemical changes involve reduction in acteylcholine and choline acetyl transferase. Microscopically we find marked reduction of neurons, neurotic plaques with amyloid core in which aluminium silicate is present as mature plaques.
- It comprises progressive loss of memory and cognitive function in middle age. This is an important cause of dementia, the problem is serious between the age of 65-85 years.
- It is the superior parietal cortex which suffers inadequate blood supply. There is loss of cholinergic nerve fibres in cerebral cortex (neocortex, nucleus basalis of meynert, hippocampus, amygdala).
- Drug physostigmine is of some value since it inhibits enzyme acetylcholinesterase, → decreased breakdown of acetylcholine. But it cannot resist the main degenerative process.
- Nicotine also produces improvement by stimulating nicotinc receptors. Drugs inhibiting receptors of GABA improve the memory.
- Patients with Down syndrome who are having chances to develop this disease have an extra-chromosome 21 (trisomy 21).
- Amyloid protein is toxic to nerve cells; is contained by "neuro-fibrillary tangles" which is made up in parts of altered forms of protein associated with micro-tubules and extra-cellular senile plaques. This β amyloid protein is having its precursor as "APP"—(amyloid precursor-protein) which is located on chromosome-21.

RAS: AT A GLANCE

- Its main driving component is an excitatory area—the "bulbo-reticular facilitory area" lying in reticular substance of middle and lateral pons, and mesencephalon. It transmits facilitatory signals downward to spinal cord to maintain tone in antigravity muscle and also to control activity level of spinal cord reflexes.
- The signals are also passing through thalamus which falls into two groups: The first type is exciting cerebrum by rapidly transmitting action potential. These nerve endings are releasing acetylcholine, which is an excitatory neuro-transmitter. Second type of neurons are spreading throughout reticular formation and then pass to intra-laminar and reticular nuclei of thalamus and from here fibres are directed to cerebrum.
- So we can understand that fibres are not only directed to cerebral cortex but are again synapsing back in this excitatory area. This arrangement helps to establish positive feedback or vicious cycle of functions.
- Similar reverberating circuits are also seen between thalamus and cerebral cortex; then back from cerebral cortex to thalamus.
- Located medially and ventrally to excitatory area is a reticular inhibitory area in medulla. This area when excited will decrease activity in superior as well as inferior portion of brain.
- There are inhibitory systems which cuts off the inputs to these facilitatory ascending activating system
  - *Diencephalic inhibitory system:* Sleep is produced if posterior hypothalamus (pre-optic nuclei) and its adjoining thalamus nuclei (intra-laminar etc.) are stimulated
  - *Medullary inhibiting system:* Sleep patterns in EEG are noticed if medullary region at the level of tractus solitarius is stimulated.
- Basal forebrain inhibitory area—Sleep patterns in EEG is noticed on stimulating suprachiasmatic, preoptic and diagonal band of brain.

Descending reticular activating system: It receives fibres from motor cortex, caudate nucleus, vestibular nucleus and cerebellum. It sends fibres to spinal cord and influence motor neurons.

1. *Descending inhibitory reticular projection*
   a. If areas 4S, 2S, 8S, 9S, 24S, caudate nucleus or ventromedial part of medullary reticular formation area stimulated, then inhibition of movements which has stimulated cortical areas or pyramidal tracts, occurs.
   b. This pathway is also influenced by inhibitory projection fibres from cerebellum through nucleus fastigius.
   c. The bulbar inhibitory areas are under control of cortical or strial inhibitory areas.

d. This pathway is functioning to inhibit the movement already initiated, and reduces the muscle tone. It is inhibitory to extensors and facilitatory to flexor muscles.
e. If it is damaged, decerebrate rigidity results due to release phenomenon.
f. These pathways are organised in cortico-bulbo-reticular, caudato-spinal, cerebello-reticular, reticulo-spinal tracts.

2. *Descending facilitatory reticular fibres:*
   - It is confined to lateral region.
   - It is quite independent of inhibitory pathway. It relays to spinal motor neurons through reticulo-spinal and vestibulo-spinal tracts, running in lateral funiculi of spinal cord.
   - On its stimulation, there occurs increased discharge of gamma efferent neurons.
   - Damage to its central part leads to atonia, paucity of movements etc.
   - On its stimulation, there occurs exaggerated movements and increased muscle tone of extensor muscles, decreased tone of flexor muscles, increased tendon reflexes mediated by extensors.
   - It is confined to tegmentum of mid-brain, pons, hypothalamus, bulbar area outside the inhibitory pathway.

NEURO-HUMORAL SYSTEM: BRAIN

1. *Nor-epinephrine* secreted by locus ceruleus which is a small area located bilaterally and posteriorly at junction between pons and mesencephalon. It is an excitatory substance as well as causative agent of dreaming type of REM sleep.

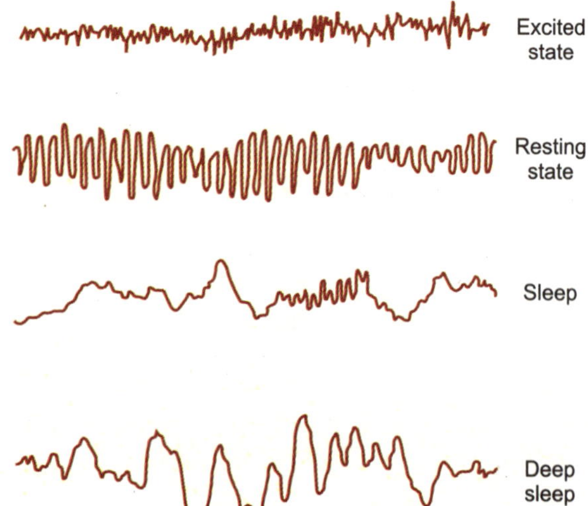

Fig. 109.1: Electro-encephalogram (EEG)

2. *Dopamine* is secreted by substantia nigra. It is an inhibitory transmitter. Their destruction leads to Parkinson's disease.
3. *Serotonin* is secreted by raphe nuclei located in mid-line of lower pons and medulla. It plays an inhibitory role in causation of sleep. Their fibres also descend to spinal cord which has ability to suppress pain.
4. *Acetylcholine* is secreted by giant cells of reticular excitatory area of pons and mesencephalon. The fibres go to both direction—upwards and downwards to spinal cord. It is an excitatory transmitter.
5. Others include—GABA, glutamate, vasopressin, ACTH, enkephalins, endorphins, angiotensin II, neurotensin etc.

EEG (ELECTRO-ENCEPHALOGRAM) (Fig. 109.1)

- The recording of electrical activities of brain is EEG. Its activity is complicated owing to large number of neurons and synapses.
- *Different waves:*
  a. *Alpha*: Frequency 8-12 waves per second, amplitude 50 μV. Most marked in parieto-occipital area. Obtained in inattentive brain, e.g. drowsiness, light sleep/closed eyes and so diminished on opening of the eye. On their diminution, they are replaced by fast irregular low voltage activity without any dominant frequency. This is called alpha block or desynchronization which can also occur on mental concentration/sensory stimuli.
  b. *Beta*: High frequency - 15-60/second; low amplitude i.e. 5-10 μV. Not affected by opening the eyes. They can be recorded during mental tension/arousal state.
  c. *Delta*: Frequency 1-5 per second; amplitude 20-200 μV occurs during deep sleep in adults, and in childhood. Their presence suggestive of epilepsy, increased intra-cranial tension, depression etc.
  d. *Theta*: Frequency 4-8/second, amplitude 10 μV. Seen in children below 5 years of age.
- *Significance:* EEG pattern is altered in epilepsy, mid-brain diseases involving ascending RAS, subdural hematoma etc.
- *Method:*
  a. Scalp electrodes are placed over un opened skull or over the brain after opening it, or by piercing.
  b.
     - *Unipolar electrode:* Active on cerebral cortex while indifferent one—away from it.
     - *Bipolar:* Both terminals are placed in different parts of the brain.

EPILEPSY (SEIZURES)

- It is a brain disorder characterised by convulsive seizures with loss of consciousness (sudden uncontrolled involuntary muscular contractions). In between the attacks the person is normal. It is mainly because of increase of excitability of neurons which causes excessive discharge.
- *Types:*

  a. *Grand mal:*

   i. Just before the attack one feels warning signals like hallucinations (epileptic aura) then convulsion starts. First is tonic stage—characterised by tonic contractions of muscle leading to spasm twisting facial features, flexion of arm and extension of lower limbs. Tonic and spasmodic contractions collectively called tonic-clonic-contraction. Patient bites the tongue, may be urination or defecation and cyanosis. After the attack is over, the patient remains in stupor/depression/severely fatigued.

   ii. Causes are hereditary, emotions, loud noise, flashing lights, alkalosis/over breathing, traumatic lesion, fever, drug induced.

   iii. It is because of extreme neuronal discharge in all areas of the brain and massive activation of many reverberating pathways throughout the brain.

   iv. The attack stops because of neuronal fatigue + active inhibition by inhibitory neuron.

   v. High voltage synchronous discharge occurs from every part of brain.

b. *Petit mal:*

   i. Characterised by unconsciousness of 3-30 seconds during which patient demonstrates twitch like muscular contractions (blinking of the eyes, i.e. in head region) and then the consciousness is returned.

   ii. EEG assumes spike and dome pattern which tells that entire brain is involved. The patient may have one such attack monthly.

c. *Psychomotor seizures (Focal epilepsy):*

   i. Sequence is—short period of amnesia, attack of rage, anxiety/discomfort/fear, incoherent speech, motor act to attack some body. Both the things exist, i.e. sometime the patient remembers the activities during attack while sometimes he does not remember. Limbic system is usually involved, i.e. hippocampus- Amygdala etc.

   ii. *In EEG* low frequency rectangular waves, frequency 2-4/second, super imposed by 14/second wave.

d. *Focal epilepsy:*

   - It results from some local organic lesion or functional abnormality, e.g. congenital deranged local circuit, brain tumour, scar tissue in brain.
   - These lesions leads to rapid discharge from neurons. Along with it a wave also appears at adjacent cortical area. This constitutes epileptic zone. When such discharge covers entire cortex (motor), it causes contraction throughout opposite side of body, i.e. from mouth to legs. This is Jacksonian epilepsy.
   - It may cover brainstem/localised region of cerebral cortex or their deeper structures.

BIBLIOGRAPHY

1. Berkovic SF, et al. Progressive myoclonal epilepsies: specific causes and diagnosis. New Eng J Med 1986;315:296.
2. Branes DM. Debate about epilepsy: what initiates seizures. Science 1986;234:938.
3. de Reuck AVS, O'connor M (Eds). Disorders of Language. Ciba Foundation Symposium, Boston: Little Brown. 1963.
4. Dichter MA, et al. Cellular mechanism of epilepsy: A status report. Science 1987;237:157.
5. Hanna Damasio, Antonio R Damasio. The Anatomical basis of conduction aphasia. Brain 1980;103:337-350.
6. Head H. Aphasia : disorders of speech. New York: Macmillan. 1926.
7. IRIS R, Bell, Diane Amend, Alfred W. Kaszniak, Gray E. Schwartz. Memory deficits, sensory impairment and depression in elderly. Lancet 1993;341:63.
8. Scheuer ML, et al. The evaluation and treatment of seizures. New Eng J Med 1990;323:1486.
9. Ward C, Halstead. American physiological society - Thinking - imagery and memory. Handbook of Physiology Neurophysiology 3:1669.
10. Weisenberg T, McBride KE. Aphasia—A clinical and psychological study. New York Common Wealth Fund. 1935.

110 Index of Emotions: Limbic System

It includes part of brain constituted by a rim of cortical tissue around the hilus of cerebral hemisphere. The other associated structures are amygdala, hippocampus and septal nuclei. Along with hypothalamus, it subserves many other functions.

CONNECTIONS/AFFECTIONS

As told above, this system responsible for emotions and behaviour, is connected with frontal and temporal lobes as well as with thalamus. Sensory informations from sensory pathways are fed to limbic system. It is neocortex which exerts a great influence on this limbic system.

FUNCTIONS

i. It is chiefly concerned with emotions which is a hallmark in human behaviour. The single word emotions is constituted by many components viz. fear, rage, love, joy, hope, anxiety etc.

In series of experiments conducted on animals in cages, where a lever is placed at the side of cage, arranged in a way that depressing the lever makes electric contact with a stimulator. Electrodes are placed successively at different areas in brain so that animal is capable of stimulating the area by pressing the lever. On this ground of experimental studies it was found that *reward centre* is there located in ventromedian hypothalamic nuclei with secondary centres in amygdala, septum, thalamus, basal ganglia etc. Its counter part *punishment centre* has been found to be located in mid-brain—periventricular area of dorsomedial tegmentum which extends to periventricular structures of hypothalamus and thalamus.

ii. *Fear:* Fear reactions are being produced on stimulating 'hypothalamus or amygdaloid nucleus.' As taken a natural event that normally monkeys are afraid of snakes but this fear is lost on temporal lobectomy, which indicates that this procedure (temporal lobectomy, surgical removal of temporal lobe) abolishes fear reactions. ACTH increases the excitability which leads to an increase in generalised fear while corticosterone counteracts this influence because it acts to restore a normal level of excitability.

FEAR: SOME MORE ASPECTS

- It is to be recalled here that afferent sensory inputs which excite the conditioned fear response go directly to amygdala without reaching neocortex. When this long-term potentiation is disrupted then this fear learning is blocked. So it is said that amygdala encodes the memory which produces fear.
- If blood supply of anterior end of each temporal lobe is increased, then anxiety is produced.

iii. *Rage* (fighting or attacking reaction): For example, in cat, it is characterised by hissing, spitting, biting, pilo erection, clawing. Opposite of rage is placid. Experimental evidences suggest that stimulation of a wide area from lateral hypothalamus to central greymatter of mid-brain is eliciting this rage phenomenon. This can occur in decorticated animals. There are two distinct areas in hypothalamus and limbic system which evoke rage or placidity.

RAGE-PLACIDITY—SHAM RAGE

- If an individual is irritated repeatedly, he will lose his temper or will react badly—this is rage and its opposite is placidity. Normally there is a balance between the two but sometimes it is altered.
- If neocortex is removed; or when ventro-medial hypothalamic nuclei are destroyed then rage response to minor stimuli are observed. Abnormal placidity has been observed in some animals on destructing

amygdaloid nuclei bilaterally. There is a specific area reported for rage reaction also, i.e. extending from lateral hypothalamus to central grey area of mid-brain.

- Sham rage term is inadequate one and requires to be dropped. It means physical and motor manifestation of anger as explained before in monkey's experiments. It is noticed on lesion of diencephalon and forebrain, and are noticed on minor stimuli and are directed with great accuracy at the source of irritation. It is also unpleasant to animals because of conditioning.
- *Examples:* In patients with brain damage rage attacks are common in response to stimuli, they are seen after pituitary surgery because of damage to the base of brain; the agitated patients became placid after bilateral lesion of amygdala.
- Sham rage can occur in decorticate animals also. It is due to release of hypothalamus from cortical control.

iv. *Sexual behaviour:* The sexual behaviour consists of sexual urge, efforts made for its completion and finally the act itself. For all this fulfilment, Neocortex is playing a dominant role. Its removal inhibits the sexual behaviour along with the fact that partial decortication or specific frontal lobe lesion puts a check on it, and is true for both the sexes. On having lesions in cingulate and retrosplenial portion of limbic cortex, the maternal feeling is lost.

v. Of course less specific one; the libmic system is also said to influence *sleep*.

vi. It is concerned with *olfaction*.

vii. It integrates higher *intellectual* functions.

viii. Of course less, it is also concerned with *thirst*.

ix. *Hippocampus* is associating the different incoming sensory signals in the way that is capable of exciting hypothalamic reactions. Then these signals are exposed as punishment or reward when its different regions are stimulated. Involuntary tonic or clonic movements in different body parts along with rage or other emotional reactions are seen. It is also having a dominant role in determination of one individual's *attention*.

x. *Limbic lobe and its ablation*
   - Limbic lobe is the ring of cerebral cortex surrounds the subcortical limbic structures. So it is believed to be the cerebral association cortex controlling the lower centres which are primarily related with behaviour.
   - Intense motor restlessness is observed on ablation of posterior portion of fronto-orbital cortex (bilateral removal).
   - *Kl̦ ver- Bucy syndrome* is characterised by loss of fear, excessive tendency to examine objects, changes in dietary habbits, psychic blindness, decreased aggressiveness etc. It is caused by removal of entire anterior tip of temporal lobe.
   - Increased tameness, lack of social consciousness, loss of fear has been observed in animals in whom operation of bilateral removal of anterior portion of cingulate gyri has taken place.

xi. *Amygdala*: It is located immediately below ventral surface of cerebral cortex in the pole of each temporal lobe. It is normally controlling the overall pattern of behaviour. Bilateral lesions of these nuclei is producing placidity in some animals while its stimulation leads to rage.

Amygdala and Memory

- It has no concern in encoding the declarative memory. It is concerned chiefly with emotions. So it can give emotional coloration to memory.
- In lower animals, it is concerned with olfaction, since major division of olfactory tract terminates into a portion of it called cortico-medial nuclei in temporal lobe. But in human beings, its another portion baso lateral nuclei has become more prominent which is concerned with behavioural activities.
- It transmits signals to (a) hippocampus, (b) back to cortical areas, (c) thalamus, (d) hypothalamus.
- It receives signals from all parts of cortex viz temporal, parietal, occipital including audio visual areas.
- It justifies the correct status of an individual in relation to thoughts and surroundings. It is classed as a behavioural awareness area which operates at a semi-conscious level.
- On stimulation, it causes—alteration in arterial pressure, heart rate, GIT motility and secretion, micturition, defecation, piloerection, pupillary dilatation, licking/chewing/swallowing, clonic rhythmic movements, rage pattern, sexual activities like erection/ejaculation/ovulation/premature labor/uterine activity etc.

HYPOTHALAMUS (Fig. 110.1)

It is formed by the grey nuclei of diencephalon which forms the floor of third ventricle. Laterally, it is continued with subthalamic area (subthalamic nuclei of Luys, capsula interna, cerebral peduncle); it is separated medially from thalamus by hypothalamic sulcus; anteriorly it is continued into para-olfactory region of telencephalon.

The Afferents

i. The mammillary nuclei is receiving fibres from brain stem forming spino-bulbar and ponto-bulbar

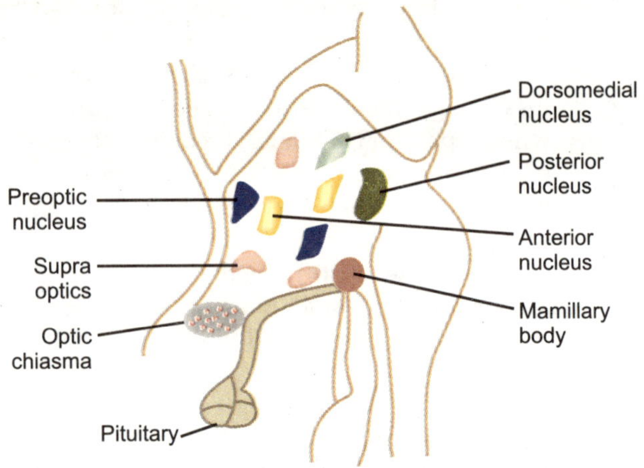

Fig. 110.1: Hypothalamus (Nuclei)

hypothalamic tracts. These are conducting impulses from the receptors of general sensibilities.

ii. Supra-optic nucleus is connected with vagus.

iii. Median forebrain bundle arising in ventro-medial centres of cerebral hemispheres is permeating the lateral pre-optic nucleus, and passes to hypothalamic nucleus, ending in tegmentum.

iv. Fibres from the fornix, from hippocampus to mamillary bodies.

v. Fibres coming from striatum by way of median forebrain bundle and from globus pallidus by way of subthalamus.

vi. Median lemniscus is sending fibres to hypothalamus.

viii. Fibres also from cerebral cortex (area 6, 113; ill-defined bundle).

The Efferents

i. Mamillothalamic tract (from medial mamillary nucleus to anterior thalamic nucleus and to cingulate gyrus).

ii. From posterior hypothalamic area fibres are passing into dorsal longitudinal bundle (periventricular system). These fibres are situated in tectal part of pons and laterally in reticular formation of medulla and in spinal cord. They are forming part of antero-lateral column. These fibres are terminating in visceral centres of mid-brain, pons, medulla, spinal cord after decussating at different levels.

iii. Supra-optico-hypophyseal tract is formed by fibres from the supra-optic paraventricular nuclei and cells in anterior part of infundibular eminence; and it passes into hypophysis.

iv. A profuse network of fine myelinated fibres passing to frontal cortex.

HYPOTHALAMIC NUCLEI: CLASSIFICATION—ENUMERATION

1. Periventricular region
   a. Periventricular system.
   b. N. preopticus periventricularis
   c. N. arcuatus periventricularis.
2. Lateral region
   a. Lateral hypothalamic area
   b. Lateral nuclei of tuber
3. Medial/supra-optic region
   a. N. supra-opticus
   b. N. paraventricularis
   c. N. suprachiasmaticus
   d. N. supra-opticus diffusus.
4. Medial tubular/Infundibular region
   a. N. hypothalamicus ventromedialis
   b. N. hypothalamicus dorso-medialis
   c. Posterior hypothalamic area
   d. Perifornical area
5. Caudal/Mammillary region
   a. N. paramammillaris
   b. N. supramammillaris
   c. N. mammillaris medialis
   d. N. mammillaris lateralis
   e. N. intercalatus

It includes subthalamic tegmental region, structures forming floor of third ventricle and, anterior part of lateral wall of 3rd ventricle.

Functions

i. It is having a leading role in *regulation of body temperature*. It is said to possess a heat conserving centre caudally while rostrally heat dissipating centre has been reported. Warming of anterior hypothalamus leads to decreased rectal temperature, cutaneous vasodilatation while its cooling results into vasoconstriction in skin if they are dilated. Destructive lesions in caudal part of lateral hypothalamus are resulting into fall in temperature due to damage to centres regulating the reactions to cold.

ii. *It controls water balance*. There are osmo-receptors present in rostral region. When they get stimulation by raised blood osmotic pressure, the supra-optic - neuro-hypophyseal system is triggered to secrete ADH which acts on renal tubular cells. Polyurea results if supra-optic nucleus is damaged.

iii. As regards emotions, it should not be considered as a mechanism for production of emotions, but *it is acting as a part of effector mechanism of emotional expression.*

- If it is damaged patient represents maniacal character, absence of control of behaviour, anxiety, fear, hallucinations.
- On destructing area near mammillary nuclei, patient becomes somnolent, apathetic having tendency for hypothermia.
- Stimulation of caudal region in cats produces pattern characteristic of rage.
- Cerebral cortex exerts inhibitory effect over hypothalamus towards its control over emotional behaviour and sympathetic effect.

iv. Lesion in near vicinity of para-ventricular nucleus is said to stimulate hypoglycaemia and hypersensitivity to insulin. So *it is said to participate in regulation of carbohydrate metabolism* via sympathico-adrenal-glycogenolytic mechanism.

v. On bilateral destruction of ventromedial nuclei, hyperphagia and obesity have been reported while lesion more laterally leads to hypophagia. Metabolic rate falls on removal of central hypothalamus while adiposity has been reported on destruction of ventromedial and tuber nucleus.

vi. A neuro-humoral factor is said to be secreted from hypothalamus which is absorbed into portal system of adeno-hypophysis to trigger the secretion of its hormones. Suprachiasmatic lesions derange circadian rhythm in secretion of ACTH, interruption of oestrous cycle.

vii. Its stimulation leads to cardiac arrhythmias owing to stimulation of both sympathetic and parasympathetic system. *So it controls the cardio vascular activities being a regulating centre of ANS.*

viii. It is designated as head ganglion of ANS (Sherrington) on stimulation. Dorsomedial and posterior hypothalamus via emotions (limbic system), secretion of catecholamines results.

- Posterior hypothalamic nuclei concerned with control of sympathetic activity; while stimulation of posterior and dorsomedial nucleus leads to increased secretion of adrenaline and noradrenaline from adrenal medulla. Stimulation of middle hypothalamic nuclei leads to raised parasympathetic activity. Sympathetic and parasympathetic over reactions are reported on its damage or lesions.

ix. Lesions of ventral part of hypothalamus changes sexual behaviour in animals. Lesions affecting caudal part of hypothalamus leads to inhibition of oestrous cycle in animals. Stimulation of median forebrain bundle and its near vicinity leads to senile erection and emotional attachments for females by male animals. So it is clear that there are sensitive areas in hypothalamus which respond to circulating androgen and oestrogen to initiate sexual behaviour pertaining to individual sexes. Genital dystrophy and adiposity is there in lesions involving ventromedial and tuberal nucleus.

x. If posterior hypothalamus is damaged, the animal undergoes sleep which is prolonged; while stimulation of dorsal hypothalamus leads the animal to go for sleep and somnolence. So it can be said that *there exists sleep and waking centre in it.* Disorders of sleep and wakefulness have been reported in lesion involving posterior hypothalamus.

The magnitude and time course of sympathetic nerve activity during its stimulation is varying with stimulus area, stimulus frequency, combinations of area stimulated and baroceptor reflex effects.

Hypothalamus and Neurotransmitters

i. Mammillary nuclei have lowest concentration of all neurotransmitters.

ii. Highest concentration of dopamine, GABA found in its preoptic area. High levels of dopamine also found in infundibular and supra-optic nuclei and dorsal area.

iii. Catcholamines - being high in more centrally located nuclei and lower in lateral and pre-optic area. Highest concentration of both adrenaline and noradrenaline is in dorsomedial nucleus.

iv. GABA found in high concentration throughout hypothalamus, of course, posterior area and infundibular nuclei having lower concentration than adjacent ventromedial nucleus.

Hypothalamus Disorders

- Its lesions occur due to tumours, ischaemia, encephalitis etc.
- On damage to ventromedian nuclei—disturbed carbohydrate and fat metabolism.
- On damage to mamillary body and anterior hypothalamus—disturbed sleep.
- On damage to anterior, posterior and lateral nuclei—disturbed sympathetic and parasympathetic functions.
- On damage to ventromedial and posterolateral part-sham rage, emotional disturbance.
- On damage to mid-hypothalamus—disturbed sexual functions.

- They may lead to diabetes mellitus, diabetes insipidus, Laurence-Biedl-Moon syndrome narcolepsy and cataplexy.
- *Narcolepsy:* Abnormal sleep pattern due to hypothalamic damage. Person suddenly falls asleep even in day time which may resemble the normal sleep. It is of short duration (from few seconds to 20 minutes). In night insomnia is found.
- *Cataplexy* is sudden uncontrolled outbursts of emotions with narcolepsy. The person is exhausted with muscular weakness. It is a brief attack in which one does not become unconscious.

LIMBIC SYSTEM—AT A GLANCE

- It is chiefly responsible for behavioural pattern. It is the limbic cortex which is functioning as a cerebral association area.
- *Kluver-Bucy syndrome* is observed on ablating temporal cortex which is described elsewhere.
- Motor restlessness is observed in an animal along with insomnia; on ablating posterior orbital-frontal cortex bilaterally.
- In anterior temporal gyrus there are gustatory and olfactory associations; in posterior cingulate cortex there is sensori motor association; in parahippocampal gyri there exists complex auditory + thought association.

Lesions of Amygdala, piriform lobe or both are not essential substrates for elicitation of savage behaviour. There is no evidence that hippocampal damage contributes significantly to development of aggressiveness. Behavioural changes ascribed to bilateral removal of amygdala and piriform lobe specially angry behaviour has been studied in cats. Two animals with incomplete removal became moderately hostile as indicated by hissing and growling.

Function of prefrontal cortex: It is essential for important inhibitory capacities. Its ablation is associated with removal of inhibition and with regression to primitive forms of motor and motivational behaviour patterns. Its relation is reflected to limbic subcortical structure via caudate subthalamic hippocampal complex and hypothalamic amygdaloid complex. It is involved in somatomotor and sensory functions, autonomic functions, learning and discrimination and in highest psychical functions.

An interaction between hypothalamus and amygdala has been investigated. Electrical stimulation in lateral hypothalamus of adult cats led to an effective well directed attack on a rat. Amygdaloid stimulation alone did not elicit any apparent fixed behaviour patterns. However, during simultaneous simulation, electrical stimulation in some regions of amygdala (medial portion of lateral nucleus and suppressed the hypothalamically elicited attacks response, while in other regions, (dorsolateral portion of lateral nucleus) electrical stimulation facilitated the attack response.

There are two intimately related mechanisms in the hypothalamus and limbic system; one promoting placidity and the other rage. Emotional state is determined probably by afferent impulses between them. In epidemics of influenza and encephalitis there occurs destruction of neurons in limbic system and hypothalamus.

HIPPOCAMPUS AND MEMORY

- The mamillary bodies project to anterior thalamus through mamillo-thalamic tract; and from thalamus, these fibres (carrying memory) are projecting to prefrontal cortex and thence to forebrain and from here the fibres are diffusely settled in entire neocortex/amygdala and hippocampus from nucleus basalis of Meynert. It is recalled here that these fibres are damaged in Alzheimer's disease.
- It is involved in encoding the short-term memories while long-term memories are stored in neo-cortex. So when neo-cortex is stimulated, then detailed memories of remote past which is beyond the power of voluntary recall are remembered.

HIPPOCAMPUS—A VIEW

- It is elongated medial portion of temporal cortex folding upwards and inwards to form the ventral surface of inferior horn of lateral ventricle.
- It has got numerous connections with many portion of cerebral cortex as well as amygdala, septum, hypothalamus, mamillary bodies etc. Any sort of sensory experience will activate it and this in turn will give outgoing signals to thalamus, hypothalamus, through fornix to other parts of limbic system. So it is an additional channel through which such behavioural reactions are occurring. It is composed of only three layers histologically as compared with six layers of cerebral cortex.
- Very weak electrical stimuli over this region results into seizures which persists even after the stimulation is over plus psychomotor disturbances like hallucinations of auditory visual/tactile/olfactory etc.

HIPPOCAMPUS AND FUNCTIONS: INTERESTING VIEW

- If an immediate memory is to be converted into short-term or long-term memory which can be recalled after weeks, months or years, then the main thing required is its consolidation. This is achieved by physical, chemical or anatomical changes for its imprinting. Generally 5-10 minutes are required for short-term and an hour or so is needed for long-term storage.

- Rehearsal of same information again and again will accelerate/potentiate this consolidation. This is the reason that person under mental fatigues cannot consolidate as compared with a person in alert state.
- The persons in whom, hippocampus is removed, are having very little capacity for storing verbal and symbolic types of memories in long-term memory. So such persons are unable to establish new long-term memories of those informations which are basis of intelligence. This is *anterograde amnesia*.
- On the contrary, *retrograde amnesia*—means—inability to recall memories from the past. The degree of amnesia for recent event is much greater than for events of distant past. This is because of the fact that distant memories have been rehearsed many times. Hippocampal damage can cause both types of amnesia of course the persons with hippocampal damage don't feel any difficulty in learning physical skills.

SUMMARY AND HIGHLIGHTS

Limbic system is index of emotions. Punishment and pleasure centres have been investigated in animals. It will be an epoch discovery if we can discover such centre of pleasure in human beings, so that we may stimulate it whenever we are not happy.

Hypothalamus being the highest centre of ANS extending axially from lamina terminalis to a vertical plan caudal to mammilary bodies together with dorso-ventrally from hypothalamic sulcus to pial surface of floor of third ventricle. It has got various nuclei viz. (i) Supra-optic, (ii) Pre-optic, (iii) Para-ventricular, (iv) Posterior group, (v) Tuber cinereum, (vi) Dorsomedial and Ventro-medial.

On its destruction following disorders have been reported viz. (i) Obesity (Laurence-Moon-Biedl syndrome), (ii) Diabetes insipidus, (iii) Sexual disturbances (precocity or even impotency), (iv) Sleep disturbances (Narcolepsy, somnolence), (v) Hyperglycemia and glycosurea, (vi) Upper GIT ulceration, (vii) Diencephalic autonomic Epilepsy (sweating, flushing, tachycardia, salivation, lacrimation, slowing of respiratory rate, unconsciousness).

BIBLIOGRAPHY

1. Cingulate, posterior orbital and temporal pole cortex. Birger R Kadda in handbook of physiology: Neurophysiology II: 1345.
2. David Egger, John P. Effects of electrical stimulation of amygdala on hypothalamically elicited attack behaviour in cats. Flynn J Neurophy 1963;26:705.
3. Eugene S Boyd, Leonard C Gardner. Effect of some brain lesions of intracranial self stimulation in rat. Am J Phy 1967;213:1044 No. 4.
4. Functions of prefrontal cortex Stefan BrutKowski. Phy Rev 1965;45:725.
5. Hippocampus by John D. Green. In Handbook of Physiology: Neurophysiolog II p. 1373.
6. Hillon M, Zbrozyna AW. Amygdaloid region for defence reaction and its efferent pathway to brain stem. J Phy 1963;165: 160.
7. James olds. Hypothalamic substrates of reward. Phy Rev 1962;42:554.
8. Jay M, Weiss BS, Mcewen MT, Silva, Kalkut M. Pituitary-adrenal alteration and fear responding. Am J Phy 1970;218:864, No. 3.
9. Olds A, Yuwiller ME. Neurohumors in hypothalamic substrates of reward. Olds and Co. Yun. Am J Phy 1964;240:242.
10. Summers TB, Kaelber WW. Amygdalectomy: Effect in cats and a survey of its present status. Am J Phy 1962;203:1117.
11. Thomas Dunwiddie, Gary Lynch J Phy 1978;276:353-367.

111 Fluid of Mind: Cerebrospinal Fluid (CSF)

A special type of blood supply, the choroid plexus found in ventricles, is involved in production of this CSF filling the brain ventricles and space between brain and skull.

INTRODUCTION

COMPOSITION	
Amount	Wide variation. Total amount is 150 ml (0.3 ml/minute). Average normal volume must not exceed 1500 ml per day Specific gravity ... 1.007;
pH	7.35 (alkaline)
Consistency	Clear, colourless, transparent, no clotting on standing
Total protein	Lumbar 15-45 mg/100 ml
Glucose	65 mg/100 ml
Chlorides	720 mg per 100 ml
Total base	157 m Eq/L
Water	99.13%,
Solids	0.87%
Lymphocyte	5/cubic mm

FORMATION

It is formed in lateral ventricles in majority while remainder is formed in third and fourth ventricle. The principal sources are choroid plexus. Much of CSF is formed by dialysis across the walls of the choroid plexuses. It cannot be a simple physical force but an active process since energy is expanded on its formation (13 calories are needed for one litre CSF production).

ABSORPTION

Subarachnoid villi are site of its greatest absorption which are projecting into dural venous sinuses. Along longitudinal sinuses are large arachnoid villi called Pacchionian bodies. The mechanism of absorption is pressure gradient between the hydrostatic pressure in subarachnoid space fluid and that exists in dural sinus blood, resulting in filtration. The colloids pass very slowly and cystalloids more rapidly.

CIRCULATION

Major amount, is formed in lateral ventricles and passes into third ventricle through foramen of Monro, and from here, it passes to fourth ventricle through aqueduct of Sylvius. From here, through foramen of Magendi and foramen of Luschka it enters into cisterna magna and cisterna lateralis. Greater part of fluid passes upward over the brainstem to the surface of cerebral hemispheres.

FUNCTIONS

i. It acts as a cushion for brain, preventing or diminishing the transmission of jarring or shocking forces to the brain and spinal cord. It is a fluid buffer protecting neural substances.
ii. It might convey nutritive materials to central nervous system and carry away the metabolites.
iii. Changes in intra-cranial volume are occasionally compensated by production of CSF.

PRESSURES

- In lateral recumbent position—100-200 mm water.
- In sitting position 300 mm of water.
- Coughing, crying, compression of internal jugular vein raises pressure.

Concentration of substances

	Substances	*CSF*	*Plasma*
1.	Protein (mg/dl)	20	6000
2.	Glucose (mg/dl)	64	100
3.	Urea (mg/dl)	12	15
4.	Na^+ (mEq/kg H_2O)	147	150
5.	K^+ (mEq/kg H_2O)	2.9	4.6
6.	Cl^- (mEq/kg H_2O)	113	99
7.	pH	7.33	7.40
8.	Cholesterol (mg/dl)	0.2	175

Source: Ganong WF, Medical Physiology Review, Lange Publication.

CSF PRESSURE—AT A GLANCE

- It is regulated by absorption through arachnoid villi.
- Villi functions like a valve (gatekeeper) which allows the fluid to flow into venous blood of sinuses and not backwards in opposite direction. If the pressure rises higher the valves open very widely which prevents excessive increase in the pressure.
- The pressure rises in abnormal states, e.g. brain tumour—by decreasing rate of absorption of the fluid.
- In certain infections or haemorrhages occurring in cranial vault, there appears large number of cells in CSF which lead to severe blockage of small channels for absorption through arachnoid villi.
- Sometimes the babies are born with increased CSF pressure. Sometimes the number of arachnoid villi is very few or they are having abnormal absorptive properties.
- When pressure rises in CSF, it also rises in optic nerve sheaths. It is to be recalled here that retinal artery and vein pierce this sheath a few millimetre behind the eye and then passes with optic nerve into the eye itself. High pressure in optic sheath pushes fluid along optic nerve fibres to interior of eyeball. The high pressure in the sheath resists the blood flow in retinal vein which increases retinal capillary blood vessels throughout the eye which causes retinal oedema. The optic disc becomes more oedematous because it's more distensible. This constitutes *papilloedema*.

BRAIN OEDEMA

- Brain concussion → increased cerebral blood pressure → increased capillary pressure → oedema.
- Oedema → compression of vasculature → decreased blood flow, i.e. ischaemia → arteriolar dilatation + increased capillary pressure → more oedema fluid. Thus, a vicious cycle sets in. Furthermore, decreased blood flow means diminished oxygen delivery, which increases capillary permeability which further causes more leakage causing oedema. This factor also blocks sodium pump which results into swelling of cells.
- Mannitol (I.V. infusion) is helpful which pulls fluid by osmosis from brain tissue and so this circle is broken.

LUMBAR PUNCTURE

- A device to draw either CSF or to introduce some drugs is called lumbar puncture. The puncture is usually made opposite the median plane in the interspinous space between third and fourth lumbar spines by lumbar puncture needle.
- It is performed with the patient lying down. In this position the pressure is 70-200 mm water. If sitting upright the fluid will rise up to mid cervical and subsequent fall in pressure is noticed on straining owing to congestion of spinal veins.
- The above mentioned site is selected because of two reasons; firstly, there is no chance for spinal cord for injury and secondly, here we get wide subarachnoid space.
- It should be done with a great care in the patient of brain tumour (specially of posterior fossa) because herniation of cerebellum and medullary compression may follow removal of fluid.
- Severe headache is an untoward effect of this procedure which is due to leakage of fluid through site of puncture. This lumbar puncture headache is reduced on lying down while it is aggravated upon raising the head.
- Routine examination of CSF includes cell counts, total proteins, colloidal gold curve, Wassermann reaction.
- The aims/objectives/purposes of lumbar puncture are for diagnostic and therapeutic purposes, production of spinal anaesthesia, measurement of CSF pressure, replacement of CSF by contrast media.
- Froin's syndrome is characterised by having high globulin content and free from cells; standing. It may be linked with subarachnoid block.

VENTRICULOGRAPHY

- A hole is made in temporal region of skull for passing a needle through it into ventricular cavity through which fluid is replaced by air. It gives good information for localisation of space occupying lesion. So it is a diagnostic aid.
- Any obstruction to the normal passage of CSF causes the fluid to back up in the ventricles leading to a general increase of intra-cranial pressure. *Hydrocephalus* is an excessive accumulation of CSF. Fluid sometimes collects in the subarachnoid space over the external surface of the brain following meningeal trauma, but most cases of hydrocephalus are the blockage along the passage ways and the extra-fluid brain ventricles.

CSF—AN OVERVIEW

- It is a part of extracellular fluid.
- It is contained in spinal cord/central canal, subarachnoid space and cerebral ventricles.
- The choroid plexus (forming CSF) are tuft of capillary projections present inside the ventricles covered by pia mater and ependymal covering.

- It contains more sodium than potassium.
- Factors affecting formations are:
  1. Stimulated by pilocarpine, ether and pituitary extracts through exciting choroid plexus.
  2. Injecting hypotonic saline → increased capillary pressure plus increased intra-cranial pressure + fall in osmotic pressure → increased formation of CSF.
  3. Hypertonic saline reduces its formation. The increased intra-cranial pressure is reduced by administrating 30-35 per cent NaCl or 50 per cent sucrose.
- Since specific gravity of brain and CSF is the same so brain floats in CSF. It also regulates the volume of cranial contents.

BLOOD-BRAIN BARRIER

- Many years ago, it was demonstrated that when acidic dyes (trypan blue) are injected into living animals, it was failed to stain most of the tissues of brain and spinal cord. This was probably the beginning of concept of blood-brain barrier. According to one established fact which seems to be true that, exchange across the cerebral vessels is so different that in other capillary beds and rate of exchange of most of the physiologically important substances is slow.
- So, two possibilities are existing one is material from the blood into brain enter either from capillaries into cellular space of brain (blood-brain barrier) or they are passing the capillaries via the choroid plexus into cerebrospinal fluid which a small amount may pass into the brain tissue (blood cerebrospinal fluid barrier).
- As regards penetration of substances into brain; substances readily crossing are water, CO_2 and O_2; while more slowly crossing is glucose. Bile salts and catecholamines don't enter the adult brain in more than minute amounts. Dopamine, serotonin penetrate to a very limited degree but their corresponding acids (α-dopa and 5-hydroxytryptophan) enter with ease. Intravenous injection of hypertonic solutions cause movement of water from the ventricles to the blood, resulting in a decreased brain volume, of course a temporary effect.
- The barrier effect is due to astrocytic surrounding many capillaries of brain. Their mechanism to be by two ways; first by modifying permeability of capillary membrane or by completely covering the capillary restricting the area available for penetration.
- This system functions to maintain the constancy of environment of the neurons in CNS. The milieu interieur of the neuron is extra-cellular space and rapid changes in this environment may be injurious. This additional defence has been provided to CNS because cortical neurons are highly sensitive towards ionic changes.
- As regards clinical physiology of this is concerned there are two things. One is about drugs, i.e. among antibiotics penicillin and chlortetracycline enter the brain to a limited but among readily entering drugs are erythromycine and sulfadiazine. Second fact is that blood-brain barrier breaks-down in areas of the brain which are irradiated, infected of tumours.
- Blood-brain barrier develops during early year while cerebral capillaries are much more permeable at birth than in adulthood.
- This barrier is not well developed in infants, so bile pigments can enter the brain tissue (kernicterus).
- This prevents brain from injurious effects of many substances which cannot cross them. It also maintains a neuronal environment within. CNS by preventing escape of neuro-transmitters into the blood.
- The cellular tight junctions are formed between endothelial cells of capillaries as childhood cell membranes are oily, so only lipid soluble materials (anaesthetic agents viz. nitrous oxide, ether) can cross them since they are lipid soluble.
- It also protects the brain from blood toxins—whether they are exogenous or endogenous in origin.

BIBLIOGRAPHY

1. Bradbury M. The concept of blood brain barrier, Wiley. 1979.
2. Cserr HF. Physiology of choroid plexus. Phy Rev 1971;51:273.
3. Fishman RA. CSF in diseases of Nervous system. 2nd ed. Saunders 1992.
4. Leusen I. Regulation of CSF composition with reference to breathing. Phy Rev 1972;52:1.
5. Wood JH (Ed). Plenum. Neurobiology of CSF, 1980.

112 Visceral Control: Autonomic Nervous System (ANS)

(Vegetative or Involuntary Nervous System)

Autonomic nervous system (ANS) is chiefly controlling the viscera; and reactions in this system are prompt, unwilled, inborn and purposive.

INTRODUCTIVE OUTLINES

Nervous system is having two aspects to be considered namely somatic and visceral and both of them are controlled by higher brain centres. Visceral reflexes may be initiated by impulses entering the brain from somatic fibres.

GENERAL PLAN OR CLASSIFICATION

I. *Anatomical:*
   a. Cranio-sacral (cranial nerve nuclei III, VII, IX, X; sacral 2, 3, 4)
   b. Thoraco-lumbar (Thoracic 1-12; Lumbar 1-3)

II. *Physiological or Functional*
   a. Sympathetic or thoracolumbar
   b. Parasympathetic or cranio-sacral

III. *Chemical:* According to liberation of chemical substances:
   a. *Adrenergic:* Producing adrenaline or noradrenaline at nerve endings, e.g. post-ganglionic fibres of sympathetic except to sweat glands.
   b. *Cholinergic:* Producing acetylcholine; e.g. both pre- and post-ganglionic fibres of parasympathetic system, post-ganglionic sympathetic fibres supplying sweat glands. Acetylcholine is produced both at synapses (ganglia) as well as at the nerve endings.

ARRANGEMENT

Autonomic reflex arc is constituted by afferent, connector, and efferent. Afferent neurons are located in posterior root ganglia while lateral horn cells constitute the connector and efferent neurons are present outside the CNS in the form of ganglia which are hallmark of ANS and are a composition of aggregation of nerve cells lying between CNS and visceral structures. Ganglia are arranged in three systems. (a) paravertebral, (b) prevertebral or collaterals and (c) terminal or peripheral. Ganglion cells are motor or secretory in function having no afferent connections from periphery.

NERVOUS SYSTEM (BROAD CLASSIFICATION)

a. Central
   i. Brain
   ii. Spinal cord
b. Peripheral
   i. Craniospinal nerves (12 pairs cranial + 31 pairs spinal)
   ii. Visceral—sympathetic and parasympathetic

PARASYMPATHETIC OR CRANIOSACRAL DIVISION

a. *Cranial nerve III:* (Edinger-Westphal nucleus) Preganglionic fibres terminate in ciliary ganglia while post-ganglionic fibres are going to ciliary muscles and iris sphincters. It causes pupillary contraction and sets accommodation to near and distant vision. This nerve is included within mid-brain or tectal outflow.
b. *Cranial nerve VII:* Some preganglionic fibres terminate in spheno-palatine ganglia while few in submaxillary ganglia. Postganglionic fibres are distributed to lacrimal gland, glands of mucous membrane of nose and palate and also to submaxillary as well as sublingual salivary glands. It is supposed to increase their secretion.

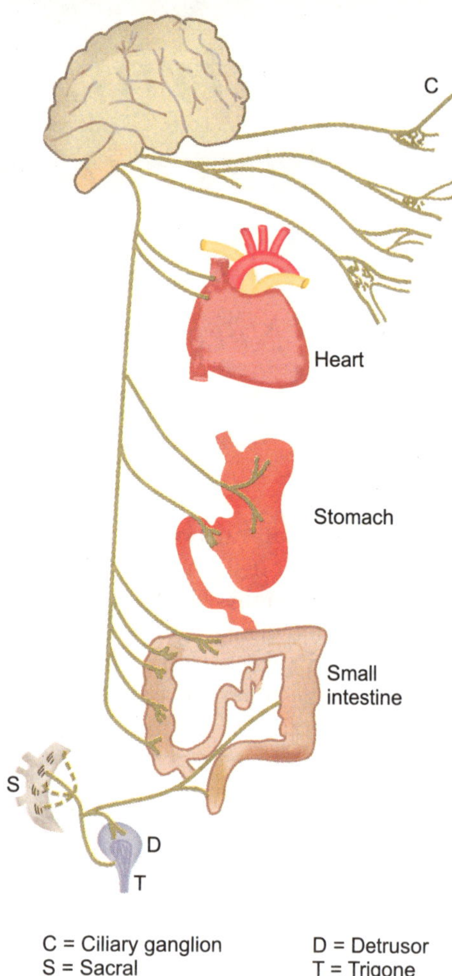

Fig. 112.1: Parasympathetic nervous system

c. *Cranial nerve IX*: It is the otic ganglia where the preganglionic fibres are terminating. Post-ganglionic fibres are terminating to parotid gland. It is said to provoke its secretion.

d. *Cranial nerve X (Vagus)*: It arises from dorsal vagus nucleus. Connector fibres are arising from 'nucleus inter calatus'; fibres then pass out in vagus trunk, ending in ganglia in or very near to viscera; meaning that preganglionic fibres are long while postganglionic fibres are short. Supply is as follows -
   i. Constrictor fibres to bronchial muscles.
   ii. Inhibitory fibres to junctional cardiac tissues and dilatory fibres to coronaries.
   iii. Fibres causing secretion from pancreatic tissues.
   iv. Excitation of peristalsis of GIT including gallbladder along with an increase in their secretion.

Sacral Outflow

Preganglionic fibres are arising from cells in lateral part of anterior horn of 3rd and 4th sacral segments. These are emerging from spinal cord in corresponding ventral roots to form *nervi erigentes* to synapse on cells in ganglia of pelvic plexus or on walls of bladder and rectum. Postganglionic fibres are running to hindgut, bladder, blood vessels of uterus and penis. The distribution is:

Bladder: Musculature receiving motor fibres while sphincter gets inhibitory fibres.

External genitalia: Vasodilator fibres responsible for erection. Sympathetic vasoconstrictors are also there which are responsible for orgasm.

Large Bowel: They receive motor fibres while sphincters receive inhibitory fibres.

SYMPATHETIC OR THORACO-LUMBAR DIVISION

The mother cells are present in grey matter of lateral horn of spinal cord extending from first thoracic to third lumbar segments. The cord is left by preganglionic fibres of these cells and they enter sympathetic ganglia.

The axons of lateral horn cells of spinal cord are passing out through anterior root and enter anterior division of mixed spinal nerve. These fibres are medullated/white, leaving the nerve in the form of a branch called *white ramus communicans* which is found only from first thoracic to first three lumbar segments.

Postganglionic/effector fibres are arising from ganglia and are non-medullated (grey). In the form of a branch called *grey ramus communicans*, they run back to join the spinal nerve and are distributed to (vasomotor) blood vessels, sweat glands, arrector pili muscles.

Sympathetic Ganglia

i. Twenty-two in number, extending from base of skull to coccyx. Lying by side of vertebral bodies are vertebral ganglia.

   Superior, middle and inferior cervical ganglia are constituted by fusion of eighth cervical ganglia. Stellate ganglion is formed by union of first thoracic with inferior cervical ganglion.

ii. Prevertebral ganglion lie in or near the heart, lungs and other thoracic viscera.

iii. Coeliac, mesenteric (superior and inferior) are others, lying in close relation with aorta or its branches.

iv. Terminal ganglia is small collection of cells lying in close relationship to pelvic organs, e.g. rectum and bladder.

Sympathetic Outflow

i. *Limbs*
   - *Upper limb:* Fibres arise in 4-8 thoracic segments; synapsing in lower cervical as well as first thoracic ganglia. Supply structures of skin and skeletal muscle's vessels which respond by dilatation.
   - *Lower limb:* Fibres arising from T_{12} to L_2 segments. Postganglionic fibres are emerging from lumbar as well as sacral ganglia (L_4 - S_3), reaching the limb either along perivascular network in adventitia to main arteries or through gray rami to nerves of limb.

ii. *Gastro-intestinal tract*: Splanchnic nerves are supplying, emerging in lower five or six thoracic nerves and upper two lumbar nerves, synapsing in coeliac and superior mesenteric ganglia. Post-ganglionic fibres are running with blood vessels to alimentary canal.

   They lead to sphincter contraction, mucus production reducing tone and peristalsis as well as secretion of digestive juices. No sympathetic supply to oesophagus.

iii. *Heart:* Fibres are arising from lateral horn cells (upper five thoracic segments), synapsing in respective thoracic and cervical ganglia (upper, middle, lower). Post-ganglionic fibres are emerging from these ganglia and supply cardiac musculature along coronary vessels.

   Accelerated heart (increased rate and force of ventricular contraction) and dilatation of coronary vessels are their principle effects.

iv. *Pelvic structures* : Fibres are emerging in last thoracic and upper two lumbar nerves and synapse in hypogastric ganglia.

   It constricts glomerular arterioles of kidney, contraction of prostatic muscles as well as smooth musculature of epididymis, ejaculatory ducts, seminal vesicles. Both motor and inhibitory fibres are going to supply uterus, fallopian tube, ureters. Movements are inhibited but constricted sphincters are reported in urinary bladder.

v. *Skin:* Postganglionic fibres are passing from superior cervical ganglion to upper four cervical nerves. They pass along cutaneous nerves by joining brachial plexus.

   Fibres of sweat glands are cholinergic. Blood vessels and plain muscles (arrectores pile, anal sphincters and vagina) are other structures supplied by them. It controls amount of sweat.

vi. *Respiration*: Fibres arise in upper four thoracic segments and synapsing in ganglia (inferior cervical and upper thoracic).

   It relaxes bronchial muscle along with dilatation of bronchi. Pulmonary vessels get constricted.

vii. *Others*

   Liver—Mobilisation of glycogen
   Spleen-Gall bladder—Contraction
   Eye—Pupil dilated, lesser tone of ciliary muscles, accommodation to distant vision.
   Adrenal—Controls amount of secretion
   Uterus—Smooth muscles in pregnancy contract while inhibited in non-pregnant state.

ACTIONS OF PARASYMPATHETIC AND ITS MODE

- The preganglionic fibres of both systems viz. sympathetic and parasympathetic are cholinergic. In general, the post-ganglionic fibres of parasympathetic system are cholinergic, while post-ganglionic sympathetic fibres are adrenergic. However, exceptions are also existing like sweat glands have an excitatory cholinergic innervation supplied by sympathetic system and there exists adrenergic cardio-accelerator fibres in vagus nerve.
- Anyway, parasympathetic acts by releasing *Acetylcholine* at nerve endings which is destroyed by enzyme *cholinesterase* found in RBC along with in motor plate endings and synaptic junctions. Its actions are:

i. *Heart:* Cardio-inhibition and decrease in strength.
ii. *Blood vessels:* Vasodilatation
iii. *GIT:* Regulation and increasing secretion of saliva, gastric juice, pancreatic glands. Motility of stomach, relaxation of pyloric sphincter.
iv. *Eye:* Pupillary constriction, accommodation to near vision.
v. *Lungs:* Contraction of smooth muscles of bronchi or constriction of bronchi.
vi. *Smooth muscle:* Contraction of digestive tube and gallbladder is excited, relaxation of muscular capsule of spleen.
vii. *Others:*
   - Contraction of urinary bladder
   - Control of secretion of posterior pituitary lobe
   - Regulation of emotions and behaviour
   - Contraction of skeletal muscles.

MODE OF ACTION

a. *Sympathetics*: Act by releasing nor-adrenaline and adrenaline (3:1) at postganglionic nerve endings. Exceptions: postganglionic sympathetic nerve fibres to sweat glands and preganglionic sympathetic nerve fibres release acetylcholine.
b. *Parasympathetic*: Act by releasing acetylcholine at nerve endings; which is destroyed by choline-

esterase—an enzyme present in RBC, motor plate endings and synaptic junctions. It is inhibited by eserine (physostigmine).

CONTROL OF ANS

a. *Cortical representation*: There exists cortical control and cells are believed to be in premotor cortex and in its vicinity. It is evident that autonomic representation of cardiovascular, pilomotor, respiratory system are found in grey matter near third ventricle. The area 24, 23, 29 in cingulate gyrus and areas 13, 14, in inferior orbital gyri are its representatives. Area 4, 6, 8, 47, 38, 24 are representing both motor and autonomic centres.

b. *Hypothalamus*: It is highest centre for ANS. It is having nuclei which are sending fibres down into spinal cord. Fibres make synaptic connections with cells of origin of thoracolumbar nervous system. Adrenergic response is obtained.

   Anterior hypothalamic nucleus is representing parasympathetic while posterior hypothalamic nucleus is representing sympathetic and parasympathetic reflex centre. Efferent hypothalamic tracts descending to mid-brain, pons, medulla are sending collaterals to brainstem parasympathetic nuclei and intermediolateral column cells of cord segments.

c. *Others*:
   i. *Cortico-hypothalamic efferents*: From area 6 to medial mammillary nucleus. Also from area 8, 10 to supraoptic nucleus; from area 10, 47, 46 to paraventricular nuclei; from area 13 to ventromedial nucleus of hypothalamus.
   ii. *Hormonal control* is also existing through adrenaline, noradrenaline and acetylecholine via hypothalamus.
   iii. Vital centres are also having their existence which are medullary centres for autonomic reflex control of body activities, like vasomotor, cardiac, pupil dilating centre etc.

PHARMACOLOGY OF ANS

i. Drugs called sympathomimetics are producing similar effects as that of sympathetic while drugs producing similar effects as that of parasympathetic stimulation are called parasympathomimetics. Drugs suppressing effects of sympathetic or of parasympathetic are called sympatholytic and parasympatholytic respectively.
ii. Sympathomimetics—adrenaline, noradrenaline.
iii. Parasympathomimetics—acetylcholine (it acts as a chemical mediator in synaptic transmission in ganglia, skeletal muscle end plate. It plays a role in conduction of nerve impulse as well as in central synaptic transmission); choline, pilocarpine, muscarine.
iv. Atropine (belladona alkaloid) is parasympatholytic drug, active at peripheral junction.
v. Drugs enhancing cholinergic effects by inhibiting enzyme cholineesterase include eserine, prostigmine, di-isopropyl fluorophosphate
vi. Quarternary ammoniums (tetramethyl ammonium) 'hexamethonium ions,' 'pentolinium' are said to block impulse transmission from pre- to post-ganglionic neurons. Curare and its alkaloids are blocking impulses by competiting with acetylcholine for receptor substance on which acetylcholine acts to produce depolarisation.
vii. Drugs causing autonomic effects by stimulating post-ganglionic neurons are named as nicotinic drugs. Nicotine is capable of stimulating both sympathetic (vasoconstriction in limbs and abdominal organs) as well as parasympathetics (heart slowing, enhanced GIT activity). Acetyl-choline, carbamylcholine, methacholine are said to create both type of actions namely—muscarinic and nicotine one. In large doses, nicotine paralyses all autonomic synapses.
viii. Reserpine is said to prevent synthesis and storage of noradrenaline in sympathetic nerve endings, while its release is blocked by guanethidine.
ix. • Drugs blocking alpha receptors: Dibenamine, phenoxy benzamine, phentolamine.
   • Drugs blocking beta receptors: dichloro-isoproterenol, nethalide butoxamine, propranolol metaprolol.

AUTONOMIC REFLEXES

a. *Cardiovascular:* Example is functioning of baroreceptors in controlling blood pressure and heart rate.
b. *GIT:*
   - By smell or sight of food or even by placing the food in mouth, initiates signals to vagal, glossopharyngeal, salivary nuclei of brainstem. These through parasympathetic division transmit signals to secretory glands of GIT to secrete digestive juices.
   - Similarly, when rectal wall is stretched with faecal matter; the information is sent to sacral part of spinal cord. From here signals are coming through

parasympathetics to colon to perform peristaltic contractions to evacuate the intestine.

c. *Others:*
   - Stretching of urinary bladder with urine → impulses to spinal cord → contraction of bladder + relaxation of urinary sphincters → promoting micturition
   - Sexual stimulation → sacral cord gets the impulse → erection penis (parasympathetic action) + ejaculation (sympathetic action)
   - Pancreatic secretion regulation, emptying of gall bladder.

DENERVATION SUPER SENSITIVITY

- If sympathetic or parasympathetic nerve is destroyed; then during first week of this episode the innervated organ becomes more and more sensitive to injected noradrenaline or acetylcholine.
- It is thought that number of receptors in post-synaptic membrane of the effector cell increases tremendously when these chemicals (noradrenaline/acetylcholine) are not released at synapses.

THE TONE: SYMPATHETIC; PARASYMPATHETIC

- Both these systems are continuously active.
- Tone, allows a single nervous system to increase or to decrease the activity of a stimulated organ.
- Immediately after cutting sympathetic or parasympathetic nerve, the innervated organ loses its respective tone.
- *Example:*
  - Parasympathetic tone is dominant in GIT. If this nerve supply of gut is removed then gastric and intestinal atony results which terminates into disturbed gastro-intestinal propulsion and so constipation.
  - Sympathetic tone is maintained by basal secretion of epinephrine (0.2 µg/kg/minute) and norepinephrine (0.05 µg/kg/minute). This amount is in addition to tone resulting from direct sympathetic stimulation.
  - All systemic arterioles are constricted by sympathetic tone. If they are stimulated more and more, vasoconstriction can also be increased in proportion. But a stage can come that they may cause vasodilatation, by inhibiting normal tone.

SOME DISORDERS

a. Symptom complex characterised by meiosis, ptosis, facial flushing and dryness of same side, enophthalmos, ipsilateral vasodilatation and anhidrosis are constituting ***Horner's syndrome***. It is resulting due to paralysis of cervical sympathetic chain or upper thoracic cord.
b. Due to interruption in peripheral sympathetic innervation of blood vessels the symptoms begin with local vascular changes in which toes and fingers first of all becomes cold and pale, followed by bluish grey discoloration of skin and finally terminating in gangrenous changes affecting both sides. It is ***Raynaud's disease***.
c. Sometimes parasympathetic ganglia in gut wall is absent with birth (congenital). This causes enormous dilatation of colon with constipation. This is ***Hirschsprung's disease or congenital megacolon***.
d. Other conditions due to ANS disorder include: angioneurotic oedema, scleroderma.

OTHER FUNCTIONS

i. It is concerned with smooth muscular activities like peristalsis, size of pupil and lens position, controlling cardiac muscles etc.
ii. The activity of all secreting glands of digestive tract, lacrimal and sweat glands, along with blood sugar level is also controlled.
iii. Temperature control system is also performed.
iv. The importance of catecholamines lies in regulation of metabolic processes through increasing the rate of cellular metabolism and stimulating the conversion of complex fuels into readily usable substrates. Fasting suppresses and overfeeding stimulates the sympathetic nervous system since during fasting suppression of sympathetic activity conserves calories by diminishing metabolism and heat production while during over feeding its stimulation expends calories by accelerating metabolism and producing heat.
v. By reflex responses, vital functions of body are controlled, e.g. digestion, circulation, secretion, etc.
vi. It participates in somatovisceral and viserosomatic reflexes, e.g. respiration, vomiting, swallowing, coughing, sudomotor etc.

BIBLIOGRAPHY

1. Burnstock ME. Smooth muscle autonomic nerve transmission. Holman Ann Rev Phy 1963;25:61-90.
2. Dale Purves, Jeff W. Lichtman. Formation and maintenance of synaptic connections in autonomic ganglion. Phy Rev 1978;58: No. 1.
3. Julius Axelrod. The fate of norepinephrine and effect of drugs. Physiologist 1968;11(1):63.

4. Mauskopf M, Gray SD, Renkin EM. Transient and persistent components of sympathetic cholinergic vasodilatation. Am J Phy 1969;216:92, No. 1.
5. Malmejae. Activity of adrenal medulla and its regulation. Phy Rev 1964;44:186.
6. Ulf Soderberg. Neurophysiological aspects of homeostasis. Ann Rev Phy 1964;26:27-288.

NERVOUS SYSTEM — GLOSSARY

CNS: Brain + spinal cord.
ANS: Nerves and ganglion arising from ventral part of spinal cord.
PNS: Cranial nerves + spinal nerves.
Forebrain: Cerebral hemisphere. Olfactory lobe, diencephalon.
Midbrain: Optic lobes + cerebral peduncle.
Hindbrain: Cerebellum + medulla oblongata
Cerebral hemisphere: Have folds and grooves called gyri and sulci. Outer layer is cerebral cortex made up of grey matter containing nerve cells in it. Controls activities like auditory, premotor, motor, sensory etc.
Spinal cord: Centre of reflex action, and forming link between brain and spinal nerves. White matter surrounds grey matter. Wing like ridges of grey matter called dorsolateral and ventro-lateral horns. Lateral horns also found in thoracic and lumbar region. Sensory tract is ascending while motor tract is descending one.
Afferent nerve (sensory): Nerve transmitting impulses from receptor to CNS.
Efferent nerve (motor): Nerve transmitting impulses from CNS to effector muscles.
Mixed nerve: Having both sensory + motor fibres.
Neurons: Morphological + physiological unit of nervous system. Each consists of a cell body (perikaryon), dendrites (afferent fibres) and axons (efferent fibres). The terminal part of axon has got buttons (swollen structure) which forms the connection with dendron of another neuron.
Unipolar: Neuron having single process dividing into dendron and an axon (site-dorsal ganglia of spinal cord).
Bipolar: Neurons having two processes arising from opposite poles of cyton (site retina of eye).
Multipolar: Many processes arising from cyton. Single axon and many dendrons. Majority are of this type.
Nerve impulse: A nerve cell is highly irritable. Can be excited by stimulus. A stimulus disturbs the equilibrium of living protoplasm. The energy of stimulus is transformed into electric energy by neurons and this electric energy initiates a series of events which travel along neuron. The conduction wave of electric charge constitute a nerve impulse.
Synaptic delay: Delay in the transmission of nerve impulse at each synapse due to time taken in releasing neurotransmitter and stimulating next neuron is synaptic delay.
Neurotransmitters: These are chemicals stored in synaptic vesicle meant for transmitting nerve impulse across synapse. Nerve impulse is one way conduction.
Resting potential: is determined by K^+ concentration within cell and outside cell. It is about 60-70 mV.
Action potential: A wave like change in membrane's electrical properties. It is the mean for transmitting nerve impulse along neurons.
All or none principle: The stimuli with strength below threshold don't cause any impulse, while stimuli having intensity above threshold induce the same action potential.
Reflex action: Automatic and rapid response to a stimulus.
Reflex arc: Path through which impulse travels during reflex action.
Receptors: A specialised ending of a sensory neuron that receive the stimuli from environment and generate nerve impulse.
Isotonic contraction: When a muscle contracts with a constant load that it can lift, it is said to be isotonic. There is a change in shape of muscle and they maintain tension.
Isometric contraction: When a muscle contracts against a weight that it cannot lift, it is called isometric contraction. No change in shape of muscles as it maintains length.

QUESTION BANK—CNS

1. **Short notes:**
   a. Aphasia
   b. Conditioned reflex
   c. Parkinsonism (Raj Univ 1989, MD, Raj Univ First MBBS, 1995)
   d. Brown sequard syndrome
   e. Decerebrate rigidity
   f. Lumbar puncture and hydrocephalus
   g. Blood-brain barrier
   h. Righting reflex
   i. Inverse stretch reflex
   j. Paradoxical sleep
   k. Functions of hypothalamus
   l. Electroencephalogram (E.E.G.) (Raj Univ First MBBS, 1995)
   m. Lateral motor System (Raj Univ First MBBS, 1995)
2. **Discuss**
   a. Mechanism of propagation of impulse
   b. Complete transection of spinal cord
   c. Write an assay on synaptic inhibition (Raj Univ 1980, MD)
   d. Length servo system in muscles
   e. Lesion of parietal lobe
   f. Neurotransmitters
   g. The functions of thalamus and changes in person having thalamic syndrome (Raj Univ 1988, 1990, MD)
3. **Describe Physiological basis of**
   a. A patient enters your clinic with stamping gait. Describe disorder underlying?
   b. A patient enters your clinic with short steps but running along with flexion attitude. Describe disorder underlying?
4. **Explain**
   i. Babiniski sign is positive in upper motor neuron lesion. Why?
   ii. Final common pathway of motor impulses.
5. **Discuss patho-physiology of pain?** (Raj Univ 1986, 1994, 1996, MD). **Write in short about physiological basis of referred pain?** (Raj Univ First MBBS, 1995)
6. **What is reflex. Classify it and give differences among themselves?**
7. **Describe origin, function, course of corticospinal tracts.**
8. **Differences between**
   a. Upper and lower motor neuron lesion
   b. Decerebrate rigidity and rigidity seen in Parkinsonism.
   c. Somatic pain and visceral pain
9. **Discuss physiology of sleep and wakefulness.** (Raj Univ 1980, 1991, MD)
10. **Discuss vestibular and non-vestibular factors in maintenance of equilibrium.** (Raj Univ 1990, MD)
11. **Name different proprioceptors. Describe the path of kinesthetic (proprioceptive) impulses.** (Raj Univ First MBBS, 1995)
12. **Describe functions of cerebellum in control of voluntary motor activity. (Raj Univ First MBBS, 1995)**
13. **Describe Physiological basis of short-term memory.** (Raj Univ First MBBS, 1995)
14. **Discuss the functional importance of extra-pyramidal nervous system and neurological deficits produced by its disorders.** (Raj Univ 1990, MD)
15. **Describe cerebral speech mechanism and effect of its disruption.** (Raj Univ 1989, MD)
16. **How CNS regulates cardiac activity. Describe ventricular function curves.** (Raj Univ 1976, 1979, MD)
17. **Discuss physiology of learning and memory.** (Raj Univ 1986, MD)

MULTIPLE CHOICE QUESTIONS : CNS

1. **Pain sensitive structures in brain are:** (AIIMS-1983, PGI-1987)
   a. Pia arachnoid
   b. Grey matter
   c. Venous sinuse
   d. Cerebellum
   e. Dura mater [ ]
2. **Which of the following is *not* a feature of mid-brain lesion:** (AIIMS-1987)
   a. Upper gaze palsy
   b. Pupillary dilatation
   c. Crossed hemiplegia
   d. Extension of arm [ ]
3. **Which of the following is *not* a normal CSF value:** (UPSC-1983, 1987, Delhi - 1982, AIIMS - 1984)
   a. Pressure 60-80 mm CSF
   b. Protein 20-40 mg%
   c. Sugar 20-40 mg%
   d. Chloride 750 mEq/L [ ]
4. **Negri bodies are most often found in:** (AIIMS-1985, UPSC-1991)
   a. Mid-brain
   b. Basal ganglia
   c. Frontal cortex
   d. Hippocampus [ ]
5. **Mask like face is seen in:** (PGI-1986)
   a. Parkinsonism
   b. Disseminated sclerosis
   c. After stokes
   d. Pseudo-bulbar palsy [ ]
6. **Blood-brain barrier is maximum permeable to:**
   a. Na^+
   b. K^+

c. Chloride
d. CO_2 [ ]

7. **Kinaesthetic sensations are detected mainly by what type of receptors?** (AMC-1984, Delhi - 1984, 1986)
   a. Muscle spindles
   b. Golgi tendon apparatus
   c. Skin receptors
   d. Joint receptors [ ]
8. **Cerebrospinal fluid is:** (AIIMS-1985)
   a. Protective in nature
   b. Pressure is less than venous pressure
   c. Ultrafiltrate of plasma
   d. None of above [ ]
9. **Slow waves during sleep in EEG are:** (Delhi-1986, 1989)
   a. Beta
   b. Delta
   c. Reticular activation
   d. None of above [ ]
10. **CSF pressure in lying down posture is:** (Delhi - 1984, 1986, UPSC-1984, 1987)
    a. 20 - 50 mm
    b. 50 - 150 mm
    c. 150 - 200 mm
    d. 200 - 300 mm [ ]

ANSWERS

1. c, e 2. d 3. c 4. d 5. a 6. d 7. d 8. c 9. b 10. c

VIVA VOCE : CENTRAL NERVOUS SYSTEM

1. **What are the major levels of nervous system function?**
   i. *Spinal cord level:* Sensory signals are transmitted through spinal nerves into each segment of spinal cord which are capable of causing localised motor response. All such spinal cord motor responses are automatic occurring instantaneously in response to sensory signal.
   ii. *Lower brain level:* It lies in medulla, pons, hypothalamus, thalamus and basal ganglia. It controls subconscious co-ordinate function of body like arterial pressure, respiratory, emotions, sexual activities, reaction to pain and pleasure, feeding reflexes etc.
   iii. *Higher level*: It is cerebral cortex; and is vast information storage area.
2. **Enumerate the effects of section of posterior nerve roots?**
   i. Loss of all forms of sensations from supplied site.
   ii. Loss of reflex activity.
   iii. In co-ordinated limb movement.
   iv. Vasodilatation.
   v. Complete loss of tone of muscles of affected area.
   vi. Weakness and muscular incoordination.
3. **Enumerate the ascending tracts.**
   A. In anterior funiculus
      i. Anterior (ventral) spinothalamic tract
      ii. Inter-segmental tract
   B. In lateral funiculus
      i. Posterior spino-cerebellar tract
      ii. Anterior spino-cerebellar tract
      iii. Lateral spino-thalamic tract
      iv. Spino-tectal tract
      v. Spino-olivary tract
      vi. Spino-reticular tract
      vii. Spino-vestibular tract
      viii. Spino-pontine tract
      ix. Spino-cortical tract
   C. In Posterior funiculus
      i. Tract of Goll (Fasciculus gracilis)
      ii. Tract of Burdach (Fasciculus cuneatus)
      iii. Comma tract (Posterior intersegmental)
4. **Enumerate the descending tracts of spinal cord.**
   a. Corticospinal tract (cerebrospinal tract)
   b. Vestibulo spinal tract
   c. Tectospinal tract
   d. Rubrospinal tract
   e. Olivospinal tract
   f. Reticulospinal tract
5. **Enumerate the functions of tract of Goll and Burdach.**
   i. They carry proprioceptive somatic sensation.
   ii. They are carrying discriminatory impulses of fine touch.
   iii. They carry vibration sensation along with deep pressure sensation.
   iv. They carry sensation to arouse spatial discrimination.
   v. They are also said to carry nonsensory impulses arising through cutaneous stimulation.
6. **What is Basal ganglia?**
   These are submerged masses of grey matter in subcortical level of each cerebral hemisphere. They include structure like corpus striatum (lentiform and caudate nucleus), claustrum, red nucleus, substantia nigra, amygdaloid body, subthalamic body of Luys.
7. **Enumerate functions of Basal ganglia?**
   i. Originator of useful voluntary muscular activity.
   ii. Production of automatic associated movements.

iii. Control reflex muscular activity.
iv. Striate body helps to control gross intentional movements which are performed unconsciously.
v. Principal function of globus pallidus is to provide background muscle tone for intended movements.

8. What is Thalamus?

They are two large, oval convex cell mass located below cerebral hemisphere. The thalami are joined across the midline by an isthmus called 'massa intermedia'. Below it are subthalamic nucleus as well as forepart of red nucleus, and in front lies head of caudate nucleus; above it is lateral ventricle whose floor is constituted by it.

9. Enumerate functions of Thalamus?

i. It is a great relay station.
ii. It is a conscious centre for cruder sensation.
iii. It is concerned with arousal and alert reaction.
iv. It behaves like emotional reflex centre.
v. It is linked with personality and social behaviour.
vi. It acts as a link between cerebellum, basal ganglia and cerebral cortex (area 4 and 6).
vii. It differentiates modality of sensation.
viii. It is concerned with visceral sensation.

10. What is Thalamic syndrome?

The chief features are

i. Astereognosis and sensory ataxia
ii. Some loss of tactile and thermal sensation over body and face.
iii. Over reaction : Spontaneous paroxysmal pain may occur and threshold for it may be increased (hyperalgesia)
iv. Intention tremors
v. Hemiparesis and defects in visual fields.
vi. Thalamic hand (moderate flexion of wrist with hyperextension of fingers with extension of whole hand).

11. Enumerate the functions of reticular formation?

i. It maintains conscious alert state.
ii. It controls sleep.
iii. It generates sensory impulses or controls their transmission through specific sensory pathways.
iv. It is said to be highest centre for glucostatic mechanism.
v. It is also responsible for feeding, satiety, and thirst.
vi. It is related with controlling viscero vascular system like heart rate, respiration, GIT, metabolism, blood pressure etc.
vii. It regulates tone of muscles, and posture giving a background for execution of purposeful movements.
viii. It is responsible for postural reflexes and righting reactions.

12. Enumerate the main functions of Hypothalamus.

i. Regulation of water balance.
ii. Formation of oxytocin and vasopressin.
iii. Concerned with sleep and wakefulness.
iv. It regulates body temperature.
v. It is also concerned with hunger, feeding, satiety and thirst.
vi. It is concerned with sexual functions.
vii. It influences autonomic activities (both sympathetic and parasympathetic).
viii. It secretes releasing hormones for pituitary activation.
ix. It is also concerned with metabolism of fat, protein and carbohydrates.
x. It also regulates cardio-vascular activities.

13. Enumerate functions of prefrontal region of cerebral cortex.

a. In human beings it is the seat of mind.
b. It is seat for planned action.
c. It is seat for emotions.
d. It influences autonomic reactions associated with emotions.
e. It is said to be a faculty for emotional stability, judgement, planned actions, intelligence etc.

14. What is meant by end organs?

These are specially organised bodies located at end of either a motor nerve or at peripheral end of a sensory nerve. They function to transmit the impulse to effector organ or to receive a particular stimulus from periphery.

15. Enumerate characteristics of stretch (myotatic) reflex?

a. Short latent period.
b. It is abolished on any damage to reflex arc.
c. As stimulus is over the response also goes off.
d. If brainstem is sectioned through mid brain the response is augmented.
e. The response is directly proportional to amount of stretch and there occurs relaxation of antagonists as response starts which is due to reciprocal innervation.
f. It is highly localised.
g. The inhibitors are painful stimulation of skin, stretching of antagonistic flexor muscles, applying noxious stimuli to extremity, excessive stretching of responding muscles.

16. Name the speech centre.

Four centres :

i. Lower frontal area (area 44) Broca's area.
ii. Upper frontal motor cortex (paracentral lobule).
iii. Parietal cortex posterior to lower part of postcentral gyrus.
iv. Temporal cortex (posterior part).

17. Mention the characteristics of REM sleep (paradoxical sleep).

i. Rapid eye movements.
ii. Reduction of skeletal muscle tone.
iii. Inhibition of stretch reflexes.
iv. Teeth grinding occasionally.
v. Associated dreams.

18. What are upper motor neuron?

Cortical, subcortical or brainstem nuclei are these structures which are sending impulses to lower motor neurons. They are said to provide origin to pyramidal and extrapyramidal tracts.

19. **What are lower motor neurons?**
These are nothing but anterior horn cell of spinal cord and their cranial homologues. They supply the muscles at peripheral end through ramifications.

MULTIPLE CHOICE QUESTIONS: AUTONOMIC NERVOUS SYSTEM

1. **Following are the structures supplied by sympathetics alone *except:***
   a. Adrenal medulla
   b. Most arterioles
   c. Ureters
   d. Gastric glands [ ]
2. **Following are the structures supplied by parasympathetics alone *except*:**
   a. Oesophagus
   b. Pancreas
   c. Gastric glands
   d. Uterus [ ]
3. **The substance responsible for destruction of catecholamine is:**
   a. Bradykinin
   b. Cholinesterase
   c. Amino-oxidase
   d. Sympathin [ ]
4. **Acetylcholine is hydrolyzed quickly by:**
   a. 5 HT
   b. Amino-oxidase
   c. Cholinesterase
   d. Bradykinin [ ]
5. **Beta receptors are strongly blocked by:**
   a. Adrenaline
   b. Noradrenaline
   c. Di-chloro-iso-proterenol
   d. Acetylcholine [ ]
6. **The characteristic feature of ANS is:**
   a. Presence of efferent neurons in posterior root ganglia.
   b. Location of connector neurons in posterior horn cells.
   c. Presence of peripheral ganglia.
   d. Location of effector neurone on lateral horn cells [ ]
7. **The concept of receptors first proposed by:**
   a. Abel
   b. Dale
   c. Euler
   d. Pavlov [ ]

ANSWERS

1. d 2. d 3. c 4. c 5. c 6. c 7. b

VIVA VOCE : AUTONOMIC NERVOUS SYSTEM

1. **What is Autonomic nervous system?**
Nervous system controlling visceral activities and its actions are independent of 'will'. Because of its effects on viscera it is also called 'visceral or vegetative nervous system'. It is under central control coming from cortex as well as hypothalamus.
2. **What are the main functions of ANS?**
   a. It governs the activities of cardiac and smooth muscles of sweat and digestive glands, adrenal medulla and other endocrine glands. On the whole, it is concerned with those processes which are normally beyond voluntary control and for most part beneath consciousness.
   b. It helps in maintaining and stabilising internal environment called homeostasis (milieu internee of Claude Bernard and Canon).
   c. Through its companion adrenal medulla; it prepares the animal and human being against stress (general adaptation syndrome).
   d. Vital body processes like circulation, digestion, secretion, excretion are controlled by ANS by reflex response.
   e. It also takes part in many somato-visceral and viscerosomatic reflexes like respiration, lachrymation, sneezing, coughing, swallowing, genital, pilomotor reflexes, etc.
3. **What is Homeostasis?**
Life began as unicellular organism in primordial sea. Air was the 'external environment' and salt water was 'internal environment' without which individual cell could not exist. The mechanism by which constancy of internal environment is maintained and ensured is called homeostasis (canon). It is the mechanism which serves to maintain constancy of acid-base balance, osmotic pressure, body temperature, blood sugar, blood volume. The chief instrument in this orchestra is kidney but posterior pituitary (ADH), adrenal cortex and thyroid are also playing a leading role. When the mechanism breaks down clinical picture is noticed called a 'disease' which

leads to 'death' if it becomes prolonged, profound and uncontrolled.

4. **Describe general arrangement of ANS?**
The reflex arc in autonomic system is composed of three neurons viz. afferent, connector and efferent. Afferent lies in posterior root ganglia; 'connectors' located in lateral horn cells and 'efferent' (or effector) lies outside central nervous system as 'ganglia' which constitutes the characteristic feature of ANS.

5. **What is 'white and grey ramus communicans'?**
Sympathetic outflow originating from thoraco-lumbar segments and the connectors of which are located in lateral horn cells in thoracic and upper two lumbar segments. Now since effectors are situated outside CNS; so axons of leaving fibres passing out through anterior root; entering anterior division of mixed spinal nerve; the fibres are white so medullated; leaving the nerve in form of a branch called 'white ramus communicans'.

   The effector fibres arising from ganglion of sympathetic chain are non-medullated (so grey), running back to join spinal nerve in the form of another branch called 'grey ramus communicans'.

6. **Describe sacral outflow of parasympathetics.**
   a. Sacral 2 and 3 are said to be connectors.
   b. They are coming out through respective anterior roots and unit to form single nerve known as 'nervi erigentis'.
   c. It is relayed in hypogastric ganglion from where post-ganglionic fibres are arising which are supplying urinary bladder, prostate and large intestine except caecum.
   d. Vaso-dilatation in erection of penis, stimulated movements and inhibition of sphincters are its main actions.

7. **What are adrenergic receptors?**
'Dale' (1906) was the first man who proposed the concept of specific receptors. 'Ahlquist' divided it into two—Alpha and beta. Alpha are associated with vasoconstriction, myocardial excitation, myometrial contraction, nictitating membrane contraction, intestinal relaxation, iris dilator muscle contraction, pilomotor contraction and glycogenolysis; while beta receptors are concerned with vasodilatation, cardio-acceleration, myometrial relaxation, bronchial relaxation, myocardial strength etc. Beta receptors are influenced by activation of adenylcyclase; leading to increase in cyclic AMP.

8. **What are nicotinic drugs?**
Drugs causing autonomic effects by stimulating post-ganglionic neurons are nicotinic drugs. Examples—Acetylcholine, methacholine.

9. **What are muscarinic drugs?**
'Muscarine' derived from toad stool was among the first drugs of type causing parasympathomimetic effects. They are acetylcholine, methacholine, carbamycholine.

10. **Name the drugs blocking beta receptors.**
Di-chloro-iso-proterenol; nethalide, propranolol.

11. **How transmission occurs in sympathetic ganglia?**
   a. Initial depolarisation is produced by acetylcholine through a nicotinic receptor.
   b. Slow IPSP (inhibitory post-synaptic potential) and prolonged EPSP (excitatory post-synaptic potential) are two factors regulating transmission through sympathetic ganglia.
   c. Slow 1 PSP is created by 'dopamine' which is secreted by an interneuron located within ganglion.

12. **What is Horner's syndrome?**
Over constriction of pupil, ptosis (narrowing of palpebral fissure) (overactivity of third cranial nerve) due to drooping of eyelid results on severing cervical sympathetics, constitutes Horner's syndrome.

UNIT A

Chalte-Chalte

“There are many other things which we come across while reading the subjects. Many of them are under research, while many of them have become history. Some are of undergraduate, while some are of postgraduate, while some are of research interest. Any way let us see them all by running across the way, i.e. chalte-chalte.”

Appendices

APPENDIX 1

Medical Statistics

AVERAGES

"For a given data, a single value of the variable representing the entire data, which describes the characteristics of the data, is called average of the data."

Mainly we are interested in two types of averages: viz. mean and median.

ARITHMETIC MEAN

"The average of numbers in arithmetic is known as arithmetic mean of these numbers in statistics."

If marks obtained by 12 students in an examination are 7, 3, 5, 8, 3, 7, 3, 6, 4, 4, 7, 3 respectively then average of marks is:

$$\frac{7+3+5+8+3+7+3+6+4+4+7+3}{12} = \frac{60}{12} = 5$$

Thus, if the n values of the variable quantity are denoted by $x_1, x_2, ... x_n$ respectively, the arithmetic mean is expressed by the formula.

$$\text{Arithmetic mean} = \frac{x_1 + x_2 + x_3 + ... + x_n}{n} \text{ or } \bar{x} = \frac{\Sigma}{n}$$

Symbol sigma (Σ) is a letter of Greek alphabet and used to denote the process of addition. Arithmetic mean denoted by $\bar{x} - (x\ bar)$.

MERITS : ARITHMETIC MEAN

- Simple and easy to calculate.
- Affords a good standard of comparison.
- Least affected by fluctuations of sampling.
- Reliable.
- Mathematical analysis is possible.

DEMERITS : ARITHMETIC MEAN

- Unduly affected by extreme values.
- Cannot be computed unless all timings are known.
- Fallacious results may be drawn in non-availability of actual figures.
- Cannot be used in the study of rates.

MEDIAN

- *"The value of the middle most observation when the data are arranged in ascending or descending order of magnitude, is called median."*
- If all n values of a variable are arranged in ascending or descending order then the value of middle most item of the arranged series is called median.
- Thus, if all 15 students of a class are made to stand in a row according to their height then the height of 8th student standing in middle most part of the row will denote the median height of the student.
- If there are 10 persons, then median is worked out by taking the average of two middle values, e.g. blood pressure of ten persons is as 71, 75, 75, 77, 79, 81, 83, 84, 90, 95. Then $\frac{79+81}{2}$ will be the median.

MEDIAN : MERITS

- Easy for calculation.
- Can be located graphically
- Not affected by extreme values
- Best measure for qualitative data like intelligence, honesty etc.

MEDIAN: DEMERITS

- May not be a true representative of a given data, when items vary greatly in magnitude.
- Not based on all the observations in given data.
- Not very useful in further analysis.
- Becomes very tedious when number of items are large.

MODE

- By saying that most prevailing daily wages of labourer for whitewashing is Rs. 80, we mean that such labourers get Rs. 80 per day, OR in other words the rate/rates of labour are not so common as the figure 80 per day. Here, Rs. 80 per day denotes the mode of labour rate.

- So mode is the value of the variable in a given distribution which has the maximum frequency.
- There can be more than one mode in a given distribution, e.g. if 500 students of a school wear shoes of Bata company; and suppose 150 of them require size of 6, and 150 of them require size of 7. So size 6 and 7 are equally prevalent, so here there are two modes (6 and 7).
- It is most commonly occurring value.
- It is not often used in medical statistics since its exact location is uncertain, so not clearly defined.

DISPERSION

- The measures that are constructed to indicate the spread of the data with respect to the average in a set of observations are called measures of dispersion.
- The measure of dispersion about the mean is variance.
- The square root of the variance is standard deviation; the measure of dispersion about the median is the mean deviation.

MEAN DEVIATION (M.D.)

- Expressed as M.D. $= \frac{\Sigma (x-\bar{x})}{\eta}$

For example

Name of person	*Diastolic B.P. (x)*	*Arithmetic mean ($\bar{x}$)*	*Deviation from mean ($x-\bar{x}$)*
1. Ramesh	83	81	2
2. Radha	75	81	-6
3. Ajay	81	81	0
4. Asha	79	81	-2
5. Mohan	71	81	-10
6. Monika	95	81	14
7. Madan	75	81	-6
8. Meena	77	81	-4
9. Mukesh	84	81	3
10. Meera	90	81	9
Total	810		56

Σ = sign of mean. So the mean deviation is $\frac{56}{10} = 5.6$

η = number of observation (10 is total No. of persons)

STANDARD DEVIATION (S.D.): Most frequently used measure of deviation. Denoted by Greek letter σ (sigma).

$$\text{S.D.} = \sqrt{\frac{\Sigma (x-\bar{x})^2}{\eta}}$$

For example

Name of person	*Diastolic B.P. (x)*	*($x-\bar{x}$)*	$(x-\bar{x})^2$
1. Ramesh	83	2	4
2. Radha	75	6	36
3. Ajay	81	0	-
4. Asha	79	-2	4
5. Mohan	71	-10	100
6. Monika	95	14	196
7. Madan	75	6	36
8. Meena	77	4	16
9. Mukesh	84	3	9
10. Meera	90	9	81
n = 10	X = 81		482

When the sample size is more than 30, the above formula is correct. For smaller samples, the formula needs correction as:

$$\text{S.D.} = \sqrt{\frac{\Sigma (x-\bar{x})^2}{\eta-1}} = \sqrt{\frac{482}{10-1}} = \sqrt{\frac{482}{9}} = \sqrt{53.33} = 7.31$$

Mean: Individual observations are first added together and then divided by number of observations. This adding together is called summation (denoted by S or Σ). Mean is denoted by sign $\bar{x}$ (*x* bar).

Median: Dates are first arranged in ascending or descending order of magnitude and then value of middle observation is located called median.

Mode: Means most commonly occurring value in distribution of a data. Easy to locate and not affected by extreme items.

APPENDIX 2

Yoga and Meditation

- Yoga is complete mastery of mind and emotions - *3rd century B. C. Maharshi Patanjali*
- Yoga establishes mind over body.
- Yoga is derived from sanskrit word *"Yuj"* meaning control or unite.
- Yoga is a science which enables us to learn to make union of individual soul (*Jeevatma*) with universal soul (*Parmatma*).
- Yoga-sadhna leads to hormony and perfection of body, mind and spirit.
- Yoga is defined as a state of steadiness with control of senses and mind and intellect - *Kathopanishad* (X 1, 3, 10-11).
- The first step is *Dharana*, which leads to meditation or *Dhyana* and through this one may enter the holy destination of *Absolute.*

YOGI IN AN AIR TIGHT BOX

He was Ramanand Yogi who was studied by Dr. B. K. Anand et al. He was kept in an air tight box for 8 to 10 hours. His oxygen utilisation was reduced to 13.3 litres per hour in contrast to his basal requirement of 19.5 litres per hour. Same behaviour was given by carbon dioxide output. No tachycardia or hyperpnoea was reported. In EEG low voltage fast activities was observed suggestive of early stages of sleep (B.K. Anand et al, 1961).

- Following are the steps of *Hath Yog* namely - Abstention (Yama), Observance (Niyama), posture (Asana), Control of Prana (Pranayam), Sense of withdrawal (Pratyhara), Concentration (Dharana), Meditation (Dhyana), Sublimated super consciousness (Samadhi).
- Persons indulged in Yogic exercises have slower heart rate, slow respiratory rate, low serum cholesterol, low fasting blood sugar level, increased lymphocyte count.
- Types are: Shirshasna (Standing on head), Halasna (plough pose), Sarvangasana (standing on shoulder), Matsayasana, Paschimatsana.
- Yoga has been described as a three-fold path of development—physical, mental and spiritual. Its purpose is to bring man to the highest state of advancement on all these planes.
- The word Yoga means union/joining. Its ultimate aim is—liberation of spirit, the union of the soul with universe.

YOGI ON VOLUNTARY CONTROL OF THE HEART AND PULSE

Four Yogis were studied by M. A. Wenger et al. Two of them claimed to stop the heart and the fourth claimed to slow the heart. Their method involved retention of breath and considerable muscular tension in abdomen and thorax with glottis closed. The data indicate strong increase in vagal tone of unknown origin (M.A. Wenger et al, 1991).

- Hath yoga—is the beginner (ha = sun, tha = moon), i.e. flow of breath through right nostril is controlled by sun, while that through left is controlled by moon.
- Every age is the right age to start yoga.
- Yoga will not disrupt the normal sexual life but on the contrary, by toning up the whole body it increases poise, magnetism and joy in living.
- Half of stomach should be filled with food, one quarter with water and quarter should be kept empty for Pranayama—excellent rule for health.
- Yoga person should eat food which is digestible, agreeable and cooling—to nourish the humours of the body.

EEG CHANGES IN YOGIS

Four yogis were studied by B.K. Anand et al. on EEG aspects. Their resting record showed persistent alpha activity with increased amplitude modulation during samadhi. The alpha activity could not be blocked by various sensory stimuli during meditation (B.K. Anand et al, 1991).

- A physiologist is sometimes unable to explain the changes before and after the exercise. He thinks that during

Pranayam there is better oxygenation of the blood since prana means oxygen which is essential for life.

- A neuro-physiologist thinks that there is some toning and stimulating effect of these asanas upon the higher centres of brain—the cerebrum.
- Bronchial asthma and yoga:

(Asthma = Aazein Greek word means breathe with open mouth)

Normally:

Gas	*Inspiration*	*Expiration*
O_2	21%	16.5%
CO_2	0%	3.5%
N_2	79%	80%

- *Kapalabhati* (the process of cleansing frontal air sinuses: with air) regularly practised leads to decrease in CO_2 per cent in blood, and CO_2 is a regular stimulant of respiratory centre in medulla. Decreased CO_2 concentration will not abnormally stimulate the respiratory centre. The carotid body plays a similar role which are very much sensitive to chemical changes. This decreased CO_2 exerts a sedative effect on these sensitive centres which play a major role in relief from asthma.
- Yoga recognises the need for health. All yogic exercises aim at nervous control, purification and co-ordination rather than at muscular display and strength. Therefore, they encourage poise and control of the body and mind through a non-violent and non-fatiguing type of physical education.

HATH YOGA—PHYSIOLOGY

1. *CVS:* With few months of training there is improvement in fitness. Improvement has been also noted in vagal tone as shown by decrease in heart rate.
2. *Nervous system:* Relative increase in parasympathetic activity within 2-3 months of training. Dominant EEG wave is alpha initially which is then replaced by low voltage + high frequency action.
3. *Locomotion:* Relaxation of concerned muscles; provided particular asana is done in correct way in presence of "Guru," otherwise muscular activity may be exaggerated. Postural equilibrium is achieved at a new resting muscle length. It is sign of fitness and improves flexibility of joints.
4. *Respiration:* Physiological reserve is increased with repeated practice of yogic actions. It causes increase in vital capacity, increase in resting tidal volume, decrease in resting respiratory rate and an increase in breath holding time.

MEDITATION

- Reduction in O_2 consumption, reduction in CO_2 elimination—arterial lactate concentration
- Decrease in heart rate and respiratory rate
- Rise of serum amino acid—phenylalanine
- More alpha wave and occasional theta wave (EEG)
- Decrease in plasma cholesterol
- Decrease in arterial pH
- Decrease in cardiac output, blood pressure
- Meditation is having a therapeutic effect. It is of utmost importance in psychosomatic diseases (peptic ulcer, hypertension, migraine, psychiatric disorders etc.) which are increasing day by day with the advancement of civilisation.

KUNDALINI OR SHAKTI YOGA

Shakti = Life energy as power
Kundalini = Nervous system
Shakti yoga = Awakening of nervous system by power.
Mooladhar chakra = Sacral plexus
Components are: Mantra yoga, hatha yoga, laya yoga, raja yoga, tantra yoga.

BIBLIOGRAPHY

1. A retrospective on yoga research. Indian J Phy and Pharm 1991;35:79-83.
2. Anand BK, et al. Studies on subjects staying in an air tight pit. Indian J Med Res 1968;46:1282.
3. Anand BK. Yoga and medical science. Indian J Phy and Pharma 1991;35:84-87.
4. Anand BK, et al. Studies on Ramanand Yogi during his stay in an air tight box. Indian J Med Res 1961;49:82.
5. Anand BK, Chhina GS, Baldev Singh. Some aspects of Electroencephalographic studies in Yogis. Indian Journal of Physiology and Pharmacology, 1991;35:(I).
6. Augustus T. Miller. Physiology of Exercises. The CV Mosby Co. St Louis: 1959.
7. Instant yoga for every busy persons by Pd. Shiv Sharma and Kailash Sharma, Arnold Heinemann Publisher 1977.
8. Jayadeva Yogendra, J Clement Vaz (Eds). Yoga today. The Macmillan Co. India (P) Ltd. 1977.
9. Kundalini yoga by R.K. Karanjia. Arnold Heinemann Publisher 1977.
10. Mazumdar S. Yogic Exercises, Orient Longmans 1960.
11. Nancy Phelan and Michail Volin. Yoga for woman - Stanley Paul London 1963.
12. Wenger MA, Anand BK. Experiments in Indian Yogi on Voluntary Control of heart and pulse. Circulation 1961;24:1319-25.
13. Wenger MA, Bagchi BK, Anand BK. Indian Journal of Physiology and Pharmacology 1991;35(I).

APPENDIX 3

Evolutionary Differences: Comparative Aspects

PHYSIOLOGY OF DIGESTION

There are various species in animal kingdom. Some are living on restricted foodstuffs while others are having wide field of foodstuffs. Broadly speaking nature of feeding mechanism is certainly dependent upon habitat and availability of food, and on this basis their digestive tract is also framed. Let us briefly study this part too.

STRUCTURAL VARIATIONS

Here are some fundamental structural variations

a. *Salivary glands:*
   i. These are reduced or absent in whales.
   ii. In frog and toad lingual glands tend to secrete a viscous fluid material which help in insect capturing.
   iii. Venom of snakes is, in fact coming from labial gland of upper jaw which is considered as homologous with animal's parotid gland.
   iv. Anterior and posterior sublingual gland are only present in birds.

b. *Tongue:*
   i. In birds it is covered with some horny material and provided with thorn like projections and strangely it cannot be protruded.
   ii. In turtles and crocodiles tongue is not prehensile lying in floor of mouth.
   iii. Snakes and lizards has well developed tongue capable of extension and retraction.
   iv. In fishes primary tongue is a non-muscular one.

c. *Oesophagus*
   i. Amongst mammals, giraffe has got largest Oesophagus.
   ii. Short oesophagus together with cilia is found in amphibians and this ciliated epithelium produces 'propepsin' which actively works in acidic media in stomach.
   iii. Its lining is covered with backward directing cornified papillae in marine turtles.

d. *Stomach*
   i. Cardiac and fundus are two parts of this organ in frog.
   ii. It assumes sac like appearance by bending upon itself in reptiles and as it appears spindle shaped in snakes and lizards.
   iii. In birds, two regions are seen in stomach named as proventriculus and gizzard, former is secreting a digestive enzyme while later is a thick muscular structure.
   iv. Hourglass stomach is found in monkeys, rodent and some other mammals where a line of constriction separates cardiac and fundus regions.
   v. In blood sucking animals like bats, an elastic pouch is constituted by drawing out of pyloric region.

e. *Liver*
   i. Amphibias are having large lobulated liver.
   ii. Reptiles are also having well-defined organ.
   iii. Birds are though having well-defined liver but their gall bladder is absent.
   iv. The mammals lacking gall bladder includes rodents, whales, perissodactyla, rats and certainly these animals have very little affection with fats.

f. *Pancreas*
   i. It is absent in amphioxus while widely diffused in teleosts and bony fishes.
   ii. Pancreatic bladder is representation of this organ in cats.
   iii. It is also well-defined in lamprey.

g. *Intestine*
   i. The length of whole gut is short in carnivorous as compared to herbivorous animals, the division of small and large intestine is unclear even in cyclostomes.

ii. No jejunum is well marked in amphibians.
iii. A structure called colic caecum is developed at the junction of small and large intestine in reptiles while it is not seen in crocodiles and turtles.
iv. In rabbits ileum and caecum are well differentiated.
v. In birds the structure colic caeca is developed.
vi. Rectum with specialised salt secreting glands (NaCl) is seen in sharks playing a leading role in osmoregulation.
vii. Rectum opens into cloaca in amphibias while it opens outside through a separate anus in cyclostoms, teleosts etc.

RESPIRATORY SYSTEM

In frogs:

a. Cutaneous respiration is the accessory. During their hibernation period they respire by this route. They take O_2 as 50 ml/kg body wt/hour.
b. *Bucco-pharyngeal*: Mucosa is ideally adapted for gaseous exchange. During this mouth, glottis and gullet remain closed but nares are open. The floor of the cavity is alternatively raised and lowered. Atmospheric air is sucked into cavity through nares when the floor lowers and is forced out when floor rises.
c. *Pulmonary ventilation:* Accounts for 65 per cent of total O_2 intake. It is by lungs. Gaseous exchange between atmospheric air and blood in the lungs takes place across the thin and highly vascularised wall of alveoli. Lungs also help the frog in quietly floating at water surface. They inflate their lungs with air. So becoming buoyant in this way, they rise up to water surface and keep passively floating until undisturbed.

CENTRAL NERVOUS SYSTEMS

1. Birds have a large cerebellum; less olfactory sense but powerful eyesight.
2. In cockroach it is composed of brain, nerve cord and nerve fibres.
3. Developed brain with ten pairs of cranial nerves in amphibia.
4. There are twelve pairs of cranial nerves from the brain, in reptile.
5. In camel, eyelids are modified having big eyelashes. Nostrils are reduced to small holes, because of dusty/stormy environment. Organs of special senses are well developed.

CARDIOVASCULAR SYSTEMS

1. In birds (class Aves) heart is four chambered.
2. In cockroach; blood vessels are absent. The blood filled body cavity is called haemocoel. Due to absence of haemoglobin blood is colourless. The blood has fluid filled plasma and blood cells called haemocytes.
3. In amphibia, heart is three chambered. RBC are oval, biconvex and nucleated.
4. In reptiles, three chambered heart with incomplete ventricular partition.
5. The Giraffe's blood pressure may be highest 300/200.
6. The only fish of species of "Antarctic fish," have white blood. No red pigment.
7. Nereis and Amphioxus don't have heart. Blue whale has the largest heart.

REPRODUCTION

1. In amphibia, sexes are separate and fertilisation is external. A larval stage is present in life history. Eggs are mesolecithal.
2. In reptiles, sexes are separate and fertilisation is internal. They are oviparous having cleidoic eggs.
3. In birds (Aves), right ovary and right oviduct are rudimentary. Birds are oviparous, eggs are large, megalecithal and cleiodic. During development embryo is surrounded by amnion, allantois, yolk sac and chorion.
4.

Species	*Kind of cycle*
Dog	mono-oestrus
Sheep	poly-oestrus
Cow	poly-oestrus
Horse	poly-oestrus
Monkey	menstrual cycle

EXCRETION

1. In amphibia kidneys perform the function of excretion. Skin is scaleless, soft, slimy and moist.
2. In reptiles, skin has no glands.
3. In cockroach, excretory system is made up of malpighian tubules which are excretory organs. They are 70-90 in number in six bundles. It excretes uric acid.
4. Excretory system is a tube-like canal in roundworms.

5. Animals living in dry conditions (e.g. land reptiles like lizard and snakes, most insects, birds etc.) have to conserve water in their bodies. So they synthesise crystals of uric acid from ammonia (uricotellic excretion).
6. In camel, colour of skin is similar to dust to protect from other hunter animals.

CIRCULATION AND CLIMATE

- The heart of a hibernating animal (ground squirrel) can beat effectively at 5-10 beats/minute rate at low temperatures. It will continue to beat even after removing from the body and placing in un-oxygenated saline.
- The heart of a non-hibernating animal stops beating within few minutes.
- With decreasing the body temperature heart rate decreases in dogs (At 18-20°C temperature—20 beats per minute), blood pressure also decreases. This causes an increase in duration of systole and isometric relaxation + duration of diastole.
- The cardiac output of dogs at body temperature of 20°C is about 15 per cent of normal. Though coronary blood flow is reduced but is adequate for usual needs of myocardium.
- In dogs, on hypothermia, ventricular fibrillations exist. Here calcium shifting in the heart while potassium is leaving.

LOCOMOTION

1. *Fishes:* With the help of fins and muscles. Tail also help.
2. *Reptiles:* Creeping with the help of legs (except snakes). Wall lizards are provided with cup like pads. Snakes move with help of ribs and scales.
3. *Camel:* Long limbs, feet are covered with furs and are fleshy at basal part forming a pad like structure.

APPENDIX 4

Normal Values—Serum

Albumin	3.0 - 5.5 gm/dl	
Amylase	2 - 20 U/litre	
Bilirubin	Total	0.2 - 1.2 mg/dl
	direct	0 - 0.4 mg/dl
Calcium	8.7 - 10.6 mg/dl	
Chloride	95 - 105 mEq/litre (m mol/litre)	
Creatinine	0.7 - 1.5 mg/dl male adult	
	0.5 - 1.3 mg/dl Female adult	
Glucose	80 - 120 mg/dl	
Total Iron	40 - 150 µg/dl	
Iodine	3 - 6.5 µg/dl	
Protein bound iodine	4 - 8 µg/dl	
Lipase	4 - 24 IU/dl	
Inorganic phosphorous	2 - 4.3 mg/dl	
SGOT	5 - 40 IU/litre	
SGPT	5 - 30 IU/litre	
Sodium	135 - 145 mEq/litre	
Vitamin A	0.15 - 0.60 µg/ml	
Vitamin B_{12}	200 - 850 Pg/ml	

APPENDIX 5

Conversion Units

Length

One km	=	0.62 mile
One mile	=	5280 feet or 1.61 km
One inch	=	2.54 cm
One meter	=	100 cm or 39.37 inches
One millimeter	=	0.1 cm (10^{-1})
One micron	=	0.0001 cm (10^{-4})
One millimicron	=	0.0000001 cm (10^{-7})

Weights

One pound	=	453.6 gm or 16 ounces
One kg	=	1000 gm
One mg	=	0.001 gm
One grain	=	65 milligrams

Respiration

a. *Alveolar gas (partial pressure)*

Po_2	=	104 mmHg
Pco_2	=	38 mmHg

b. *CO_2 to O_2 gradients (ml/100 ml)*

	Ambient air	*Expired air*	*Alveolar air*	*Arterial blood*
O_2	20.94	16.3	14	20.0
CO_2	0.04	4.4	5.6	48.0
N_2	79.02	79.07	80.4	0.8

APPENDIX 6

Paying Honour: Historical Review

Great persons and their great works are just like foundation bricks or stone of this attractive building so-called human body. Let us give tribute/honour to all of them who may be called as pioneers in specific field.

- The first great gift to medicine came from the mind of Greek genius ***Hippocrates*** (C. 460 BC - C370 BC) - the father of medicine. He rescued medicine from clutches of superstitions and placed it on podium of scientific reasoning. His keen eye at bedside and his nimble brain laid foundation for modern clinical medicine.
- Another Greek ***Asclepiades*** (C-124 BC - 40 BC) recognised and stressed the importance of rest, message, diet and exercise.
- (1676) ***Antony Van Leeuwenhoek*** (Amsterdum) is credited as early discoverer of microscope. Father of Bacteriology.
- Physiology in its present form is a relative newcomer on the stage of biological science. Physician of Roman Empire Claudius, ***Galen*** (Greek Physician 131-210?) performed many experiments. In that time it was thought that all living things were controlled by a mystical influence called *vital force.*
- After passing this era of vital force, there was a trend towards logic approach. ***Theophrastus Hopenheium*** (1490-1541; wrote under the name of ***Paracelsus***, German) attempted to study the actions of body in much the same way as we do today. He developed methods which actually form the basis of many modern concepts.
- Greatest contribution was made by ***William Harvey*** (1578-1657; Englishman) who published a book in Latin entitled *"Exercito anatomica de motu cardies et sanguinis in animalibus"* of 72 pages only (commonly translated as "Anatomical dissertation on the movement of the heart and blood in animals). He demonstrated clearly that the flow of blood around the body is really a circulatory movement in which arteries, veins and capillaries form the conducting channels.
- Since microscope was not fully developed up to that time Harvey had to imagine that the smallest vessels capillaries are present. Their presence was demonstrated by Italian anatomist ***Marcello Malpighi*** (1632).
- Harvey's work did not receive any attention for sometime. It was only after Descartes and others who made it popularised.
- ***Claude Bernard*** (1813-1878) published his book "The way of a medical investigator" which appeared in 1865 and heralded the dawn of a new era in physiological science.
  Galen constructed an incorrect scheme of blood circulation with liver as the central organ.
- Physiology as an independent science was founded in 17th century and it was by William Harvey. The middle ages were characterised by stagnation in science, including medicine.
- ***I. Sechenov*** (1829-1905) was founder of Russian physiology. He discovered phenomenon of inhibition in CNS. He was first to study composition of gases in blood, elucidated the role and importance of haemoglobin in transportation of O_2, CO_2 etc.
- ***I. P. Pavlov*** (1849-1936) was a brilliant materialistic scientist and invented conditioned reflex and lot of work has been done on gastric physiology.

GREAT CONTRIBUTORS IN DIGESTIVE SYSTEM

1. *William Prout (1785 - 1850)*: English physiologic chemist, educated at Edinburg University, got M.D. in 1811. His contribution is really classic in the world of physiology and that is, in 1823 he found that stomach contains free HCl. He is also famous for his speculation that atomic weights of all the elements are exact multiples of that of hydrogen or half of it.

2. *Theodor Schwann (1810 - 1882)*: Basically a zoologist. The credit goes to him for discovering enzyme pepsin of gastric juice, confirming the fact that acid of gastric juice is HCl not lactic acid. He is also famous for his famous Schwann sheath, yeast cell theory of putrefaction, neurophysiological concept of neuron theory.
3. *Ivan Petrovitch Pavlov (1849 - 1936)*: Great Russian physiologist educated at St. Petersburg, got M.D. in 1883. Worked on gastric secretion, discovered psychic phase and got Nobel prize in 1904. All this further gave him success to discover conditioned reflex. He was professor in military medical academy.
4. *Watter Bradford Cannon (1871-1945)*: He is the discoverer of method of study of normal GIT movements, diagnosis of ulcer, malignancy etc. The techniques we do everyday in hospital laboratories are actually derived from his work. Educated at Harvard University and got MD in 1900 and was professor there.
5. *William Maddock Bayliss (1860 - 1924) and Ernest Henry Starling (1866 - 1927)*: Together they discovered hormone secretin, electrical phenomenon of heart beat, arrangement of vasomotor phenomenon in sympathetic nervous system. Bayliss was professor at university college London, was first man to got Copley Medal of Royal society in 1919.
6. *William Beaumont (1785-1853)*: A United States army physician. He studied the digestive process through a permanent gastric fistula which was produced in young French Canadian voya geur Alexis St. Martin by a gunshot wound. Inspite of his repeated dressings he could not prevent a permanent opening into stomach which opens the doors of further research for him and due to it, he confirmed the presence of HCl and pepsin in gastric juice.

GREAT CONTRIBUTORS IN EXCRETORY SYSTEM

1. *Lorenzo-Bellini (1643-1704)*: Italian anatomist. Famous for his classical description of gross anatomy of the kidney in which he announced the discovery of renal secretory ducts known after his name Bellini's ducts. He showed that kidneys are not merely flesh like spleen, liver etc. but consist of minute ducts, and he elaborated a mechanical theory for the formation of urine.
2. *Marcello Malpighi (1628-1694)*: The discovery of Bellini was important for Malpighi because it showed him that kidney had a minute structure analogous to that of secreting glands. He hence sought for the glandular unit in which urine might be formed from arterial blood.
3. *Richard Bright (1789-1858)*: Born at Queen square-Bristol, studied medicine at Edinburg. He was assistant physician to Guy's Hospital where he performed his greatest work upto death. He correlated the appearance of certain kinds of dropsy with albuminous urine and with a diseased state of kidney. He also studied functions of kidney. He established the relation of kidney and with hypertension.
4. *Sir William Bowman (1816-1892)*: Ophthalmic surgeon of King's College Hospital, London. He was eminent physiologist, histologist and morbid anatomist. He reached to zenith of his career before the age of 26th. He was made a fellow of royal society on his work entitled, "On the minute structure and movement of voluntary muscle." He also published his theory of urinary secretion and his discovery of capsule surrounding the Malpighian body is remarkable. He thus established for the first time the anatomical frame work within which any theory of kidney function must be placed.

   Bowman: Water alone was separated at Malpighian body while the dissolved constituents of urine was secreted by epithelium of urinary tubules.

   Ludwig: A filtrate containing all water soluble constituents of the blood was separated at glomerulus and that a process of selective reabsorption occurred in urinary tubule.
5. *Carl Friedrich Wilhelm Ludwig (1816-1895)*: Greatest physiologist of 19th century. He became professor of physiology at Leipzig where he has established an institute for physiology.

GREAT CONTRIBUTORS IN ENDOCRINOLOGY

1. *George Redmayne Murray (1865-1939):* Born in England. Educated at Cambridge. He was professor of comparative pathology at Durham university and later on he shifted to Manchester university where he was professor of systemic medicine until 1925. He decided to attempt the treatment of myxoedema by thyroid extract when he was a young houseman at university college hospital London. It was he who introduced the term 'testosterone.' This male sex hormone was first isolated in crystalline form by Adoeph F. J. Butenandt (1931) who was awarded Nobel prize.
2. *John Jacob Abel (1857-1939)*: A pioneer worker in development of physiology and experimental medicine in America (a native of ohio). After two years as professor of pharmacology at university of Michigan, he went in 1893 to John Hopkin university

where he remained long. His most important contribution is crystallisation of insulin in 1926 and his early studies on adrenal medullary hormone.

3. *Henry Hallett Dale (1875)*: Educated at Trinitty College Cambridge. He continued to work at Cambridge in physiology under John Newport Langley (1852-1925). He also worked with E. H. Starling at university college London and in laboratory of Paul Ehrlich at Frankfurt.

    He shared the Nobel prize with *Otto Loewi* (1873-1936) for their discoveries relating to chemical transmission of nerve impulses. Dale has demonstrated the production of acetylcholine at the end plates of motor nerves in skeletal muscle. Loewi showed that acetylcholine was also identical with 'vagustuffe' which he had found to be produced at the nerve endings of the vagus. Otto Loewi occupied the chair of pharmacology at Graz since 1909. He studied nuclein metabolism, diabetes, renal function, digitalis and ANS.

4. *Alfred Erich Frank (1884)*: Born in Berlin, graduated in medicine. He showed in 1912 that diabetes insipidus was associated with a disturbance of pituitary.

5. *Friederick Grant Banting (1891-1941)*: Born near Alliston Ontario, educated at Toronto where he completed the medical course in end of 1916 and joined army medical corps. He was oversea medical officer from 1917-1919. He worked as an orthopaedician at Sick's children hospital Toronto. While remaining at London he became interested in diabetes.

    His work on isolation of insulin was in limelight in 1921, and he was assisted by C. H. Best and J. B. Collip. The first diabetic patient were treated successfully in 1922. Banting along with JJR Macleod got Noble prize in medicine for 1923. He was appointed as professor of medical research at university of Toronto and awarded as an annuity for life by parliament of Canada. At university of Toronto Banting institute was established for medical research in 1930. In 1941 on a war time mission to Britain he died of injuries and exposure following an air crash in New found land.

6. *Charles Herbert Best:* Born at west Pembroke, Maine and was educated at university of Toronto. He assisted Banting in his work on insulin. He became professor of physiology since 1941 at university of Toronto.

7. *Bernardo-Alberto Houssay (1887):* Born at Buenos Aires where he got his education too. In 1911 he got M.D. degree for a thesis on pituitary body. He was appointed as professor of physiology at school of veterinary medicine. Later on he became professor of physiology at medical school and director of institute of physiology. In 1944, he shifted to a private institute of experimental biology and medicine where he continued to study functions of hypophysis and in 1947 he shared nobel prize in medicine with C.F. and G.T. Cori, and with Biasotti (1931). "On role of anterior pituitary in sugar metabolism."

8. *James Bertram Collip (1892-1965)*: Born at Belleville, ontario, educated at university of Toronto. He became professor of biochemistry at McGill university in 1928; In 1947 Dean of medical faculty at university of western Ontario upto 1961. His important work is on adreno-cortico tropic hormone.

9. *Edward Calvin Kendall (1886)*: Emeritus professor since his retirement in 1951. Educated at Columbia university. He succeeded in isolating pure crystalline thyroxine from extracts of thyroid. Before it pure crystalline adrenaline was isolated by Abel and Crawford in 1897. Then in 1934, he and his co-workers succeeded in isolating crystalline from the physiologically active hormone of suprarenal cortex. This was announced on 13th April. In 1950 Kendall, Philip S. Hench (1896-1965) and Tradeus Reich Steen (1897) were jointly awarded the nobel prize for their work on adreno corticotropic hormone.

GREAT CONTRIBUTORS IN REPRODUCTORY MEDICINE

1. *Gabriele Falloppio (Fallopius, 1523-1562)*: Anatomist of Venice. Favorite pupil of *Andreas Vesalius (1514-1564)*. Discoverer of Fallopian tube, seminal vesicles in male, named placenta, ovaries, hymen, clitoris etc. He published two books.

2. *Charles Edouard-Brown-Sequard (1817-1894)*: French American neurophysiologist-endocrinologist and clinician. (a) In 1856 he proved that excision of both adrenal glands invariably prove fatal; they are indispensable for life; (b) He proved that sexual power of ageing human male could be restored and a man rejuvenated through injection of testicular extract; (c) In 1852 he noted that stimulation of cervical sympathetic chain evoked contraction of the small vessels of rabbit's ear accompanied by a fall of temperature where a simple section of sympathetic trunk led to vasomotor paralysis, dilatation and increased temperature of ear, (d) He observed that when a lateral hemisection of the cord is performed, there follows Brown-Sequard paralysis characterised

by loss of motor power and position sense on the side of lesion, with loss of pain and thermal sensibilities on the side opposite to lesion. This was published in three instalments in Journal de-physiologic in Paris.

GREAT CONTRIBUTORS IN VASCULAR SYSTEM

1. *Aristotle of Stagira (384-322 B.C.)*: Greek philosopher, biologist. His interests were on sex, growth, heredity, nutrition etc. He made some errors like intelligence lies in the heart, the arteries contain air as well as blood etc. Born as son of a court physician in hamlet of Stagira in Thrace. His teachings spread to every corner of the world and during twenty-five centuries since his death he exerted a profound and determining influence on medical and biological thought.
2. *William Harvey (1578-1657)*: He announced his discovery that blood circulates; on 17th April 1616 at a lecture to the college of physicians in London. He also popularised the presence of valves in the veins. He was born in English coastal town of Folkestone on 1st April 1578. Got M. D. degree in 1602 while working under eminent professor of anatomy Fabricius of Aquapendonte.
3. *Stephen Hales (1677-1761)*: He took the next step after Harvey and Malpighi in describing the physiology of circulation. The determination of blood pressure made it possible to calculate the work done by the heart and to estimate for the first time the magnitude of peripheral resistance. He made critical microscopic observations on capillaries in living state.
4. *Friedrich Hermann Stannius (1808-1883)*: Born at Hambarg; studied at Berlin with Helmholtz, and Dubois Reymond. His experiments are striking because they illustrate vagal inhibition of the heart beat and indicate the existence of a pacemaker.
5. *Wilhem His Jr. (1863-1934)*: Anatomist and cardiologist. His research on embryonic heart led to the discovery of auriculo-ventricular bundle, was first announced in 1893. He also showed that following section of A-V-bundle the auricular and ventricular beats become dissociated.
6. *Ernest Henry Starling (1866-1927)*: He postulated his law in 1915.

GREAT CONTRIBUTORS IN MUSCLE AND PERIPHERAL NERVE FUNCTIONING

1. *Galen (131-201 A-D)*: Suggested the significance of reflex action. His simple experiments on action of individual muscle and muscle groups.
2. *Arachibald Vivian Hill (A V Hill) (1870-1943)*: Biophysicist, educated at Trinity College, Cambridge. He was appointed professor of physiology at university college in 1923. He with William Hartree contributed extensively to knowledge of thermodynamics of muscle. He continued to persue the elusive problem of heat production in muscle and nerve (for which he got nobel prize in 1922 shared with Otto Meyerhof). Since his first paper on the action of nicotine and curare as determined by temperature co-efficients and form of contraction curves of muscle twitch. In coming days he could increase both the speed and sensitivity of his heat detecting thermo-couples.
3. *Alan Loyd Hodgkin (1914) and Andrew Fielding Huxley (1918):* These were the first persons to succeed in the difficult task of inserting electrodes into a living giant nerve fibres, and thereby measuring directly the action potential within nerve fibre. They have further shown that generation of nerve impulse was accompanied by a leakage of potassium ions across the membrane with a resulting marked change in membrane conductance and during recovery that potassium ions are reabsorbed. In 1952, they were able to publish equations which accurately predicted the form of the conductance changes and the form and amplitude of action potential during impulse transmission and allowed them to restrict the number of possible kinds of ionic events which might produce these changes. This work was recognised in 1963 when both of them shared the nobel prize with *Sir John Carew Eccles* in physiology.

   Hodgkin born at Danbury near Oxford England educated at Trinity College Cambridge. In 1952, he was appointed Foulerton Research Professor of the Royal society.
4. *Edgar Douglas Adrian (1889):* Shared nobel prize with Sir Charles Sherrington on his fundamental discoveries concerning the mechanism of sense organs and motor nerve cells and structure of nerve messages.

GREAT CONTRIBUTORS IN BLOOD CAPILLARIES

1. *Marshal Hall (1790-1857):* A well known contributor to the physiology of nervous system. He has gone through a series of observation on capillary circulation in such membranous structures, e.g. web of frog's foot; a fish tail and mesentery. He clearly distinguished the true capillaries from the arterioles.
2. *Ernest Henry Starling (1866-1927)*: British physiologist, eminent teacher held the chair at University College London — made series of works with W. M. Bayliss- like hormone control of pancreas,

nature of lymph, functional significance of osmotic pressure of proteins of the blood. He first of all pointed out that since capillaries were permeable to the blood crystalloids the effective osmotic pressure is exerted by serum proteins and that this is responsible for absorption of fluid from the tissues, a point of particular significance to the physiology of kidney.

3. *Thomas Lewis (1881-1945)*: Cardiologist.

GREAT CONTRIBUTORS IN RESPIRATION

1. *Joseph Priestley (1733-1804)*: Born at Field head, Yorkshire. His isolation of O_2 has been the subject of much dispute. He also studied the relationship between air and blood. Full credit of discovery of oxygen was given to *Lavoisier*.
2. *John Scott Haldane (1860-1936)*: Oxford physiologist for respiration with methods of gas analysis. His apparatus was described in 1892. He told that CO_2 tension served as normal stimulus for respiration centre. The explanation of apnoea following forced breathing was a direct corollary to their observation upon the influence of CO_2 tension.
3. *Yandell Henderson (1873-1944)*: Professor of applied physiology at Yale University (1921-38). He recommended administration of CO_2 in shock (anaesthesia, drowning, co-poisoning).
4. *Joseph Barcroft (1872-1947)*: Professor of physiology at Cambridge. He is well known for his studies of haemoglobin and physiology of life at high altitudes. Later he concerned himself with functions of spleen and physiology of developing foetus. He believed that exchange of substances through lung epithelium and tissues occur by virtue of simple process of diffusion.
5. *Friederick Gowland Hopkins (1861-1947)*: Professor of biochemistry at Cambridge, studied medicine at Guy's hospital qualifying in 1894. He became a fellow of royal society in 1905. He shared a Nobel prize with Christian Eijkmann (1929) for his discovery of growth stimulating vitamins. Finally he discovered glutathione — a respiratory enzyme of tissues which shed light upon metabolic processes occurring peripherally.

GREAT CONTRIBUTORS IN CENTRAL NERVOUS SYSTEM

1. *Wilder G. Penfield (1891)*: Born at Spokane Washington, M. D. from John Hopkins Medical School in 1918. He was pioneer in electrical stimulation of cerebral cortex of human subjects during brain operation. He discovered thought pattern including vivid recall of past experience.
2. *Sir Charles Bell (1774-1842)*: Anatomist, born in Edinburg; a beautiful writer. Discoverer of functions of anterior and posterior roots of spinal cord.
3. *Francois Magendie (1783-1855)*: Pioneer experimental physiologist of France. Functions of roots of spinal nerves.
4. *Errist Heinrich Weber (1795-1878) and Edward Friedrich Weber (1806-1871)*: Shared the discovery of inhibitory power of vagus nerves upon the beating of the heart. The Weber induced inhibition at first by connecting one pole of an electromagnet apparatus to nostril of a frog and other to mid region of the spinal cord and they deserve great credit for finally tracing the pathway of effect which they observed to the vagus.
5. *Sir Charles Scott Sherrington (1857-1952)*: Professor of Physiology at Oxford from 1913-1955, born at London, educated at Gonville and Caius College Cambridge. After M. B. he studied pathology at Berlin with Koch and Virchow. He shared the Nobel prize with E.D. Adrian in 1932 for discoveries regarding the functions of neurons. The present day knowledge of neuro physiology, e.g. nature of Knee jerk, reciprocal innervation of motor area, focal epilepsy, proprioceptive system, final common pathway etc. has emerged from his work.
6. *Harvey Cushing (1869-1939)*: Professor of surgery at Harvard medical school and surgeon in chief of Peter-Bent Brigham hospital for two decades (1912-1932) born in Cleavland, educated at Harvard medical school. He established the direct evidence that irritation of the post-central gyrus gives rise to sensation.

REFLEXES: HISTORY

1. In 1830, ***Bell*** in England, and ***Magendi*** in France established the functions of dorsal and ventral roots of spinal cord.
2. *Sherrington* at oxford had begun a detailed investigation of properties of extensor and flexor reflexes.
3. Spanish histochemist ***Ramon y cajal*** argued that sensory and motor neuron were contiguous and not continuous.
4. In 1920-26 by ***Gasser*** and ***Erlanger*** electro physiological studies were introduced, i.e. cathode ray oscilloscope for the study of electrical responses of nerve and spinal cord.
5. By the same techniques, ***Adrian*** investigated the receptor response.

6. ***Lloyd*** made a definite study of spinal reflexes in 1940.
7. ***Eccles*** (1946) examined the events of excitation and inhibition at the neuronal level.
8. Action potential was analysed in 1950-55 by ***Huxley, Hodgkin*** and ***Katz***.

LABYRINTHINE REFLEXES

- 1924- *Magnus* observation was that if change in position of labyrinth takes place, then there occurs increased tone in the muscles of all forelimbs.
- After few years, *Roberts* has done experiment on cat. Neck reflexes were eliminated by denervation of first three inter-vertebral joints in cervical region. He noted that when head was tilted to nose down position, there occurs extension of forelimbs and flexion of hindlimbs. When head was tilted to right side down position, there was extension of right forelimb. Lateral rotation of head produced no effect and he explained that it cannot stimulate otolith organs.

CLASSICAL EXPERIMENT FOR CORPUS CALLOSUM FUNCTION IN MONKEY

Corpus callosum was cut and optic chiasm was split longitudinally so that signal from each eye can go only to cerebral hemisphere on the side of the eye. The animal is taught to recognise different types of objects with its right eye while left is covered. Next the right eye is covered and animal is tested to determine whether or not its left eye can recognise the same object. The left eye cannot recognise the object. The experiment was repeated in another monkey with optic chiasma split but corpus callosum intact. So it was thought that recognition in one hemisphere of the brain creates recognition in opposite hemisphere.

CLASSICAL EXPERIMENT—LIMBIC SYSTEM

A lever is placed at the side of a cage. It is arranged so that depressing the lever makes electric contact with a stimulator. At different areas of the brain electrodes are placed so that animal is able to stimulate the particular area by pressing the lever. If particular area gives reward it will continuously press it. By this *reward and punishment centres* are discovered. Reward centres are said to be located in lateral and ventromedial nuclei of hypothalamus.

BIBLIOGRAPHY

1. Best and Taylor, Physiological Basis of Medical Practice, Williams and Wilkinson Co. 1967.
2. David A. Myshne. Human Anatomy and Physiology. Translated from Russian - MIR Publishers, Moscow 1971.
3. Guyton AC, Medical Physiology. W.B. Saunders Co.
4. Hill AV. The absence of temperature changes during the transmission of a nervous impulse. J Phy (London), 1912;43:433-40.
5. Hill AV. The mode of action of nicotine and curaris determined by the form of contraction curve and method of temperature coefficients. J Phy (London) 1909;39:361-73.
6. Hodgkin AL, Huxley AF. Resting and action potential in single nerve fibre. J Phy (London) 1945;104:176-95.
7. Hodgkin AL, Huxley AF. A quantitative description of membrane current and its application to conduction and excitation in nerve. J Phy (London) 1952;117:500-44.
8. Selected Readings in History of physiology compiled by John. F. Fulton and Leonard G. Wilson Second edition, Charles C. Thomas - Publisher Spring Field - Illinois - U.S.A. 1966.

	Name	Year	Work	Country
	NOBEL PRIZE WINNERS			
1.	RONALD ROSS	1902	MALARIA	U. K.
2.	IVAN PETROVICH PAVLOV	1904	PHYSIOLOGY OF DIGESTION	RUSSIA
3.	ROBERT KOCH	1905	DISCOVERY OF TUBERCULOSIS	GERMANY
4.	CAMILO GOLGI	1906	STRUCTURE OF NERVOUS SYSTEM	ITALY
	S. R. CAJAL			SPAIN
5.	ELIE METCHNIKOFF	1908	IMMUNITY	RUSSIA
	PAUL EHRLICH			
		1908	IMMUNITY	SILESIA
6.	THEODOR KOCHER	1909	THYROID - PATHOPHYSIOLOGY AND SURGERY	SWITZERLAND
7.	ALLVAR GULLSTRAND	1911	DIOPTRICS OF THE EYE	SWEDEN
8.	CHARLES RICHET	1913	ANAPHYLAXIS	FRANCE
9.	ROBERT BA 'RA' NY	1914	PATHOPHYSIOLOGY OF VESTIBULAR APPARATUS	AUSTRIA
10.	ARCHIBALD-VIVIAN HILL	1922	PRODUCTION OF HEAT IN MUSCLE	ENGLAND
	AND OTTO MEYERHOF		CONSUMPTION OF OXYGEN AND METABOLISM OF LACTIC ACID IN MUSCLE	GERMANY
11.	FREDRICH GIANT BANTING	1923	INSULIN	CANADA
	JOHN JAMES			ENGLAND
12.	WILLIUM EINTHOVEN	1924	ELECTROCARDIOGRAM	DUTCH EAST INDIES
13.	KARL LANDSTEINER	1930	BLOOD GROUPS	AUSTRIA
14.	CHARLES SHERRINGTON	1932	FUNCTION OF NEURONS	ENGLAND
	EDGER-DOUGLAS-ADRIAN			
15.	HENRY DALE	1936	TRANSMISSION OF NERVE IMPULSES	ENGLAND
	OTTO LOEWI			GERMANY
16.	BERNARDO-ALBERTO	1947	ANTERIOR PITUITARY LOBE	ARGENTINA
	HOUSSAY AND CARL F. CORI		GLYCOGEN CATALYSIS	CZECHOSLOVAKIA
17.	WALTER RUDOLF HESS	1949	ORGANISATION OF INTER BRAIN AS A CO-ORDINATOR OF ACTIVITIES	SWITZERLAND
18.	EDWARD CALVIN KANDALL	1950	SUPRA RENAL CORTEX HORMONES	USA
	PHILIP SHOW WALTER HENCH			PITTSBURGH
	TADEUS REICHESTEIN			POLAND
19.	HANS ADOLF KREBS FRITIZ	1953	CITRIC ACID CYCLE CO-ENZYME A	GERMANY
	ALBERT LIPMANN			
20.	GEORGE VON BE 'KE' SY	1961	MECHANISM OF STIMULATION IN COCHLEA	HUNGARY
21.	A. L. HODGKIN	1963	NERVOUS FUNCTIONING	USA
	A.F. HUXLEY			
	JOHN ECCLES			
22.	RANGER GRANIT	1967	VISUAL MECHANISM	SWEDEN
	H. K. HARTLINE			GERMANY
	GEORGE WALD			
23.	SIR BERNARD KATZ (FRS)	1970	NEUROMUSCULAR AND SYNAPTIC TRANSMISSION	ENGLAND
24.	ROGER GUILLEMIN	1977	PEPTIDE HORMONE OF THE BRAIN	SAN DIEGO
25.	G. N. HOUSFIELD (FRS)	1979	COMPUTERISED TOMOGRAPHY	HAYES, ENGLAND
	ALLAN CORMACK			BOSTON, USA
26.	ROGER, SPENY	1981	CEREBRAL HEMISPHERE	CALIFORNIA, USA
	DAVID HUBEL		VISUAL STIMULI	HARVARD

27.	SUNE BEGSTROM BENGT SAMUELSSON	1982	PROSTAGLANDINS IN HUMAN METABOLISM	SWEDEN
28.	STANLEY COHEN RITA-LEVI-MONTALCINI	1986	EPIDERMAL GROWTH FACTOR NERVE GROWTH FACTOR	USA, ROME, ITALY
29.	HAROLD E. VARMUS	1989	CANCER GENETICS	USA
30.	ERWIN NEHER BERT SAKMANN	1991	FUNCTION OF SINGLE ION CHANNELS IN CELLULAR MECHANISM	GERMANY
31.	STANLEY PRUSINOR	1997	BIOCHEMICAL ASPECTS OF AND MAD COW	AMERICA
32.	SYDNEY BRENNER H. ROBERT HERVITZ SIR JOHN E. SUSLTON	2002	GENETIC REGULATION OF ORGAN DEVELOPMENT AND PROGRAMMED CELL DEATH	SALK INSTITUTE WELLCOME TRUST SANGER INSTITUTE MASSACHUSETT'S INSTITUTE OF TECHNOLOGY
33.	PAUL C. LAUTERBUR SIR PETER MANSFIELD	2003	MAGNETIC RESONANCE IMAGING	UNIVERSITY OF ILLINOIS UNIVERSITY OF NOTTINGHAM
34.	RICHARD AXEL AND LINDA B. BUCK	2004	ODORANT RECEPTORS AND ORGANIZATION OF OLFACTORY SYSTEM	
35.	BARRY MARSHAL ROBIN WARREN	2005	THE BACTERIUM H.PYLORI AND ITS ROLE IN GASTRITIS AND PEPTIC ULCER DISEASE	AUSTRALIA

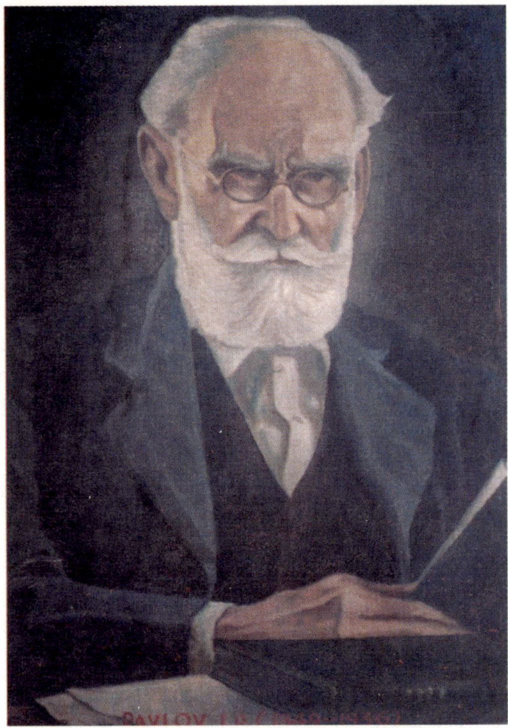

Fig. 1: I.P. Pavlov (1849-1936)

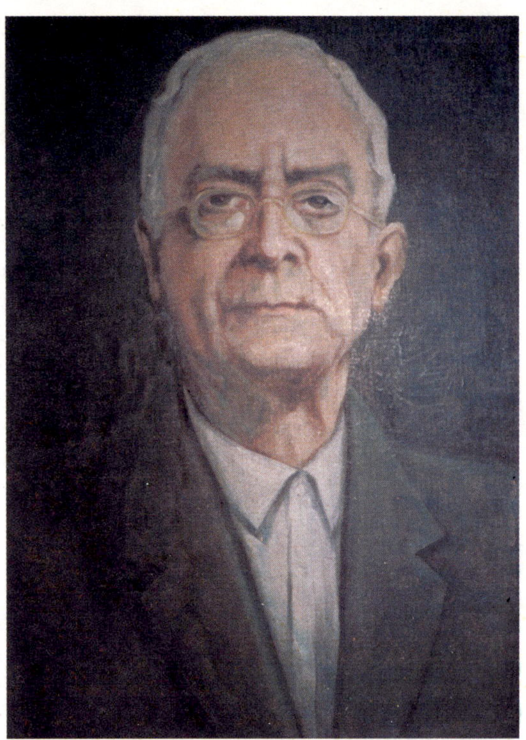

Fig. 2: Sir Charles Scott Sherrington (1857-1952)

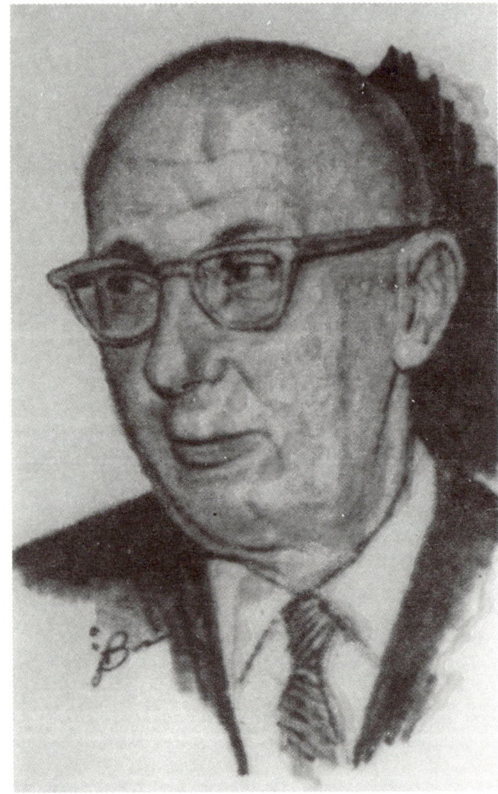

Fig. 3: Bekesy, Georgevon
Nobel Prize (1961) American

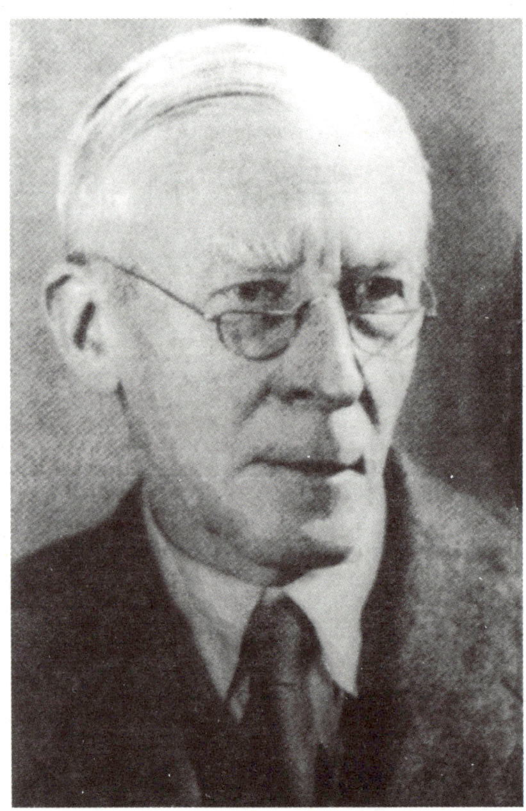

Fig. 4: Adrian Edgar Douglas
Nobel Prize (1932) British

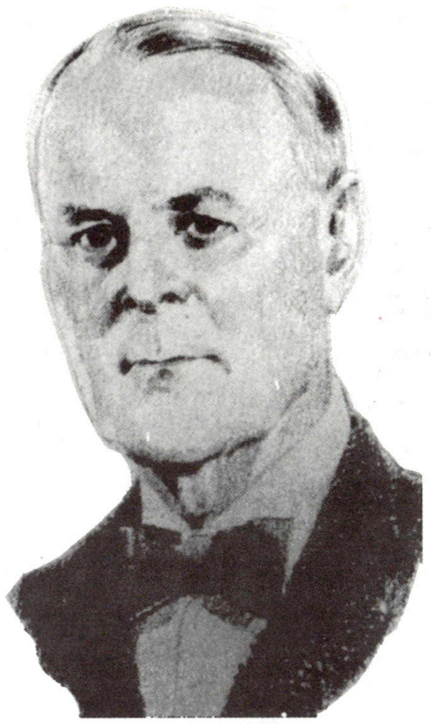

Fig. 5: Granit R. Arthur
Nobel Prize (1967) Swedish

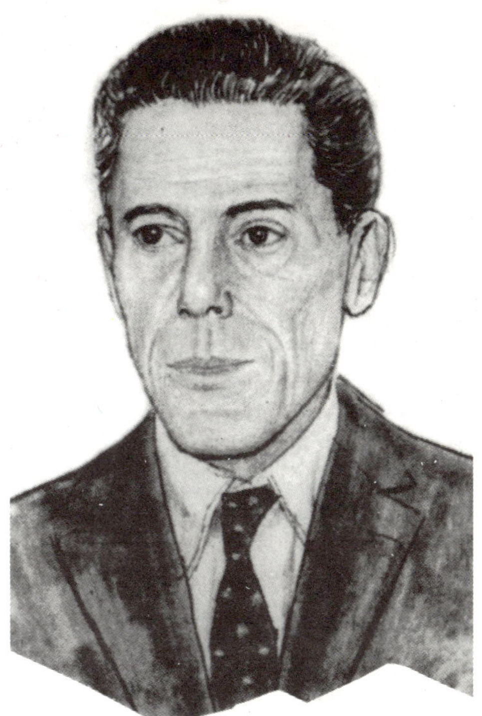

Fig. 6: Monod Jaqueus
Nobel Prize (1965) French

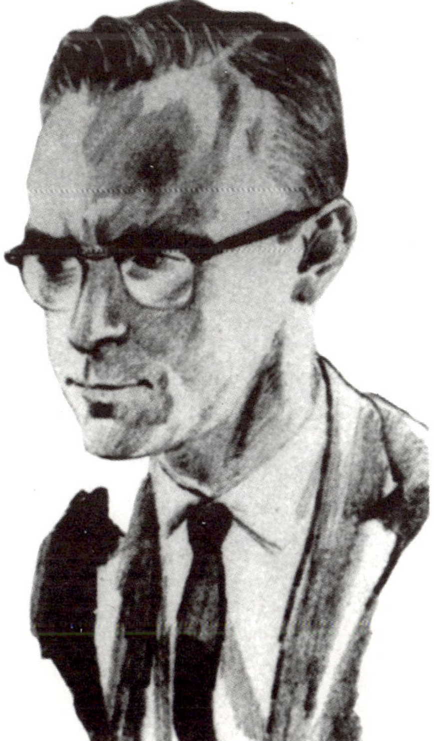

Fig. 7: Holley Robert Willium
Nobel Prize (1965) American

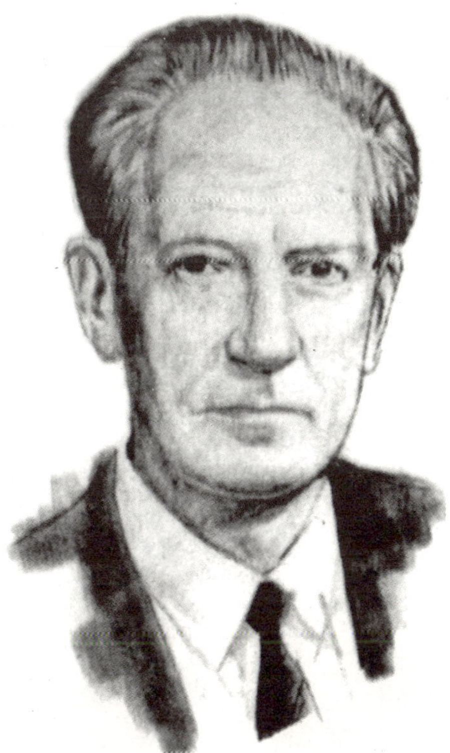

Fig. 8: Cori Ferdenand
Nobel Prize (1947) American

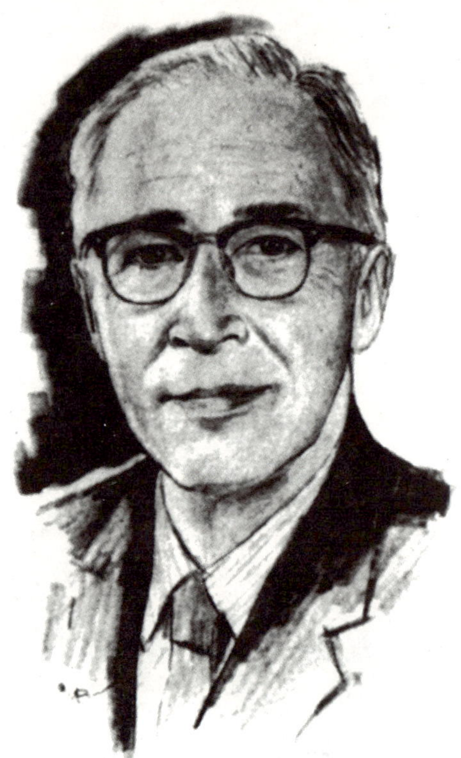

Fig. 9: Wald, George (1906-1967)
Nobel Prize – American

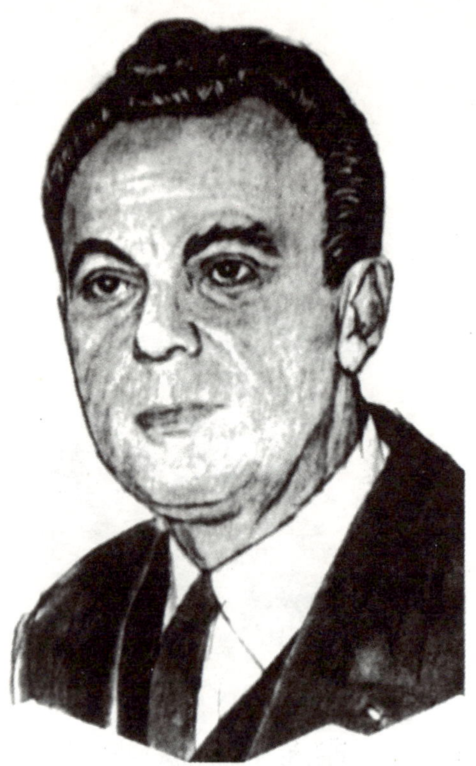

Fig. 10: Jacob Francois
Nobel Prize (1965) French

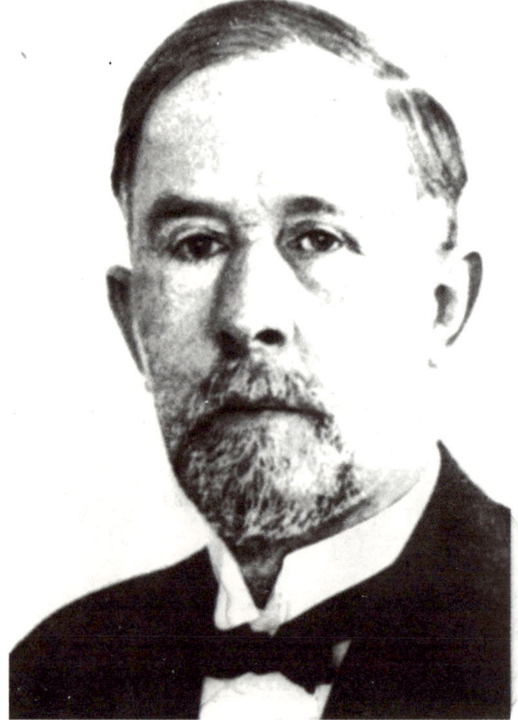

Fig. 11: Hess-Walter Rudolf
Nobel Prize (1949) Swiss

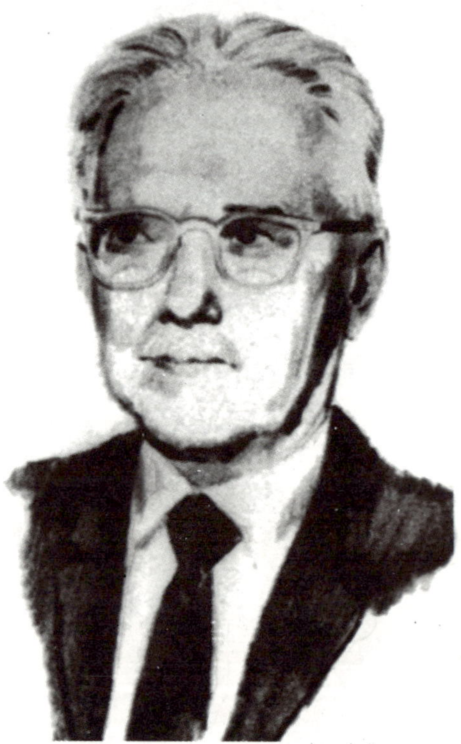

Fig. 12: Hartline Haldane
Nobel Prize (1967) American

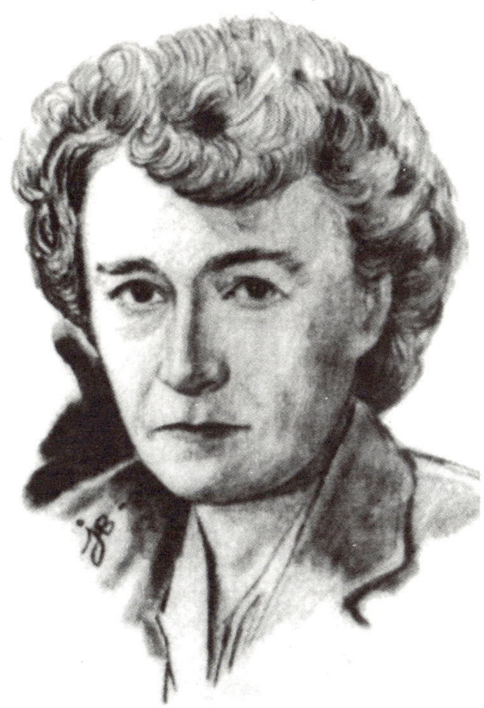

Fig. 13: Cori (1896-1957)
Nobel Prize (1947) American

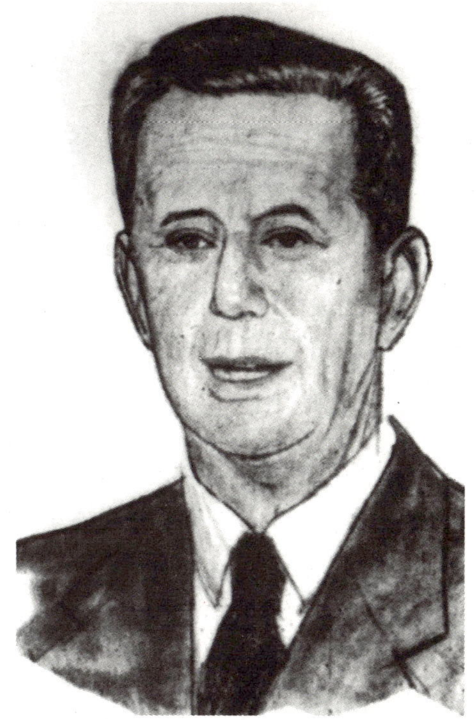

Fig. 14: Lwoff-Andrc
Nobel Prize (1965) British

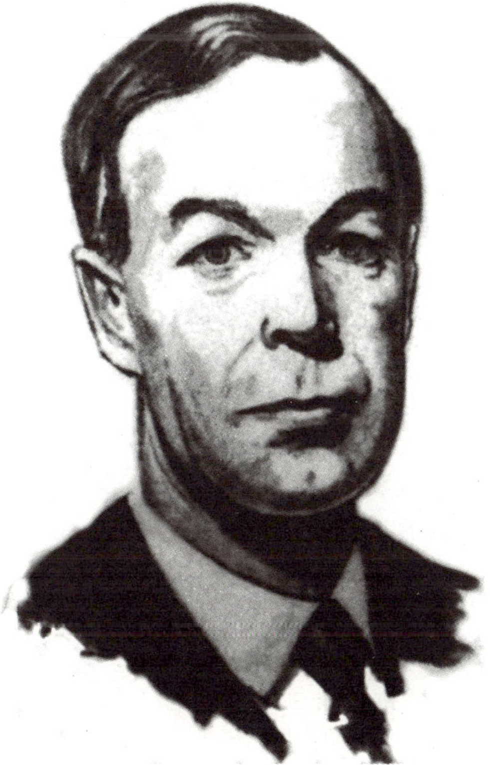

Fig. 15: Hodgkin-Allen Loyd
Nobel Prize (1963) British

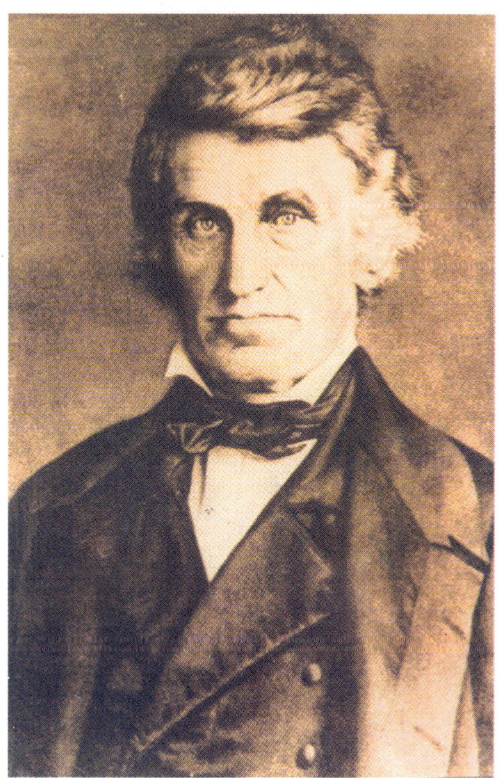

Fig. 16: Beaumont Willium
American Gastrophysiologist

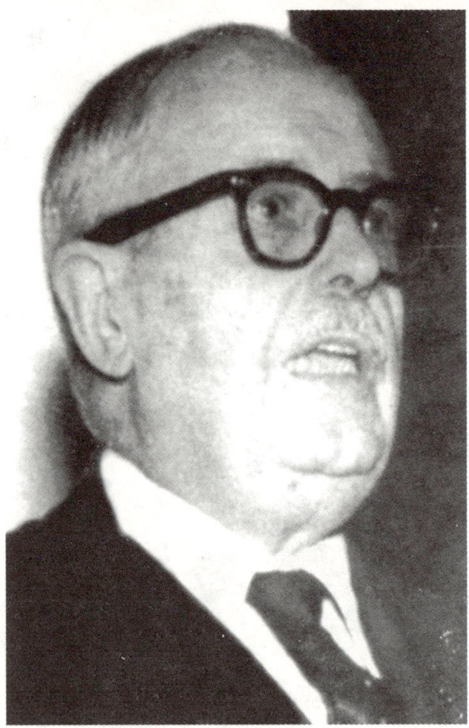

Fig. 17: B.A. Houssay (1947) Argentenee

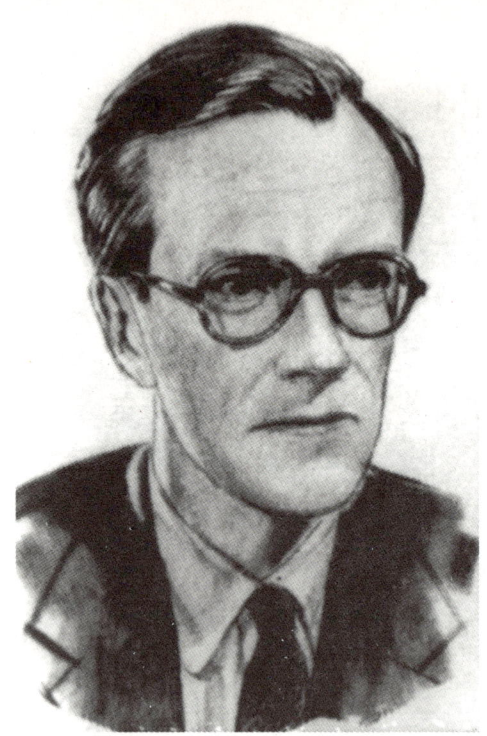

Fig. 18: Wilkins, M.H. Frederck (1962) English

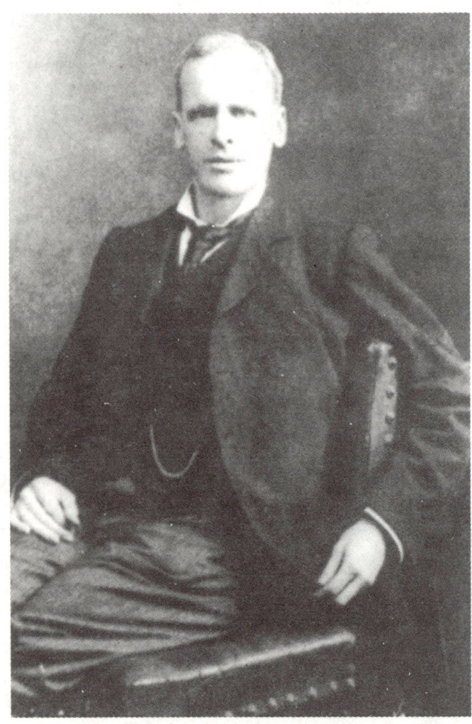

Fig. 19: Starling, Ernest Henry
Eminent English Physiologist (1866-1927)

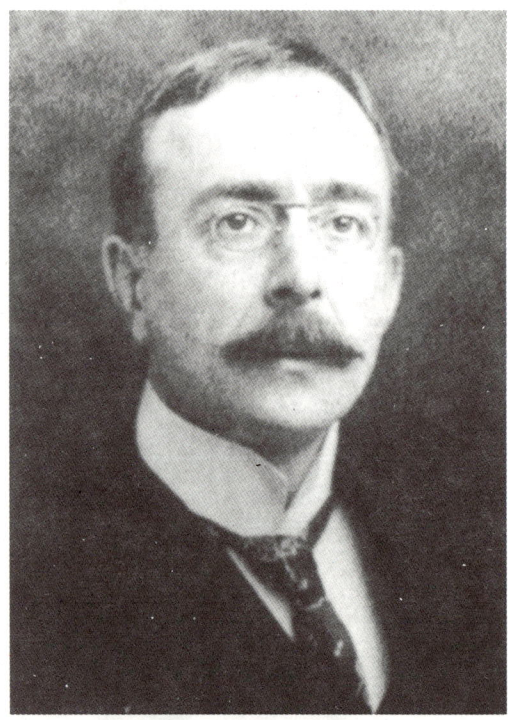

Fig. 20: Sherrington Charles
Nobel Prize (1932) British

Figs 1 to 20: Nobel Prize Winner
(*Courtesy:* Department of Physiology, S. P. Medical College, Bikaner)

Glossary

A

Absorption	The transfer of materials from free surface into blood.
Acapnia	A marked decrease of CO_2 in the blood.
Acidosis	Condition in which concentration of bicarbonates in the blood is below normal.
Action potential	A change in electric potential of an active cell or tissue.
Acidaemia	A relative increase in H ions in blood.
Adequate stimulus	Stimulus most efficient for a given structure to produce a desirable action.
Aerobic	Growing in air or oxygen.
Afferent nerve	A nerve which carries impulses to central nervous system.
Alkali reserve	The amount of bicarbonate in blood or body available for neutralizing acids.
Alveolus	One of the terminal air pockets of the lungs.
Anaemia	A lack of proper number of RBC/cu. Mm. Of blood or of proper Haemoglobin percentage.
Anorexia	Lack of appetite.
Anoxaemia	Lack of proper amount of O_2 in the blood.
Apnoea	The temporary cessation of breathing.
Asthenia	Lack of loss of strength.
Astigmatism	A refractive error of the eye in which the various meridians of the cornea or lens don't have the same radius of curvature.
Ataxia	Lack of muscle co-ordination.
Atrophy	A wasting away of a tissue or organ due to a decrease in protoplasm.
Axon	One of the protoplasmic process of a neurone.

B

Basal metabolism	The minimum expenditure of energy compatible with life.
Bilirubin	Yellow pigment found in bile.
Blind spot	An area of retina where the optic nerve leaves the eye ball; it is insensitive to light.
Blood pressure	The force which the blood exerts against the walls of the vessels or heart or lateral pressure produced by blood on walls of arteries during systole and diastole of heart.
Buffer	A compound which has the power to combine with either acid, or base, thus helping to maintain acid base balance.
Base change	An effect on DNA caused by ionisation of a base (purine or pyramidine) such that the base forms normally forbidden pairs during DNA replication and results in heritable changes in genetic code.
Basilar membrane	A membrane in cochlea on which the organ of corti rests. The membrane separates cochlea duct from scala tympani.
Beer's law	The assertion that the absorption coefficient of a substance is proportional to the concentration of that substance at lower concentration.
Benign	Of mild character; not malignant.
Binaural beat	A sensation of variation in loudness perceived when two sounds of slightly different frequencies are introduced into different ears of same person.
Biogenesis	The doctrine that all living things come only from pre existing living things.

C

Calorie	The unit of heat energy.

Carb haemoglobin	The compound formed by union of Haemoglobin with CO_2.
Carboxy-haemoglobin	A compound formed by union of haemoglobin and CO.
Cataract	An opacity of crystalline lens; sign of advanced age, producing diminution in vision by obstruction.
Centrosome	One of the constituent of cell playing a part in cell division.
Cerebellum	A part of hind brain; silent brain.
Cerumen	Ear wax
Chemotaxis	The property of a motile cell or organism to move toward or away from a chemical agent.
Chromatin	A deeply staining material of nucleus; it gives rise to chromosomes.
Chromosomes	The cellular elements regarded as the carrier of hereditary characteristics.
Chyme	The partially digested food, leaving the stomach; like paste.
Coagulation	The transformation of a soluble into an insoluble protein.
Colloid	Substance that diffuses and dialyses slowly or not at all and give rise to but a small amount of osmotic pressure; opposed to crystalloid.
Commissural fibres	Nerve fibres connecting one lateral half of brain or cord with the other.
Complementary colours	A pair of colours that, on mixing, physically or physiologically, produce white.
Conduction	The passage of an impulse along a protoplasmic structure.
Crenation	The shriveling of a RBC due to withdrawal of water.
Cretinism	A dwarfed and malformed condition of the body caused by hypofunction of thyroid in infancy.
Crystalloid	A chemical compound which, in solution, gives rise to osmotic pressure and dialyses through a semi permeable membrane.
Cytoplasm	The protoplasm to the exclusion of the nucleus.
Cyanosis	A bluish discoloration of the skin caused by presence of excessive venous blood.
Cerebro-vascular	Pertaining to blood vessels of cerebrum of the brain.
Congenital	Existing at birth.
Contraception	The prevention of conception.
Cryptorchidism	Undescended/hidden testes.
Canaliculi	Small canals extending between lacunae in the matrix of the bone.
Cardiac vector	The direction of the net polarisation wave that progresses through the heart during the cardiac cycle.
Cell	The fundamental unit of a living system. It consists of protoplasm and a nucleus enclosed in a cell membrane.
Centriole	A small body near the nucleus of a cell which in the process of cell division forms the centre about which it is rotating.
Centromere	A constricted region of a chromosome that marks the junction of the arms of the chromosome.
Chromatin	The filamentous form of DNA which in cell division forms the substance of chromosomes.

D

Decibel	A unit of sound pressure level, expressing the relationship between two sound levels in terms of logarithm of the ratio of level.
Decussation	Crossing over like an X.
Defecation	Elimination of waste matter from intestine; act of passing the stool.
Dendrite	A short branch of a neurone that conducts impulses from the cell body of a neurone.
Deglutition	Swallowing.
Diffusion	The spreading of molecule of a gas or of a substance in solution. OR the process by which particles suspended in a fluid medium spontaneously move from a region of high to low concentration.
Dentition	Teething; arrangement of teeth.
Diastole	The relaxation phase of the cardiac cycle during which heart chambers dilate and fill with blood, of systole. OR relaxation of heart muscles and dilation of heart cavities.
Diploid	Having double the number of chromosomes present in a gamete.
DNA	(De-oxyribonucleic acid) The substance in the cell nucleus containing genetic information in the sequence of its structural units. It regulates and specifies the protein synthesis process.
Dialysis	Separation; the separation of crystalloids from collids by the faster diffusion of the former through a membrane.
Dosimetry	The measurement of ionising radiation.
Distal	Toward the end of a structure. Opposite of proximal, remote.
Dose	The quantity and type of radiation directed at or absorbed by a biological system.

Diapedesis	Passage of blood cells (WBC) through intact blood vessel wall.
Diarthrosis	Freely movable joint.
Dyspnoea	Difficulty in breathing; laboured breathing.
Diplopia	Double vision; seeing one object as two.
Dystrophy	Faulty nutrition; malnutrition.
Diencephalon	Parts of the brain between the cerebral hemispheres and midbrain.
Dead space	The amount of space of respiratory tract in which no, or very little respiration takes place (nasal passage, trachea, bronchi, bronchioles).
Depolarisation	Destroying the polarised state of a body.
Detoxifying	Destroying the poisonous action.
Dick's test	A test for susceptibility of an individual to scarlet fever.
Dropsy	Edema; an excessive amount of lymph in a part of the body.

E

Effectors	The responding organs (muscles, glands etc.)
Efferent nerve	A nerve which carries impulses out of CNS.
Electrolyte	A substance which ionises in solution and aids in conduction of an electric current.
Embolism	A condition in which floating aggregate of a matter blocks a blood vessel (blood clot).
Emesis	Vomiting; (emetic = agent causing vomiting).
Emmetropia	The condition of un-accommodated eye in which principal focus lies in Retina.
Enterokinase	Enzyme transforming trypsinogen into trypsin.
Ergograph	An instrument for recording mechanical work done by a muscle or a group of muscles.
Erythroblast	A red bone marrow cell which gives rise to RBC.
Eupnoea	Normal quiet breathing.
Exteroceptor	Receptor stimulated by changes in the external environment.
Exudate	The material transferred from blood stream into the tissue spaces.
Eclipse	That phase of virus reproduction during which the host cells contains no visions.
Electrocar-diogram	The recorded pattern of an electrocardiograph.
Electrocardio-graph	An instrument for recording the changes in potential on the surface of the body that results from polarisation changes on and within the heart.

F

Fatigue	Tired/exhaustion; The gradual weakening of tension in a muscle contracted for an extended period OR loss of irritability or of the normal function of a structure due to previous work.
Foetus	Unborn offspring of a mammal during later stages of development, in man third month to parturition.
Fibrillation	The inco-ordinate contraction of muscle fibres.
Fibre	Threadlike structure.
Flaccid	Soft, limp.
Fovea	An indentation in the retina of the eye on the axis of eyeball. It is rich in cone cells having power of discriminating details.
Follicle	A small sac.
Fissure	A groove.
Fluorescent antibody	A group of atoms, coupled to certain location in specimens that becomes luminous when excited by ultra violet light.
Funiculus	A bundle of axons and their covering.
Frontal plane	A plane that divides the body of an organism into anterior and posterior portion.
Fibrin	Insoluble protein in clotted blood.

G

Ganglion	Collection of nerve cell bodies; cluster of nerve cell bodies outside CNS.
Gene	One of the units of which chromosomes are composed; carrier of hereditary characteristics; a specific region on a DNA molecule capable of determining a specific trait.
Genotype	The genetic constitution of an individual, in contrast to the appearance or expressed characteristic of that individual.
Gustatory	Pertaining to taste.
Gyrus	Convoluted ridge.
Graffian	Graaf-17th century Dutch anatomist.
Glycolysis	The breakdown of carbohydrates into pyruvic and lactic acid in the metabolic processes of cells.
Glycogenesis	The manufacturer of glycogen from glucose.
Glycolysis	
Genetics	The science of heredity.

H

Hemiplegia	Paralysis of one side of the body.

Hemopoiesis	Formation of blood.
Hemocytometer	An instrument for counting number of blood cells.
Hemolysis	Blood destruction.
Haemophilia	A condition in which CT is prolonged.
Haemorrhage	The escape of blood from the blood vessels.
Hoemostasis	Arrest of bleeding.
Homeostasis	The maintenance and ensurance of internal environment i.e. maintaining a constant state.
Hormone	A chemical compound formed generally by endocrine glands, which is absorbed in blood stream and influences the growth, development or function of some other parts of body.
Hyperglycaemia	An excessive amount of glucose in blood.
Hyperpnoea	Increased rate and depth of respiration.
Hypertrophy	An increase in size of an organ due to an increased amount of protoplasm.
Hydrophilic	Having an affinity for water.
Hydro cephalus	Enlargement of head due to an abnormal accumulation of fluid.
Hysterectomy	Surgical removal of uterus.
Hematoma	A tumour/swelling filled with blood.
Hyperchromic	Highly coloured.
Heterogenous	Composed of different substances.
Hypodermic	Below the skin or dermis.
Hydrophobia	Fear of water.

I

In vivo	In a living system.
In vitro	In a laboratory situation; outside the normal environment of a living system.
Isometric	A condition of muscle contraction in which no change in length of muscle occurs.
Isotonic	A condition of muscle contraction in which muscle shortens while maintaining constant tension OR of the same tension/pressure.
Ischaemia	A temporary and local deficiency of blood; local anaemia.
Ion	Electrically charged atom or group of atoms.
Irritability	The ability of a living matter to respond to a stimuli; excitability.
Intima	Innermost.
Intercellular	Between cells/interstitial.
Internuncial	Like a messenger between two parties; internuncial neurone is one which conducts impulses from one neurone to another.
Involuntary	Not willed. Opposite of voluntary.
Involution	Return of an organ to its normal size after enlargement.
Inhalation	Inspiration or breathing in.
Impulse-nerve	A change in nerve fibre induced by stimulation and traveling throughout the fibre.

J

Jaundice	Presence of bile in blood.
Joint	Point of union between two bones.

K

Kinaesthetic sensation	The proprioceptive sensation by which we judge of the position and movement of our limbs (kinaesthesia = muscle sense).
Karyoplasm	The material within the nucleus of a cell.
Keratin	A highly insoluble, indigestible scleroprotein found in skin, nails etc.
Karyotype	The shapes of the individual chromosomes of a set of chromosomes within the nucleus of a cell.
Karyokinesis	Cell division by mitosis.
Kinase	A ferment of ferments; it activates proenzyme.

L

Lachrymal (Lacrimal)	Pertaining to tears.
Lactation	Secretion of milk.
Latent period	The length of time elapsing between stimulus and the response.
Lesion	A pathologic change in a tissue; hurt; wound.
Leukocyte	White blood cell.
Lipase	A fat splitting enzyme.
Lymph	The fluid found in lymph vessels and spaces.
Lymphocyte	A type of white blood cell which forms antibodies.
Lateral	Away from median plan of body.
Lysozyme	An enzyme which causes lysis; i.e. destruction of cells by enzymes that cause bursting of the plasma membrane of the cell.
Luminance	The brightness of a source of light.
Lipid	A group of organic compound which are insoluble in water; includes fats, oil, waxes, sterols etc.
Lead	A pair of electrodes used as detectors of potential difference at two points on the surface of body in electro-cardiography.

Lambert's law	A mathematical statement of the relationship between intensity of electromagnetic radiation and the thickness of an absorbing material through which it passes.

M

Macrophage	A cell of loose connective tissue having the power of phagocytosis; a resting wandering cell; histiocyte.
Manometer	An instrument for measuring pressure, filled with mercury and having graduations.
Mastication	Chewing.
Menopause	The cessation of the periodic menstruation climacteric.
Menstruation	The periodic changes in the uterus during sexual life, monthly bleeding from uterus.
Micron	1/100th of a millimetre.
Miotic	A drug which causes constriction of pupil.
Motor areas	The areas of cerebral cortex which on stimulation give rise to muscular action.
Morphology	The study of form and structure of the things.
Malnutrition	Lack of necessary food substances/nutrients.
Mega karyocyte	Giant cell of bone marrow.
Melanin	Black/dark brown pigment found in skin and hair.
Myaesthenia	Weakness of skeletal muscles.
Malleus	A hammer; one of the ossicles of middle ear.
Meatus	A natural opening in the body.
Metaphase	The phase of cell division (mitosis) in which the chromosome pairs are arranged with their centromeres along the equatorial plane.
Mitosis	Cell division in which the daughter cells have the same number of chromosomes as the parent cell.
Myocardium	The heart muscle.
Myopia	Near sightedness, person is unable to see distant objects clearly.

N

Neuroglia	The supporting, non nervous cells of nervous system.
Neuron	A nerve cell.
Node of Ranvier	One of the series of constrictions in the myelin sheath that surrounds some axons.
Numerical aperture	A measure of the light gathering power of a lens.
Nyctalopia	Night blindness.
Neurilemma	Nerve sheath; outermost covering of a nerve fibre.
Nystagmus	Involuntary and abnormal oscillatory movements of the eyes.
Nuclein	A compound protein found in the nucleus.

O

Obesity	The state of being excessively fat.
Occipital lobe	The hinder most lobe of cerebral cortex.
Osmosis	The diffusion through a membrane of solvent (or water) from a lower to a more concentrated solution.
Ovulation	The setting free of ovum from the ovary.
Oxy-haemo-globin	Haemoglobin united with oxygen.
Osmotic pressure	The pressure required to prevent water from passing into a solution from which it is separated by a membrane permeable only to water.
Ovum	An egg cell.
Objective lens	The lens of a microscope closest to object being viewed.
Oval window	A membrane between the middle and inner ear against which the stapes transmits pressure signals which are carried into cochlea through a fluid.
Optic disc	The blind spot on retina; the passageway through which nerves exit the retina.
Optic nerve	The nerve from the eye to the brain, originating at optic disc.
Organelle	Any of the specialised structures within a cell.
Oxygen debt	The state of muscles which have performed work at a rate such that insufficient oxygen has been supplied to the muscles and lactic acid has accumulated.

P

Paralysis	Loss of motion or sensation in a part of body.
Parturition	Childbirth; delivery
Pathogenic	Disease producing
Pepsin	The proteolytic enzyme of gastric juice.
Phagocyte	A cell able to engulf solid particles; process is phagocytosis.
Plasmolysis	The shrinkage of protoplasm due to withdrawal of liquid from the cell by a hypertonic solution.
Plenthysmo-graph	An instrument for measuring or recording the changes in the volume of an organ.
Poikilothermic animals	Animals with a variable body temperature: cold blooded animals.

Presbyopia — Loss of accommodation due to hardening of the crystalline lens: sign of old age.

Propricoceptive impulses — Impulses received from muscles, tendons and joints.

Psychic — Pertaining to mind.

Ptyalin — A starch splitting enzyme of saliva.

Pulse pressure — The difference between systolic and diastolic pressure.

Puberty — The period of life at which young of either sex becomes capable of reproduction.

Pyramidal fibres — The cortico-spinal nerve fibres extending from pyramidal cells (Betz cells) in pre central convolution and extending into spinal cord.

Q

Quantum — A photon; a discrete packet of electromagnetic energy.

R

Rachitis — A disturbance in bone formation; rickets.

Receptor — An organ for the reception of stimuli; sense organ.

Refractory period — The period of reduced irritability during the activity of a protoplasmic structure, time interval between height of contraction and completion of relaxation.

Reflex action — An action induced by the stimulation of a receptor and carried on without the intervention of the will.

Rennin — A milk clotting enzyme.

Rheobase — The threshold, or liminal.

Rhodopsin — A pigment in the rods of retina held to be necessary for vision.

Rigor mortis — The stiffening or hardening of the muscles soon after the death.

Rod — One of the visual cells of retina.

Rheumatism — Inflammation specially of muscles and joints.

Reisner's membrane — One of the major membranes in the cochlea that separates two of cochlear chambers.

Resolution — A measure of the ability of a microscope to resolve, or visually separate two closely spaced points.

Respiration — The series of chemical reactions by which a living cell obtains energy from nutrients, taking oxygen in and discarding carbon dioxide out.

Retina — The layer of nervous tissue on inner posterior surface of the eye ball upon which images are focused.

Ribosome — Small bodies, usually attached to endoplasmic reticulum within a cell that are rich in RNA and function in synthesis of protein.

S

Sarcomere — A contractile unit of striated muscle.

Schwann cell — One of the cells that form myelin sheath around axons of nerve cell.

Sinus — Cavity

Serum — Yellowish liquid that separates from a clot of blood; the plasma of blood from which fibrin has been removed.

Synapse — Joining; point of contact between adjacent neurones. The connection between axon of one neurone and dendrite of another.

Spike potential — The largest of the series of peaks within the action potential of an axon.

Sematic — Pertaining to the body.

Sphygmograph — An instrument for recording the pulse.

Senescence — Old age, ageing.

Semen — Male reproductive fluid (latin for seed)

Syncope — Fainting

Sebum — The oil secreted by oil glands

Sensation — A change in consciousness caused by stimulation of a sensory surface.

Stimulus — Agent that causes a change in activity of a structure; a change in environment which modifies the activity of protoplasm.

T

Telophase — The final stage of mitosis, characterised by the appearance of two new nuclei.

Tetanus — A sustained contraction of muscle produced by complete fusion of twitches.

Tonus — The state of light tension in muscles; a subdued continuous contraction of a muscle by which it resists stretching.

Transducer — A device that converts energy from one form into another.

Twitch — A single contraction of a muscle in response to a stimulus of short duration.

Tympanum — Drum

Tunica — Covering

Trauma — A wound, injury.

Transudate — The material passing through the capillary wall from blood into surrounding spaces.

Translation — The process in which an amino acid chain is formed at the direction of the coded information on mRNA.

Transcription	The process by which mRNA is produced from DNA bearing encoded genetic information.
Toxin	A poisonous compound of animal or vegetable origin.

U

Umbilicus	The navel.
Ultracentrifuge	A high speed centrifuge; a device for rapidly spinning suspensions to separate the materials of different densities.
Uvula	(Latin-from grapes; a projection hanging from soft palate).
Utricle	Little sac.
Urinometer	An instrument for determining the specific gravity of urine.
Uro-genital	Pertaining to urinary and genital organs.
Urea	A nitrogenous waste product found in urine.
Uterus (Womb)	Sex organ in which egg and foetus develop.
Ureometer	An instrument for determining the amount of urea in urine.

V

Vacuole	A cavity within a cell usually filled with a fluid.
Viscera	Internal organ.
Vasoconstriction	The reduction in diameter of blood vessels.
Vasodilatation	The relaxation of blood vessels with an accompanying increase in diameter.
Visual acuity	The ability to distinguish details of an object (e.g. letters of a printed page) or to see objects clearly with naked eye.
Vitellin	A protein of egg yolk.
Vertigo	dizziness; giddiness.
Valve	One or more flaps that open to permit flow of blood in one direction, but not in opposite direction, gate keeper.
Vaso	A prefix referring to a blood vessel.
Voluntary muscle	Striated muscle.
Vertebrate	An animal possessing a back bone.
Vermiform	Worm shaped.
Volar	Pertaining to palm of hand or sole of foot.
Vernix-caseosa	The fatty substance on the skin of new born (vernix = varnish, caseus - cheese).
Vasa vasorum	The small blood vessels supplying the walls of larger arteries.

W

Wave	A cyclic disturbance in a medium that propagates through the medium without bodily moving the particles of the medium along with the wave itself.
Wave length	The distance between successive disturbance maxima in a wave.
Willis	English Anatomist (17th century).
White matter	That part of central nervous system characterised by neurones having medullary sheaths.
White blood corpuscles	Large nucleated blood cell called loyal soldiers of our body.
Wisdom tooth	One of the four molar teeth that erupt very late from 18th-23rd year; it is third molar on each side of upper or lower jaw.
Wharton's duct	The duct of sub maxillary gland.
Whitlow	Inflammation of soft tissue in the neighbourhood of nail; paronychia.

X

X-ray	High energy electromagnetic waves that originate in extra nuclear electrons of atoms.
Xerophthalmia	A pathologic condition of cornea of eye due to lack of vitamin A.
Xiphoid	Sword shaped.

Y

Yolk	Non living material in cytoplasm of an ovum. It serves as food for developing embryo.
Yellow bone marrow	Marrow in medullary cavities of long bones, containing many fat cells.

Z

Zygoma	Yoke
Zymase	The alcoholic enzyme present in yeast.
Zymogen	The material from which an enzyme is formed.

Index

B

C

D

R

S

T

U

V

W

Y